THE HEALING PRESENCE OF ART

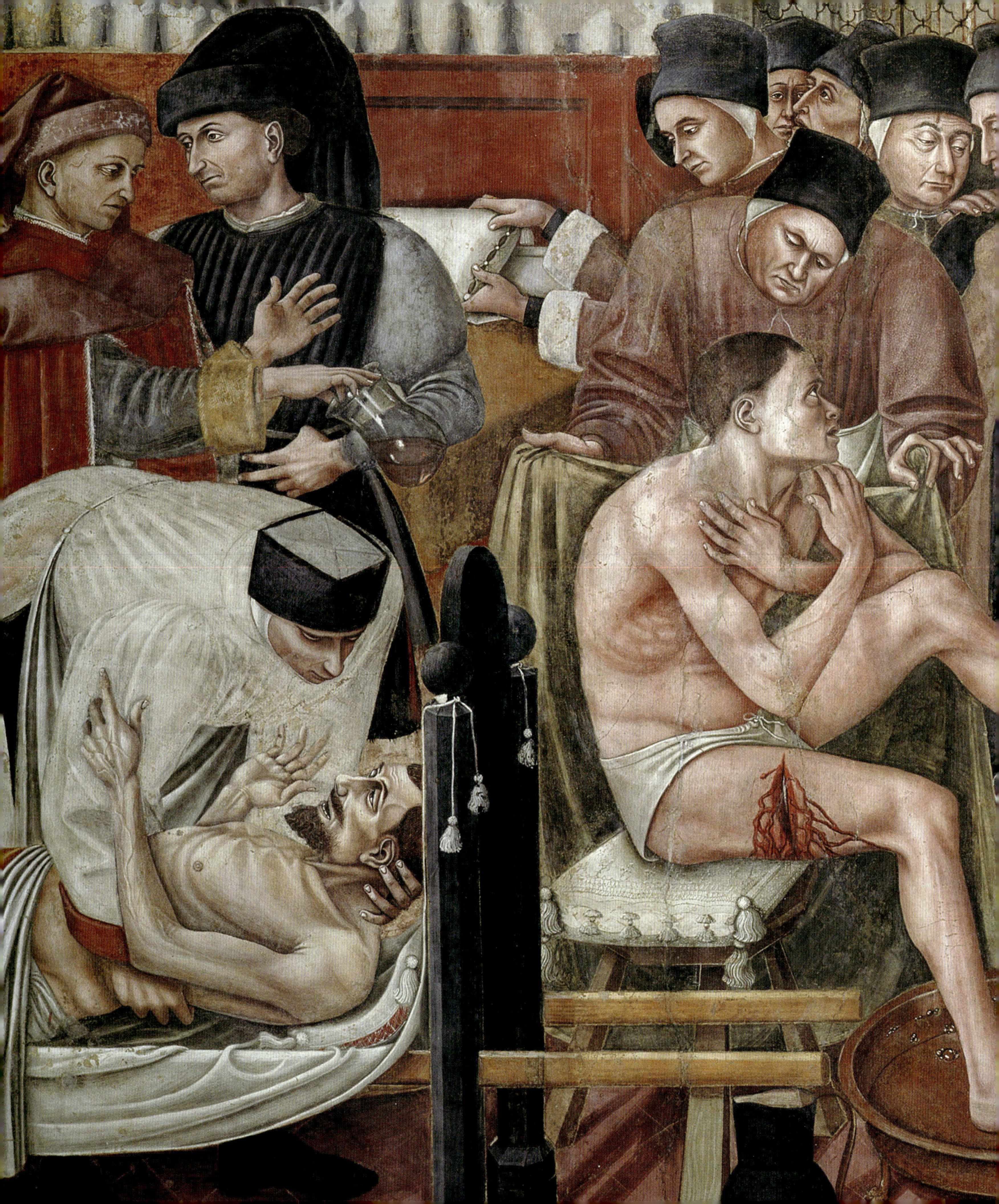

THE HEALING PRESENCE OF ART

A History of Western Art in Hospitals

RICHARD CORK

YALE UNIVERSITY PRESS • NEW HAVEN AND LONDON

Designed by Elizabeth McWilliams

Printed in China

Library of Congress Cataloging-in-Publication Data

Cork, Richard.
The healing presence of art : a history of western art in hospitals / Richard Cork.
p. cm.
Includes bibliographical references and index.
ISBN 978-0-300-17036-8 (cloth : alk. paper)
1. Art in hospitals–History. 2. Hospital buildings–Decoration--History.
I. Title. II. Title: History of western art in hospitals.
RA967.C617 2012
725'.51–dc23

2011042293

A catalogue record for this book is available from The British Library

Frontispiece Detail of pl. 6

In loving memory of my mother, Betty, and my father, Hugh, who never forgot the crucial role played by French and English hospitals in his recovery from a machine-gun wound suffered soon after D-Day, 1944

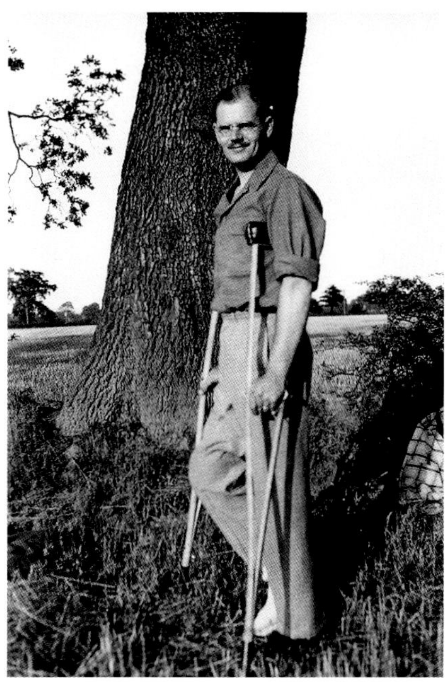

DONORS

This publication would not have been possible without the generosity of the following donors:

Wellcome Trust

Guy's & St Thomas's Charity

Portrack Charitable Trust

Saffery Champness Trust Corporation

Paul Mellon Centre for Studies in British Art

Nicholas and Diana Baring

CONTENTS

ACKNOWLEDGEMENTS

The task of writing my book was kick-started by a timely and very welcome invitation to deliver the Durning-Lawrence Lectures in the History of Art at University College London, in 1987. Preparing those six lectures proved an excellent way of ordering my thoughts and I was further encouraged by the response they elicited. Special thanks are due to Professor John White and his colleagues at the University's Art History Department for making the Durning-Lawrence lectures so enjoyable and thereby helping to push this book forward.

Soon after, I was delighted to participate in an 'Art For Hospitals' seminar at the Whitechapel Art Gallery, where a range of speakers illuminated the issues at stake in this complex endeavour. Subsequently, I delivered a talk at the Royal Society of Medicine's symposium on 'Art in Hospitals: Past, Present and Future', while Roy Porter provided further encouragement by inviting me to give a lecture on the history of art in European hospitals at a major Wellcome Trust conference. I have benefited from subsequent invitations to lecture on various aspects of the subject at Chelsea Royal Hospital, Bart's Hospital, St Thomas's Hospital, St Mary's Hospital, Chelsea and Westminster Hospital and Charing Cross Hospital. I had the pleasure of giving the 2008 Marlay Lecture on the subject at the Fitzwilliam Museum, Cambridge. More recently, I was delighted to give the 2010 De Ferrieres Lecture to the Friends of Cheltenham Art Gallery & Museum. Martin Daunton, the Master of Trinity Hall, my old Cambridge college, very generously invited me to deliver a Milestones talk on the subject. I also contributed a paper to the Art and the Health Service Conference, organised by South East Wales Arts Association and Artworks Wales.

I likewise learned a great deal when working with the BBC producer Judith Bumpus on 'A Picture for Health', our 1985 Radio 4 programme about contemporary art in hospitals. As well as interviewing a number of authorities in the field, we were able to talk to a range of patients and staff members who offered honest assessments of the artists' work from the vantage of people who lived with it on an everyday basis. More recently, I much enjoyed being invited to Oslo in 2011 by Gavin Jantjes, to give a lecture at the National Museum on Edvard Munch's crisis in the Copenhagen clinic.

One of the participants at the Whitechapel Art Gallery seminar was Lesley Greene, the Director of the pioneering Public Art Development Trust where I served as a trustee for a number of years. I want to offer Lesley my particular gratitude. She worked with the King's Fund on many hospital schemes and I am also grateful to her for asking me to join the committee who acquired art for the new building at St Mary's Hospital, Paddington. Bridget Riley's two commissioned installations are among the highlights of the work now installed there. I was delighted that the committee meetings brought me into contact with the hospital's architect John Weeks, whose earlier collaboration with Mary Martin is discussed in the final chapter of this book.

At an early stage in my research, I was also stimulated by the 1983 conference on 'Art and the NHS' staged by the King's Fund and admirably chaired by Sir Patrick Nairne. It helped to clarify the value of art in hospitals from the viewpoint, respectively, of a writer, consultant physician, administrator and artist. More recently, I was delighted when Charles Jencks invited me in 2009 to become a member of the Maggie's Art Group, formed to consider the role played by artists in the inspirational network of Maggie's cancer caring centres as they continue to grow throughout the UK.

I am particularly grateful to all those who contributed very generous grants towards the production costs of this book. Without their crucial help, we would not have been able to illustrate the text as beautifully and comprehensively as possible. The invaluable donors are: the Wellcome Trust; Guy's & St Thomas's Charity; the Portrack Charitable Trust; the Saffery Champness Trust Corporation; the Paul Mellon Centre; and Nicholas and Diana Baring. The importance of these grants cannot be exaggerated.

For assistance either with enquiries or the stimulus of conversation, I must thank the following as well: Patricia Allderidge, the archivist and curator of the Bethlem Royal Hospital Museum; Marjorie Allthorpe-Guyton; R. Aquilla Clark, the Keeper of Visual Arts at the Herbert Art Gallery, Coventry; Dr Ken Arnold; Robert Baldock; Dr Hugh Baron, for his pioneering role in researching the history of art in many London hospitals; Elisabeth Bell of the Tate Library; Dr Jonathan Black; Kate Bland; Alan Borg; Bruce Boucher at University College's History of Art Department; Robert Breen of Art in Partnership Scotland Ltd; Richard Burton, the architect of St Mary's Hospital, Isle of Wight; Fiona Byrne-Sutton, formerly of the Midland Group, Nottingham; Sir Roy Calne; Helen Chadwick; Peter Coles, the psychologist and author of several important reports on aspects of contemporary art and the NHS; Hannah Collins, who produced art for Colindale Hospital; Graham Cooper, an artist at the Whittington Hospital; Michael Craig-Martin, who has made outstanding work for hospitals; Francis Creed of Manchester University; Graham Crowley, who executed a commission for the Brompton Hospital; Elizabeth Cumming, who kindly showed me Traquair's mortuary murals at the Royal Hospital for Sick Children in Edinburgh; Claire and Martin Daunton; Stuart Davie; Celina Fox of the Museum of London; Terry Friedman at Leeds City Art Galleries; Michael Ginsborg, who made work for St Charles Hospital; Kathleen Goff; Camilla Goslett; Simon Granger, an artist at Aycliffe Hospital; Keith Grant of the Froebel Institute; Belinda Harward at St George's Hospital, Tooting; Sally Hawkesworth at St Charles Hospital; David Holliday, the General Services Manager of the Robert Jones and Agnes Hunt Orthopaedic Hospital, Oswestry; Carolyn Hopkins of the Victoria and Albert Museum's Sculpture Department; Camilla Hornby; Charles Jencks; Peter Joyce at the Brompton Hospital; Anish Kapoor; Balraj Khanna; Laura Lee, Maggie's Chief Executive; Hilda Lobelle-Caluwe, the Director of the O.C.M.W. Musea, St John's Hospital, Bruges; Dr Adrian Locke; Jenni Lomax; Richard Long; Susan Loppert at Chelsea and Westminster Hospital; Gillian Malpass, the eminent Art and Architecture publisher at Yale University Press; Robert Maxwell, the Chief Executive of the King's Fund; Grace McDonald at Paintings in Hospital; Bruce McLean; Janet McLean at St Charles Hospital; Lucy Milton of the Artists' Agency, Sunderland; Paul de Monchaux; Alison Moon at St Thomas's; Victor Morrison, the Publishing and Press Secretary of the King's Fund; Dr Linda Moss at Manchester Polytechnic; Patricia Mowbray of the Special Trustees at St Thomas's Hospital; Anne Mullins, the Director of Vital Arts for Barts and the London NHS Trust; Sir Patrick Nairne, former Permanent Secretary at the Department of Health; Sandy Nairne; Rabbi Julia Neuberger; Robin Nicholson, the architect with Cullinans for the Lambeth Community Care Centre; John Nicoll; Simon Olding, London Museums Officer; Therese Oulton; Michael Phillips at Bethlem Royal Hospital Museum; Rosie Anne Pinney, the art historian for the Special Trustees at St Thomas's Hospital;

Bridget Riley; Eugene Rosenberg, the architect responsible for installing Naum Gabo's *Revolving Torsion: Fountain*, at St Thomas's Hospital; Moira Rudolf, the art historian at St Thomas's Hospital; Rebecca Salter; Charles Saumarez Smith; Dame Cicely Saunders, the Medical Director of the St Christopher's Hospice; William Schupbach and the staff of the indispensable library at the Wellcome Trust; Robert Scott; Peter Senior of Manchester Hospitals' Arts Project; Geoff Shepherd; Moira Sinclair of Vital Arts at Bart's Hospital; Charlotte and Dennis Stevenson; Cecil Symons at the Royal Free Hospital; Lisa Tickner; Isabel Vasseur; Kate Whiteford; Iden Wickings, the Deputy Secretary of the King's Fund; and Sarah Wilson at the Courtauld Institute, who at a crucial moment during my Henry Moore Fellowship at the Courtauld in the early 1990s urged me to complete this book. I am also grateful to all those who, attending my Courtauld Institute Summer School courses on the history of art in hospitals, gave me such stimulating experiences with their thoughtful responses to the images we explored.

As ever, my wife Vena and my children Adam, Polly, Katy and Joe sustained me immeasurably with their love and support during the long period of researching and writing. They also provided hugely enjoyable and perceptive company on visits to many of the places explored in this text, from Siena, Sansepolcro, Florence and Toledo to Greenwich, Venice, Beaune, Bruges and Barcelona. I have also benefited from the wisdom of my book's excellent editor, Elizabeth McWilliams. Above all, though, I want to thank Geoffrey Phalp. His seminal contribution to this book is explained in my Introduction. Sadly, he did not live to see its publication but I will never forget the enthusiasm, warmth and sensitivity with which he encouraged its initial stages, giving me free rein to pursue the historical course that, in the end, engaged me most closely. Geoffrey loved art and fully understood that the spirit, as well as the body, needs sustaining in hospital.

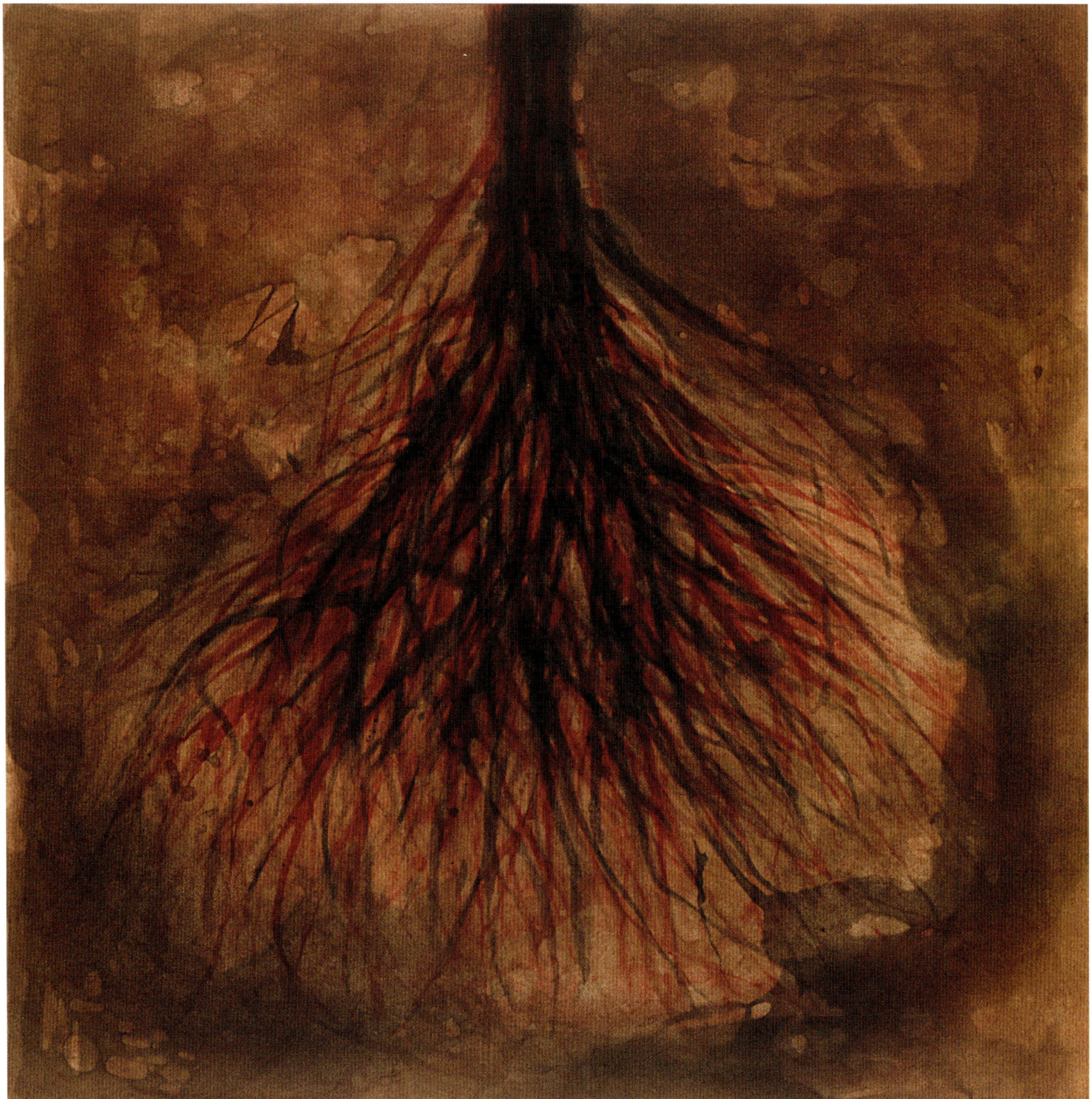

INTRODUCTION
MERCY, MADNESS, PESTILENCE AND HOPE

The importance of hospitals became clear to me at a very early age. Looking at the extensive damage inflicted on my father's slender and carefully swathed leg, I grew conscious of just how close he had come to death in June 1944. Soon after D-Day he was shot by a German machine-gunner near Bayeux, captured and sent eventually to a large hospital in Rennes. For two months he was dealt with by French medical students under the supervision of a doctor almost overwhelmed by caring for an immense number of wounded and dying soldiers. My mother, who had only got married in May 1944, did not know if her husband was dead or alive until August. But then the American army attacked Rennes and all the Germans fled. My father and the other patients were moved to what he called a 'USA Evac. Hospital' and he was soon flown back to the Royal Air Force Hospital in Wroughton. Hearing at last that he was alive, my mother conveyed her relief in a telegram she sent to him at Burntwood Emergency Hospital, Lichfield: 'Such joy. Coming tomorrow. All love, Betty.' Her delight increased once she realised just how well he had been treated by medical teams who succeeded in their determination to save his leg.

My childhood awareness of this episode intensified when I was contacted, suddenly and quite unexpectedly, by Geoffrey Phalp, the former Chief Executive of the King's Fund. Knowing of my interest in widening the boundaries of contemporary art, he asked me whether I would be prepared to consider writing a book about art and hospitals. As a lifelong hypochondriac, I was initially taken aback by the whole notion of exploring such a subject. But my curiosity was aroused. I had already become aware of the artists' projects which the King's Fund, collaborating with the Public Art Development Trust, had recently helped to finance for various hospitals in the National Health Service (NHS). On a personal level, too, I knew how much my young family had appreciated the outstanding Edwardian tile decorations in the old Paddington Green Children's Hospital, encountered during visits to its Outpatients' Department. My realisation that the presence of such images alleviated the stress and alienation of hospital life was reinforced when our eight-year-old son, Adam, was rushed to St Mary's in Paddington for an emergency appendix operation. He found himself in the Lewis Carroll Ward, where the walls are enlivened with tile illustrations of scenes from *Alice in Wonderland*.

Once I met Geoffrey and got to know him, my interest quickly deepened. At that stage, hoping I would write principally about contemporary developments, he asked me to spend a few months looking at new enterprises and talking to a range of

1 (*facing page*) Anish Kapoor, *Untitled*, 1989, Tate, London

architects, curators, physicians and hospital authorities already engaged in experimental ventures with art. Geoffrey also invited me to commission a special set of six *King's Fund Prints*, offered at well below market value to NHS hospitals and health authorities.[1] All the artists who accepted my invitation, including Helen Chadwick, Anish Kapoor, Richard Long and Kate Whiteford, responded to the venture with great enthusiasm and flair (pls 1 and 2). Their work now enhances medical interiors throughout the country, helping to counter the clinical bleakness that often confronted me on visits to institutions across Britain.

At that time, the appearance of many hospitals was utterly forbidding. I often found myself agreeing with Florence Nightingale's forthright assertion that 'hospitals are a curse to civilisation'.[2] But other visits disclosed the existence of inspiriting alternatives. At St Thomas's in London, I was fascinated to discover the statues of infirm patients carved by the little-known Thomas Cartwright for the original hospital exterior late in the seventeenth century. These remarkable images are now displayed indoors, only a modest distance from the grounds where Naum Gabo's final public sculpture, the graceful *Revolving Torsion, Fountain*, performs its aquatic choreography with inimitable precision and poise.

The sense of continuity I found here, binding together these otherwise disparate works created for St Thomas's at either end of a three-hundred-year period, helped me to appreciate that present-day attempts to humanise hospitals belong to a rich, complex and largely overlooked tradition. So while continuing to visit individuals recommended by Geoffrey, I found myself drawn to exploring the prodigious wealth of paintings and sculpture produced for the great historic institutions by artists of the past. London is particularly well endowed with impressive paintings and sculpture, from Caius Gabriel Cibber's compassionate *Madness* carvings for Bethlem Hospital and James Thornhill's monumental Painted Hall at Greenwich to the Court Room embellished by William Hogarth, Thomas Gainsborough, Michael Rysbrack and many others at the Foundling Hospital. With Sebastiano Ricci's visionary *Resurrection* enlivening Wren's Royal Hospital at Chelsea in the early eighteenth century, and 'Mad' Richard Dadd producing intense images while incarcerated at Bethlem and Broadmoor asylums during the Victorian period, London alone contained enough to convince me that a history of the finest art in hospitals was well worth attempting.

My subsequent explorations, of outstanding work produced in Western Europe and America from the Renaissance to the mid-twentieth century, amply reinforced this belief, for the completed book is replete with major commissions which enabled leading artists to produce images on the most ambitious scale imaginable. The healing power of Piero della Francesca's *Madonna of Mercy*, his first surviving commission as an individual painter, originally enhanced a major hospital in his home town of Sansepolcro. Hugo van der Goes painted his last and most profound work for the high altar of the church of Sant'Egidio in Santa Maria Nuova, Florence's major hospital. Many of Hans Memling's most impressive achievements can still be found at St John's Hospital in Bruges, filled with references to the friars and sisters who looked after the patients. The Antonites of Isenheim gave Matthias Grünewald the opportunity to reveal the full extent of his formidable abilities in a complex, multifaceted and overwhelmingly powerful altarpiece. Murillo's finest cycle of paintings was created for the church of the Hospital de la Caridad in Seville, while several of El Greco's most original and impassioned canvases were commissioned by the enlightened governors of hospitals in Illescas and Toledo.

Although some of the work discussed in the following pages is unfamiliar and deserves to be better known, plenty of these images have long been ranked among the outright masterpieces of Western art. But their redemptive relationship with hospitals has often been minimised or overlooked. By restoring them to their initial social, religious, medical and political contexts, I hope that even the most celebrated of these works will be seen in a different light. They possess inextricable connections with the *raison d'être* of the institutions for which they were produced. And since the artists who made them were fired by a fascinating variety of intentions, it is important to distinguish between them. The elaborate *Last Judgement* altarpiece produced by Rogier van der Weyden and his workshop for Chancellor Rolin's Hôtel-Dieu at Beaune was displayed at the end of a ward, iremarkably near patients lying in their beds. Hogarth's paintings on the Grand Staircase of St Bartholomew's Hospital,

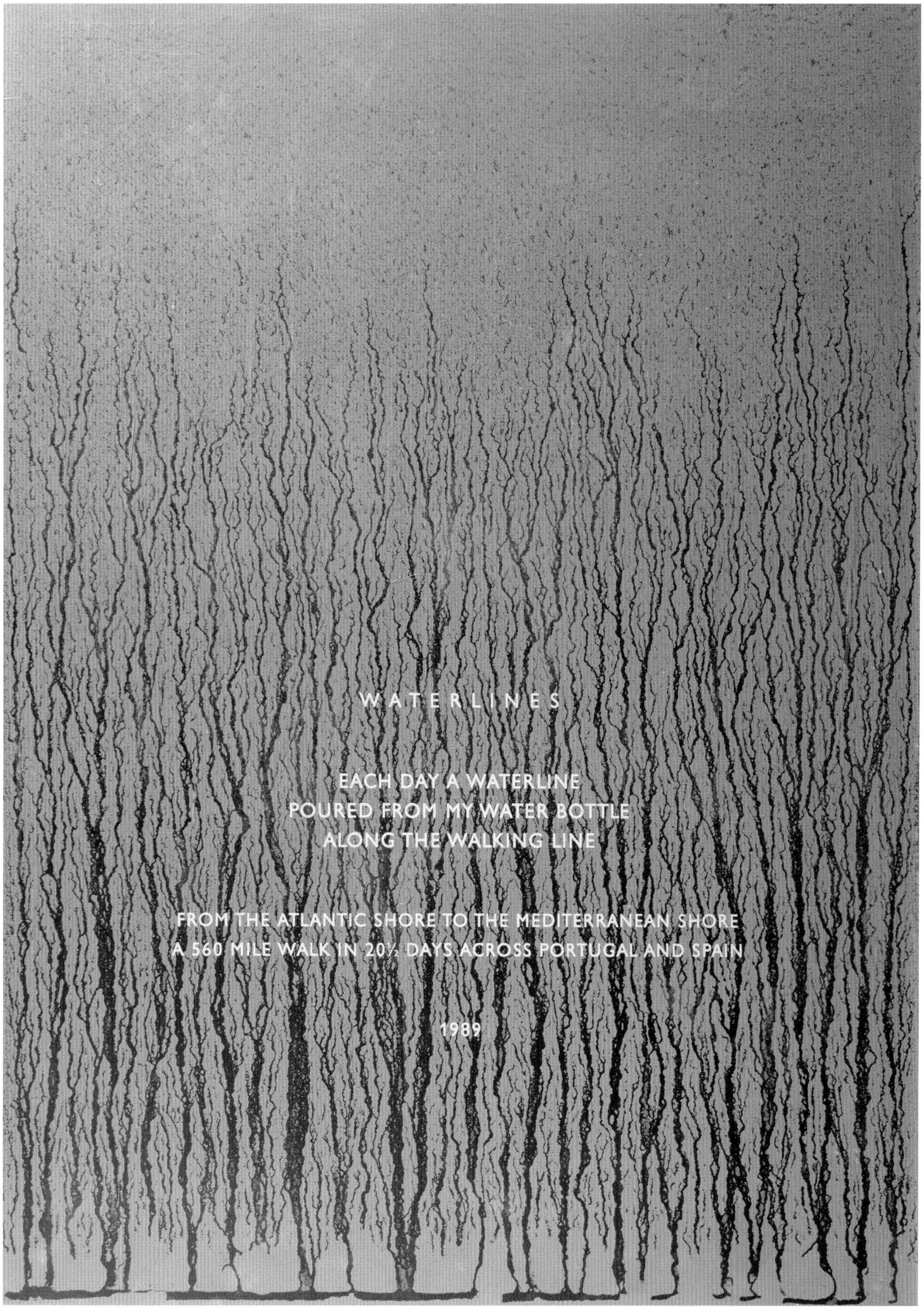
W A T E R L I N E S
EACH DAY A WATERLINE
POURED FROM MY WATER BOTTLE
ALONG THE WALKING LINE
FROM THE ATLANTIC SHORE TO THE MEDITERRANEAN SHORE
A 560 MILE WALK IN 20½ DAYS ACROSS PORTUGAL AND SPAIN
1989

2 Richard Long, *Waterlines*, 1989, Imperial College Healthcare Charity Art Collection, London

by contrast, were more distanced from the everyday life of the institution. So were the extensive frescoes embellishing Hardouin-Mansart's Church of the Dome in Paris, conceived at a symbolic and highly political remove from the pensioned soldiers who inhabited the Invalides building. But the major schemes painted in successive centuries for Siena's Spedale della Scala, the Crociferi Oratory in Venice and the chapel of Paris's Hôpital des Enfants-Trouvés all contained prominent and specific references to the inhabitants of the institutions themselves. Indeed, many of the artists discussed in this book must have carefully studied patients while preparing for their commissions, Jacques-Louis David notable among them in his major altarpiece at Marseilles. The work they produced afterwards gained significantly from their willingness to acquire first-hand knowledge of life and death in the hospitals concerned.

My emphasis on context also led me to consider how the medical profession has been depicted by artists during this period. It is an enormous and absorbing subject in its own right, ranging from Rembrandt's profoundly meditative *Anatomy Lesson* canvases to Thomas Eakins's dramatic *The Gross Clinic* and corrosive caricatures by James Gillray and Hogarth of ruthless, lethal quacks. Toulouse-Lautrec, who often claimed that 'if I were not a painter, I would like to be a doctor',[3] painted two of the most outstanding images of surgical operations. He became so fascinated by observing the celebrated doctor Jules-Emile Péan that he gave his friends excited and vivid descriptions of the operating theatre, with 'all the gore, the aluminium table worth ten thousand francs, raised and lowered by piston . . . the patient being operated on who slides on the table and has to be pulled back, by Péan's strength: he can move anything: the aides, the patient, the table in one go; he can pull a molar with his fingers; and while butchering talk graciously to his audience.'[4] Although I have been sparing in my use of such material, major paintings of operations by artists like Vuillard facilitate a greater understanding of work executed for hospitals themselves. So do Leonardo da Vinci's astonishing studies of human anatomy, many of which were carried out in Italian hospitals where he was able to study patients, talk to them and, after death, dissect their bodies in a spirit of pioneering enquiry. Similarly, I examine non-commissioned paintings by Elsheimer and Goya of hospital interiors, for they illuminate in contrasting ways artists' attitudes towards the whole notion of medical care.

I also find room for images intimately linked with the attitudes of enlightened doctors towards the hospital patients in their charge. Donatello was so appreciative of the expert medical help provided by Giovanni Chellini that he gave this eminent Florentine doctor a unique, heartfelt bronze roundel of the *Virgin and Child with Four Angels*, now known as *The Chellini Madonna*. Géricault's profound portraits of sufferers from 'monomania' are the most outstanding manifestations of such work, while van Gogh's wholly unprompted readiness to combat his trauma by depicting doctors, staff, patients and their surroundings at both Arles and Saint-Rémy is the product of an unusually intense involvement with the hospital world – especially at Saint-Rémy which, he declared, 'it would be splendid to hold an exhibition in, the empty rooms, the large corridors'.[5] Soon afterwards, Munch executed an immensely revealing series of images connected with his shooting injury, operation, nervous breakdown and subsequent treatment in a Danish psychiatric clinic under the care of Dr Daniel Jacobsen, who became the subject of a powerful full-length portrait. During the twentieth century Frida Kahlo even managed to paint some of her finest work when confined to a hospital bed with a severely damaged body. She had wanted initially to become a doctor, and testified in particular to the expertise and sensitivity of the eminent surgeon Juan Farill, whose double portrait with the convalescent Kahlo can be compared with Goya's far more turbulent, intimate *Self-portrait with Doctor Arrieta*. As for Antonin Artaud, his wartime struggle with chronic mental illness led him, with a doctor's help, to produce the brilliant if unnerving 'Cahiers de Rodez'.

While attempting to provide a reasonably comprehensive account of my subject, I have tried throughout to concentrate on ventures that seemed most rewarding to analyse. If, by emphasising these landmarks, I have omitted or underestimated other schemes and images which readers expect to find here, the fault is mine alone. Any history of art in hospitals is bound to be selective, however. It is astonishingly rich territory and I make no apology for limiting myself to work carried out within the geographical and chronological confines of this book. The wealth of projects created outside these boundaries certainly deserve examination but they must await another author. So must the burgeoning developments of the past few decades, which cannot be included in a historical study of this kind. Nevertheless, I hope that many of the achievements discussed in these pages will stimulate everyone involved in developing art for hospitals today. Across the world, there is an ever-increasing awareness that art can do an immense amount to humanise our hospitals, alleviate their clinical harshness and leave a profound, lasting impression on patients, staff and visitors. Hospitals can undoubtedly do more to look after the *whole* person, not just the patient's bodily ailment. Many critical moments in our lives occur there, from birth through to death, and they deserve to take place in surroundings that honour their true significance.

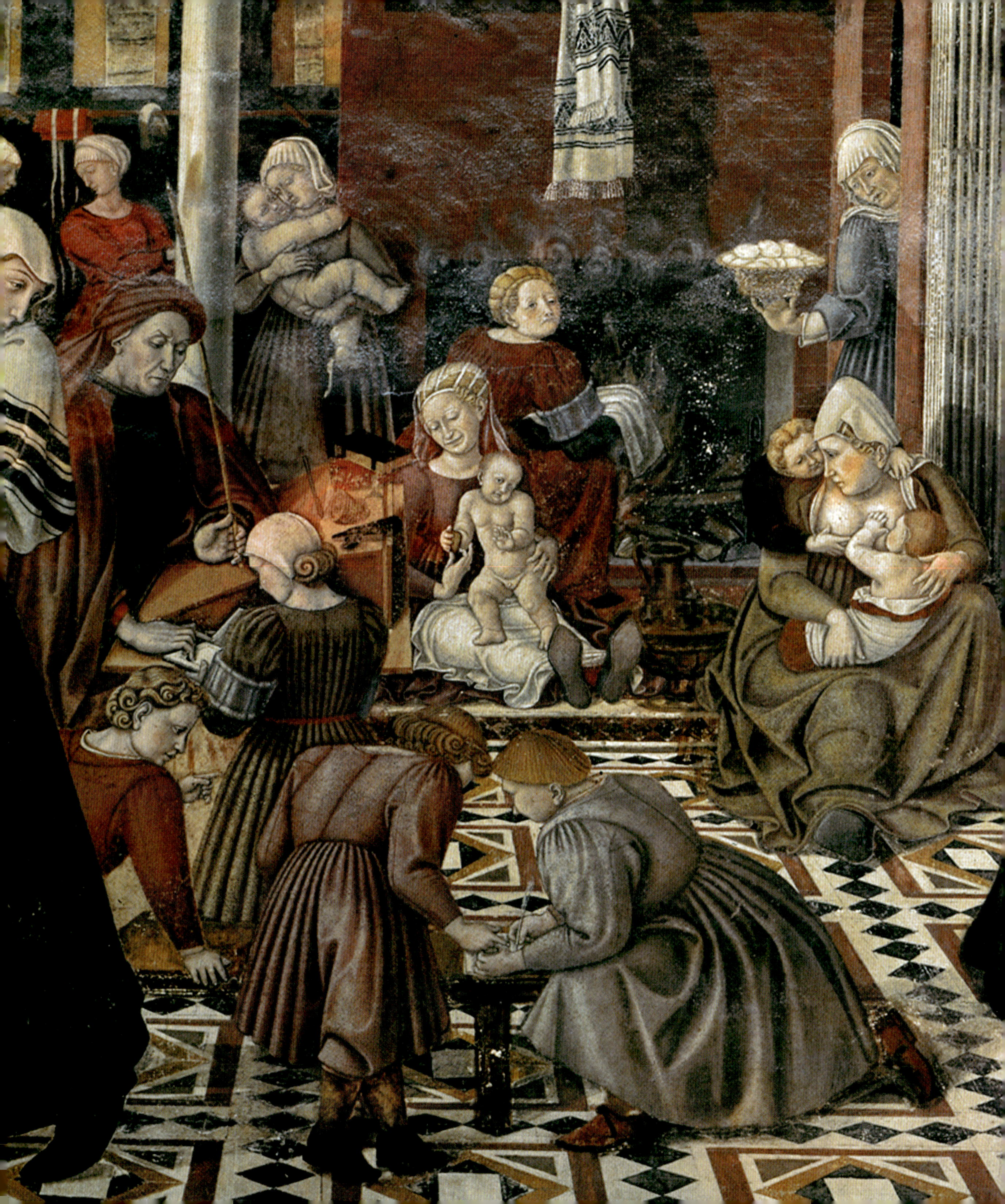

ONE
SALVATION IN SIENA

The idea that hospital patients might benefit from redemptive surroundings is far from new. Even in ancient Greece, where priests took their cue from patients' dreams when devising therapeutic treatment, large and handsome halls called Asklepieia were built to provide suitably soothing contexts for nursing. During the fifth century BC, Athenian dreamer-patients were able to sleep in a majestic double hall, opened to the south with a portico of pillars positioned to take the best possible advantage of the sun's healing force. The whole concept of medicinal care based on the implications of dreams may seem bizarre, especially since a number of 'patients' were acting on behalf of people so ill that they could not be sent to the Asklepieia themselves. Sometimes, too, dreams obliged the priests to permit treatment of the most extraordinary kinds. One man with a groin tumour was allowed to undertake a lengthy ride on horseback, simply because the god Asklepios had issued this agonising prescription in a dream. Apparently the patient thereby gratified a masochistic impulse and overcame his illness.[1] It sounds at once misguided and far-fetched; but the seriousness with which patients' inner needs were attended to, in a building that enhanced their existence while waking and sleeping, compares very favourably with the personal abruptness and environmental degradation offered by so many hospitals today.

Western civilisation took a long time to recover the notion that patients' surroundings should be places of dignity and calm. After Christians were responsible for introducing hospitals in late antiquity, as 'dormitories for travellers, vagrants and derelicts', they soon became identified with pest-holes. Medical expertise gradually infiltrated some, at least, of these unsavoury shelters, and Ivan Illich pointed out that 'physicians began to visit hospitals regularly at the time of the crusades, following the example of the Arabs. During the late Middle Ages, as charitable institutions for the custody of the destitute, they became part and parcel of urban architecture.'[2] Even so, John Summerson was right to stress that the history of hospitals 'is necessarily rather complicated', because for many centuries there was 'a variety of meanings for the word. A "hospital" might mean an almshouse, a school, a place for the healing of the sick or a home for the incurable, an asylum for lunatics or a place of reception for illegitimate children.'[3] All these diverse purposes were served by the buildings examined in this book, and sometimes a single hospital was enterprising enough to carry out a wide range of services under its capacious vaults. The quality of care on offer varied alarmingly but there was no doubt about the excellence of an outstanding Tuscan institution that managed, during the early

3 (*facing page*) Detail of pl. 7

years of the fourteenth century and beyond, to revive the Greek idea that a hospital should be beautiful.

Prominently positioned opposite the cathedral in the very centre of Siena, the Spedale di Santa Maria della Scala was admired throughout Europe as a model of how a great hospital should conduct itself. The cathedral's canons had founded the institution as a lodging-house for pilgrims but the Spedale soon took on a curative mission. By the end of the eleventh century, when its surviving records begin, the building had become a hospital dedicated to nursing anyone apart from lepers. Aided by munificent gifts and bequests, the Spedale acquired immense holdings of land in the local area (*contado*). Embracing granaries as well as a cluster of smaller subservient hospitals, their ample income rapidly proved a source of tension between Siena's sacred and secular authorities – exacerbated by the fact that the Spedale's original charter could not be found.

Determined to bring such a powerful body under their control, the city's General Council ordered in 1309 that a substantial plaque, adorned with the communal arms, be installed on the building's entrance doors. For the Spedale was by then a major Sienese corporate body, a focus for pride and venerated above all other civic institutions by the community at large. The burgeoning resources and status of the hospital were reflected in its decision to commission two major frescoes for the facade from Simone Martini, widely considered the most outstanding Sienese painter of his day.

Completed some time before Simone left the city for ever around 1335, the frescoes have long since disappeared. But Ghiberti, who greatly admired Simone's work, recorded that they depicted a *Marriage of the Virgin* and a subject he described, with tantalising obliqueness, as 'how [the Virgin] is visited by many ladies and virgins'.[4] Another fifteenth-century witness asserted that the scene represented the *Return of the Virgin to the House of her Parents*[5] and Ghiberti also related that Simone's frescoes were accompanied by paintings carried out by Ambrogio and Pietro Lorenzetti. Since they depicted the *Birth of the Virgin*, the *Presentation of the Virgin in the Temple* and the *Assumption*,[6] Simone and the Lorenzetti brothers presumably contributed to a unified cycle of frescoes on the hospital's front wall. It must have amounted to a stirring and substantial proclamation of the Spedale's commitment to the finest, most innovative Sienese artists of the time. And their enduring fame was demonstrated when, in 1448, Sano di Pietro was commissioned to paint an altarpiece elsewhere in the city with five scenes from the Virgin's life 'like those on the facade of the hospital.'[7]

Since the Virgin was Siena's principal patron saint, the frescoes on the Spedale's facade were part of a larger determination to place Marian images in major locations throughout the city. Duccio's *Maestà* altarpiece in the cathedral, and the fresco of the Virgin in majesty on the wall of the Palazzo Pubblico's great council chamber, testified to a concerted campaign. So the images painted by Simone Martini and the Lorenzettis for the Spedale, which acquired a sacred relic of the Virgin's girdle in 1359, should be seen in this wider civic context. Diana Norman, whose book *Siena and the Virgin* explores the city state's art and politics in the late medieval period, is confident that

> such a programme of interrelated Marian images would, in itself, have been a potent and effective means of proclaiming and reiterating the devotion of the Sienese to the Virgin. In addition, however, the Virgin was also celebrated on altarpieces on the altars of the most important churches within the city and in other public locations, including the city gates and a number of street tabernacles.[8]

Although nothing remains of this once spectacular scheme on the Spedale's frontage, the frescoes were still intact in 1404 when civic control over the hospital tightened. The new Sienese government decreed that responsibility for electing the institution's rector should pass from the cathedral canons to the Consistory. Aspects of the Spedale's religious origins remained, still symbolised by the building's position in the Piazza del Duomo. But from now on the rectorship became a city office electable in its councils, and Carlo d'Agnolino Bartoli became the hospital's first outstanding *quattrocento* rector after he was appointed in 1410.

An instinctive expansionist, Bartoli was so determined to assume direct administrative control of the satellite hospitals that he pushed the Spedale itself into debt. The financial difficulties enabled the commune to strengthen its power over the

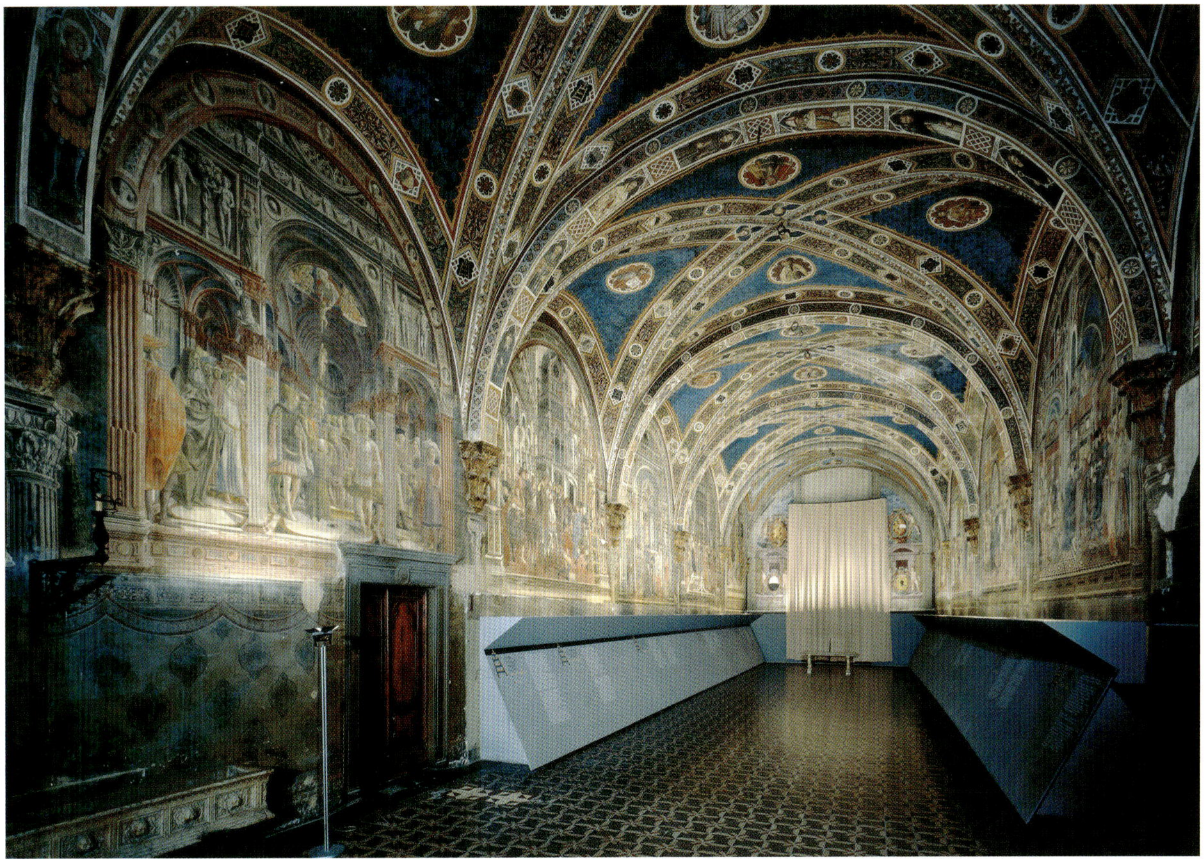

4 Frescoes by Lorenzo Vecchietta and Domenico di Bartolo, 1441–4, Sala Pellegrinaio, Spedale di Santa Maria della Scala, Siena

troubled institution, ordering a review of the fiscal crisis in 1428 and then, five years later, reiterating the importance of the role played by the hospital throughout Siena. 'The ancient governors of this city have always had an eye to the conservation and growth of the pious and religious House of the Hospital of Santa Maria della Scala', declared a civic ordinance in 1433, 'because that gives great honour to our city, and has in times past enjoyed good and great fame among all Christian nations.'[9]

The commune was not exaggerating: at the beginning of the fifteenth century Gian Galeazzo Visconti had decreed, after studying the Spedale's constitution, that Milan's hospital ought to base itself on this distinguished Sienese precedent. The Emperor Sigismund was equally impressed in 1413, and Saint Bernardino reminded congregations in his highly influential sermons that the Spedale 'is one of the eyes of your city, and the other eye is the Bishopric: they do well tied one to the other. The right eye is the Bishopric, and the left is the Hospital: and the nose is the piazza in between. See how long is the nose. O, citizens, take care of the Hospital! Do so that it can maintain its charities continually.'[10]

As if in response to Saint Bernardino's impassioned plea, the commune decided that continuing financial problems at the Spedale necessitated a new rector. Niccolo di Galgano Bichi, who had taken over the post when Carlo d'Agnolino Bartoli became bishop of the city in 1427, resigned six years later. And his enterprising successor, Giovanni di Francesco Buzzichelli, lost no time in commissioning an ambitious sequence of frescoes dedicated to celebrating the hospital's distinguished history while depicting its impressive range of charitable initiatives. Past and present were therefore brought together on the walls of the city's wealthiest institution, with a pictorial splendour that reflected the commune's new-found pride in controlling not only the Spedale's landholdings but its responsibilities to the citizens of Siena as well.[11]

The principal site of the elaborate fresco cycle devised by Buzzichelli was the Pellegrinaio, a spacious vaulted interior traditionally regarded as a pilgrims' hospice but used in the early *quattrocento* as a

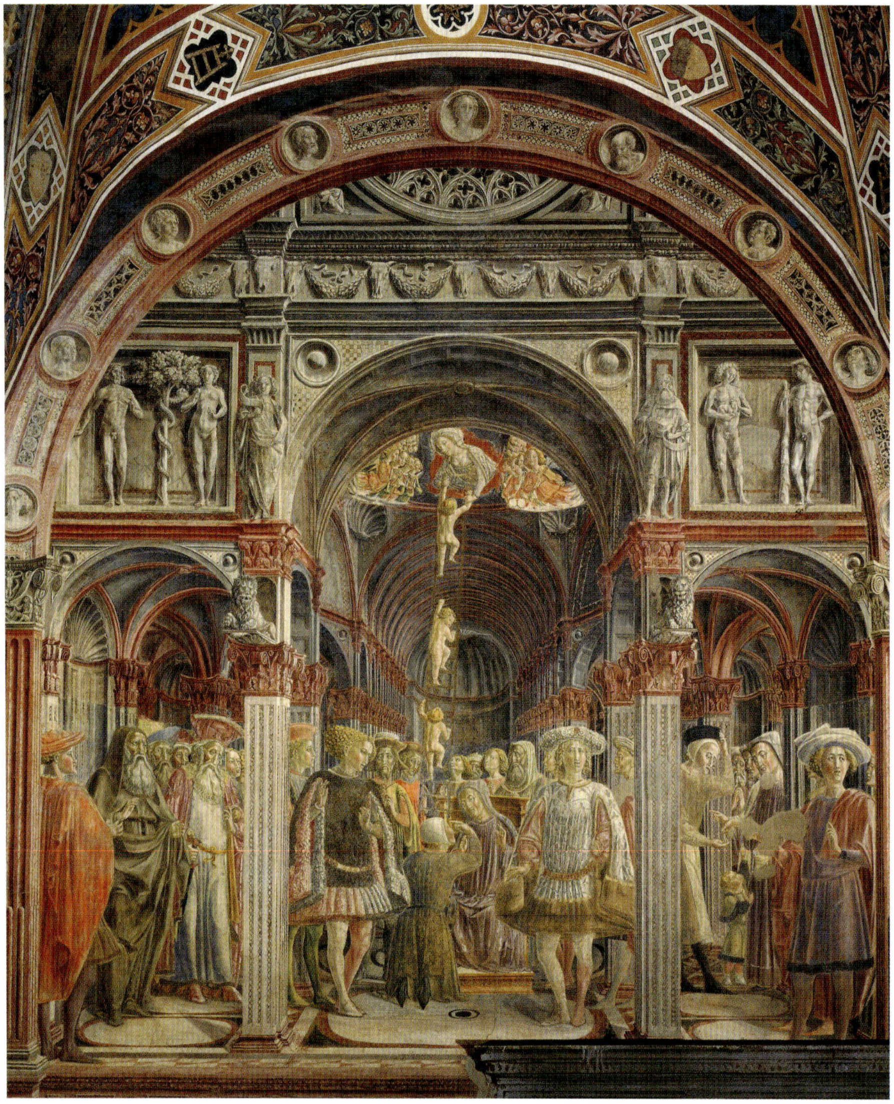

5 Lorenzo Vecchietta, *The Legend of the Foundation of the Hospital*, c. 1441, Sala Pellegrinaio, Spedale di Santa Maria della Scala, Siena

reception area and infirmary for male patients. If the hospital had still been run by the cathedral authorities, a conservative artist would probably have been entrusted with the commission. Religious painting in Siena was aimed at a devout public who preferred images based on home-grown *trecento* precedents rather than the new realism of the Florentine Renaissance. Now that the Spedale was regulated by a secular body, however, progressive artists found themselves favoured for the Pellegrinaio. Just as Ambrogio Lorenzetti's robust, forward-looking images had been commissioned for the secular Sienese fresco cycle devoted to *Good* and *Bad Government* a century earlier, so the enterprising Spedale now furnished itself with a major sequence of wall-paintings between 1441 and 1444 (pl. 4).

The scheme, justly described by John Pope-Hennessy as 'the most important fresco cycle executed in Siena during the fifteenth century',[12] was probably initiated by Lorenzo Vecchietta. He painted three frescoes in the Pellegrinaio, but only one remains in the room today: *The Legend of the Foundation of the Hospital* (pl. 5). It reflects the shift in power at the Spedale from religious to civic control. Pious the legend may be, yet it offers a decidedly communal interpretation of the truth by maintaining that the hospital was founded by a ninth-century cobbler called Sorore. After nursing pilgrims who passed through Siena en route to Rome, he handed on responsibility for the continuation of his work to the hospital friars. Vecchietta, however, concentrates on the dream of a woman, probably identifiable as the Blessed Sorore's mother. She saw, on the site where the Spedale would be erected, a ladder extending to Heaven. Infants were climbing up its steps into the welcoming embrace of the Virgin, and the legend maintains that the hospital started looking after foundlings as a result of the dream. The ladder duly forms the centrepiece of Vecchietta's fresco, his first documented work. But this Florence-orientated artist framed the mystical vision of the children's ascension in a highly rational context, with an exact perspectival rendering of the heavily ornamented architecture. Its proliferation of swags, statues and medallions threatens to detract from the representation of the woman's dream, and so does the solemn congregation of richly attired figures who attend the event. Since many of them gaze outwards rather than contemplating the ladder, their worldliness militates against the religious meaning of the scene. Such an emphasis accorded well with the secular bias of the hospital, and Vecchietta was doubtless selected because of his strong affiliation with recent Florentine developments in art. He had probably just returned from a spell of collaboration with Masolino on the frescoes in the Collegiate Church at Castiglione d'Olona. The legend fresco in the Pellegrinaio proclaims the influence of this formative period in a distinctly programmatic way, and Vecchietta learned how to shed much of this stiff elaboration in his later work for the Spedale della Scala.

After completing these initial frescoes, however, he found that the rest of the scheme in the Pellegrinaio had been assigned to Domenico di Bartolo

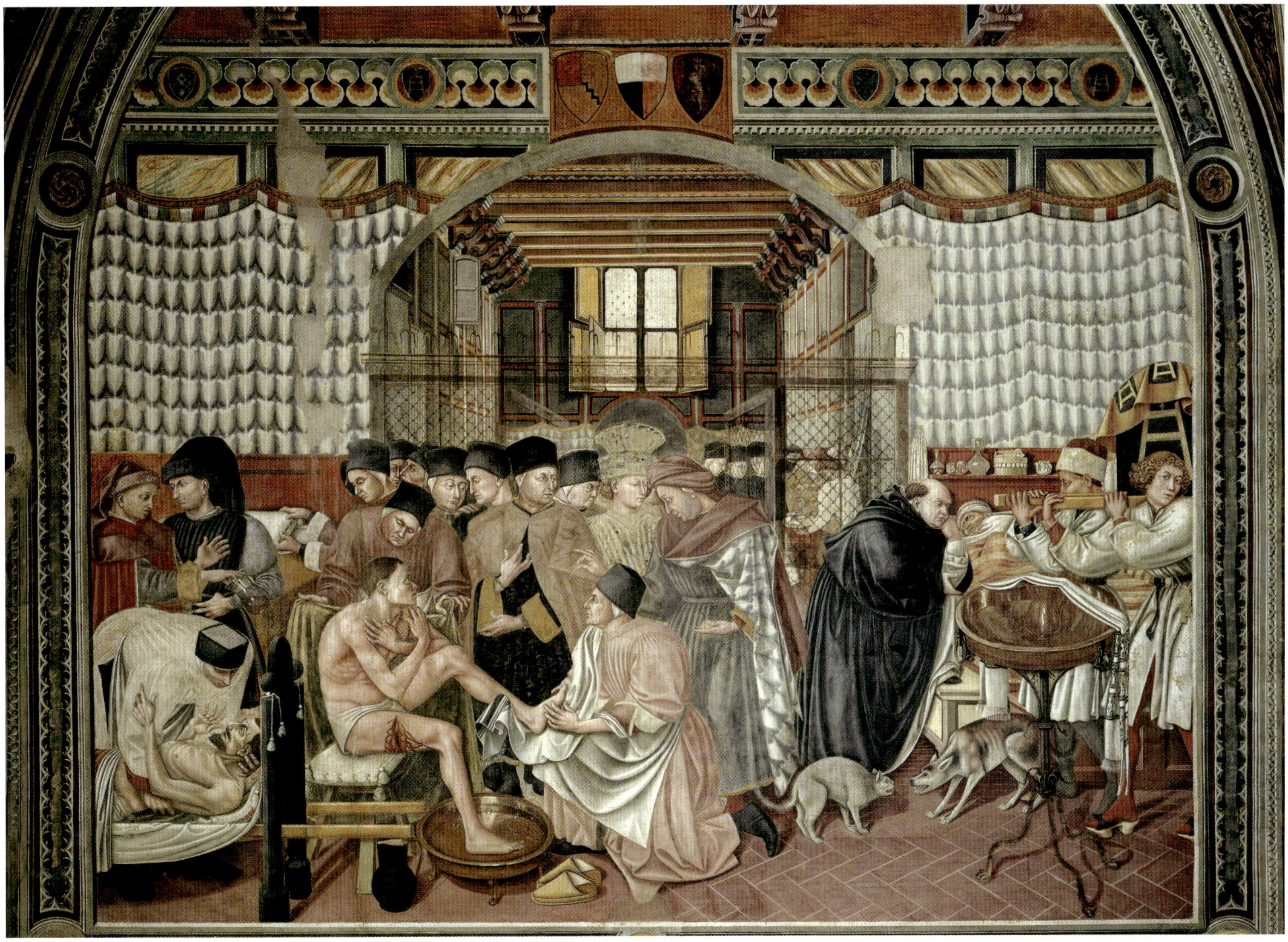

6 Domenico di Bartolo, *Care of the Sick*, 1441–4, Sala Pellegrinaio, Spedale di Santa Maria della Scala, Siena

and his pupil Priamo della Quercia. Perhaps Buzzichelli felt dissatisfied with the congestion evident in Vecchietta's work. At all events, Domenico di Bartolo was invited to complete an ambitious cycle recording the history and contemporary functions of an immensely busy institution dedicated to the foundlings' care, the burial of the dead, nocturnal shelter for homeless adolescents, the apprenticeship of orphans, distributing free bread during famines and much else besides. Buzzichelli commissioned an extensive scheme defining, in a sequence of detailed scenes, subjects as important as the growth of the building, the moment when Pope Celestine III granted him privileges, and the admission of patients in the very room where the frescoes were painted.

Domenico di Bartolo was uniquely qualified, among his Sienese contemporaries, for such a task. He commanded a degree of naturalism that marked him out from his more mystical counterparts and allied him even more clearly than Vecchietta with recent developments in Florentine painting. That must be why he was chosen by the Spedale, for the rector clearly wanted people entering the Pellegrinaio to find themselves surrounded by an authentic and comprehensive testimony to the building's curative activities. Patients were able to discover, in Domenico's frescoes, consoling evidence of a building dedicated to their well-being. A physician and a surgeon with pincers in *Care of the Sick* (pl. 6 and frontispiece) tend to the needs of grievously suffering men with skill, patience and stoical compassion.

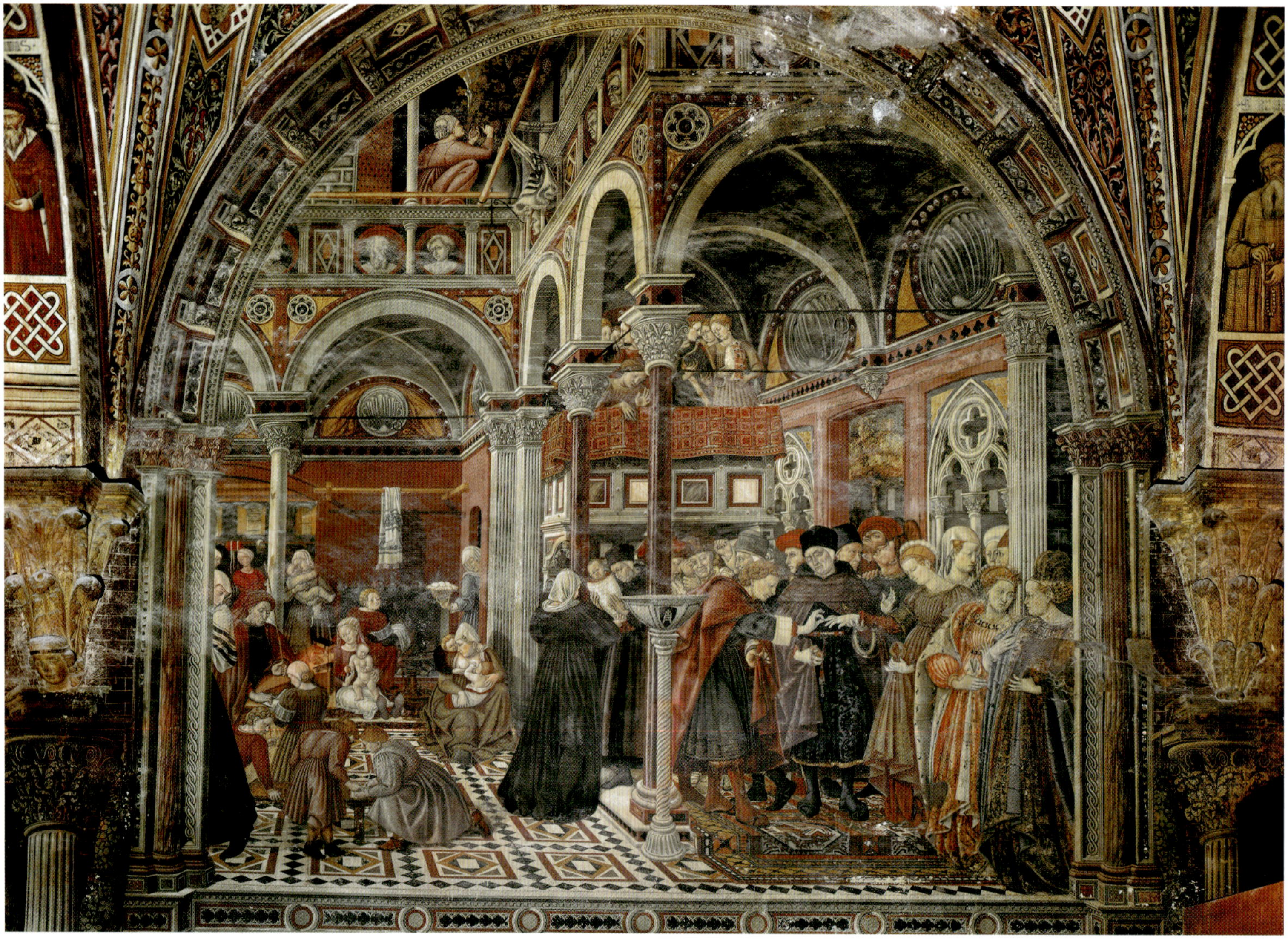

7 Domenico di Bartolo, *The Nurture and Marriage of the Foundlings*, 1441–4, Sala Pellegrinaio, Spedale di Santa Maria della Scala, Siena

The paintings were above all a celebration of the hospital's charitable aims, and orphans would have received particular confirmation of its long-term commitment to their needs in the scene entitled *The Nurture and Marriage of the Foundlings* (pl. 7). The Spedale's statutes made clear that it recognised an obligation to fund the care of foundlings by nurses whom the hospital chose for the purpose. It also felt duty-bound to assist the marriage of girl foundlings when they reached a suitable age, giving each of them *cinquanta libri de denari senesi* from the institution's coffers when the wedding occurred. Both these aspects of the Spedale's work are represented in the fresco and they gain very movingly from Domenico's decision to place them under the same pictorial roof.

The left half of *Nurture and Marriage* is given over to the nurses, who tend the foundling babies with vigorous affection (see pl. 3). One nurse grins as she encourages the little boy to stand up on her lap, and no trace of formality prevents the women from establishing remarkably close maternal relationships with the infants in their charge. The nurse standing by the fireplace hugs her baby with unbridled feeling, and the depth of their love for each other is conveyed with the sculptural grandeur that distinguishes the same artist's *Madonna and Child* paintings.[13] But the hospital staff are no less devoted in their attitude towards the foundlings. In the most powerful section of the fresco, an elderly official is shown clasping an orphan with tender solemnity as he passes over the small, swathed body

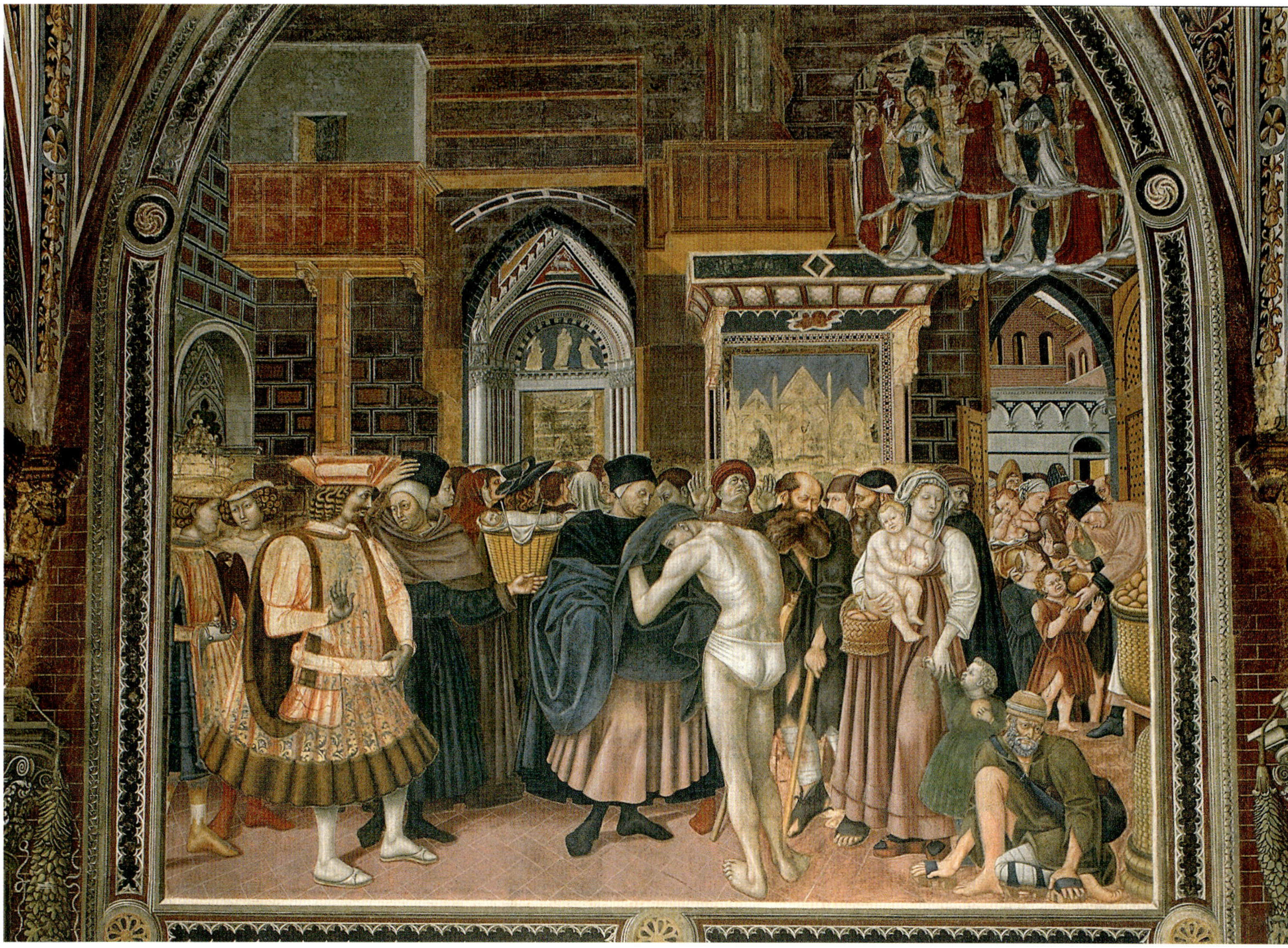

to a nurse's outstretched hands. He appears saddened by the plight of the child. And there is nothing in the least bureaucratic or indifferent about the way his fingers press hard against the baby, even as he prepares to relinquish his hold on the helpless body.

Although the other half of this fresco is marred by Domenico's tendency to crowd his pictorial space with an excess of figures and architectural detail, the marriage of the foundling girl is depicted with a similar depth of feeling. Viewers examining the picture were left in no doubt about the solemnity with which the Spedale officials regarded such a ceremony, marking as it did the moment when the children whom they had nurtured finally entered an existence beyond their immediate responsibilty.

In the most clearly organised of the Pellegrinaio frescoes, however, the hospital's involvement with the world beyond its boundaries received unequivocal affirmation (pl. 8). The composition this time is dominated by the dramatic figure of a near-naked novice, about to clothe himself in the robes of a hospital official. The religious significance of this event, with its overtones of monastic dedication and spiritual regeneration, is confirmed by the sober concentration of the man who supervises the clothing ritual. He stares down at the novice with great sobriety, absorbed in an awareness of the momentous decision taken by the figure who now dedicates his life to the care of others.

As if to counter any suggestion that the Spedale was an inward-looking institution, the right half of

8 Domenico di Bartolo, *Clothing of Novice and Distribution of Alms*, 1441–4, Sala Pellegrinaio, Spedale di Santa Maria della Scala, Siena

9 Domenico di Bartolo, *Madonna della Misericordia*, 1444, Sacristy, Spedale di Santa Maria della Scala, Siena

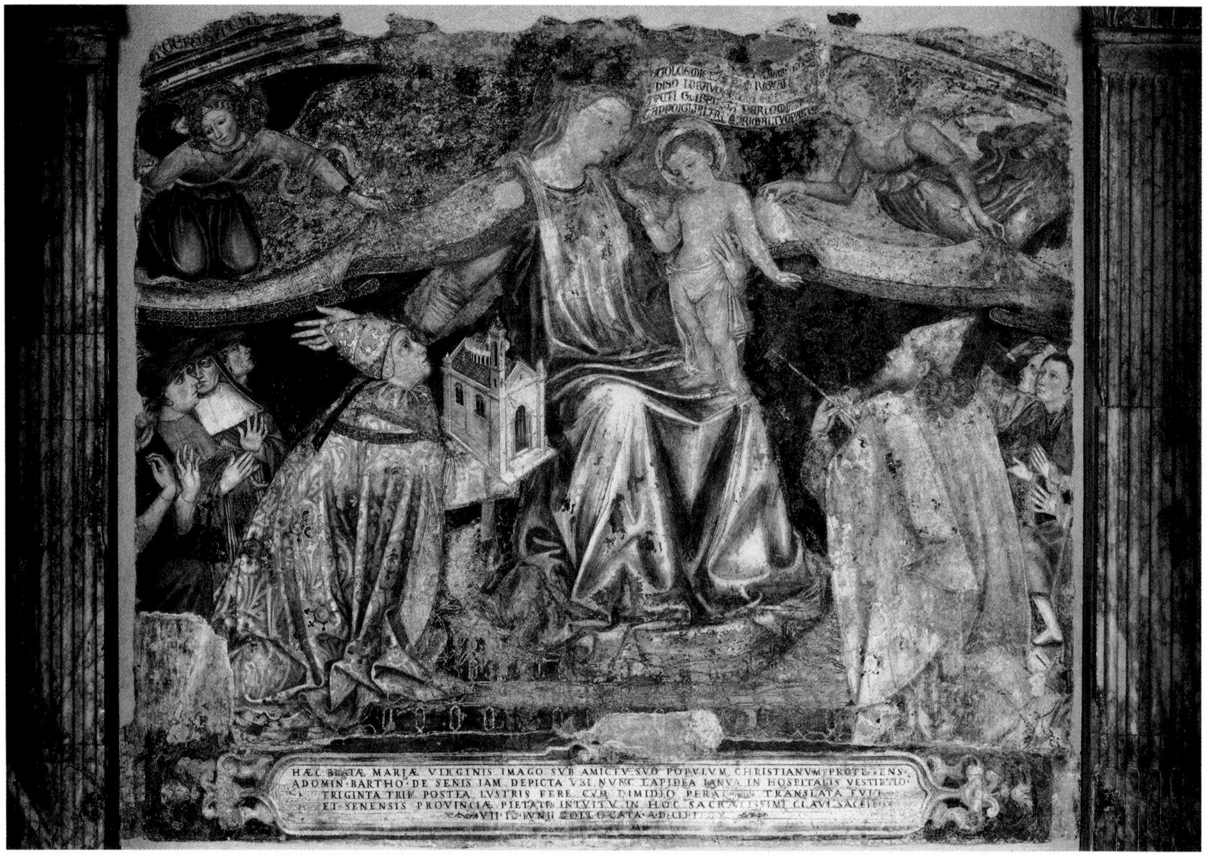

the fresco is taken up with the distribution of alms. Rather than carrying out their responsibilities solely within the hospital's confines, the staff are shown dispensing gifts to the poor who throng Siena's streets and squat, like the ailing beggar, on its paving stones. Prominent among them is the mother standing in symbolic proximity to the novice. Holding one of her children by the arm, she carries a baby boy whose nakedness implies her inability to afford clothes for him. Instead, the child relies on the sustenance provided by the breast he so greedily bares and grasps with both hands. It is a surprisingly frank gesture, and occupies an important place in this fresco because of the Spedale's overriding concern for the well-being of those least able to look after themselves.

The presence of such an elaborate and carefully planned fresco scheme argues that the hospital hoped its foundlings and staff would both benefit from surveying the images painted on the Pellegrinaio's walls. But the scheme's completion in 1444 did not mark the end of the hospital's involvement with art. In the very same year, Domenico was also commissioned to paint a fresco of the *Madonna della Misericordia* (pl. 9) for the chapel.[14] The Virgin, seated with her child, is besieged by a crowd of supplicants. As if in response to their devotion, angels part her mantle so that the kneeling multitude can shelter underneath its capacious folds. Domenico must have finished the fresco around the time that Piero della Francesca began thinking about his commission, from a confraternity in Sansepolcro, for an ambitious *Misericordia Polyptych*. Compared with Piero's innovatory boldness, especially in the central panel (see pl. 22), Domenico's fresco lacks audacity. But it is still a heartfelt image, and the scroll positioned near his Madonna's head adds to the aura of spiritual intensity with an impassioned plea to Jesus: 'O my sweet son, look upon this people who hasten beneath the mantle of she who is their advocate and you, their salvation, and for the love I bear grant them all good things, and above all your guidance.' Viewers would have found immense reassurance in such sentiments and consoled even more by the inscription beneath: 'Here is an image of the Blessed Virgin Mary.

Under your mantle the Christian populace is protected.'[15]

While Domenico was at work on this fresco in 1444, Buzzichelli died. But the new rector, Urbano di Pietro del Bello, soon began to commission work for the sacristy. Rather than continuing to favour Domenico, he turned back to Vecchietta.[16] Possibly dissatisfied with the awkward blend of Gothic and Renaissance styles in the later Pellegrinaio frescoes, with their frequent spatial confusions, Urbano invited Vecchietta in 1445 to produce a painted chest or *armadio delle relique* (pl. 10) for a space specially reserved in the sacristy wall. Since the reliquary was given to the Siena Pinacoteca for safe keeping in the early twentieth century, its original purpose is often overlooked. Initially, though, Vecchietta's painted front served to seal off the space in the wall, and the presence of an altar below it suggests that his work was intended as an altarpiece as well. The finest images on the reliquary certainly have a devotional aura. Shorn of the architectural excess that clogged his Pellegrinaio fresco four years before, they rely for the most part on isolating saints and blessed figures against simple backgrounds. The panel most closely associated with the hospital's history is situated in the middle row, where the Blessed Agostino Novello invests the Spedale's rector with the habit of the Augustine Tertiaries. Novello, highly popular among the Sienese for his involvement with their everyday lives, is guided by the whispering of a diminutive angel as he hands over the habit of his own order to the wizened man kneeling before him.

The austerity of the scene enhances its religious conviction, like the other panels where Vecchietta isolates equally revered figures like the Blessed Ambrogio Sansedoni or Saint Bernardino. Doubtless inspired by the example of Sassetta, he knows precisely how to convey the sober intensity of their faith and belief in the potency of prayer. Ultimately, though, all these embodiments of solitary conviction are placed in the context of God's crucifixion and resurrection, both represented in the lunette above the saints. Bordered by the participants in an annunciation, these two unostentatious scenes bring the reliquary paintings to a quiet yet heartfelt climax.

Urbano must have been immensely gratified by the work, for the following year he entrusted Vecchietta with the whole of a grand fresco scheme on the sacristy's walls and vault. The artist and his assistants laboured on the project until 1449, producing a sequence of paintings that elucidated a theological programme more complex and monumental than anything achieved in Siena before. The grievous damage inflicted on the frescoes hampers the task of evaluation, and several areas of the cycle are completely ruined. Enough survives to prove, however, that the erudite Vecchietta interpreted a series of parallel stories from the Old and New Testaments with considerable suppleness and gusto. He is able to invest the figure of Christ the Saviour, presiding over the sacristy from the centre of the decorated vault, with an appropriate gravity of bearing. The saints hovering round this focal figure are similarly imposing and dignified, but elsewhere in the room Vecchietta displays his command of very different moods. In one of the wall frescoes he gives the Angel Gabriel a lyrical delicacy, whereas the deliverance from the snake plague is handled with an alert understanding of danger and alarm. The most disturbing fresco reveals his grasp of leering violence, as the devils carry off naked chil-

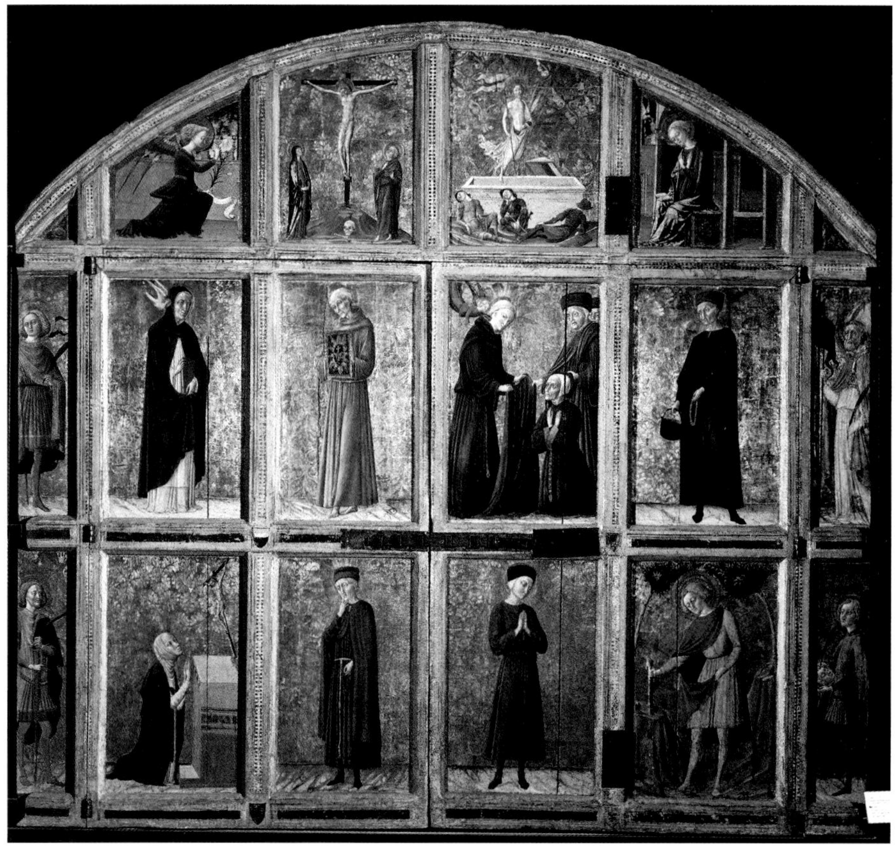

10 Lorenzo Vecchietta, painted chest, c. 1445, Pinacoteca Nazionale, Siena

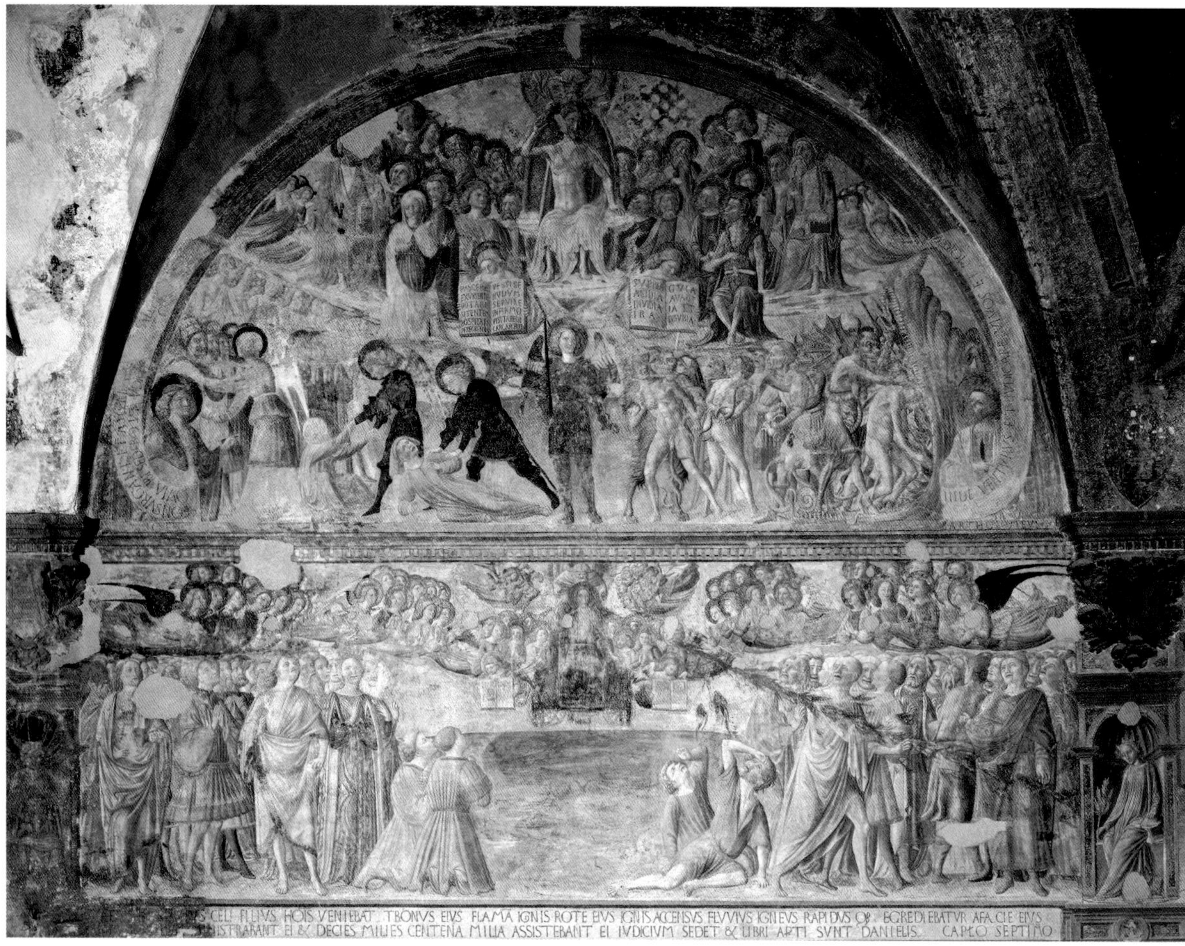

11 Lorenzo Vecchietta, *Devils in Limbo*, 1449, fresco scheme for Sacristy walls and vault, Spedale di Santa Maria della Scala, Siena

dren from Limbo (pl. 11). This gruesome scene is dramatised with a conviction that shows how much Vecchietta may have learned from medieval paintings of the same theme. He is, nevertheless, equally adept at conveying ethereal splendour in the frescoes where figures kneel adoringly in Solomon's Temple or gather to witness the funeral of Saint Lawrence.

The hospital church likewise became a showpiece of Sienese art, especially after Guidoccio d'Andrea supervised its rebuilding in 1466. Even so, one of its most distinguished paintings had by then been installed in the church for more than a decade. In April 1447 the Guild of Grocers commissioned Giovanni di Paolo to produce an altarpiece for its chapel in the Spedale's church (pl. 12). The painting, which he undertook to complete by November 1449, was strictly controlled by the Guild's contract: as well as specifying the subject, the rectors of the guild claimed the right to dictate the work's composition and treatment. They probably went so far as to insist that Giovanni di Paolo base his picture on Ambrogio Lorenzetti's *Presentation in the Temple*, painted just over a century before. In other words, it was a conservative commission, and the painting received by the guild declared an obvious debt to Lorenzetti's example.

All the same, Giovanni di Paolo was sufficiently independent as an artist to stamp his own identity on the picture he produced. While remaining faithful to the disposition of figures in Lorenzetti's painting, and their relationship with the temple architecture, he felt at liberty to introduce an array of small yet telling changes. The octagonal structure presiding over Lorenzetti's *Presentation* is transformed into a domed alternative, and he enlarges the row of ascending dragons above the principal arch. Their vivacity affects Giovanni di Paolo's handling of the temple floor, where Lorenzetti's steady receding tiles are replaced by a more

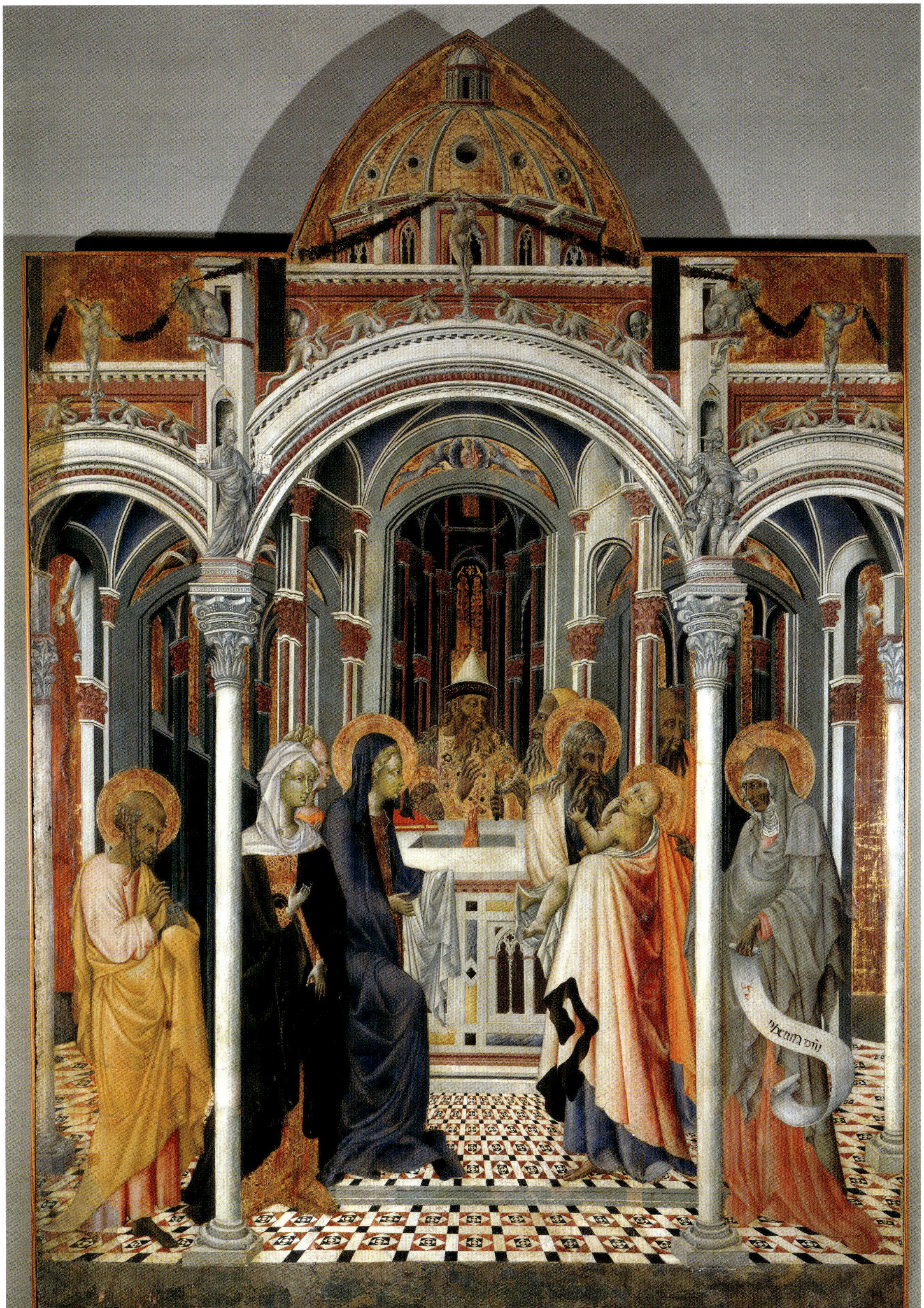

12 Giovanni di Paolo, *Presentation in the Temple*, 1447–9, Pinacoteca Nazionale, Siena

complex and dizzying pattern. The floor's solidity and spatial recession no longer seem so reassuring. Nor do the figures themselves, who lack the measured confidence of Lorenzetti's group. Influenced by the frankly linear rhythms of Gentile da Fabriano, the new version flattens its participants' bodies and raises the emotional temperature by clothing them in draperies of sharp lemon and puce.

An access of nervous urgency results, heightened still further by the intensity of the haunted faces attending the ceremony. Simeon, now looking towards the right, stares down with an air of troubled enquiry towards the baby gathered in his voluminous robe. The Virgin herself seems agitated, extending her hand as if to safeguard the child against a possible fall. Giovanni di Paolo seems bent on prophesying, through the apprehensive mood, the tribulations to be suffered by this cossetted little boy in later life. The picture's eeriness is confirmed not only by the openly alarmed head peering out from a pillar above Christ's head, but also by the cowled woman on the right of the scene. Carrying a scroll more twisted by far than its predecessor in Lorenzetti's picture, she stares grimly towards the vibrating floor and broods over the most sombre implications of the child's destiny.

Although this introspective painting was later moved to the Accademia, it stayed in the Spedale longer than the elaborate bronze tabernacle commissioned for the church in 1467 (pl. 13). Vecchietta, whose sculpture was esteemed just as highly as his painting, once again found himself entrusted with this important project. He was promised 1200 florins for the complex execution of the ciborium, completed just over five years later. A lesser artist might have found its demands oppressive, and produced a dutiful work that testified merely to his capacity for dogged labour. Vecchietta, however, carried out his task with deftness, agility and finesse. A preliminary drawing for the tabernacle shows how delicately he prepared himself for the feat of orchestrating so many bronze statuettes in a coherent ensemble, and the final figures are characterised by their consummate refinement.

Technical skill is never allowed to overshadow inner vitality in this *tour de force* of sustained inventiveness. The putti at the ciborium's base twist their limbs in a display of uninhibited *élan*, contrasting effectively with the poise of the music-making angels above them. Their elegance does not prevent them from performing with exultation, and the same dignified fervour can be found in the figures who inhabit niches around the central drum. Seated and constrained by their surroundings they may be, but these exquisite statuettes are still capable of conveying the most subtle and tremulous of emotions. Vecchietta has ensured, however, that they remain restrained in comparison with the uppermost part of the reliquary. Here, progressively freeing himself from the limits imposed by the receptacle below, he arrives at a climactic group perched triumphantly on a globe-like dome. The two attendant angels appear to be enjoying their liberty as they brandish wings and convoluted drapery beneath the lithe deity, who balances on top of the ciborium with acrobatic panache and extends a beneficent hand into space. With hindsight, this culminating figure can be seen as an unconscious preparation for the greater eloquence of *The Risen Christ* (see pl. 15), made by Vecchietta for the Spedale four years later.

The hospital greeted the arrival of the completed reliquary with understandable delight, paying its maker 1,500 florins and giving him a rent-free house for the duration of his life. The tabernacle, claimed Vecchietta's ecstatic patrons, was 'a most notable work, and more beautiful, and more ornamental, and greater than he had promised'.[17] The very success of the commission meant, however, that the ciborium was taken away from the church of Santa Maria della Scala little more than thirty years after its installation there. In 1506 the 'Magnificent' Pandolfo Petrucci, a powerful member of the Sienese government, decreed that the high altar of the city's cathedral be moved from under the cupola to the place it occupies today. Scorning tradition and the achievements of earlier Sienese art, he took the astonishing decision to oust Duccio's cherished *Maestà* from its original position and relegate it to a side aisle. Petrucci replaced the painting with the Vecchietta reliquary, and it was never returned to the Spedale. It remains one of the masterpieces of the cathedral to this day, accompanied on either side of the high altar by two bronze angels made by Francesco di Giorgio nine years before the ciborium was carried, in triumph, across the Piazza del Duomo to its present exalted location.

Ironically enough, the selfsame Francesco di Giorgio had already carried out significant embell-

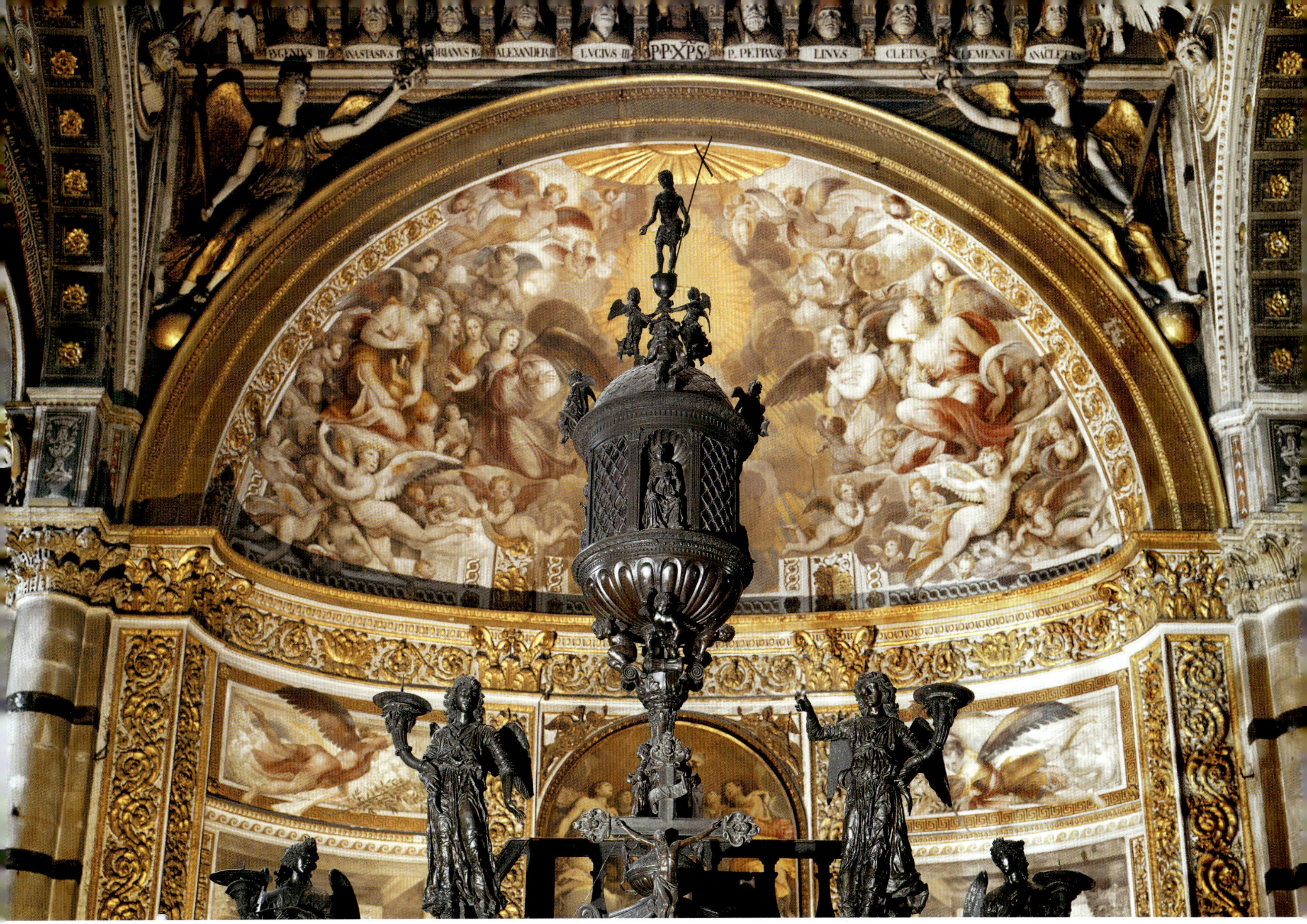

ishments of his own for the hospital. An accomplished painter, military engineer and architect as well as a sculptor, this Leonardo-like all-rounder was invited in 1471 to construct a new choir and ceiling for the Spedale church. Working in collaboration with Guidoccio Cozzarelli, he also executed a substantial painting, *The Coronation of the Virgin*, probably on the wall behind the high altar. The space is now occupied by a Baroque fresco of *The Pool of Bethesda* painted by Sebastiano Conca in 1732, and no trace remains in the church of Francesco's picture. But it has often been confused with another version of the Coronation that he painted, in 1472–4, for the monastery of Monte Oliveto Maggiore (pl. 14). Since this panel is supposed to have been brought to Siena later and installed in the Spedale, the confusion is forgivable. But the surviving picture is surely identifiable as the monastery version, which was taken to the hospital possibly in order to compensate for the obliteration of the church's version. At any rate, the painting is now in the Pinacoteca at Siena, and offers some notion at least of the image produced by Francesco for the Spedale's high altar wall.

The composition is packed with figures to a claustrophobic degree, and their sheer proliferation threatens to smother the significance of the coronation ceremony. Its spatial organisation seems bewildering at first, for Francesco is not at pains to clarify the positions occupied by his ranks of attendant saints. The perspectival recession established in the floor is counteracted, almost eccentrically, by

13 Lorenzo Vecchietta, Bronze Tabernacle of the High Altar, 1467–72, Cathedral, Siena

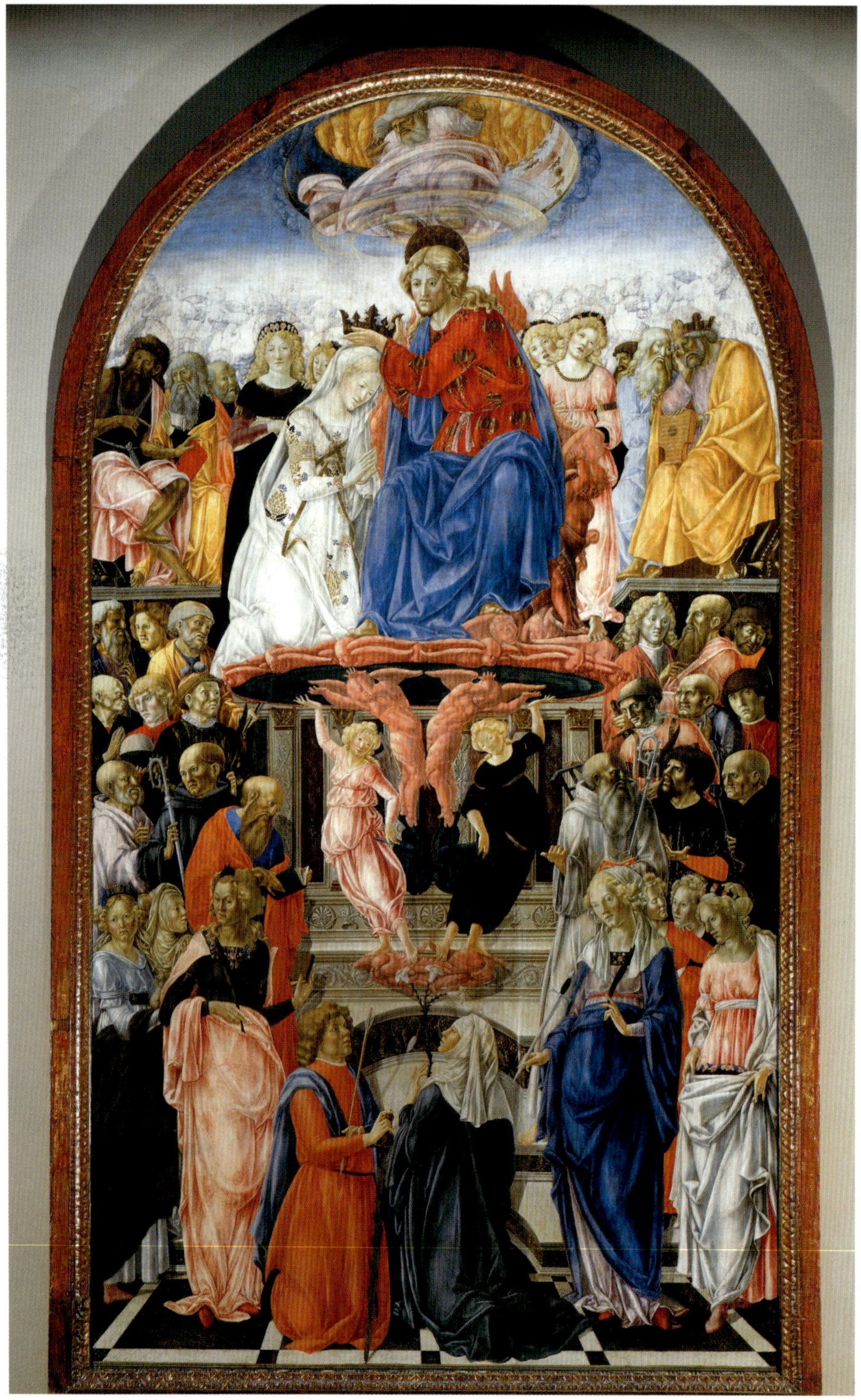

14 Francesco di Giorgio Martini, *Coronation of the Virgin*, 1472–4, Pinacoteca Nazionale, Siena

a typical Sienese desire to emphasise the decorative flatness of the picture surface as well. That is why the figures ascend towards the Virgin with such an apparent disregard for the spatial propriety found in contemporary Florentine painting. The strangeness is further enhanced by the exceptionally outspoken brightness of the colours, for Francesco relies on an unusual, obsessive range of red and blue variations.

In the end, though, all these idiosyncratic strategies contribute to the painting's charged emotion. Unlike so many saints who witness religious ceremonies with blatant unconcern, these figures are intensely absorbed in the coronation. Their faces react ardently to the ritual crowning, and the Virgin is a beatific young woman so engrossed in the event that she remains oblivious of all the cosmic whirling in the sky overhead.

The most impassioned of the remarkable *quattrocento* works created for the Spedale della Scala, however, is Vecchietta's *The Risen Christ* (pl. 15). A life-size statue, it was originally intended by its maker for the chapel he asked the hospital to let him build near the close of his life. Vecchietta was by then the artist most intimately associated with the institution, where he had produced all his most outstanding paintings and sculpture over several decades. As a final expression of his relationship with the Spedale, he arranged to be buried in this chapel. And by 1476 the *Risen Christ* was completed for the same cherished location.

It is a memorable swansong. Four years before his death, the elderly artist managed here to embody in the bronze figure his most profound feelings about mortality and regeneration beyond the grave. Spurred no doubt by his admiration for Donatello's anguished *St John the Baptist* in Siena Cathedral,[18] which must have taught Vecchietta a great deal about the expression of vehement emotion, he gave his *Risen Christ* enormous power. This is a figure who has undergone a depth of suffering declared, not just by the brazenly exposed wounds gouged in his side, hands and feet, but throughout his body. Swaying as he struggles to retain his stance on the ground, and haggard with exhaustion after his terrible travail, Vecchietta's Christ still bears disquieting signs of the extinction he endured. But this frailty makes his determination to transcend death all the more moving. His outstretched arm acts as a defiant affirmation of immortality. And after the *Risen Christ* was installed on the high altar in the hospital church, it must have extended an invaluable amount of redemptive hope to all the patients who worshipped there.

15 (*facing page*) Lorenzo Vecchietta, *The Risen Christ*, 1476, Spedale di Santa Maria della Scala, Siena

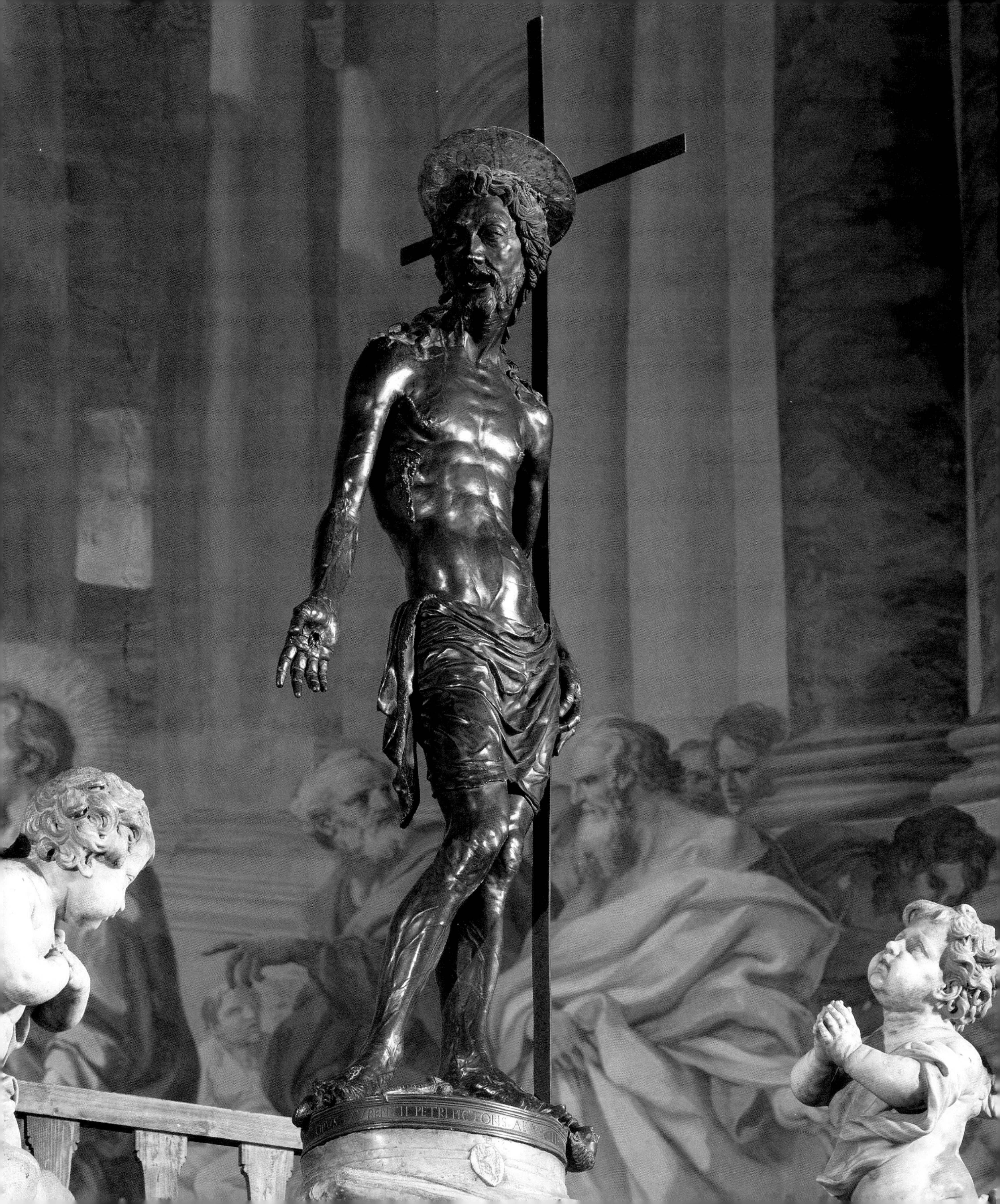
OPVS
PETRI PICTORIS

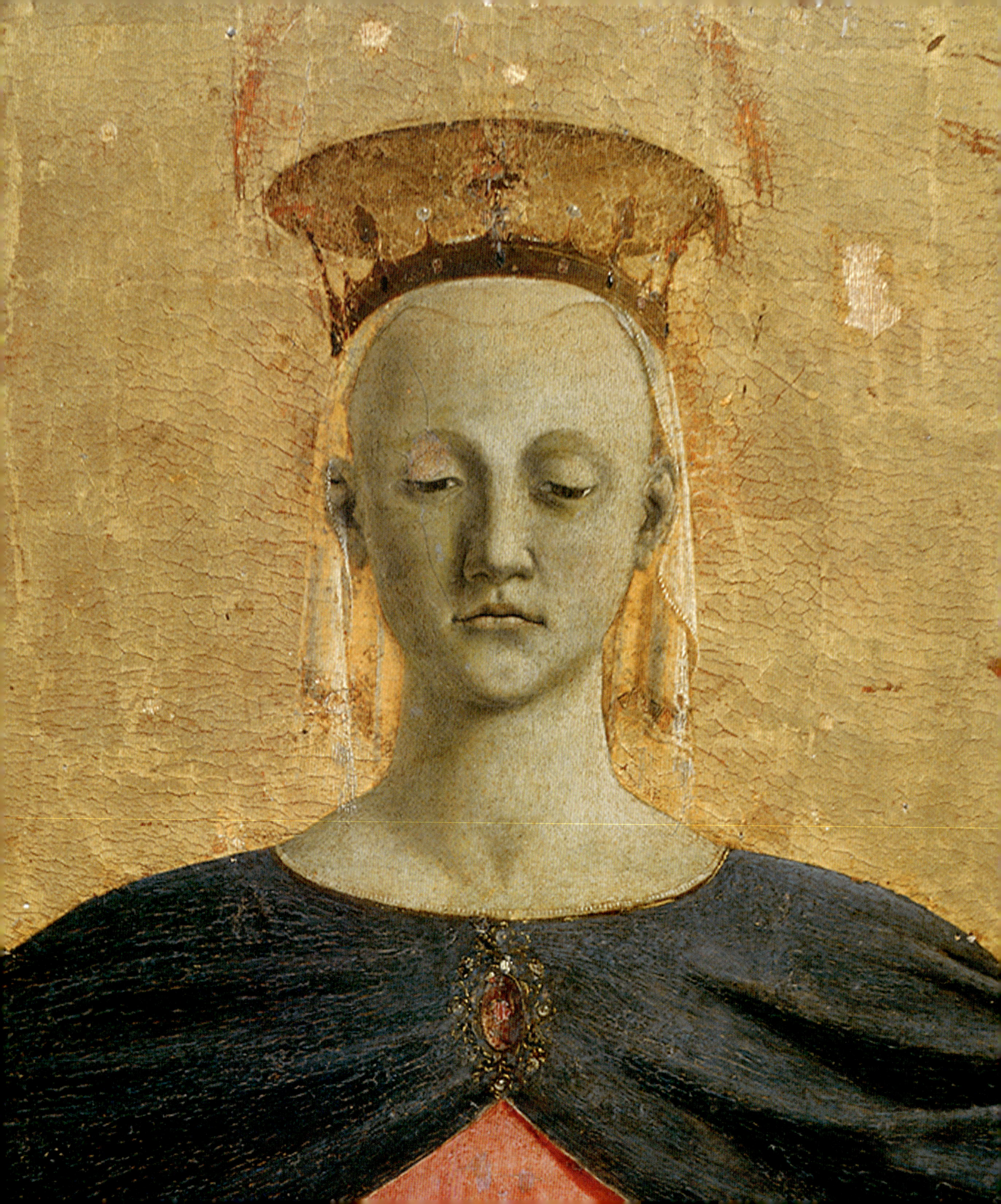

TWO
MADONNA OF MERCY

Piero della Francesca must have been immensely gratified to receive, in 1445, a commission for a major altarpiece in his home town of Sansepolcro. The invitation came from the Compagnia di Santa Maria della Misericordia, one of the oldest and most powerful confraternities devoted to the community's welfare. Piero's own family, who belonged to the town's affluent merchant class, had been associated with the Misericordia since the late fourteenth century. His father, who rose to become one of Sansepolcro's four governors in 1444, probably helped to procure the commission for Piero.[1] One of his brothers, the Camaldolite monk Don Francesco, was the confraternity's chaplain.[2] And another one worked as an administrator for its hospital, a major institution founded in 1348 soon after the Black Death began decimating the citizens of Sansepolcro. Dedicated to the Madonna of Mercy, the hospital occupied an ample site on the north-east side of the town's defensive walls. A church was built alongside, as well as a private oratory, administrative quarters and a garden for medicinal herbs. The entire complex, now deserted and in ruins, played a vital role in sustaining the local populace for many centuries.

The advent of the Black Death transformed the confraternity's aims. Before then, the Misericordia had focused its works of mercy on impoverished people and housed them, rent-free, in 'hospices for the poor'.[3] But when the plague struck, the confraternity realised that they should learn to encompass the needs of the community as a whole. Aided by hundreds of bequests from Sansepolcro's wealthier inhabitants, the Ospedale della Misericordia swiftly expanded to cope with the town's accelerating economic problems in the early decades of the fifteenth century.[4] By the time Piero began work on the Misericordia commission, hardship within the town was approaching crisis-point. In response, the confraternity strove to perform the seven acts of mercy defined by Christ as a necessary preparation for salvation.[5] Diane Cole Ahl has described how the Misericordia 'distributed alms and food to the poor and provided medicine to the sick. It succoured foundlings, ministered to condemned prisoners, and provided lodging and food to indigent pilgrims who came to Sansepolcro. Perhaps a new altarpiece for its church was deemed essential to serve the Misericordia and its growing constituencies within the town.'[6]

Confraternity members were prepared to go to surprising lengths in their quest for divine mercy at the Last Judgement. The central act of devotion among the Misericordia fraternity was flagellation, performed by *disciplinati* who willingly imitated Christ's suffering before the crucifixion. Since Jesus

16 (*facing page*) Detail of pl. 22

had been stripped, spat on and scourged with whips, the *disciplinati* were prepared to undergo the same gruelling punishment. Here, in the privacy of the oratory near the hospital and its church, they strove to expiate humanity's sins.[7] But the pain of flagellation was complemented by singing sacred songs of praise and mourning to the Madonna, Jesus and the saints. A book of these songs, still surviving in Sansepolcro and sharing a strong Marian emphasis, probably belonged to the Compagnia di Santa Maria della Misericordia.[8] They implore Mary to bestow her compassion, and songs dating from the period when Piero commenced work on his altarpiece plead in particular for assistance from Saint Sebastian, identified as the protector against plague. The confraternity hoped he would ask God to ensure that 'the pestilence be lifted by your clemency and give us rest'.[9]

Piero, who had grown up in Sansepolcro and knew the Misericordia's members, would later make flagellation the subject of his finest and most mysterious painting. But in 1445, when he signed the contract committing him to paint the altarpiece for the hospital church, Piero was already considering how to reflect the confraternity's priorities in this complex and demanding work. It must have constituted a great challenge to the young artist, whose reputation was based principally on work he had carried out with an older and more experienced artist, Domenico Veneziano. In 1439 they had collaborated on a series of choir frescoes for Sant'Egidio, the chapel of the hospital of Santa Maria Nuova in Florence. The paintings' subsequent destruction constitutes one of the most grievous losses in *quattrocento* art. But Piero's contribution to this scheme must have been impressive in the eyes of the Misericordia fraternity, even if the innovatory boldness of Veneziano was too advanced for provincial tastes in Sansepolcro. They honoured tradition more fervently than the forward-looking Florentines, and the Misericordia's contract makes clear that Piero's altarpiece must be made 'according to the size and type of the painting on wood . . . there at present'.

In other words, the valued precedent established by the older image (doubtless a *Madonna of Mercy*) would be honoured. At the same time, the eight confraternity officers who witnessed the contract also insisted that 'no other painter put his hand to the brush' apart from Piero himself. They cherished his individual contribution, even if the contract also stressed that he would only paint 'the images, figures, and adornment . . . expressly detailed by the above Prior and council, or their successors in office'. They would control the overall content of the altarpiece, and their presence would be duly reflected in the figures who pray to the Madonna in the main panel.

Although Piero duly agreed to execute the entire altarpiece, and complete the ensemble within three years using only the finest materials 'especially ultramarine', the terms of the contract were soon flouted.[10] The commission stemmed from a bequest made by Urbano di Meo dei Pichi, who belonged to one of the richest families in Sansepolcro. Sixty florins had been bequeathed to the Misericordia by Urbano back in 1422, for 'an ornamented altarpiece for the high altar' of its 'church or oratory'.[11] But the payment promised by the Pichi was not handed over, even after the confraternity tried several times to obtain it. So when Piero was awarded the commission, well over twenty years after Urbano's bequest, the monetary problems continued. The contract promised that he would receive fifty florins immediately, as a mark of 'good faith'. But the Pichi did not pay him for at least five years, and their failure to do so may well explain why the artist delayed his work on the altarpiece. He does not appear to have finished the work until the early 1460s, when the Misericordia was obliged to take action against the Pichi and obtain compensation for payments it had made to Piero. As late as 1467 the artist was still waiting for a final instalment of the 150 florins promised as the total sum in his original contract.

It is a wonder, then, that the *Misericordia Polyptych* was ever brought to completion at all (pl. 17). The original buttressed frame was destroyed in the seventeenth century and the altarpiece sawn into separate panels in a thoroughly misguided attempt to make it look less old-fashioned. Some of the side paintings have suffered from fading and extensive cracking, doubtless because they were executed more quickly than the carefully handled, well-preserved central panels. But the ensemble is still intact in Sansepolcro's Palazzo Communale, where it has long been honoured as Piero's earliest surviving work.

Although the admiration it arouses is wholly justified, the altarpiece was not, in the end, his work

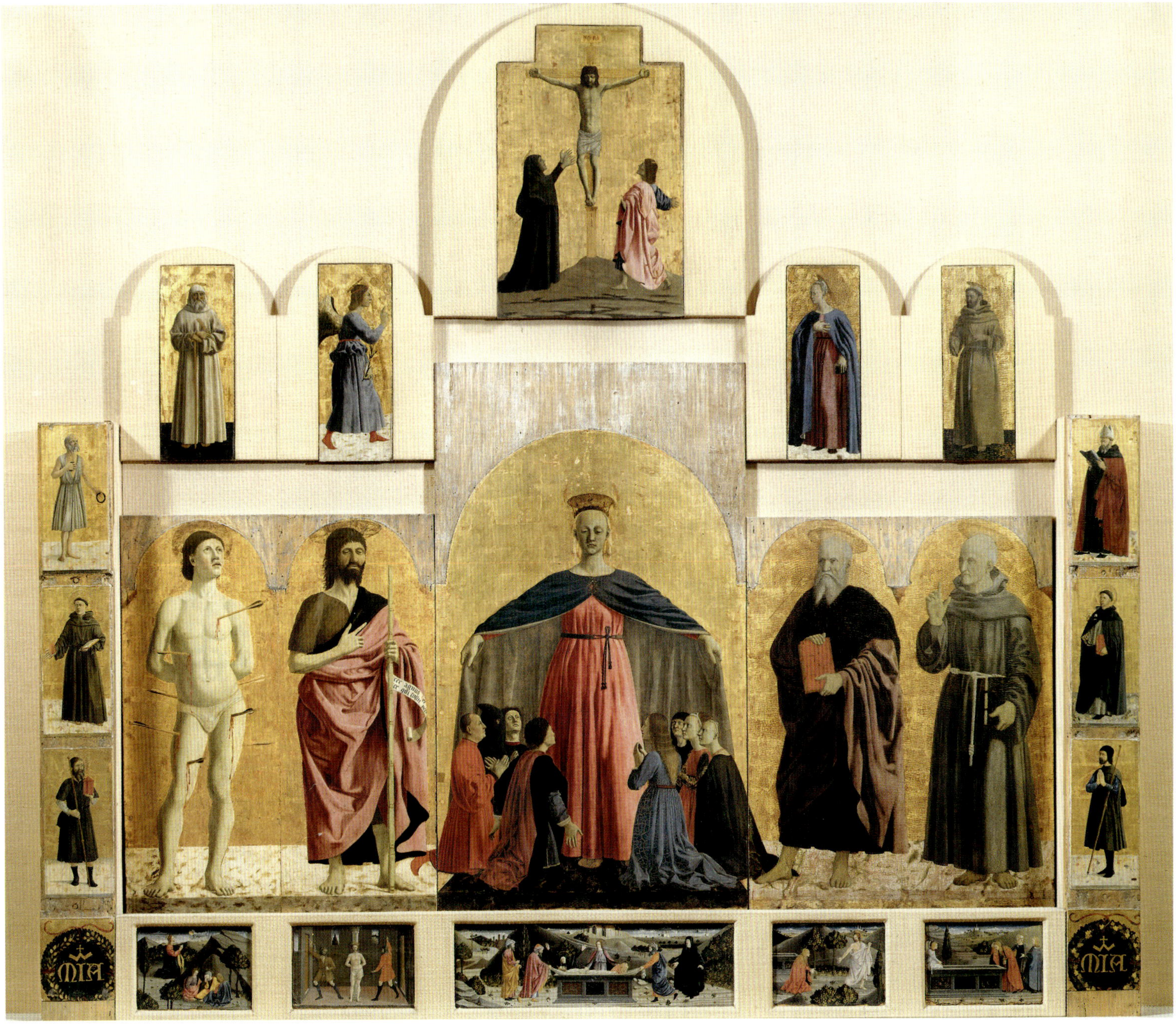

17 Piero della Francesca, *Misericordia Polyptch*, 1445–61, Pinacoteca Comunale, Sansepolcro

alone. The flanking pilasters, each one terminating in a base painted with the confraternity's insignia 'MIA', were probably executed by the Camaldolite monk Fra Giuliano Amedei. And the predella panels are by the same hand, following Piero's conception. Amedei was a miniaturist and the images in the predella lack the potent physical presence as well as the spiritual intensity so evident elsewhere in the polyptych. All the same, the subjects of these small panels remain crucial in any attempt to understand the confraternity's aims. The flagellation is here, a curiously dance-like image reflecting the performances enacted by the *disciplinati* in the oratory. So are other episodes from Christ's passion: the agony in the garden, the empty tomb and Christ's miraculous encounter with the Magdalen. But the central panel, the largest piece in the predella, tackled the most important theme of all: the *Entombment of Christ* (pl. 18). For the reverence with which his corpse is lowered into the sepulchre, watched by grief-

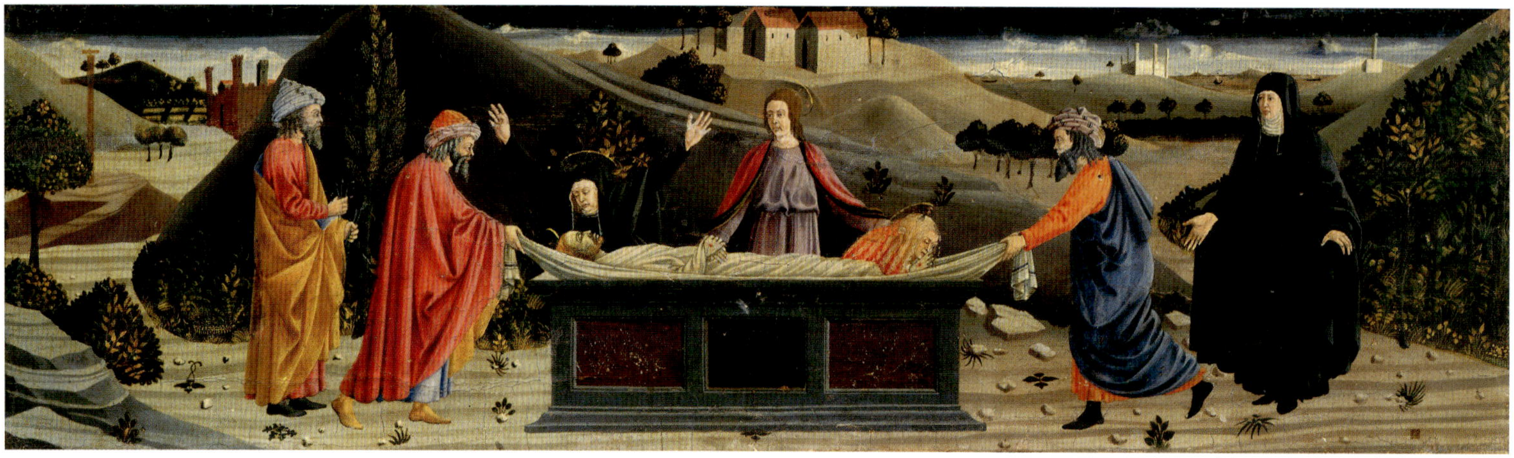

18 (*above*) Piero della Francesca and Giuliano Amedei, *Entombment of Christ*, predella of *Misericordia Polyptych*, 1445–61, Pinacoteca Comunale, Sansepolcro

19 (*facing page*) Piero della Francesca, *Annunciation*, detail of *Misericordia Polyptych*, 1445–61, Pinacoteca Comunale, Sansepolcro

stricken women, honours the special significance of the tomb in Sansepolcro's history.

The town was named after the Holy Sepulchre of Jerusalem, where Jesus had been laid in the tomb and ultimately achieved resurrection. Supposed fragments of the stone from the Sepulchre were among the holy relics brought back to Sansepolcro by Saints Arcanus and Giles, who are depicted in the *Misericordia Polyptych* (see pl. 17). They returned from a pilgrimage to the Holy Land with wood from the cross, drops of Christ's blood, cloth from his burial shroud and even specimens of the Virgin's hair and milk. All these curious trophies became so venerated that pilgrims converged on Sansepolcro in substantial numbers, eager to attend the Feast of the Holy Sepulchre at the beginning of each September. Among the celebratory masses and processions, the giving of alms became increasingly significant as the Renaissance era approached. And Fra Giuilano Amedei, as well as executing the predella of the Misericordia's polyptych, painted the confraternity's insignia on a stone plaque attached to the facade of its church. The papal indulgence inscribed on the plaque offered remission of punishment for sin to 'every person, male or female, young or old, confessed and contrite' who presented alms to the church, especially on the Feast of the Annunciation.[12]

The cardinal importance of that day, 25 March, is acknowledged in the upper reaches of the altarpiece. Here, the Archangel Gabriel advances with scarlet-stockinged feet and fingers raised in blessing on one side while, on the other, the Virgin Mary places hand on breast as she receives the momentous news (pl. 19). The heavily cracked paint has obscured her expression. But she appears as solemn as the two saints flanking the scene, Benedict and Francis. They both look burdened by a sense of foreboding. And well they might: the two annunciation panels are separated by the base of a larger painting lodged at the altarpiece's apex. There, the tragic outcome of the Virgin birth is dramatised in a stark, uncompromising *Crucifixion* (pl. 20).

Unlike so many other artists who painted this harrowing scene, Piero reduces it to a simple, severe encounter between three people. No sign of other crosses can be detected, let alone the figures who often accompany them. Calvary is nothing more than two planks of wood thrust into a single mound of mud-coloured earth. All distracting incidents have been jettisoned, by an artist determined to concentrate our attention on the plight of Jesus and his two helpless, traumatised mourners. They realise, now, that all hope has gone. Christ is no longer capable of registering their presence. His eyes are closed, and his slender body seems unable to muster any more resistance to the inevitable onset of death. His emaciated arms, stretched painfully by the nails hammered through his open palms, testify to the starvation he must have endured. Although blood smears his hands and courses brightly from the wound in his side, Jesus's flesh is pallid. All his former vitality has drained away, leaving behind a bleached body motionless on the cross.

At some point in his ill-documented early life, Piero must have studied with avidity Masaccio's great Pisa Altarpiece.[13] For the connections between the *Crucifixion* in Masaccio's polyptych (pl. 21) and Piero's version are clear enough. The scene in Masaccio's painting is likewise stripped of everything save Christ and his grief-stricken attendants, one of whom collapses before the cross and thrusts up protesting arms in a gesture of inconsolable distress. The young Piero would have learned the expressive power of pictorial economy while he looked at Masaccio's *Crucifixion.* But when the two paintings are compared, Piero's version seems all the more raw. For one thing, Masaccio's Jesus is a more muscular, powerfully built figure. Despite the extreme duress he suffers, this man still seems fortified by an inner resilience. By contrast, Piero's Christ seems even more wan and etiolated. He lacks the elaborate, burnished halo glowing around the head of Masaccio's Saviour. The latter's hands extend to the very edges of the arched panel, whereas the hands belonging to Piero's Jesus stop well short of the painting's sides. In Masaccio's *Crucifixion*, Saint John stares down at the weeping woman slumped at the base of the cross. With clasped hands unable even to support the weight of his sagging head, he seems momentarily oblivious of the crucified figure above. In Piero's painting, however, the collapsed woman has been eliminated. And Saint John, like the Virgin opposite him, looks up in open-mouthed dismay at Christ marooned in emptiness above him.

Judging by the position of his legs, John has been walking forward to get as close to Jesus as possible. But the sight of the blanched, paralysed body has arrested him in mid-stride. Flinging out both arms in a frantic gesture of despair and incomprehension, he stares at the Saviour and, very probably, lets out a yell. This is a painting bent on making the viewer feel at once bereft and indignant. John appears to be asking why such torture should have been inflicted on an innocent victim. He deplores the waste involved in losing his inspirational leader, and he cannot, finally, believe that Christ has gone.

John's anguish is shared by the hooded Virgin, wrapped in a funereal black cloak almost silhouetted against the gold ground. Unlike her monumental counterpart in Masaccio's altarpiece, who wrings her hands as she contemplates death on the cross, Piero's Virgin exercises no such restraint. She reaches up impulsively and imploringly towards her son, raising both arms as high as the stiffness in her bones will allow, thumbs and fingers thrust out-

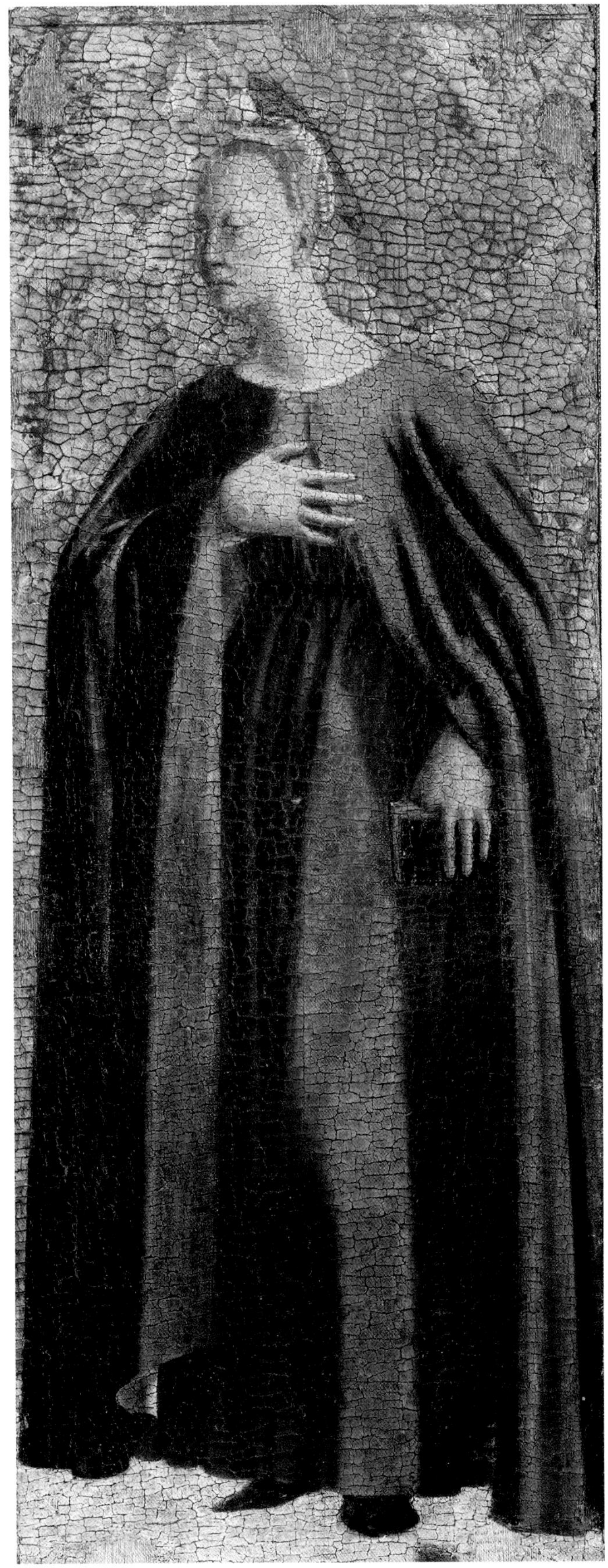

20 Piero della Francesca, *Crucifixion*, detail of *Misericordia Polyptych*, 1445–61, Pinacoteca Comunale, Sansepolcro

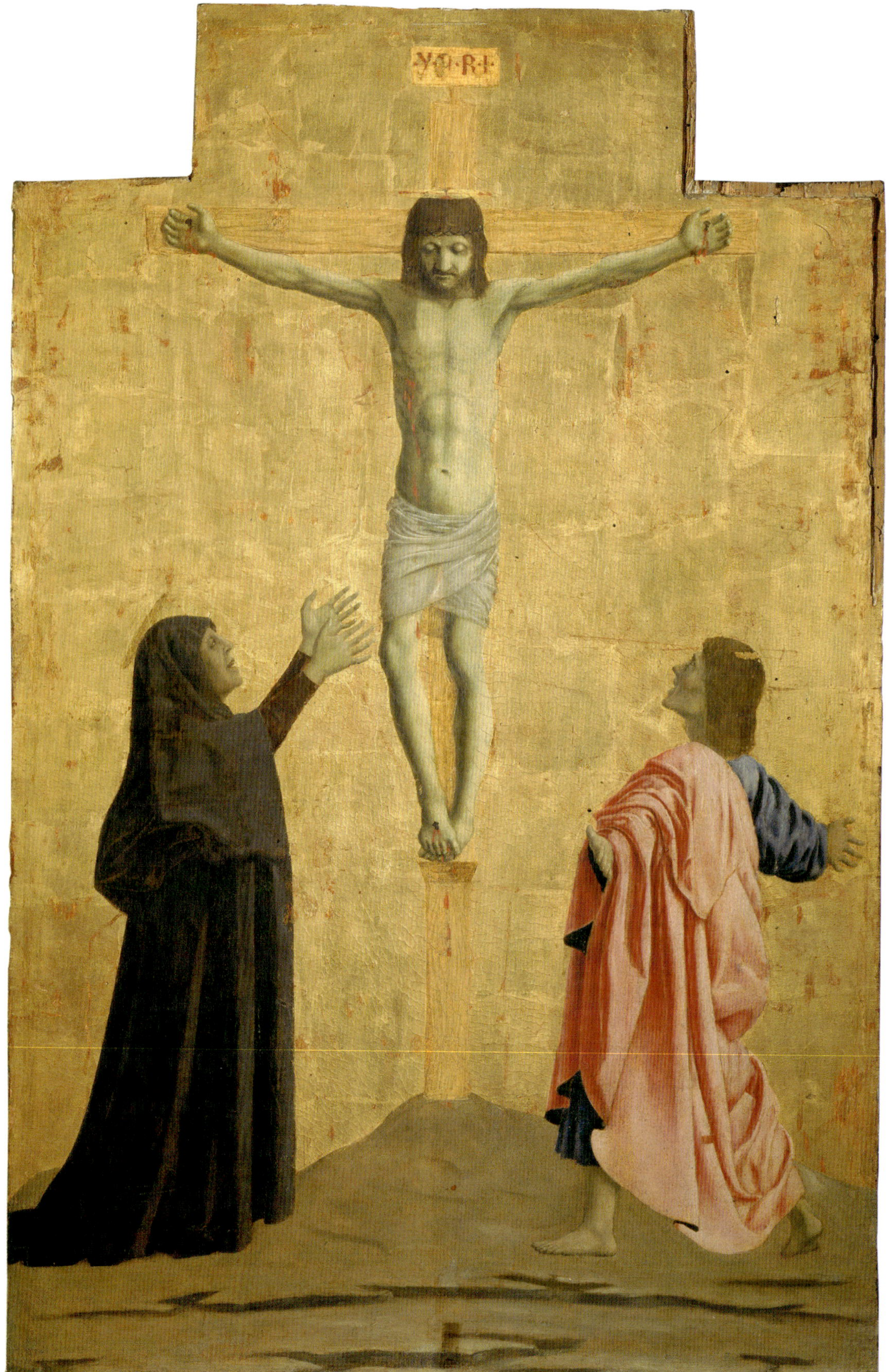

wards, desperate to touch him. But she is unable to do so. A tantalising gap remains between mother and offspring, possibly reflecting the Virgin's grim realisation that his flesh is now cold. Unwilling to confirm it for herself, she remains frozen like a figure from a Greek tragedy doomed to lament her loss. Clawing the air, this inconsolable matriarch sums up the visceral force of a panel where the anguish caused by Christ's martyrdom is conveyed with heart-wrenching immediacy.

Directly below this harshness, however, Piero and his patrons ensured that the principal painting offered immense spiritual solace. For the panel is dominated, not by a corpse on a cross, but by the Madonna della Misericordia herself (pl. 22). Capped by a crown and a halo suspended perspectively in space, the Virgin this time is a young woman free from the agony of bereavement. Her outstretched arms may contain an echo of Christ's crucified pose, and she too lowers her eyelids. But rather than closing her eyes altogether, the Madonna trains her compassionate gaze on the mortals assembled below. And her arms are lowered in their direction as well. Clasping the sides of her voluminous blue cloak, she seeks to encircle all the kneeling figures in a protective, tent-like embrace.

No sentimentality is permitted to impair her encompassing gesture. The Virgin, whose pale beauty is akin to Domenico Veneziano's Madonnas, does not smile. She remains strikingly grave, and her statuesque serenity suggests that Piero has been impressed by Sassetta's celebrated *Sansepolcro Polyptych*, where Saint Francis takes up a similarly commanding position at the heart of the central panel (pl. 23). This consummate altarpiece, the most expensive ever commissioned in *quattrocento* Italy, had arrived at the church of San Francesco in Sansepolcro only a year before Piero signed his contract for the *Misericordia Polyptych*. He would have been able to scrutinise Sassetta's work with ease, and doubtless concluded that a single figure with arms held out in a simple gesture of love could be far more eloquent than a complex, heavily populated alternative.

Even so, Piero went much further in the direction of pared-down simplicity. Sassetta had made Saint Francis look up at airborne angels, and enclosed him in a gleaming mandorla where haloed heads reside. Piero, wanting no doubt to compete with the much-revered Sassetta, places his

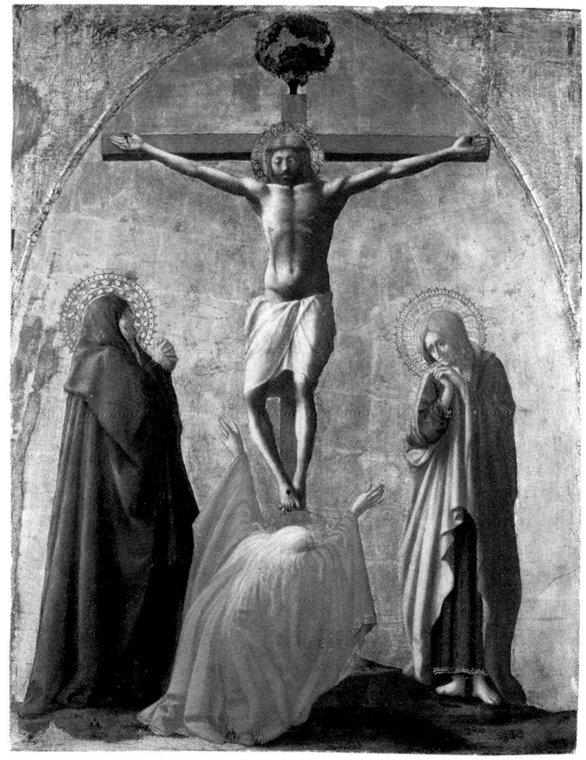

21 Masaccio, *Crucifixion* from *Polytych of Pisa*, 1426, Museo di Capodimonte, Naples

Madonna against a plain gold backdrop. He makes the Sienese master seem fussy by comparison, and the complete absence of visual incident beyond the Virgin adds to her aura of calm, redemptive stillness. Piero models the folds in her cloak with a feeling for sculptural fullness, and the Madonna's red dress takes on an even greater palpability. It lends her an extraordinary sense of tactile substance, and must have persuaded awed contemporary onlookers that the Virgin herself truly stood before them in the hospital church.

The carved quality of the Madonna's garments suggests that Piero had also been looking at sculptural precedents in Sansepolcro. He would have learned a great deal about investing a female image with gravitas from a *Madonna and Child* statue in the church of the Badia. Carved by Presbyter Martinus in 1199, its deeply undercut drapery and solemn facial expressions may well have persuaded Piero to invest his own Madonna with its stern, volumetric intensity. The inscription on the base of Martinus's sculpture declared that 'from the lap of the mother shineth the wisdom of the Father'. And Piero undoubtedly wanted his Virgin to embody a comparable god-like authority.

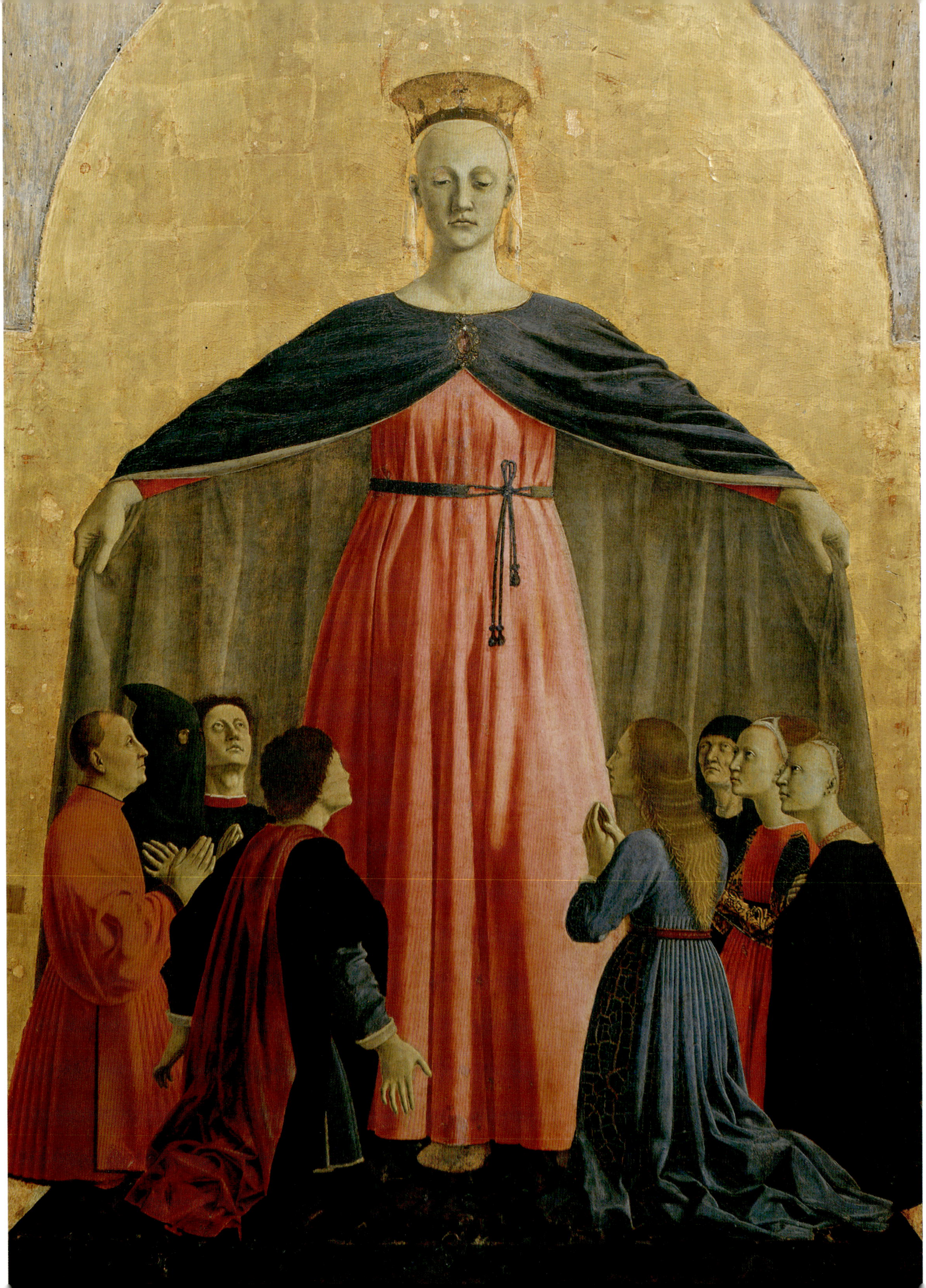

The lessons provided by sculpture must have helped him move away from the most familiar and widely admired painted precedent for his panel. Around 1445, when Piero finally received the commission for the altarpiece, a *Madonna della Misericordia* by Parri Spinelli was installed to great acclaim in Santa Maria delle Grazie, a small chapel in nearby Arezzo. Commissioned by Saint Bernardino of Siena, it excited immense veneration among the adoring populace. But compared with Piero's panel, it looks strangely cluttered. The angels swinging their censers of incense beside the Virgin's head seem awkwardly crammed into the composition. Since she stares straight ahead rather than gazing down at the worshippers, her enveloping gesture with the mantle appears less sincere than Piero's Madonna, who gazes directly at the supplicants and holds her cloak with a firmer, more convincing grasp. Spinelli's Virgin has a flattened air. She lacks substance, and the crowd of figures kneeling around her look uncomfortably claustrophobic. A pope and a monarch can be detected here, elbowing each other for room with the citizens of Arezzo. And the fact that all the figures clasp their hands in identical attitudes of prayer gives the painting an air of monotony.

When he appraised this painting in Santa Maria delle Grazie, Piero must have vowed to avoid such tiresome clutter. Only eight figures kneel before his Madonna, and each of them has enough space to establish an individual identity. All of them were, no doubt, specified by the eight officers of the confraternity who formally witnessed the contract for the altarpiece, and some – particularly the elderly woman wearing a black mantle and the plump, balding man in a crimson tunic – may well be portraits of Pichi family members. But their status as patrons does not enable them to enjoy greater prominence than the other figures. The young man kneeling in front of the Virgin, with arms held out in devotion and wonder, is painted with all the formidable plasticity at Piero's command (pl. 22). As for the fair-haired young woman whose curling tresses tumble right down to her waist, she is rendered in her full sensuous vitality. Rather than jostling for room like the beleaguered supplicants in Spinelli's painting, she seems utterly transfixed by her proximity to the beneficent Madonna.

Everyone who came to view Piero's altarpiece must have felt equally spellbound. Here, at last, was

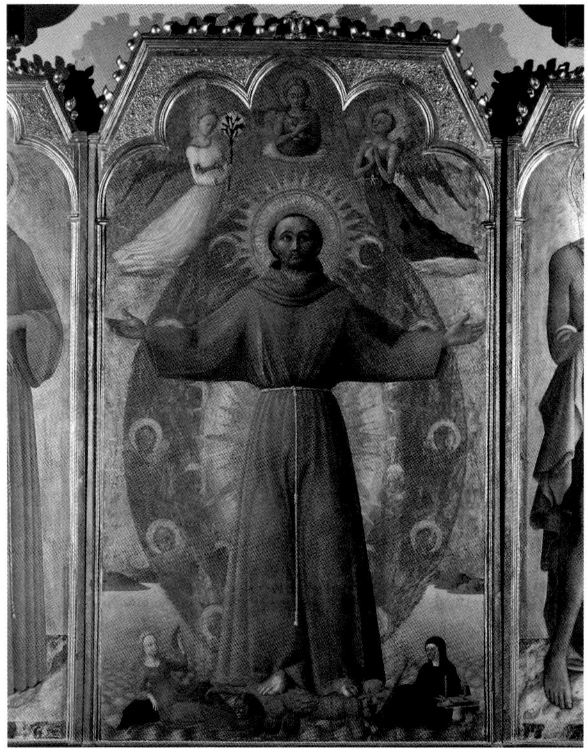

23 (*left*) Sassetta, *Saint Francis in Glory*, central panel of *Sansepolcro Polyptych*, 1437–44, Berenson Collection, Florence

22 (*facing page*) Piero della Francesca, *Madonna della Misericordia*, detail of *Misericordia Polyptych*, 1445–61, Pinacoteca Comunale, Sansepolcro

an altarpiece that presented the Madonna della Misericordia as a fully graspable presence rather than a remote figure from a dream. She seems, in an earlier Florentine fresco painted for the Bigallo, to rear far above the Confraternity of Mercy praying below. Beatific yet impersonal, the Bigallo Madonna inhabits a different realm and appears sublimely unaware of the kneeling figures straining to attract her attention. In Piero's painting, however, she has become a flesh-and-blood reality. The Madonna occupies the same space as the humans around her, and they feel confident in their ability to be enveloped by her consoling protection. In this respect, the panel is closer in feeling to the scaled-down *Madonna della Misericordia* painted by Domenico di Bartolo for the hospital chapel of Santa Maria della Scala in Siena (see pl. 9). But few of the worshippers who viewed Piero's altarpiece can ever have seen Domenico's fresco, and the sheer approachability of the *Misericordia Polyptych* must have come as an outright revelation to the people of Sansepolcro.

To our eyes, the hooded man on the left may appear somewhat sinister as he stares through pierced eye-holes. But his black sackcloth robes identify him as a brother of the confraternity. Members would don these hoods to confer

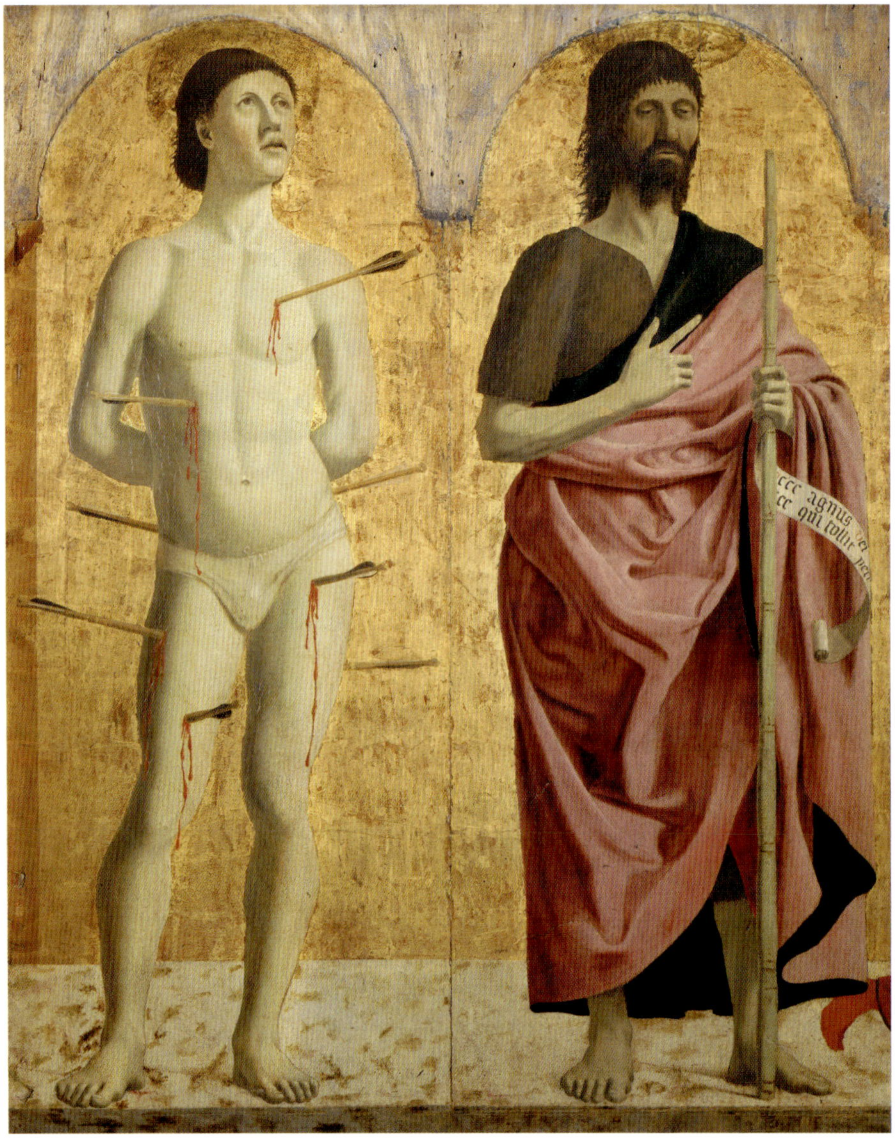

24 (*above*) Piero della Francesca, *Saint Sebastian and John the Baptist*, detail of *Misericordia Polyptych*, 1445–61, Pinacoteca Comunale, Sansepolcro

25 (*facing page*) Piero della Francesca, *Saint John the Evangelist and Bernardino of Siena*, detail of *Misericordia Polyptych*, 1445–61, Pinacoteca Comunale, Sansepolcro

anonymity on themselves while carrying out their acts of charity. Piero depicts the brother with hand on chest, like the Virgin Mary in the *Annunciation* panel above. This gesture is also related to the sign made by the priest as he celebrates Mass. So it becomes easy to imagine confraternal members adopting a similar pose when they kneel in front of the *Misericordia Polyptych*, submitting themselves to God's will and beseeching his grace.

All the figures kneeling in Piero's panel probably belonged to the confraternity. Its statutes never mention women, and they would later be excluded from El Greco's great *Madonna of Charity* painted for the Illescas hospital church (see pl. 103). But women are equal in number to men in Piero's painting, and would undoubtedly have made a vital contribution caring for patients in the hospital. Their costly clothes and jewellery identify them as women of wealth, able to make substantial donations and expand the efficacy of the charitable work in the Sansepolcro community. So when the town's poorest citizens came to pray in front of Piero's altarpiece, they felt confident that the Madonna's merciful cloak would extend over them as well as the confraternal members already sheltering under her generous robe.

Worshippers would also have felt heartened by the tall panels flanking Piero's central image. They contain the four saints most venerated within Sansepolcro. The near-naked Saint Sebastian, far sturdier than he often appears in paintings of his martyrdom, defies the arrows wounding his blood-smeared flesh (pl. 24). Although very pale, he stands erect on the marble floor and looks up at the painting of ultimate sacrifice personified by the crucified Christ. Alongside Sebastian, John the Baptist offers a dramatic contrast: bearded, elaborately draped and looking down as if absorbed in his own prophetic thoughts. The patron saint of Florence, the city that now ruled Sansepolcro, John clasps a staff with an inscription bearing the prominent word *agnus*. It must refer to the lamb of God, whose sacrifice takes away the sins of the world.

Such a message would have been approved by the two saints on the other side of the Madonna. Sansepolcro's patron saint John the Evangelist stands next to Bernardino of Siena, the newly canonised Franciscan preacher who was an impassioned champion of the Madonna of Mercy (pl. 25). Unlike Sebastian and John the Baptist, they are painted on a single panel and thereby inhabit a more unified space. Far more conscious of the Madonna, towards whom they turn, Bernardino and John the Evangelist occupy a part of the altarpiece that heralds a move away from archaic, multi-panelled flatness. Instead, they belong to a new kind of altarpiece popularised in recent years by Fra Angelico, where the attendant saints seem to engage in a *sacra conversazione* with the Virgin.[14]

The townsfolk of Sansepolcro, along with pilgrims who had journeyed there from distant regions, likewise wanted to feel close to the Madonna. Looking at Piero's altarpiece, they could easily imagine themselves kneeling under her heavy, fur-lined mantle. They might also be fortunate enough to hear the confraternity's members singing one of its favoured songs:

> Mercy, we are crying out,
> Mercy, do not abandon us,
> Mercy to God, we implore you,
> Mercy to the sinner.[15]

The controlled clarity displayed by Piero in his depiction of the Misericordia's supplicants should not be mistaken for lack of emotion. On the contrary: the figures sheltering beneath her immense, reassuring cloak are fervent in adoring their protector. Eager for the closest possible contact with this redemptive mother, they enjoy more of her attention than do the saints ranged at either side.

But there is no selfishness involved in their ability to gain such an unprecedented amount of intimacy with the Madonna. The men and women of the confraternity are aware that they belong to the body of Christ. And as Saint Paul pointed out to the Corinthians, 'a body is not a single organ, but many . . . the eye cannot say to the hand, "I do not need you" . . . if one organ suffers, they all suffer together'. Piero, who was himself subsequently elected prior of a confraternity in Sansepolcro, must have understood why Saint Paul emphasised God's insistence 'that there might be no sense of division in the body, but that all its members might feel the same concern for one another'.[16] Hence the Misericordia members' determination to build a hospital, enabling as many stricken people as possible to realise that they would not die abandoned and alone.

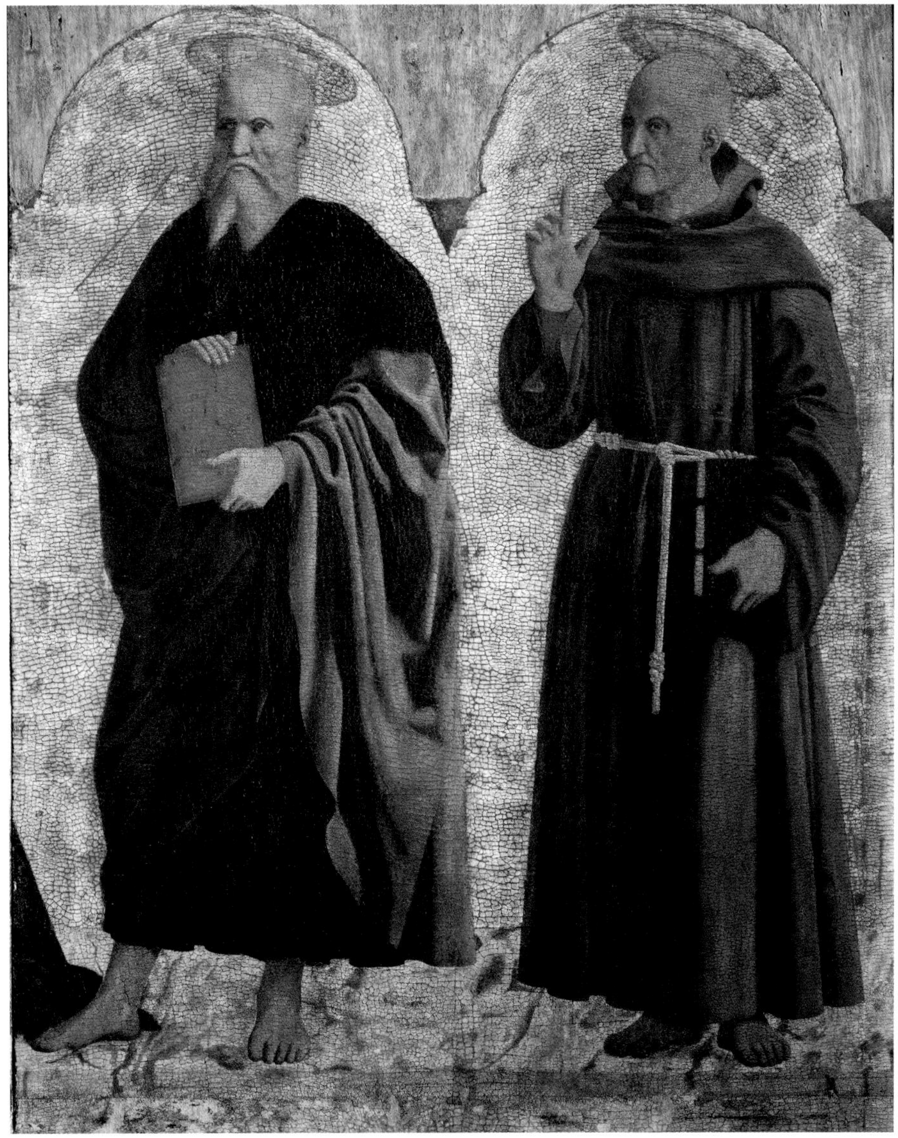

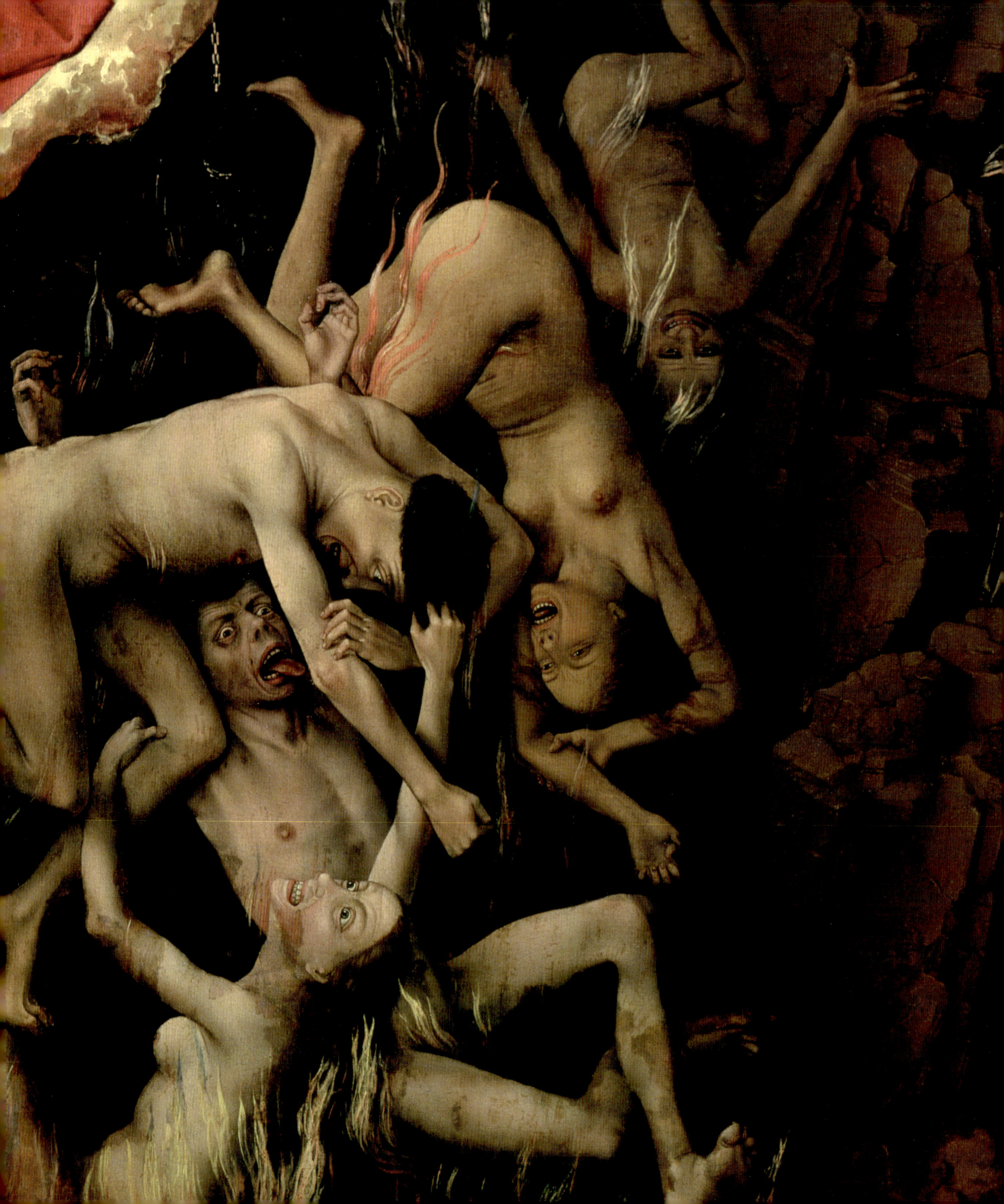

THREE
THE HARROWING OF HELL

No biblical subject is more fearsome than the Last Judgement, and hospital patients today would never be expected to confront it from their sick-beds. But Nicholas Rolin, Chancellor of the Duchy of Burgundy, decided in 1443 that the Hôtel-Dieu hospital he had founded at Beaune 'to take in, care for and lodge sick paupers'[1] would contain an altar-piece on this harrowing theme. He approached Rogier van der Weyden, the widely esteemed master based in Brussels, to tackle this immense challenge for the hospital chapel. It was a daring commission: van der Weyden had gained his justified reputation as a radical painter, escaping from pious medieval stereotypes in order to give his work an often disconcerting amount of profound, forceful and persuasive emotion. Rolin's choice of setting was equally audacious. Unlike most art commissioned for hospitals in the fifteenth century, this *tour de force* of northern European painting was placed in a patients' ward at the very heart of the building's curative quarters.

Death was inescapable at the Hôtel-Dieu. It was a house for the dying, and probably originated in Rolin's horrified reaction to a severe outbreak of plague that decimated the population of Burgundy after the Hundred Years War came to an end. He had been born a lawyer's son in Autun, and nearby Beaune was stricken with particular severity by the pestilence. Hence Rolin's decision, around 1440, to 'found, build, equip and then donate to the city of Beaune in the diocese of Autun a hospital'.[2] After receiving permission from Pope Eugenius IV to set up just such a charitable institution attached to a monastic community, he bought land for the new building in 1441. 'I am constructing this hospital with my own means', he proudly declared in August 1443, 'on land that I have acquired near the markets of Monseigneur le Duc, from the orchards of the monastery of St Francis to the Bouzaise River.'[3] Impressed by Rolin's promise 'from this moment and for all time' to 'irrevocably endow' the hospital, the Duke of Burgundy granted him letters patent exempting the Chancellor from all taxes. In the same year, the deed of foundation was pronounced and greeted with delight by the plague-beleaguered citizens of Beaune. But Louis XI, the King of France, reacted with sarcasm: 'It is entirely fitting that the man who made so many people poor during his life should create an asylum for them before he died.'

Nobody, however, could have predicted just how resplendent the hospital would turn out to be (pl. 27). Inspired above all by the Hôtel-Dieu in Valenciennes, Rolin made sure that his building outstripped its predecessor in sheer magnificence. From the street it looked austere and defensive,

26 (*facing page*) Detail of pl. 33

27 (*right*) Inner courtyard, Hôtel-Dieu, Beaune, built 1443–51

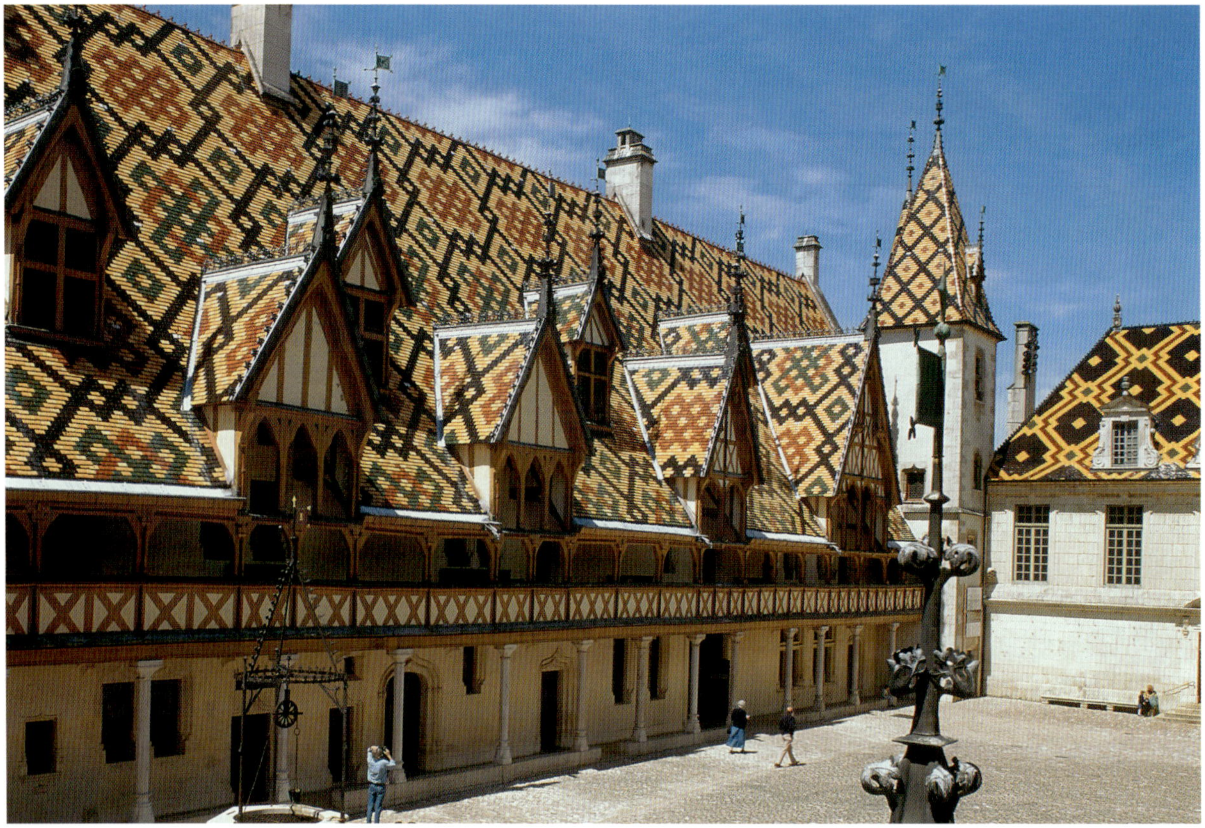

28 (*below*) Rogier van der Weyden, *The Last Judgement*, 1443–51, Musée de l'Hôtel-Dieu, Beaune

reflecting his determination to erect a fortress-like structure capable of warding off attack from armed groups still terrorising the area. Even here, though, dramatic carvings enlivened the porch roof, while the entrance door boasted an elaborate knocker decorated with a predatory lizard stalking a fly. The International Gothic style revelled in surprising encounters of this kind, between humans and

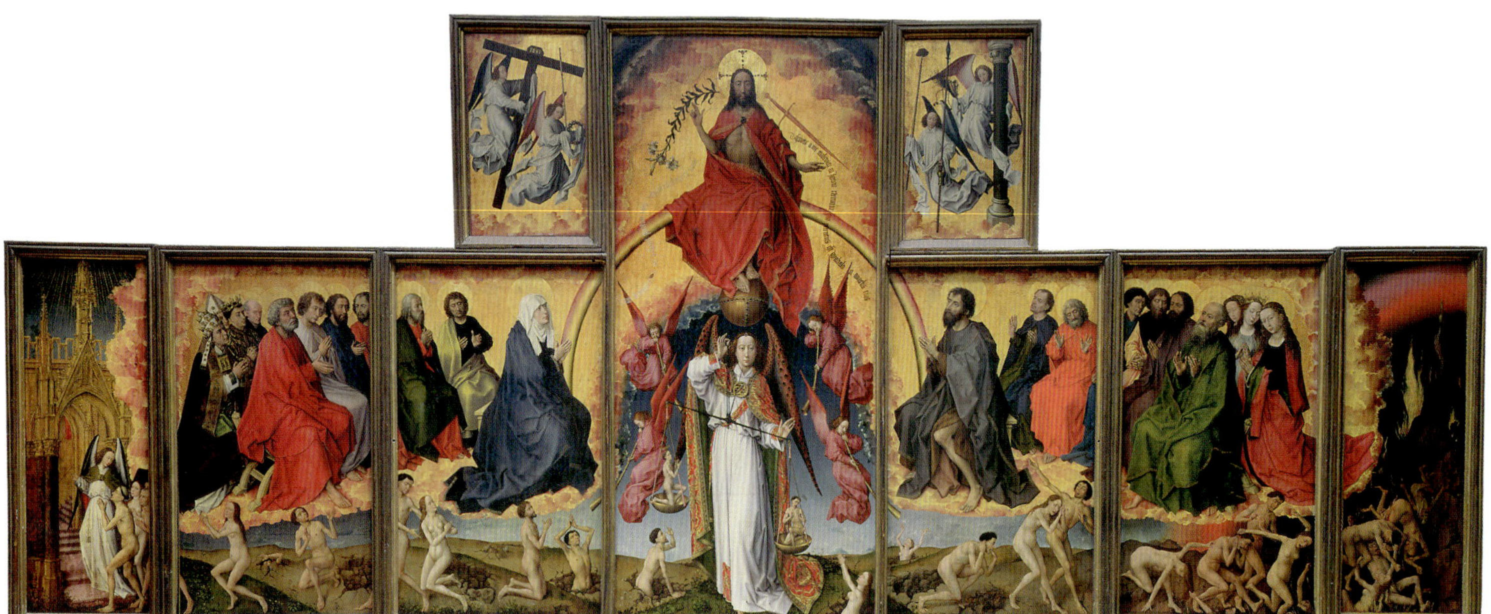

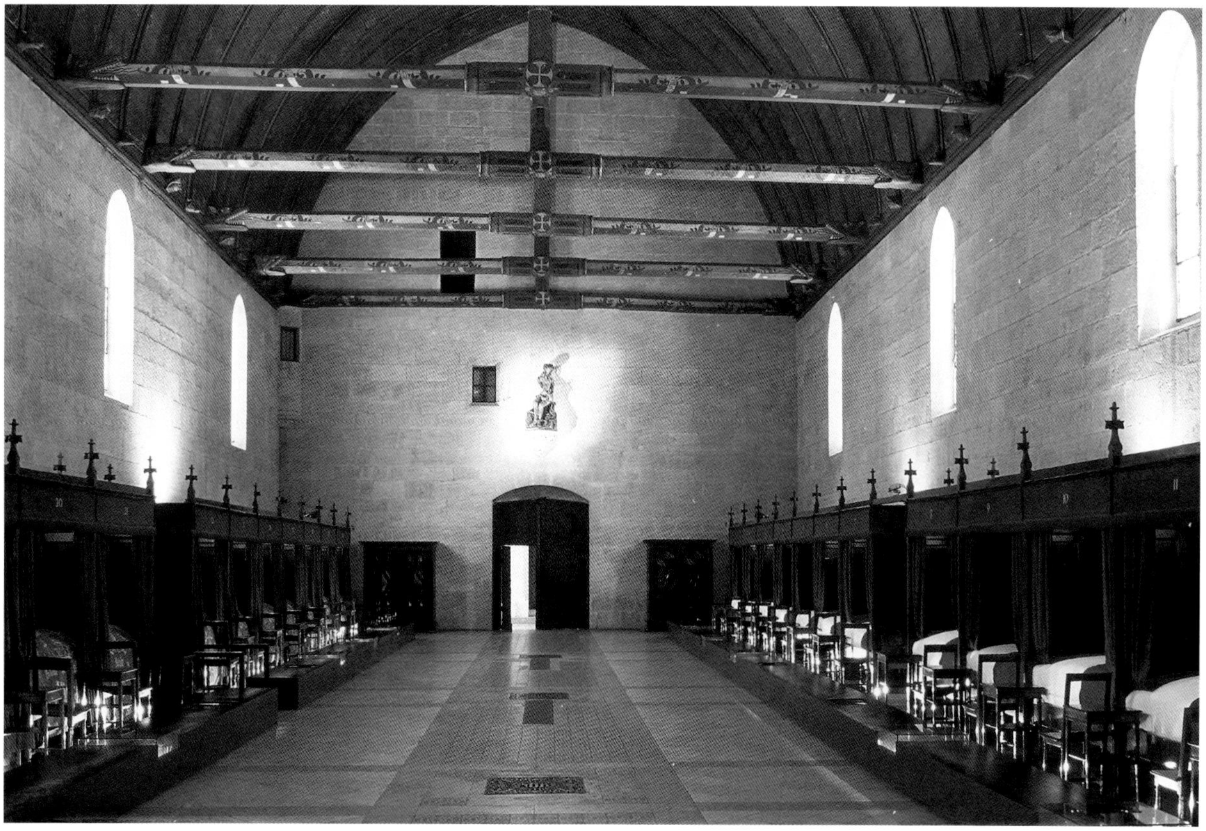

29 Salles des Pauvres, Hôtel-Dieu, Beaune, built 1443–51

animals alike. Winged gargoyles sprouting horns confronted visitors when they entered the courtyard within. But the main impact of this 'Palace of the Poor' was delivered by the spectacular roof. Designed by Denis Goet, its glazed multi-coloured tiles create arresting geometrical patterns. Along with the carvings and lead decorations on the gable windows, the dynamic yet shimmering roof prepares us for the even more powerful emotions generated inside the hospital by the *Last Judgement*. No early documents connect the altarpiece to van der Weyden, and it has in the past been wrongly attributed to Jan van Eyck.[4] But the painting was probably commissioned from Rogier around 1443. Extensive contributions by the artist's assistants, prompted no doubt by pressure of other work in the large Brussels studio, affected the quality of its execution.[5] So did subsequent damage, yet the overall organisation and inventive power of the altarpiece remain profoundly impressive (pl. 28).

The *Last Judgement*, the largest and most complex surviving work produced by Rogier and his workshop, was probably completed in time for the dedication of the chapel in December 1451 to the all-powerful God and his glorious mother, the Virgin Mary.[6] But its ecclesiastical setting was in no sense distanced from the daily lives of the patients. As in so many medieval hospitals, most dramatically at Tonnerre where an enormous barrel-vaulted hospital opened as early as 1293, the chapel of the Hôtel-Dieu at Beaune was placed at the end of the great 'Salle des Pauvres' where inmates' beds occupied most of the space (pl. 29). Bryan Little has described how

> the patients' accommodation in the hospitals of the Middle Ages, whether in monastic infirmaries or in public charities . . . was arranged in long, aisled buildings whose basic design was that of a nave of a church, the chapel in some instances being in an eastward building which corresponded to the chancel. The patients' beds were all on one level, without any subdivision into upper floors.[7]

This was the system adhered to at Beaune, but no medieval hospital had ever furnished its chapel with a painting as spectacular or compelling as the van der Weyden altarpiece. Although a light screen

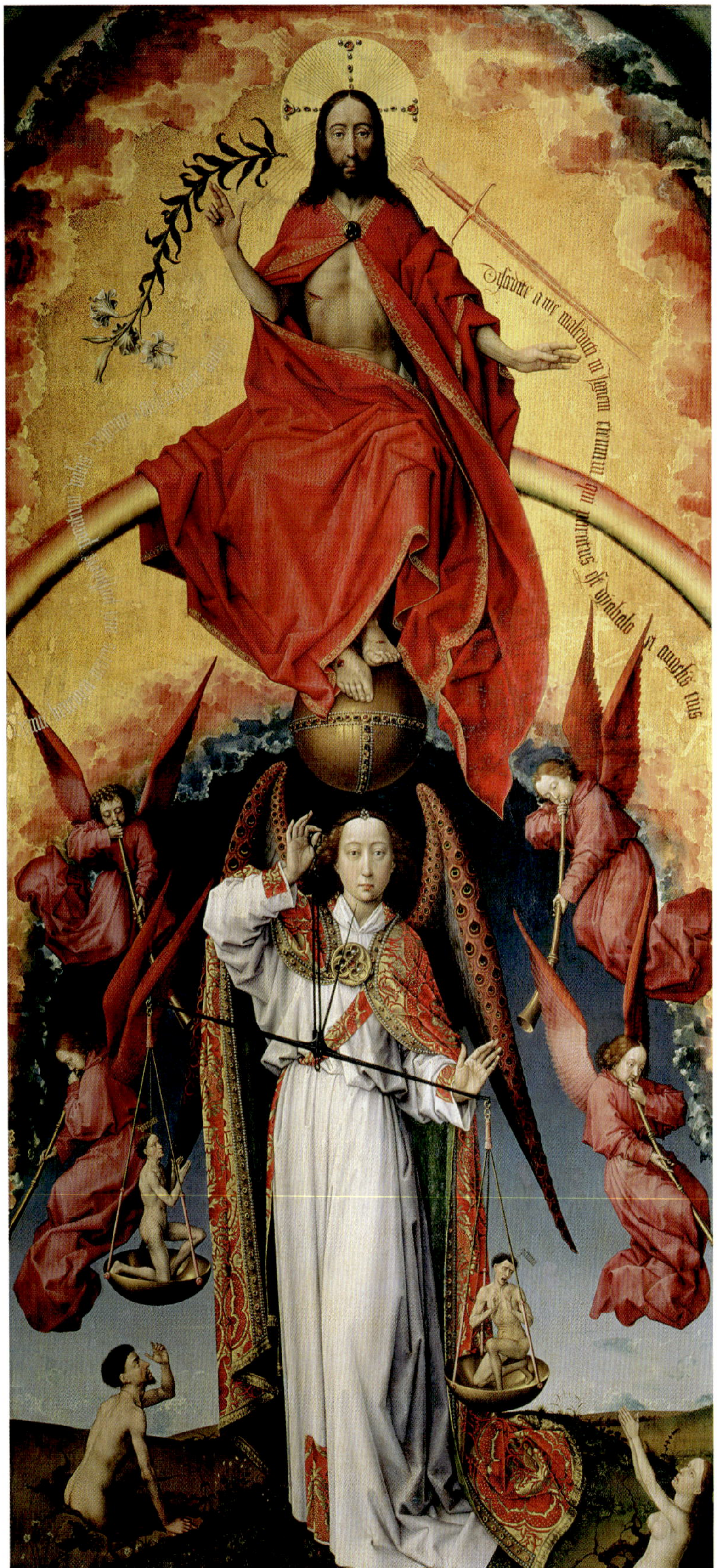

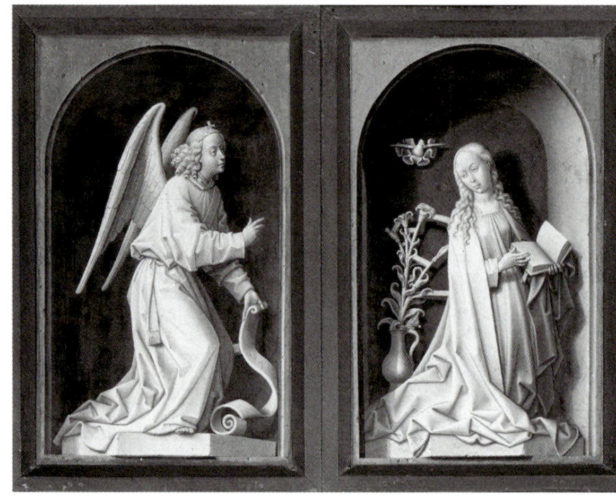

divided the hall from the chapel, and cubicles gave each patient privacy, the beds were positioned carefully enough to guarantee that their occupants could see the awesome work provided for their contemplation.

Chancellor Rolin formally founded the hospital in a 1443 document where he vowed to 'set aside all earthly concerns to turn my thoughts wholly to the salvation of my soul. Through a happy transaction, I hope to exchange the temporary possessions granted to me by divine bounty for heavenly goods – the transient for the eternal'.[8] But he also insisted on exposing the hospital's inhabitants to a painting that shows no sign of minimising the fate meted out to sinners on judgement day. When the altarpiece was closed during the week, patients could see *The Annunciation* painted in grisaille on two upper panels (pl. 31). Presenting the first announcement of Christ's advent, these restrained paintings offered hope to the patients by looking forward to the second coming at the end of time. On Sundays and religious holidays, however, the altarpiece was opened to reveal the *Last Judgement* in all its apocalyptic force.

The Christ who presides with such commanding authority over the central panel wears an expression of uncompromising melancholy (pl. 30). Rogier, whose intense religious convictions stamp everything he produced, did not alleviate the solemnity of the occasion with any hint of benign smiles. Although the Latin inscription on the left side of Christ declares 'Come ye blessed of my Father, inherit the kingdom prepared for you from the foundation of the world', the other side carries a very different and more vehement message: 'Depart from me, ye cursed, into everlasting fire, prepared for the devil and his angels.' The sky is irradiated with an apocalyptic glow, and neither Christ nor Saint Michael beneath intends to be deflected from the gravity of his duties.

Like his divine master, the saint stares directly out of the picture as he weighs the figures on massive scales bearing the words 'Virtues' and 'Sins' respectively. The virtuous soul is raised higher than his erring counterpart, who reacts with horror as he sinks towards the region of the damned.[9] Saint Michael's eyes seem directed at the onlooker, as if to remind the patients lying in the great hall that they will all be subjected to the evaluation ceremony over which he inexorably presides. Four angels reinforce the momentousness of his task by blowing vigorously on trumpets so elongated that two of them jut into the side panels with conspicuous force.

The stricken occupants stretched out in the hospital beds at Beaune would have found nothing to comfort them in the right half of the altarpiece, where naked sinners cower and weep as they wander across a barren, benighted landscape towards hell (pl. 32a). One figure thrusts up a beseeching arm towards the circle of saints above, who raise their hands in acknowledgement of the terror awaiting the damned. For all their concern, however, they can do nothing to stop the progress of the bodies approaching the abyss (pl. 32b). A hapless woman is tugged violently downwards by her hair, while her companions scream with anguish as they plummet to their doom.

Rogier reserves the full horror of divine retribution for the outermost panel, where the saints are represented only by the tail-end of some crimson drapery. The heavenly clouds move to one side, and reveal a terminal blackness envenomed by flames

30 (*facing page, left*) Rogier van der Weyden, central panel of *The Last Judgement*, 1443–51, Musée de l'Hôtel-Dieu, Beaune

31 (*facing page, right*) Rogier van der Weyden, *The Annunciation*, from reverse of *The Last Judgement*, 1443–51, Musée de l'Hôtel-Dieu, Beaune

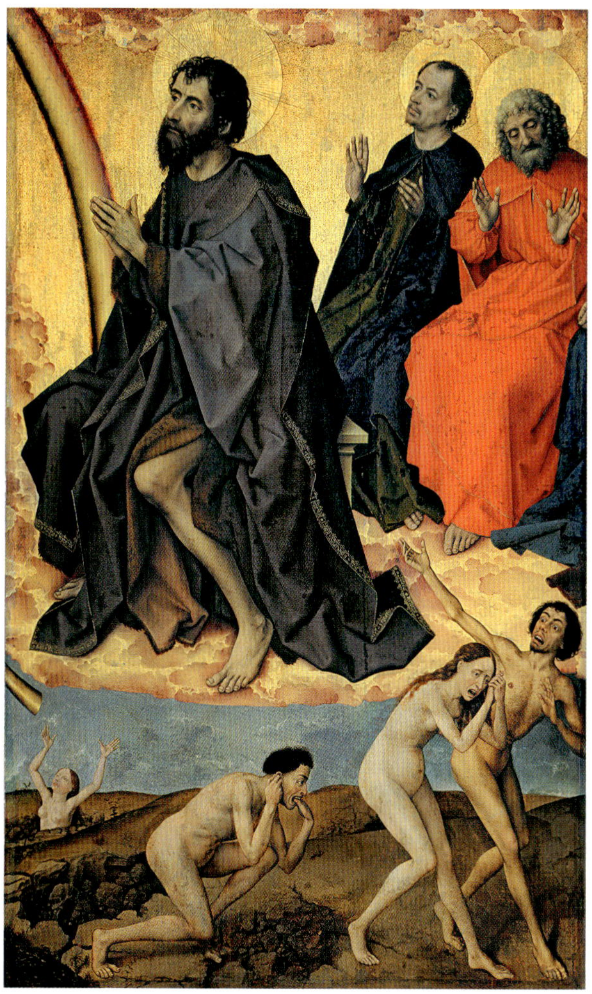

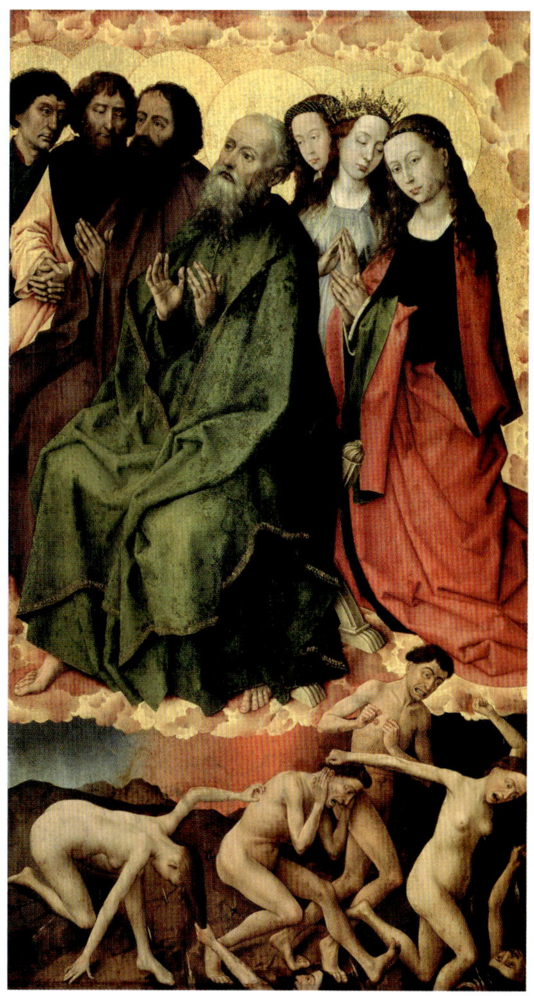

32a and b Rogier van der Weyden, details from right half of *The Last Judgement*, 1443–51, Musée de l'Hôtel-Dieu, Beaune

33 Rogier van der Weyden, *Hell* panel of *The Last Judgement*, 1443–51, Musée de l'Hôtel-Dieu, Beaune

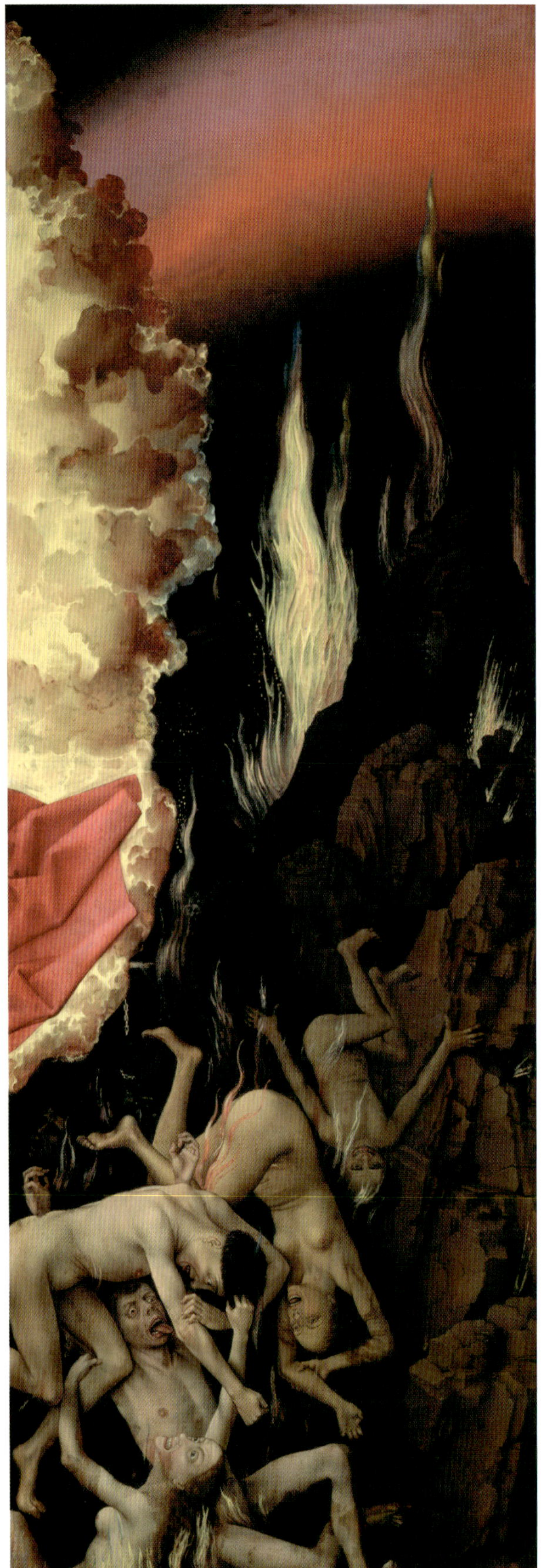

erupting viciously from the rocks below (pl. 33). Into this inferno tumble the howling victims of God's displeasure, their flesh already ignited in places by the heat that will perpetually assail them. Their scalding agony is presented in explicitly physical terms, thereby ensuring that everyone who viewed Rogier's visceral polyptych could grasp the most gruesome implications of the scene. Only the absence of devils mitigates the pain in this otherwise searing and relentless panel (see pl. 26).

Might the Hôtel-Dieu's patients have felt unduly distressed by the immediacy and frankness of the *Last Judgement*? It is difficult to tell, but Rogier's main composition would have been familiar to them from the Gothic tympanum reliefs that provided him with precedents. The truth is that citizens of fifteenth-century France were accustomed to scrutinising images of the harrowing of hell. Such visions could be found in the stained-glass windows embellishing medieval churches, and religious education necessitated a prolonged meditation on the significance of the *Dies Irae*. It was regarded as a salutary experience, and many of the invalids in the 'Salle des Pauvres' might even have found comfort when they gazed at Rogier's masterpiece. Looking up in prayer at the terror confronting the people God rejected, they may well have been prompted to conclude that their own plight entailed less suffering than hell's victims endured. Besides, they undoubtedly appreciated their proximity to the chapel where services were held, for religious feelings were at their most heightened among those confronted by the prospect of death. 'To see the host lifted was paramount', explained Thompson and Goldin, 'or at the very least to hear the words of the Mass.'[10] The whole altarpiece could be equated with a religious service, in fact: Martin Davies wrote of the *Last Judgement* that 'It is not a violent scene; rather a rite, conducted by the priestly figure of Saint Michael'.[11] Hence the eucharistic character of the painting's iconography, where Michael resembles a deacon helping Christ to achieve mystical manifestation in the course of the Mass.

Moreover, if patients had already made peace with their God, they could probably identify with the optimistic scenes on the other side of the *Last Judgement*. For here, aided by the intercession of the Virgin seated at the rainbow's base, figures approach the full redemptive grace of a Christian

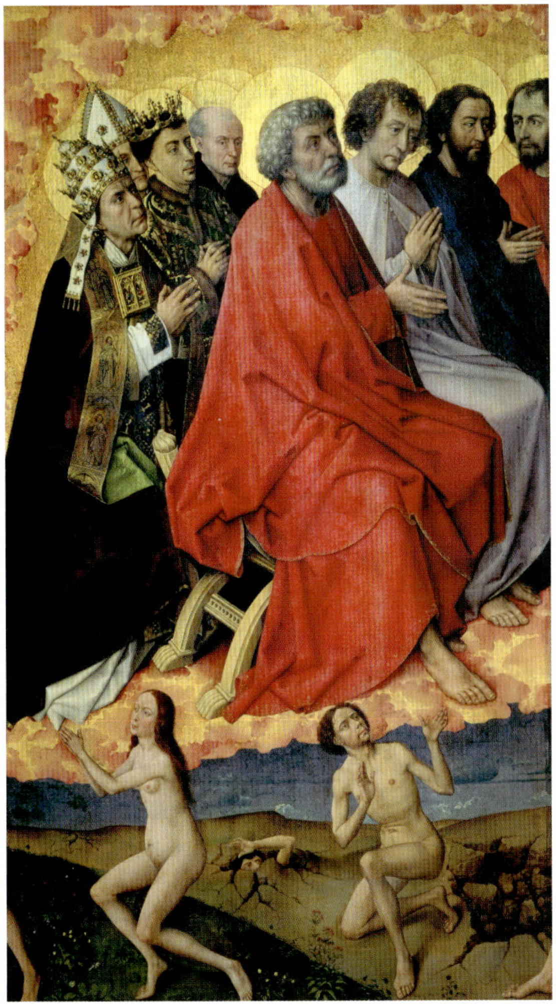

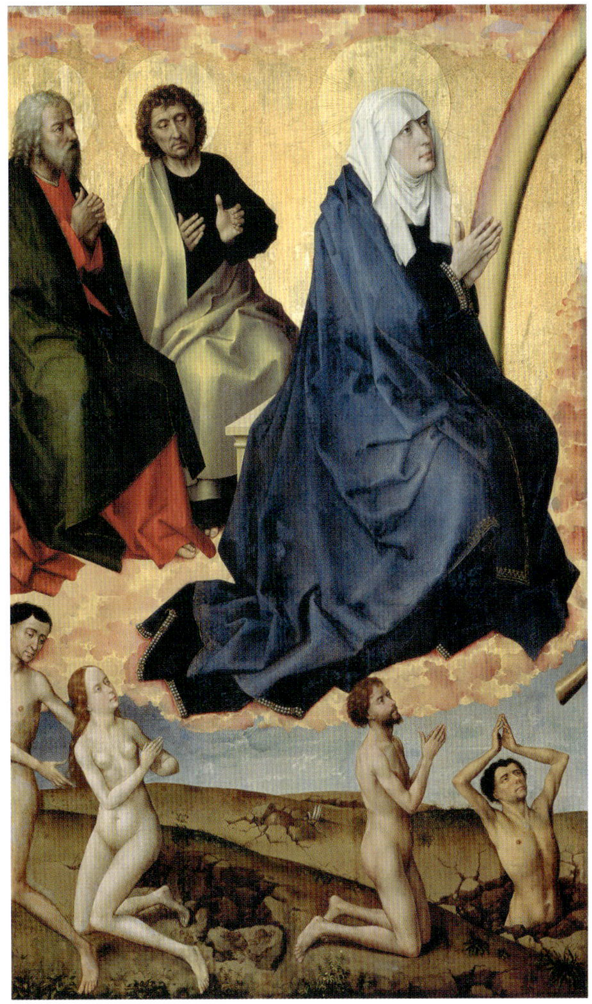

34a and b Rogier van der Weyden, details from left half of *The Last Judgement*, 1443–51, Musée de l'Hôtel-Dieu, Beaune

heaven (pl. 34b). Even though Rogier invests their attenuated bodies with as much northern vulnerability as their counterparts in hell, they emerge from the graves with an unmistakeable sense of wonder. One woman is so eager to kneel and offer thanks to God that she has to be coaxed gently towards paradise by a companion, whose foot has already crossed over a frame into the next panel. Resurrecting figures are still emerging from the cracked earth even there (pl. 34a). But only a few steps are needed to reach the ministering attentions of a guardian angel at the gates of heaven, where the entrance columns are embellished with ripe grapes (pl. 35). The contrast between the gleaming gold architecture of this panel, and the flame-filled void at the other end of the *Last Judgement* could hardly be more poignant. While the penumbral depths promise nothing but despair and excruciating torment, the Gothic archway leading to heaven offers shelter, light and aesthetic magnificence.

However much sustenance the patients may have derived from such an imposing altarpiece, whose site provides such 'a striking example of the part played by religious art in human life',[12] Rogier's vision is in the end undeniably grave. His stern emphasis on the ultimate moment either of absolution or retribution has an uncompromising finality, and on the outer wings both his donor portraits likewise assume expressions of the utmost solemnity. Identifiable from their coats of arms, each held by an angel floating behind, Chancellor Rolin and his third wife Guigone de Salins pray before devotional texts. Rolin, who died ten years after the consecration of the Beaune chapel at the reputed age of eighty-six, was already an old man by the time

35 (*right*) Rogier van der Weyden, Gates of heaven in *The Last Judgement*, 1443–51, Musée de l'Hôtel-Dieu, Beaune

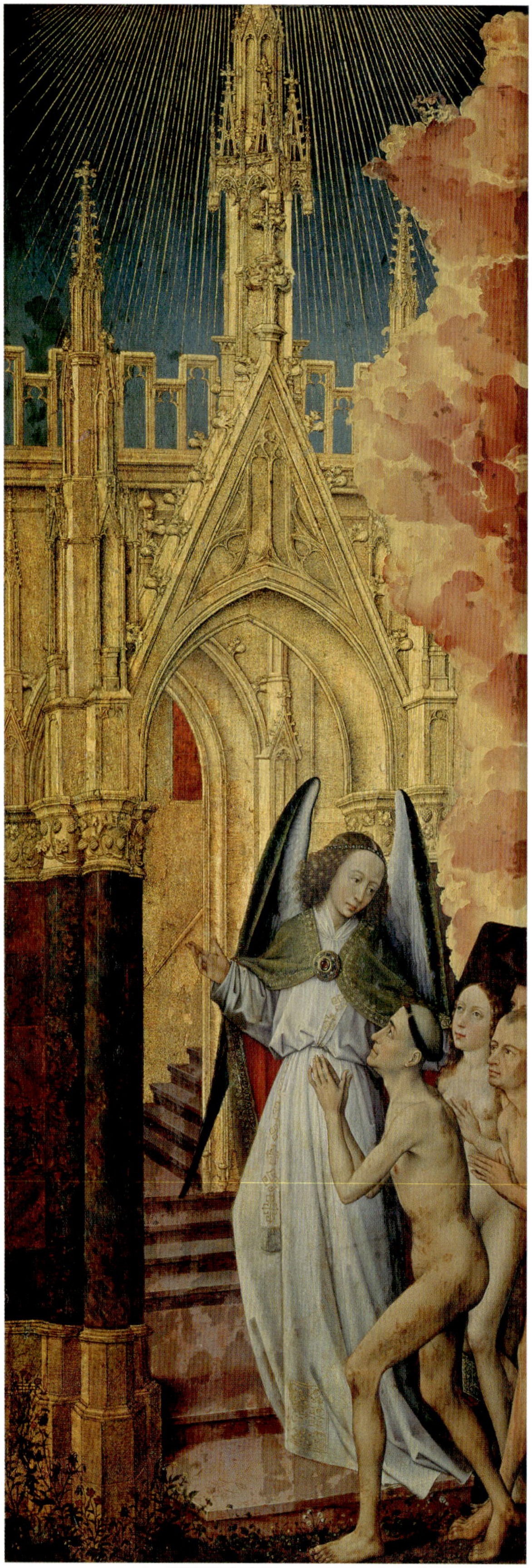

36 (*far right*) Rogier van der Weyden, portrait of Nicolas Rolin, from reverse of *The Last Judgement*, 1443–51, Musée de l'Hôtel-Dieu, Beaune

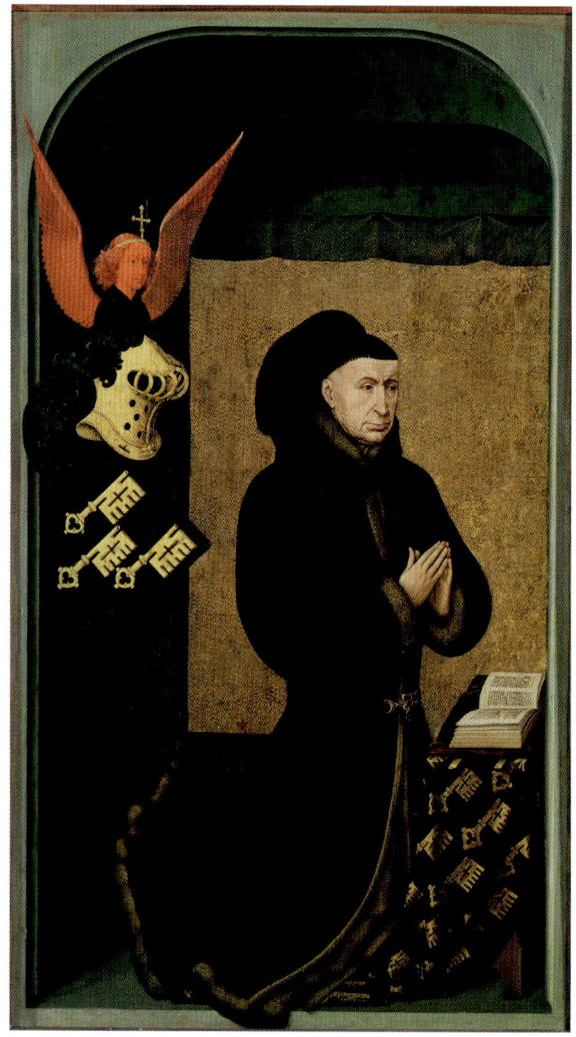

Rogier and his assistants painted him here (pl. 36). Sporting the same semi-shaven hair that also characterised his earlier portrait by Jan van Eyck, in *Virgin and Child with the Chancellor Rolin*, he creases his ascetic brow with a frown as he contemplates his own mortality. Perhaps he is meditating in particular on the biblical passage in Matthew,[13] where the division between the damned and the blessed on Judgement Day is linked with the charitable works they had managed or failed to carry out during their lives on earth.

Rolin was originally a more sumptuous figure in the painting, for a scarlet pattern once covered the gold cloth behind him. It would have accentuated the contrast between the donor portraits and the *grisaille* paintings of Saints Sebastian and Anthony, whose resemblance to sculpture echoes the exterior of an earlier altarpiece that profoundly influenced

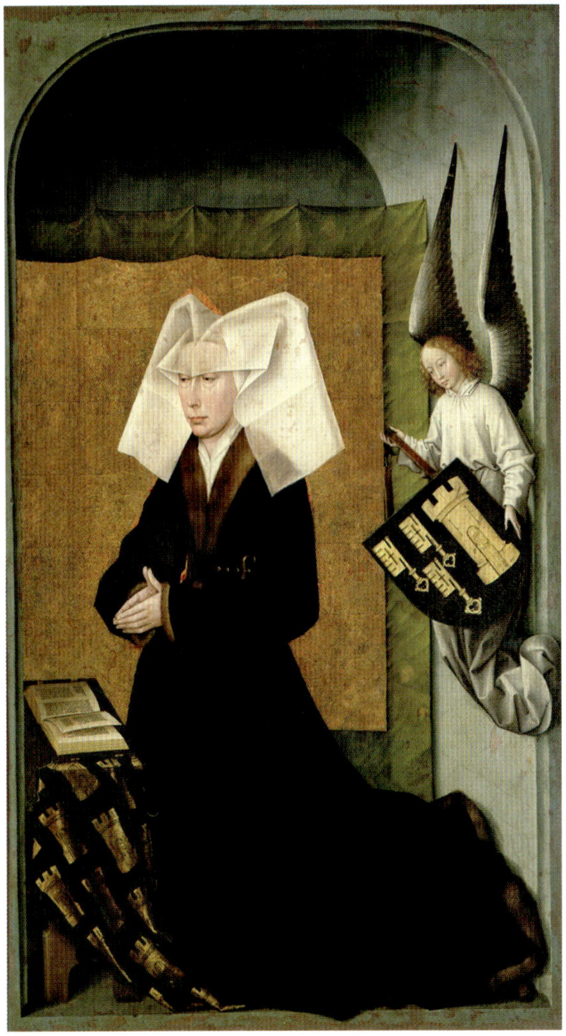

Rogier at Beaune: van Eyck's *Adoration of the Lamb*. But damage and alteration in pigments have made both Rolin and his wife more blanched than they would initially have appeared. As for the 'excellent and generous lady' Guigone (pl. 37), she retired to Beaune after her husband's death at Autun in 1462. A strong personal involvement with the Hôtel-Dieu led her to join its monastic community. Eight years later she died there, and demonstrated her abiding respect for Rogier's painting by asking to be buried before the altar where the *Last Judgement* was displayed. So it became a funerary monument, and a Requiem Mass had to be sung there twice daily along with the recitation of prayers for the souls of both Rolin and his wife. In her eyes, as well as the patients who gazed at the painting from their beds, it must have offered the positive and indispensable hope of salvation to come.

37 Rogier van der Weyden, portrait of Guigone de Salins, from reverse of *The Last Judgement*, 1443–51, Musée de l'Hôtel-Dieu, Beaune

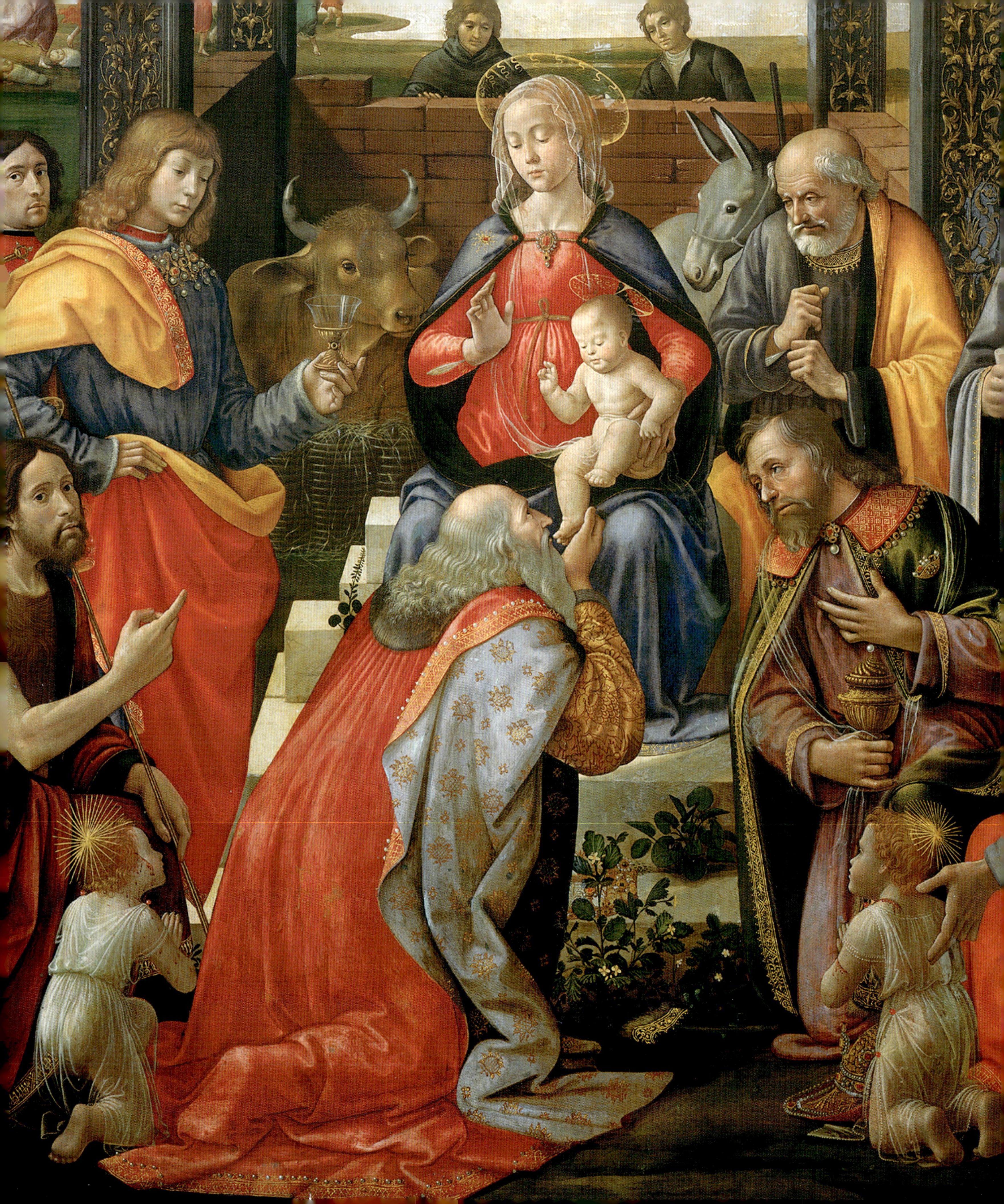

FOUR
RESCUING THE ORPHANS

Little time was lost before the full resources of early Renaissance architecture were devoted to ensuring that the first hospital exclusively devoted to foundlings, anywhere in the world, was a building of sublime proportions. In 1410, the great Florentine Spedale di Santa Maria Nuova had been bequeathed a thousand florins by the well-known Prato merchant Francesco di Marco Datini, who wanted a special hospital to be constructed for *gittadelli bambini*. Nine years passed and Santa Maria Nuova failed to honour Datini's dying wishes. So the consuls of the Silk Guild, the Arte della Seta, eager to embark on another major building after the completion of Orsanmichele, took over the project. They entrusted a forty-two-year-old member of their guild, Filippo Brunelleschi, with the task of designing the Spedale degli Innocenti in 1419.[1]

Whereas Brunelleschi remained faithful to the Gothic tradition in his contemporaneous dome for the city's cathedral, the Innocenti commission gave him the opportunity to provide Florence with the first building to apply the new classical ideas to the Tuscan style (pl. 39). As a result, full-blown Renaissance architecture was effectively inaugurated in the Piazza SS. Annunziata. Like the double halls built for the Asklepieia in ancient Greece, Brunelleschi's hospital made every effort to let the sun warm and illuminate its structure. The graceful ground-floor colonnade deploys arches wide enough to allow the maximum amount of heat and light into the loggia. And the notably slender columns, crowned by delicate Corinthian capitals, do little to impede the sun's penetration.

The hospitable mood created by this exquisitely harmonious arcade can be fully appreciated by comparing it with the facade of San Miniato al Monte, the great Florentine church from the eleventh and twelfth centuries where several of Brunelleschi's Innocenti motifs can be found. For the rounded arches of San Miniato do not open into a loggia, and the central window above them is embedded in an upper frontage where sternly patterned decoration displays its brazen geometry. The similarly pedimented windows on the Innocenti's first floor are ranged along its generous width, and nothing disturbs the expansive spaces left between each window. Modest and companionable, the Foundling Hospital has an inviting air wholly in keeping with its pioneering purpose.

Established to care for infants 'deserted by their parents contrary to the law of nature',[2] the building gains enormously in symbolic meaning from the loggia behind its columns. By opening the Innocenti out into a great city square, Brunelleschi implied that it should not be regarded merely as a

38 (*facing page*) Detail of pl. 45

39 Filippo Brunelleschi, Spedale degli Innocenti, 1419–27, Piazza SS. Annunziata, Florence

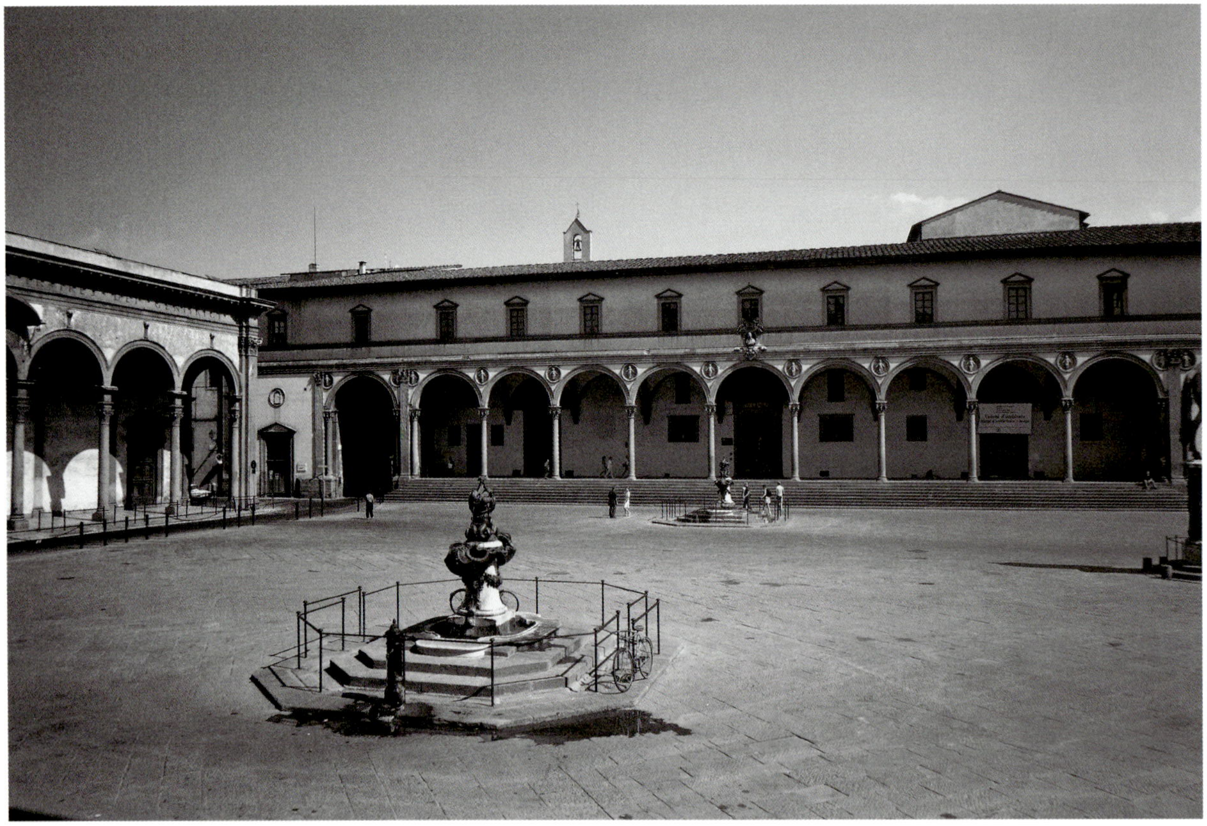

40 Andrea della Robbia, terracotta medallion of child, *c.*1487, Spedale degli Innocenti, Florence

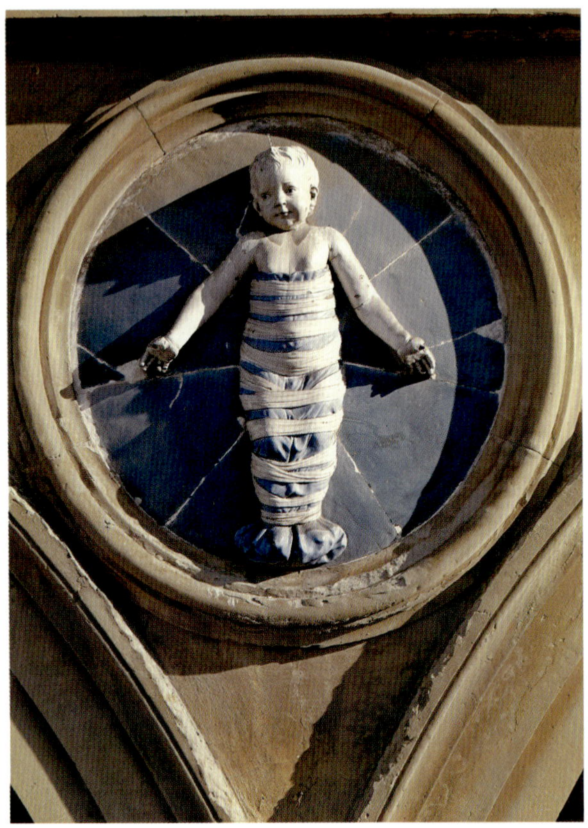

home for shameful outcasts, fit only to be hidden from view. Instead of finding themselves shunned by society, the foundlings were granted a sun-filled gathering point where other Florentines could also laze on the steps and savour the life of the city around them. Indeed, the institution played such an important part in the population's development that it came eventually to be seen as a central, indispensable part of Florence's social structure. 'The statistical role of the hospital in the evolution of the Florentine people', Frederick Hartt noted, 'may be attested by the presence, in a recent edition of the Florentine telephone directory, of nearly eight columns of persons called Innocenti, or its derivatives.'[3]

The loggia's all-important air of welcome is confirmed by the coloured terracotta medallions installed around 1487 in the spandrels of the colonnade by Andrea della Robbia (pl. 40).[4] Another sculptor might easily have disrupted the harmony of Brunelleschi's refined equilibrium, for he had intended that his ten concave roundels should remain empty.[5] Their circular geometry was devised as an integral feature of his design, and Eugenio

Battisti maintained that Brunelleschi would have made the stonecutters 'sweat over their compasses'[6] in order to fit the roundels precisely between arches and architrave. After he finished work on the building in 1427, to be replaced by the altogether more controversial Francesco della Luna, nothing was added to the decoration of the facade for sixty years – apart from a fresco over the door to the church in 1459 and the coat of arms of the Arte della Seta, the powerful silk guild responsible for the welfare of the foundlings. So the eventual advent of Andrea della Robbia, who made an image of a swaddled baby for each of the medallions, could have resulted in a jarring intrusion that wrecked Brunelleschi's original design.

Despite the arbitrary nature of his addition, della Robbia managed to avoid disrupting the harmony of the facade. His glazed images chime with the architecture while confidently reinforcing the hospital's commitment to the care of the children in its charge. Far from producing sculptural embellishments so neutral that they pass unnoticed by anyone entering the Innocenti, della Robbia made his medallions declare the building's aim in a robust and open manner. The children's outstretched arms offer a warm-hearted greeting to their flesh-and-blood counterparts approaching the hospital for the very first time.

The chronic financial troubles afflicting the Innocenti for a while after its completion might have led some visitors to conclude that the 'terracotta babies', as they are called in the record of payment, were holding out their arms to plead for generous donations. But the truth is that their gestures are profoundly ambiguous, encompassing both affirmation and melancholy. Their most prominent and positive meaning was memorably defined in E.M. Forster's *A Room with a View*, where young Lucy Honeychurch sums up the reaction of many visitors to Florence after she drifts 'through a series of those grey-brown streets, neither commodious nor picturesque, in which the eastern quarter of the city abounds'. Lucy becomes discontented, but then for 'one ravishing moment Italy appeared. She stood in the Square of the Annunziata and saw in the living terra-cotta those divine babies whom no cheap reproduction can ever stale. There they stood, with their shining limbs bursting from the garments of charity, and their strong white arms extended against circlets of heaven. Lucy thought she had never seen anything more beautiful.'[7]

Her response to the Innocenti's children has been shared by so many that the popularity of these images extended far beyond the hospital's boundaries. As Nikolaus Pevsner once wrily observed, 'the famous babies in swaddling clothes are sold in cheap copies of all sizes by the souvenir-dealers of Florence'.[8] But the truth is that the infants' outspread arms also carry a distinct suggestion of suffering. Like many images of the Christ Child in Renaissance paintings and sculpture, emitting intimations of the tragedy ahead, they convey the pain of martyrdom as well as the joy of birth. Their arms, defined so clearly against a brilliant blue ground redolent of the sky, are spread out in positions subtly prophesying the crucifixion to come.[9]

Before the medallions were installed, a distinguished contribution had already been made to the Innocenti by another member of the prolific della Robbia dynasty. Luca, the oldest and most impressive of the family's three sculptors, made a delightfully intimate enamelled terracotta group of the *Madonna of the Innocents* (pl. 41). Although smaller

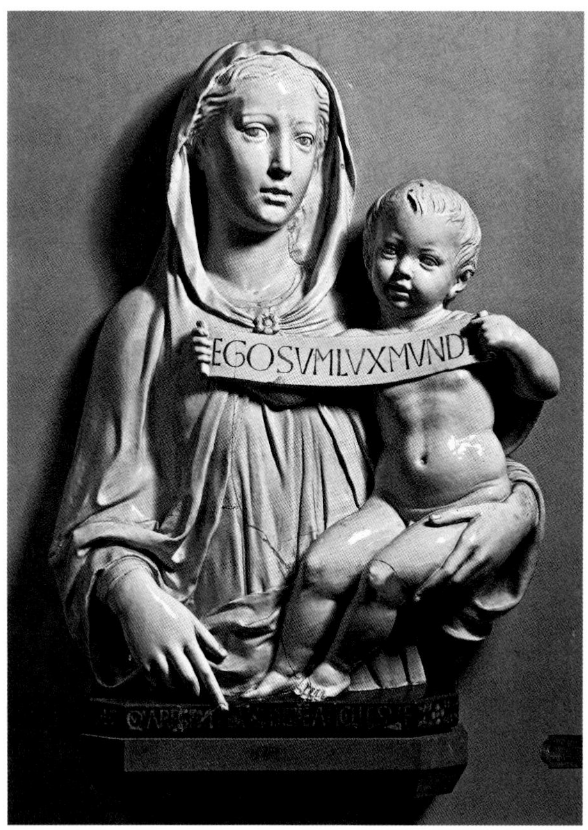

41 Luca della Robbia, after 1450, *Madonna of the Innocents*, Spedale degli Innocenti, Florence

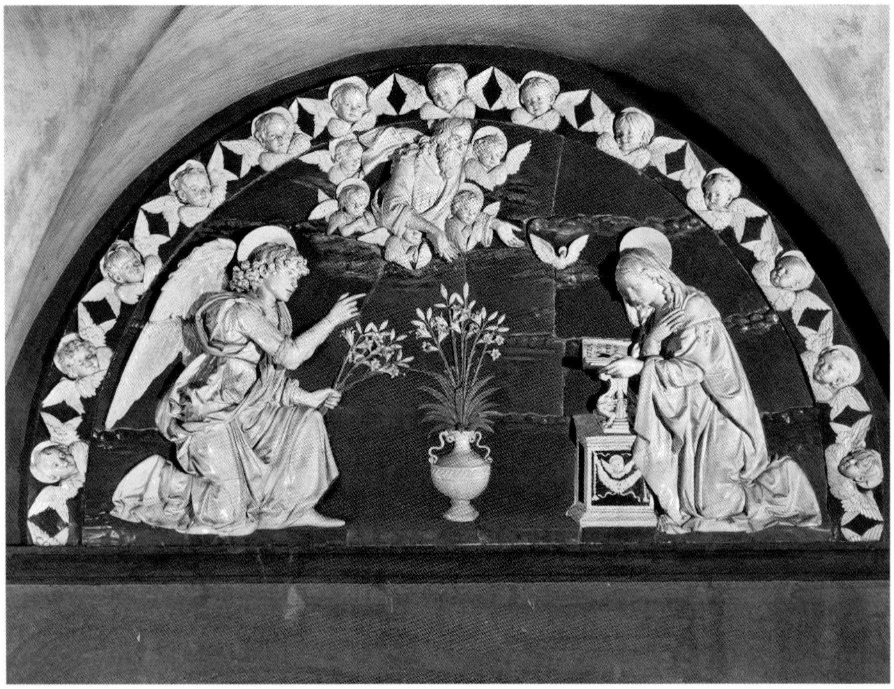

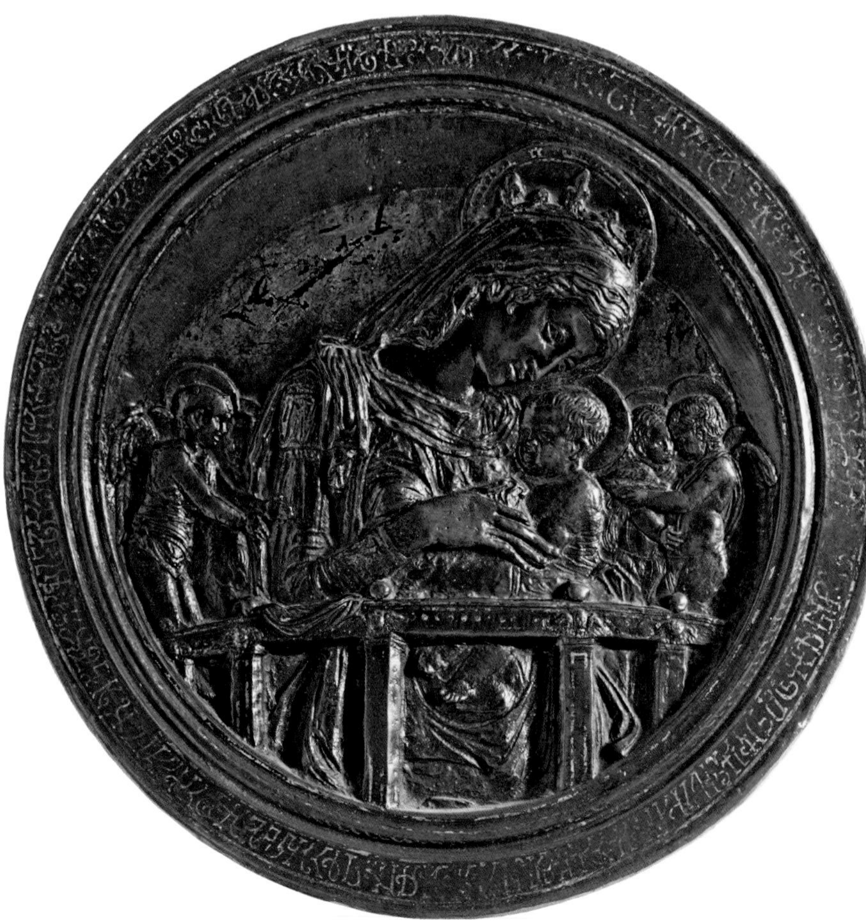

than Andrea's babies, it makes a virtue out of modest dimensions by presenting the relationship between mother and child with the utmost freshness. Dignified she may be, but the Virgin's chubby features denote a very young woman who has no intention of stressing her divine authority in an aloof manner. On the contrary: she seems a simple, approachable individual, unfettered even by a halo. The hood defining an oval around her face is graceful enough to provide the Madonna with an aura, after all, and the little rose brooch attached to the cloak at the base of her neck is more captivating than a thousand elaborate jewels.

The baby held familiarly in her arm enjoys a close rapport with his mother, too. Instead of the clothed and formally posed infant who looks so self-conscious in Luca's roughly contemporaneous *Madonna of Santa Maria Nuova*, he appears quite naked and lolls against his mother's body with a conspicuous and persuasive air of relaxation. Even though he holds out a scroll, announcing that 'I am the light of the world', there is nothing didactic or sanctimonious about his stance. The holy child brandishes the inscription in a disarmingly playful manner, pointing at the words with his finger and yet managing to imply that they convey a meaning as festive as a welcoming banner at a party. Luca was adept at this beguiling informality, and even managed to retain it when he made the unexpectedly spirited *Emblem of the Guild of Doctors and Apothecaries* for the Orsanmichele in 1466.

The far larger *Annunciation* (pl. 42) made by Andrea for the Innocenti makes no attempt to vie with Luca's engaging spontaneity. The Virgin this time is portrayed with solemnity as a withdrawn and bookish woman, overcome by the visitation from the lily-bearing angel. The distance between the two figures accentuates the momentousness of the occasion, but Andrea's innate light-heartedness prevents him from investing the event with too much gravity. A vase of lilies gives a lively, expansive flourish to the centre of the image. And the God floating in a reassuringly blue sky is a benevolent presence, who releases the dove with immense tenderness. Above all, though, Andrea seasons the mood of this elaborate *Annunciation* by framing the terracotta's arc with a chorus of cherubs' heads. Surrounded by wings waving cheerfully in space, they smile down on the scene beneath like the Innocenti's foundlings, delighted to behold the genesis of the baby whose Christian example would inspire the charitable motives behind the establishing of their own hospital.

An even greater intensity of feeling enlivens Donatello's *Virgin and Child with Four Angels* (pl. 43), an outstanding bronze roundel given by the sculptor to his doctor Giovanni Chellini in return for medical treatment. Like Luca della Robbia's carving for the Innocenti (see pl. 41), Donatello's unique roundel shows the humanity of the Virgin as an ideal mother. But now she bends over her baby with heartfelt care, having received a tray of sweetmeats like those donated to many new mothers in Renaissance Italy. Donatello's Virgin, the embodiment of compassion, is supported in her devotion by all the little anxiously gesturing angels attending the mother and child. Perhaps the artist realised that her tender concern was paralleled by the care he had himself received from Chellini, an eminent Florentine scholar and physician. In 1456 Antonio Rossellino carved a remarkable marble bust of Chellini, whose austere face and almost forbidding hauteur is countered by a very kindly smile filled with affectionate concern (pl. 44). Chellini's sympathy and expertise clearly won Donatello over as well, for the doctor later described in his account book how, 'on 27 August 1456, Donato, called Donatello, the singular and outstanding master of bronze, wood, and terracotta figures . . . generously presented me, in consideration of the medical care I had been giving him, with a bronze roundel the size of a trencher.' It became known as the *Chellini Madonna* and its owner proudly recorded that 'the other side is hollowed so that molten glass can be cast in it to make the same figures as those on the other side'.[10] After the Victoria & Albert Museum acquired the original bronze roundel in 1976, Chellini's intriguing claim was put to the test. The Glass Department of London's Royal College of Art, together with the Venini glass firm of Murano, made coloured-glass impressions which suggest, in their transparent eloquence, that Donatello had fully intended to make this unexpected metamorphosis possible.

The Prior of the Spedale degli Innocenti subsequently ensured that his institution continued to employ other artists with the most scrupulous care. Antonio Rossellino produced the holy water basin for the hospital church, and in 1480 Giuliano da Sangallo built a new altar for its interior. The Prior's enlightened initiatives meant that triumph attended the most spectacular of the paintings commissioned for the Innocenti's church. In 1488, soon after the installation of Andrea's medallions, the Prior devised an immensely detailed contract for a large 'altar panel' by Domenico Ghirlandaio. The document, still preserved in the hospital's museum, was drawn up by 'the Jesuate Brother' Fra Bernardo di Francesco. It insisted that Ghirlandaio should

> colour and paint the said panel all with his own hand in the manner shown in a drawing on paper with those figures and in that manner shown in it, in every particular according to what I, Fra Bernardo, think best; not departing from the manner and composition of the said drawing; and he must colour the panel at his own expense with good colours and with powdered gold on such ornaments as demand it, with any other expense incurred on the same panel, and the blue must be ultramarine of the value about four florins the ounce.[11]

The contract's zealous attention to quality and materials alike received its reward in the final painting, where Ghirlandaio produced an exceptionally rich, complex and appropriate interpretation of the

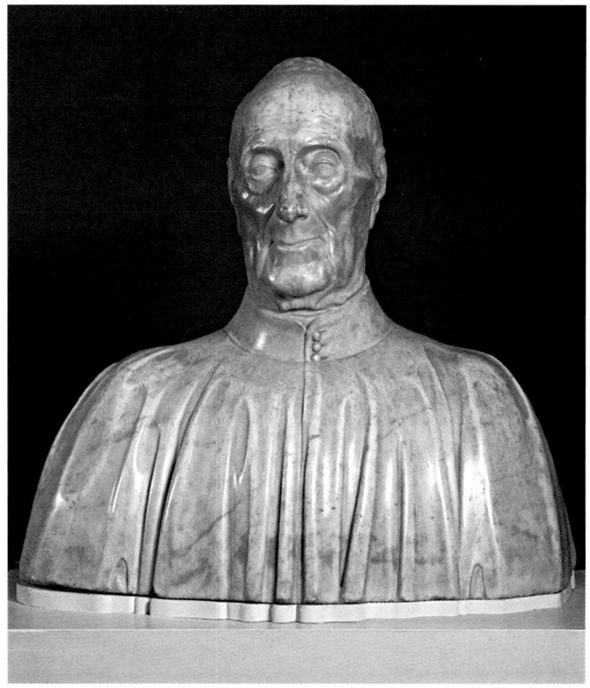

44 (*left*) Antonio Rossellino, *Giovanni Chellini*, 1456, Victoria and Albert Museum, London

42 (*facing page, top*) Andrea della Robbia, *Annunciation*, *c.*1470, Spedale degli Innocenti, Florence

43 (*facing page, bottom*) Donatello, *Virgin and Child with Four Angels* (*Chellini Madonna*), 1456, Victoria and Albert Museum, London

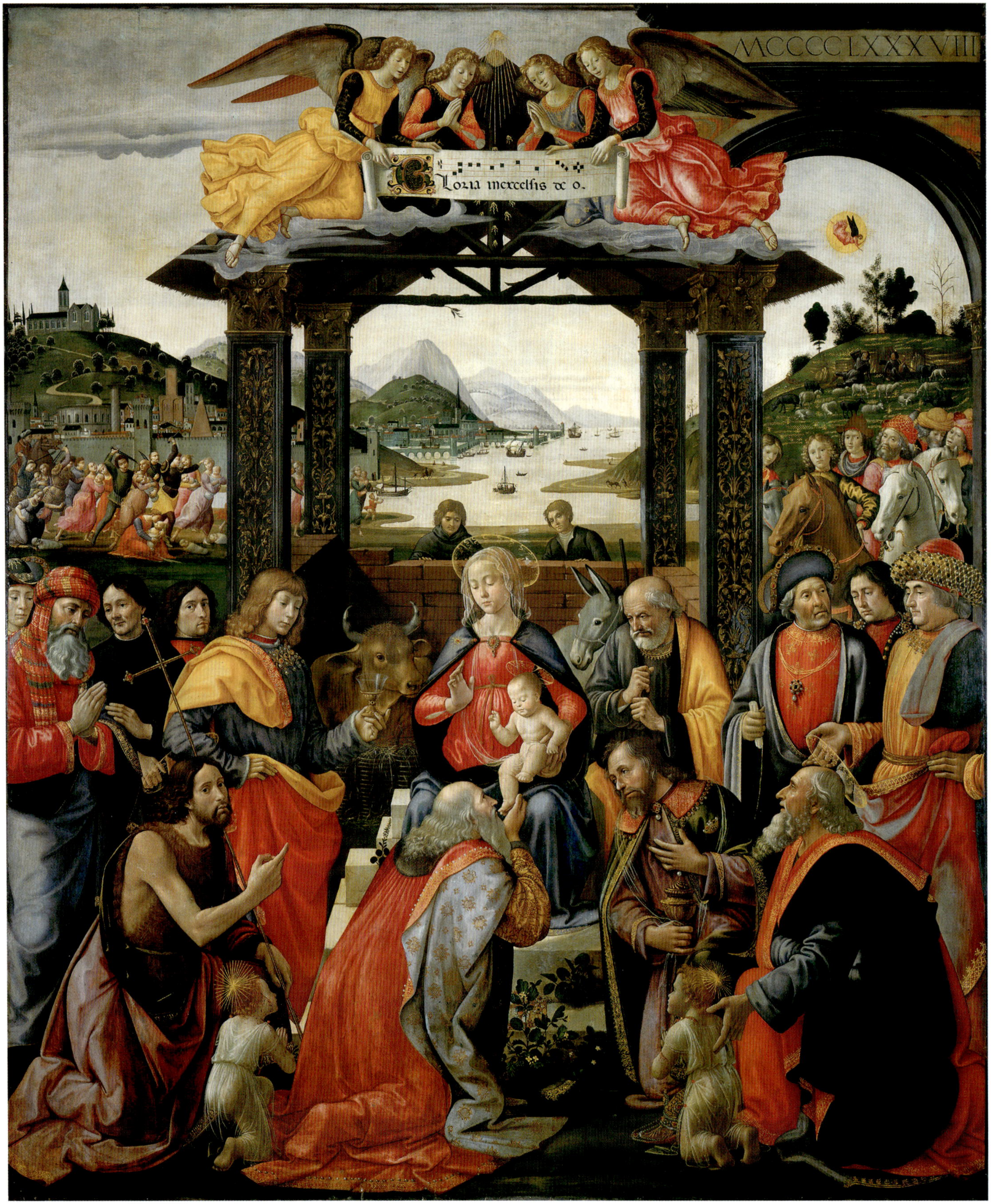
MCCCCLXXXVIII
GLoria inexcelsis deo

Adoration of the Magi theme (pl. 45). Still in astonishingly good condition, it hangs in the hospital today as the finest work of art commissioned by the institution. Ghirlandaio, one of the leading painters in late *quattrocento* Florence and the head of a workshop where the young Michelangelo became an apprentice while the *Adoration of the Magi* was being painted, took several years to complete the altarpiece. The Innocenti's function is prominently acknowledged, doubtless at Fra Bernardo's bidding, by the inclusion of two children kneeling at the forefront of the composition. Both seem to be protected by the voluminous robes of the figures nearby, and one bearded magus draws attention to the child in his charge with the wave of an avuncular hand. As if in response, the other magi leave a space between them, thereby enabling the child to look past the cluster of meticulously painted flowers and see the Virgin and offspring beyond (see pl. 38).

More formal than their counterparts in Luca della Robbia's sculpture, they are nevertheless flanked by the stable's earthbound animals rather than ethereal saints. Both mother and son raise their hands to bless the awed figures gathered eagerly around them. The central magus is so overcome that he leans forward, clasps the Christ Child's foot and kisses his toes. But the spirit of beneficence permeating the central group is contrasted with an agitated scene beyond painted by Bartolomeo di Giovanni (pl. 46). There, the luminous serenity of a Tuscan landscape is violated by the Massacre of the Innocents in all its brutality and despair. Mothers scream and clutch their babies as the soldiers' swords descend and lunge, while several infants are already left to die on the ground like the foundlings so often abandoned in the streets of Florence.

By taking the unusual step of incorporating this earlier biblical episode in the altarpiece, Bartolomeo and Fra Bernardo emphasised the danger threatening any foundling who failed to find a home in an institution like the Innocenti. Its redemptive role is affirmed above all by the building above the Virgin and Child. Instead of a makeshift stable, nobly proportioned pillars rise up to a roof where singing angels hover on clouds. The notable sturdiness of this structure, coupled with the placid waters of the lake it frames, ends up implying that substantial shelter is available for every unwanted child who needs support, protection and sustaining love.

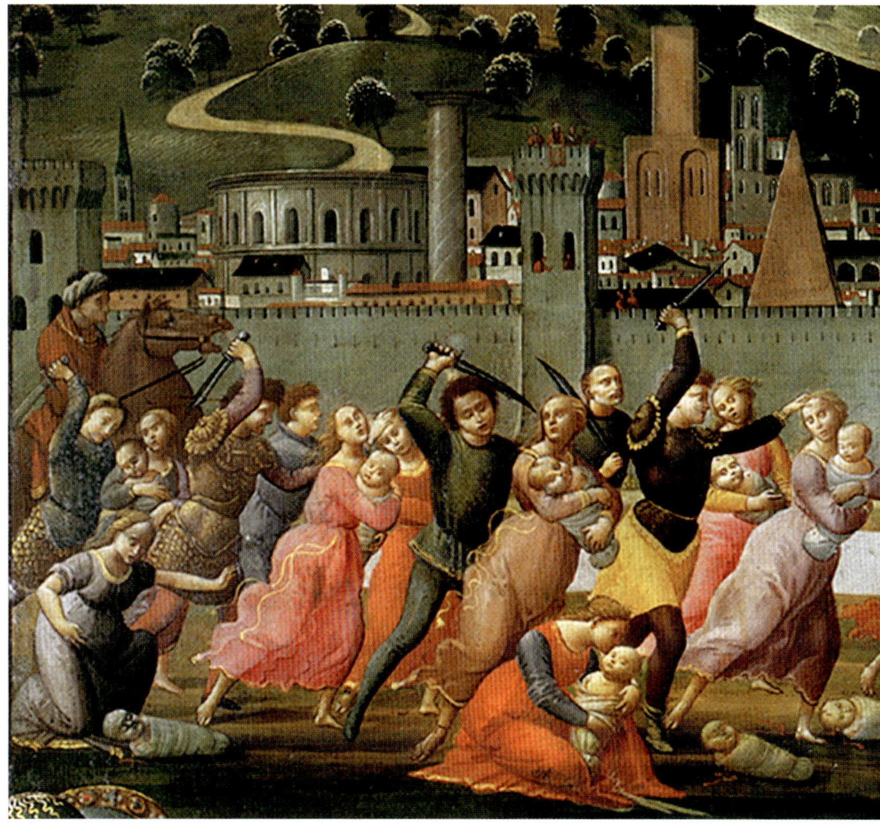

46 (*above*) Bartolomeo di Giovanni, *Massacre of the Innocents* (detail of pl. 45)

The intensity of feeling in Ghirlandaio's altarpiece undoubtedly benefited from his admiration for another outstanding Florentine hospital commission: *The Adoration of the Shepherds* by Hugo van der Goes (pl. 47). When this great Netherlandish triptych arrived in 1483, it was positioned on the high altar of the church of Sant'Egidio in the hospital of Santa Maria Nuova.[12] It was in excellent company: Domenico Veneziano and the young Piero della Francesca had earlier executed a major sequence of frescoes in the choir. Although later destroyed, they proved widely influential. So did the van der Goes altarpiece. Florentine artists like Ghirlandaio, as well as painters from the rest of Italy, were impressed by its radical blend of outspoken realism and devotional intensity.

Santa Maria Nuova, the city's major hospital, had been sustained by the Portinari family's patronage since the final years of the thirteenth century when it was founded by Folco Portinari, the father of Dante's Beatrice. Tommaso Portinari continued this bountiful tradition, promising in 1472 that

45 (*facing page*) Domenico Ghirlandaio, *Adoration of the Magi*, 1488, Spedale degli Innocenti, Florence

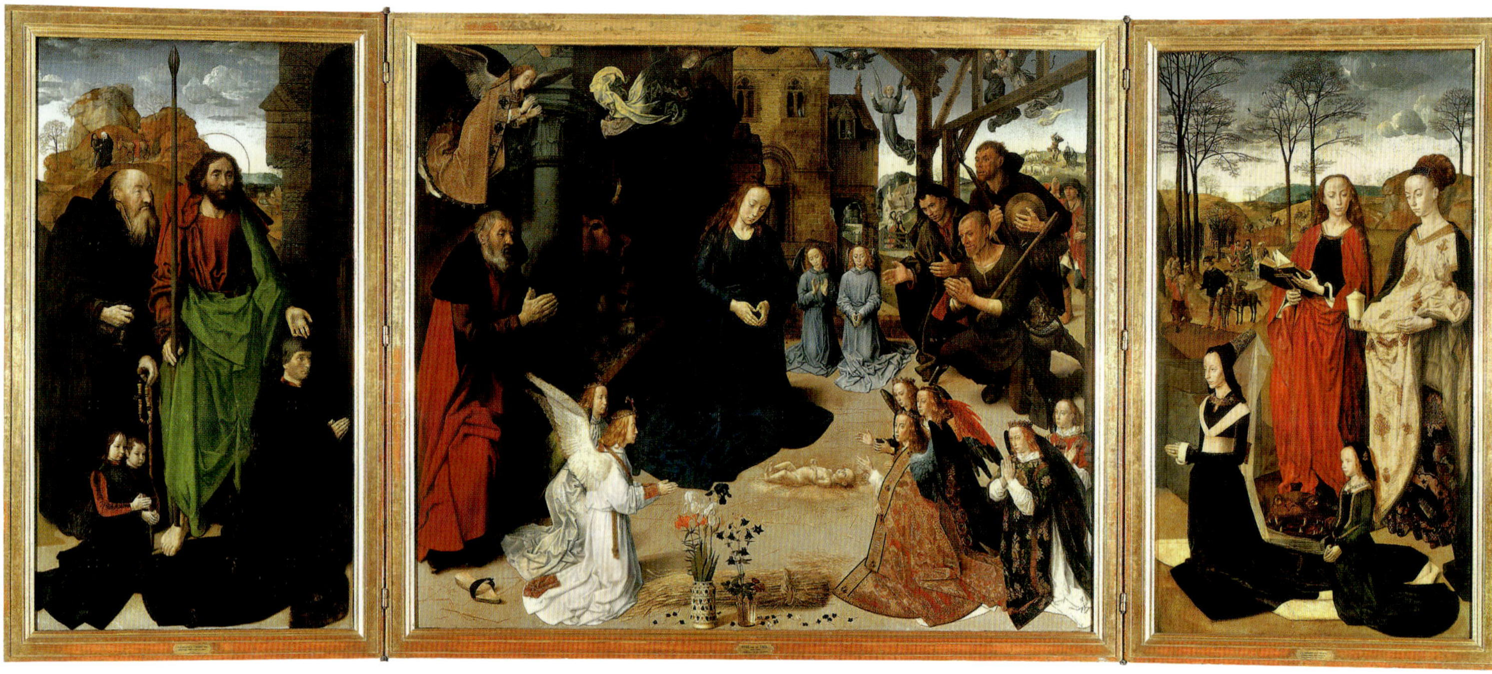

47 Hugo van der Goes, *Portinari Triptych*, 1475–82, Galleria degli Uffizi, Florence

seven hundred gold florins would be endowed for daily masses offered in perpetuity on the high altar of Sant'Egidio and at SS. Annunziata. Almost thirty years later Portinari would die in the family hospital, and he was very probably buried in front of the altar where the van der Goes painting had been installed. No location could have been more appropriate. For Portinari had himself commissioned the triptych while running the Medici bank's branch in Bruges. He was long believed to be guilty of chronic mismanagement there, expending so much energy on pleasing the Dukes of Burgundy that the bank eventually suffered financial disaster.[13] But Margaret L. Koster's recent research in Portinari's family archives has established that he did not end his career in penurious disgrace.[14] He went on working for Lorenzo de Medici after his bank career had terminated. And Portinari certainly showed exceptional discernment in choosing van der Goes, a brilliant yet profoundly disturbed artist who seems to have died from acute melancholy in an Augustinian monastery near Brussels.

The commission must have taken years to complete, and includes a central panel considerably larger than any executed by a northern painter before. Van der Goes knew that this altarpiece would be judged by the most innovative and discerning artists after its arrival in Florence. So he must have striven hard to ensure that the *Adoration of the Shepherds* did justice to his formidable abilities. He succeeded in full measure, but the struggle to complete this showpiece may well have proved arduous. According to a chronicle written by Gaspar Offhuys of Tournai, a novice when van der Goes entered the monastery of Roode Klooster (the Red Cloister), the artist underwent severe fits of depression, amounting on occasion to outright delirium. He also tried to combat the manic delusion that he was 'doomed to perdition',[15] and by the late nineteenth century Emile Wauters had mythologised his predicament in a popular painting called *The Madness of Hugo van der Goes*. Vincent van Gogh became preoccupied with this image of the deranged artist, often referring in letters to his fear that 'not just my pictures but I myself have become especially haggard of late, almost like Hugo van der Goes in the painting by Emile Wauters'.[16]

If Margaret Koster is right, van der Goes included his own self-portrait in the Portinari altarpiece's central panel.[17] Behind the shepherd who hurries forward to catch up with his three companions, a face in near-profile trains sharp, watchful eyes in the direction of the stable (pl. 48). Although sliced off just below his nose, this face bears a resemblance to the probable self-portrait in van der Goes's *Lamentation*. But he is far less prominent in the *Adoration of the Shepherds*, possibly because the artist was very conscious of the need to portray Portinari, his wife and children in the triptych's wings. Not that the banker insisted on enjoying an ostentatious presence in the painting. Far from it: he is depicted in dark, almost funereal robes, and looks strangely diminished compared with the saints towering above him (pl. 49). By flouting the laws of naturalistic proportion in this deliberate way, van der Goes disregards the prodigious realism he explores in his depiction of the shepherds, animals and flowers. The disparity between Portinari and his saints prompted Erwin Panofsky to find 'a contrast of almost frightening intensity: gigantically looming up behind their protégés and foiled by the scenery of arid hills and leafless trees inhabited by jackdaws, the saints appear austere to the verge of forbidding'.[18]

But the truth is that van der Goes and Portinari must have agreed on the supremacy of the saints. After all, Thomas was the patron saint of the Magistrato dei Sei della Mercanzia in Florence, and his namesake Tommaso Portinari would become one of the 'Sei' towards the end of his life. Moreover, Saint Anthony Abbot has the same name as Portinari's firstborn son Antonio, portrayed directly beneath with his brother Pigello. Anthony Abbot often appeared in altarpieces commissioned for hospitals: as Mathias Grünewald and his patrons realised when they planned the Isenheim polypytch (see pl. 71), the bearded saint with his emblematic stick and bell was widely regarded as a crucial figure in fighting the pestilential spread of Saint Anthony's Fire.[19]

In the right-hand wing, where Maria Maddalena Portinari kneels with her daughter Margherita, the saints perform similar roles (pl. 50). The Magdalen, a statuesque and imperious presence with auburn hair piled dramatically high on her head, echoes the mother's name. She personifies hope, having successfully changed her status from sinner to saint. And Saint Margaret, standing further back to make room for her gruesome dragon's-head attribute snarling on the ground below, chimes with the name of the daughter. Little Margherita appears remarkably unconcerned about the proximity of the dragon's voracious teeth, gaping in a mouth of hell as if determined to swallow up the little girl entirely. Perhaps she feels especially reassured by

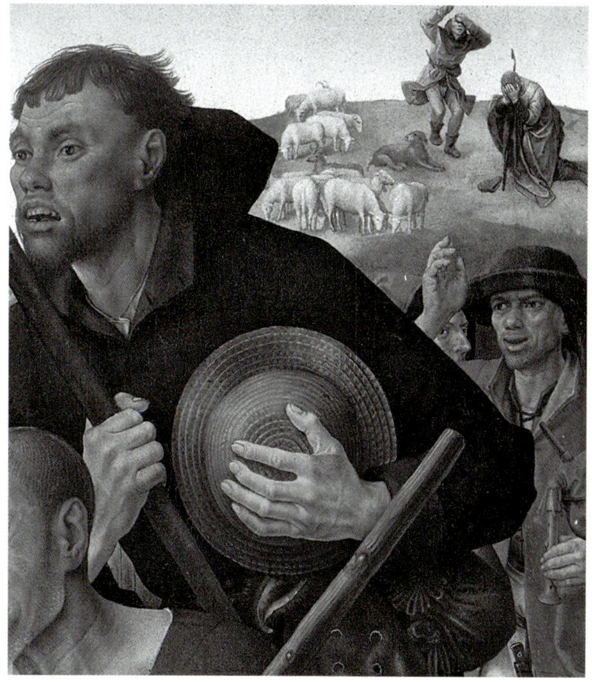

48 Detail of pl. 47

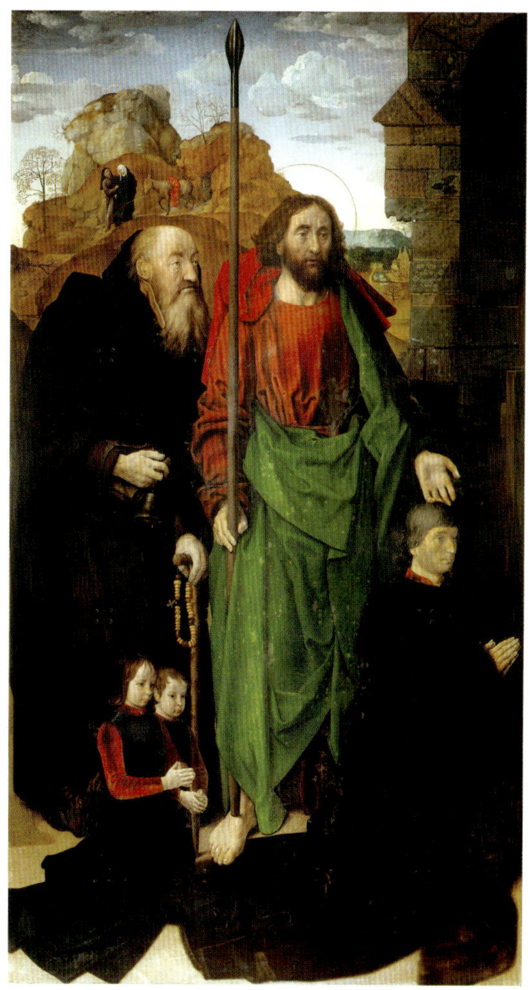

49 Hugo van der Goes, *Tommaso Portinari, his Sons, and Saints Thomas and Anthony Abbott*, left-hand shutter of *Portinari Triptych*, 1475–82, Galleria degli Uffizi, Florence

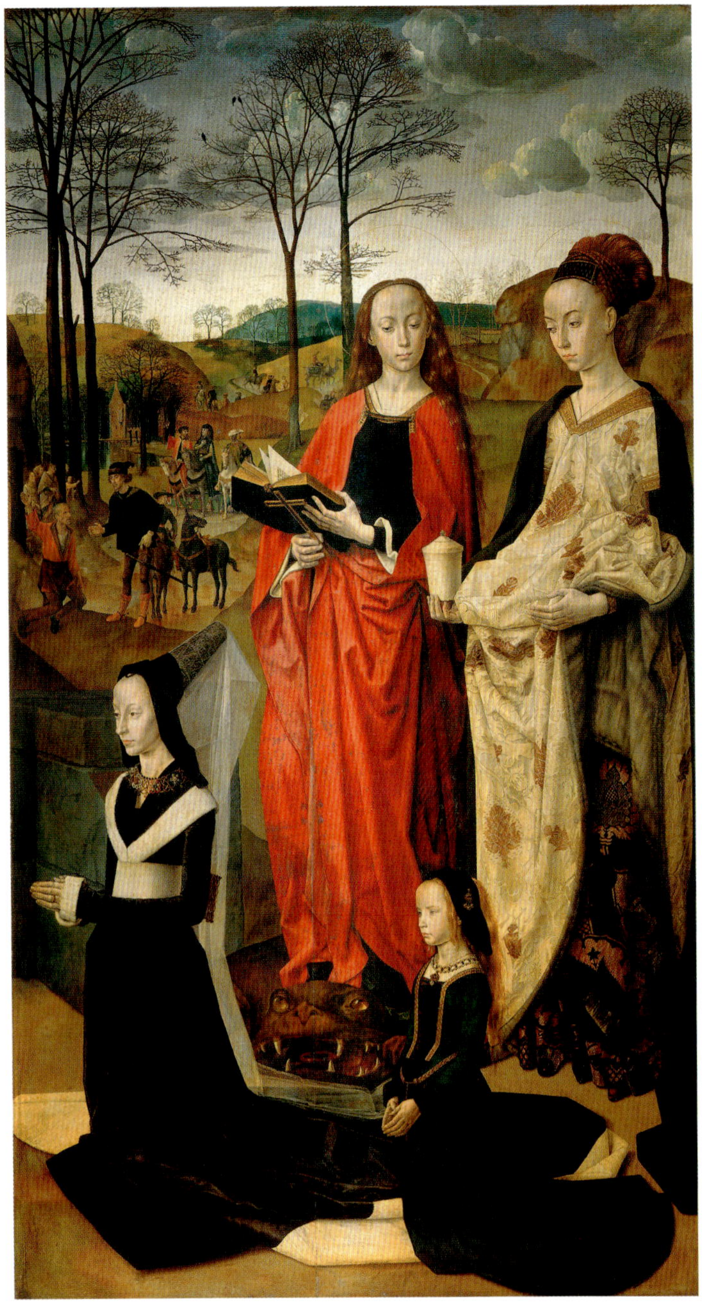

50 Hugo van der Goes, *Maria Maddalena Portinari, her Daughter, and the Magdalene and Saint Margaret*, right-hand shutter of *Portinari Triptych*, 1475–82, Galleria degli Uffizi, Florence

the presence of Saint Margaret, who was the patroness of pregnant women. Maria Maddalena Portinari would have been equally gratified, for she spent much of her married life in a pregnant state. And this emphasis on the welfare of children prepares the viewer for the central panel's climactic meditation on the plight of the holy infant.

The originality of the *Adoration of the Shepherds* becomes clear once the Nativity scene is examined. For the first time in any painting of this subject, a demon is depicted. It may be Lucifer himself, lurking so menacingly in the darkness just above the cow's horned head. He is difficult to discern, but careful scrutiny reveals his sinister presence. And van der Goes's decision to include such a diabolic creature, in a painting celebrating the miracle of divine birth, has disturbed many art historians. Robert Walker wondered whether, for van der Goes, 'the demon of the Portinari altarpiece did not have a particular meaning . . . at a time when the mental torments that sent him to his death in the Roode Klooster may have begun their critical intensity.'[20] But *The Golden Legend* discloses another, more devotional and positive way of interpreting the devilish presence. By attending the Nativity, the demon implicitly declares his belief that the Virgin's baby was indeed the son of God. And the fact that he is so indistinct in the shadows, just below a far more visible and flamboyant angel flying towards the Virgin, may reflect the widely held belief that Christ's birth was intended 'to confound the demons'.[21]

More important still, from the vantage of the Santa Maria Nuova hospital and its patients, the birth of Christ was in Augustine's view 'an example, a sacrament, and a medicine. A most fitting example it was for man's imitation, a high sacrament by which we were delivered from the bonds of sin, and a most powerful medicine, which heals the tumour of our pride.'[22]

Even so, van der Goes ensures that the forces of darkness have not faded completely from view. Their representative is still there, and his obstinate, spectral presence lends an extra dimension of meaning to the intense scene unfolding in the central panel (pl. 51). Here, van der Goes deploys the flair of a theatrical director as he makes every element in this complex drama converge on the infant. All the participants, whose expressions range from pity to foreboding, seem mesmerised by the compelling sight of this small, blanched child lying alone on the stable floor. Even the animals, so often oblivious of Christ's advent in other Nativity paintings, stop munching. They look up, arrested and alert. The two angels hovering above them may not share the surprise felt by the cow and donkey, but they are equally enthralled. One clasps his hands in fervent prayer, while the other makes a more open gesture filled with wonder.

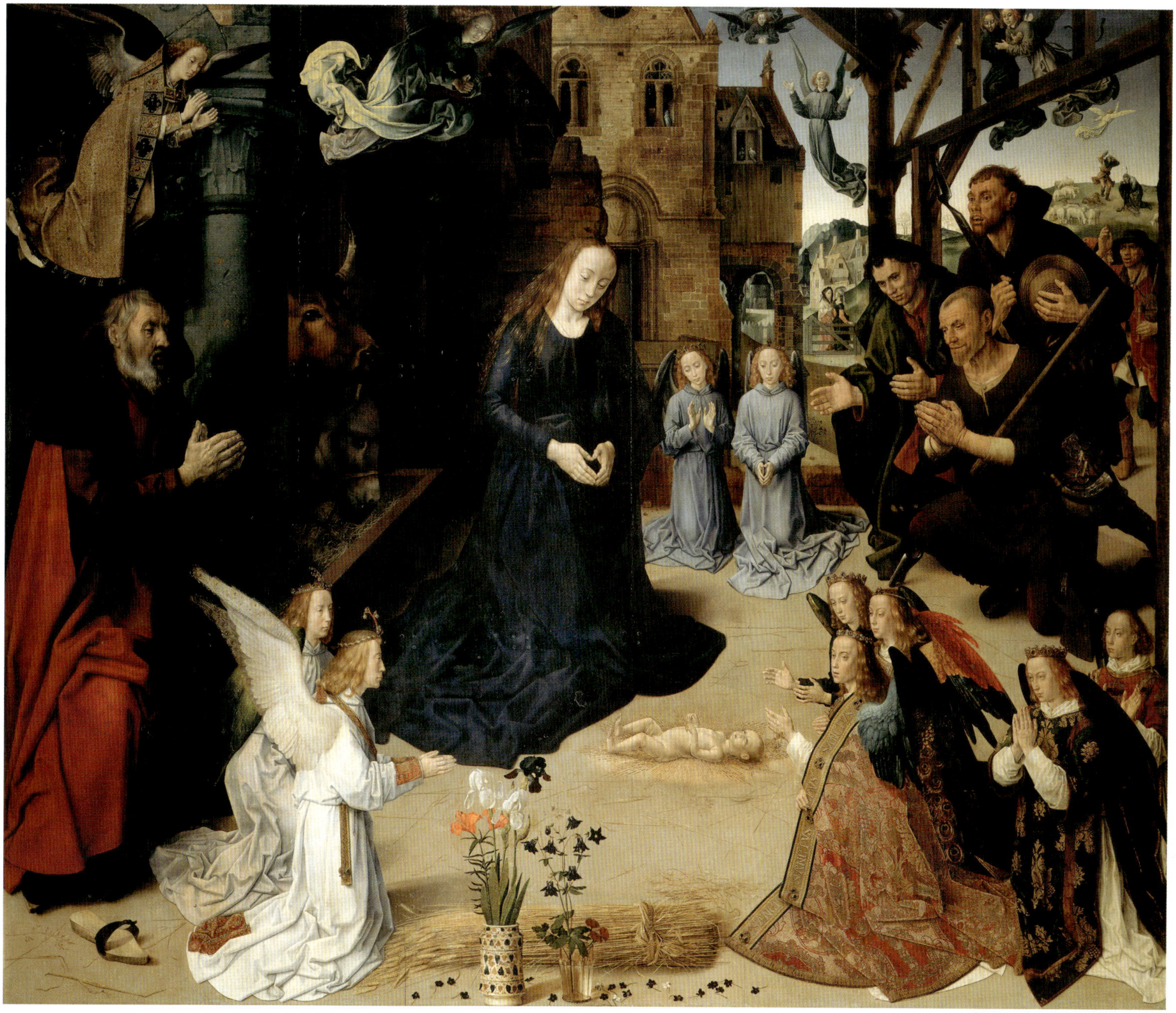

51 Hugo van der Goes, *The Adoration of the Shepherds*, central panel of *Portinari Triptych*, 1475–82, Galleria degli Uffizi, Florence

Directly beneath, a far older figure stands by a ruined column. He is Saint Joseph, and his furrowed face appears almost stunned as he stares in awe towards the space where the infant rests. One of his wooden shoes has become detached from his left foot, and he seems unsteadily caught between the desire to remain standing and the urge to kneel. Van der Goes accentuates his hesitancy in the convoluted structure of the robes heaped awkwardly around his thighs. All the same, Joseph's trenchantly delineated hands are clasped with complete assurance, as if to echo the praying gesture of the angel kneeling in front of him. Joseph's gravity is shared by the angel, too. Dressed in pale, simple raiments, the winged visitor seems concerned about the infant. He extends his praying hands as if wanting to reach forward and alleviate the Christ Child's loneliness.

Beside his hands, however, a piercingly observed still life of flowers dominates the foreground (pl. 52). It is a *pièce de résistance*, demonstrating the artist's

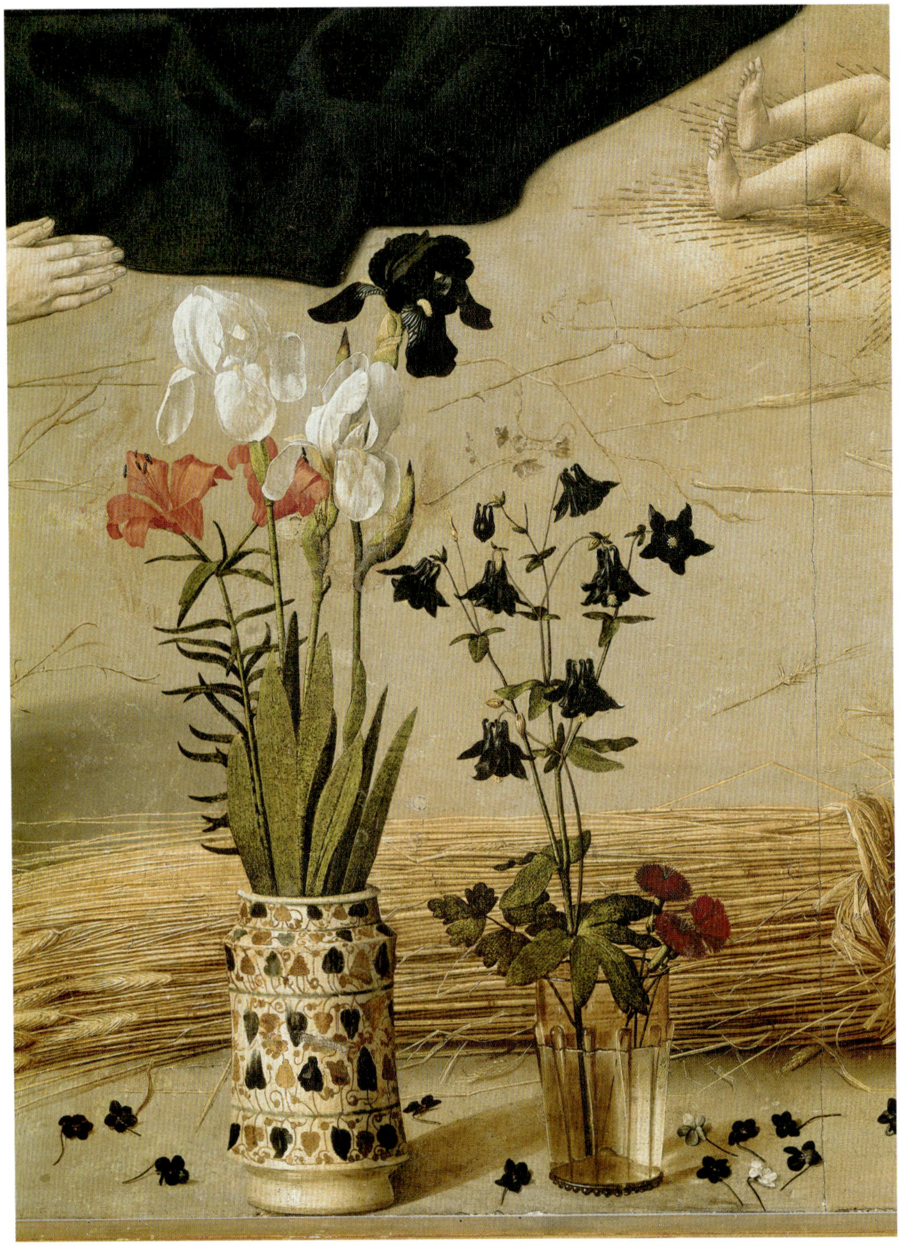

52 (*above*) and 53 (*facing page*) Details of pl. 51

ability to deploy oil paint with beguiling assurance. On one level, van der Goes must have intended the flowers as a demonstration of his consummate skill. The freshness and precision of these leaves, stalks and petals would have astounded many of the Florentines who viewed the altarpiece in its original location. The angels on the other side of the panel certainly find their attention distracted by the blooms, gazing at them rather than the baby. Dressed with far greater splendour than their austere counterparts on the left, they brandish multicoloured wings and robes so sumptuous that their textures glisten in the light. The repeated word 'SANCTUS' runs like a sacred chant all the way up the edge of the garment worn by the most prominent angel. He has clearly come to honour the sacred baby, yet his eyes are diverted by the sight of the flowers. Although his companions follow suit, van der Goes does not simply want them to admire his still life. He also intends them to be struck by a sense of dread. After all, they would realise that the red lily symbolises the blood of the Passion. They also know that the wheat laid out beside the flowers refers to the bread of the Eucharist. As for the petals scattered so inescapably across the foreground, they must signify transience. Snapped off and left to die without water, these scattered blooms transform the still life from a celebration of birth into a *vanitas*.

Nothing could be further removed from the angels' refined and exquisite melancholy than the boisterous shepherds grouped above them (see pl. 51). Unaware of the *memento mori* in the vases, they have eyes only for the Christ Child. Bending eagerly forward, they are depicted at the moment of recognition. While the oldest shepherd sinks to his knee and prays, his younger companion holds out both hands in a gesture of delight. As for the shepherd immediately behind them, he clutches his hat and implement while attempting to lean over his friends' heads and gain a closer look. The effort involved in this impulsive manoeuvre gives him a wild intensity (see pl. 148). While his companions smile at the infant, he lets his mouth fall open in big-toothed, gaping amazement. Van der Goes dramatises his robust urgency with the flair he expends on the smaller, red-coated figure running in from the field, where two more shepherds leap and fall to the earth as they listen to the miraculous news announced by the airborne messenger above them.

The vigour conveyed by the shepherds' reaction fills this section of the panel with life-affirming buoyancy. Van der Goes's unprecedented naturalism is persuasively rendered, and the angels floating over their heads are the most joyful of all the heavenly observers. Even here, however, intimations of the suffering to come can also be detected. The makeshift wooden beams of the stable entrance, so rudimentary compared with the grandeur of King David's ruined palace nearby, prophesy the structure of the cross where Jesus will be martyred. And the bare, wintry trees in the wing where Maria Portinari kneels are equally forbidding. Ravens perch on the black branches while the Magi, journeying from the East, struggle to find the right way forward. It is an ominous, frozen landscape, making us wonder how the newborn offspring can possibly withstand the coldness of the earth where he has been laid.

Mary makes no attempt to hold him (pl. 53). She looks as overcome by the sheer momentousness of the occasion as the Virgin Annunciate painted by van der Goes's workshop on the exterior wing of the altarpiece.[23] Far from seeking to warm the baby or feed him, she maintains a respectful distance. Perhaps Mary feels inhibited by the advent of this miraculous infant. Her projecting hands suggest that she would like to touch the child or even pick him up. But shyness prevents her, so she stares down devotedly while her fingertips press against each other in a paralysed act of reverence.

As a result, the Christ Child is left helplessly on his back. Gilded rays fan out from his slender body, signifying holy radiance. But he looks pallid and etiolated. More akin to a sacrifical offering than the son of God, he is all too mortal. However heartening his advent may be, he appears ominously reminiscent of a corpse laid out for burial. In this respect, he seems far more vulnerable than the smiling infant in Ghirlandaio's *Adoration of the Magi* (see pl. 45). Although van der Goes makes sure that the hem of Mary's voluminous dress is only inches away from the baby's upturned feet, Jesus cannot touch his mother. The child remains as alone and apart as the Florentine orphans had been before the Innocenti Hospital was founded. And van der Goes, the haunted artist who died a year before his altarpiece arrived in Florence, makes it impossible for onlookers to forget that the life of this newborn infant would end in a premature grave.

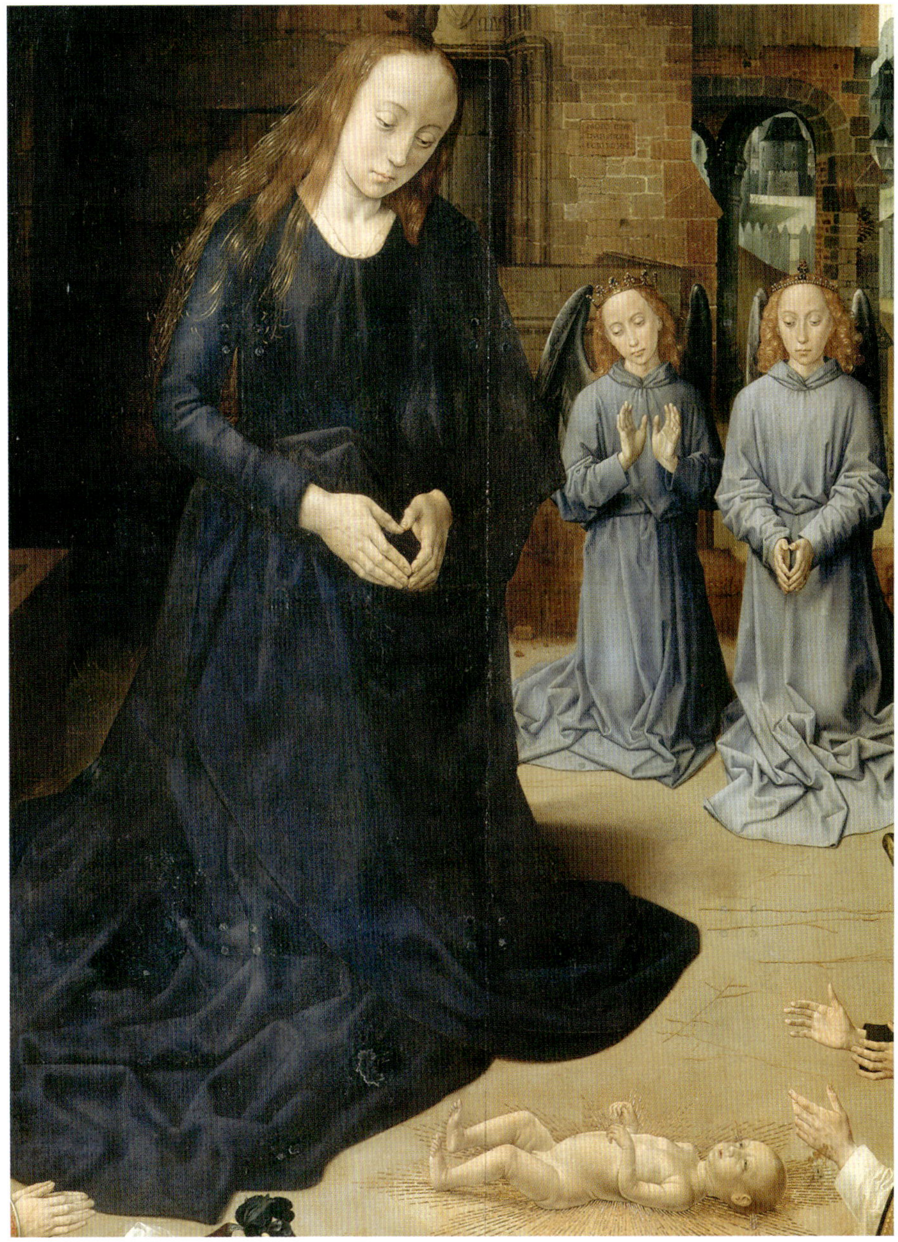

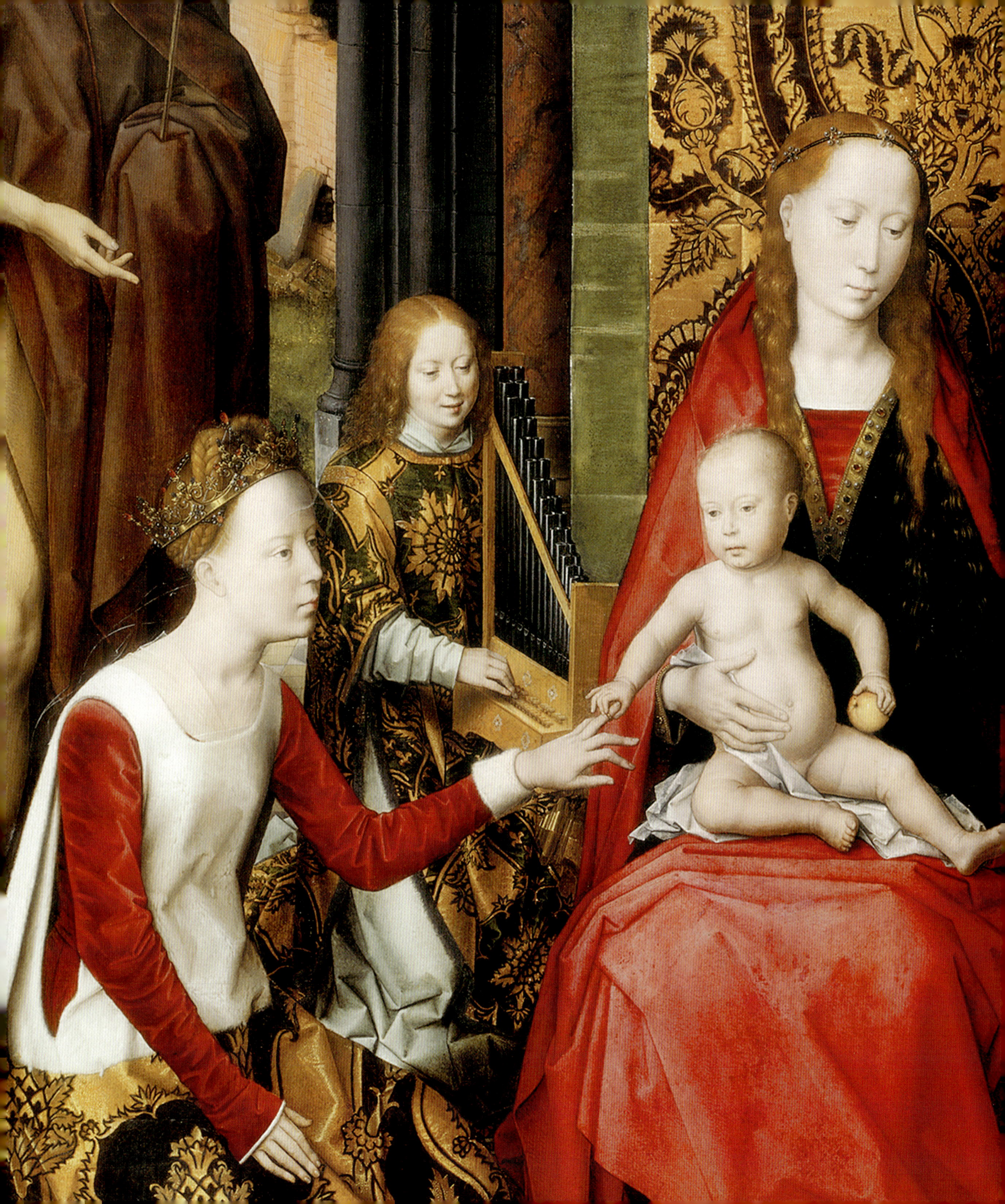

FIVE
THE BLOOD OF THE MARTYRS

Within the medieval entrance arch of Saint John's Hospital in Bruges, the conflict between life and death is fought out with great ceremonial intensity. The two lay orders of monks and nuns responsible for commencing the building, in the second half of the twelfth century, inspired their successors to commission an ambitious *Virgin Mary Porch* around a century later (pl. 55). Built against the street frontage of the middle sick-ward, it contains elaborate sculptural groups in the pointed arches directly over the doors. Probably executed by a local workshop aware of French High Gothic precedents, these carvings were extensively restored in the early twentieth century when additional sculpture was installed in the tympanum.[1] But enough survives of the medieval scheme to prove that the elaborate carvings above the entrance were devoted to dramatically contrasted scenes focused above all on the Virgin *in extremis*.

Such a theme was inevitable, for Saint John's stands to this day in the shadow of the Church of Our Lady. But the monumental emphasis on mortality in the entrance-arch sculpture also reflects an awareness of the ever-present struggle enacted within the hospital's walls. Some of the Virgin's deathbed carvings convey an almost relentless sense of grief and loss. On the left, angels line the side of her bed and look down with stoical resignation on the woman stretched out before them. Even so, they are countered on the right by a row of grieving apostles flanking Christ. The mood here is far more anguished: the mourning figures are gathered in open consternation alongside her body, and some are scarcely able to continue gazing at the Virgin's corpse. But their suffering is countered by a serene *Coronation of the Virgin* above, where the beatific scene is further enhanced by more apostles witnessing it from the archivolts overhead. Hovering with serene affirmation above the Virgin, they seem to ensure that she is guided above all by divine grace.

Although Saint John's also served as a lodging house for travellers, its all-important curative role extended as far as coping with periodic outbreaks of the plague. Whenever Bruges suffered an epidemic, its victims were taken to the most isolated quarters of the hospital along the water's edge. We do not know how much everyday contact any of the patients had with the hospital's outstanding collection of paintings. But Jan Beerbloch's fascinating view of the interior in the late eighteenth century, when the nuns had been running Saint John's on their own for around 150 years, indicates that most of its inhabitants did not enjoy a familiar relationship with the images owned by the institution (pl. 56). Shut off from each other by wooden cubi-

54 (*facing page*) Detail of pl. 62

55 Entrance Arch of Saint John's Hospital, Bruges

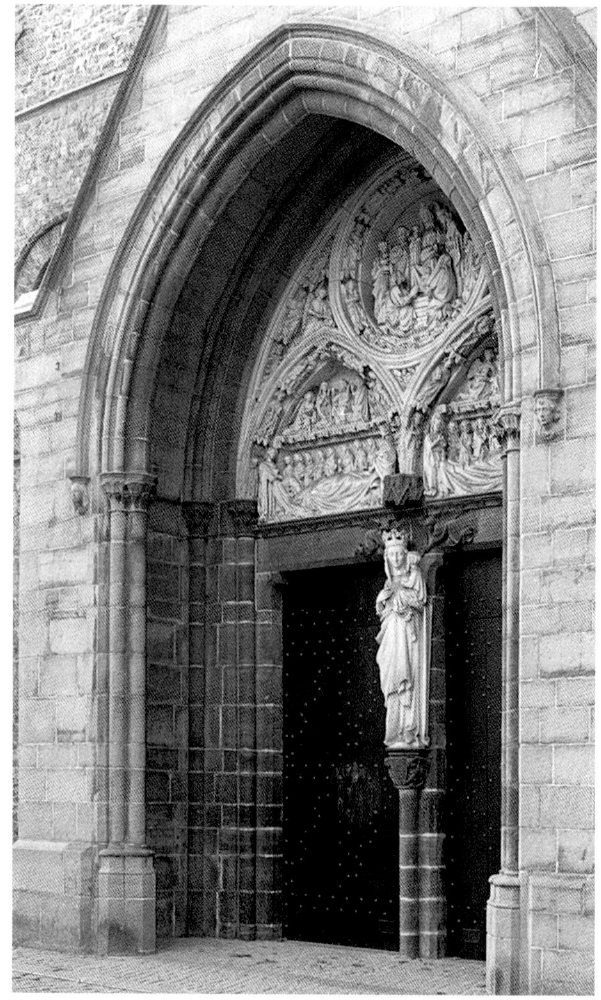

cles equipped with curtains, the patients were clearly encouraged to retreat into their own worlds. An awareness of the ward as a whole was not easy to cultivate here, probably because the authorities considered that it might prove unduly disturbing.

Nevertheless, the chapel at Saint John's was open to the ward until the 1970s[2] and the placing of beds belonging to the terminally ill in the aisles of the ward would have given their occupants a clearer view of the surroundings. The plentiful presence of both staff and visitors in Beerbloch's picture demonstrates that they could move around the building with a freedom denied to the patients themselves, and that they would have appreciated the paintings and sculpture clearly displayed on the building's ample walls. Beerbloch shows images hanging on the far left of the hospital interior and on the extreme right, where a crucifixion scene appears to act as an introductory devotional panel for anyone entering the hall.

By far the finest paintings at Saint John's can be found in the outstanding collection of Hans Memling's work. Having made Bruges his home in 1465, only a year after Rogier van der Weyden's death, he quickly became the city's leading artist. Comparisons with van der Weyden, who may for a while have employed the young Memling in his workshop, tend to be unflattering. But Memling's mild-mannered disposition should not blind us to

56 Jan Beerbloch, *View of the Sick Ward of St John's Hospital*, 1778, Memling Museum, Bruges

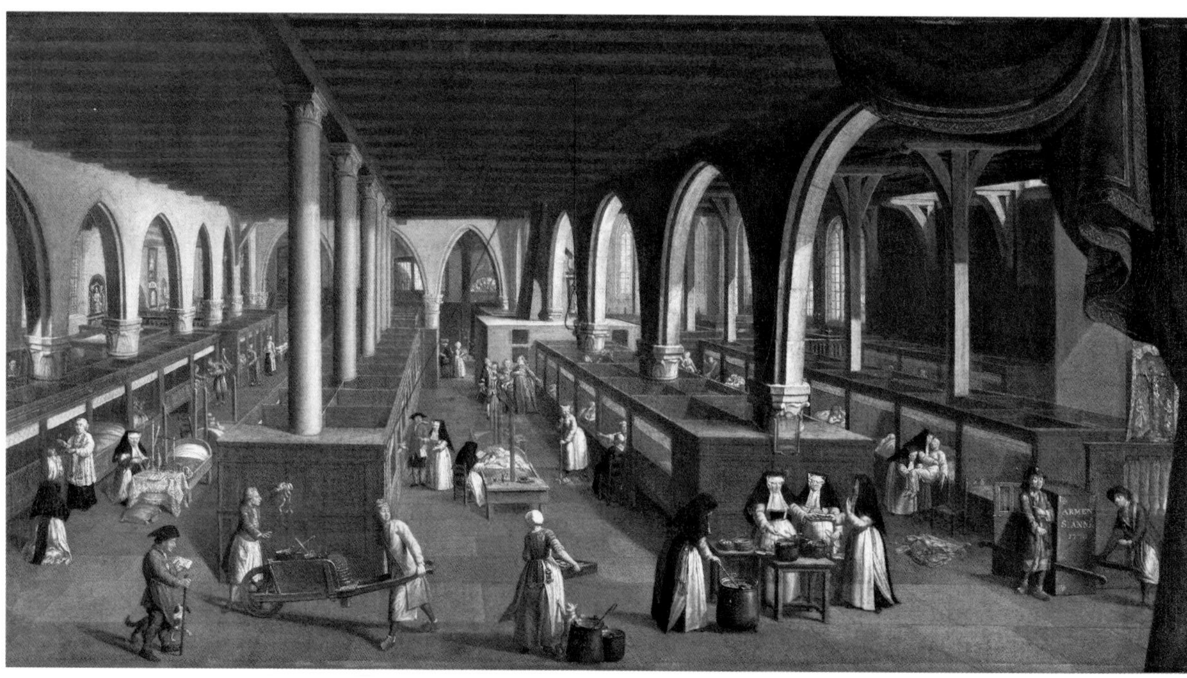

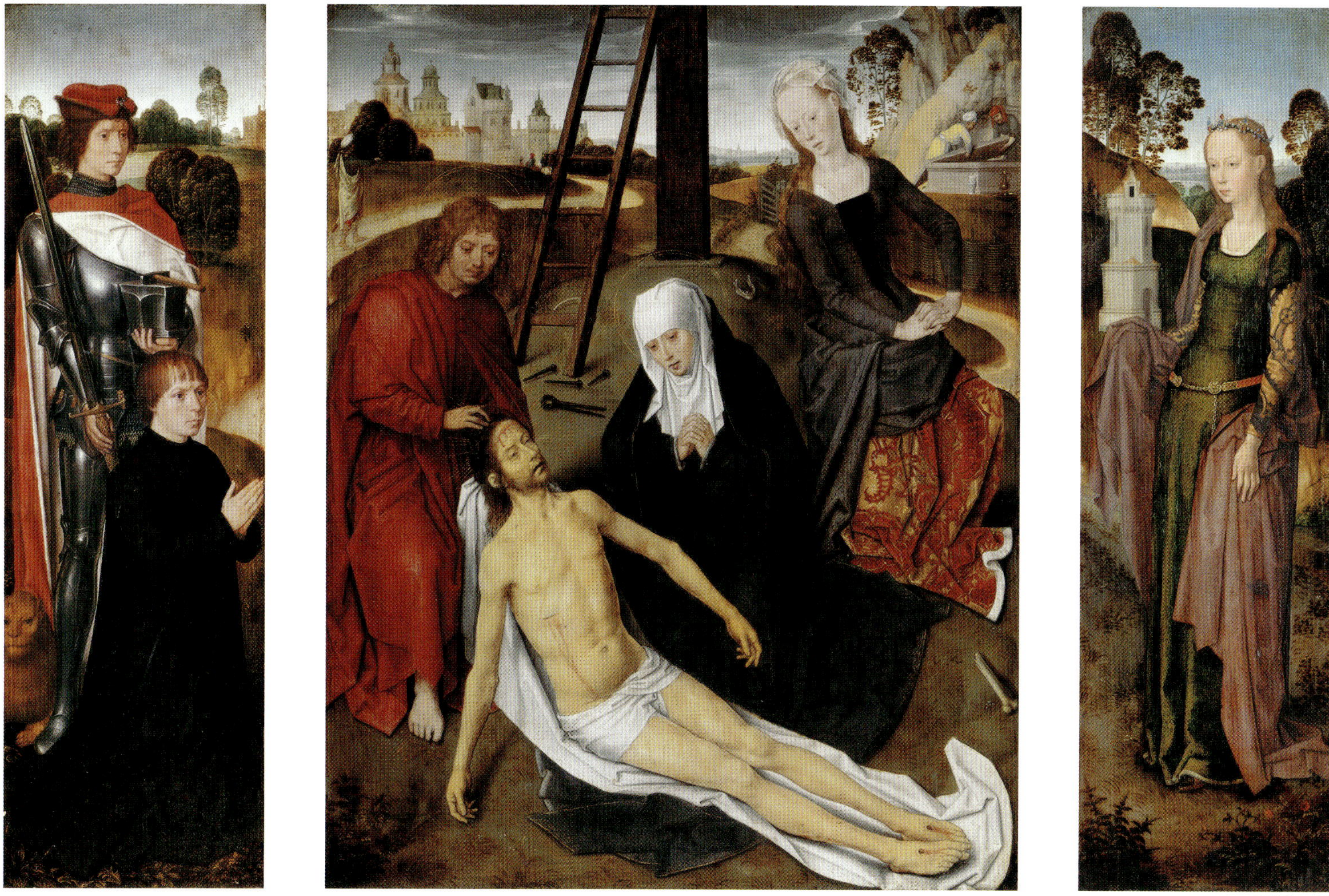

57 Hans Memling, *Reyns Triptych*, *c.*1480, Memling Museum, Bruges

the eloquence of his work. Although he lacks Rogier's tragic depth, Memling is an impressive painter in his own right. Just how inventive he could be, within the striking diversity of his commissions, is evident in the works preserved now in one of the hospital's old wards.[3]

The reason why Saint John's should harbour such an extraordinary collection remains tantalisingly unclear. The hospital's historians do not know precisely how the principal paintings arrived there,[4] even though an attractive if unverifiable account of Memling's life maintains that he received treatment at Saint John's for wounds sustained at the Battle of Nancy in 1477 while serving as a soldier for Charles the Bold. There is probably no truth in this story,[5] and yet the fact remains that a significant proportion of his finest achievements came to rest in the hospital. Since Saint John's was often in financial difficulties during the second half of the fifteenth century, its ability to procure these paintings remains puzzling. No documents recording payments or contracts survive in the archives, but the bishop of Bruges may have exerted a decisive influence. He established his authority within the hospital in 1459, when it formed a canonical community to partly distance itself from the city magistrates who had always supervised the institution. And the four works[6] by Memling most closely associated with Saint John's all include portraits of individual donors who must have played central roles in the commissioning process. These paintings also prove that Memling was capable of commanding a greater emotional range than he is often given credit for.

The small *Reyns Triptych* (pl. 57) is the starkest of the four important paintings made for Saint John's. Although it bears the date 1480 on top of the central panel's frame, the inscription may refer

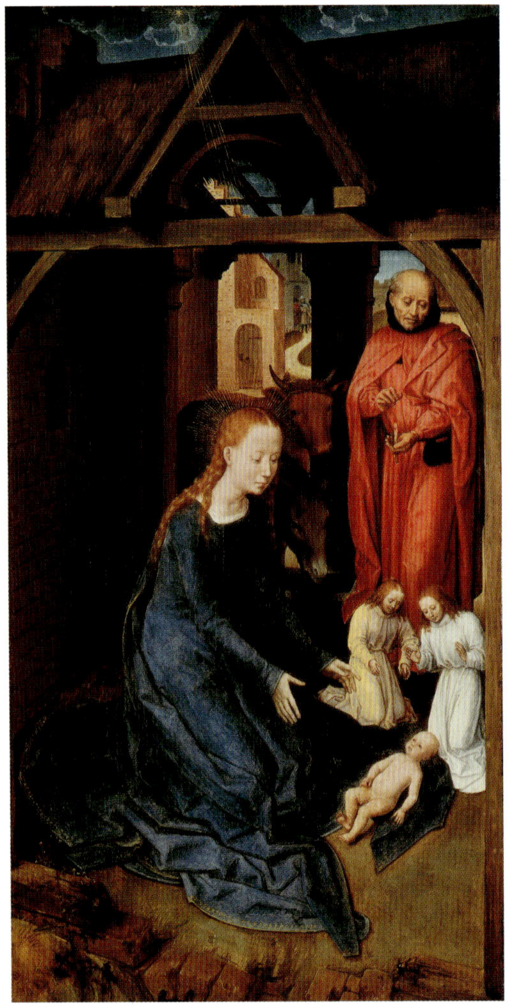

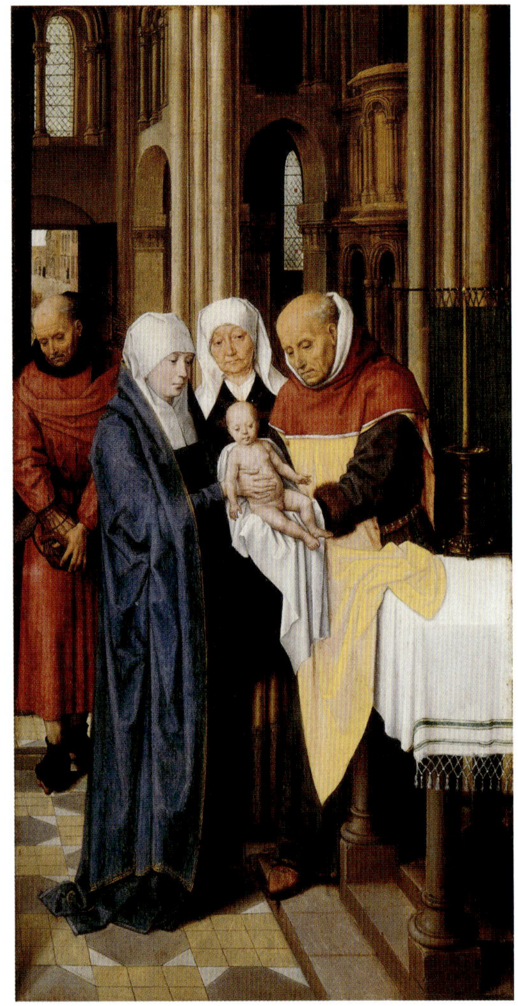

58a and b Hans Memling, *Floreins Triptych*, left and right panels, 1479, Memling Museum, Bruges

to the year of donation rather than execution. For this painting appears, on stylistic grounds, the earliest of the major Memlings in the hospital. Sweet amiability is displayed on the outer wings by Saint Wilgeforte,[7] the bearded princess who symbolises consolation for the oppressed and holds the cross of her own martyrdom. A similar placidity characterises Mary of Egypt on the other lateral panel, and she allows long tresses to flow over her breasts in one of Memling's most sensual images. But Mary was supposed to have survived in the desert for forty years with only the three small loaves she holds before her, and an austere mood prevails in the main triptych panels themselves. Adriaen Reyns, a friar in the community of Saint John's, is accompanied by the sober, frowning figure of Saint Adrian holding an ominous anvil. They both gravely contemplate a central *Lamentation* dominated by the blood-smeared corpse of Christ, and the anvil's metallic grimness is echoed by the large, cruel nails lying so forcibly on the ground beneath the cross. The serenity with which Saint Barbara looks on from the other side of the triptych does little to ameliorate the tragic atmosphere.

A far gentler temper prevails in another altarpiece, the *Floreins Triptych* definitely painted by Memling in 1479 (pls 58a–c). Originally intended for the hospital chapel in honour of the Nativity, it flanks the central *Adoration of the Magi* with narrower images of the holy birth and the presentation in the temple. Heavily indebted to van der Weyden, they combine an awareness of the event's exalted significance with Memling's typical sense of humility. Although the ruined stable in the nativity scene is supported by two symbolic columns, it is modest enough in structure; and the Virgin's

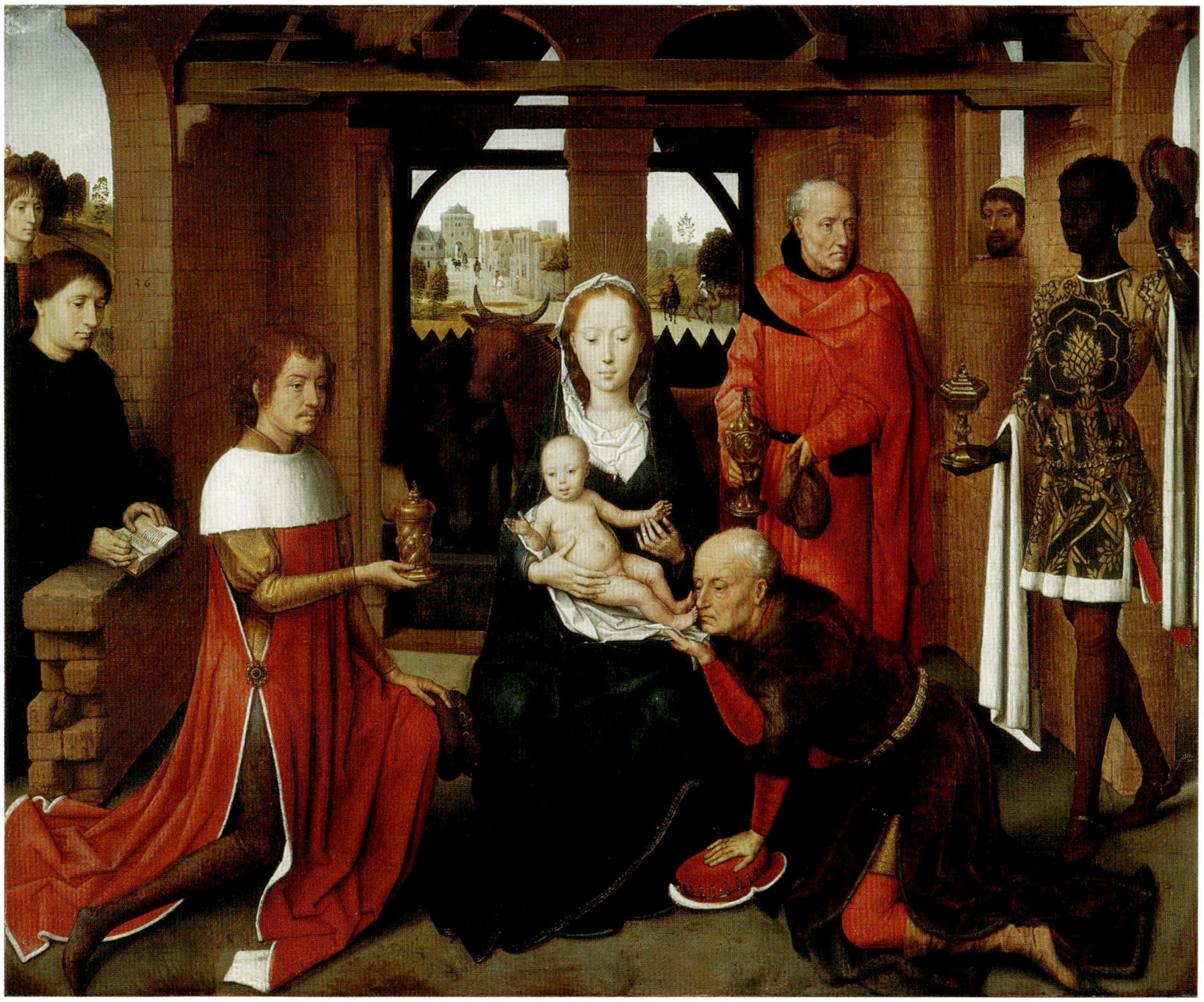

58c Hans Memling, *Floreins Triptych*, central panel, 1479, Memling Museum, Bruges

joyful relationship with her baby is delightfully unaffected. The temple presentation, probably situated in the historic Bruges church of Saint Donation, likewise fuses its elevated setting with an aura of simple grace. Saint Joseph is shown reaching into his homespun basket to take out some turtle doves, the offering of the poor. The mood of blessedness, so removed from the agitation of Giovanni di Paolo's *Presentation* in the church of the Spedale della Scala (see pl. 12), is movingly defined in the elderly features of Anna the prophetess, as she bears calm witness to the proceedings in front of her.

The largest panel of the *Floreins Triptych* continues the theme of tender devotion. Here the thirty-six year-old hospital friar Jan Floreins kneels behind a broken wall to meditate, as donor, on the adoration of the kings (pl. 58c). Although he is part of the principal scene, Floreins plays a far more modest role than his brother Jacob claimed for himself in a later Memling altarpiece (now owned by the Louvre). Jacob, a prosperous member of the corporation of merchant-grocers in Bruges, insisted on occupying a place next to the Virgin in a hall filled with all nineteen of his children – seven sons on one side, twelve daughters on the other. Jan, by contrast, shies away from such presumption. Accompanied by an equally reticent youth, thought to be a portrait of Memling's own son Jan, he quietly reads a religious text and leaves most of the picture-space to a scene of heartfelt celebration. Although the Magi are arrayed with magnificence in the monarchical robes of Spain, Arabia and Ethiopia respectively, one of the kings demonstrates the extent of his sincerity by casting grandeur aside, kneeling on the stable floor and

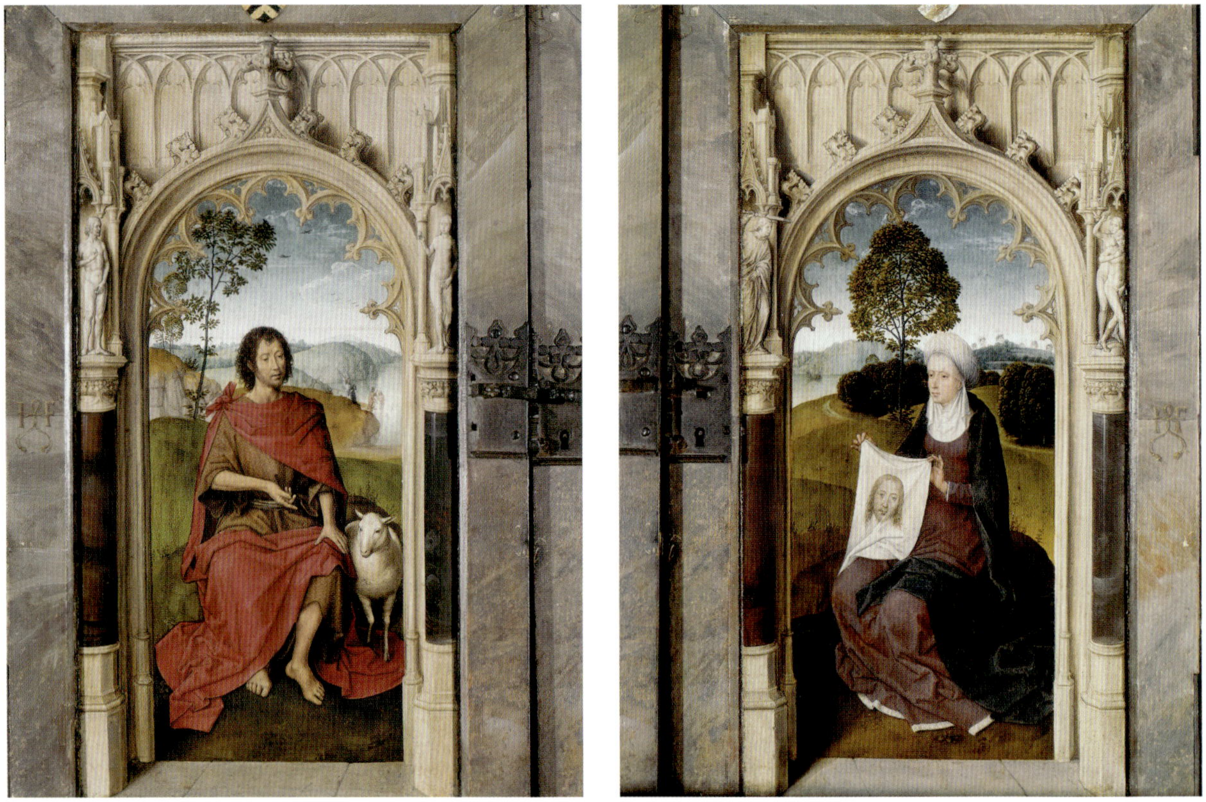

59a and b Hans Memling, *Floreins Triptych* (closed), outer panels, 1479, Memling Museum, Bruges

kissing the holy infant's feet. The very antithesis of an ostentatious grandee, this solemn and respectful old man personifies Memling's consistent preference for an art of stillness, humanity and restraint.

In reality, Floreins himself turned out to be rather less sensible than his devout portrait might suggest. Surviving a plague epidemic that decimated the hospital's other brothers, he became Master of Saint John's in 1488, nearly a decade after the Floreins triptych was painted. But his time in the post soon became marred by controversies. He had a weakness for employing 'unsuitable staff',[8] and the chronic problems they caused finally led to his summary dismissal in 1497. Although Floreins remained at the hospital as a friar until his death around 1505, the disgrace he suffered had been severe. In this respect, the outer panels of his tripytch contain some strangely prophetic images. For Memling placed the figures of Saints John the Baptist and Veronica inside simulated marble porticoes, enclosing sculpture that dramatises the expulsion of Adam and Eve from their earthly paradise (pls 59a and b). With supreme irony their fleeing, humiliated bodies are placed next to Jan Floreins's initials painted so proudly on the frame.

All Memling's finest qualities as an artist are exquisitely conveyed in the most important altarpiece owned by Saint John's. Inscribed with the date 1479 on the frame of the central panel, the *Altarpiece of Saint John the Baptist and Saint John the Evangelist* was surely commissioned for the high altar. The presence of both these figures in the central panel must indicate a desire to honour the hospital's patron saint.[9] And the exceptional significance of this triptych is also conveyed by the portrayal on the outer panels of no less than four devout hospital community members, all praying below their patron saints. On one side Antonius Seghers, the master of Saint John's, kneels with Jacob de Keuninc beneath Saints Anthony Abbot and James of Compostela. Its companion piece depicts the equally pious figures of Agnes Casembrood and sister Clara van Hulsen, accompanied by Saints Agnes and Clara who holds the monstrance in her pale hands. All the donors' sincerity is convincingly defined, and the close relationship they enjoy with their chosen saints must have provided hospital patients with a reassuring vision of similar companionship in the hereafter.

What a shock, then, to find this quiet, intent mood overturned by a disturbing alternative when

60 (*facing page*) Hans Memling, *Martyrdom of St John the Baptist*, left-hand panel of *Altarpiece of St John the Baptist and St John the Evangelist*, 1479, Memling Museum, Bruges

the outer panels were opened. There, on the left wing of the main painting, the *Martyrdom of Saint John the Baptist* is depicted in all its butchery (pl. 60). The victim's severed neck lies openly exposed in the foreground, where it spurts blood next to the massive weapon responsible for the savage slicing. As if to demonstrate the full extent of his callousness, the oddly dandefied executioner twists away from both the corpse and the viewer in order to present his gory trophy to Salome. She greets his triumphant gesture with utter detachment, holding her plate out to collect the martyr's head with no sign either of triumph or disdain. Three bystanders observe the proceedings thoughtfully yet without overt emotion. And Memling makes this entire group even more eerie by investing it with absolute calm.

Only in the distance, where a diminutive Saint John baptises Christ in the Jordan, does a more lyrical mood assert itself. For this pellucid landscape is soothingly removed both from the murderous frigidity of the martyrdom and from the macabre festivities in the middle distance, where Salome dances for Herod in a luminous Gothic interior. Accompanied by musicians playing shawms and a trumpet, the cunning temptress performs for her monarch while he relishes a sumptuous meal with his guests. Seated before a glistening tapestry, Herod raises his hand – perhaps for more wine from the goblets displayed on a nearby dresser, but more probably as a sign of approval directed at the treacherous dancer herself.

Memling makes sure that the mood of deceptive sweetness persists in the right panel as well (pl. 61). Although Saint John the Evangelist is here supposed to be contemplating his apocalyptic vision from the island of Patmos, he remains wholly undisturbed by the revelation. With placid hands folded on his book, the equable saint manages to ignore a panorama of destruction in the landscape beyond. While armed riders maraud the coastal scene, flames erupt and ships are sunk at sea by airborne dragons. High in the sky, even a Virgin-like 'apocalyptic woman'[10] and child encircled by the sun are menaced by a seven-headed monster extending its rapacious orange necks towards them. And down below, the horseman of the Apocalypse who symbolises starvation holds the future grimly in balance with his scales. Next to him a voracious beast of hell breathes fire behind Death, a skeletal figure on

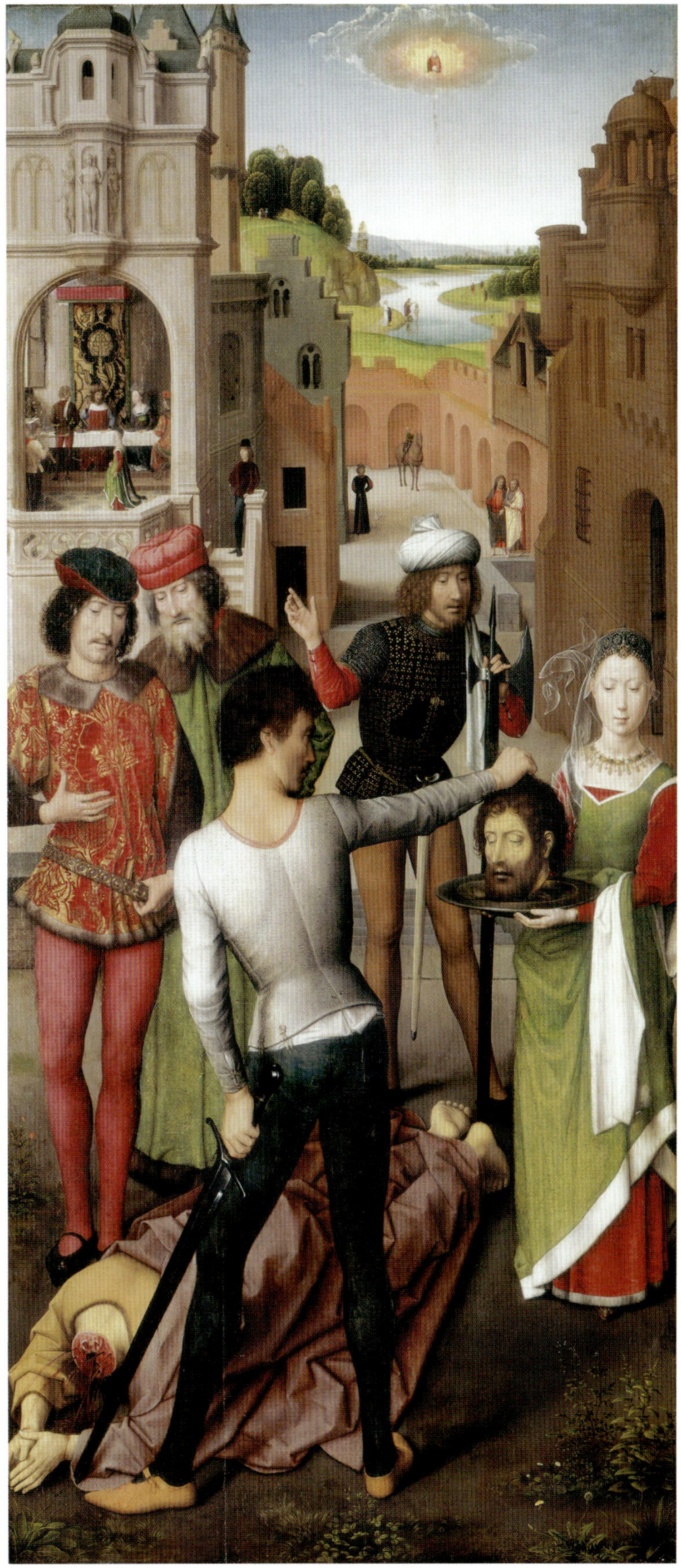

61 Hans Memling, *St John the Evangelist on the Island of Patmos*, right-hand panel of *Altarpiece of St John the Baptist and St John the Evangelist*, 1479, Memling Museum, Bruges

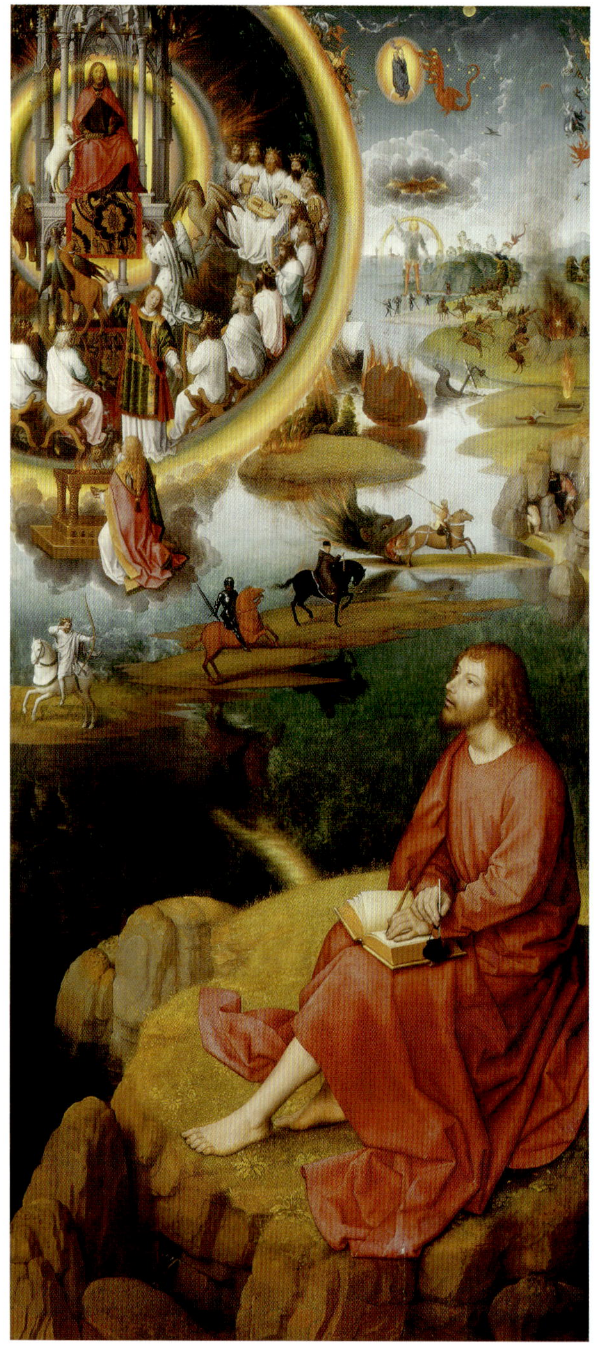

horseback who aims his spear at a cave where a naked figure appears to be hiding from persecutors.

Even so, the Evangelist remains oblivious to all this mayhem. He reserves his attention for a mystic gathering in the sky, filled for the most part with adoring ranks assembled to celebrate God with music. Memling's innate quietism did not equip him to interpret the vision of Saint John with the headlong conviction and dynamism that El Greco brought to the subject over a century later, when he painted one of his most ecstatic late canvases for the Tavera Hospital in Toledo (see pl. 109). But Memling's airborne musicians gaze at the enthroned deity with a palpable sense of awe, and they play their carefully specified instruments in rapt concentration while circular, rainbow-like beams of light enclose them in heavenly brightness.

The limitations of Memling's vision become outright strengths in the superbly wrought central panel of the altarpiece, focusing on the mystic marriage of Saint Catherine (pl. 62). Glimpses of contemporary Netherlandish buildings and countryside are included in thin vertical slices between the Gothic pillars punctuating the central group. And one historian has maintained that the hospital's 'gauger' Jodocus Willems is portrayed in a distant scene where wine is delivered in barrels from an immense crane standing on the Kraanplaats in Bruges.[11] While 'crane children' are shown running in the crane's wheel, Willems gauges the casks sent from Bordeaux to a hospital whose wine-measuring rights had been granted as a civic privilege back in the fourteenth century. Dressed in black, Brother Jodocus supposedly reappears in the distant scene on the right, but this attentive figure has also been identified as a self-portrait of Memling himself. Whatever the truth, no uncertainty surrounds the identity of the saint above him, plunged in boiling oil. He is Saint John the Evangelist, naked this time and praying grimly as the scalding liquid is poured onto his defenceless head. After miraculously surviving this ordeal, John is also shown in the background stepping gingerly into the boat that took him to exile on Patmos.

Throughout this complex and intricately organised painting, the respective textures of dresses, cloaks, flesh, carpet and tapestry are realised with beguiling virtuosity. Memling's command of perspectival recession, accentuated by the slightly aerial vantage he adopts, also gives the image an aura of realism. In every other respect, though, his panel asserts the priority of spiritual experience. Just as its title suggests, we are witnessing a mystical union between the Christ Child and a saint whose recent martyrdom is openly declared in the foreground of the design. A sword and broken wheel, viciously festooned on its outer edge with hooked blades, introduce an element of gruesome violence to the otherwise placid scene. But no blood is detectable

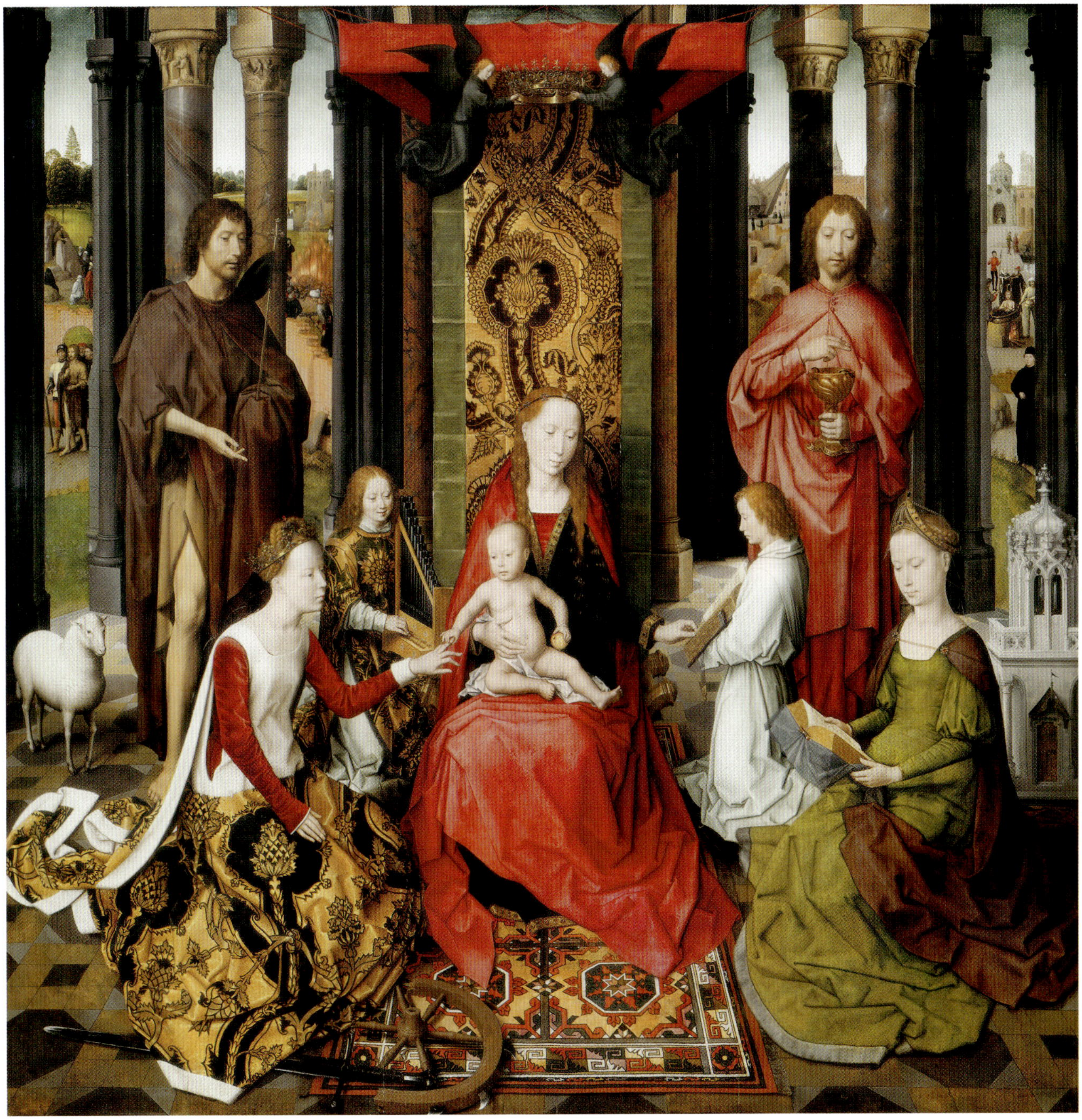

62 Hans Memling, *Mystical Marriage of Saint Catherine*, central panel of *Altarpiece of St John the Baptist and St John the Evangelist*, 1479, Memling Museum, Bruges

on these symbols of Catherine's travail, and she has likewise been restored to unblemished serenity by the redemptive ritual enacted here.

Wearing an expression of tense concentration, Catherine stretches out her hand to receive the ring proferred by the divine infant (see pl. 54). The delicacy with which he pushes the gold circle onto her upturned finger is a measure of the ceremony's heightened significance, and Catherine is so overcome that she cannot bring herself to look at the baby who bestows this honour upon her. Even so, the music-making angel nearby has no hesitation in smiling as she witnesses this felicitous event, and Saint John the Baptist above her gestures sympathetically while staring down at the momentous meeting of hands. Miraculously restored to life after her terrible suffering, and brought now into an intimate relationship with her God, Catherine could be seen by patients of the hospital as a heartening embodiment of the salvation that might await them after death.

The ceremonial splendour of the altarpiece must have made it the most compelling image in the hospital until the arrival of the *Saint Ursula Shrine* (pl. 63). This heavily gilt reliquary, adorned with a proliferation of paintings by Memling and his workshop on most available surfaces, was consecrated on 21 October 1489, when the chapter clerk of Saint Donation's in Bruges certified the deposition in the shrine of relics connected with Saint Ursula and her legendary eleven thousand virgins. The Memling decorations remain astonishingly well preserved to this day, even though until 1869 the shrine was carried every October in procession to the hospital church during the octave of Saint Ursula. Its bejewelled riches presumably reflect the legend of the hapless abbot who once kept a martyred virgin's body on his abbey altar. Having promised to instal it in a silver shrine, he settled for an oak receptacle instead. Since the dead virgin then rose up in protest and returned to Cologne, the embellishments on the *Saint Ursula Shrine* were probably meant to ensure that its relics never disappeared. But by the time it was formally opened up some years ago, they had indeed been stolen.[12]

63 Hans Memling, *St Ursula Shrine*, 1489, Memling Museum, Bruges

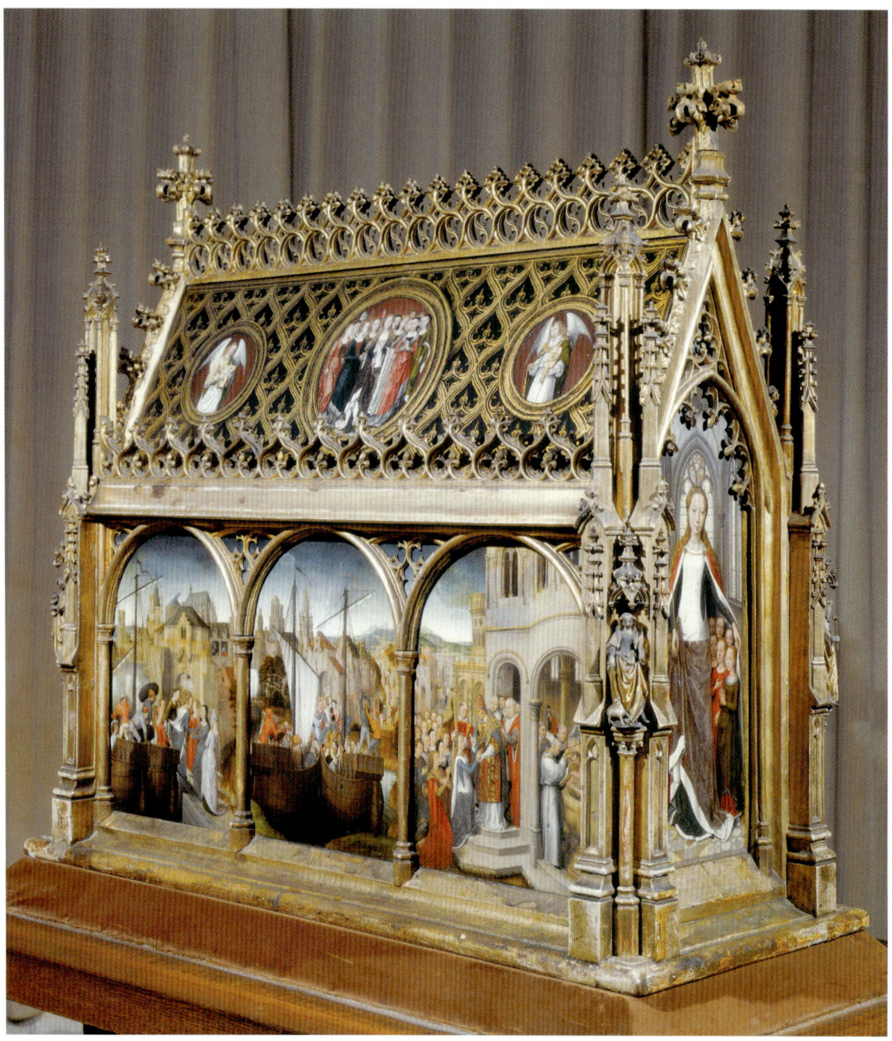

Memling himself can hardly be blamed for failing to provide adequate protection. Pieter Pourbus 'never tired of praising the workmanship'[13] whenever the reliquary was shown off on feast days, and the paintings alone add up to a resplendent pageant. Moreover, Memling does everything in his power to counter the violence of the martyrdom with more reassuring alternatives. The three arched scenes on each side of the shrine are largely taken up with pacific subjects. Above them, set into the sloping roof, the beatific mood is intensified by an exquisite oval of Saint Ursula in glory with a group of virgins, all savouring their proximity to each other in an intimate, harmonious gathering. And the four tondos set into the painted tracery depict angels playing a viol, a lute, a psaltery and a portable organ.

Most of the Ursula story illustrated by Memling was harmless enough (pls 64a–c). Based on the thirteenth-century *Legenda Aurea* by Jacob de Voragine, it described how the Breton princess Ursula was invited by the King of England to marry his son. She agreed, but only on condition that she would be allowed to make an epic pilgrimage to Rome beforehand. Accordingly, she persuaded ten other virgins to go with her, and they in turn each brought a thousand more virgins along on the journey. Memling shows them, in his first panel, disembarking gracefully from their vessels in Cologne and moving through a Gothic entrance to the city beyond. A great deal of the image is taken up with closely observed architectural details of identifiable landmarks in Cologne, ranging from the Church of Saint Severinus to the east end of the incomplete Cathedral. But through a small, darkened window on the right, Memling finally allows an ominous element to enter the otherwise optimistic scene. A spectral angel can be seen flying into Ursula's bedroom and, with both arms stretched out urgently towards her, predicting the martyrdom to come. With a dismayed expression Ursula clasps her hands in prayer, while realising

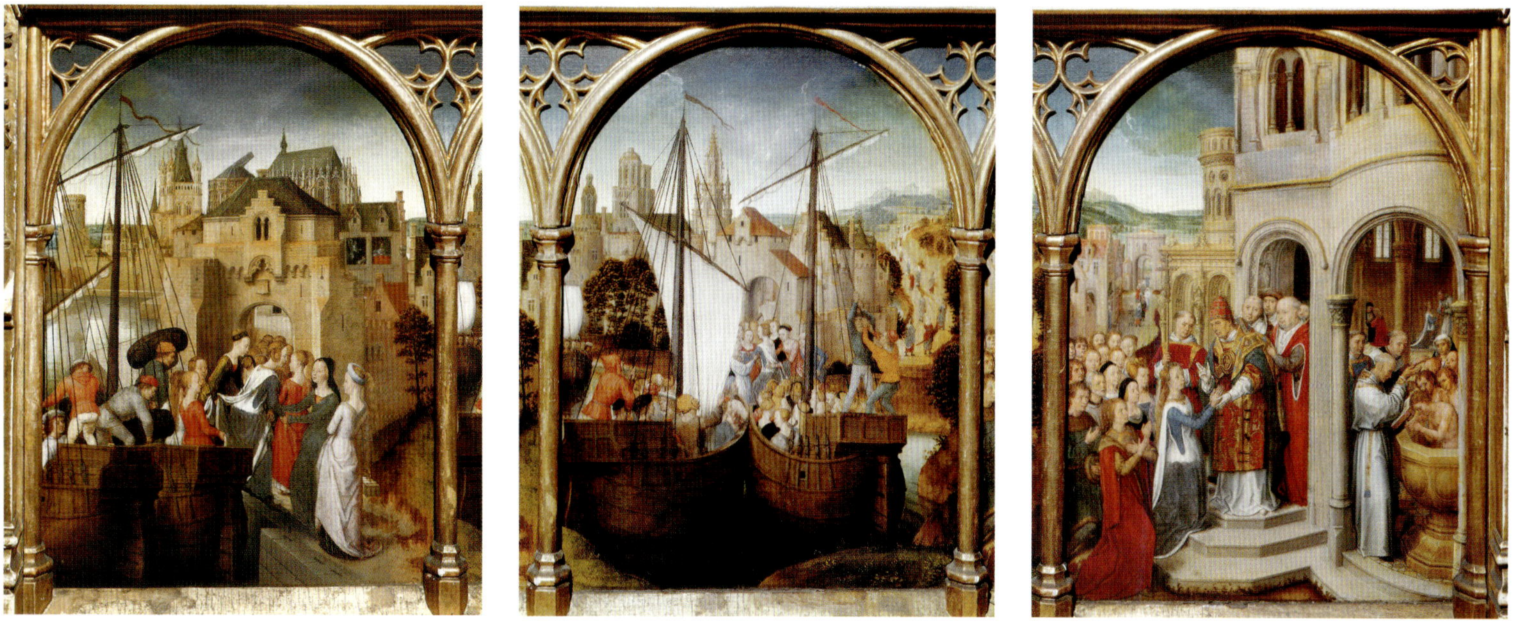

64a, b and c Hans Memling, first three panels on one side of *St Ursula Shrine*, 1489, Memling Museum, Bruges

that she can do nothing to stop the tragic momentum of an expedition organised with such faith and care.

It is a remarkably tense and gloomy portion of the painting. But this window is easily overlooked, and does little to spoil the air of liveliness and optimism animating the rest of the scene. The same vitality dominates the second panel, where Ursula and the virgins arrive in Basle, disembark and enter the city. Once again Memling makes us aware of Gothic architectural splendour, its towers and spires contrasting with the wooden masts of sailing vessels in the harbour. But a more melancholy note is sounded on the right, where the virgins seem oddly incommunicative after their communal energy at the quayside. Making their way by foot on a winding path to the Alps, each of the young women appears vulnerable and essentially alone.

They must have taken a long time to reach Rome. In the third panel, Memling shows the diminutive figures walking into the Holy City from the epic landscape beyond. Weary yet still resolute, one of them is obliged to lean on a stick for support. But a heartening spectacle encourages them ahead, where a cluster of virgins led by Ursula finally reach their goal. Kneeling on a stone staircase, she holds out clasped hands to Pope Cyriac. He blesses her, and his benediction is echoed by the gesture of the priests within the other arch who pour water on naked pilgrims gathered in the font. Behind them, Ursula can be seen kneeling to receive the sacrament below a window. Unaccompanied this time by any of the virgins, her isolation subtly prefigures the moment of martyrdom ahead.

On the other side of the shrine, the return journey leads inexorably towards death (pls 65a–c). At first, everything appears positive as Pope Cyriac and his retinue accompany Ursula and her company boarding vessels outside Basle's city gate. The emphasis here is on purposeful activity, enhanced by mutual respect: the Pope is given a helping hand both by a cardinal behind him and a white-haired supporter in front. Down on the water, oarsmen strain as they take a rowing-boatful of virgins to their destination. Ursula beams while she raises two praying hands and gazes in gratitude at her papal champion.

But the mood of peaceful fulfilment does not last long. In the penultimate panel, the virgins arrive in Cologne to find themselves assailed by Huns who were occupying the city. Two helmeted archers stand on the grassy shore, disconcertingly close to the virgins who cower and shield their faces in a boat. Although one of the arrows has struck a sail, the other pierces the upflung arm of a woman who desperately lifts her clasped hands as she falls towards the deck. Below her, at the side of the vessel, three more terrified virgins plead with the archers. Their bowed heads recall the poses of the pilgrims receiving holy water in Rome, yet here the women seem doomed to be slaughtered without mercy. In a neighbouring ship, arrows have already entered two of the passengers' bodies, while a golden-tressed virgin reels back from the brutal impact of a sword thrust straight into her heart by a scowling soldier. Blood spurts from her dress and spills down towards an equally crimson expanse of drapery. Behind her, Ursula reaches out with uncanny calm to embrace the dying woman. Yet nothing can save her – not even the graceful turrets and pinnacles of medieval Cologne forming a helpless backdrop to the butchery.

Ursula even retains her composure in the final scene, where she is taken to the chief's tent and rejects a bizarre offer of marriage. The executioner Dschem, brother of the Sultan Bajazet II, is aiming his arrow at her breast. But as she sways back a little, Ursula is still able to raise her hand in a gesture of proud independence. While a distraught, veiled companion prays behind her, Ursula remains poised as she prepares for the inevitability of death. Soldiers jostle nearby, preparing to assault more of her companions. But she lowers her eyes and appears as stoical as the dog gazing up at her from his docile, unprotesting position on the flower-strewn grass. Above Ursula's head, the choir of Cologne Cathedral asserts its magnificence, and yet the building's unfinished state may also reflect Ursula's inability to complete her own natural lifespan.

The utter imperturbability of the saint's bearing, undefiled by any sign of a wound, is confirmed by the narrow painting installed at one end of the shrine (pl. 66). Delicately holding the fatal arrow between finger and thumb, Ursula here stands in coolly triumphant resurrection before the clear illumination provided by the windows of a Gothic oratory. Taller by far than in the oval painted for the reliquary's roof, she towers over ten of her upright virgins and offers them shelter beneath an enveloping cloak. The gesture, similar to Piero della Francesca's *Madonna of Mercy* and to the *Madonna of Charity* later painted by El Greco for the Illescas hospital (see pls 22 and 103), seems wholly appropriate for Saint John's. Patients who gazed at the shrine would have drawn particular comfort from the gesture of the virgin on the far left, who pulls Ursula's cloak and presses it firmly against her own dress. At the same time she stares towards the luminous tip of the arrow, wondering at the terrible infliction of pain that led to martyrdom and eventual salvation.

At the other end of the shrine, Memling provided formal confirmation of the hospital's commitment to the values celebrated in the reliquary. He painted another, equally heartfelt vertical panel, this time showing two of Saint John's sisters kneeling and praying beside the Virgin and Child (pl. 67). Identifiable as Anna van der Moortele and Jossine van Dudzele, the latter of whom became

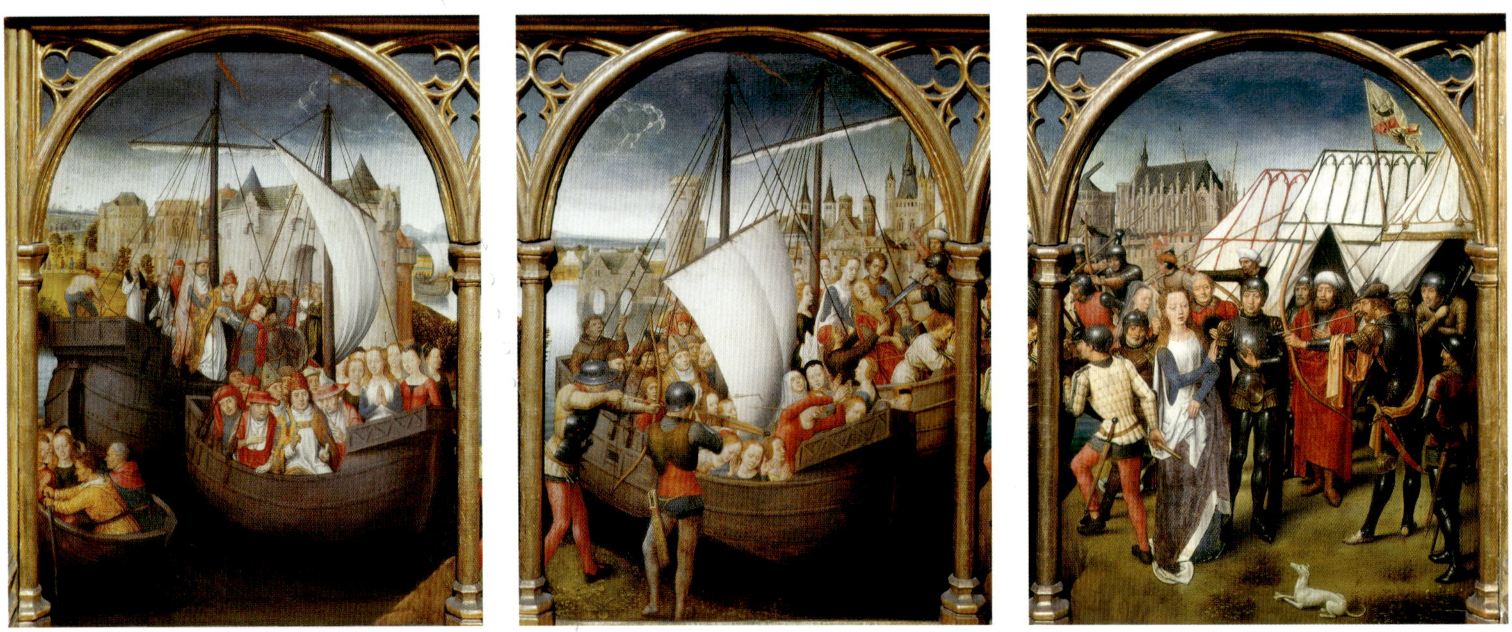

65a, b and c Hans Memling, last three panels on other side of *St Ursula Shrine*, 1489, Memling Museum, Bruges

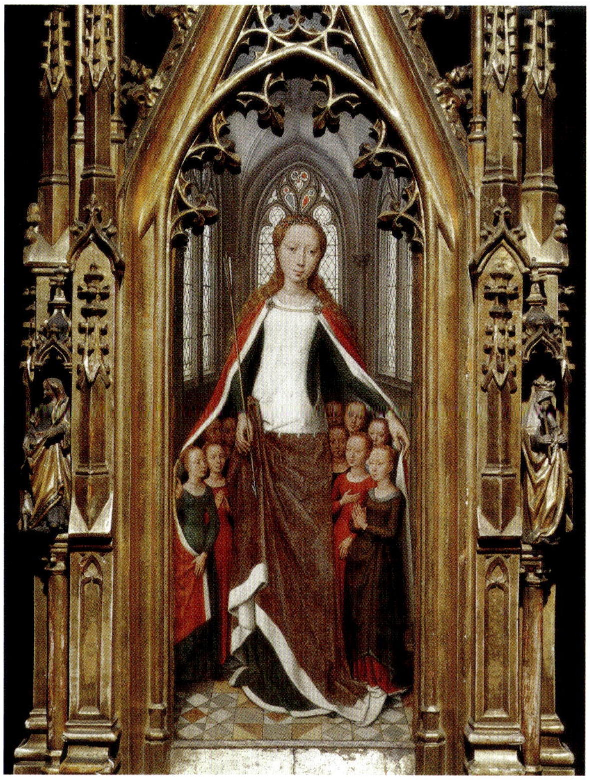

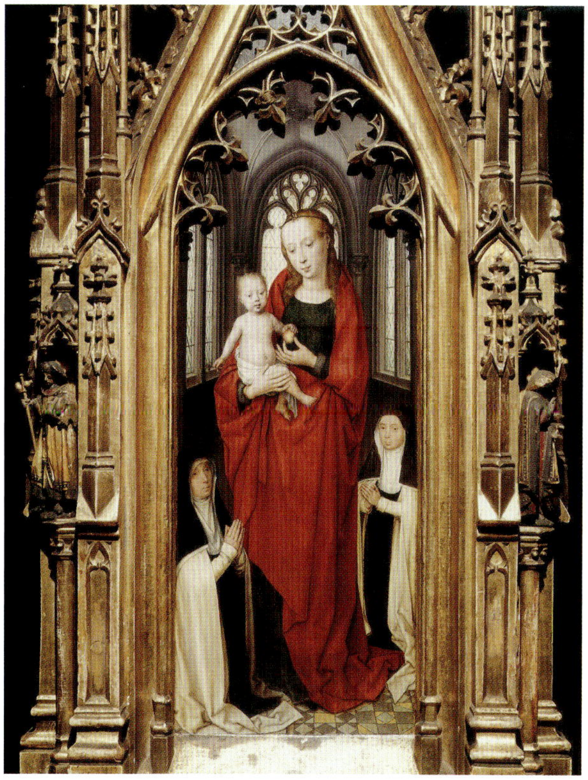

66 (*far left*) Hans Memling, *Ursula with Ten Virgins*, at end of *St Ursula Shrine*, 1489, Memling Museum, Bruges

67 (*left*) Hans Memling, *Virgin and Child with Anna van der Moortele and Jossine van Dudzele*, at end of *St Ursula Shrine*, 1489, Memling Museum, Bruges

Mother Superior in 1489, they could hardly be positioned closer to the holy pair. Clearly subservient to the deities they honour in this Gothic choir, and unwilling to claim any more substantial place for themselves, these composed women seem to associate themselves with the equanimity shown by Saint Ursula in the face of death.

They would doubtless have attempted to instil the same attitude in the people who ended their lives at the hospital, and Memling's art is ideally suited to conveying such an aim. He was able in his Saint John's paintings to give memorable and persuasive expression to the religious ideals informing the care provided by the institution. Max Friedländer, while remaining quite frank about Memling's shortcomings as an artist, was right to assert that his 'faith is completely trusting, serenely confident, with no trace of fanaticism, melancholy or sentimentality, no feelings of guilt, no doubts, yearnings or driving ambition.'[14] In a hospital context, where suffering and death were an ever-present reality, such an outlook would have been supremely consoling.

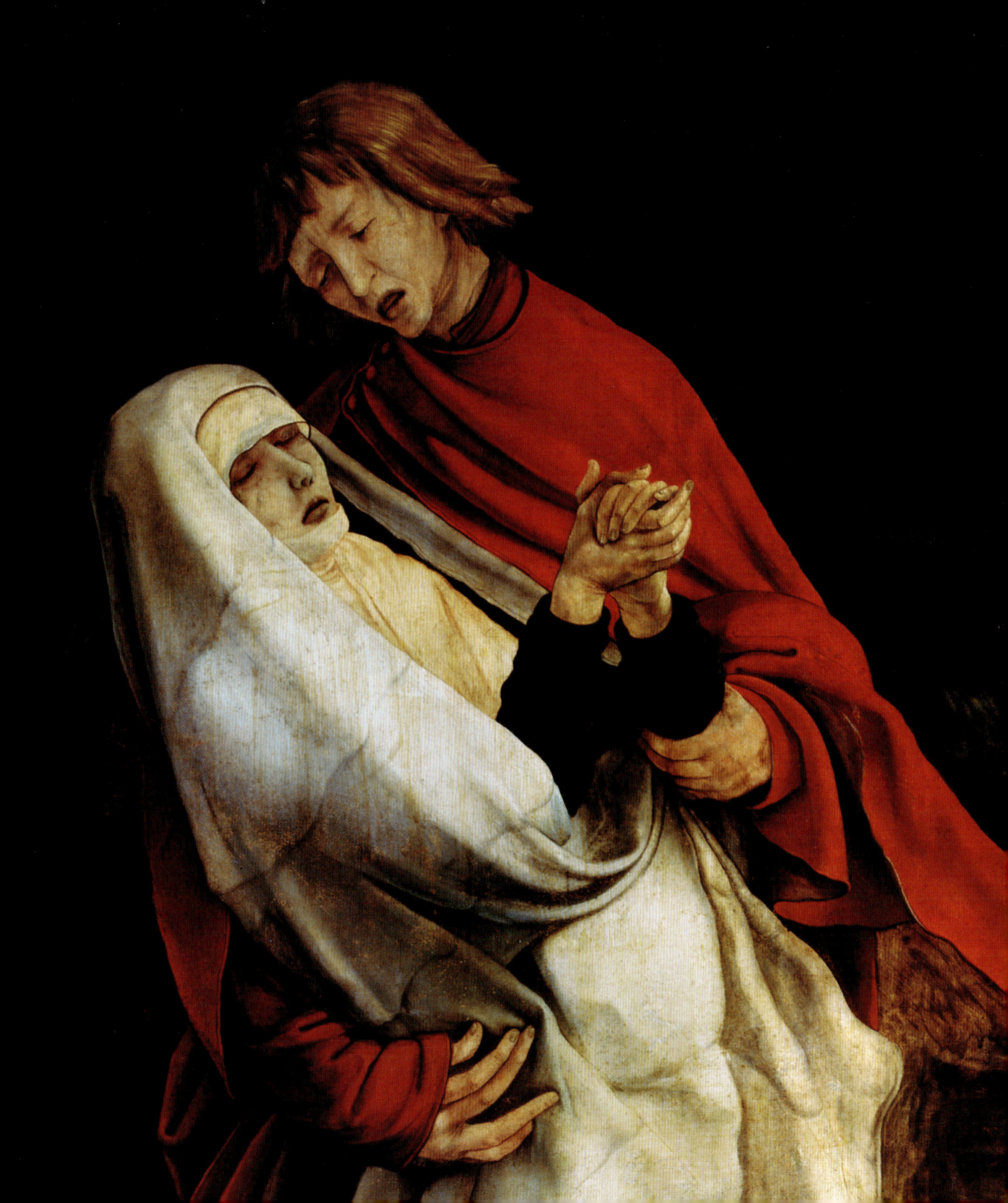

SIX
THE BURNING SICKNESS

By the advent of the sixteenth century, some European hospitals were beginning to entertain the possibility that painting or sculpture might play an integral part in the treatment they provided. In Italy, the Scuola di San Tommaso dei Battuti was prepared to take a significant step towards realising that aim when it commissioned a major altarpiece around 1500 (pl. 69). Destined for the altar of Saint Thomas in the church of San Francesco at Portogruaro, east of Venice, the enormous panel was entrusted to one of the most important Venetian artists of the period: Cima da Conegliano. And in representing *The Incredulity of Saint Thomas*, he centred on the revelatory moment when the sceptical saint finds himself invited to touch the wound in Christ's side. The pertinence of such a theme would not have been lost on patients suffering from gashes, sores and other ailments in the hospitals supervised by the patrons from the penitent confraternity of Saint Thomas who commissioned this heartfelt painting.

Cima shows Thomas leaning forward, in a forceful diagonal motion that dramatises the strain of placing his finger within the wound under Christ's right pectoral. Only by feeling the depth of this fissure can he be convinced of his master's identity, and the other saints gather round quietly marvelling at Christ's willingness to submit his body to such probing. The interpretation of the scene is not, perhaps, as dramatic as Cima's smaller and slightly later version, where he reduces the composition to three figures and shows Christ holding Thomas's wrist in order to guide him towards the gash. But in the Scuola di San Tommaso painting, Cima made sure that all attention is concentrated on the precise moment of contact between Thomas's index finger and Christ's violated flesh. The artist's understanding of the event's psychological implications gives the painting an impressive air of wonder and suspense. All the attendant figures appear to be holding their breath, awed by their master's humility as he exposes his pierced body to this intrusive, sceptical examination.

Yet the intensity of the altarpiece does not derive solely from Cima's imaginative understanding of the event represented here. It reflects as well the policy of the confraternity of officers who commissioned the painting. For these men, recorded by name on the *cartellino* placed with such prominence on the tiled floor of Cima's picture, organised no less than four hospitals for the treatment of pilgrims who had contracted diseases in the Holy Land. The subject of the painting was therefore very apt. It commemorated a biblical episode proving that Christ, taller than his disciples and drained of all the colour enhancing their heavy

68 (*facing page*) Detail of pl. 77

robes, had no hesitation about exposing his own physical frailty to even the most unsympathetic investigation. Many of the hospitals' fearful patients would have felt wary about allowing doctors and nurses to probe their own ailing flesh. But Christ, far from being humiliated by Thomas's peremptory prodding, gains in dignity from the encounter. Indeed, he displays no hesitation in revealing at the same time the holes puncturing both his hands, thereby insisting that humanity can rise above corporeal disfigurements if the spiritual will is sufficiently resilient. By baring the gash in his side, Christ brings about an epiphany. The miraculous nature of the event is enhanced by Cima's formal lucidity, the sensuous warmth of his mellow light, and the harmonious calm permeating the two idyllic landscapes visible through windows tall enough to disclose the untroubled expanse of a gentle Venetian sky.

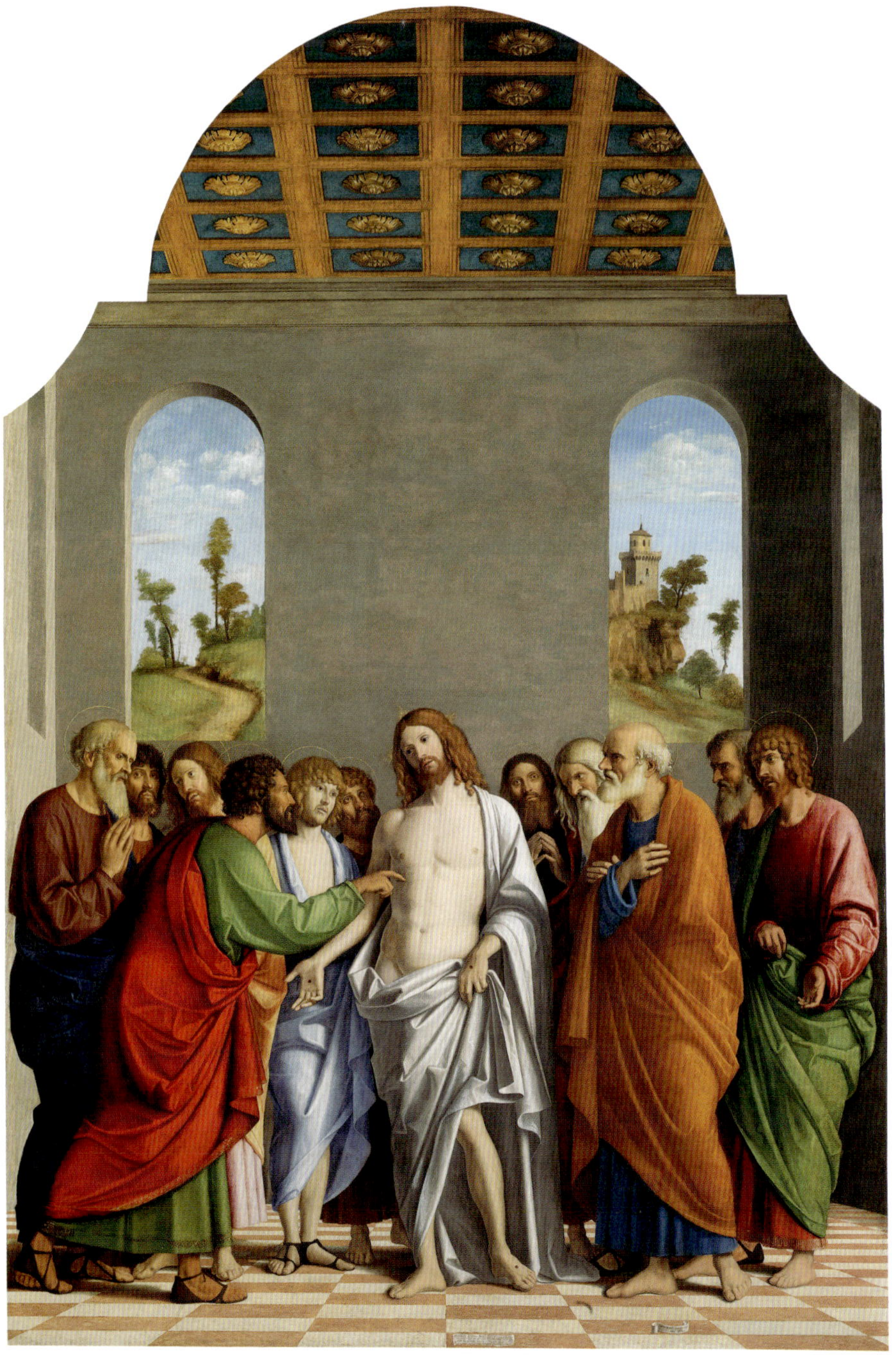

69 Cima da Conegliano, *The Incredulity of Saint Thomas*, *c.*1502–4, National Gallery, London

A few years later, Matthias Grünewald began work on his prodigious Isenheim Altarpiece. Originally installed in a hospice church belonging to the Antonite monastery, it contains the most violent and distressing image of the Crucifixion in Western art (see pl. 77). But the mendicant Order who commissioned the painting hoped that it would be able to aid healing. The Antonites dedicated themselves to the care of sufferers from the burning sickness, otherwise known as hell fire, holy fire and Saint Anthony's Fire. The nobleman who founded their European Order around 1095 wanted to celebrate his son's recovery from the horrors of this pernicious disease, and during Grünewald's lifetime the Antonites' popularity was crowned by Emperor Maximilian's decision to grant them the right to bear the imperial arms on their escutcheon. Since the burning sickness was still virulent in the early sixteenth century, the Antonite monastery in Isenheim decided to enlist a leading contemporary painter in their continuing struggle against the plague.

Johann de Orliaco and Guido Guersi, the wealthy and highly educated donors who were, successively, preceptors of the monastery, felt dissatisfied with their existing 'Lady' altarpiece. Orliaco had commissioned Martin Schongauer to paint its wings about 1475, but their unadventurous placidity soon began to pall (pl. 70). Orliaco himself is portrayed in one of Schongauer's panels, as a diminutive praying figure who kneels at Saint Anthony's feet. Although piety is conveyed effectively enough, the painting lacks intensity and any overt reference to the burning sickness. So do the other surviving wings, where Schongauer depicts the *Annunciation* and the *Virgin Adoring the Christ Child* in a similarly bland manner.

An older Orliaco reappears in the sculpture he went on to commission as the first stage of a new, far larger and more complex altarpiece in the hospice church (pl. 71). Executed by Nikolaus

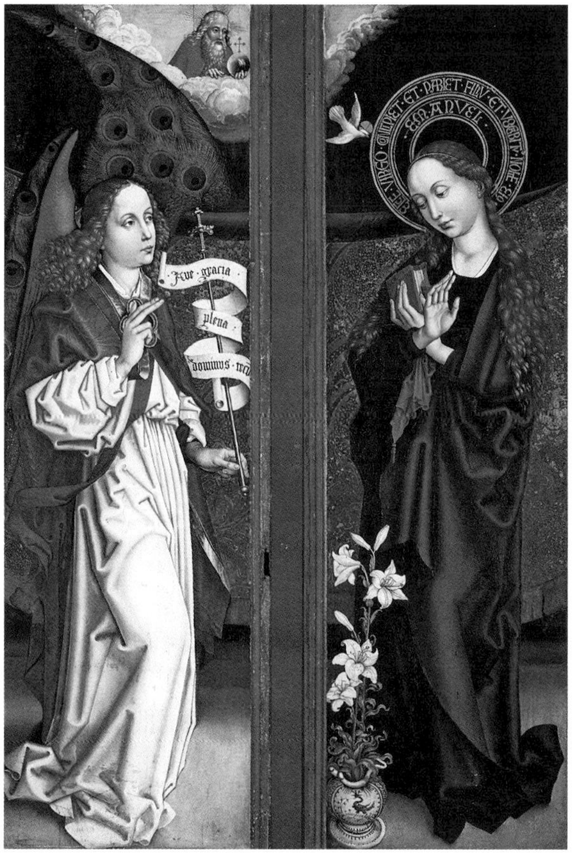

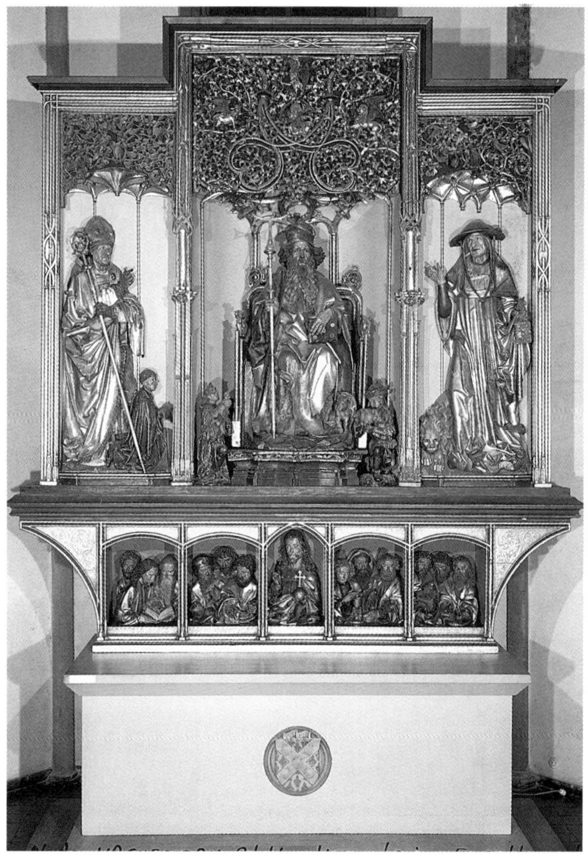

70 (*far left*) Martin Schongauer, *'Lady' Altarpiece*, *c.*1475, Musée d'Unterlinden, Colmar

71 (*left*) Nikolaus Hagenauer, *Altarpiece with enthroned Saint Anthony*, from the *Isenheim Altarpiece*, *c.*1490, Musée d'Unterlinden, Colmar

Hagenauer, these limewood carvings focus at their centre on an enthroned Saint Anthony. The patron saint of the Order is flanked by a kneeling freeman of the city offering up a cockerel and, on the right, a bandaged peasant who holds up a pig. This animal, Anthony's attribute, inspired the healthy food served at the Antonites' hospital where a pork-based diet was favoured. Hagenauer depicts the pig with considerable realism, and his professional competence cannot be faulted. His portrait of Orliaco, kneeling this time beneath Saint Augustine of Hippo, appears to be an incisive likeness. And he injected a certain amount of gestural energy into the crowded predella where Christ appears with the twelve Apostles, bunched together in strangely claustrophobic groups of three. But Guersi, who became preceptor after Orliaco retired in 1490, harboured altogether more audacious plans regarding the rest of this new altarpiece. After the sculpture was finished in 1505, he turned his attention to a brilliant and fiercely original talent known as 'Master Mathis the Painter'. The choice must have been controversial. Even today, the art historian Horst Ziermann finds it 'incredible that Mathis was chosen to paint an altarpiece at Isenheim. The monks of this monastery in the Vosges Mountains were, after all, French.'[1]

Guersi nevetheless went ahead with his adventurous preference. He asked Grünewald to produce a polyptych elaborate and eloquent enough to serve as the first stage of the healing programme carried out in the hospital, where patients were treated for a variety of blood and skin maladies as well as epilepsy. Daringly, Guersi believed that sufferers should be taken to the altarpiece and encouraged to examine Grünewald's images, thereby opening their minds to the possibility of participating in a miracle. Only then were they deemed receptive enough to benefit from medical treatment, so the polyptych played a crucial initiating role in the attempt to recover patients' health. Art, according to this wealthy and highly educated Antonite donor, had the imaginative capacity to exert a forceful psychological influence over the minds of the afflicted, and if they responded to its power their bodies might subsequently revive as well.[2]

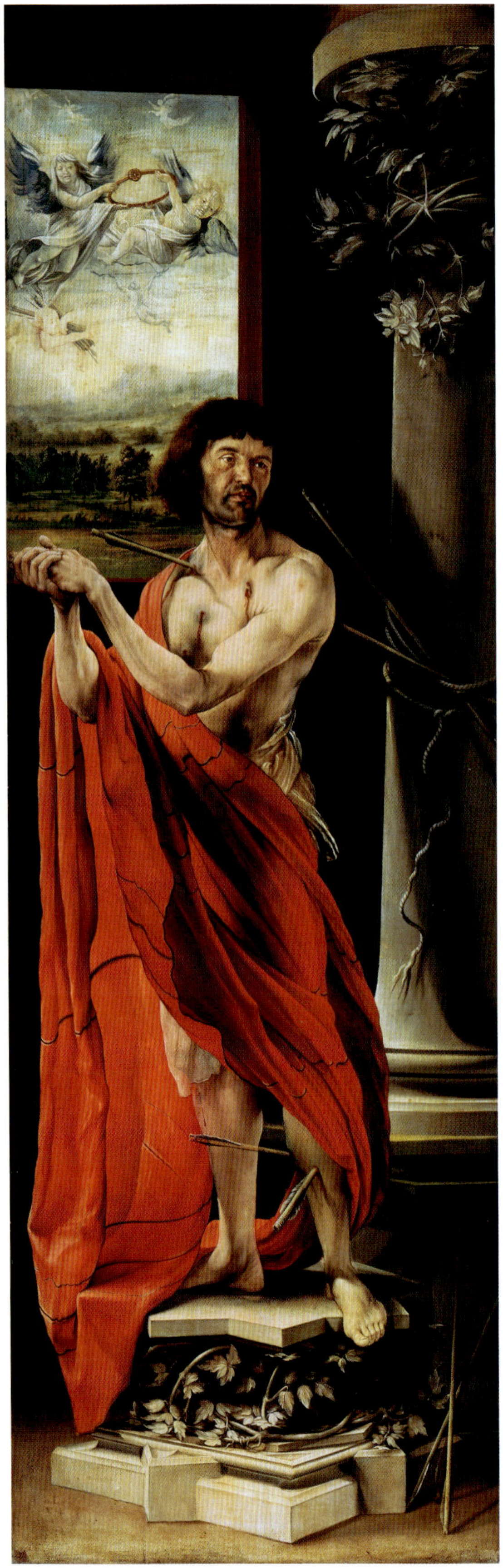

72 Matthias Grünewald, *Saint Sebastian attending The Crucifixion*, from the *Isenheim Altarpiece*, 1506–15, Musée d'Unterlinden, Colmar

Grünewald rose to the challenge with an altarpiece so potent in its depictive skills, expressive distortions and sheer visionary conviction that it must have far exceeded the donor's most heady expectations. Although it seems to issue from an intense and profoundly personal act of imagination on the artist's part, he succeeded in fulfilling the curative side of the commission as well. A luxuriantly bearded Saint Anthony, the Order's titular saint who was invoked against ergot poisoning and the fever that bore his name, took his place on one side of the great Crucifixion panel. He is accompanied on the other by Saint Sebastian, whose defiant resistance to the arrows piercing his body could be seen as an invocation against the plague (pl. 72).

But Saint Anthony also became the protagonist in a *Temptation* scene, one of the most fearful and indeed hallucinatory images to be found in the Isenheim ensemble (pl. 73). Far from maintaining a decorous distance while he contemplates his tempters, the traumatised saint is subjected to the most violent indignities. Sprawling helplessly in a macabre landscape dominated by glacial mountains, twisted mossy trees and a ruined building where devilish silhouettes run amok, he screams with pain as a cackling creature tugs at his hair. He struggles to retain his rosary on the ground while a hideous four-legged hybrid, half hen and half reptile, pecks at his clenched fingers. The main threat, however, comes from a ghoulish gaggle of demons and distorted animals who attack him from above. One fanged monstrosity pulls the saint's cloak in order to bite it with manic relish. Another grotesque winged amalgam of fish and beast snarls as he rams a clawed foot into his victim's chest. As for the outsized parrot who stands beside Anthony's feet, he raises a gnarled stick with a venom that suggests a mortal blow is about to be delivered.

Why did Grünewald here insist on portraying the titular saint *in extremis*, when Anthony was supposed to play such an important part in helping the patients who viewed the altarpiece? One answer may be that they could readily identify with the agonies suffered by a man whose entire body is subjected to pain of the most acute, flesh-wrenching kind. The sheet of paper placed in a prominent foreground position contains the inscription: 'Where were you, good Jesus, where were you? And why did you not come and dress my wounds?' This

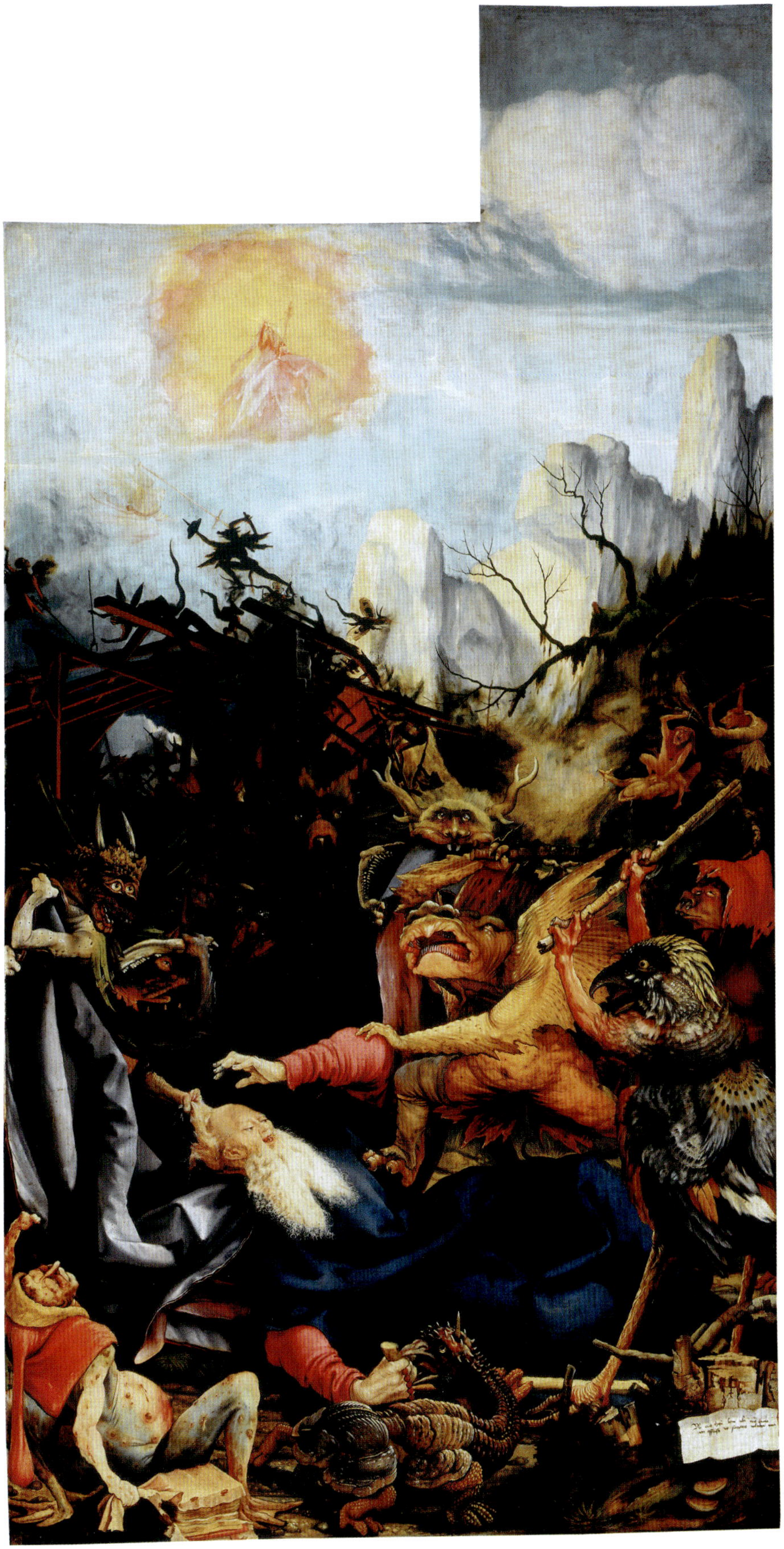

73 Matthias Grünewald, *Temptation of Saint Anthony,* from the *Isenheim Altarpiece*, 1506–15, Musée d'Unterlinden, Colmar

74 Detail of pl. 73

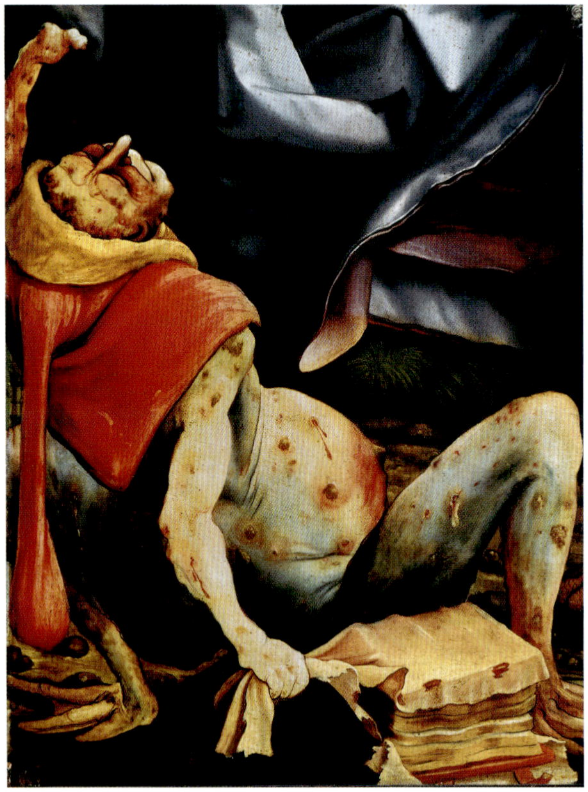

tormented cry, amounting to a bitter reproach levelled at God, could well have been uttered by the patients themselves at the height of their agony. And Grünewald ensures that the wounds refer, not just to Anthony, but also to the pathetic figure squatting in front of the beleaguered saint (pl. 74). Unlike everyone else in the panel, he refrains from attacking the old man and, despite his webbed feet, he resembles a human. But the travail he endures is just as terrible as anything Anthony experiences, for his entire body is afflicted with an excruciating rash of boils and sores.

No wonder that the *Temptation* scene was only opened up for viewing on one day each year: 17 January, the feast day of Saint Anthony. When J. K. Huysmans visited the altarpiece centuries later in the Colmar Museum, he was shocked to realise that 'no painter has ever gone so far in the representation of putrefaction, nor does any medical textbook contain a more frightening illustration of skin disease. This bloated body, moulded in greasy white soap mottled with blue, and mamillated with boils and carbuncles, is the hosanna of gangrene,

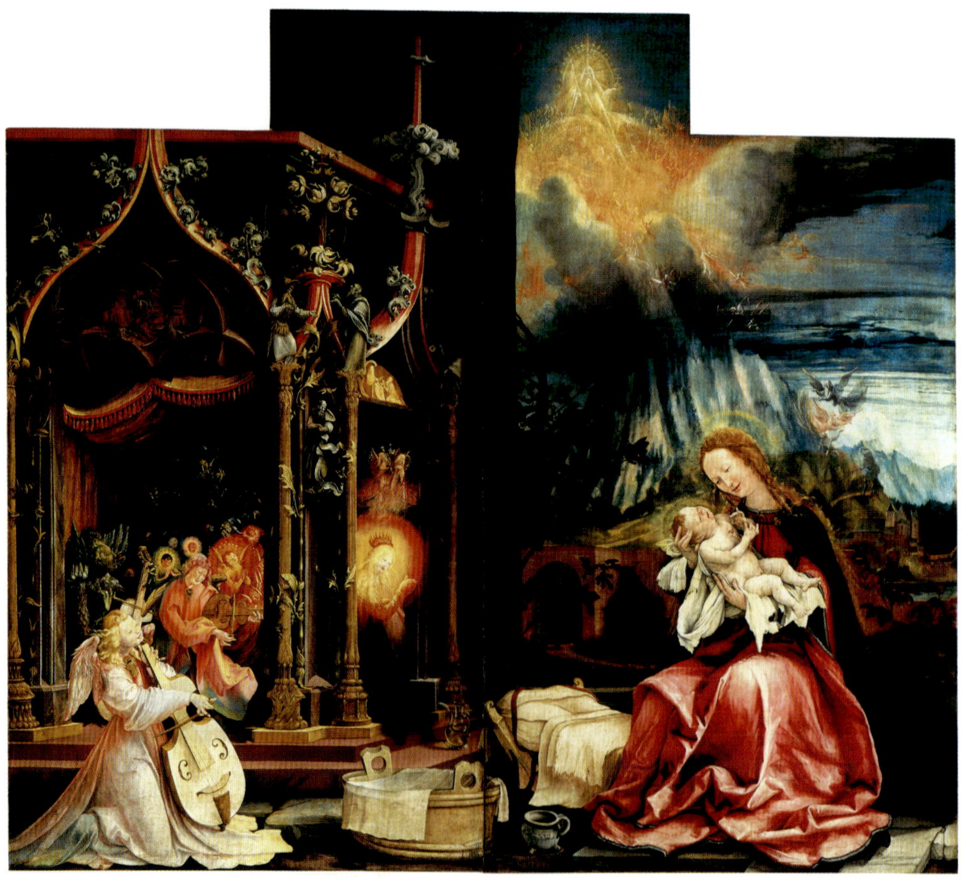

75 Matthias Grünewald, *Virgin and Child with Angelic Concert,* from the *Isenheim Altarpiece*, 1506–15, Musée d'Unterlinden, Colmar

the song of triumph of decay!'[3] Grünewald's depiction of this ravaged flesh is so authentic that Huysmans believed it was 'painted from life in the hospital ward'.[4] Only there, he thought, would the artist have been able to gain such an accurate idea of the burning sickness epidemic that gradually spread over the body in a contagion of apostems and abscesses, by degrees detaching arms and legs from their torsos. In his *History of Paris*, Dom Félibien explained that 'the victims' blood was affected by a poisonous inflammation which consumed the whole body, producing tumours that developed into incurable ulcers and caused thousands of deaths'.[5] Patients looking at the altarpiece could immediately appreciate that Grünewald had included a fellow-sufferer in *The Temptation of Saint Anthony*, and that the accusing question hurled at God from the sheet of paper was about to receive a positive response. For the sky is irradiated by an army of angels descending to free Saint Anthony – and, by extension, the hapless plague victims – from their plight.

By no means all the panels of the Isenheim altarpiece exposed onlookers to such mortifying images. As court artist to the archbishops of Mainz since 1508, Grünewald was accustomed to producing a wide range of religious images and even designing waterworks and fountains. So he was adept at painting the *Virgin and Child with Angelic Concert* (pl. 75) in a festive part of the polyptych, imbued with a desire to celebrate the joys of divine maternity in a panel animated by music-making, exuberant architecture and a burgeoning rose without thorns. Elsewhere, too, Saint Anthony is restored to equanimity in a peaceful scene where he meets Saint Paul the Hermit and converses with him while a deer rests calmly beside them (pl. 76). As Horst Ziermann has pointed out, Grünewald portrayed the preceptor as Anthony, and propped Guersi's armorial bearings against the rock where Anthony rests.[6] It was, no doubt, intended as a tribute to Guersi's bold and invaluable role in devising the iconographic programme of the altarpiece as a whole.

All the same, by far the most haunting and deeply felt part of the altarpiece is the *Crucifixion*, dated 1515 and the largest single panel in this mesmeric ensemble (pl. 77). Indeed, it is the biggest crucifixion scene to be found anywhere in European painting, and intended here as the first image viewers would encounter before the Isenheim polyptych was opened up.[7] Grünewald makes no attempt to dilute the awfulness of the martyrdom. His Christ is at the furthest conceivable remove from the noble and decorous figure who poses piously on the cross in so many interpretations by other, more circumspect artists. Exhausted by pain and degradation alike, this haggard man hangs down with such terminal heaviness that his shoulders are wrenched from their sockets. Hammered nails tear at the palms of his hands (pl. 80). Although his fingers stab the air in protest, he can do nothing to arrest the relentless process of deterioration. With head lolling forward, and mouth gaping because he no longer retains the strength to keep it shut, the defeated Christ is in a death-agony almost too gruesome to scrutinise.

Blood oozes from his gangrenous feet, the one skewered hideously on top of the other by a gleaming bolt driven through them (pl. 81). The sweaty pallor of his skin proves that the end is near, but nothing is going to hasten the last unbearable

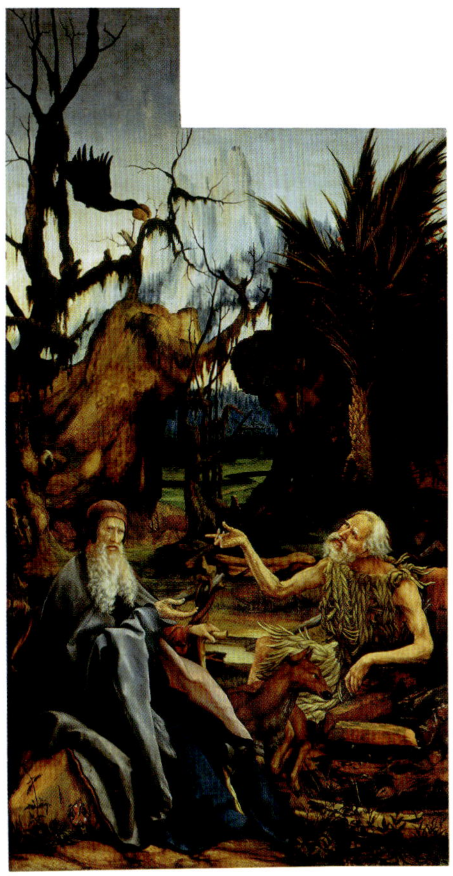

76 Matthias Grünewald, *Saint Anthony with Saint Paul the Hermit,* from the *Isenheim Altarpiece*, 1506–15, Musée d'Unterlinden, Colmar

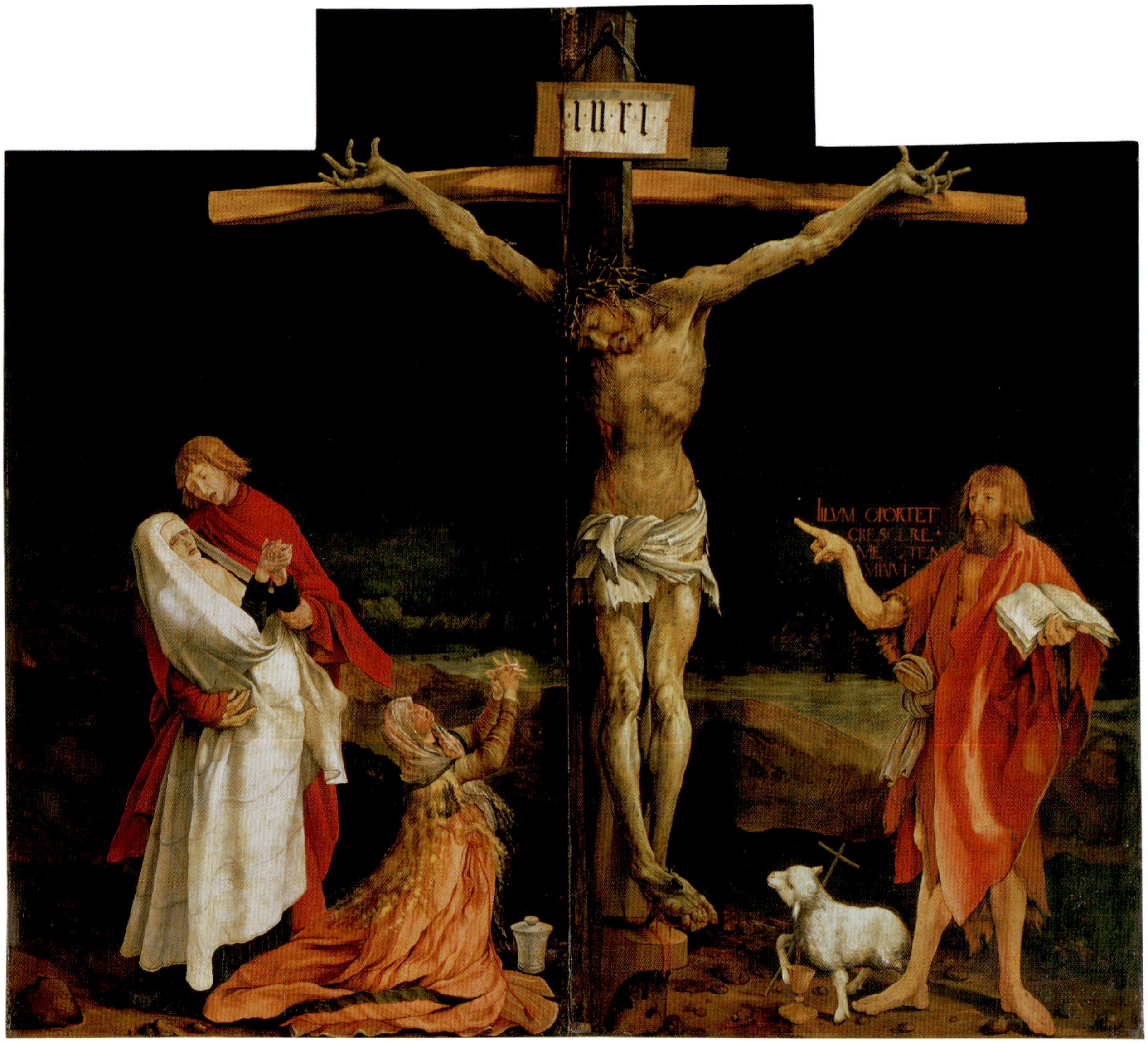
INRI
ILLVM OPORTET
CRESCERE
ME TEM
MINVI

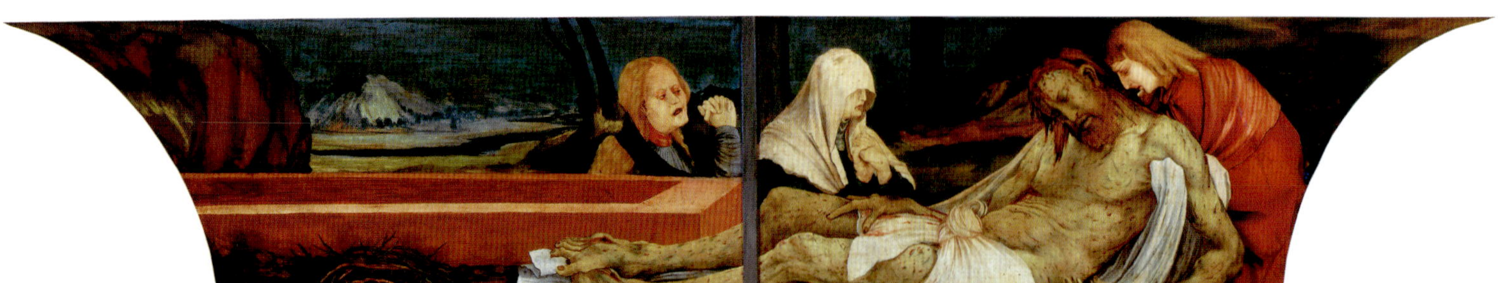

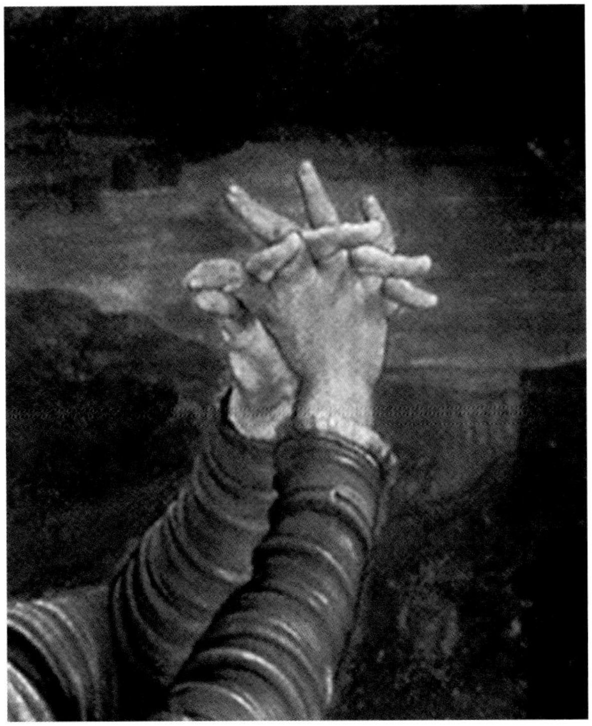

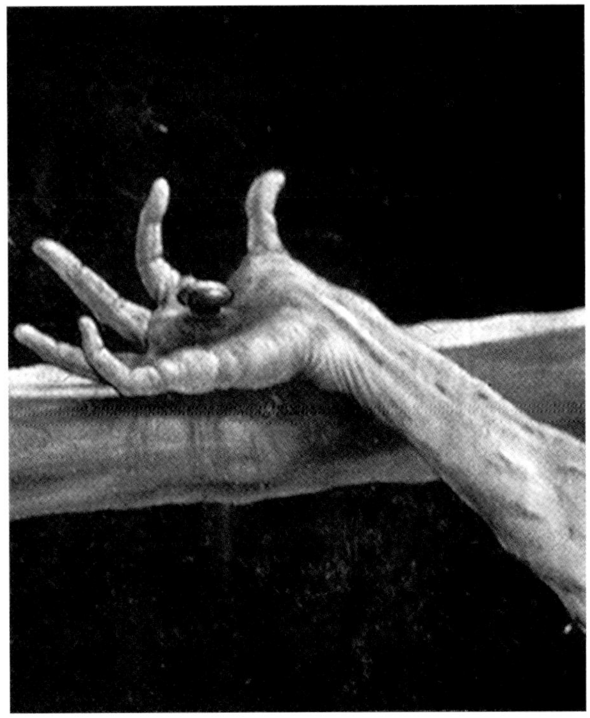

79 (*far left*) Mary Magdalene's hands (detail of pl. 77)

80 (*left*) Christ's hands (detail of pl. 77)

moments of his torture. Pitched against a dark void unalleviated by any signs of divine intervention, he is condemned to writhe and groan until his body seems unable to withstand any more punishment. The figures attending him are powerless to intervene, and his distress causes them to respond with racked, exclamatory gestures that come near to matching his own. The Virgin tilts backwards, unable to stop herself from succumbing to a swoon eerily akin to death (see pl. 68). As for Mary Magdalene, she raises her hands in an anguish that causes her to echo the twisted action of Christ's distended fingers (pl. 79).

This supremely isolated man does, nevertheless, share his torment with the onlooker. The sores erupting all over his body are as grievous as their counterparts on the figure in the foreground of the *Temptation of Saint Anthony*, and once again Grünewald shows the plague-stricken viewers that they are not alone in their predicament. But the *Crucifixion*, no less than the predella of the *Entombment* in a more visible position beneath, demonstrates beyond any doubt that Christ knew precisely how harrowing it was to suffer from the most profound and corrosive maladies of the flesh (pl. 78). One doctor maintained, after inspecting the *Crucifixion* from a medical standpoint, that 'attention to detail is carried to the point of indicating the inflammatory halo which develops around minor wounds'.[8] Grünewald had clearly gone to the most meticulous lengths to give his Christ's suppurations

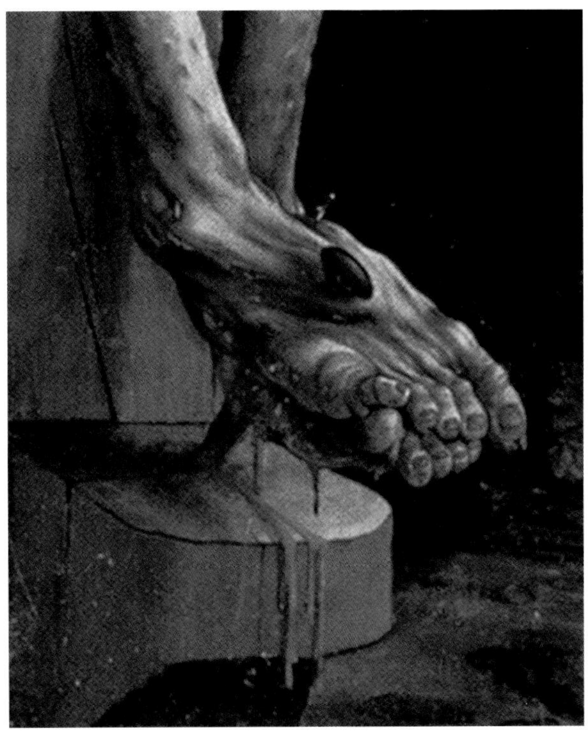

81 (*left*) Christ's feet (detail of pl. 77)

77 (*facing page, top*) Matthias Grünewald, *Crucifixion*, from the *Isenheim Altarpiece*, 1506–15, Musée d'Unterlinden, Colmar

78 (*facing page, bottom*) Matthias Grünewald, *Entombment*, from the *Isenheim Altarpiece*, 1506–15, Musée d'Unterlinden, Colmar

a clinical authenticity, and Huysmans became convinced that they were 'obviously modelled on the corpses in the hospital mortuary'.[9]

Rather than confirming the patients' despair, however, both the *Crucifixion* and its predella would surely have provided them with a cathartic experience. Confronted by the spectacle of Christ's willingness to take on even the most feared and disgusting of earthly afflictions, they might have discovered that the stigma attached to their condition no longer had the capacity to shame and humiliate them. This psychological purging was obviously of great assistance as a preparation for the medical treatment offered by the hospital. For Guersi must have realised that the recovery of patients' spiritual well-being should be regarded as an important preliminary stage in the fight to regain physical health.

Did the altarpiece prove as effective as its donors hoped? It is impossible to know, but Andrée Hayum stressed the central importance of the hospital context in her major study *The Isenheim Altarpiece: God's Medicine and the Painter's Vision*.[10] Her wide-ranging, interdisciplinary and imaginative approach is based on the belief that plague victims would have been brought before Grünewald's *tour de force* hoping that their suffering from Saint Anthony's Fire would be cured. Other historians, most notably Albert Chatelet and Christian Heck, have questioned how much access the patients were given to the choir housing the altarpiece.[11] It inhabited an area usually reserved for the monks, and a rood screen partly obstructed the view of the polyptych from the nave. Surviving ground-plans of the Isenheim buildings are deceptive, including structures that never existed. But Horst Ziermann recently had no hesitation in reaffirming the traditional view that 'the sick were led to the altar by the Antonite monks prior to medical treatment. Many of the sick were probably in such a state that they prayed more than once and at great length.'[12] If the praying was fervent enough, and arose from what the cultural philosopher Jean Gebser once described as a state of 'existential emergency', it had 'the character and function of communion'. And after the person re-emerged from 'being lost in prayer', Gebser maintained, 'he reawakens to his rational, daytime alertness, bringing healing with him from the magical depths'.[13]

If miraculous cures or relief did indeed occur in front of the altarpiece, Grünewald's exceptional intensity as an artist would undoubtedly have played a powerful role in the proceedings. Huysmans was convinced that the artist who painted the Isenheim polyptych wholly succeeded in understanding

> the religious piety of the sick and the poor. That awful Christ who hung dying over the altar of the Isenheim hospital would seem to have been made in the image of the ergotics who prayed to him; they must surely have found consolation in the thought that this God they invoked had suffered the same torments as themselves, and had become flesh in a form as repulsive as their own; and they must have felt less forsaken, less contemptible. It is easy to see why Grünewald's name, unlike the names of Holbein, Cranach and Dürer, is not to be found in the account-books or the records of commissions left by emperors and princes. His pestiferous Christ would have offended the taste of the courts; he could only be understood by the sick, the unhappy and the monks, by the suffering members of Christ.[14]

Nor would the patients of Isenheim have left the altar solely with an image of advanced putrefaction in their minds. For Grünewald produced in another panel, through an imaginative feat no less remarkable than the vision he deployed elsewhere in the polyptych, an overwhelming *Resurrection* that stressed the full, miraculous exhilaration of life after death (pl. 82). Flung forwards and sideways by the sudden, dynamic thrust of Christ's ascending body, the guards' stunned reactions testify forcibly enough to its explosive impact. The draperies following the figure out of the tomb seem almost molten as they stream, lava-like, towards a deity who no longer needs them. He hovers triumphantly against the night sky, holding up hands that still bear the red marks of the wounds inflicted on them. But now they cause pain no more, and Christ is able to raise his head from the defeated position it assumed in the *Crucifixion*. Staring straight ahead, with the utter steadfastness of a man who wants everyone to witness his newly recovered vitality, he smiles calmly out at a world that has lost its ability to defeat him. The most astounding aspect of this panel lies in its light, blinding enough to oust any doubts about the plausibility of a resurrection. Unlike a conventional halo, it encircles

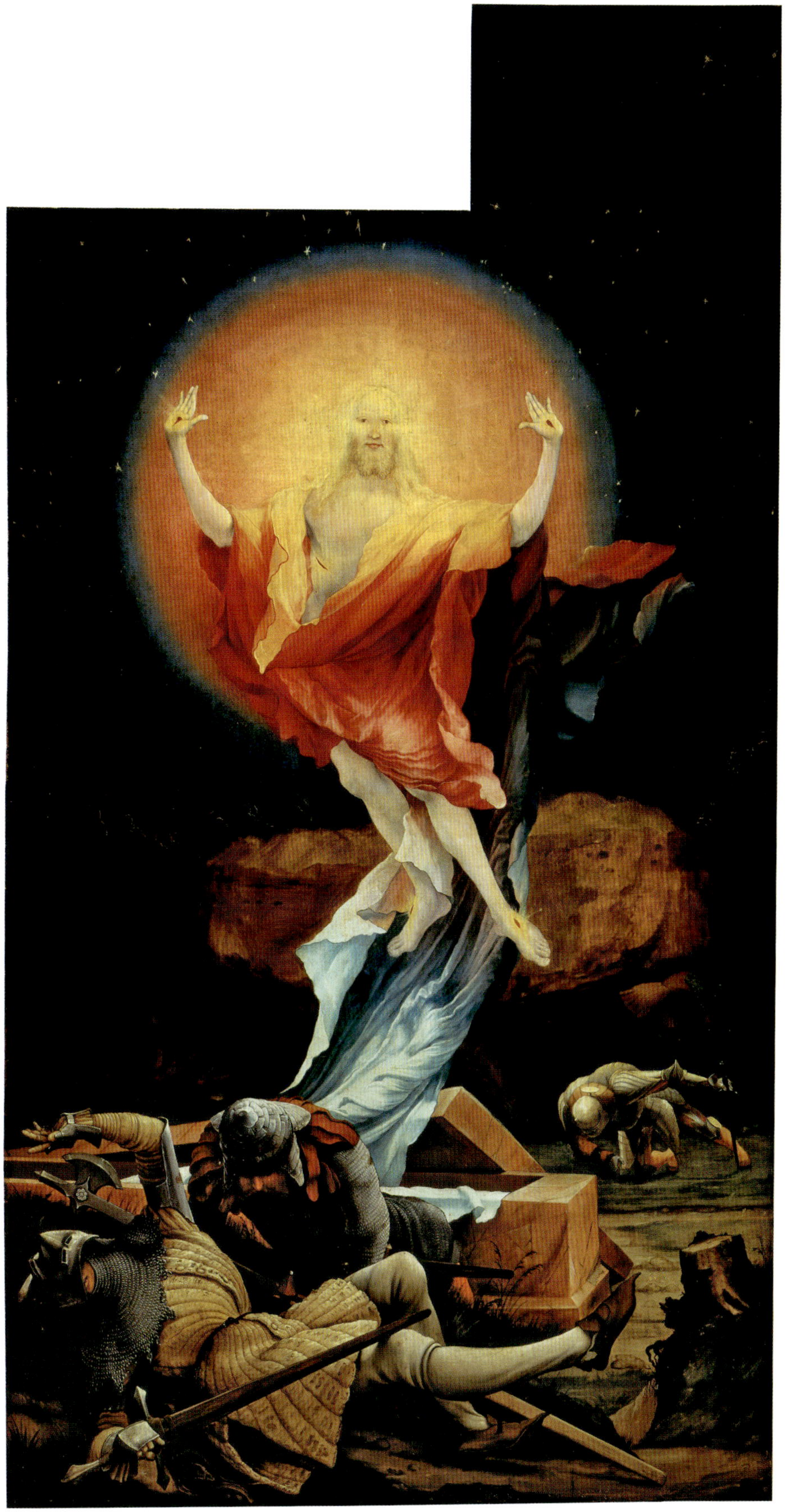

82 Matthias Grünewald, *Resurrection,* from the *Isenheim Altarpiece*, 1506–15, Musée d'Unterlinden, Colmar

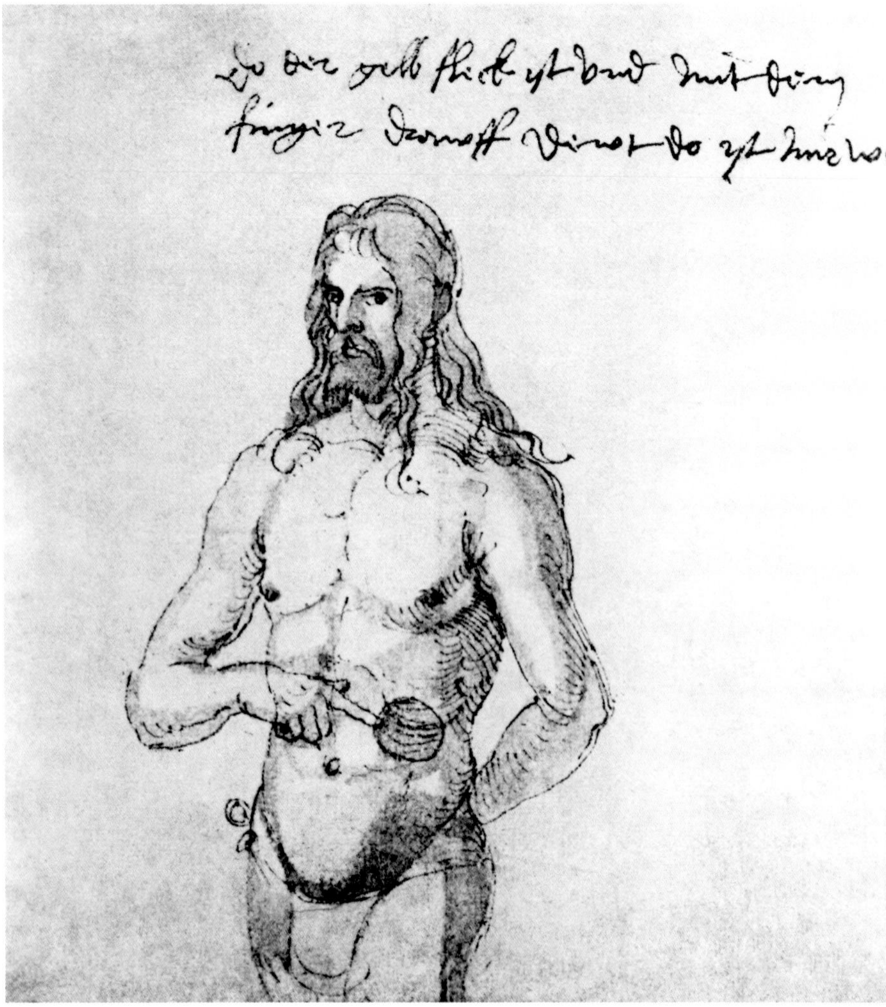

83 Albrecht Dürer, *Dürer as a Sick Man*, *c.*1510, Kunsthalle, Bremen

Christ with a pulsating orb of brightness that penetrates everything in its path. Hair, flesh and draperies are transformed by the potency of this sacred illumination, which acts as a metaphor for the regenerative event it clarifies with such blazing, hallucinatory force.

This revelatory panel would surely have offered immense reassurance to the patients who had just been identifying themselves so closely with the battered and festering body of Christ on the cross. The transformation of such an abject figure into the dazzling, purified apparition who ascends here was a thoroughly heartening spectacle. 'If the sick were in fact brought before the altarpiece as tradition says, or took part in the offices on the various feast days on which the altarpiece was opened and each of the ensembles shown,' wrote Georg Scheja, 'then they were presented with an optimistic interpretation of their physical ailments typical of the Middle Ages, since the promise of healing was extended not only by the Order's patron saints but was there to be read in the life of Christ himself.'[15]

Although Grünewald must have delighted his patrons, he could hardly have produced this formidable work without a deep personal commitment to the subject. Even if the seriousness of his dedication to the Antonites' medical aims need not be questioned, he had another compelling reason to place himself in the position of the hospital's inmates. For he knew that the burning sickness represented a threat to everyone, and Grünewald's prolonged first-hand scrutiny of the Antonites' patients would have made him appreciate still further the full, fearsome extent of their affliction.

Anyone living in those plague-ridden times could be excused for becoming preoccupied with health. Autobiographies of the period often contain very elaborate descriptions of their authors' ailments, and Grünewald's great contemporary Albrecht Dürer once utilised his own draughtsmanship to help a physician arrive at a diagnosis. Around 1510, he drew a self-portrait of *Dürer as a Sick Man* and sent it to his doctor asking for advice by letter (pl. 83). The ink and watercolour study shows a grim-faced figure, stripped for the purpose, pointing towards the offending anatomical area with an accusatory finger. In order to be more precise, Dürer has outlined the troublesome region with his pen and washed it in with colour, explaining in the inscription above that 'where the yellow spot is and where my finger points, there is pain'. The illness was, in fact, a slowly developing infection either of the spleen or the digestive organs, and yet Dürer's stark presentation of his complaint implies that he may well have harboured fears of a deadly affliction. Wilhelm Waetzoldt, who described this fascinating drawing as the 'most curious and most intimate of all self-portraits', pointed out that the artist's diary 'notes the many "stivers" which Dürer – no doubt with a heavy heart – had to spend on physicians, male and female apothecaries and all kinds of medicine'.[16]

He undoubtedly preferred to make these payments, and undergo suspect treatments devised by quacks whose ingenuity outweighed their medical knowledge, rather than rely on the even more dubious attractions of a miracle cure. In 1523 he wrote on the back of a woodcut depicting the hysteria that surrounded the cult of the Virgin in

Regensburg: 'God grant that we do not worship his worthy mother thus, but Jesus Christ himself. Amen.'[17] By that time Dürer was showing support for the Lutheran cause, and a list of books in Grünewald's Frankfurt home during the late 1520s indicates that he shared this radical new standpoint. Both artists would have felt nothing but revulsion for the charade recorded in Michael Ostendorfer's woodcut. Pilgrims can be seen crowding in their hundreds towards the aisle of the recently built Church of the Schöne Maria in Regensburg, determined to prostrate themselves before the panel painting of the Virgin and Child installed within. The two women on the far right of the procession would have been particularly anxious to implore the Virgin's assistance: they are holding a child who appears to be afflicted by total paralysis. But the pilgrims in the foreground are too impatient to join the queue. They confine their hysterical attentions to a stone statue of the Virgin standing in the square outside the church. Here, they fling themselves at the column supporting the sculpture, clutching it as they beseech the woman above to purge them of their ailments.

The aesthetic quality of the Schöne Maria images was very high. Grünewald's prominent contemporary Albrecht Altdorfer himself painted the banner of the Virgin and Child flying from the church tower, as well as designing the cult badge and producing a number of woodcuts dedicated to the pilgrimage. Altdorfer, who had approved of the expulsion of Regensburg's entire Jewish community in 1519, knew exactly how to promote the worship of the Virgin on the site of the demolished synagogue. But the truth is that a great deal of unscrupulous profit-making lay behind the creation of such a cult. Fortunes were made from booming sales in candles and badges, while many of the pilgrims ended up as forlorn as the figures in the foreground of Ostendorfer's woodcut, prostrate on the earth and wondering why the miraculous intervention had not yet occurred.

Compared with such superstitious antics, the Antonites' altarpiece at Isenheim benefited from a sustained and intense charge of imaginative conviction. Barnett Newman is among the many modern artists who have derived profound stimulus from Grünewald's masterpiece. It provided Newman with crucial confirmation for his desire to employ the Christian narrative in his great *Stations of the Cross* series. Two years after seeing the Isenheim altarpiece in 1964, he declared that

> Grünewald's Crucifixion is maybe the greatest painting in Europe, but one of the things that intrigues me about the Grünewald is the act of (active) imagination on his part. That he was not illustrating so much the Christ in terms of the legend . . . but since he was doing it for a hospital of syphilitics, that he was able to identify himself with the human agony of those patients, that he was willing to turn the Christ figure into a syphilitic. Now this of course is one of the boldest things that anybody could have done. Yet I think this is part of his genius.[18]

Determined to use Christ's Passion as a means of dealing with contemporary suffering in his own *Stations of the Cross* paintings, Newman realised that the Isenheim polyptych offered him an immensely inspirational precedent. In the end, though, the altarpiece deserves to stand in its own right. One of the most astounding achievements in European painting, it gave the hospital's patients reassurance, empathy and hope without resorting to the spurious attractions of a sudden, revelatory cure.

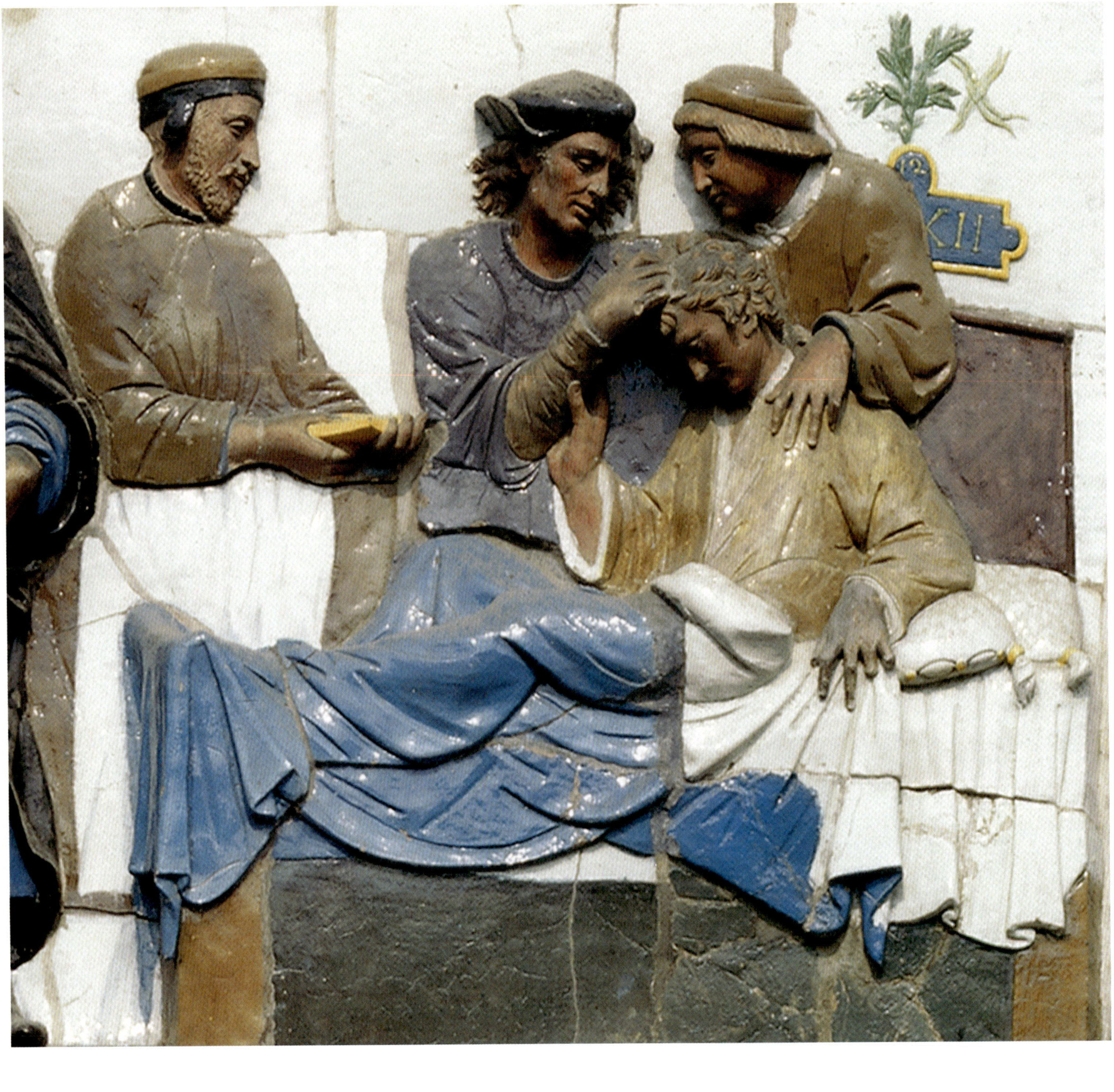
12

SEVEN
PORTRAYING THE PATIENTS

By the end of the fifteenth century, the notion of adorning hospitals with appropriate images had become more prevalent in Florence. Andrea della Robbia, who contributed so memorably to the Innocenti facade (see pl. 40), was commissioned during the final years of the *quattrocento* to carry out sculptural decorations for the loggia of the Hospital of Saint Paul in Piazza Santa Maria Novella. Although the eleven medallions of portraits and saints are relatively minor examples of his work, the lunette depicting the *Meeting Between Saint Francis and Saint Dominic* is one of Andrea's most remarkable sculptures (pl. 85). The two men grasp each other's arms with a physical intensity that gives them an unusual amount of heartfelt conviction. Far from regarding the lunette as a site suitable only for bland, routine adornment, Andrea invests the fraternal greeting with a passion that demonstrates how much it really meant to both men. As if to reinforce the strength of his commitment to the work, he restricted the use of enamel to the gleaming robes alone. On the saints' hands and faces the terracotta was left untreated, enabling Andrea to give them a harshly chiselled authenticity. The 'burnt' colour also emphasises the gaunt, weatherbeaten character of these figures, closing in an embrace that acknowledges their mutual dedication to a life of selfless concern for the welfare of others. In this respect, it was an apt image to instal on a building with similar concerns, where the staff likewise reached out to patients in an attempt to affirm the importance of their shared humanity.

But what about images of the patients themselves? So far, Italy had shown in its hospital art an overwhelming preference for saints, staff and donors. The young Pietro Torrigiano, notoriously exiled from his native Florence after attacking Michelangelo and breaking his nose, tried to counter this violent reputation by producing a lost terracotta bust of the Bolognese doctor Stefano della Torre in 1494. Soon afterwards, Torrigiano also made the marble busts of Christ and Santa Fina, as well as the terracotta bust of Saint Gregory, still preserved at the Ospedale di San Fina at San Gimignano.[1] Presented to the institution by Stefano Coppi, the rector of San Salvatore in Suburra, they reaffirmed the supremacy of religious subjects in Italian medical buildings. Apart from Andrea's children on the Innocenti frontage, who were mercifully free from the physical ailments besetting inmates of medical institutions, occupants struggling to survive hospitals rarely found themselves included in works of art. Both artists and patrons may well have been squeamish about the notion of depicting the often gruesome reality

84 (*facing page*) Detail of pl. 89

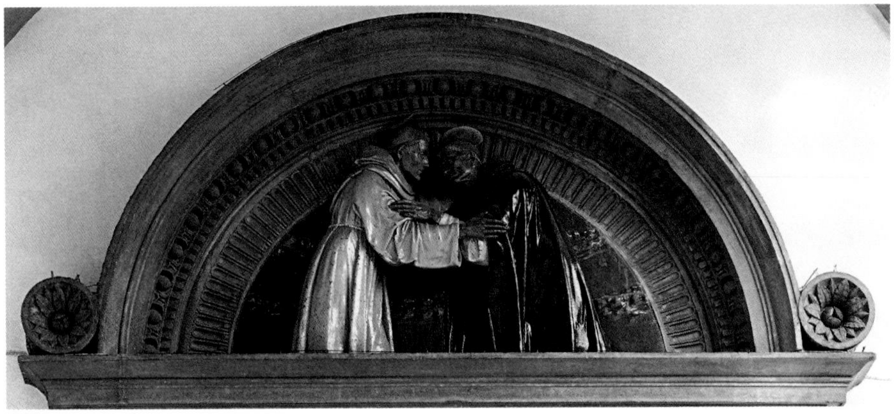

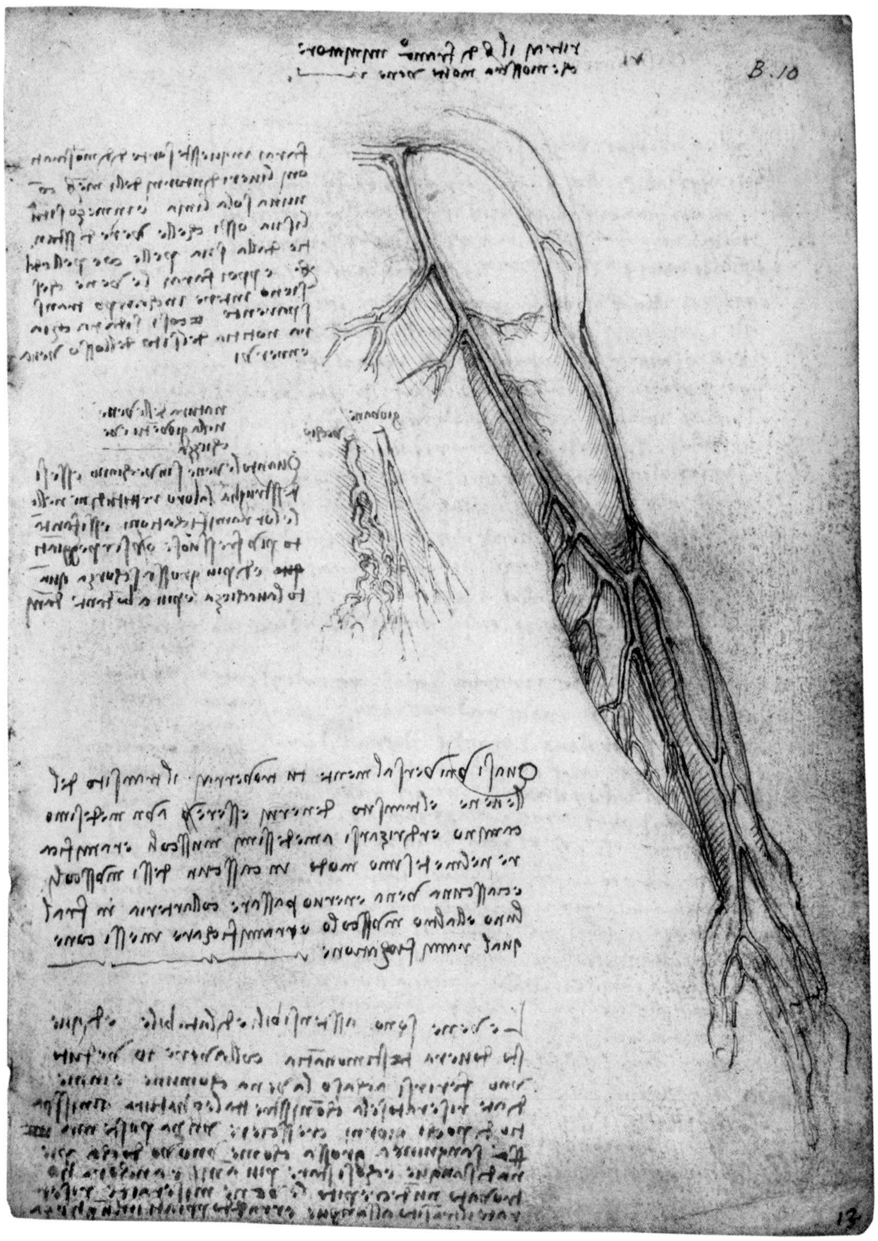

of life on a ward. After all, as George Orwell pointed out in a trenchant essay, 'if you look at almost any literature before the later part of the nineteenth century, you find that a hospital is popularly regarded as much the same thing as a prison, and an old-fashioned, dungeon-like prison at that . . . No one who was not more or less destitute would have thought of going into such a place for treatment'.[2]

Impelled by a powerful spirit of consuming curiosity, Leonardo da Vinci ignored this widespread fear of hospitals and pursued his researches among the patients he encountered in the wards. Leonardo trusted one particular Florentine institution to look after his money, books and other precious possessions: the hospital of Santa Maria Nuova, where earlier paintings had been commissioned from Domenico Veneziano, Piero della Francesca and Hugo van der Goes (see pls 17 and 47). It was here that a very elderly patient became the focus of his most zealous attention. Leonardo talked to him, conscious no doubt that time was fast running out. 'This old man, a few hours before his death, told me he that he had lived for a hundred years and that he was conscious of no bodily failure other than feebleness', Leonardo wrote with a sense of wonder. 'And thus, sitting on a bed in the hospital of Santa Maria Nuova, without any movement or sign of distress, he passed from this life. And I made an anatomy to see the cause of a death so sweet.'[3] Leonardo penned this fascinating memorandum as late as 1507 or 1508, when he was himself in his mid-fifties and just over a decade away from his own death. So he may have been driven by intensely personal reasons when taking the decision to explore the old man's anatomy.

It was probably not the first time Leonardo had dissected a corpse. He may well have done so on several previous occasions. But dissection was a highly controversial activity, and an official magistrate's permit would have been needed to perform such an invasive procedure. A few years later, when Leonardo was in Rome, a hostile observer 'hindered me in anatomy, denouncing it before the Pope and also at the hospital'.[4] But in Florence no such controversy seems to have attended his pioneering exploration of the old man's cadaver, nor, indeed, Leonardo's contemporaneous dissection of a child who had died at the age of two. Fascinated no doubt by the extreme contrast between these two bodies, he concluded that 'I found everything [in the child's corpse] to be the opposite to that of the old man'.[5]

His discovery of the differences separating youth from age would also have helped him arrive at an accurate diagnosis of the causes of death. In some notes inscribed on a drawing of veins in the arm, he speculated that the old man died from 'weakness caused by a lack of blood in the artery which feeds the heart and lower members'. Leonardo was under no illusions about the lamentable state of the patient's arteries – 'very dry, thin and withered' but he also found a paradoxical sense of vigour when describing how, 'in addition to the thickening of their walls, these vessels grow in length and twist themselves in the manner of a snake'.[6] So even in an advanced state of decrepitude, the human body yields unexpected signs of fantastical vitality (pl. 86). In Leonardo's capacious mind, the twisting arteries were linked with the equally unpredictable rhythms of rivers. He once referred to rivers as 'veins of water' and there is a strong sense in his work of the connections between the body of the earth and the body of humanity. Martin Kemp pointed out that Leonardo's

> post-mortem examination of the centenarian's blood supply was characteristically developed . . . during the succeeding months into a synoptic study of the 'irrigation' systems of the human body, not only the movement of the blood, but also the urino-genital, alimentary, nervous and respiratory systems. These systems, like the rivers of the earth and the canals of man's contrivance, ferried the vital supplies of life to all the regions of the body. They did so according to the hydrodynamic laws which he had formulated during the 1490s and confirmed in Florence during his work on the Arno canals.[7]

Although Leonardo asserted around 1508 that he had dissected 'more than ten human bodies',[8] not all of these anatomical operations were performed at the hospital of Santa Maria Nuova. At times, he seems to have kept corpses in his own studio, and once confessed to a 'fear of living at night-time in the company of these dead men, dismembered and flayed and terrible to behold'.[9] Even so, the morbid terror induced by sliced cadavers did not prevent him from pushing his investigations further. He had been fascinated by anatomy ever since his early days in Verrocchio's studio, and by the late 1480s his incessant drawings of body-parts and skulls led him to plan a full-scale treatise on the subject. Later, he called this book *Of the Human Figure*, a title indicating his belief that living, energetic bodies could only be fully understood and represented by artists willing to study the dead. Hence the proliferation of drawings, concentrating on leg and thigh muscles, executed around 1503 when he started work on the great *Battle of Anghiari* cartoon for a fresco in Florence's monumental Council Hall on the first floor of the Palazzo Vecchio. Leonardo undoubtedly wanted to give its fighting, lunging and yelling combatants the maximum amount of martial conviction. But Kenneth Clark cautioned against concluding that anatomical drawings were, for Leonardo, solely a means of making his art more convincing. 'In general', Clark argued, 'Leonardo's scientific researches were undertaken for their own sakes, and anatomy was only one manifestation of his curiosity into the workings of nature.'[10] Indeed, Leonardo went so far as to deliver a warning about the dangers of developing anatomical obsessions when painting the human figure. Probably referring to Michelangelo's work in progress on the ceiling of the Sistine Chapel, he wrote around 1514: 'O anatomical painter beware, lest in the attempt to make your nudes display all their emotions by a too strong indication of bones, sinews, and muscles, you become a wooden painter.'[11]

Michelangelo reportedly made dissections of dead bodies and, according to his biographer Ascanio Condivi, intended to publish these anatomical studies. The plan was never realised. Yet all the evidence suggests that, for at least twenty years of his career, Leonardo continued to hope his anatomical research could be channelled into what Charles Nicholl described as 'a masterwork on anatomy, suitable for publication, and offering for the first time a detailed visual description of the workings of the human body'.[12] Like so many of his prodigious projects, the plan was never realised. But Leonardo's obsessive involvement with dissection seems to have reached a climax when he attended the anatomy lectures delivered in Pavia by a brilliant young master, Marcantonio della Torre. Around the end of 1509, Leonardo began attending lectures given by this tragically short-lived pioneer. As early as 1511 della Torre succumbed to

85 (*facing page, top*) Andrea della Robbia, *Meeting Between Saint Francis and Saint Dominic*, c.1493, Hospital of Saint Paul, Piazza Santa Maria Novella, Florence

86 (*facing page, bottom*) Leonardo da Vinci, *The Superficial Veins in the Arm, and the Vessels of the Young and Old*, c.1507–8, Royal Collection, Windsor

the plague at the age of only twenty-nine. By then, though, he had given Leonardo plenty of invaluable opportunities to visit the anatomy theatre in Pavia and draw the cadavers while della Torre's assistants sliced them up with seasoned care. His pupils listened as their pioneering teacher gravely attempted to explain the internal workings of the human body. But they were also aware of the artist's eager, energetic presence. One of them, Paolo Giovio, later recalled how intently Leonardo

> dedicated himself to the inhuman and disgusting work of dissecting the corpses of criminals in the medical schools, so that he might be able to paint the various joints and muscles as they bend and stretch according to the laws of nature. And he made wonderfully skilled scientific drawings of every part of the body, even showing the tiniest veins and the inside of bones.[13]

Both Leonardo and della Torre must have benefited, in their different ways, from this collaborative relationship. According to Vasari, 'each helped and was helped by the other',[14] and maybe these thoroughgoing sessions in the medical schools enabled Leonardo to arrive at his radical belief that

> true knowledge of the shape of any body is arrived at by seeing it from different aspects. Thus to express the true shape of any limb of a man . . . I will observe the aforesaid rule, making 4 demonstrations for the 4 sides of each limb. And for the bones I will make 5, cutting them in half and showing the hollow of each of them, of which one is full of marrow, and the other spongy or empty or solid.[15]

Moving tirelessly from one vantage point to another, Leonardo built up a truly revolutionary, proto-cinematic vision of the bodies he probed with such diligence, acuity and flair.

He worked so hard in Pavia that one note, written on a sheet of anatomical drawings, proudly predicted: 'In this spring of 1510 I expect to complete all the work on anatomy.'[16] But not for the first time, he underestimated the full, infinitely demanding extent of his researches. Although della Torre's untimely death a year later meant that Leonardo could never again resume his work in Pavia, he continued the dissections during his later visits to the celebrated Roman hospital in Santo Spirito. By then, however, he was dogged by the malicious machinations of a German mirror-maker called Giovanni degli Specchi. Leonardo complained that this alarming and aggressive individual 'was in the workshop every day, wanting to see and know everything that was being done, and then broadcasting it around, and criticising whatever he could not understand'.[17] He was the dangerous man who ultimately succeeded in 'hindering' Leonardo's anatomical research, 'denouncing it before the Pope and also at the Hospital'.[18]

Vatican theologians may have been especially incensed by Leonardo's fascination with embryology. On his outstanding sheet of studies of a foetus in the womb (pl. 87), some notes and sketches dating from this Roman period claim that the foetus possessed no soul of its own, independent of its mother: 'The same soul governs these two bodies.'[19] The idea that the unborn child of a dead woman had no soul to save would have been wholly unacceptable to the church in Rome. Charles Nicholl wondered if 'this may have been the titbit of suspicion brought "before the Pope" by the mirror-man, thus "hindering" Leonardo's studies'.[20] After all, Vasari pointed out that Leonardo 'had a very heretical state of mind. He could not be content with any kind of religion at all, considering himself in all things much more a philosopher than a Christian.'[21] Such a man could easily have incurred the disapproval of the Vatican, where Aristotelian heresies were denounced and purged in a vehement book-burning of 1516.

Perhaps it contributed to Leonardo's sudden decision, in the very same year, to leave Rome and make the long journey to retirement in France. The patronage of François I, whose enthusiasm for the elderly artist was limitless, proved irresistible. But in 1517, only two years before his death, the unrepentant Leonardo was still prepared to boast to a visiting cardinal about his controversial work as an anatomist. According to the prelate's chaplain and secretary, Antonio de Beatis, who recorded the visit in his diary, 'Master Leonardo' made clear to the cardinal that he

> has written a great deal about anatomy, with many illustrations of the parts of the body, such as the muscles, nerves, veins and the coilings of intestines, and this makes it possible to understand the bodies of both men and women in a way that has never been done by anyone before. All this we saw with our own eyes, and he told

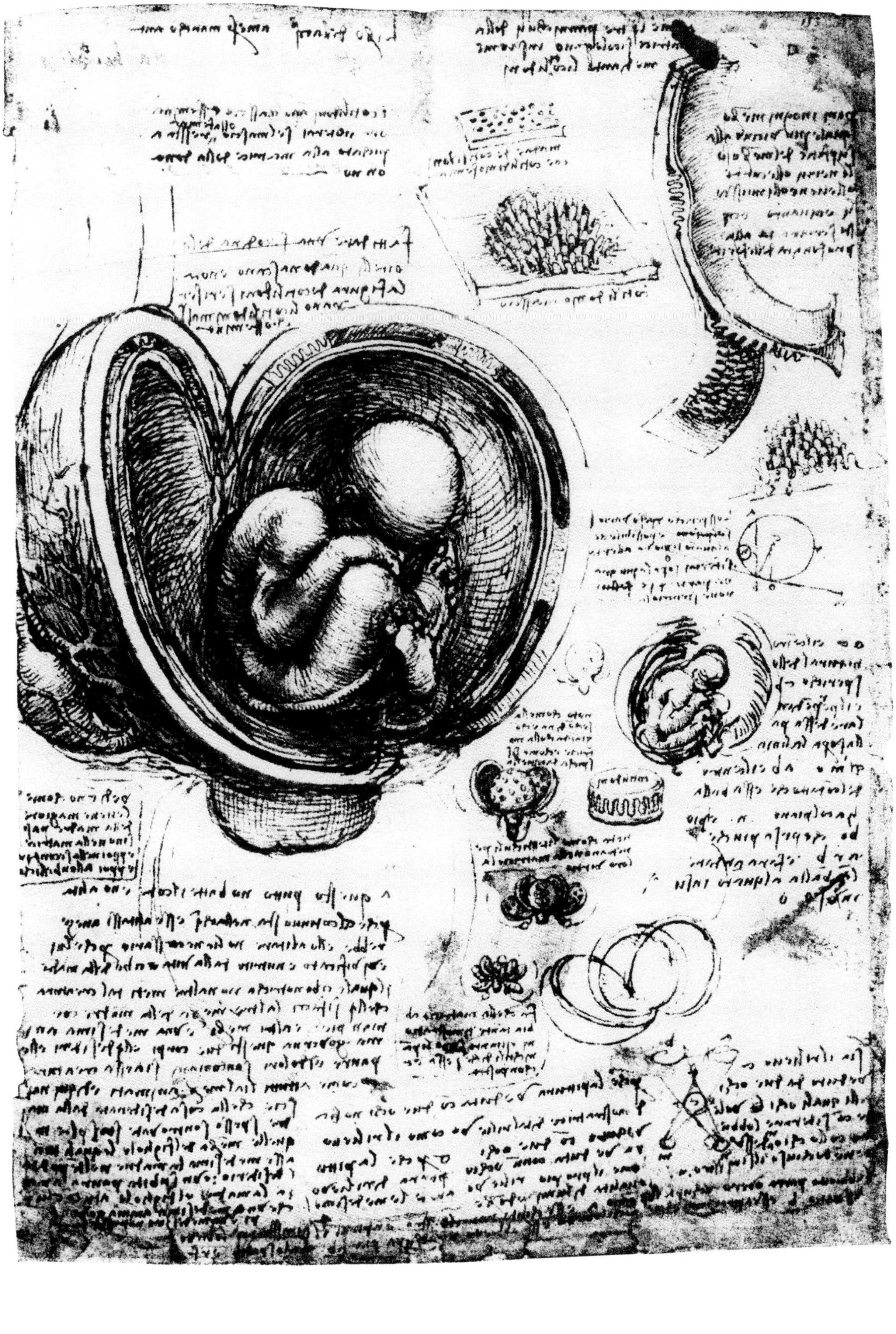

87 Leonardo da Vinci, *Studies of Foetus in Womb*, *c.*1510, Royal Collection, Windsor, facsimile, Ann Ronan Picture Library, London

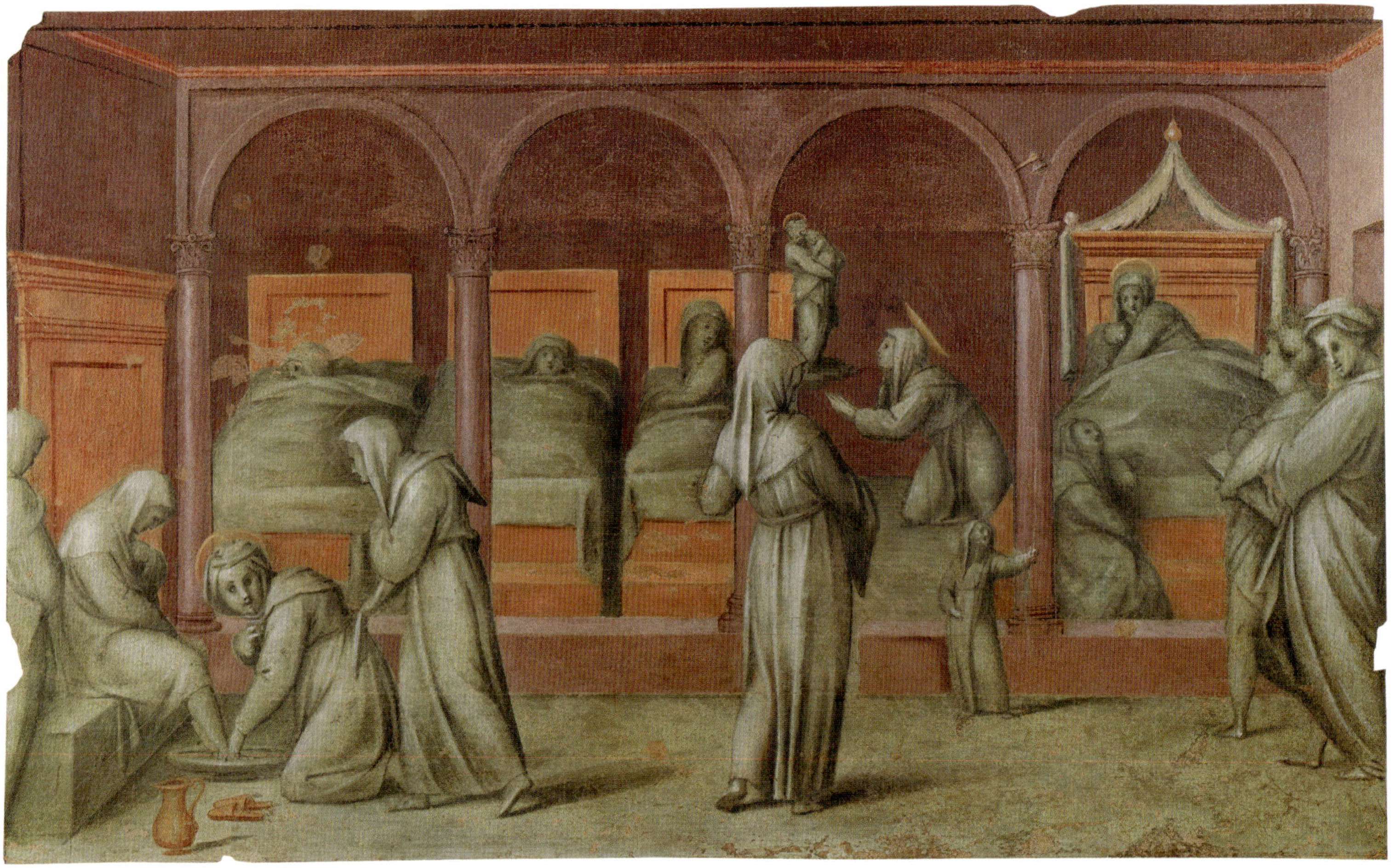

88 (*above*) Jacopo Pontormo, *Fresco from Women's Ward of Saint Matthew Hospital*, c.1514, Accademia, Florence

us he had already dissected more than thirty bodies, both men and women, of all ages.[22]

Although Leonardo spent so much time probing the interior workings of patients who had died in hospitals, he never drew or painted the interiors of the medical institutions themselves. But Jacopo Pontormo was prepared to do so in one of his earliest surviving works, a remarkable fresco from the women's ward in the former Florentine hospital of Saint Matthew (pl. 88). Painted by the precocious Pontormo around 1514, when he was no more than

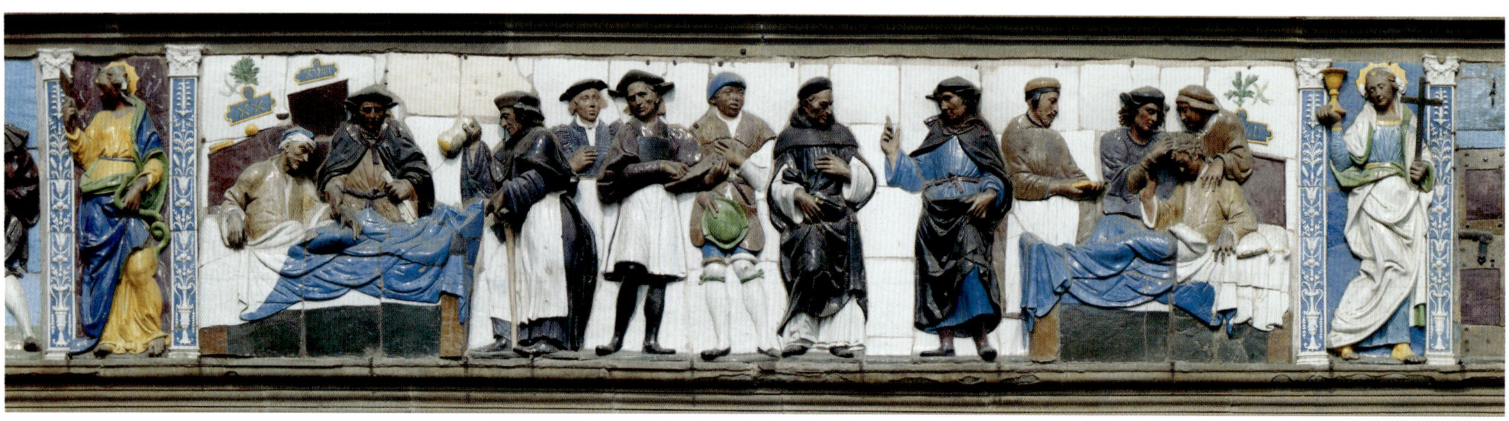

twenty years old,[23] it does not shirk from depicting the interior of a Renaissance ward with unusual realism. The two patients in beds on the left of the painting are clearly experiencing considerable distress, a feeling accentuated by the green earth colour that Pontormo employed for figures and blankets alike. Yet the third patient in the group rises partially from her pillow and turns, with signs of hope, towards the saintly figure who kneels and prays by the side of the bed. The saint appears to be gesturing, not only towards the woman she hopes to cure, but also in the direction of a statuesque representation of the Madonna and Child. Whether this image is a painting, a sculpture or simply a vision summoned by the power of prayer to hover by the bed, remains unknown. But its efficacy is clear, at least to the kneeling saint.

Elsewhere in the fresco Pontormo confirms the presence of religious associations in the hospital. For the bathing scene in the foreground is accompanied by a basin and slippers reminiscent, as one historian has pointed out, of similar props in Andrea del Sarto's contemporaneous fresco of the *Nativity of the Virgin*.[24] This harmonious image, one of Andrea's most admired works, conveys a sense of quiet joy that also affects Pontormo's bathing group. In common with the graceful rhythms of the colonnade curving across the hospital ward, the woman who eagerly washes the patients' feet counteracts the grimness of suffering by embodying a more positive order of feeling, instinct with tenderness and grace.

Priorities were changing, and Italian artists began to reflect this altered attitude by making their work embrace hitherto neglected aspects of hospital life. When a new portico was erected for the Hospital 'del Ceppo' in Pistoia, Giovanni della Robbia was able to convey in his enamelled terracotta reliefs a sincere concern for the welfare of its inhabitants (pl. 89). Giovanni, the son of Andrea, spent most of his career copying both his father's work and the images originated by many other Renaissance artists. But within his prolific output, the bulk of which was 'turned out in an almost industrialised fashion',[25] the Pistoia decorations are outstanding. Executed around 1525 with the assistance of the sculptor Santi Buglioni, they employ a vein of realism that marks them out quite distinctly from the work produced by previous generations of the della Robbia dynasty. In one panel, entitled *Visit the Sick* (see pl. 84), a drooping patient is propped up by a friend in order to receive welcome ministrations. Weak though he appears, the ailing inmate musters enough strength to reach up and touch the arm of the man who lays a blessing hand on his head. The patient's gesture is a poignant demonstration of Giovanni's involvement with the scene, and the intimacy with which all three figures cluster together testifies to the warmth of feeling behind the visit.

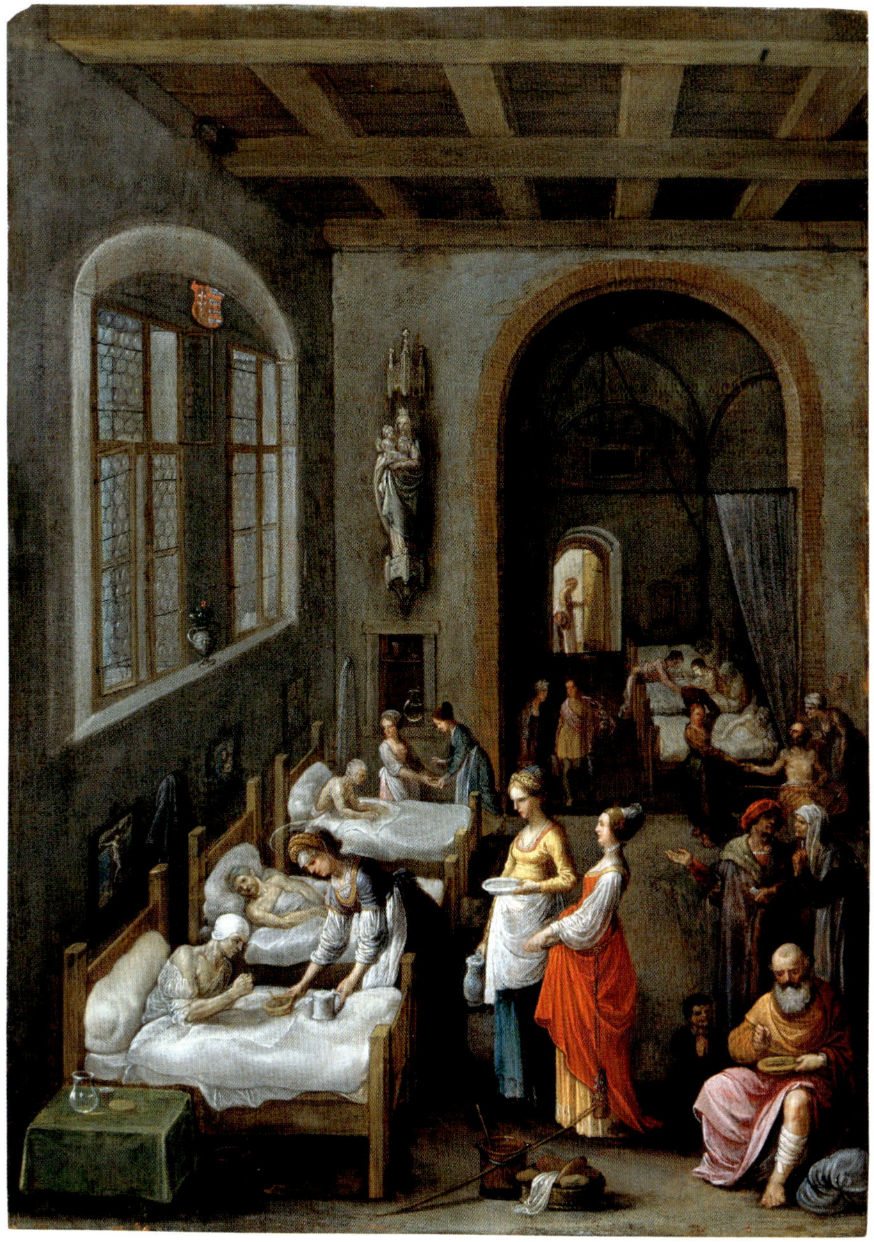

90 (*above*) Adam Elsheimer, *Saint Elizabeth visiting the Sick*, *c.*1598, Wellcome Collection, London

89 (*facing page, bottom*) Giovanni della Robbia, *Visit the Sick*, *c.*1525, Hospital 'del Ceppo', Pistoia

A similar commitment to hospital occupants characterises a small and exquisite painting executed near the end of the sixteenth century by the young Frankfurt-born Adam Elsheimer.[26] Scarcely twenty years old, he was already capable of producing the meticulously realised *Saint Elizabeth visiting the Sick* (pl. 90). Everything about this skilful oil painting on copper is redolent of the outstanding care offered to the afflicted by Elizabeth of Hungary, a thirteenth-century healing saint who used her dead husband's dowry to build a hospital at Marburg.[27] The entire ward is busy with figures attending to the patients' needs, and in the foreground no less than three women gather round a single bed. Among them is Elizabeth herself, who made it her business to nurse everyone personally. While her two companions stand ready to assist with bowls and jugs, she bends over to place food and drink in front of a haggard inmate. Elsheimer employed a red lake colour when he painted these women, giving them a glow in poignant contrast with the pallor of the patients. Such an aura was particularly appropriate in the case of Elizabeth, who became renowned during her short life for the generosity and zeal with which she gathered together ailing people on her estates, looked after them and exclaimed to her servants: 'How well it is for us, that thus we bathe and cover our Lord!'[28]

Each patient was therefore treated with the same devotion that the crucified Christ received, and throughout Elsheimer's interior there are plentiful signs of the attention enjoyed by its inhabitants. A prominent still life in the forefront of the painting consists of a pail brimming with soup and a basket containing loaves of bread assembled in fat, appetising abundance. Underneath the first bed a chamber pot and slippers can be glimpsed, while the table beside the pillow bears a carafe and a vase adorned with flowers. Hope of a life after death is provided in the ceiling rafters, where a swallow's nest symbolises the resurrection. But perhaps the most striking aspect of the room lies in the preponderance of painted and carved images housed there. A large statue of the Virgin and Child presides over the ward, handsomely enclosed in an elaborate niche. And above every bedhead hangs a painting of a religious scene, providing a constant and intimate form of spiritual sustenance to the figures enduring their fate beneath.

Did Elsheimer include these works of art on the basis of the images then to be found adorning hospital interiors in his native Frankfurt? Or was he fantasising about a lost and sentimentalised golden age, when patients enjoyed far more agreeable surroundings than they did in the late sixteenth century? The answer is difficult to determine. Elsheimer's painting may well have been commissioned by the Hospital Church in Frankfurt. According to Keith Andrews, it is very likely that the room depicted is 'indeed a [contemporary] hospital', and he also suggested that the 'old-fashioned appearance of the costumes' may be due to Altdorfer's influence on the young painter rather than any desire to imagine the clothes Saint Elizabeth would have worn in the twelfth century.[29] Moreover, Elsheimer must have known the wall-paintings of Saint Elizabeth executed around 1520 in the choir of the Hospital Church of the Teutonic Order in Frankfurt. Andrews acknowledges, however, that Elsheimer's interior may alternatively derive its character from an attempt to visualise the large building which, Jacob de Voragine maintained, was built by Saint Elizabeth at the foot of her castle. 'In this house she cared for a great multitude of the sick', Voragine wrote, 'visiting them each day . . . ministering to their needs and exhorting them to patience.'[30] The presence of the arms of Hungary, above the large windows bringing so much welcome light into the ward, tends to support the view that Elizabeth is here depicted in her own medieval hospital.

Around the same time, patients were treated with similar sympathy in several of the paintings from an ambitious and extensive Venetian cycle carried out by Jacopo Palma Giovane. His large-scale canvases, commenced in 1583 and completed nine years later, transformed the modest Oratory of the Crociferi Hospital into a blazing affirmation of philanthropic enterprise and religious conviction. The hospital itself had originated in the mid-twelfth century, when the Crociferi monks were invited to look after the poor and infirm of Venice. A munificent donation of land, buildings and funds by Doge Renier Zen in the following century assured the future of the hospital, administered with great diligence by the Procurators of Saint Mark's. In 1414 the building's inhabitants were reduced to twelve and it became a hospice for women alone, placed under the overall supervision of the 'hospitaller', a Crociferi friar. But this apparent diminution of the institution's effectiveness was followed, in the second half of the sixteenth

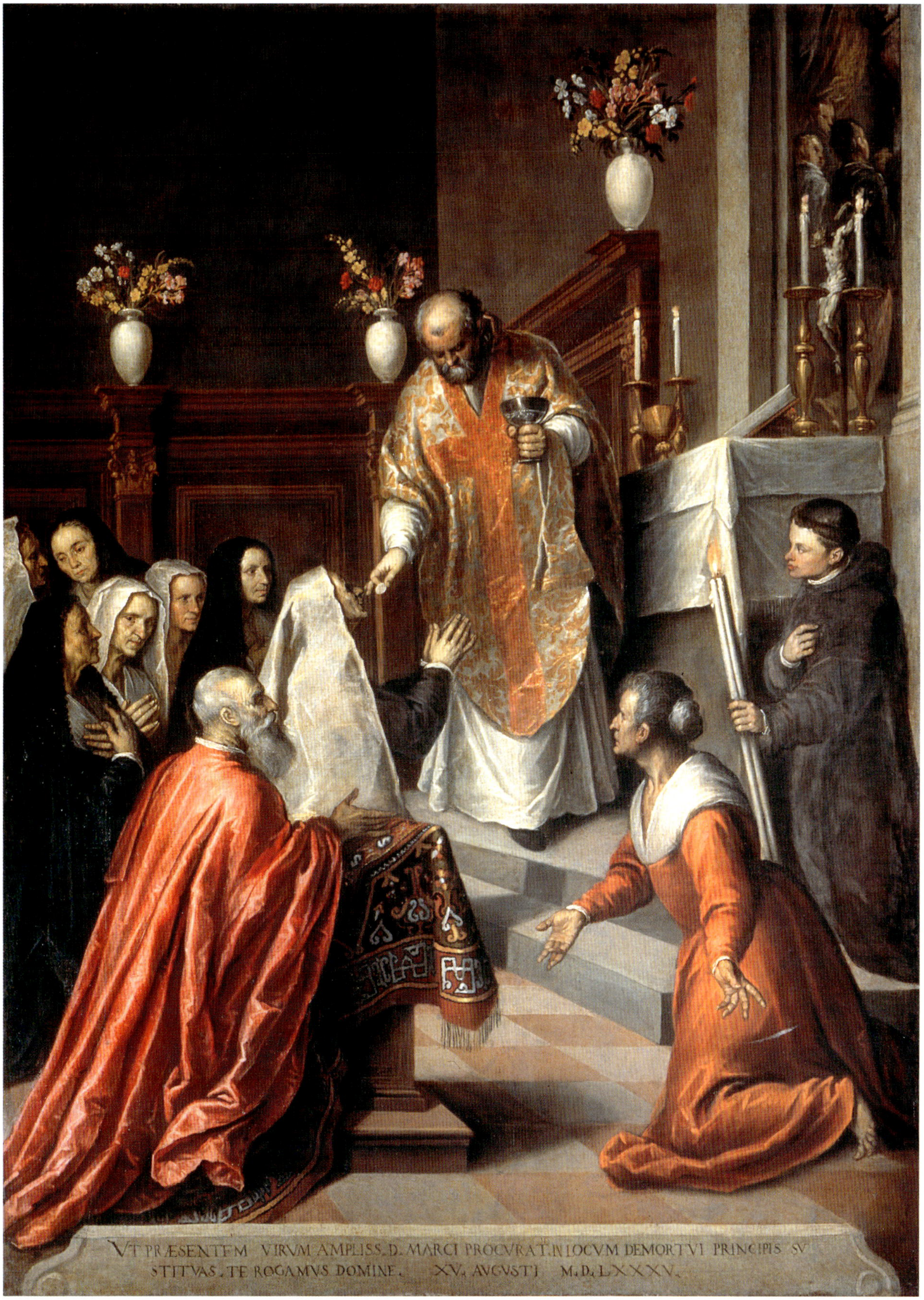
VT PRÆSENTEM VIRVM AMPLISS. D. MARCI PROCVRAT. IN LOCVM DEMORTVI PRINCIPIS SV
STITVAS. TE ROGAMVS DOMINE. XV. AVGVSTI M.D.LXXXV.

91 Jacopo Palma Giovane, *Priamo Balbi administering Mass*, 1583–92, Oratory of the Crociferi Hospital, Venice

92 (*facing page*) Jacopo Palma Giovane, *Cicogna hears of his election as Doge*, 1583–92, Oratory of the Crociferi Hospital, Venice

century, by a period of expansion and embellishment. The improvements flourished under the protection of Pasquale Cicogna, the pious Procurator of Saint Mark's who made a habit of praying in the hospital chapel. He received the momentous news of his nomination as Doge of Venice while attending a service in the church of the Crociferi and helped to ensure that the Oratory became elaborately decorated by one of the leading Venetian painters of the day.[31]

A knowledge of these landmarks in the hospital's history is a vital prerequisite in any attempt to understand Palma's cycle of paintings, which run round the walls above dark wooden panelling in this small, warmly harmonious room. For the most arresting and original canvases are directly concerned with recreating the dramatic moments that vouchsafed, in the past, the Crociferi building's security and growth. The sequence begins conventionally enough, with two paintings on either side of the Oratory altar. They depict, in a suitably solemn ceremonial manner, the foundation of the monks' Order and Pope Paul IV's subsequent concession of privileges to the Crociferi. As in the rest of the cycle, they gain pictorial conviction principally through vividly realised portraits of the individuals who attended these crucial meetings. All the same, they lack the keener sense of historical focus that Palma introduced to the most innovative trio of paintings in the series. They are placed in the position of greatest visibility, directly opposite the door where visitors to the Oratory enter from the Campo dei Gesuiti. The narrowness of the divisions between each canvas is intended to emphasise the interrelatedness of the stories they tell. But the finest of the three is undoubtedly the painting on the right, handled with a descriptive naturalism quite distinct from the neo-Mannerist style favoured by Palma's contemporaries.

The bearded figure of Priamo Balbi dominates the scene (pl. 91), administering Mass in his capacity as the Crociferi's 'hospitaller'. He was the prime mover in refurbishing the Oratory, and probably encouraged Palma to include the limpidly realised flower vases which give the painting so much of its freshness. Although the bare walls above the panelling give no indication of the canvases Balbi commissioned, Palma does include a glimpse of his own *Adoration of the Magi* over the altar, a canvas since lost and replaced by a Pieter de Coster painting.[32] Apart from the rhetorical pose of the woman kneeling in the foreground, Palma's entire picture is notable for its restraint and authenticity of feeling. Cicogna himself, a vigorously characterised presence, watches with quiet concentration as Balbi proffers the body of Christ to one of the hospital's inhabitants. He likes worshipping in the company of these simply dressed, devout old women, and Palma portrays them in all their wrinkled actuality while they pray for their protector's election as Doge. Each face is presented with a grave, dignified attentiveness that surely arises from Palma's readiness to study the hospital's inmates at first hand. They are entirely persuasive in their closely observed concentration on the service, except for the woman in a black shawl who tilts her head to hear a whispered message from her gaunt companion.

But even this exchange lends greater plausibility to a scene where everyone else's attention is directed towards the celebration of the Mass. Rather than posing for his portrait in an ostentatious manner, Balbi leans forward and involves himself with the devotional task in hand. The sense of shared intensity among the congregation is remarkable, with the old woman in the foreground accorded almost as much prominence as the distinguished Procurator. This devout man preferred their company to more elevated alternatives, and they return the compliment here by interceding on his behalf. When this painting was installed in the Oratory, the women of the hospice had good reason to conclude that Palma's cycle concerned itself wholeheartedly with their future well-being.

The central canvas on this wall is rather more formal, dealing as it does with the moment when Cicogna hears of his election as Doge (pl. 92). Palma conflates two successive stages in the service: while the central messenger delivers the tidings, the monks and novices on the right sing a *Te Deum* of thanksgiving at the news. Although it was significant that the message arrived while Cicogna worshipped at the Crociferi church, a comparison of the painting with the preliminary drawing reveals that Palma placed greater emphasis on the figures in his final canvas. Perhaps he was obliged to include more observers than the commission had originally led him to suppose, for the proliferation of portrait faces at either side of the painting ends up giving it a somewhat congested air.

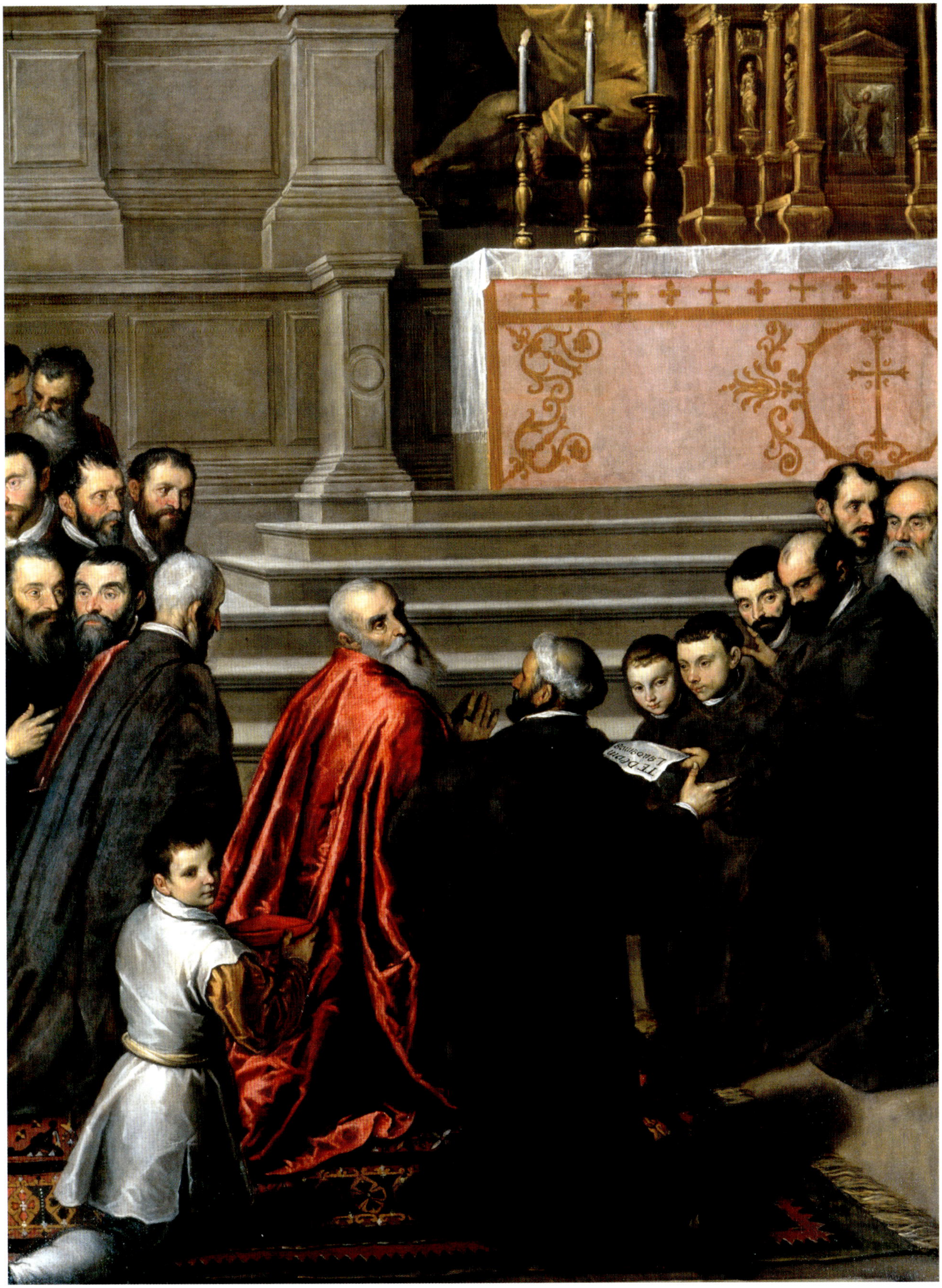
TE DEum
Laudamus

93 Jacopo Palma Giovane, *Doge Renier Zen Receiving a Document about his Hospital Benefaction*, 1583–92, Oratory of the Crociferi Hospital, Venice

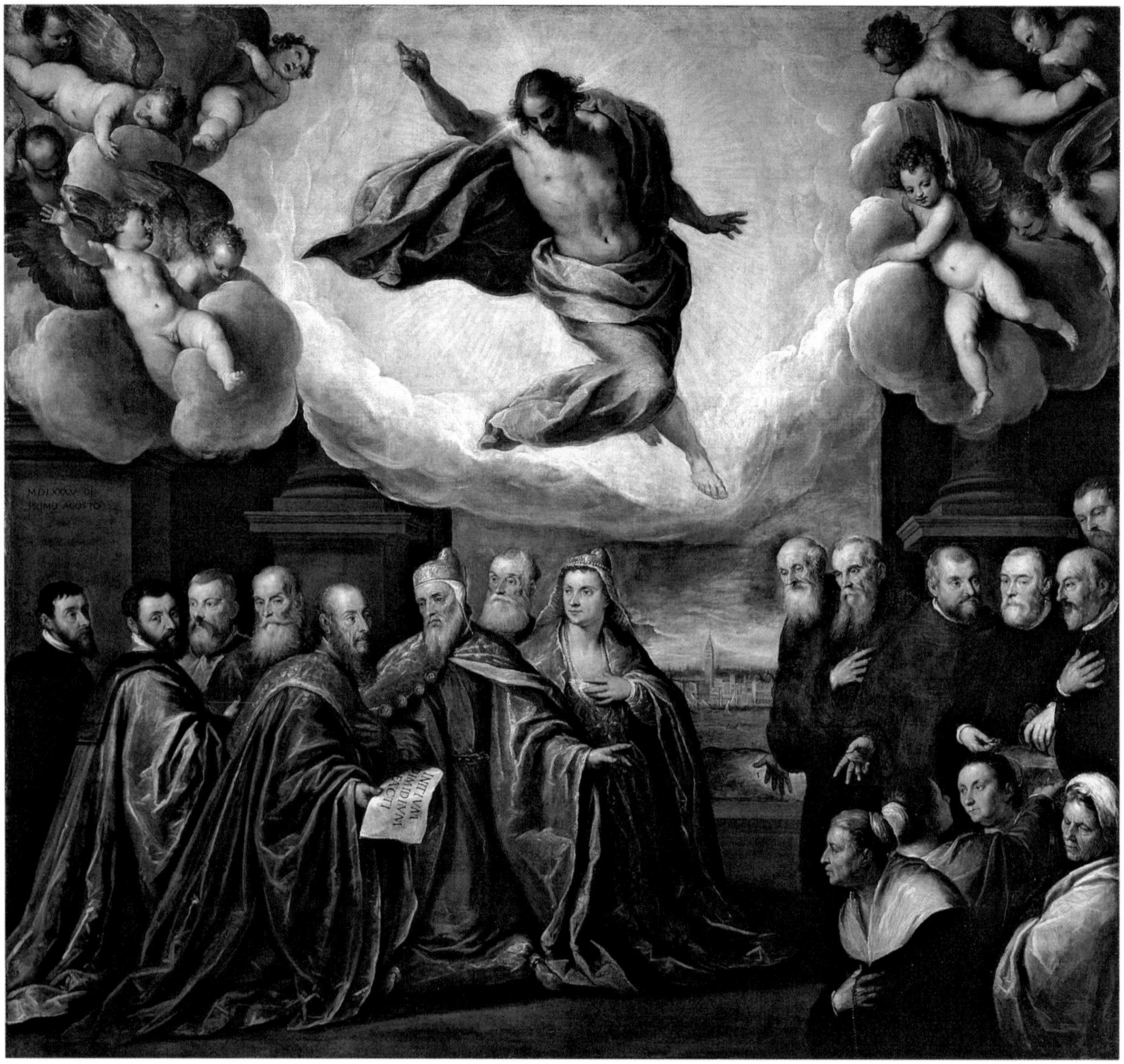

The same problem afflicts the third picture on the wall, where Cicogna returns to the hospital in ducal robes for an official visit. The Doge himself is depicted with a patriarchal grandeur suggesting how much Palma learned from Titian's even more magisterial portraits of the Republic's grandees. But the faces of the attendant dignitaries once again threaten to overcrowd the composition and the two kneeling women who receive the Doge's acknowledgement are now relegated to a very subsidiary role in the painting. The directness with which Palma treats all three of these canvases makes them stand out from their more conventional, academic counterparts in the cycle. Their almost reportorial authority points to the possibility that, as Lunardon has suggested, 'the artist himself may even have been a witness' at some of the events he depicts.[33] His own presence would help to explain why the naturalism of these pictures marks them out from the other canvases.

Palma could not, of course, have observed the scene represented in a panoramic painting on the wall opposite the altar (pl. 93). For the thirteenth-century Doge Renier Zen is shown here, accompanied by the Dogaressa Aloisia, receiving a document that refers to his hospital benefaction. Palma distances the scene still further from the actuality he achieved elsewhere by devoting half his composition to the figure of Christ in glory, blessing Zen's generosity. All the same, a substantial group of

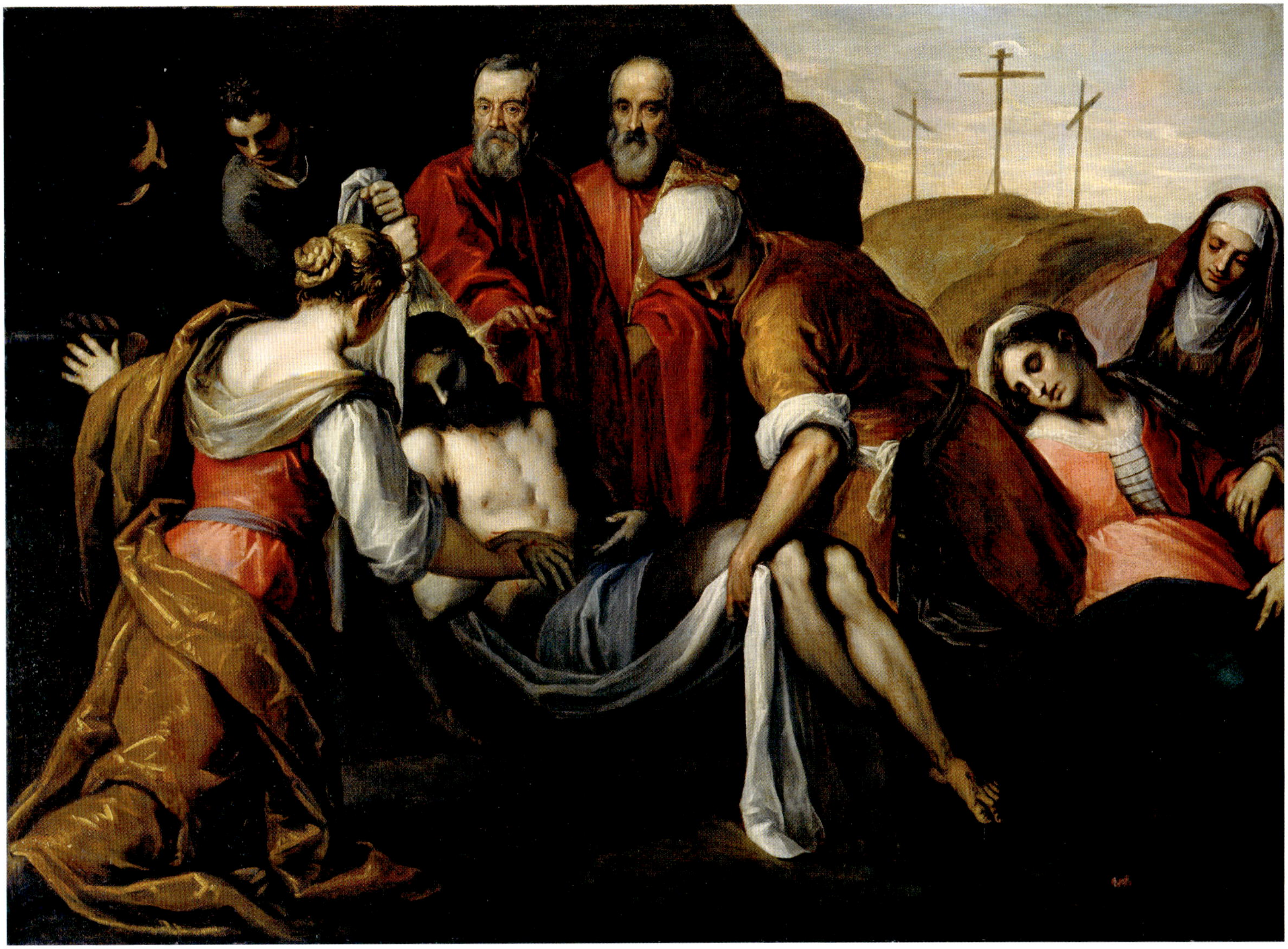

94 Jacopo Palma Giovane, *Deposition*, 1592, Private Collection, formerly Oratory of the Crociferi Hospital, Venice

monks and needy women help restore the image to the reality of hospital life. When he executed his preparatory drawing, Palma only included six figures in this area of the composition. Moreover, the women's subservient position was reinforced by stressing their proximity to the side of the dais rather than the top where all the other participants are placed. Peering over the dais, the women were relegated to the status of bystanders permitted merely to gaze at the hem of the Doge's robe. By the time the painting was completed, however, the top of the dais stretched to the very forefront of the design. If the women still occupy a lower place in the hierarchy of the event, they do nevertheless benefit from Palma's decision to accord them a more significant role.

The drawing had portrayed them as little more than ragged children, whereas the painting depicts flesh-and-blood individuals whose well-worn faces bear undisguised marks of the privation they once endured. The foremost woman clutches a rosary as she leans forward, eager yet dignified, to gaze at the Doge's extended fingers. Her neighbour looks inwards and raises her hand to receive money from the monk above. But the other two women adopt a far less beseeching attitude. While one casts her wrinkled eyes down, as if exhausted by the waiting her elderly body has been obliged to undergo, the other stares towards the august proceedings with immense stoicism. Neither overawed nor hungry for attention, she gracefully appreciates the knowl-

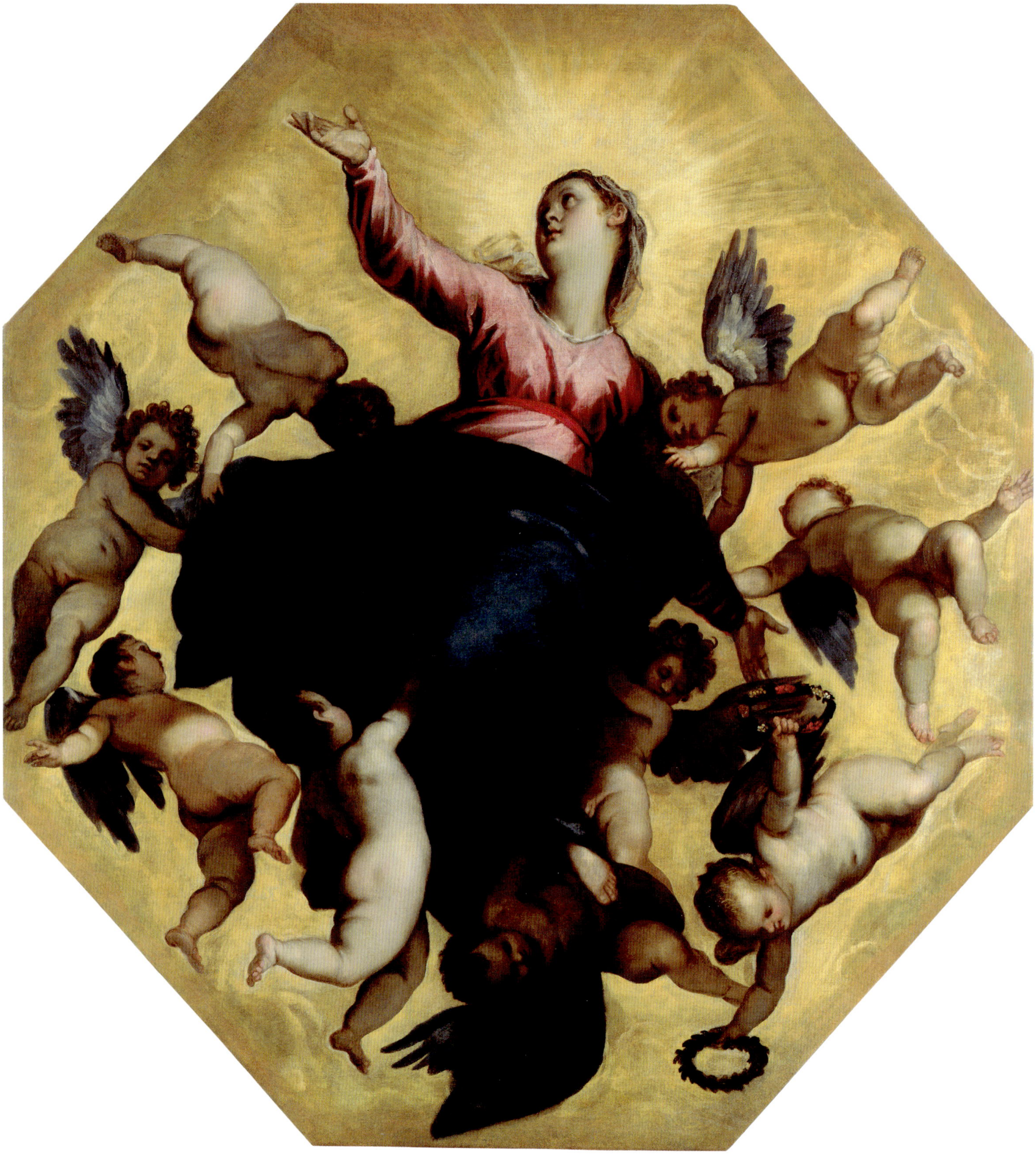

edge that her hardship will be alleviated both by the assembled rulers and the deity intervening at a dynamic diagonal far above the lagoon.

The other major paintings on the Oratory's walls refer to Christ's travail on behalf of humanity, and their exclusively biblical themes helped to persuade Palma and his patrons that a more elevated, neo-Mannerist style should now be deployed. Naturalism drops away in the *Flagellation* above the entrance, where the tormentors adopt balletic attitudes as they aim at the equally artificial figure of their victim. Since the adoption of a new manner caused Palma to lose some of the individuality he had developed elsewhere in the cycle, and ape his masters more slavishly, the outcome is less memorable. It justifies the reservations expressed by S. J. Freedberg, who observed that too often 'the élan of Palma's figures seems imposed, not really motivated, and the handling that pertains to qualities like Tintoretto's or Titian's may at times be dense, or worse, inert'.[34] These strictures apply less to the *Deposition* on the wall opposite the altar (pl. 94), where the inclusion of two contemporary portraits lends the image a greater intensity. Completed in 1592, at the end of the work Palma carried out on the cycle, the painting makes special reference to the Crociferi context by silhouetting the three crosses on Calvary's distant hillside, doubtless a deliberate repetition of the trio of crucifixes carved above the doorway on the Oratory's facade.

But the climax of the decorations, so far as their religious purpose was concerned, can be found in the ceiling (pl. 95). Like the altarpiece, the paintings installed in these heavily coffered frames honour the chapel's dedication to the Virgin. Surrounded by a choir of music-making angels, she ascends to heaven in the octagonal centrepiece. The triumphalism of her gesture, leading upwards from a foreshortened body attended enthusiastically by putti determined to hasten her progress from every side, emphasises the assurance with which Christianity offers the prospect of a life beyond death. It is no accident, perhaps, that this *Assumption* panel should be placed directly above a tombstone in the centre of the Oratory floor. Its inscription, *sepulcrum pauperum huius hospitalis*, bears witness to the fact that the hospice, as well as paying for medical services when its occupants fell ill, always subsidised last rites for the women who were never rejected by the building that had given them shelter and sustenance. Looking up at the image of Christ's mother as she rises to heaven, they would surely derive comfort from the assurance it provided. Here, on the ceiling of the Crociferi Oratory, Palma's painting was able to hold out the prospect of hope and solace alike.

95 (*facing page*) Jacopo Palma Giovane, *Assumption*, 1583–92, Oratory of the Crociferi Hospital, Venice

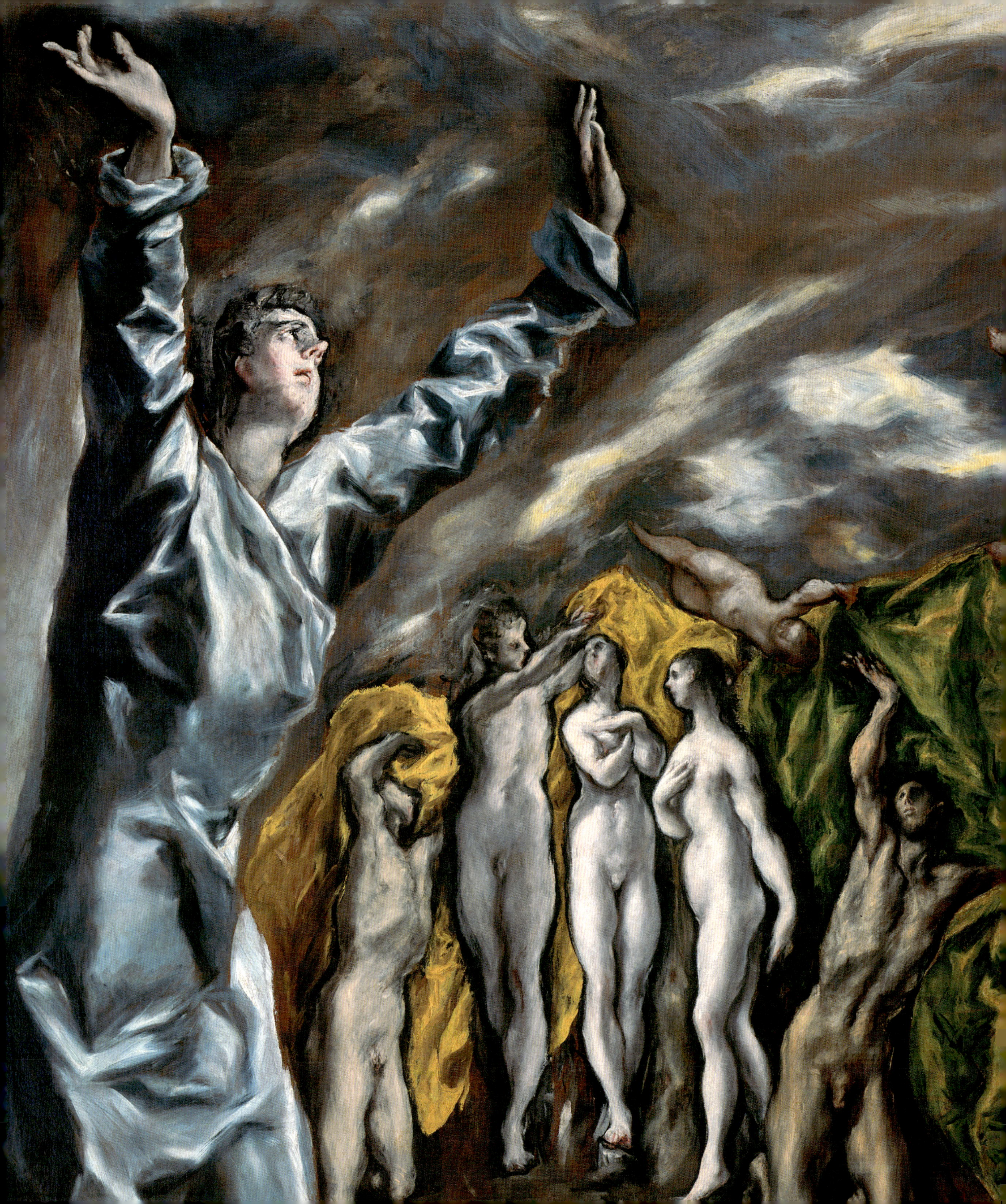

EIGHT
VISIONS OF REDEMPTION

During the course of the sixteenth century, hospital architecture enjoyed a magnificent period of embellishment in Spain. Rather than contenting themselves with adding on to medieval buildings – Saint John's Hospital in Bruges had accrued, segment by segment, from modest beginnings in the twelfth century – Spanish philanthropists ensured that resplendent structures were now erected according to newly adopted Renaissance principles. Prominent among them was the Hospital of the Holy Cross at Toledo (pl. 97), founded in 1494 by Cardinal Pedro Gonzalez de Mendoza and completed, after his death, by Queen Isabella in 1514. Enrique de Egas's splendid designs ensured that the outcome, formed in the shape of a cross, boasted a richly carved square newel staircase, wall-carvings and above all an elaborate sequence of sculpture with a Crucifixion and a cornucopia of other subjects above the entrance.

The finished building amounted to one of the most splendid examples of early Renaissance architecture in Spain and other hospitals elsewhere in the country were quick to emulate Toledo's initiative. At Santiago da Compostela, the Hospital Real, founded in 1501, displayed richly encrusted ranks of saintly statuary around and above the exuberant main entrance. Barcelona followed suit, albeit in a more restrained manner, when a doorway in the Hospital of the Holy Cross was adorned with a carving of two angels holding a coat of arms in a scalloped niche. Nor were decorations restricted to the exterior of this building. Tiled images depicting the Stations of the Cross were later installed above each bed in the ward of Nuestra Señora de los Dolores, thereby openly equating the suffering of the patients with the agony experienced by Christ before his crucifixion.

No wonder that El Greco, the most impressive painter at work in late sixteenth- and early seventeenth-century Spain, found himself invited to undertake major hospital commissions. During the final stage of his career an increasing amount of El Greco's prodigious energy was devoted to hospital work, commencing very dramatically with the *Saint Francis's Vision of the Flaming Torch* executed for the Hospital de Nuestra Señora del Carmen in Cadiz around the turn of the century (pl. 98). With characteristic audacity, El Greco seizes on the moment of most intense revelation. Staring up at the vision of a flaming torch, which explodes in a cataclysm of lightning flashes, Saint Francis reacts by spreading out his arms in absolute astonishment. The apocalyptic blaze irradiates his robes with an unearthly glow and picks out the contours of Brother Leo who, according to *The Little Flower of Saint Francis*, witnessed the scene with him.

96 (*facing page*) Detail of pl. 109

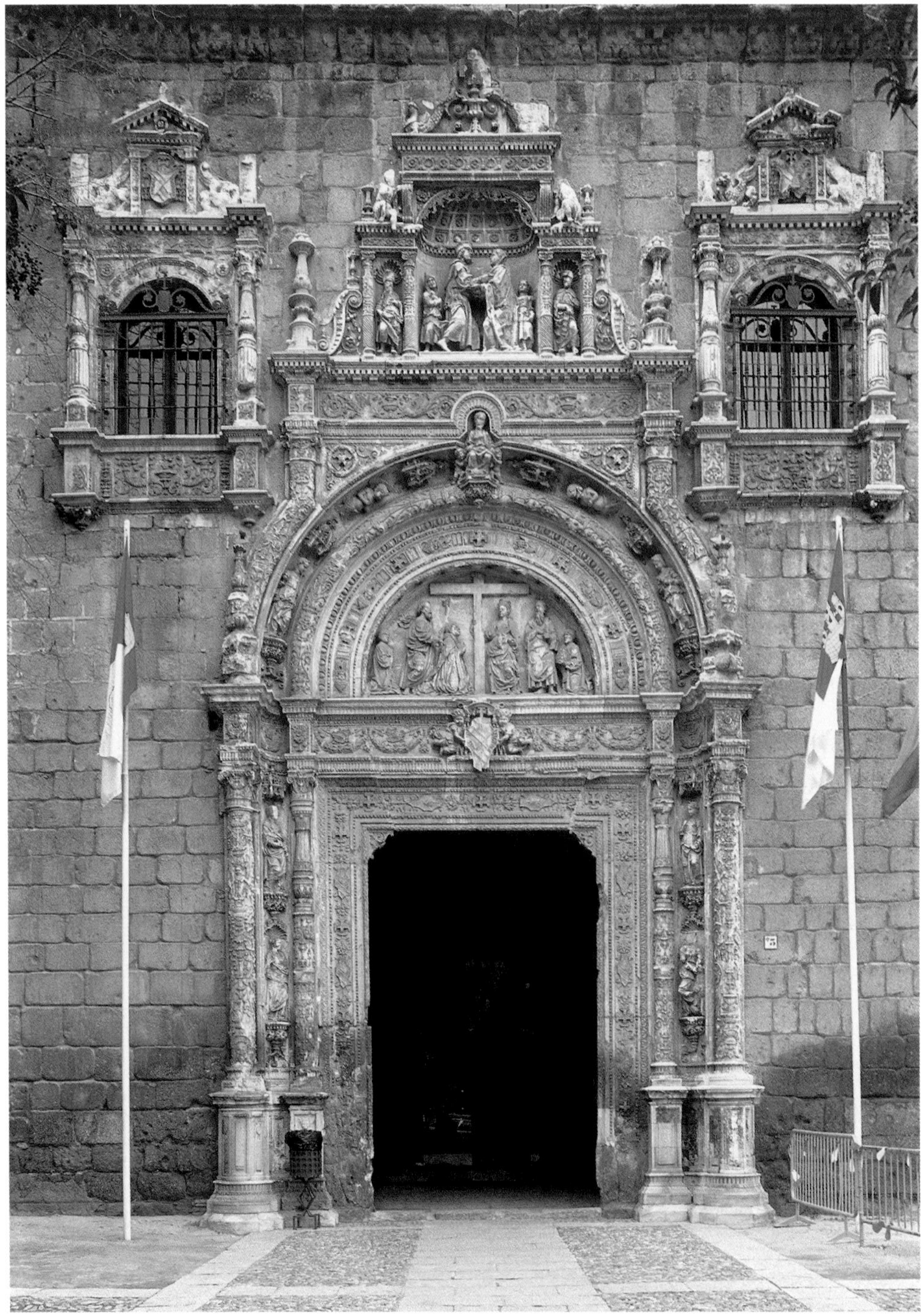

97 Enrique de Egas, Hospital of the Holy Cross, Toledo, 1494–1514

Stretching up towards the source of the vision, Brother Leo's hand typifies the ambiguity of a painting that accentuates the men's trepidation, even as it conveys the awe generated by the torch's sudden, wholly unexpected manifestation.

El Greco's fervently expressive art, centred so often on Counter-Reformation themes like the Passion of Christ, the contemplation of death, the martyrdom of saints and acts of charity, was well suited to the hospital context. His ability to invest a large canvas of *Saint Ildefonso* (pl. 99) with a dual conviction, giving him a sympathetic human presence as well as charging the scene with a mystical intensity, perhaps helped him to win an extensive commission for the general decoration of the church of the Hospital of Charity at Illescas, a small town halfway between Toledo and Madrid. Unlike conventional portraits of Ildefonso, which show him receiving the chasuble from the Virgin, El Greco's painting depicts the Toledan saint absorbed in composing his book on Mary's virginity. With one hand pressing firmly down on the pages of his manuscript, and the other arrested in mid-air with the quill stretching from his fingers like a bird in flight, Ildefonso pauses for inspiration. The account of his life given by the abbot Juan Tritemio maintains that, on completion of the saint's book, the Virgin appeared before him with his volume to display her approval of the text.[1] But El Greco elected to concentrate on the act of writing itself, probably to emphasise how much the Virgin had contributed to Ildefonso's literary labours.

The decision gives the whole scene a compelling sense of authenticity, for the saint gazes up at an image of the Virgin installed in symbolic proximity to his desk. Ildefonso's arrested pose is wholly convincing, and El Greco makes his painting even more persuasive by carefully specifying an array of sixteenth-century writing implements and furnishings in the room. He also stays as faithful as possible to the real wooden image of the Virgin that Ildefonso is traditionally supposed to have kept in his oratory, before donating it to the Illescas convent after he founded the institution. Above all, though, El Greco infuses the saint's face with enormous emotional pressure. Ildefonso is presented as an entirely credible elderly man, whose reputation as an eloquent defender of the Virgin's purity was underpinned by an ardent respect for the woman whose 'miraculous' likeness he gazes at so passionately. No painter ever succeeded in conveying the emotional strength of spirituality with more conviction than El Greco, whose pioneering iconographic image of the contemplative saint working at his desk would become immensely popular during the Baroque period.

The imaginative intensity of the Ildefonso canvas, now displayed in one of the side altars of the nave of the Hospital Church at Illescas, probably encouraged the administrators to commission from El Greco what they described as 'a retable for the altar of Our Lady of Illescas in the hospital of its sacred house'.[2] He received the invitation in June 1603, and lost little time in setting to work on the four canvases for the high altar. *Charity*, *Coronation of the Virgin*, *Annunciation* and *Nativity* were the titles given to the paintings in the commission documents.[3] Although they have remained in the hospital to this day, none occupies its original location. The dismantling of the installation is especially unfortunate, for El Greco placed them in a special setting which incorporated sculpture and may have constituted the first example of a Baroque chapel in Europe. The claim was advanced in a seminal

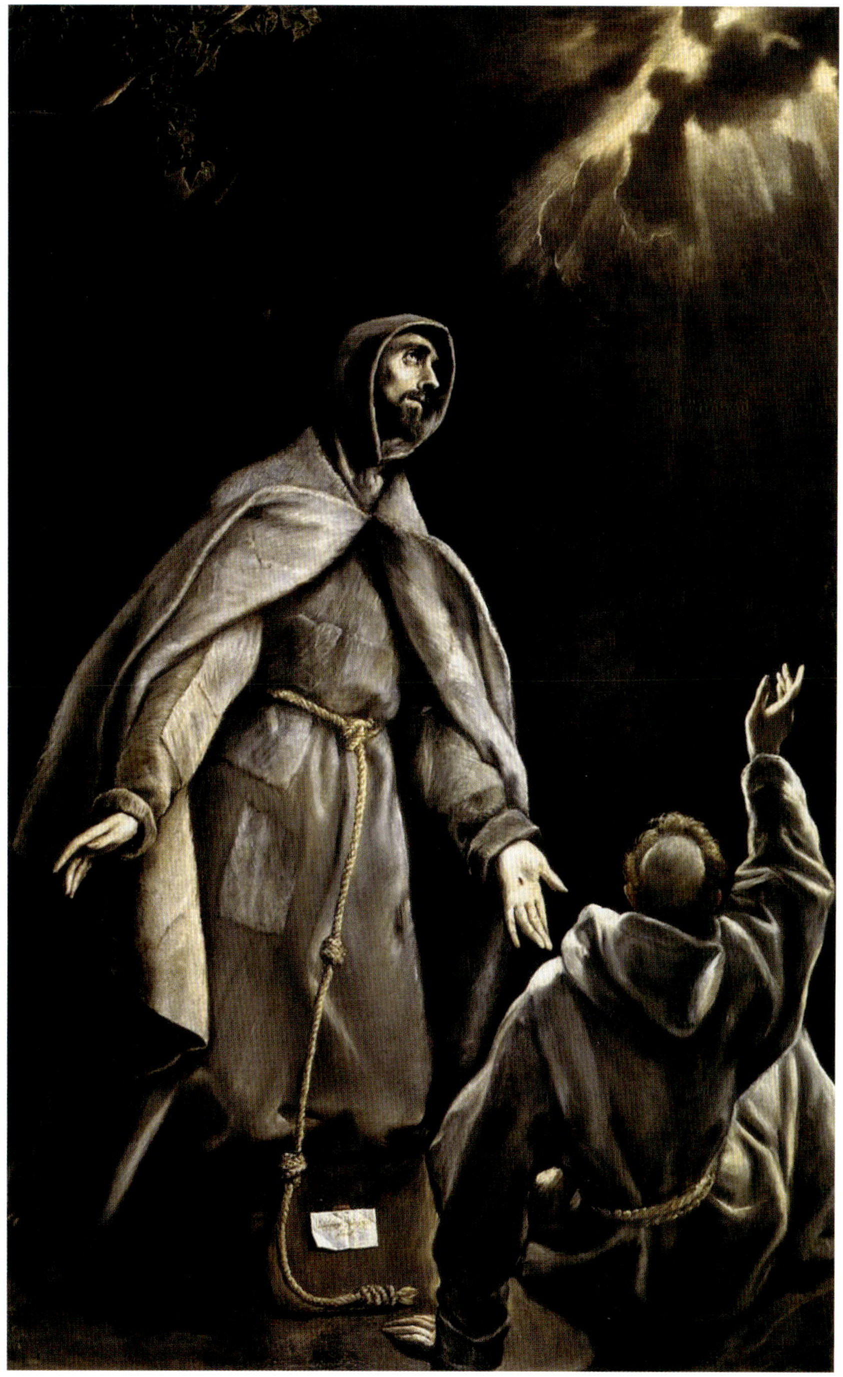

98 El Greco, *St Francis's Vision of the Flaming Torch*, 1600–05, Hospital de Nuestra Señora del Carmen, Cadiz

99 El Greco, *Saint Ildefonso*, *c*.1600–03, Hospital of Charity, Illescas

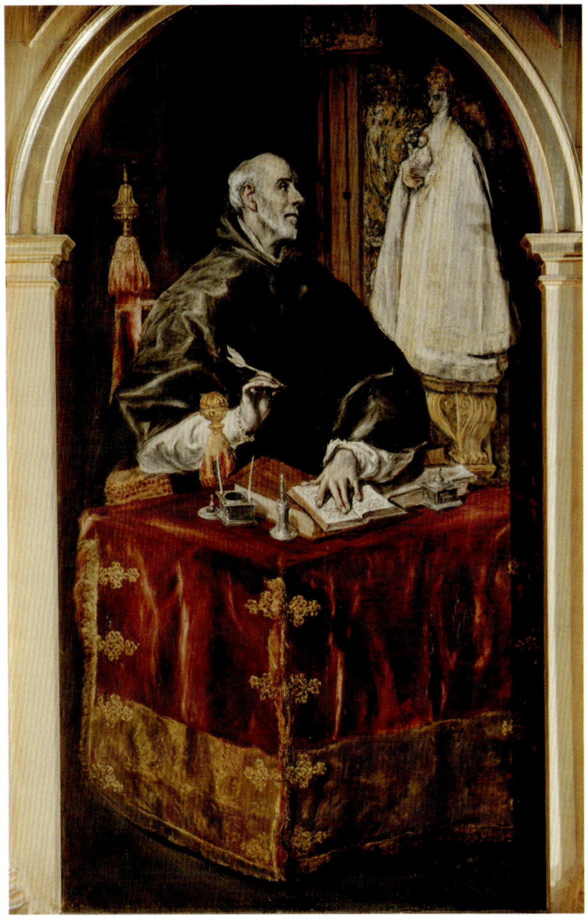

article of 1938 for the *Burlington Magazine*, where Enriqueta Harris argued that the entire scheme must have been intended to be viewed as a unity from a single, central position.[4] Ellis Waterhouse considered it a 'persuasive suggestion',[5] but the subsequent destruction of the chapel means that it remains unprovable. El Greco's innovative contribution to the development of European Baroque is unquestioned, however, and three of the Illescas canvases have been repositioned in the hospital's former reliquary to prove that he gave them an impressive poetic authority.

The vault of the confined and shadowy sanctuary where they were initially housed was occupied by a large oval painting of the *Coronation of the Virgin* (pl. 100), the same subject carved in the *Virgin Mary Porch* over the entrance to Saint John's Hospital in Bruges (see pl. 55). In place of the medieval sculpture's placid frontality, though, El Greco gives his composition a soaring dynamism. The three principal figures have an almost vertiginous quality as they perch on wildly surging clouds and participate in the sacred ceremony. The white dove this time casts a light as dazzling as the shafts of illumination that held Saint Francis so spellbound in the Cadiz canvas (see pl. 98), and aerobatic babies tumble in an ecstasy of celebration around the Virgin's swirling draperies.

It is a more fervent image in every way than the earlier version of the subject painted by El Greco for the Chapel of Saint Joseph in Toledo. There the entire composition was more bound to the earth by the presence of substantial saints in the foreground, and the Virgin herself appeared relatively stolid as she looked calmly up at Christ. In the Illescas version, by contrast, her gaze is frankly awestruck as she stares at the Holy Spirit's blazing radiance and finds herself gathered up in the irresistible rhythms created by clouds and putti alike. The outcome is an ecstatic vision, where every turbulent element in the design contributes to the feeling of sublime consummation.

This wild, electric sense of heightened rapture also infects two smaller roundels, probably placed in lunettes at the side of the *Coronation* canvas. In the *Annunciation* a dove once again provides an almost blinding amount of illumination for the gesticulating Virgin as she tilts away from an equally elongated desk (pl. 101). Although dazed by the brightness, she listens in wonder to an angel swathed in brilliant lime drapery quivering with a life of its own. The *di sotto in sù* perspective effect shared by this painting with the other two canvases gives it a more dizzying quality than it might have possessed in its original position.

But no instability affects the companion roundel of the *Nativity* (pl. 102). Even though El Greco concentrated here on an intimate moment, lacking the obvious drama of the other tondo, he managed to produce an exceptional image. This vibrant scene is his only surviving attempt to deal with the Holy Manger attended by the Virgin and Joseph alone. Taking his cue from a passage in Isaiah, which declares that 'the ox knoweth his owner, and the ass his master's crib', El Greco also included both animals in his composition. But their heads alone are shown, and the ass is half-hidden in the penumbral region behind the Virgin. The ox's head, extending its curved horn at a foreshortened angle that indicates how high the *Nativity* must initially have been sited, does not distract attention from

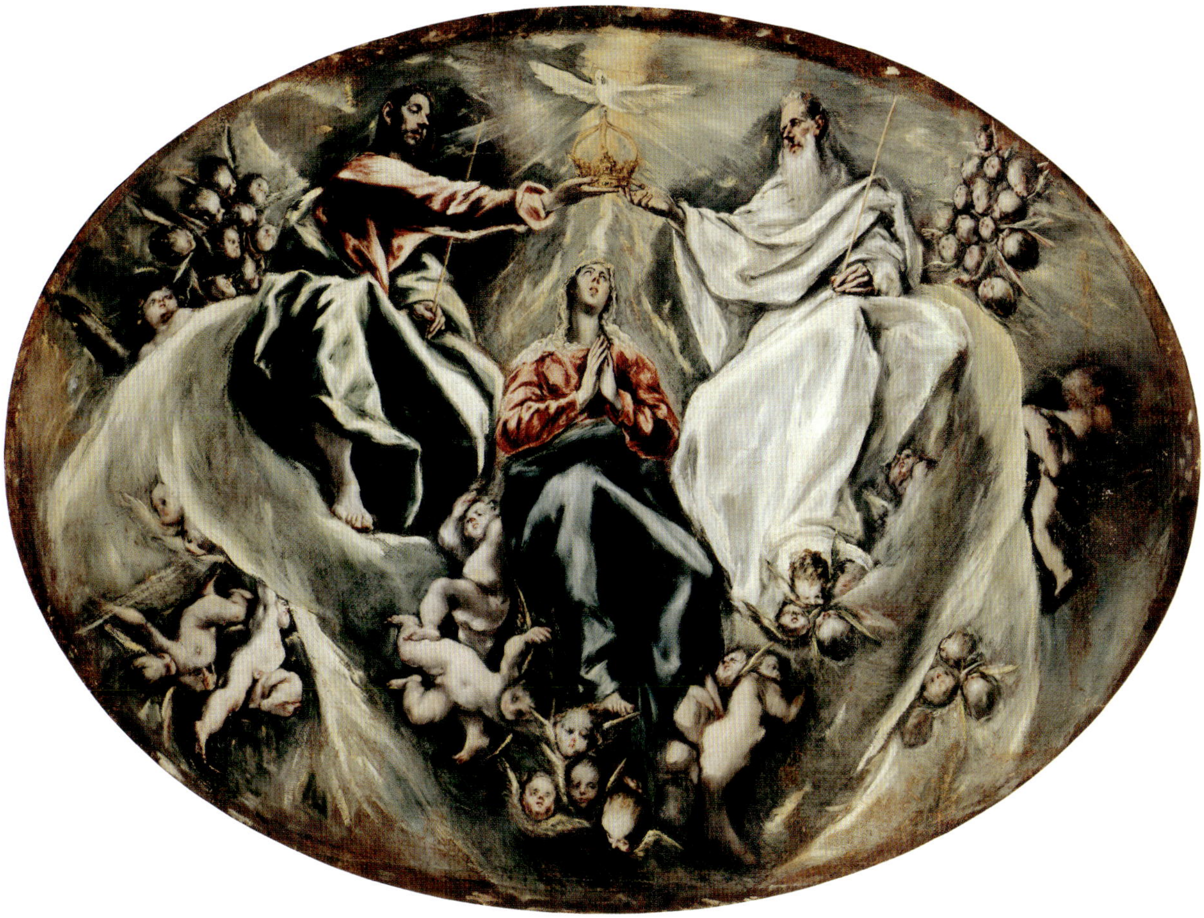

100 El Greco, *Coronation of the Virgin*, *c.*1603–5, Hospital of Charity, Illescas

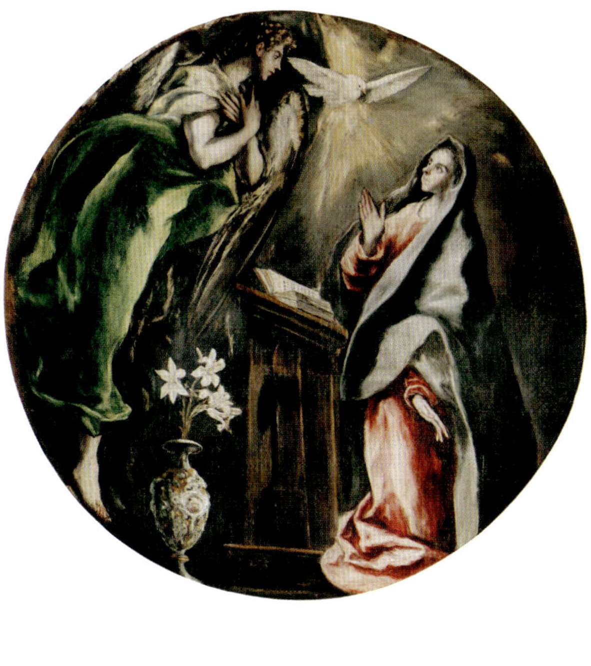

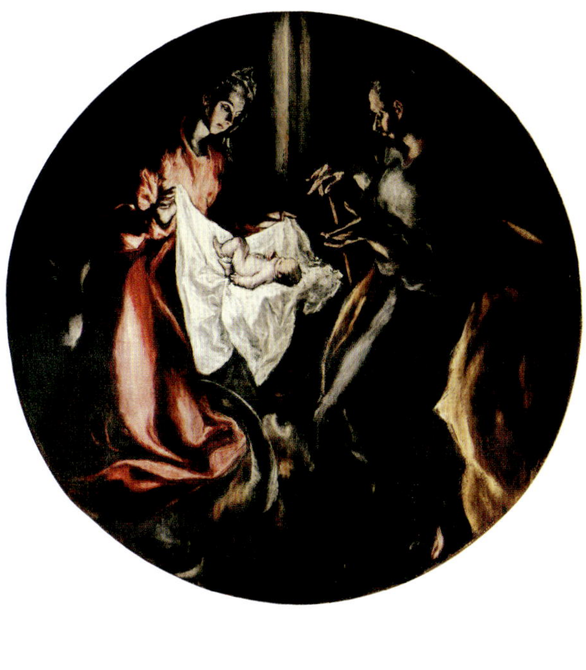

101 (*far left*) El Greco, *Annunciation*, *c.*1603–5, Hospital of Charity, Illescas

102 (*left*) El Greco, *Nativity*, *c.*1603–5, Hospital of Charity, Illescas

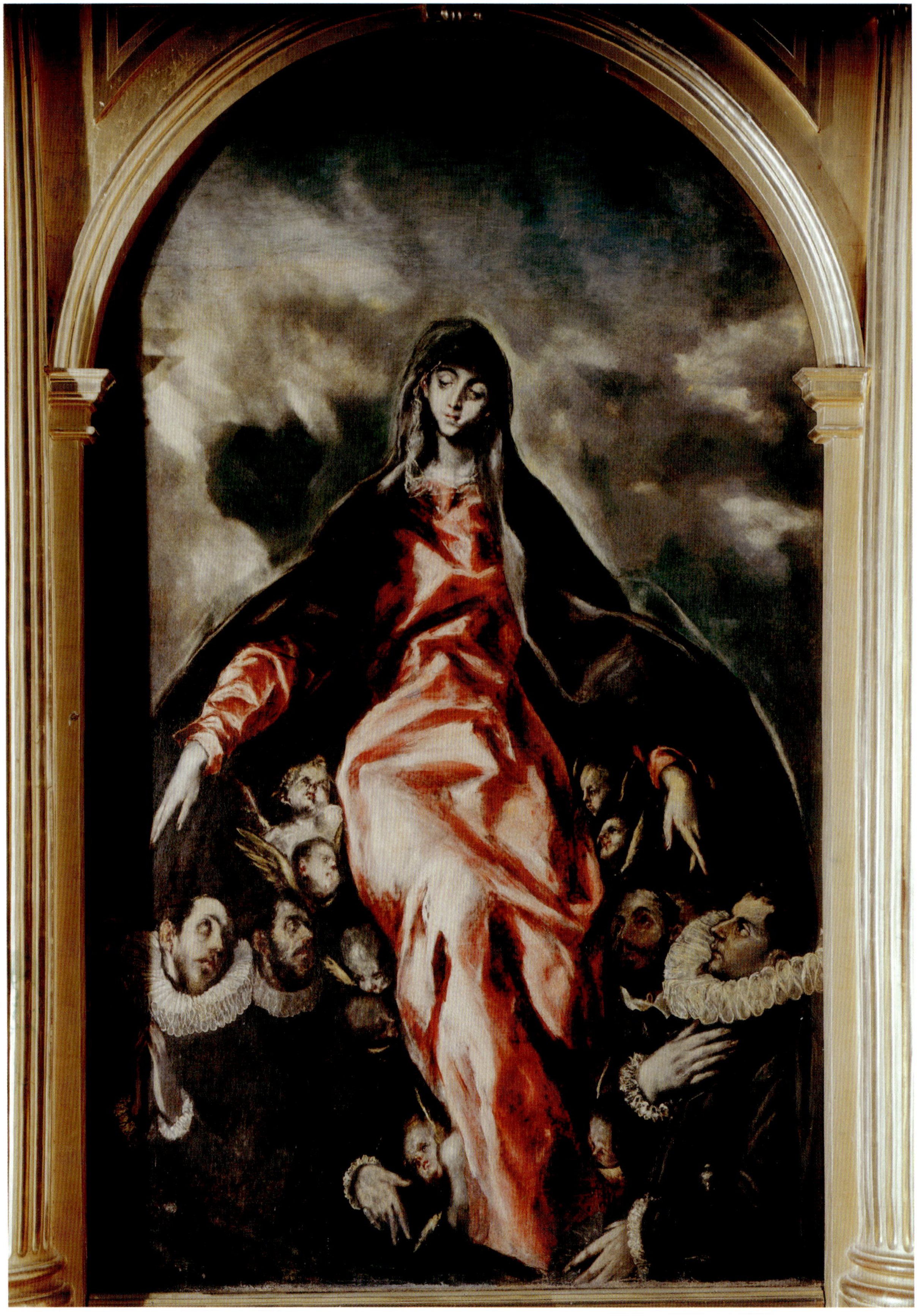

103 El Greco, *Madonna of Charity*, *c.*1603–5, Hospital of Charity, Illescas

the baby. Far from it: the animal directs our eyes towards the infant Christ with adoring insistence. Smaller and more vulnerable than in most representations of the theme, he lies on a sheet white enough for its glare to emblazon the figures staring down at him. The Virgin's gesture implies that she has just unwrapped the infant, to the evident astonishment of Joseph whose hands hang in the air as if transfixed. Both he and the Virgin are movingly aware of the child's frailty and their tender concern for his welfare outweighs any inhibition they might otherwise have felt in the presence of divinity.

Such a protective urge was, of course, well attuned to the context of a Hospital of Charity. But its priorities came fully to the fore only in the grand canvas of the *Madonna of Charity* itself, where the attenuated maternal figure counteracts signs of disturbance in the sky by directing her arms in an enfolding movement (pl. 103). Like the earlier *Madonna of Mercy* paintings made for hospitals by Domenico di Bartolo and Piero della Francesca, as well as Memling's image of Saint Ursula protecting her virgins (see pls 9, 22, 66), Greco's Virgin embraces everyone within sight. Here, gathered as if to shelter from the incipient storm above, figures and yearning putti crowd under the ample mantle flowing down from the Virgin's head. She adheres to the iconographic tradition of the *Madonna della Misericordia* and they look adoringly up at her, cheered by their proximity to the rich crimson robe. The fine clothes they wear rule out the possibility that hospital patients might be portrayed here, yet they still appear respectful enough to signify humanity's gratitude to the Virgin for her generous protection. El Greco has included his own son Jorge Manuel among the figures, thereby implying that her beneficence extends to the artist's family as well.

The painting was so powerful that it inspired Luis Tristán, who worked in Greco's studio around this time, to pay open homage to it in a picture he later executed for the Hospital de la Misericordia in Toledo. But the appraisers for the Illescas hospital took grave objection to the presence of recognisable people 'wearing ruffs' in Greco's *Madonna of Charity*. They censured him for his supposed impropriety in incorporating contemporary portraits of supplicants in equally contemporary dress, even though he had included Jorge Manuel and other individuals of the period in a number of previous paintings. Forced to defend himself, he defiantly complained that

> the job of the appraisers was to set a value on the painting but they decided to censure and correct the picture. And what they consider to be a fault – namely, that some among the crowd of people painted beneath the mantle to our Lady of Charity are wearing ruff collars like the ones that some people wear today – is a fault worth pondering, because what they hold to be indecent for that place is a practice in use throughout Christendom.[6]

Although Greco was quite justified in asserting that his painting belonged to a legitimate tradition, his defence did not prevent the drastic alteration of the *Madonna of Charity* at the hospital's behest. The offending ruffs were replaced with open Van Dyck collars until the cleaning of the canvas in 1938, and El Greco's intentions were further distorted when an arched area was added at the top to conform with the side altar it now inhabits.

Moreover, he had good reason to regret his original rash decision to agree with the hospital's proposal that appraisal for payment would be made by its nominees. For the appraisers decreed, predictably enough, that he should be paid the inadequate sum of 2410 ducats, and El Greco had no choice but to contest their verdict. Eventually, after a bitter and protracted dispute which was taken beyond the archbishop's council to the papal nuncio in Madrid, he was ordered in June 1607 to settle for a sum not far removed from the initial fee. It was a disastrous verdict, playing a substantial part in the chronic debt problems that tormented him in his final years. El Greco had protested to the archbishop's council in December 1605 that 'the delay continues to cause me much damage and loss'[7] because of frozen payments and legal costs. But nothing prevented his cash flow from faltering so badly that he relied heavily on loans from his friends to save himself from bankruptcy.[8]

He was also greatly assisted by the patronage of his friend Dr Pedro Salazar de Mendoza, a learned canon who specialised in the history of Toledo. This enthusiastic connoisseur assembled a collection that included one of El Greco's outright masterpieces, the *View of Toledo* now in New York. In Mendoza's opinion, painting was an indispensable stimulus for the historian: his biography of Saint Ildefonso even declared that painting 'excited and

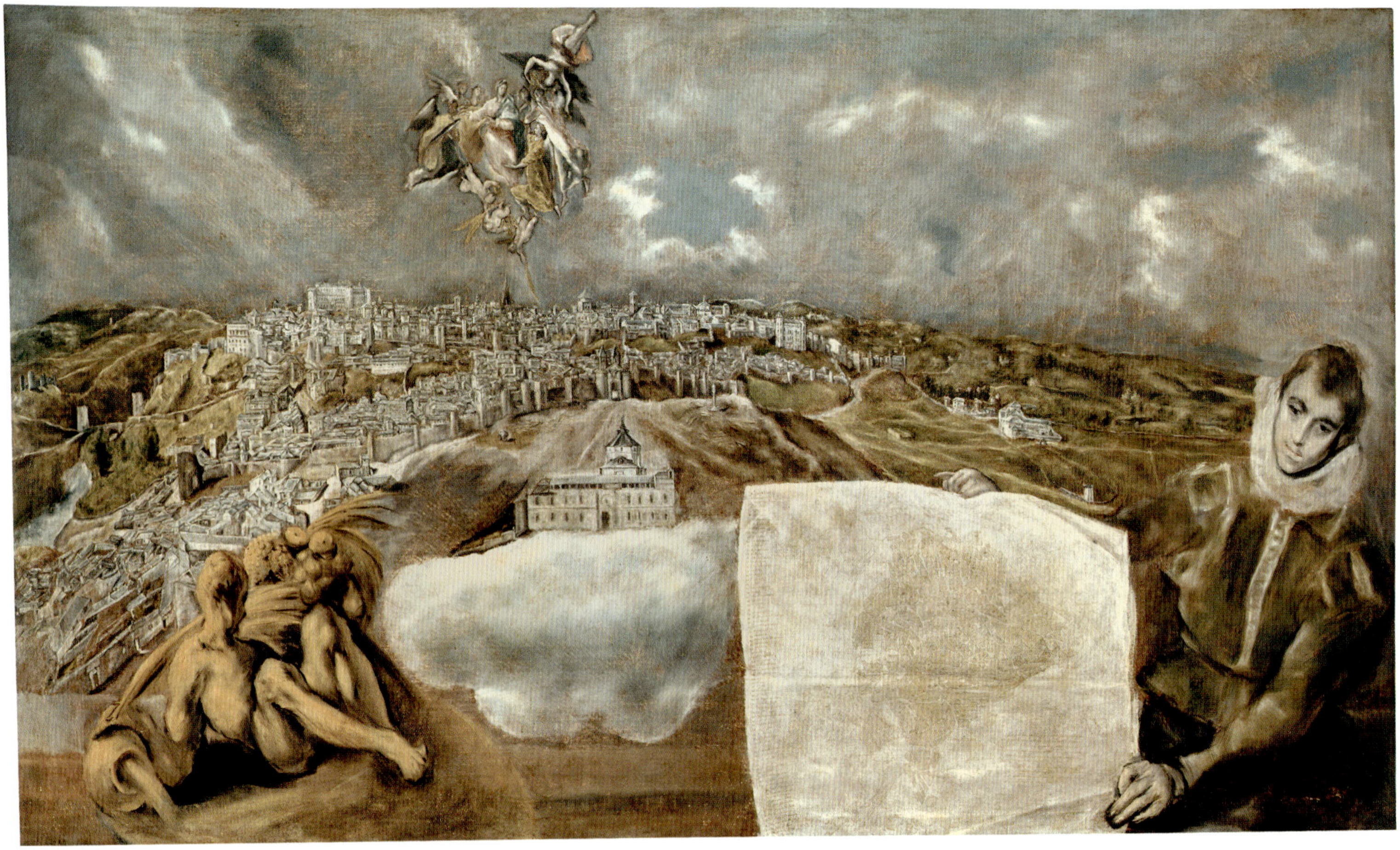

104 El Greco, *View and Plan of Toledo*, *c.*1610–14, Casa y Museo de El Greco, Toledo

roused the spirit more than writing'.[9] Mendoza was sufficiently 'roused' by El Greco's work to involve the painter in another important hospital project. As the administrator of the Hospital of Saint John the Baptist in Toledo, also known as the Hospital of Cardinal Tavera, he first asked the artist to make a gilded wood tabernacle with sculpture for the chapel. A *Risen Christ* and a section from the architectural structure survive, and Mendoza's satisfaction with the outcome of this commission probably led him to ask El Greco to paint the extraordinary *View and Plan of Toledo* (pl. 104).

Since Mendoza amassed an immense collection of maps and city views, he may well have played a considerable role in determining the content of this mysterious panorama. For the expanse of El Greco's adopted city is here juxtaposed with the explanatory map held up so surprisingly by a youth (who has often been identified as Jorge Manuel). The presence of the holy group in the sky confirms the importance attached by the artist to a pervasive religious presence, even when painting a canvas with no overt ecclesiastical subject-matter. He has defined the figures of the Virgin and angels bringing their chasuble to Saint Ildefonso with a prominence that defies aerial perspective, explaining in an inscription on the map that 'in order to justify making the figures large, I made use of the fact that they were in a certain way like celestial bodies and treated them like lights that, when seen from afar, appear to be large no matter how small they may really be'.[10] A different passage in the same inscription accounts for the other hallucinatory element in the painting – the inclusion of the Hospital of Saint John the Baptist, detached completely from the city itself and appearing to float on a cloud. This bizarre device was employed, according to El Greco, because the hospital would have obscured the view of the Bisagra Gate if represented in its true position. The decision to place the hospital on a cloud then prompted him, according to the inscription, to alter its position and present the facade to the viewer. These ingenious explanations should not obscure the fact that both Mendoza and El Greco were by this time united in their special concern for the hospital. Although represented in the painting as a building still under construction, it is depicted with great accuracy by an artist who had received in 1608 his final large commission for the main and side altars of the hospital's chapel.

Cardinal Juan de Tavera, whose posthumous portrait El Greco painted around this period with the aid of a death mask (pl. 105), was the founder of this charitable institution dedicated to the destitute sick.[11] He had died at the age of seventy-three, four years after founding the hospital in 1541. But as his portrait testifies with such mesmeric intensity, the Cardinal was also a powerful, determined and highly intelligent politician. While rising in the hierarchy of the Church to become primate of Spain in 1534, he acted as chief Counsellor to the Emperor Charles V and effectively ruled the country during his master's frequent absences.

Tavera, a noted humanist and patron of the arts, had ordained that part of his hospital should become a palace, and inside the massive, imposing building a suite of splendid rooms leads off the vestibule. Here, in surroundings where heads of state were often entertained, a collection of important paintings still bears witness to the role played by artists in the hospital's creation. The contribution of the architect Bramante was enriched by the participation of many other notable Spanish artists, including Berruguete, Covarrubias, the Vergeras, Villalpando and El Greco himself, working not only as a painter but also as sculptor and architect. In the hospital chapel Berruguete's portal, and above all the resplendent tomb of the Cardinal placed directly beneath the light-filled octagonal dome, are especially memorable. But El Greco's canvases constitute the finest single body of work commissioned by the hospital, for he intended the chapel to contain his last and most personal cycle of paintings.

Death prevented him from completing the project and most of the canvases he did produce have long since been dispersed to museums elsewhere in the world. The inventory drawn up when he died in 1614 provides some insights into the nature of the scheme, however, especially when taken in conjunction with a related document produced seven years later at the time of Jorge Manuel's second marriage. He had agreed to finish the venture and, although he never fulfilled his promise, the inventories prove that a *Baptism of Christ* was supposed to be installed in the chapel's high altar as 'the principal Baptism of the Hospital'.[12] Furthermore, references to 'two large sketched paintings for the side altars of the Hospital'[13] confirm that El Greco had commenced before his death an *Annunciation* and an *Apocalyptic Vision* which Jorge Manuel intended at one stage to complete. He never fully achieved that aim, becoming embroiled in a protracted lawsuit with the Hospital culminating in a lien against his assets. The paintings for the side altarpieces were cut down into separate pieces and sold, but he did finish his father's *Baptism of Christ* (pl. 106). It inhabited one of the side altars for several centuries, and the tumultuous composition induces a sense of exaltation that permeates the cycle as a whole.

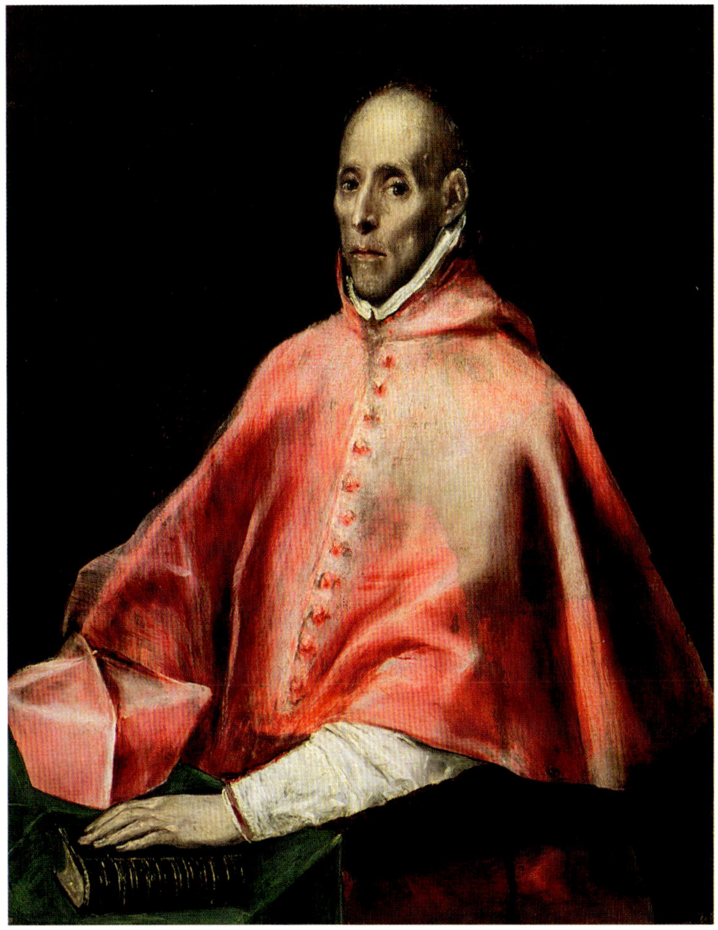

105 El Greco, *Cardinal Juan de Tavera*, c.1604, Hospital de Tavera, Toledo

The colour-tests clearly visible on both upright sides of the canvas provide a reminder that El

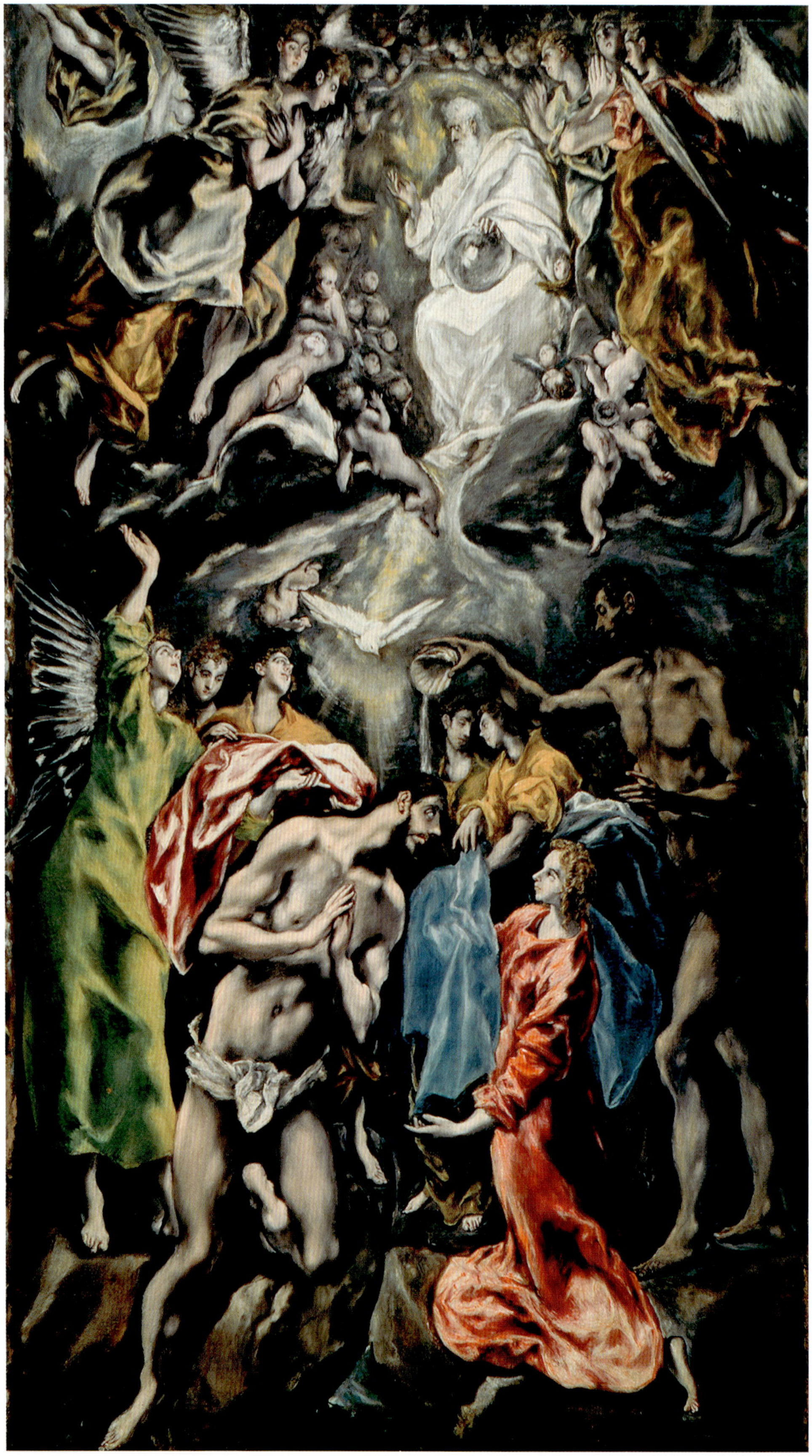

106 El Greco and Jorge Manuel, *Baptism of Christ*, *c.*1608–22, Hospital de Tavera, Toledo

Greco left the canvas incomplete at his death. Even so, these feathery strokes of paint also signify the extraordinary freedom and lightness of touch pervading El Greco's final productions. His quivering brushmarks dart and flicker with restless energy over the crowded canvas, where God and his angels fill the air with a motion that seems to press down on the scene below. The same *horror vacui* is evident there, for Christ and Saint John are surrounded by ecstatic attendants and burgeoning draperies that threaten to distract attention from the act of baptism itself.

A comparison with El Greco's earlier treatment of the theme, painted for the altarpiece of the College of Doña Maria de Aragon in 1596, discloses that the two principal figures in the hospital canvas are based on the first version. But the upper and lower halves of the design are now brought into greater unity by the dramatically upflung arm of the angel standing behind Christ, and God the Father in the sky adopts a more active role in the hospital picture. The earlier *Baptism* presents him as a kindly yet removed figure, quietly raising his finger in blessing, whereas he is subsequently transformed into a more vigorous agent of benediction who appears to drop a shower of light on the scene below.

No crowding affects the *Annunciation* (pl. 107), where an angel delivers the fateful message to the Virgin with nothing to impede their encounter. Desk, platform and receding floor-tiles are depicted with as much stark economy as the wall behind, and the whole room is handled in a manner so sparse that it must have been left in a very incomplete state at El Greco's death. Unlike the roundel of the same subject executed for the Illescas hospital (see pl. 101), the angel is now earthbound, and the Virgin leans towards her visitor as if impelled by the magnetic force of the arm gesturing in her direction. Moreover, the dove hovering above them seems to be attended by a retinue, and El Greco has also included seated figures of the Virtues in all their celestial magnificence at the top of the fragmented picture. Faith and Prudence can be discerned among this refulgent company, but the most important from the hospital's point of view is the personification of Charity.

They were originally joined to an upper section, which now forms a separate segment called *Concert of Angels* (pl. 108). Even in its sadly severed state it exudes the vitality of El Greco's final style, imparting to the throng of divine musicians a quicksilver exuberance. Variously absorbed in singing from choir books and playing a harpsichord, violin, flute and harp, the heavenly figures perform with such rapt expressiveness that even the garments clothing their bodies swirl and leap in flame-like transports of feeling. Compared with the far more solid, matter-of-fact angelic players painted by Memling for the *Saint Ursula Shrine* just over a century

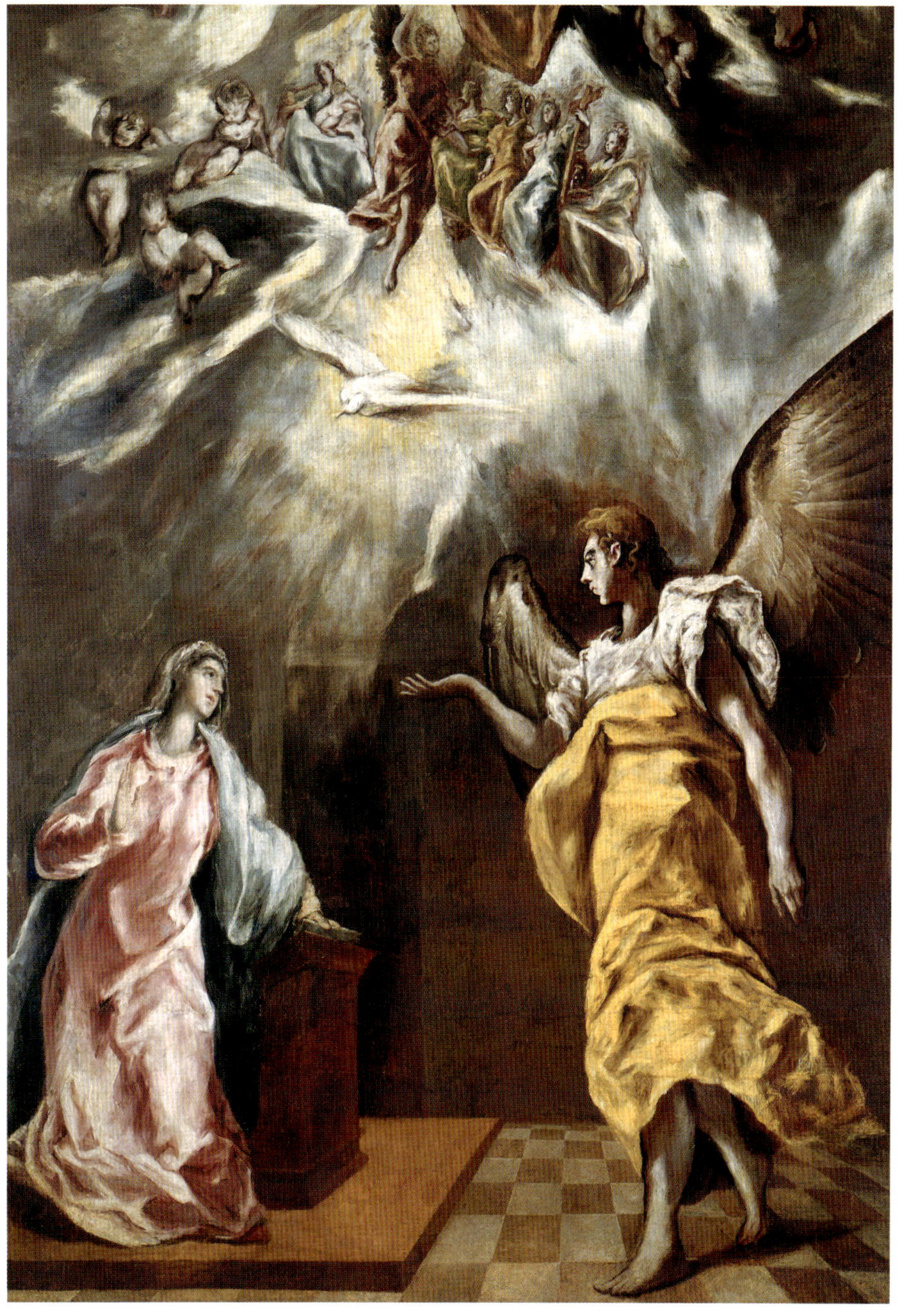

107 El Greco, *Annunciation*, *c.*1608–22, Private Collection

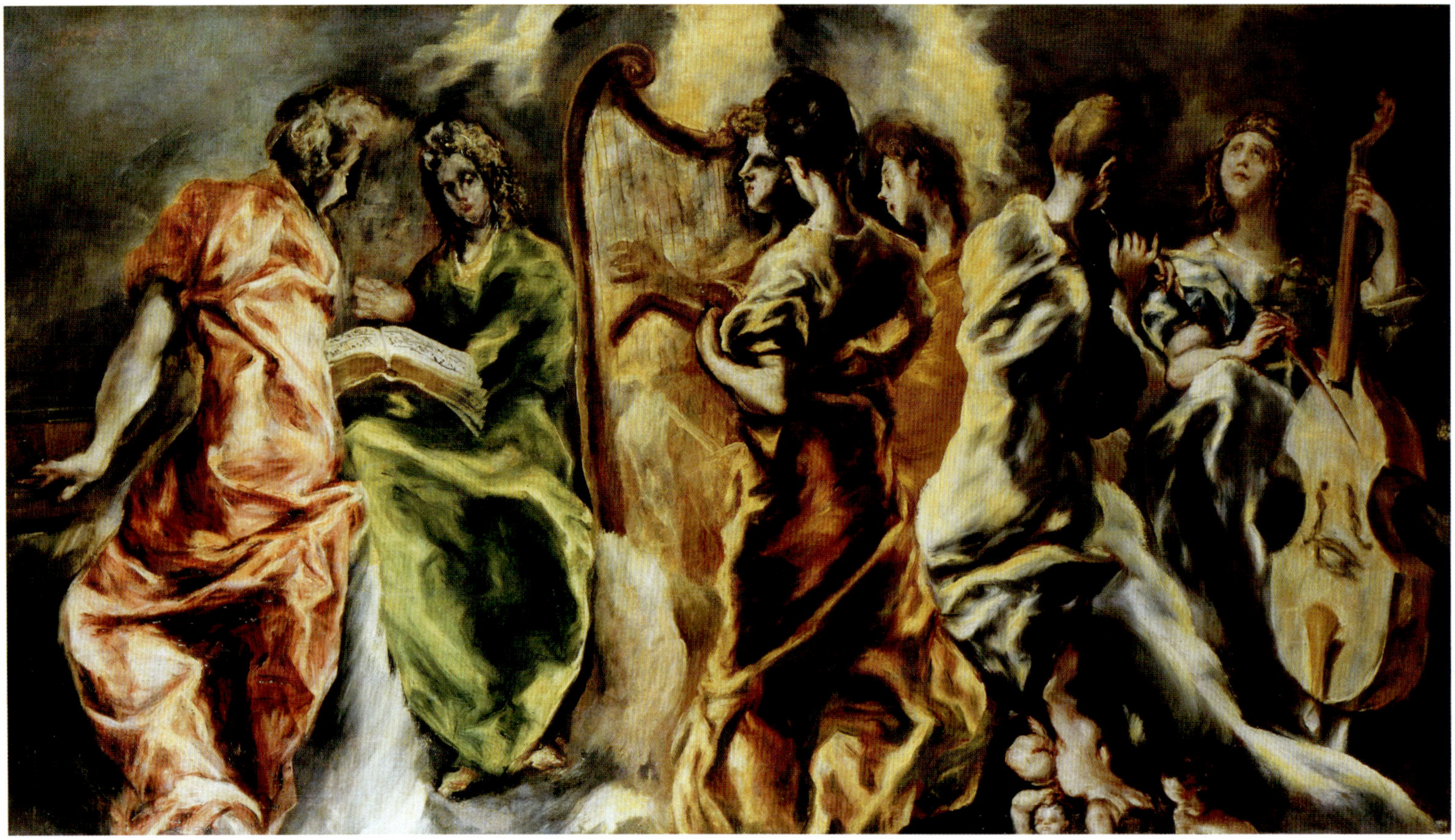

108 El Greco, *Concert of Angels*, *c.*1608–22, National Art Gallery, Athens

before (see pl. 63), these wraith-like apparitions seem to transcend all earthly constraints and inhabit a celestial realm.

A still more convulsive emotion charges the outstanding masterpiece of the cycle with an almost seismic fervency (pl. 109). *The Opening of the Fifth Seal (The Vision of Saint John)* may likewise have suffered the loss of its topmost section, as well as a narrow strip from the left side,[14] but the remaining canvas is still the most enthralling of all El Greco's late paintings, and profoundly impressed a whole range of radical twentieth-century artists from Picasso to Pollock.[15] The principal figures in both the *Baptism* and the *Annunciation* were weakened by Jorge Manuel's pedestrian intervention, but he does not seem to have worked on the *Opening of the Fifth Seal* at all. So, despite the cutting down of the canvas and extensive damage, this *tour de force* retains its original and arresting dynamism.

El Greco probably took as his starting point the passage in the Book of Revelation where the Lamb commands Saint John to witness the breaking of the seven seals:

> when he had opened the fifth seal, I saw under the altar the souls of them that were slain for the word of God, and for the testimony which they held: and they cried with a loud voice, saying, 'How long, O Lord, holy and true, does thou not judge and avenge our blood on them that dwell on the earth?' And white robes were given unto every one of them; and it was said unto them, that they should rest yet for a little season, until their fellow servants also and their brethren, that should be killed as they were, should be fulfilled.[16]

This heightened passage inspired the feverish emotion that gives El Greco's canvas its wild and unearthly excitement. Swaying with mystical rapture, his arms flung upwards in utter abandonment, Saint John's outsized presence dominates the event. His draperies possess a near-molten energy as they flow down his body and then rush in a crimson flood towards the arising martyrs. Their call for revenge on the world that slaughtered them can be counted among the most disturbing passages in the Bible, and El Greco gives the forms of the naked men on the right a flailing fury. Lit as much by inner passion as by the tempestuous white flashes streaking across the sky, their eerie whiteness gives the picture the unsettling quality of a nightmare. The rasping character of this phantasmal painting is envenomed by the acid-green sheet with which El Greco, in defiance of the 'white robes' described by Revelation, surrounds the tormented men. Only at the side of this drapery does one male figure stretch up to receive a white garment bestowed on him by a hovering putto. It is by no means clear that the man will be able to swathe himself in this purified clothing, and El Greco revels in the acute psychological tension generated by the air of uncertainty.

But beyond the writhing limbs, a far more consoling spectacle is defined at the centre of this turbulent canvas (see pl. 96). For here, positioned against a great curtain of gold, two women have been liberated from their graves. Gazing towards a male companion who seems about to clothe them in the glowing material, they embody the sense of astonishment that attends a rebirth. Rather than calling for the destruction of their oppressors on earth, they advance into the new life with shyness. It prompts them to place arms and hands over their breasts. Vulnerable and halting, like denizens of the dark dazed by their sudden emergence into the radiance and commotion surging all around them, they nevertheless succeed in asserting their newfound resilience with poised dignity.

El Greco gives their blanched yet shining bodies a greater brightness than any of the other figures in his painting, thereby ensuring that it is permeated, in the end, by a spirit of miraculous hope and wonder. For all the heady freedom of his galvanic painting, it remains very faithful to the beliefs governing a hospital where salvation was vouchsafed to the dying patients. Mendoza, who took an unusually close interest in the paintings he commissioned, and reserved the right to halt any unsatisfactory work in progress,[17] also gave his patients special indulgences allowing them to join the ranks of the resurrecting elect. No affirmation could be more heartening either for the artist, conscious no doubt of his own imminent death, or for the Tavera's stricken occupants as they gazed at his uncanny yet inspiriting vision.

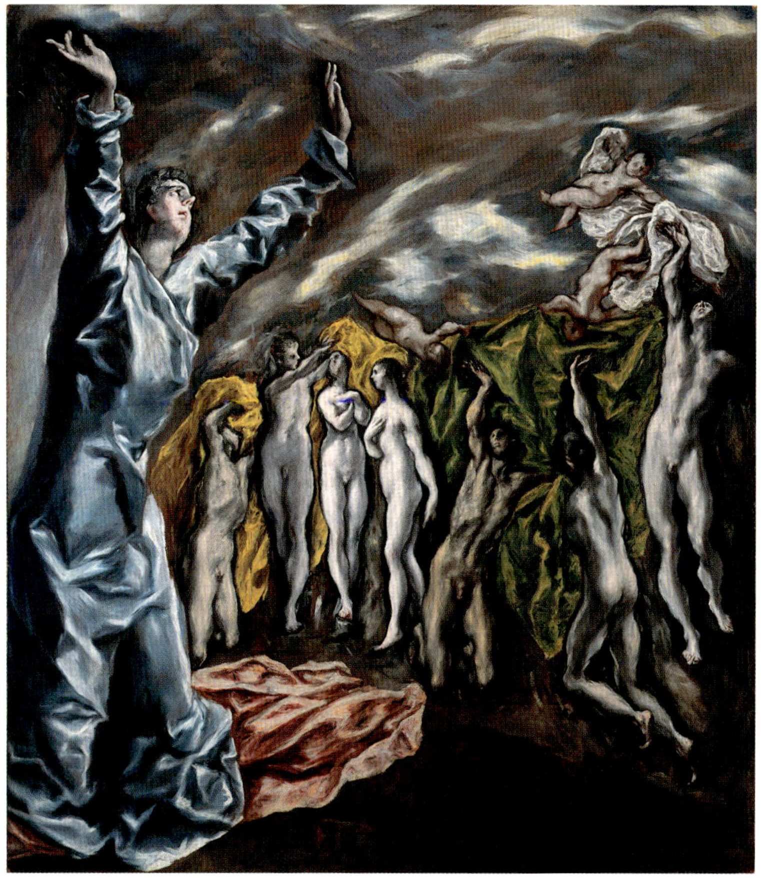

109 El Greco, *The Opening of the Fifth Seal (The Vision of Saint John)*, 1608–14, Metropolitan Museum of Art, New York, Rogers Fund, 1956

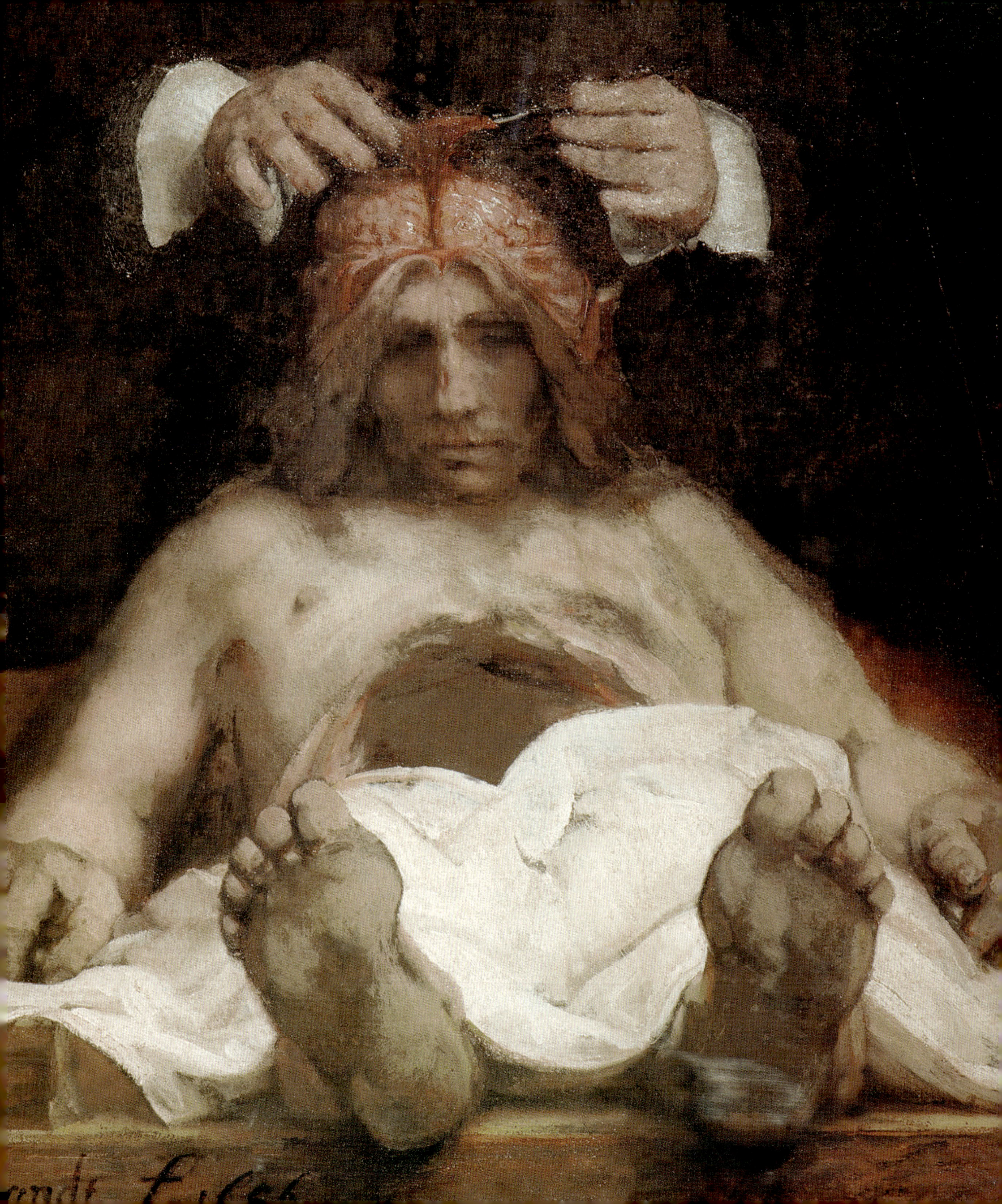

NINE
THE ANATOMIST'S KNIFE AND REGENTS' CHARITY

In seventeenth-century Holland, paintings and sculpture were displayed in many of the almshouses created to shelter and care for the destitute. Joost-Cornelis Droochsloot's large canvas, showing the halt and blind summoned to the rich man's feast (pl. 111), is typical of the pictures still to be found on display in these buildings. Droochsloot identifies himself as a member of the unfortunate crowd in this painting, thereby implying his awareness that ill-health or financial ruin might oblige him, one day, to rely on the largesse of a wealthy philanthropist. He would have drawn reassurance from the fact that there were an increasing number of such sources to choose from. Simon Schama has described how 'the profusion and magnificence of charitable institutions in the Netherlands' derived part of its momentum from the realisation that, 'where elites governed by suasion rather than coercion, philanthropic donation on a large and obligatory scale was a small price to pay for cushioning themselves against the threat of popular revolt'.[1]

The prodigious flowering of Dutch painting during the century enabled many artists to convey a variety of conflicting atttitudes towards the medical profession. The most positive aspect of physicians' burgeoning status was celebrated in their official group portraits. As Jakob Rosenberg explained, 'no other country in Europe developed this type of portraiture and this fact makes it a strong national manifestation of Holland's culture'.[2] Over in London Holbein had, admittedly, provided an imposing precedent for a large-scale portrayal of the medical establishment in his iconic late painting, where Henry VIII grants the Royal Charter to representatives of both the Barbers' Company and the Guild of Surgeons who united in 1540 (pl. 112). But the stiffness of the image, probably completed after Holbein's untimely death and then damaged in the Great Fire of London,[3] stresses the Barber-Surgeons' collective subservience to their overweening monarch.

Holland lacked an absolute sovereign, so Rembrandt was able to concentrate on the surgeons as an autonomous group when he painted, almost a century after Holbein, *The Anatomy Lesson of Dr Nicolaes Tulp* (pl. 114). In this ambitious canvas, commissioned by the Amsterdam Guild of Surgeons, he broke away resoundingly from the rigid, conservative format adhered to not only by Holbein but also by Dutch artists like Aert Pietersz, Thomas de Keyser and Michael Janszen van Miereveldt. Painted as early as 1601–3, Pietersz's *The Anatomy Lesson of Dr Sebastian Egbertsz* is a crude affair, showing row upon row of attendant figures who threaten to block the view of the corpse. Perhaps, at such a formative stage in the

110 (*facing page*) Detail of pl. 116

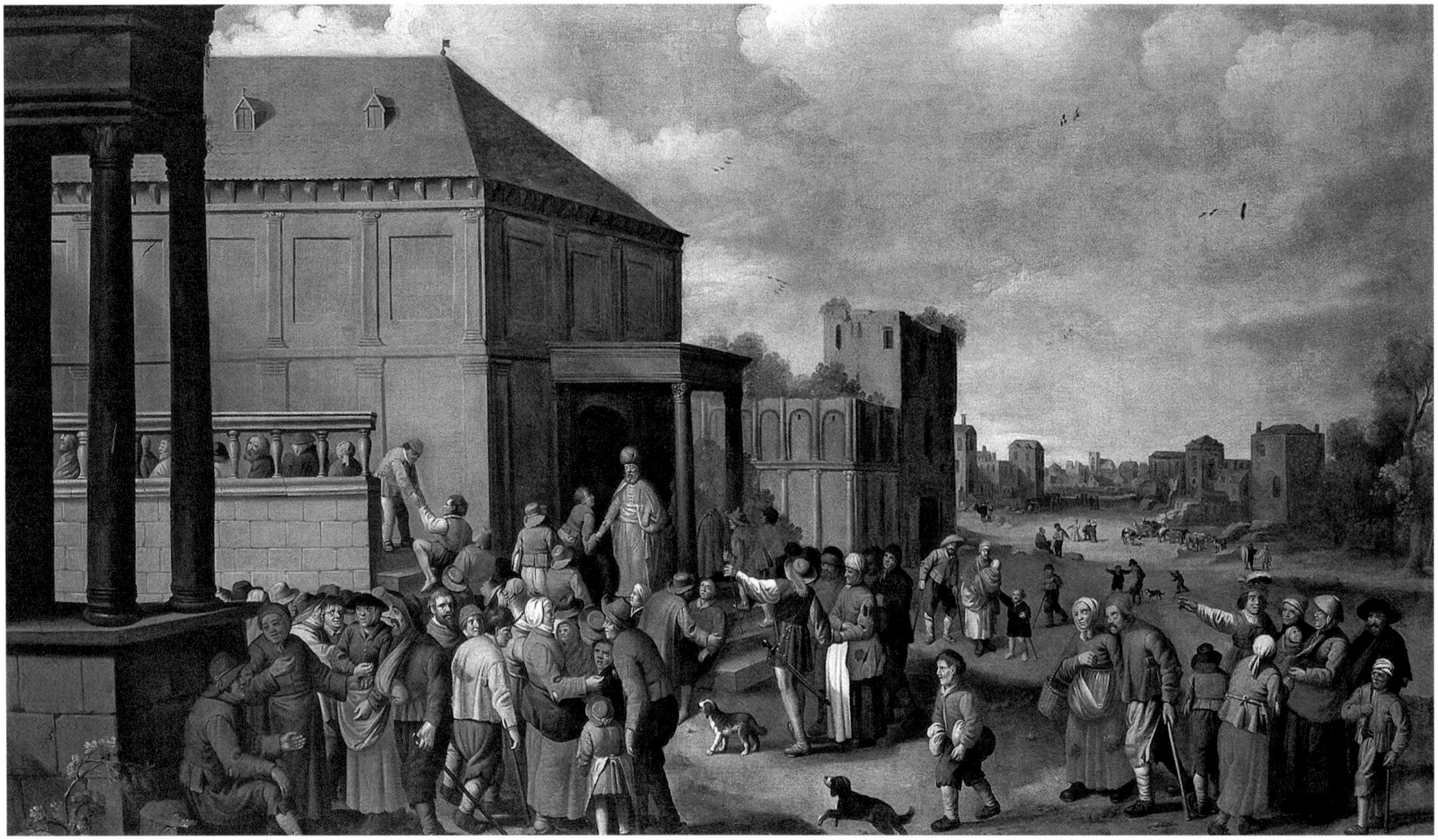

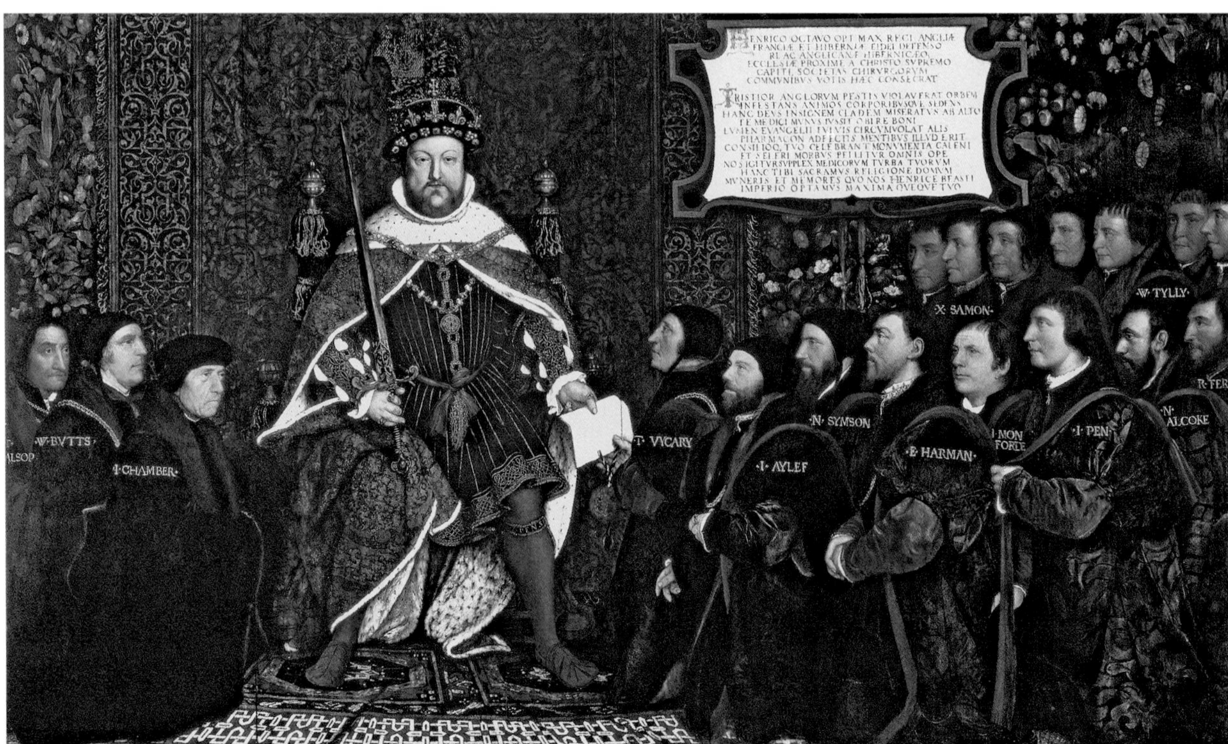
HENRICO OCTAVO OPT MAX REGI ANGLIÆ
FRANCIÆ ET HIBERNIÆ FIDEI DEFENSO
RI AC ANGLICANÆ HIBERNICÆQ
ECCLESIÆ PROXIME A CHRISTO SVPREMO
CAPITI SOCIETAS CHIRVRGORVM
COMMVNIBVS VOTIS HÆC CONSECRAT
TRISTIOR ANGLORVM PESTIS VIOLAVERAT ORBEM
INFESTANS ANIMOS CORPORIBVSQVE SEDENS
HANC DEVS INSIGNEM CLADEM MISERATVS AB ALTO
TE MEDICI MVNVS IVSSIT OBIRE BONI
LVMEN EVANGELII FVLVIS CIRCVMVOLAT ALIS
PHARMACON ADFECTIS MENTIBVS ILLVD ERIT
CONSILIOQ TVO CELEBRANT MONVMENTA GALENI
ET CELERI MORBVS PELLITVR OMNIS OPE
NOS IGITVR SVPPLEX MEDICORVM TVRBA TVORVM
HANC TIBI SACRAMVS RELIGIONE DOMVM
MVNERIS ET MEMORES QVO NOS HENRICE BEASTI
IMPERIO OPTAMVS MAXIMA QVEQVE TVO
W. BVTTS
I. CHAMBER
T. VICARY
I. AYLEF
N. SYMSON
E. HARMAN
I. MONFORDE
I. PEN
N. ALCOKE
X. SAMON
W. TYLLY
R. FEREIS

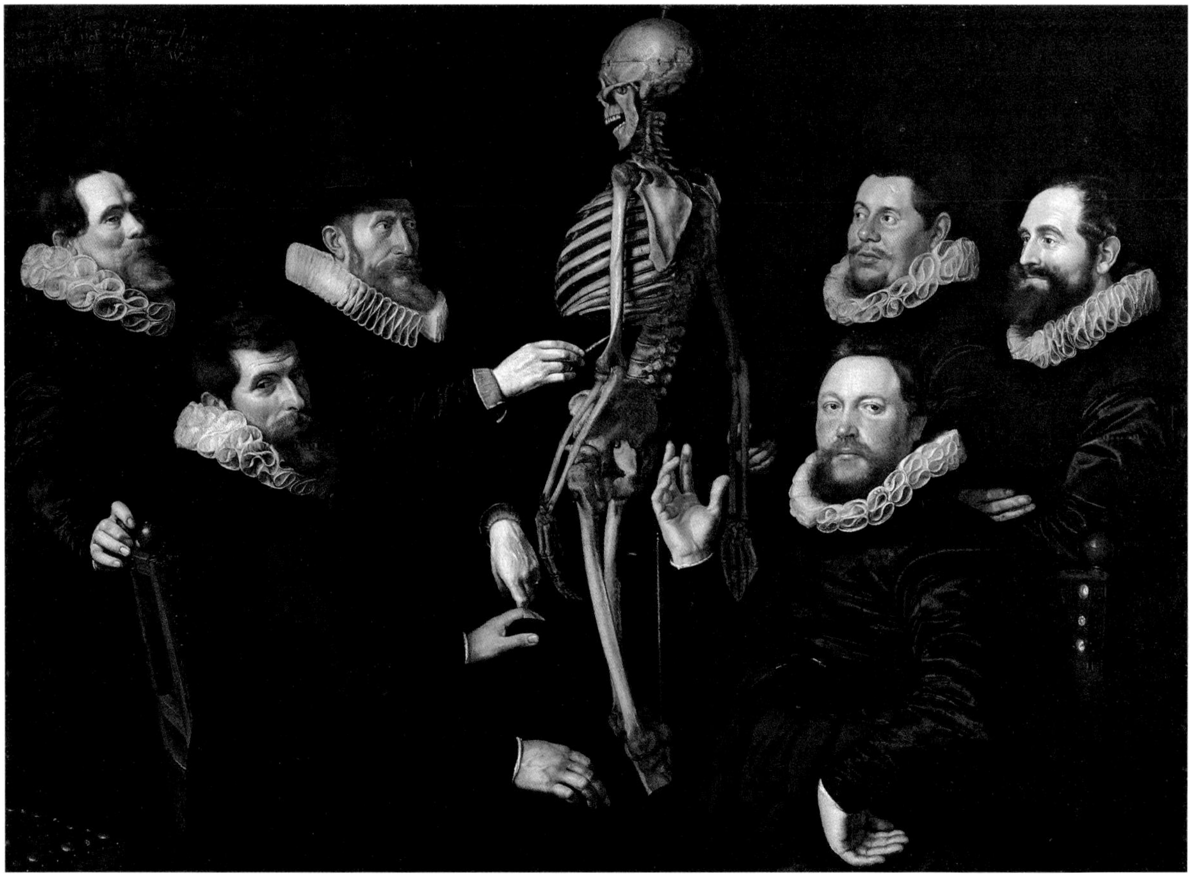

113 (*left*) Nicolaes Eliasz Pickenoy, *Osteology Lesson of Dr Sebastian Egbertsz*, 1619, Amsterdam Museum

development of these group portraits, surgeons and artists alike felt wary of exposing the dead body in too much unsettling detail. Nicolaes Eliasz Pickenoy was less inhibited when dealing with a skeleton in his dramatic *Osteology Lesson of Dr Sebastian Egbertsz* (pl. 113) where the same doctor expounds the mysteries of human bone structure to a far smaller and incisively portrayed audience. But most of them are smiling, devoid of the astonishment and awe that Rembrandt uncovered in his painting. He would never have made the mistake perpetrated by van Miereveldt, whose *Anatomy Lesson of Dr Willem van der Meer* in Delft Hospital dissipates the potential drama by allowing too many of the observers to stare out at the painter, posing blatantly for their portraits rather than attending to the gruesome slicing of the corpse.

Rejecting such stiffness, Rembrandt transformed the learned medical lecture into a momentous event (pl. 114). Dr Tulp's audience gathers eagerly, and almost breathlessly, around the corpse of Adriaen Adriaensz. (Aris) 't Kint of Leiden, a multiple offender who had been found guilty of stealing a coat and executed at the end of January 1632. Tulp was pre-eminent in his field as Praelector Anatomiae in the Guild of Surgeons, so the sense of expectation would have been high. The onlookers' expressions, ranging from curiosity to the most devouring wonder, emphasise the excitement attending a mesmeric demonstration only held once or twice a year. Even the man occupying such a prominent place in the foreground, turning away from the cadaver to acknowledge the viewers' gaze, seems unwilling to take his attention away from the lesson for long. The blanched, curiously shining corpse possesses a magnetic and eerie fascination. But the calm figure of Dr Tulp, demonstrating with his instrument the actions of the arm-muscles revealed in the dissection, conducts the lesson with the solemnity of a priest performing a religious ceremony.

The theological implications of the scene were by no means a fanciful interpretation on Rembrandt's part. As Gary Schwartz has shown, Tulp

111 (*facing page, top*) Joost-Cornelis Droochsloot, *Halt and Blind at the Rich Man's Feast*, c.1625, Wellcome Collection, London

112 (*facing page, bottom*) Hans Holbein, *Henry VIII Granting Royal Charter to the Barbers' Company and the Guild of Surgeons*, 1541, Barber-Surgeons' Hall, London

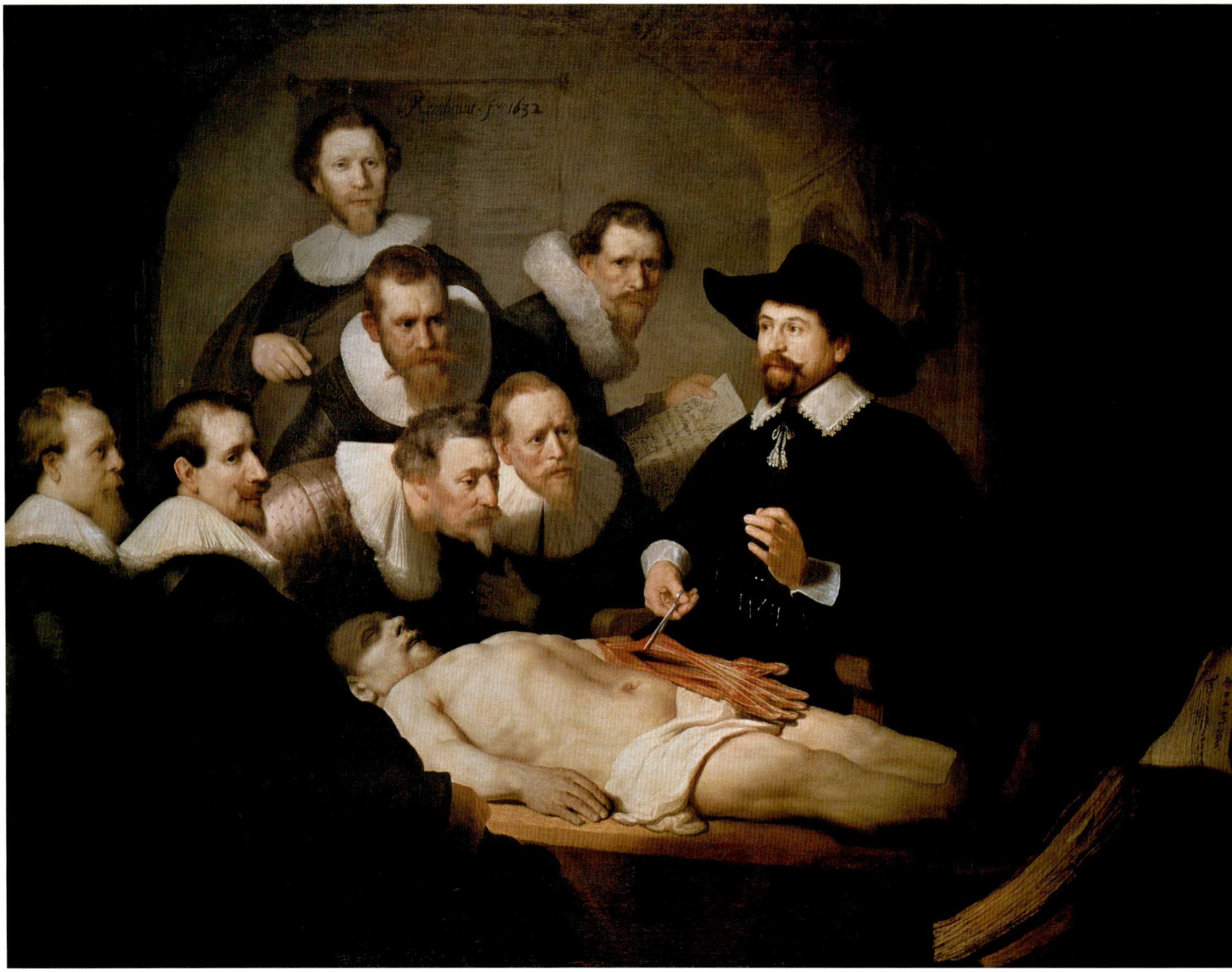

114 Rembrandt, *Anatomy Lesson of Dr Nicolaes Tulp*, 1632, The Hague, Mauritshuis

himself considered public dissection to be a demonstration 'of the sympathy between body and soul'.[4] The surgeon was even seen as a man capable of providing humanity with a greater insight into God. When a Dutch translation of an anatomical treatise by Bartholomaeus Cabrious was published, Joost van den Vondel wrote a poem in 1633 declaring that the book would enlighten '[Him] who seeks to comprehend / From beginning until end / What our human skins encase, / What keeps all our parts in place, / How the wisdom of the Lord obtains / Throughout our nerves, throughout our veins.' The poem concluded that Cabrious's treatise should help the reader / 'To know himself and then proceed / To knowledge of God's nature too.'[5]

In this respect, leading medical practitioners were almost as close to religious truth as church authorities, and they were portrayed in the seventeenth century as men of formidable learning. Rubens, whose *Tribute Money* had provided Rembrandt with the starting point for *Anatomy Lesson of Dr Nicolaes Tulp*, painted Lodovicus Nonnius as a distinguished sage around this time (pl. 115).[6] An Antwerp doctor and antiquarian of Portuguese descent, Nonnius wrote several books including the *Diaeteticon*, now considered to be the earliest work to discuss diet as a crucial factor in the maintenance of health. Rubens places him in an elevated architectural setting where his head is framed by an impressive niche, and places a shelf of books very prominently by his side. A marble bust of Hippocrates dignifies the sitter still further, investing him with a classical *gravitas*, and Nonnius is shown holding a conspicuously large volume on his lap. Rather than regarding it complacently, however, he engages in an active dialogue with the words it contains. Caught in a moment of animated exposition, the eminent doctor gestures towards the book so vigorously that it seems in danger of falling from his grasp.

No such dynamism can be found in the hands of Dr Joan Deyman (pl. 116), who succeeded Tulp as Praelector Anatomiae of the Amsterdam surgeons' guild in 1653. Three years later, when Rembrandt applied for a form of bankruptcy, the guild commissioned him to paint Deyman conducting an anatomy lesson. The fragment that survived a disastrous fire in 1723 shows how steadily his fingers carried out the delicate task of dissecting the corpse's brain with a scalpel. Deyman's head and the figures who once gathered round him were destroyed in the fire, yet Rembrandt's preliminary drawing (pl. 117) reveals that the doctor was originally attended by an audience as rapt as the figures peering at Tulp's demonstration. This time, however, Rembrandt presented the whole event in a formal and symmetrical way, emphasising the high seriousness of Deyman's actions. With the audacity and directness of a painter far more radical than he had been twenty years before, Rembrandt allowed the cadaver to extend towards the spectators. We are granted a wholly disconcerting view of his hollowed-out stomach and, above all, the brain itself spreading like strands of matted hair down either side of the dead man's face (see pl. 110).

It should be a grim spectacle, yet Rembrandt succeeds in giving the whole macabre scene a sacramental dimension. The corpse, that of a criminal called Joris Fonteijn of Diest who had been hanged for breaking into a draper's shop and pulling a knife on his apprehender,[7] is ultimately based on Mantegna's *Dead Christ*.[8] In Rembrandt's painting the foreshortening is equally steep, the feet even more prominent. But the most important outcome of Rembrandt's reliance on a *quattrocento* prototype lay in the religious dimension it gave to his painting. The inert, partly dismembered Fonteijn takes on the pathos of the crucified body in a Lamentation. Deyman's assistant, Gysbrecht Matthijsz. Calcoen, a Master of the Guild of Surgeons, stares down at the corpse with the sadness of a man meditating on the transience of human life. Holding the upper dome of the skull in his left hand, while taking care to turn his right palm and fingers away from the blood-spurting corpse,[9] he reflects like Hamlet at Yorick's grave on the final frailty of man.

If Deyman's entire figure had survived, he would surely assume a hieratic significance. Since the

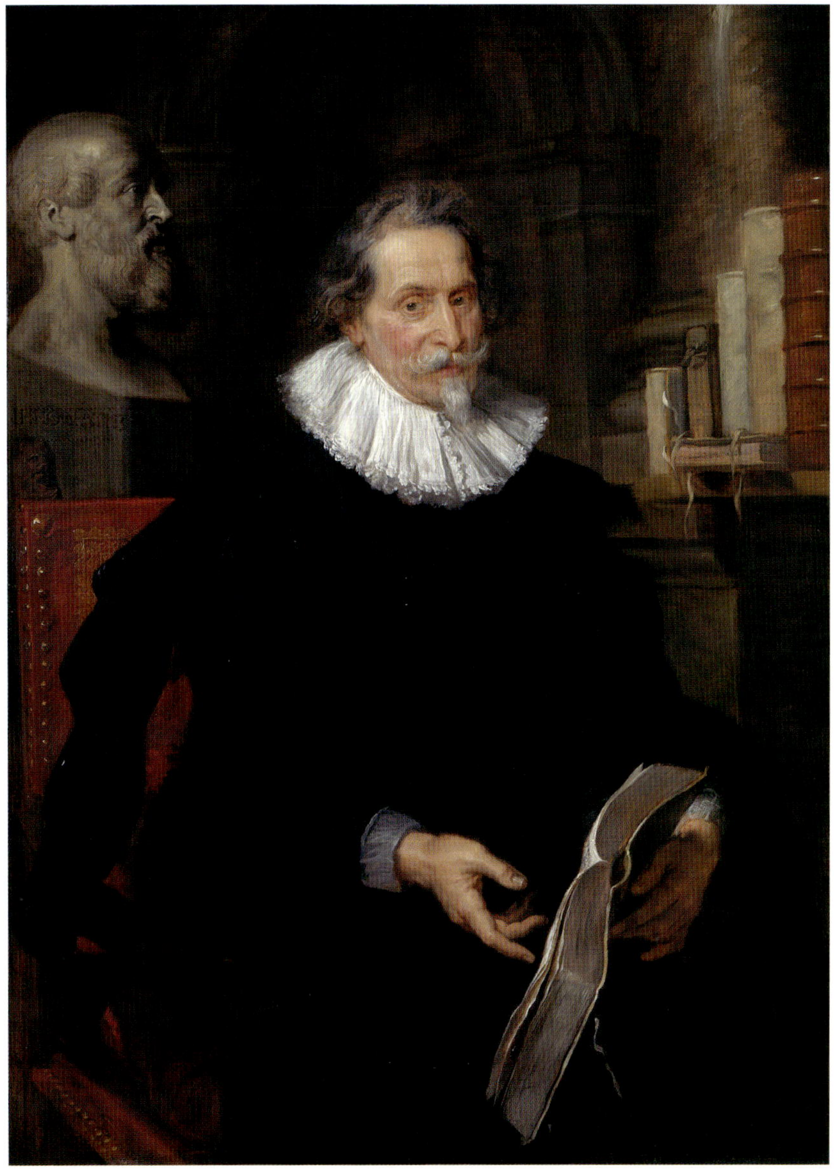

115 Rubens, *Lodovicus Nonnius*, *c.*1627, National Gallery, London

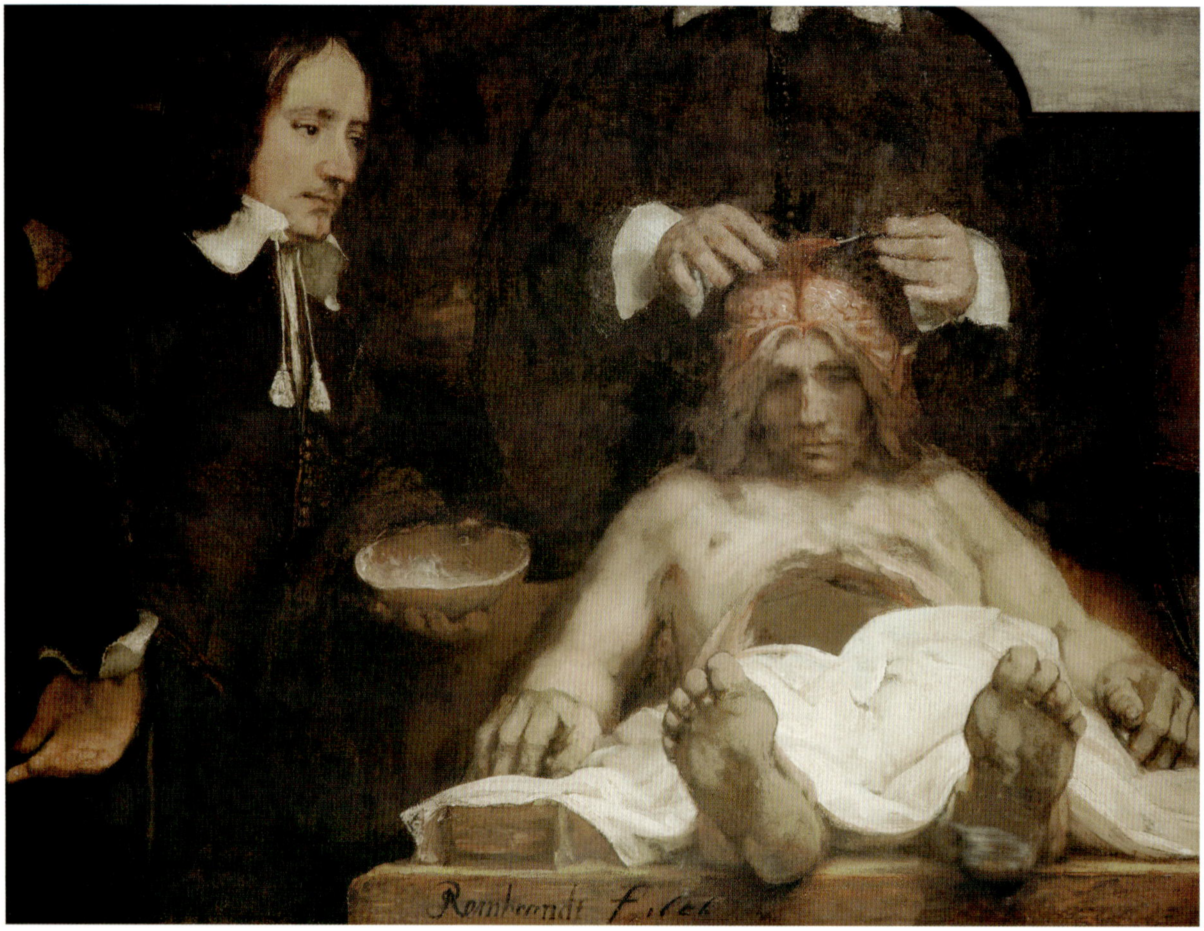

116 Rembrandt, *Anatomy Lesson of Dr Joan Deyman*, 1656, Amsterdam Museum

Dutch believed that dissection engendered a greater awareness of God's identity, an examination of brain tissues was tantamount to probing the very workings of His mind. Brain dissections were rare and the only other Dutch painting of the event is Nicolaas Rijnenburg's *The Anatomy Lesson of Dr Theodore Hoogeveen*, where the anatomist carries out his lesson in front of seventeen colleagues. But Rembrandt may well have been able to observe the dissection at first hand. He also had probable access to a copy of Vesalius's *De Humani corporis fabrica, Libri septem*, for the edition published in Basle by Joannes Oporinus contains an extensive sequence of cranial illustrations delineated with clinical clarity. Once complete, the Deyman painting was installed in the anatomical theatre of Amsterdam, situated appropriately enough on the upper floor of a small meat market building, formerly Saint Margaret's Church.[10] Hung on the other side of the fireplace to Rembrandt's earlier image of Dr Tulp,[11] its quietly ritualistic aura must have convinced onlookers that Deyman enjoyed a mystical ability to commune with the Holy Father and comprehend the most unfathomable enigmas of mortal existence.

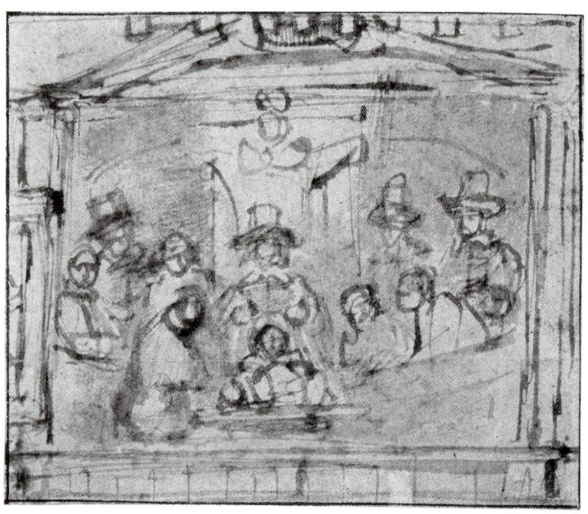

117 Rembrandt, Preliminary drawing for *Anatomy Lesson of Dr Joan Deyman*, 1656, Amsterdam Museum

Rembrandt's paintings become even more profound and compelling when compared with two

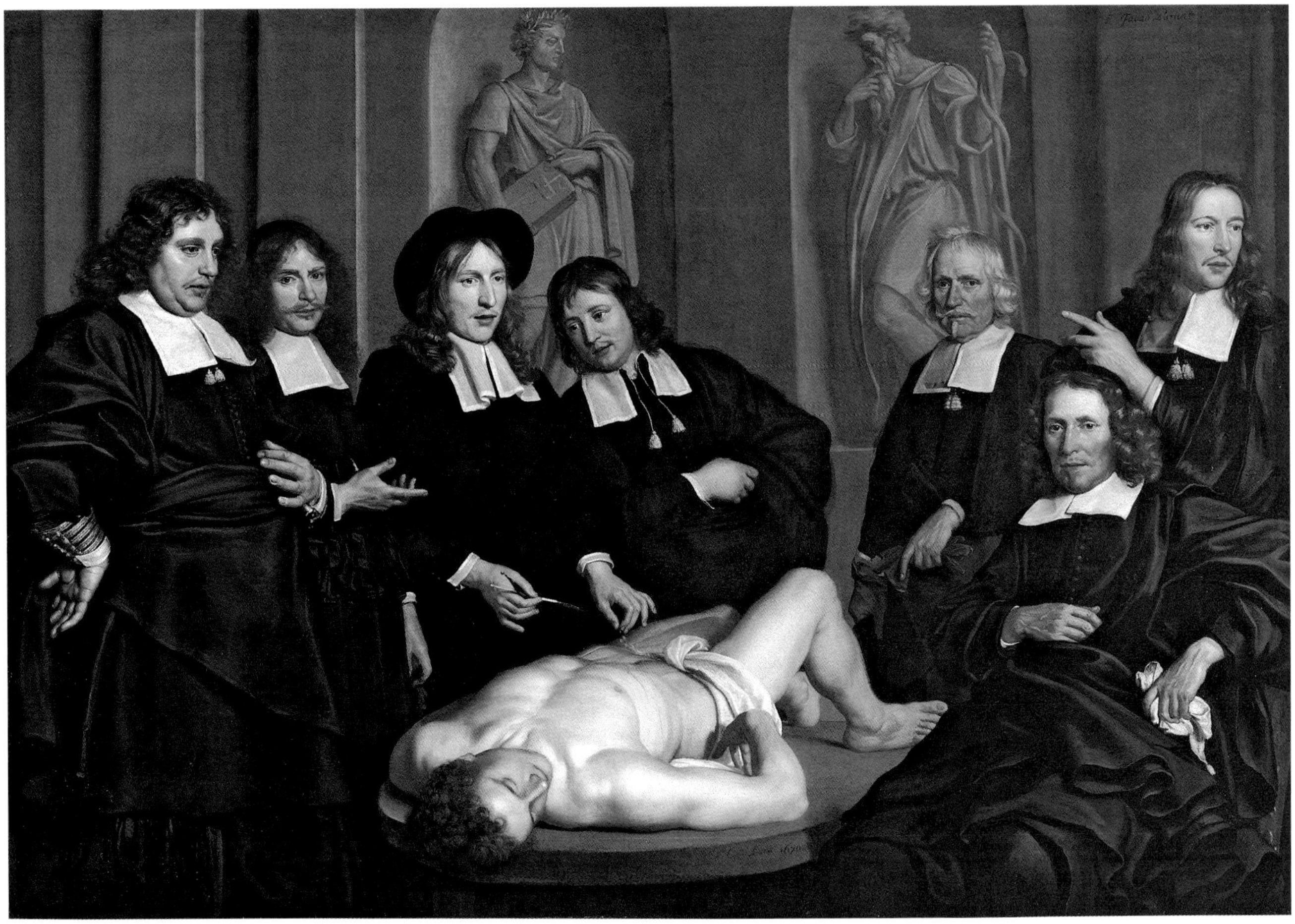

118 Adriaen Backer, *Anatomy Lesson of Dr Frederik Ruysch*, 1670, Ansterdam Museum

later attempts to paint anatomy lessons in seventeenth-century Holland. They both centre on the celebrated Dr Frederik Ruysch, the Praelector in Amsterdam between 1667 and 1731. He was particularly renowned for his preparations of 'babes in bottles', the carefully prepared remains of foetuses and babies preserved in glass jars. To our eyes they appear macabre, even ghoulish. But Ruysch's contemporaries hailed him as a doctor capable of bestowing immortality on small, defenceless humans who had died before their time. In his *Thesaurus animalium primus*, a book with painstaking yet bizarre illustrations of jars containing fish, hands and other specimens, a poem declares: 'Through thy art, O Ruysch, / a dead infant lives and teaches / and, though speechless, still speaks. / Even death itself is afraid.' When Adriaen Backer painted *The Anatomy Lesson of Dr Frederik Ruysch* in 1670 (pl. 118), he showed the young Praelector cutting with great delicacy into the leg of a strangely idealised, beautiful young man. Ruysch looks very pleased with himself and the men witnessing his feat seem more determined to pose for the painter than learn the mysteries of the human body. It is a thoroughly anodyne, self-congratulatory affair, entirely lacking Rembrandt's sense of melancholy and unfathomable mystery.

The same complacency affects Jan van Neck's *Anatomy Lesson of Dr Frederik Ruysch* thirteen years later. This time, a dead baby still attached to his placenta is the object of concern. Ruysch plucks at the umbilical cord with fastidious theatricality and everyone else appears equally smug. Only Ruysch's son appears tense as he clasps the base supporting one of his father's mounted skeletons of a baby. No wonder the boy appears somewhat haunted: he grew up dominated by the obsessions of a man who, by dint of ceaseless injections and embalming, built up a much admired cabinet of curiosities. An engraving in Ruysch's book shows his gruesome landscape tableau of injected vessels, stones and infant skeletons, two of whom touch their own

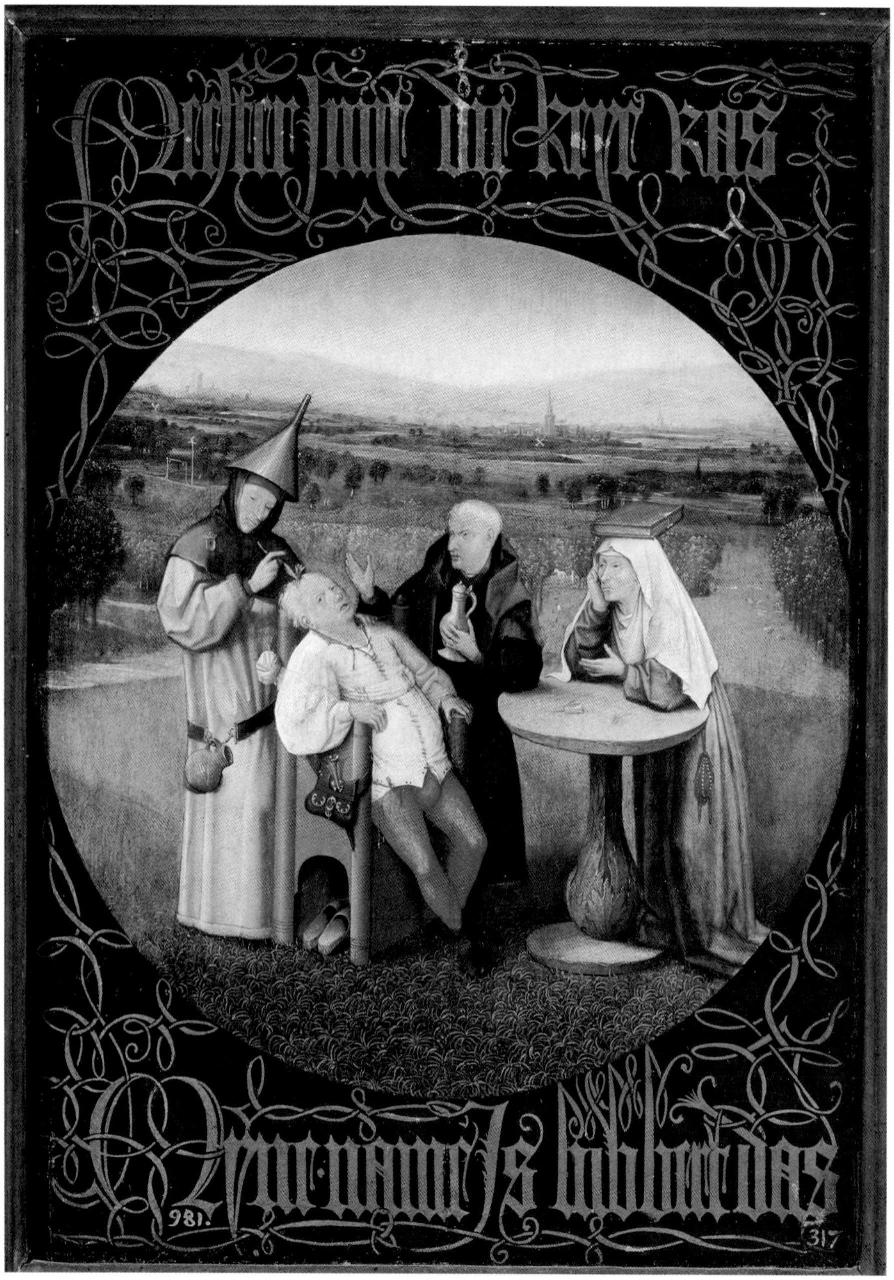

119 (*above*) Hieronymus Bosch, *The Operation for the Stone (The Cure of Folly)*, *c.*1494, Prado, Madrid

120 (*facing page*) Jan Steen, *The Doctor's Visit*, 1660–65, Philadelphia Museum of Art

skulls and eye-sockets with a mournful sense of wonder. Visitors crowded the museum he created in Amsterdam and Peter the Great had to pay Ruysch an enormous price for the whole collection before transporting it to St Petersburg in 1717.

To counter this elevated image of the medical profession, Dutch painting of the period also offers a cornucopia of genre scenes that rejoice in satirising doctors unmercifully. They follow in the tradition of earlier paintings as uninhibited as Hieronymus Bosch's *The Operation for the Stone (The Cure of Folly)* (pl. 119), where a fraudulent master-surgeon wears a preposterous funnel on his head as he slices into the skull of a man suffering from catastrophic gullibility. Foremost among the many seventeenth-century artists who regarded doctors with a similarly subversive disdain – an unrepentant array including Gabriel Metsu, Gerard Dou, Godfried Schalcken and Michiel van Musscher – one painter took a particular delight in the subject. Jan Steen, possibly prompted by motives of revenge after suffering at the hands of an incompetent physician, executed at least eighteen paintings on the theme of the doctor's visit.[12]

They all concentrate on a young woman plagued by nothing more sinister than lovesickness or pregnancy, and in the version (pl. 120) now owned by Philadelphia Museum of Art, her pulse is probably quickened by the arrival of the young man at the door. A maid beckons him in with her conspiratorial finger, while on the other side of the room a ribald figure holds up a herring. This chorus-like presence, who bears a resemblance to Steen himself, laughs lewdly as he dangles the symbol of folly and licentiousness from his fingers. The herring may well signify that the woman has been impregnated by her lover, for the piece of ribbon smouldering in the brazier was a favoured quack method of identifying pregnancy. All this Shrovetide levity seems lost on the doctor, however. A fatuously old-fashioned figure, garbed in a costume representing a weird amalgam of sixteenth- and early seventeenth-century styles, he contrasts with the other *dramatis personae* in their contemporary clothes. Moreover, the pomposity with which he leans over his patient and stares melodramatically into her face has the outsize absurdity of a character from the *commedia dell'arte*. This buffoon could have stepped onto the stage of a Molière comedy like *L'Amour médecin*, *Le Malade imaginaire* or *Le Médecin malgré lui*, plays which all provide the connection between Steen's doctor types and their Italian precedents. Rather than dignifying himself with learning, like Tulp or Rubens's Nonnius, his antiquated love of pedantic attitudes blinds him to the reality behind the maladies he pretends to diagnose.

Not that everyone in Holland relished this derisive attitude towards the medical profession. Jacob van Ruisdael, who became one of the most innovative of seventeenth-century Dutch landscapists, was encouraged by his father Isaack to study

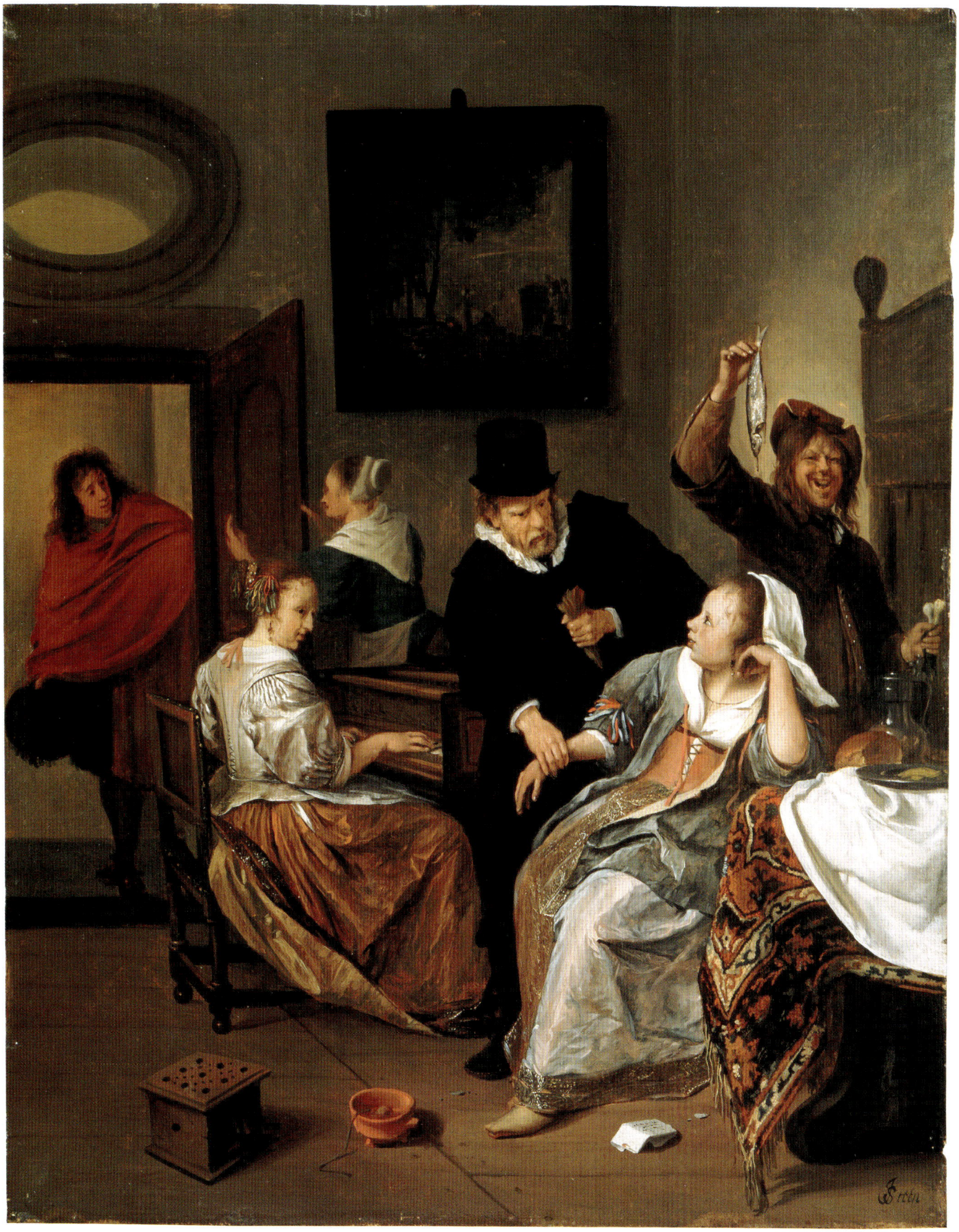

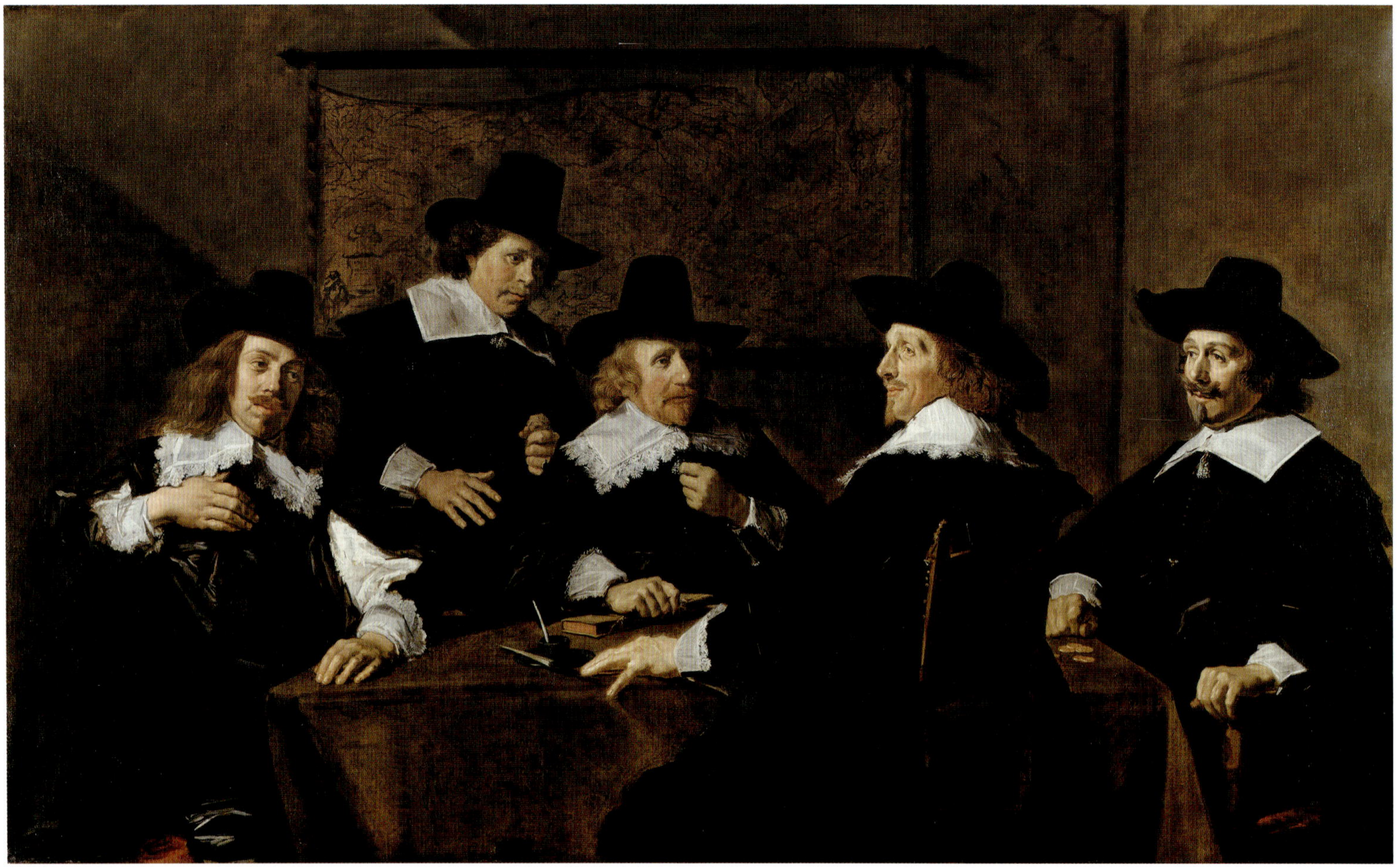

121 Frans Hals, *The Regents of the St Elizabeth Hospital of Haarlem*, 1641, Frans Hals Museum, Haarlem, on loan from the Elizabeth Hospital

medicine. Arnold Houbraken, Ruisdael's earliest biographer, recounts how Isaack's advice impelled young Jacob to pursue medicine so far that he performed several surgical operations in Amsterdam and gained a wide reputation. Isaack was an unsuccessful artist and saw medicine as a better alternative for his son.

Although Jacob did not, in the end, follow his father's advice, he probably maintained a great respect for the medical cause. And when Frans Hals painted *The Regents of the Saint Elizabeth Hospital of Haarlem* (pl. 121), he produced an image calculated to generate confidence in the acumen and nobility of the men gathered round the table. Jean Leymarie has argued that the painting marks 'a turning-point' in Hals's career,[13] and it certainly moves decisively away from the swashbuckling manner he had brandished in earlier group portraits. Instead of crowding the canvas with a plethora of banqueting officers, as he had done in the virtuoso canvases of 1616 and 1627, the sixty-year-old painter now adopts a more sober alternative. The governors' monochromatic dress encouraged an austere approach, far removed from the gaudy interplay of flags, swords, sashes and plumes that gave his youthful paintings of civic guard festivities so much of their animation. There, everything was exuberant, ostentatious and punctuated by gestures signalling the officers' consciousness of an audience. Most of them looked outwards, eager to show off their accoutrements with shameless pride, whereas the governors of the Saint Elizabeth Hospital eschew swaggering display altogether.

Even the man on the left, who places one hand rather self-consciously on his chest and seems less involved in the discussion than his companions, directs his gaze towards the table. Everyone else seems gravely absorbed in thinking about their administrative duties. The governor seen from

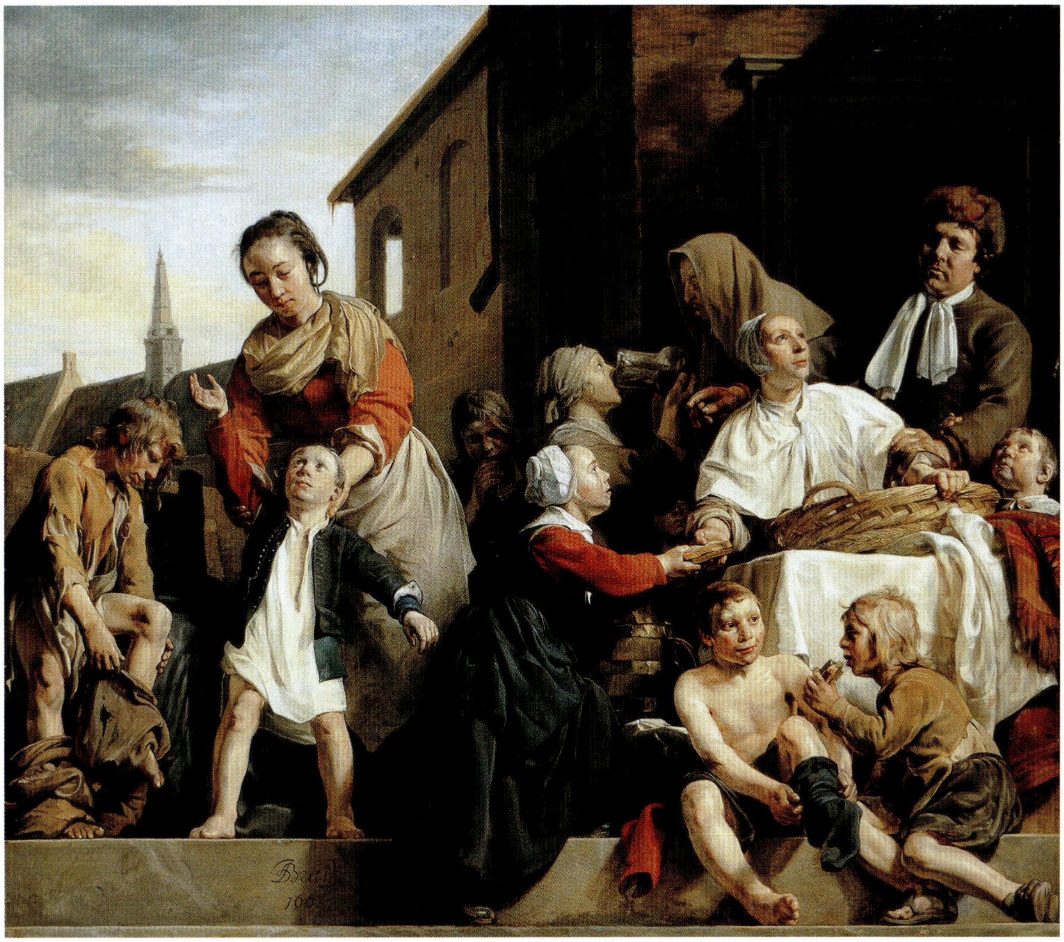

122 Jan de Bray, *Receiving children in the Children's Charity Home at Haarlem*, 1663, Frans Hals Museum, Haarlem

behind does, admittedly, turn his face as if to ensure that Hals is able to include a clear view of his profile in the final painting. But he makes no reference to a putative spectator, and the other regents respond very intently to his chairmanlike authority. Seated in front of a map signifying their sober awareness of the country as a whole,[14] these dignitaries debate the future of their hospital with earnestness and, perhaps, a hint of perturbation. They all seem conscious of the immense responsibilities involved in running the institution in their charge. No one more than the regent seen in profile, who stares away from the table as if searching for moral guidance in the source of light and, by extension, God himself.

Hals had good reason to be grateful to the Saint Elizabeth Hospital, an institution dedicated to the care of the sick and needy. In February 1637, four years before the hospital commissioned him to paint the regents, it granted his 'imbecile' son Pieter the major part of the funds needed to keep him in a special home.[15] Hals had no means of financing such a commitment himself. Records abound of his continual problems with debt after the death of his first wife in 1615, and soon after he completed the hospital painting one of his daughters was sent to live in the workhouse for the crime of fornication. During his final years, when portrait commissions dwindled and he had increasing difficulty in keeping himself and his second wife alive, the City of Haarlem granted him an annual subsidy lasting until his death in 1666. It was never sufficient and Haarlem was obliged to provide him with cartloads of fuel as a supplementary grant in winter. The penury suffered by the elderly Hals was so severe that historians used to believe that he entered the Old Men's Almshouse. R.H. Wilenski even declared that he painted his final masterpieces, two group portraits of the institution's regents and regentesses, while staying there as a recipient of

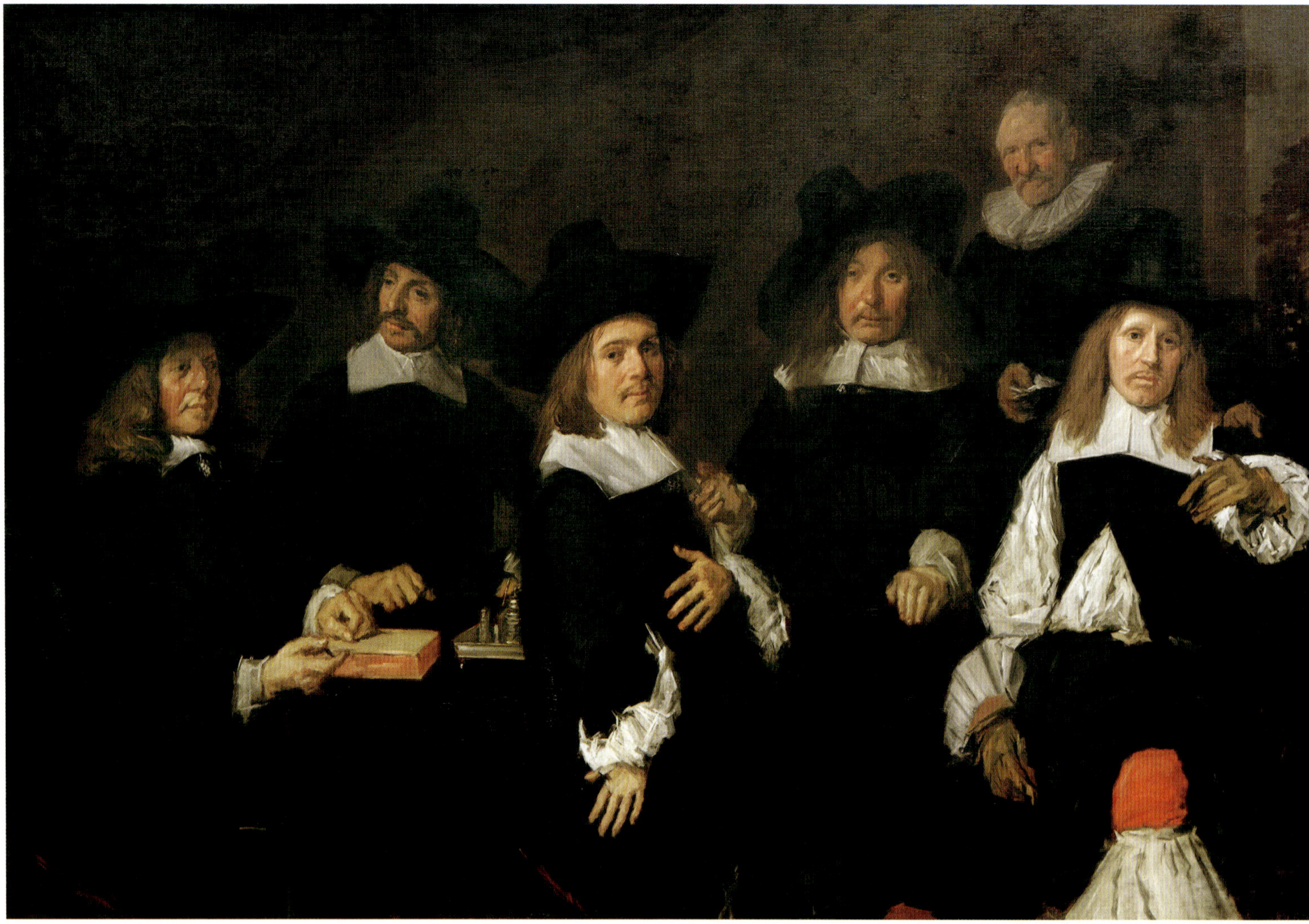

123 Frans Hals, *Regents of the Old Men's Almshouse*, *c*.1664, Frans Hals Museum, Haarlem

civic charity.[16] Although this story is apocryphal, the truth could be that only the Almshouse commission, around 1664, enabled him to escape destitution and end his life in his own home.

The Almshouse is itself a remarkable building, erected in 1608 under the supervision of the city architect Lieven de Key with funds raised by the 'Country Jewel', where orators from the entire Netherlands area took part in a celebrated literary competition.[17] Apart from its outstanding collection of Hals's work, housed in what has now become the Haarlem Municipal Art Gallery, the building contains a number of other paintings from the period. They include five canvases by Hals's near-contemporary Jan de Bray, all bearing directly on hospital administration. His two imposing group portraits of 1667 depict the governors and lady-governors of the Leper Hospital at Haarlem. The straightforward dignity with which they are portrayed is echoed by the grand *Governors of the Children's Charity Home at Haarlem*, who pause briefly for the artist before returning to the serious matters engaging their attention round the large institutional table.

The most original of de Bray's work in the Almshouse, however, records the act of *Receiving Children in the Children's Charity Home at Haarlem* (pl. 122). With true Dutch frankness, he shows them in the moment of transition between poverty and welfare. Two of the boys, tousled but by no means haggard, shed their rags in anticipation of more wholesome clothing. Another child, trouserless yet already enjoying a freshly laundered white shirt, puts on a jacket with the help of a kindly

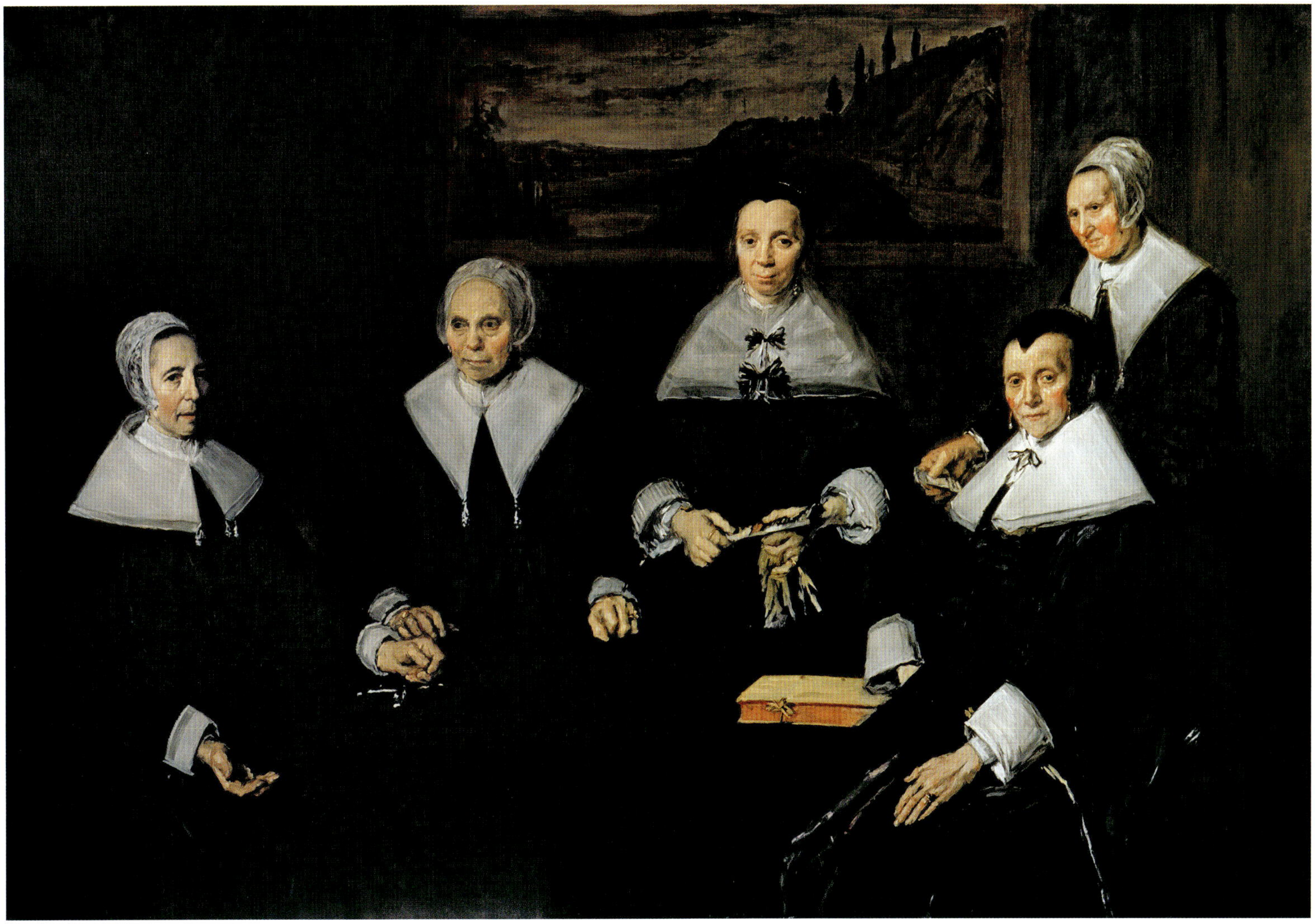

124 Frans Hals, *Regentesses of the Old Men's Almshouse*, *c.*1664, Frans Hals Museum, Haarlem

woman behind him. By depicting him with his arm raised towards the sky in order to slip on the sleeve, de Bray also implies the child's indebtedness to heavenly intervention. Nevertheless, the religious dimension is understated. The figures in the rest of the picture are vigorously engrossed in practical matters, with food and drink freely administered to grateful, greedy children by the hospital's humane staff, who exemplify what Simon Schama described as 'the almost perfervid urge with which the Dutch were commanded to honour their good fortune by sharing some of it with the less well off'.[18]

De Bray's governor portraits, for all their decency and competence, seem unexceptional when compared with Hals's group paintings of the regents and regentesses (pls 123–4), by far the most profound and searching works in the Almshouse collection. Hals was well over eighty by the time these canvases were completed, and however beholden he may have felt to his sitters, the paintings reveal a decided impatience with the approach he adopted in his hospital picture over twenty years earlier. As he grew older and his own life was darkened by hardship, the paintings acquired a greater profundity. The undoubted and often breathtaking facility of his handling never degenerates, now, into empty virtuosity. If Hals still makes us conscious of his brushwork's *élan*, it is always dedicated to enhancing the vivacity of his sitters. His crisp yet beguilingly fluent way with pigment gives each of his figures an uncanny immediacy. The very pulse of their existence seems caught on canvas, by an artist so alive to humanity that he never allowed his responses to become inert.

Unlike their counterparts in the Saint Elizabeth painting (see pl. 121), this group of regents makes little attempt to prove that they are engrossed in administrative concerns (pl. 123). They pose blatantly, and with more than a little absurdity, for the ageing painter, perhaps feeling surprised that such an old man could still manage to produce a large-scale parade of likenesses with the vivacity at Hals's command. But he misses nothing. The attempt by the two regents on the left to acknowledge each other's presence seems half-hearted, and the man in the centre gazes out with an almost preening sense of self-satisfaction.

Hals's realisation that he was desperately dependent on his sitters' charity could, at this stage in his life, have affected his attitude towards them. The smugness of the central regent must have been unpalatable to an artist who was now verging on pauperdom, and Hals regards the man on the right with equal asperity. In a passage of particular panache, brushed in crisply with a freshness of touch that no longer relies on underpainting, he shows this sitter's left hand gesturing in a lordly manner towards the artist himself. The regent seems to be giving Hals an order, and was perhaps guilty of patronising the octogenarian portraitist. Whatever the truth may be, the painter responded by treating the regent with extraordinary candour. No hint of flattery can be discerned anywhere in this outstandingly honest picture, and Hals's frank approach reaches its apogee in the figure whose hat is tilted at an extravagant angle on a head of long, unkempt hair. Although the legend that he is tipsy has been discredited, his shakiness and dishevelled appearance are undisguised. While staring straight out of the picture, his eyes are blatantly unfocused and therefore cast doubt on his capacity to carry out governorial duties with the necessary acumen.

When Hals turned his jaundiced attention to the regentesses, by contrast, he left no room for doubt of any kind about their sobriety (pl. 124). Gathered in front of an extensive yet indistinct landscape painting, which may well have hung in the almshouse itself and depicted the Good Samaritan, these five stern matriarchs appear bent on the firmest and most judicious discharge of their responsibilities. Not a trace can be detected of the maternal warmth depicted in Backer's *Regentesses of the Amsterdam City Orphanage*, where children are gently admitted to the governors' presence. In Hals's uncompromising canvas, the woman clutching a fan near the centre of the composition does manage to muster a half-smile. But her geniality is no more substantial than her white collar, painted with such subtlety that its contours seem to be melting in the air and leaving only the wispiest traces of brushstrokes behind. The paradox of this mesmerising canvas is that its evanescent handling, confined to the most fugitive and delicate of marks, nevertheless ends up affirming the women's formidable resolution.

Unlike their male counterparts, no posturing or slouching can be discerned in this grave assembly. The hand held out on the left of the picture seems to be gravely assessing rather than making a gestural flourish. And the regentess seated on the right of the table rests hand on lap with a ramrod finality that brooks no argument (pl. 125). Her iron authority is further reinforced by the jutting forcefulness of her right arm, as it drives towards her hip and terminates in a fist we do not even need to see. This blanched and cadaverous woman seems as determined as her companions to rule the old men's almshouse without a shred of sentiment. In their coldly appraising eyes, the institution's occupants require above all a disciplined rule. Alert to any sign of aberrant behaviour, they sit in deliberation over their charges like a tribunal of peculiarly unforgiving judges.

The implacable rectitude they display has prompted some critics to condemn them without reservation. 'The hypocrisy of these women', John Berger claimed, 'is not that they give while feeling nothing, but that they never admit to the hate now lodged permanently under their black clothes. Each is secretly obsessed with her own hate.'[19] The final meaning of Hals's painting is, however, too complex to sustain such a denunciatory reading. Vulpine and puritanical they may be, but these women are presented in all their considerable human frailty as governors who take their guardian-like roles with the utmost seriousness. Although their zeal has degenerated into a chilling impersonal *hauteur*, which implies a fundamental disapproval of the people they are supposed to be looking after, Hals stops short of painting them in a spirit of outright vituperation. Rather does he reveal their fallibility with the seasoned understanding of a man who may, at this late stage in his life, have been all too aware of his own failings.

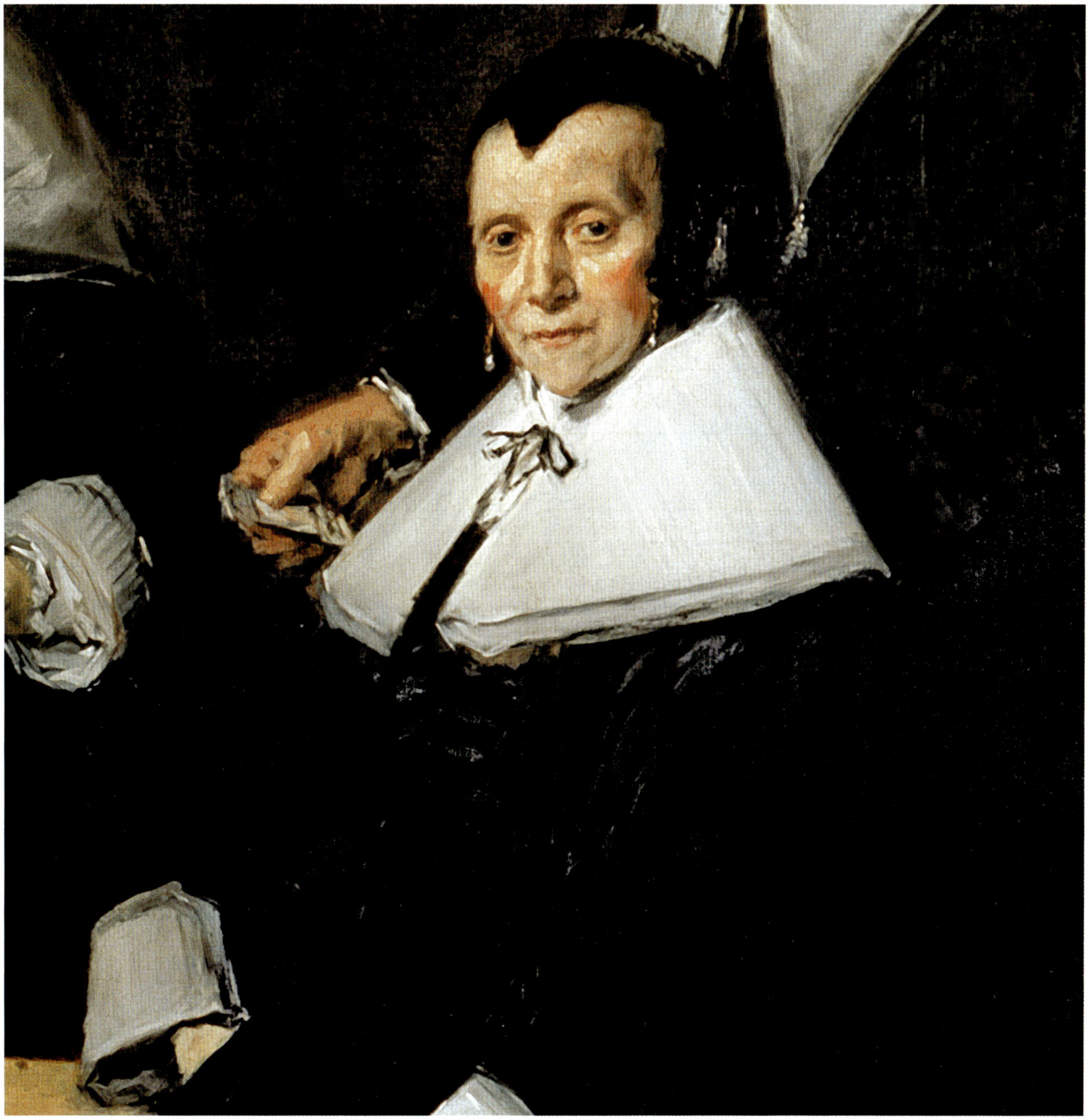

125 Detail of pl. 124

That is why each of these matriarchs is seen, ultimately, as a lonely figure, unable to draw comfort from the presence of her colleagues. Stiffened by years of stringent economising and a thankless struggle to ensure that the almshouse remains a viable institution, they are presented here as melancholy creatures marooned within their own defensive prejudices. None of the regentesses is able to break out of this rigidity and gain true fulfilment by developing a more generous, forgiving attitude towards the inmates in their charge. Within the apparent solidarity of a group portrait, isolation prevails along with a vulnerable realisation that death cannot be far away – for themselves, the occupants of the almshouse and the artist himself, who defied old age in order to complete this final meditation on mortality.

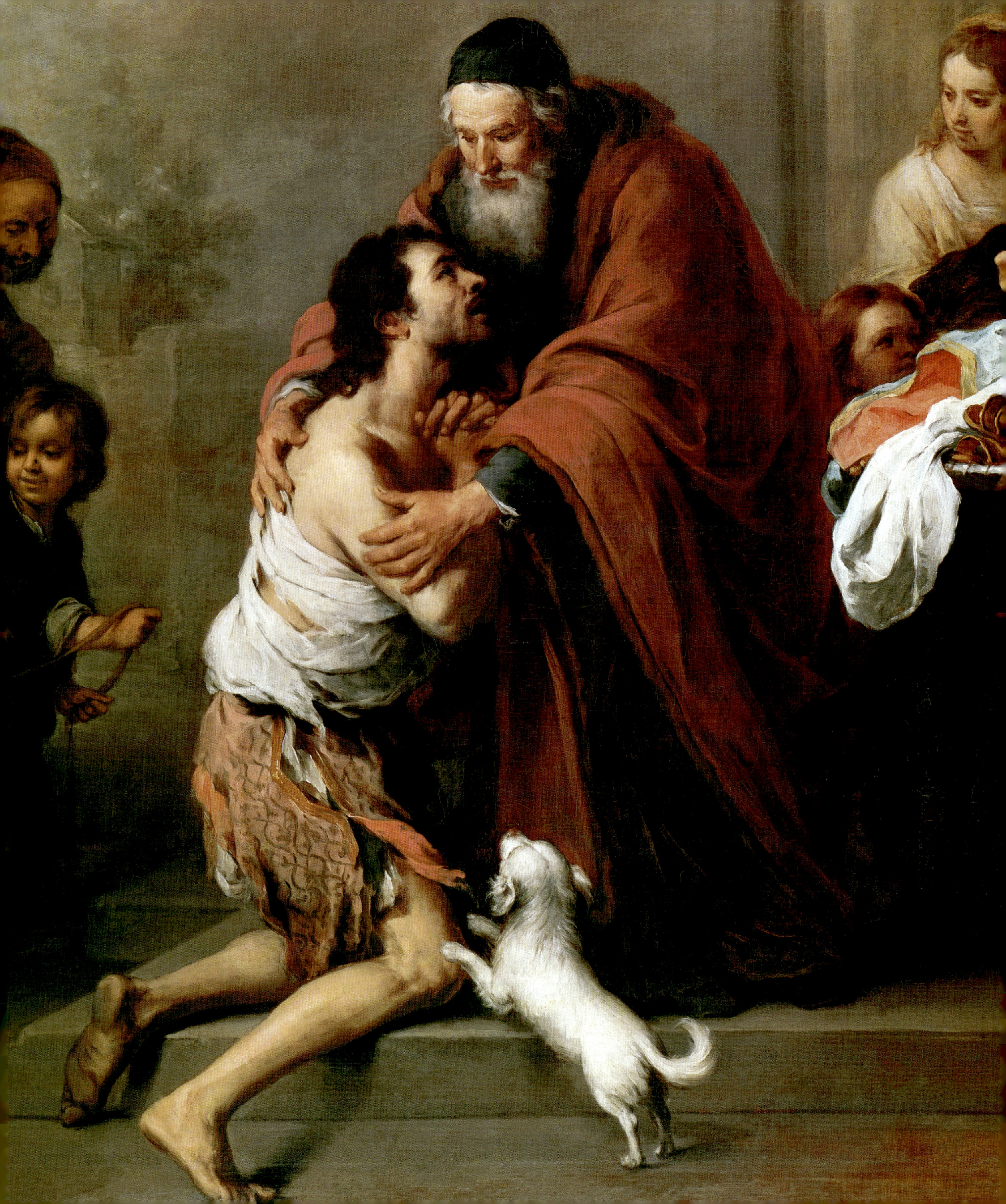

TEN
FIGHTING THE PLAGUE

A wealthy Sevillian merchant who underwent a spiritual crisis in 1661, Don Miguel de Mañara thereafter committed all his remarkable energies to helping his fellow citizens stricken by disease. With exemplary dedication, he even insisted on proper burials for the corpses of criminals who had been condemned to public execution.[1] The tragic recent death of his own young wife intensified his concern but, anyone with humane sensibilities would have realised that Seville was particularly vulnerable in this respect. Little more than a decade before, in 1649, the city's population had been decimated by a terrible plague. The anonymous artist who painted the *Hospital del Pozo Santo during the Plague* showed the scene of appalling devastation in front of the building, littered with the dead waiting to be buried by dazed citizens who pick their way through a wasteland of victims. Half Seville's population was destroyed by the epidemic, and the city took many years to recover from the catastrophe.

No wonder that philanthropists like Mañara were preoccupied with the fate of corpses. He had witnessed too much civic neglect during the years before he revived the ancient Hospital de la Caridad (Charity). The plague intensified the Sevillians' innate awareness of the fate awaiting souls after death, and the historian Antonio Dominguez Ortiz has described how this mental climate,

> in which Heaven and Hell with their attendant hopes and fears were intimately bound up with daily life, removed rather than emphasised the frontiers between life and death. In our secular society, we are intent on separating suffering and death from the living by relegating it to separate places and surrounding it with scientific 'care', while at the same time trying to make man forget that his destiny is death and that continuity and a community of ideas, feelings and interests must exist between the living and the dead. In those centuries, a corpse was not a disagreeable sight that had to be kept apart, but a being who continued living his own life and who, in exchange for prayers, offerings and remembrance, afforded his family protection and intercession.[2]

Hence the marked willingness of rich Sevillian aristocrats and merchants to make munificent contributions to the city's hospitals. The church interior of an institution like the Hospital de los Venerables Sacerdotes testifies to the decorative splendour lavished upon them with these funds. They could hardly have been more sumptuous, and Mañara ensured that his building outshone them all in the

126 (*facing page*) Detail of pl. 134

127 (*right*) Facade of Hospital de la Caridad church, Seville, built 1661–4

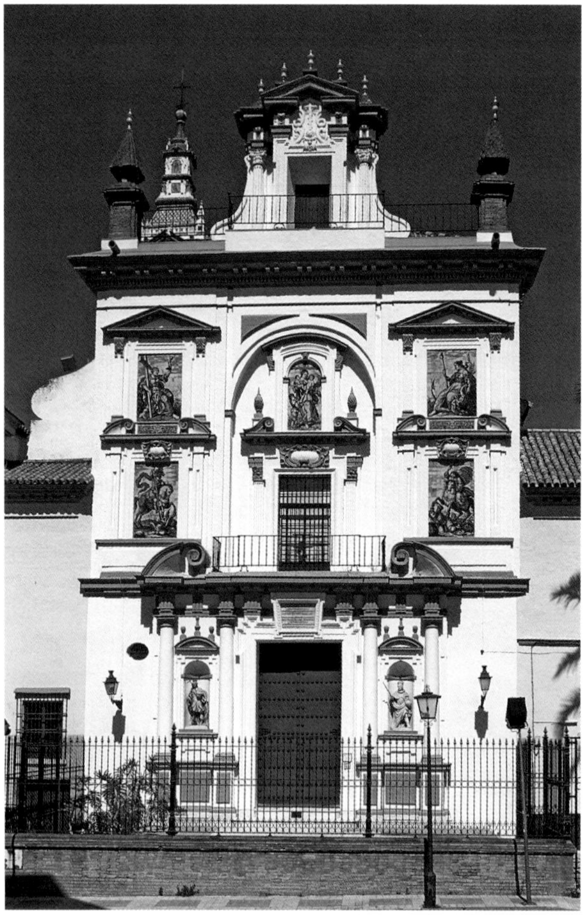

128 (*below*) Juan de Valdés Leal, *Don Miguel de Mañara*, 1681, Hospital de la Caridad, Seville

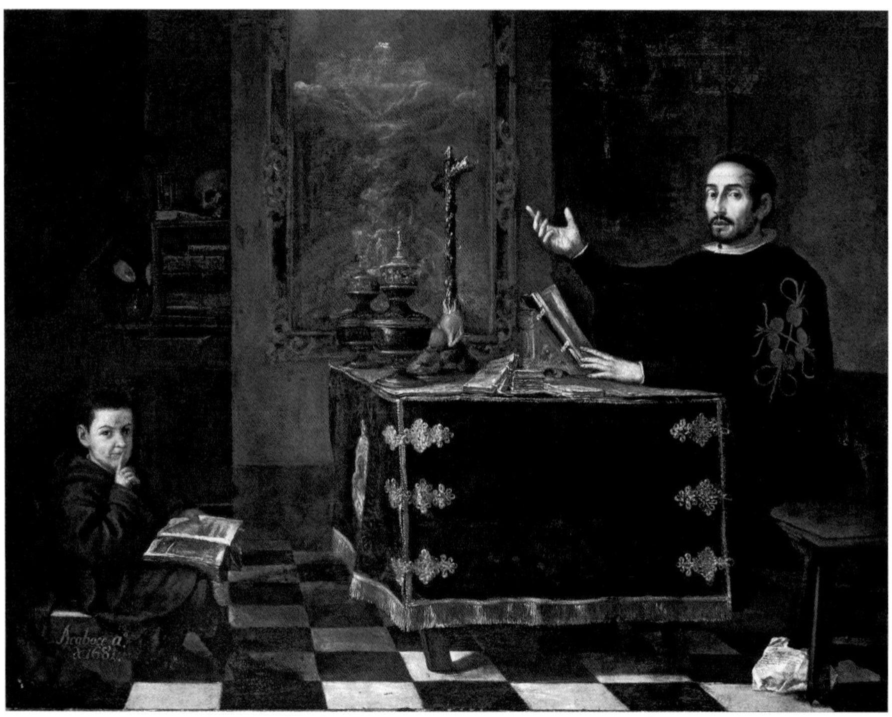

excellence of the paintings and sculpture he commissioned for its walls. The lively embellishments on the facade of the Hospital de la Caridad's church, no less than the carved fountains adorning its courtyard, demonstrated that the foundation believed in enhancing the most prominent areas of the institution with works of art (pl. 127). The funding it enjoyed was immense: Don Francisco Gómez de Castro, among the wealthiest of the Sevillians who profited so handsomely from expeditions to the Americas, bequeathed to the Caridad the whole of his vast fortune. As a result, Mañara dispensed a budget of a million ducats over the eighteen-year period when he directed the Hospital.

The money devoted to art was spent with great discernment, too. The portrait of Mañara by Juan de Valdés Leal, one of the painters he favoured, depicts a man not in the least concerned with displaying personal grandeur or ostentatious surroundings (pl. 128). His clothes are subdued, and he looks up from a devotional book to gesture, firmly yet without pretension, towards the crucifix on his desk. This is an individual who sets great store by divine guidance, and who is accustomed to seeking it in the privacy of his study. As if to emphasise the important role played by silent meditation in Mañara's life, the boy seated before his desk raises a finger to his lips. Valdés Leal's portrait may allow us to see the Hospital's director communing with God, but we are at the same time counselled to remain quiet while the devout consultation takes place.

As Mañara worked tirelessly for the relief of the afflicted poor, helping to ensure that 'although want was widespread, nobody died of hunger' in Seville,[3] he turned the interior of the Caridad church into a superb showcase for paintings and sculpture interpreting the themes closest to his charitable endeavours. The grand nave is crowned on the elaborate high altar by an impassioned *Entombment* group (pl. 129) by Pedro Roldán, the most impressive sculptor in late seventeenth-century Spain. The heartfelt care devoted to Christ's lifeless body by his grieving family was a salutary subject for a Brotherhood of Charity initially founded to bury felons whose corpses were left to rot after execution. Mañara himself regarded it as one of his Hospital's prime Acts of Mercy and Roldán's sculpture was therefore an eloquent exemplar of an activity promoted by the Caridad.

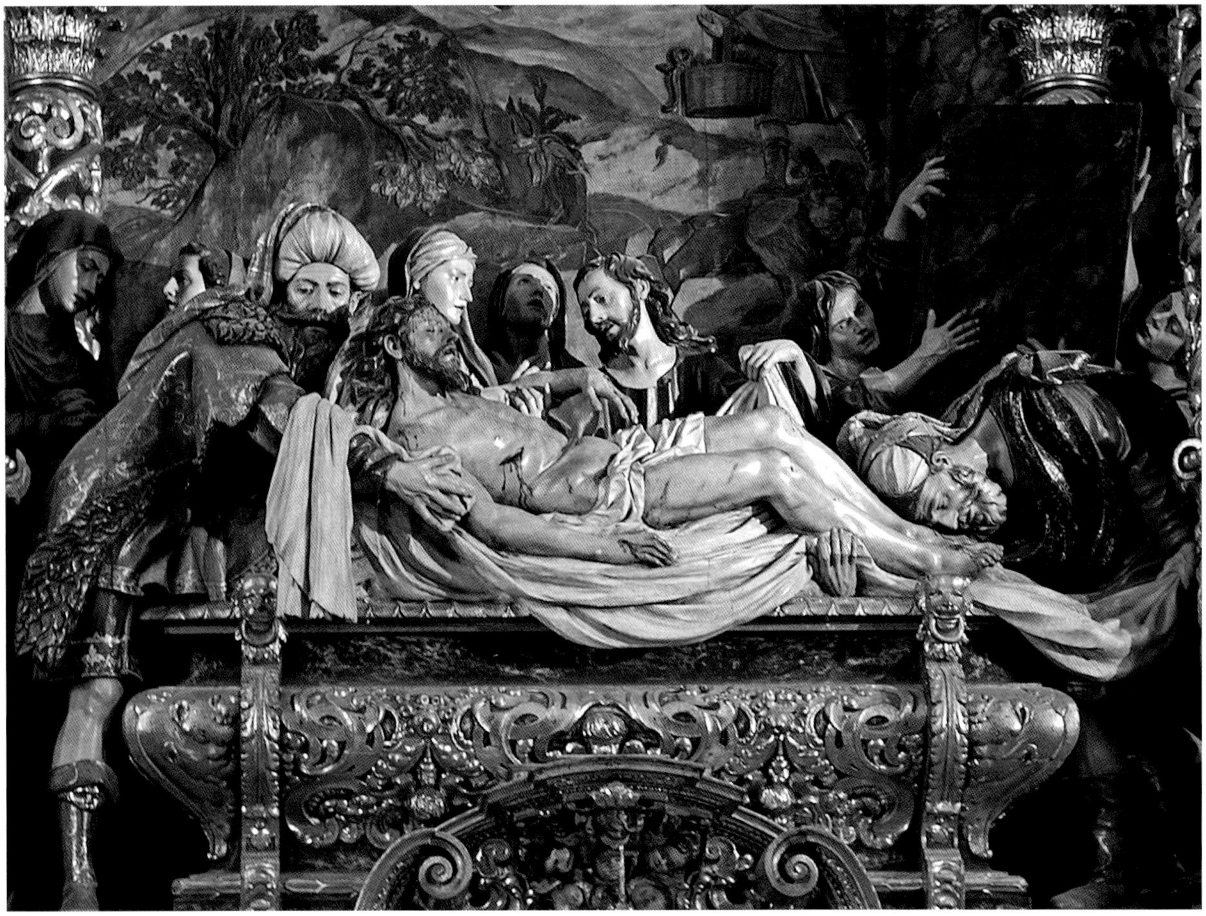

129 Pedro Roldán, *Entombment*, 1670–73, Hospital de la Caridad Church, Seville

So was the great sequence of canvases that constitute the most memorable of all Mañara's commissions. Now partly dispersed but all originally installed in the church's nave, these monumental scenes of bestowed charity mark a high point in the work of Bartolomé Esteban Murillo's maturity. Just how unusual this extensive scheme was, in terms of seventeenth-century hospital art, can be gauged by comparing it with Guercino's contribution to the church of the SS. Annunziata in the Ospedale Maggiore, Milan. Painted near the end of the 1630s, the commission consisted of a large *Annunciation* altarpiece (pl. 130). The existence of several superb preparatory drawings shows how well Guercino prepared himself for this monumental work.[4] In one study, he experimented with the idea of the angel with arms outstretched in mid-flight. Then he settled for the more conventional alternative of a kneeling position, thereby enabling angel and Madonna to face each other. This is the position they retained in the finished canvas but Guer-

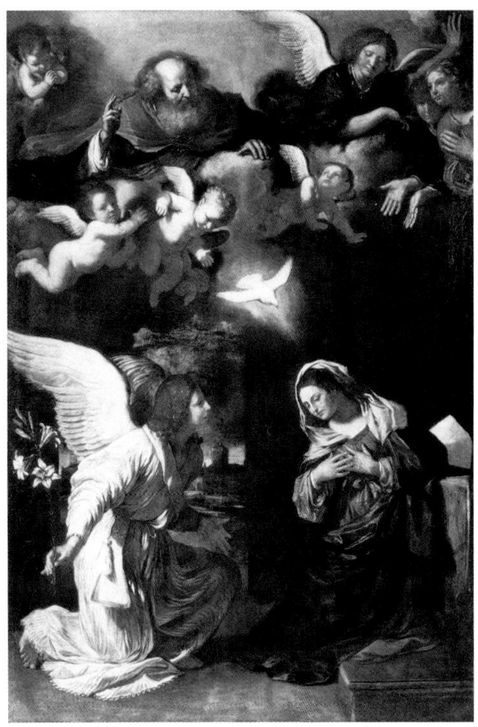

130 Guercino, *Annunciation*, 1639, Fondazione Policlinico Ospedale Maggiore, Milan

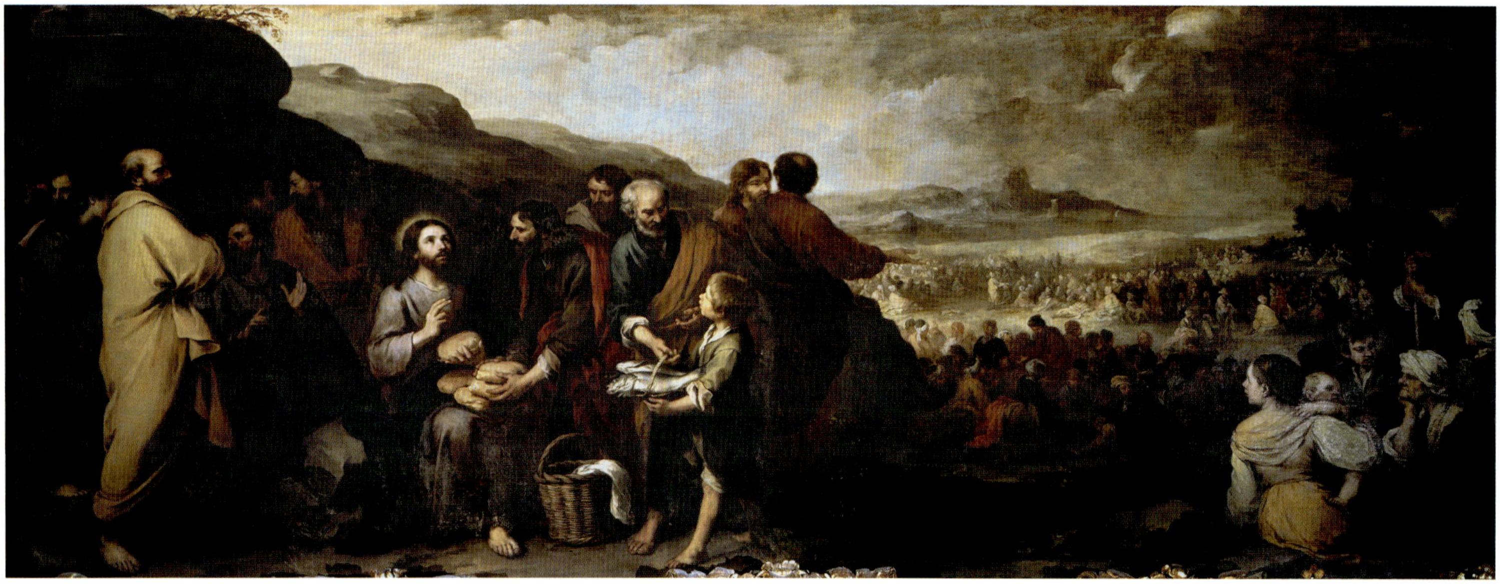

131 Bartolomé Esteban Murillo, *The Miracle of the Loaves and Fishes*, 1667–70, Hospital de la Caridad, Seville

cino, possibly under pressure from his patrons, crowded the altarpiece with an excess of figures and distracting detail. The limpidity, grace and urgency enlivening his preliminary drawings have been lost and the Ospedale Maggiore did not give Guercino an opportunity to redeem himself by commissioning any more of his paintings for the same church.

Murillo, by contrast, was able to reveal the full range of his abilities in the epic series of paintings for the Caridad church. The two widest paintings were installed below the cupola, and celebrate the alleviation of thirst and hunger. In both these panoramic canvases the emphasis is placed not so much on the protagonists responsible for providing water and food, but on the people who will receive this bounty. Almost half of the composition depicting *The Miracle of the Loaves and Fishes* is given over to the crowds gathered expectantly in the epic landscape (pl. 131). Judging by the tense faces in the foreground group, who look anxiously towards Christ, the creation and distribution of the food has not yet occurred. The figures thronging the distant countryside therefore constitute the awaiting public, as reliant on holy intervention as the people in Seville's streets who roused Mañara's conscience. The magnitude of the problem confronting him was hardly less acute than the challenge Christ confronted when the meagre extent of the loaves and fishes was first disclosed. But Mañara approached the task with the determination displayed by Jesus in Murillo's canvas, calmly looking upwards for divine inspiration while he holds the bread in his hand and waits for the miraculous transformation to take place.

In the other painting beneath the cupola, the longed-for event has just occurred (pl. 132). Murillo presents the ecstatic and indeed turbulent reaction of the figures who, having witnessed Moses' dramatic double striking of the rock, jostle for the water that 'came out abundantly', according to the Book of Numbers.[5] If the *Miracle of the Loaves and Fishes* was dominated by a spirit of suspense, *Moses striking the Rock* breaks the spell and erupts into dynamic action. Moses and Aaron are surrounded by the gesticulating eagerness of their followers, who react with a mixture of happiness and desperation to the sudden advent of thirst-assuaging liquid. At their most joyful, they are represented by the boy who points them triumphantly towards the rock from the vantage provided by a horse. He knows that the jug clutched by his fingers will soon be brimming, along with the mighty vessel slung from the horse's flank. His emotion is shared by the nearby woman who kneels to scoop up the water into an ample bucket. She seems ready to share her good fortune with the companion to whom her head is turned. And on the other side of the horse this feeling of altruism reaches a climax, as a father pours a shining stream into the pot proferred so readily by his son.

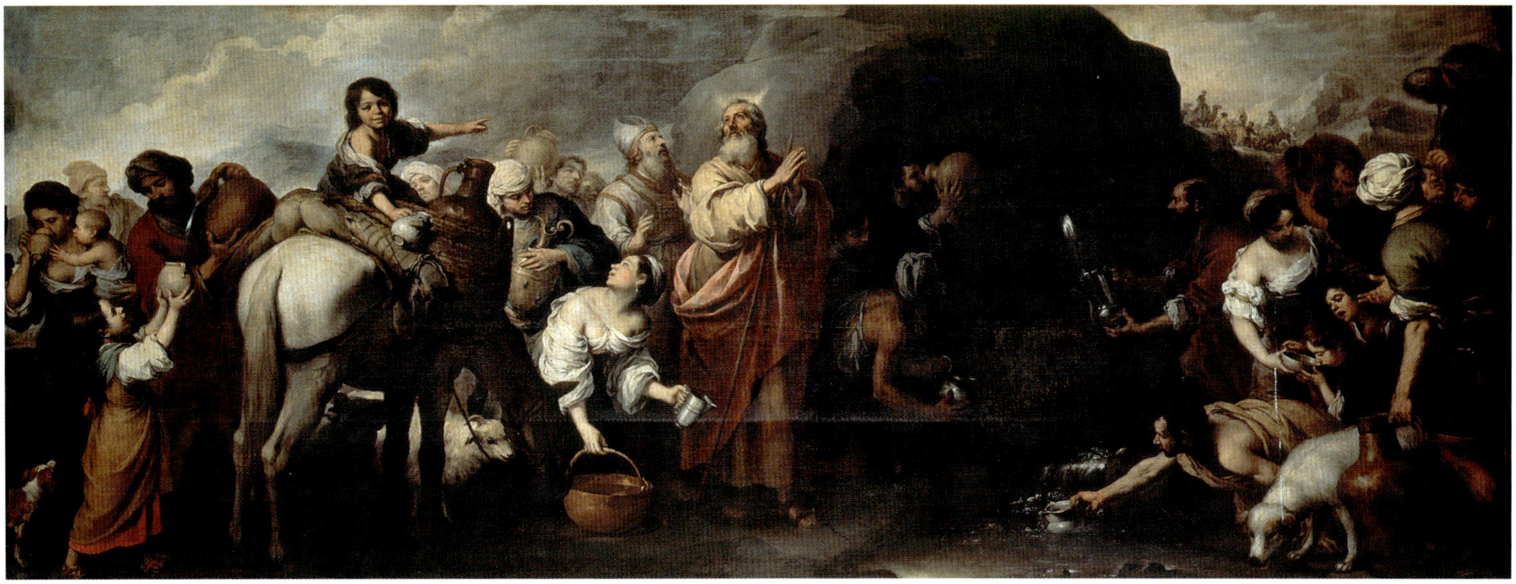

132 Bartolomé Esteban Murillo, *Moses Striking the Rock*, 1667–70, Hospital de la Caridad, Seville

Only at the far edge of the painting, beyond this gratifying spectacle, does the mood turn sour. A mother is glimpsed greedily drinking from a jug that should, ideally, have been given first to the baby whose arms stretch out with such urgency towards the same source of sustenance.[6] Murillo here seems to have relied on a precedent established by Giovachino Asseretto, a Genoese artist whose painting of the identical subject would have been known to him. The drinking mother depriving her infant of the life-giving liquid is very similar in Asseretto's canvas, where she is more prominently positioned alongside an older child who reaches up, even more protestingly, towards the vessel in her hand. But the rest of Asseretto's painting is equally clamorous, producing a composition that seems cluttered and raucous in comparison with Murillo's. He varies the design, relying on a grasp of pictorial nuance that Asseretto did not possess. The figures savouring the water in the Caridad canvas fade into the darkness of the rock next to Moses, where they relish the miracle in cool shadows. Then, on the right of this thoughtfully orchestrated design, they become far more palpable and agitated once again. A cascade of movement is set up by the two children who lunge forward, mouths gaping in anticipation, to drink from the bowl their mother offers them. The rhythm they precipitate is continued in the body of the semi-naked man who leans over the water, dipping his jug in the stream with the eagerness of a prospector looking for gold.

The two other notable paintings in Murillo's Acts of Mercy cycle deserve to be counted among his masterpieces.[7] Smaller than the cupola pictures but even more admirable in their ability to interpret acts of kindness with humane profundity, they were both stolen by Marshal Soult in 1812 and never returned to the church. The canvases survive, however, to demonstrate how seriously Murillo responded to the themes he had been invited to interpret. Unlike artists who concentrate on amassing fortunes for themselves without caring a great deal about the source of their patronage, Murillo attached enormous importance to the spiritual purpose of the work he produced. For the Convento de los Padres Capuchinos, opposite the Córdoba gate, he offered to execute paintings free of charge because the friars' work had earned his admiration. The Caridad Hospital did not need such generous gestures from artists, of course, but he still did his utmost to provide the church with images in its resplendent interior that would sustain the congregation.

One of the paintings deals with a theme of direct importance to the patients who hoped to recover their health at the Hospital. It takes as a starting-point Saint John's account[8] of *The Healing of the Paralytic at the Pool of Bethesda* (pl. 133) and contrasts the solidity of the foreground group with a

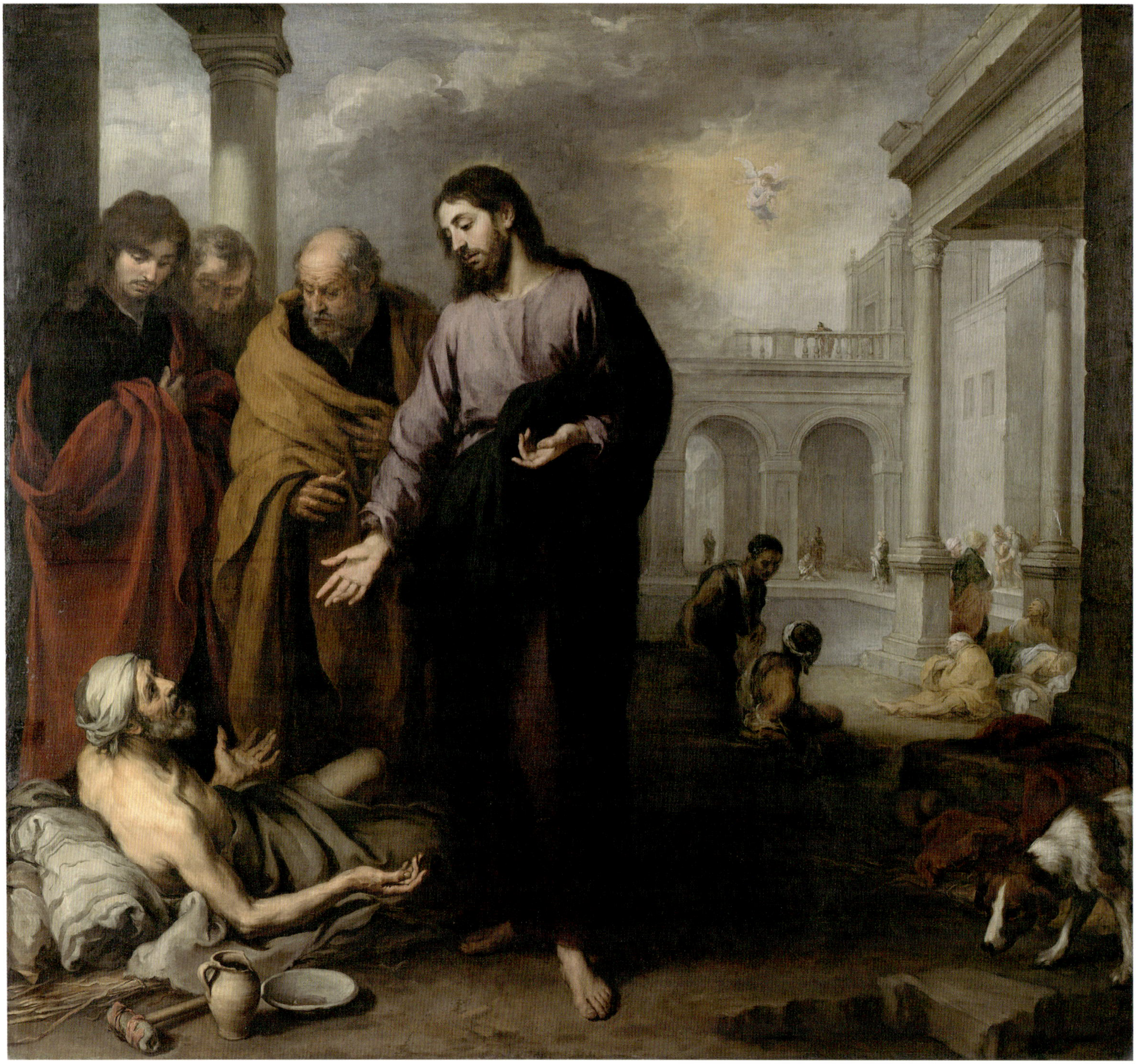

133 Bartolomé Esteban Murillo, *The Healing of the Paralytic at the Pool of Bethesda*, 1668, Hospital de la Caridad, Seville

luminous, delicately handled distant view of the healing pool. Following Saint John's reference to Bethesda's 'five porches',[9] Murillo constructs a noble edifice round the water. But he does not let the Gospel description, of 'a great multitude of impotent folk, of blind, halt, withered',[10] oblige him to festoon the pool-sides with an excess of afflicted figures. Instead, with considerable subtlety, the sufferers are arranged sparingly round the pool. Although an angel irradiates the sky, poised to trouble the pool and thereby give it the power to cure the first patient stepping into the water, everything remains becalmed. None of the figures makes an attempt to hasten towards the source of healing, and the pool itself shows no sign of any miraculous disturbance. An air of lassitude pervades the whole area, signifying that Murillo intended it to mirror the helplessness experienced by the paralytic lying on his pillow. For this abject figure has been unable to alleviate his thirty-eight year-old infirmity, lacking as he does a companion capable of immersing him in the water with the necessary speed.

Into this scene of stagnation and despair Christ makes an imposing entry. He dominates the composition with a presence so quietly masterful that it conveys, in itself, a sense of the power he will transfer to the man at his feet. Saint John reports, in one of the most arresting passages to be found anywhere in the Bible, that Jesus gave the paralytic a terse yet irresistible command: 'Rise, take up thy bed, and walk.'[11] But Murillo, rather than sharing Hogarth's urge to depict the moment of maximum physical spectacle when the ailing man discovers that he can indeed stand up and move (see pl. 186), prefers to opt for an earlier and more suspenseful stage in the drama. The paralytic is still on his back, buttressed by the makeshift pillow that has supported him for so long. He throws out his arms in apparent protest, as if to tell Christ that the divine order is impossible to obey. But even as he does so, his aggrieved and weary face registers an incipient astonishment as well. For he realises that his body, impelled by a force quite outside his control, is beginning to rise up towards the man who so confidently commands it.

Murillo contents himself with hinting at the onset of this astonishing regeneration. He shows how the paralytic's back starts to work free from the pillow, and also provides a glimpse of an upturned left thigh emerging from the blanket. But the transformation is still impending, caught very cleverly at the moment when the patient has yet to apprehend its significance. The Apostles grouped with Jesus are only just registering the momentous initiation of movement, and they scarcely dare to believe in its reality. The disciple on the left, Saint John himself, clasps hand to breast and appears to catch his breath as he gazes down. Saint Peter, standing nearer Christ and enjoying a fuller view, involuntarily thrusts his right hand out in front of him, starting at the first signs of revelatory motion in the paralytic's body.

Only Jesus, however, is wholly aware of what will happen. He stands there, with a modesty that belies his power, and holds out one hand in a straightforward yet mesmeric gesture of assistance. It causes the figure to protest that he cannot reach out to grasp the proferred help. Even as he declares this incapacity, his once-prone body begins to stir – drawn upwards by the magnetic authority invested in Christ's left hand as it beckons with such deceptive simplicity. These curling fingers, placed symbolically near the centre of the painting, are the unassuming yet decisive agent of a change that would have given enormous hope to sufferers viewing it in the church. By showing the paralytic in a wretched state, rather than upright and triumphant, Murillo helped his afflicted viewers to identify more closely with the victim and his imminent restoration to health.

The remaining Acts of Mercy canvas, *The Return of the Prodigal Son*, is a still more moving testament to Murillo's tender understanding of the story's human significance. Although he dealt elsewhere with the same subject in an extended sequence of *Prodigal Son* paintings, the dates of which are disputed,[12] the Caridad version of the 'return' theme is the larger and by far the finer of the two versions. It is also very different from the other canvas, which focuses solely on the act of reconciliation between father and son. Their meeting is, admittedly, handled with appropriate affection. The old man leans over thankfully to rest his head against the son's forehead and cheek. This sense of physical intimacy is the most impressive aspect of the picture, and Murillo reinforces it by revealing how the patriarch places his wizened hands on the prodigal's shoulder and heart as well. All the same, the son's legs are awkwardly defined and the figures observing on the side appear curiously wooden in their reaction to the encounter. As for the sacrificial calf ordered by the father to mark the prodigal's return, it is barely visible in a distant arch that seems too detached from the principal scene.

Murillo rectified these failings with admirable finality in his Caridad picture (pl. 134). By confining all the action to the forefront of his stage-like setting, he was able to give far more prominence to the calf. Led on by one of those cheerful boys who animate so many of his paintings,[13] it contributes to the festive spirit of an image also enlivened by the little white dog, joyfully displaying his excitement

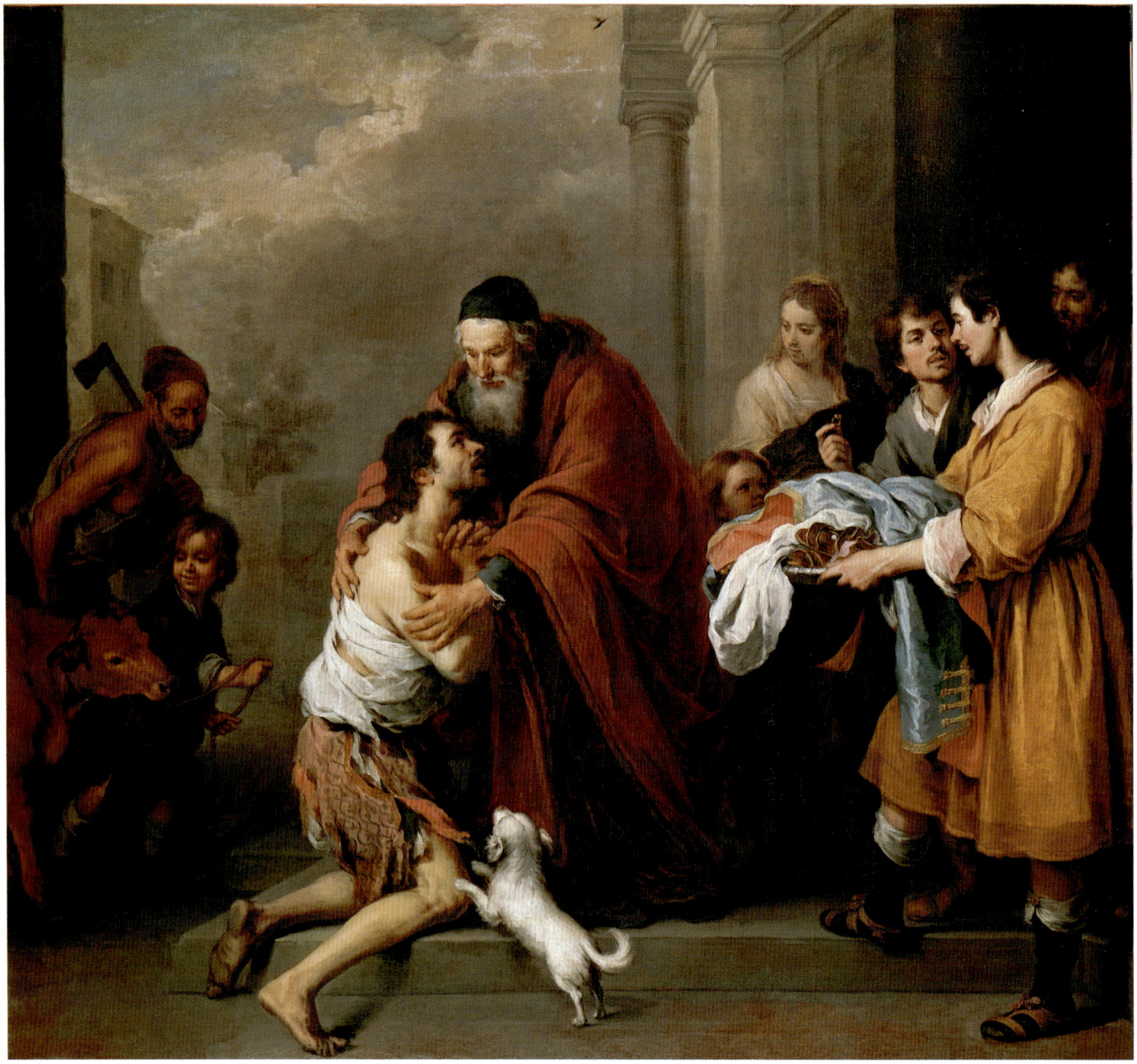

134 Bartolomé Esteban Murillo, *The Return of the Prodigal Son*, 1667–70, National Gallery, Washington D.C., Gift of the Avalon Foundation 1948.12.1

over the prodigal's arrival. But the most substantial change centres on the household servants bearing clothes. Their inclusion was probably prompted by Mañara, whose 1674 inventory of the Hospital paintings links this canvas specifically with the act of 'clothing the naked'. It was one of the Caridad's most important commitments, and in giving this element such prominence Murillo was also guided by Saint Luke's biblical account of the episode. For the Gospel reports that the father ordered: 'Bring forth the best robe, and put it on him, and put a ring on his finger and shoes on his feet.'[14]

Murillo obeyed these instructions to the letter. He allows the servant who so sturdily occupies the forefront of the design to display a trayful of garments and sandals. Lengths of linen and silk dangle invitingly over the side, almost within reach of the ragged prodigal, and they enable the artist to indulge in some of his freshest, most seductive passages of brushwork. But the attention both of the servants and the nearby boy is taken up with the ring held above the clothes like an eminently desirable trophy. They stare at it wonderingly, impressed by the patriarch's readiness to bestow such a prize on his errant offspring. Indeed, they appear to be meditating on the reason why the father should be willing to look after a son guilty of straying so far from the path he had been brought up to follow.

Mañara had his own reason for welcoming this emphasis in the painting. It lay at the core of his charitable enterprise, for the Hospital was motivated above all by the principle of Christian forgiveness and protection. Murillo gives over the entire centre of his image to the embrace between penitent and benefactor, lending the pair a resonant amount of emotional authenticity (see pl. 126). Compared with the reconciliation in his other version of the scene, where the stature of the father looks oddly diminished in relation to his son, the patriarch here is a massive presence. He bends forward to enfold the prodigal in a hug immense enough to assure him of unqualified love. The father's gnarled hands are now given a more prominent role, too, as they stretch across his son's flesh and almost succeed in encircling him with paternal tenderness.

Such an overt and generous demonstration of affection engenders an equally heartfelt response. The repentant wanderer, with his dirty upturned foot and pathetically ragged garment, clasps his hands together in a prayer of thanks and kneels before the bearded protector. Burrowing his haggard and unshaven face into the immense folds of the old man's warm-toned draperies, he looks wholly overcome with astonishment and relief at the father's welcome. Murillo's insight into the full meaning of this exorcising moment enables him to give the son's expression a profound complexity – torn between the acute sorrow of a young man who only now appreciates the extent of his misdeeds, and a concomitant gratitude to the patriarch for absolving him of the guilt that burdens his body.

As if this climactic demonstration of love's capacity for healing renewal were not enough, Murillo also carried out two impassioned altarpieces facing each other within the same church. They were the paintings addressed particularly to the Hospital's responsibility for rescuing the ill and homeless of Seville, taking them from the streets to the safety of the Caridad building where succour could be confidently relied on. One canvas was devoted to *Saint John of God* (pl. 135), the apostle of charity from Granada whose life was guided by priorities identical to the aspirations laid down in the Brotherhood of Charity's Book of Rules. The indigent poor who fall ill 'often remain on the streets until they die', declared the Book, before affirming a central commitment:

> we charge that when any of our brothers sees such a case . . . he should, with a fatherly heart, help him in his misery and seek to bring him into our house: and he should remember that beneath those rags is the poor Christ Himself, his Lord and God, and picking him up by his shoulders, he should bring him into this house; and happy is he to whom this occurs.[15]

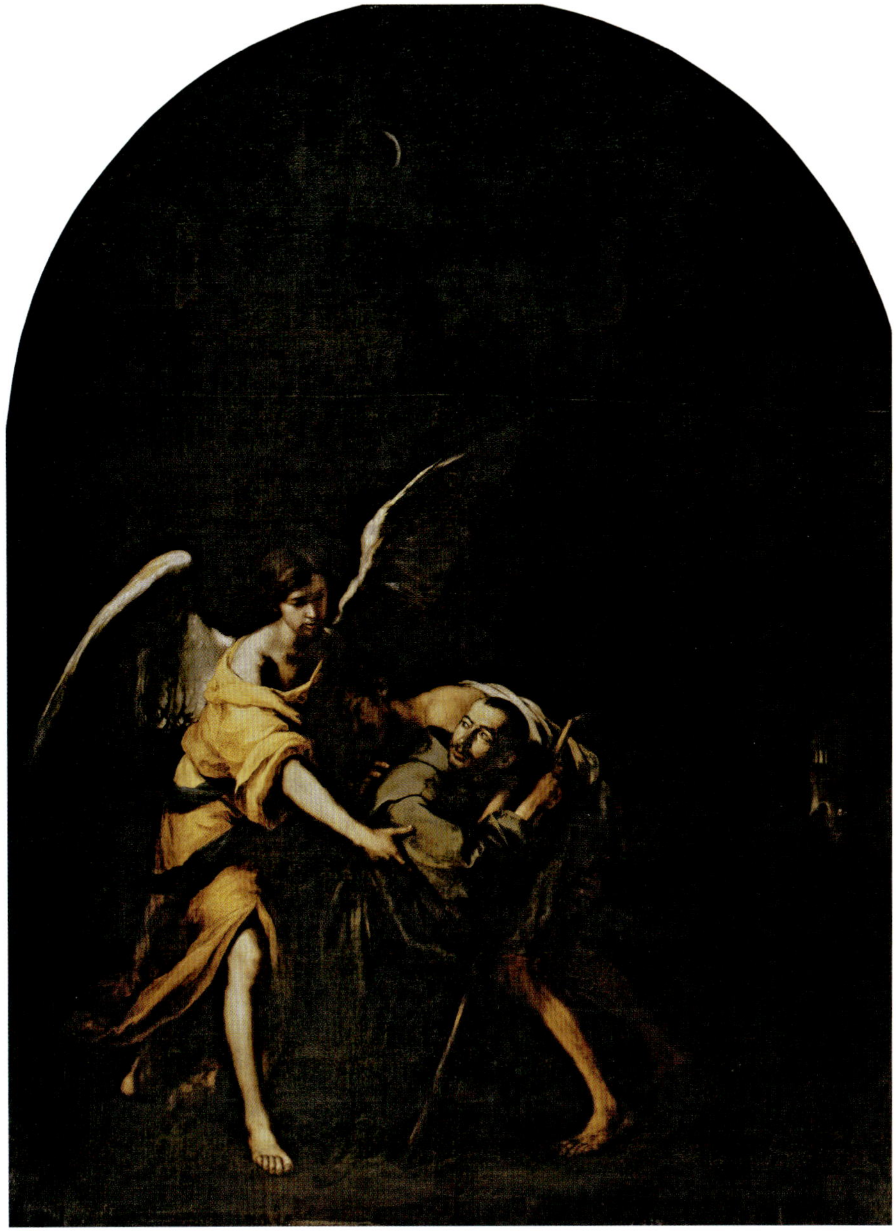

135 Bartolomé Esteban Murillo, *Saint John of God*, 1672, Hospital de la Caridad, Seville

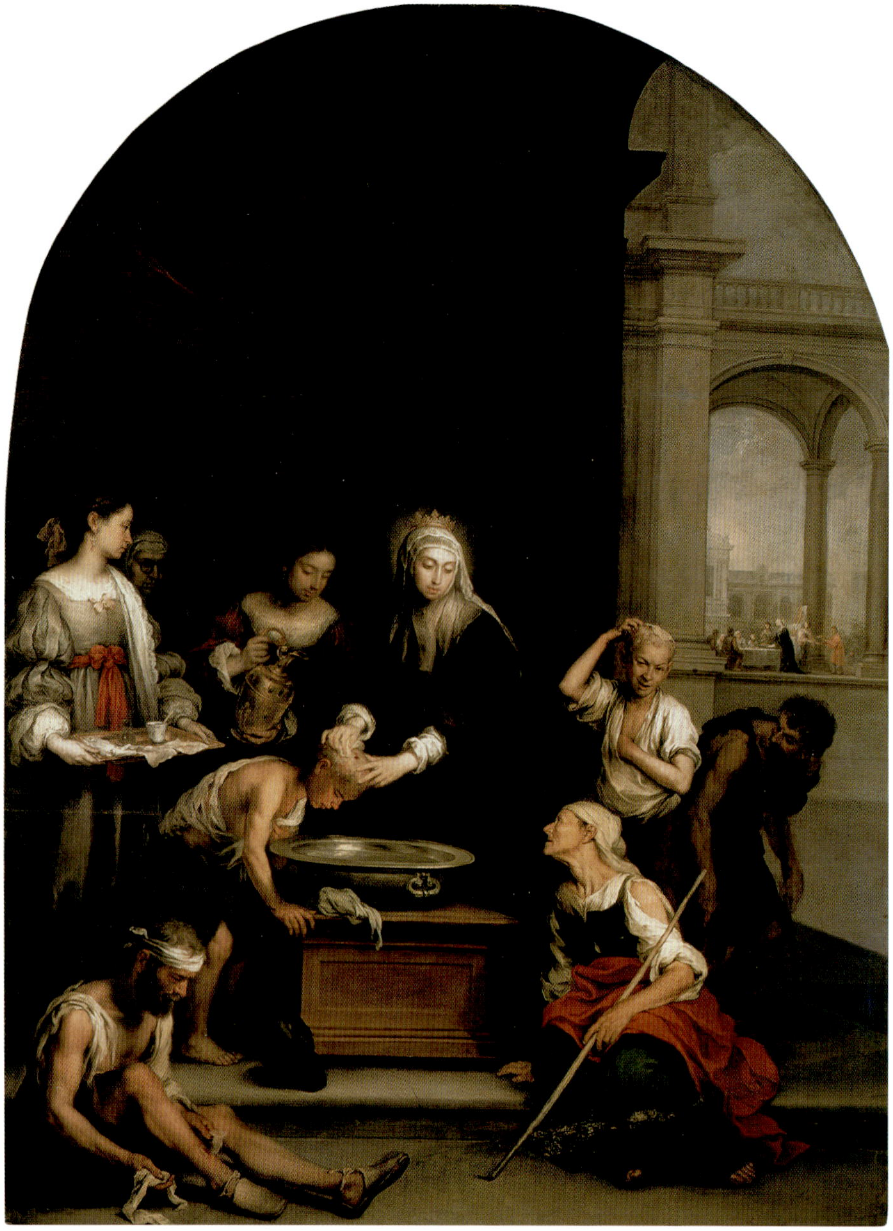

136 Bartolomé Esteban Murillo, *Saint Elizabeth of Hungary*, *c.*1671–4, Hospital de la Caridad, Seville

Such a noble passage goes a long way towards accounting for the heightened spirituality of the picture that Murillo produced. Making his way through a nocturnal street (whose gloom is now intensified by layers of grime on the painting's surface), Saint John of God staggers under the burden imposed on him by the inert body he carries. The starkness of the contrast between his strongly lit face and the surrounding dark is Caravaggesque in its moral drama. Saint John seems to personify the principle of goodness in opposition to the evil shadows around him, and he is vulnerable to assault from any villain lurking in the night. No assistance can be counted on from the figure he supports. Murillo has made sure that this ragged victim is slumped helplessly across the saint's shoulder, his head cast by the darkness into anonymity so that he ends up personifying every wretched outcast to be found in the gutters of Seville.

The strain that Saint John bears is, however, offset by the intervention of the angel. Striding purposefully forward, and equipped with wings large enough to enfold the saint and his burden alike, he extends a timely and solicitous arm towards the struggling apostle. For they both know that Saint John's task has only just begun. The Book of Rules decrees that after the patient is located and carried through the streets, members of the Brotherhood of Charity are expected to 'bring him to the infirmary and before putting him to bed, wash his feet and kiss them'.[16]

No limits were set on the extent to which nursing brothers could heal their patients through close physical contact of this selfless kind. A painting of *Saint John in Peru* specifically celebrates the act of kissing wounds. And it is no accident that the ceremony is being staged not in the privacy of a cubicle but out in the open ward where other patients can watch the symbolic ritual and gain spiritual benefit from the spectacle. Nor was Saint John the only practitioner of such intimate involvement with bodily distress. Saint Elizabeth of Hungary, already celebrated in Elsheimer's intricate little painting (see pl. 90), was likewise renowned for her readiness to take on the most repellent tasks. In doing so, she aligned herself with an ancient tradition stretching back at least as far as the fourth-century Roman matron Fabiola, who looked after patients in her own house and helped to establish a hospice in the port of Rome for pilgrims from Africa. Her achievements were lauded by Saint Jerome, who exclaimed in a letter: 'How often did she carry on her own shoulders poor filthy wretches tortured by epilepsy! How often did she wash away the purulent matter from wounds which others could not even endure to look upon!'[17]

Just such an act is depicted by Murillo in the altarpiece facing *Saint John of God*. For his image of *Saint Elizabeth of Hungary* (pl. 136), he was able to draw on knowledge of a print in his own collection by the Flemish Mannerist Raphael Sadeler. But the robust, almost homely figure who has pushed up her sleeves to bathe scab-wounds in Sadeler's image is transformed, by Murillo, into a more ethereal woman. Although the archway in the distance is reminiscent of Sadeler's architectural setting, the Caridad altarpiece is an altogether more elevated interpretation. Raised on a dais rather than kneeling on the floor, Saint Elizabeth is a graceful being who does not reveal her elbows as she administers the cleansing treatment. In this respect, Murillo is probably honouring a Spanish tradition upheld, earlier in the century, by Francisco Pacheco's *Saint Sebastian in Bed Attended by Saint Irene*, painted for the Hospital of St Sebastian outside Seville (pl. 137). Placid and statuesque, Irene points politely at the martyr's wounds and blesses him, while a view through the window beyond provides a reminder of the gruesome moment when archers pierced his body with their arrows. Similarly, Murillo ensures that Saint Elizabeth's eyes are not even directed towards the boy bending over the bowl to receive attention: she looks down instead at the elderly woman who rests on the step below, yearning for help with the ailment that obliges her to rely on a stick when hobbling.

Even so, Saint Elizabeth cannot be accused of shirking the task in hand. The sore she attends to is far more overtly depicted than anything in Sadeler's print or Pacheco's painting. And her hands show no hesitation in either clasping the head or dabbing it with a cloth. Several other figures attend this regal woman, scratching their sores and gazing in mute resignation at the limbs causing them so much distress. But the saint remains unruffled by the amount of work waiting to be done. Serene, thoughtful and above all gentle, she carries out her curative responsibilities with an unassuming dignity that gives the whole painting a sacred aura. Unlike Sadeler, who shows scant sign of wanting to stress the religious significance of the scene he represents, Murillo deliberately lifts it above the level of secular ministration. By endowing it with grace, so that the saint and her calm attendants appear to be participating in an activity akin to an ecclesiastical rite, he remained faithful once again to the spirit of Mañara's Rules, with their insistence that 'no matter how disgusting their sores, do not turn your head away but offer this mortification to God with fortitude'.[18]

Plenty of critics and gallery visitors averted their gazes from the canvas when it was taken to Paris at the beginning of the nineteenth century. At a time when neo-classical fashion dictated that restraint and idealised severity constituted the finest art, Murillo's direct representation of the complaints besetting Saint Elizabeth's patients seemed unnecessarily offensive. Today, the painting seems far from repellent, and we find the censure of the French difficult to understand. Compared with Elsheimer's version (see pl. 90) of the subject, where the hospital ward is specified in meticulous detail, Murillo's painting makes an ambitious attempt to dignify both the saint and her suppli-

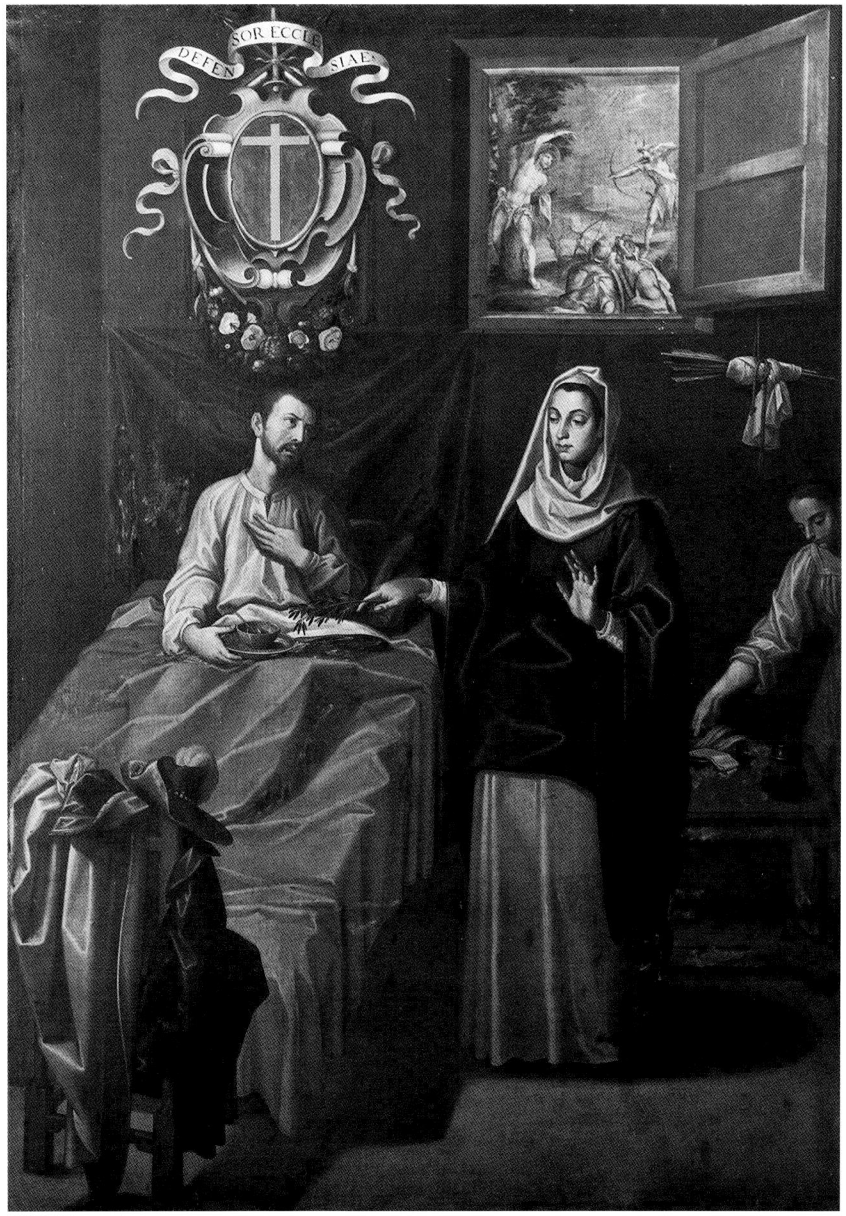

137 Francisco Pacheco, *Saint Sebastian in Bed Attended by Saint Irene*, 1616, Alcalá de Guadaira, Seville

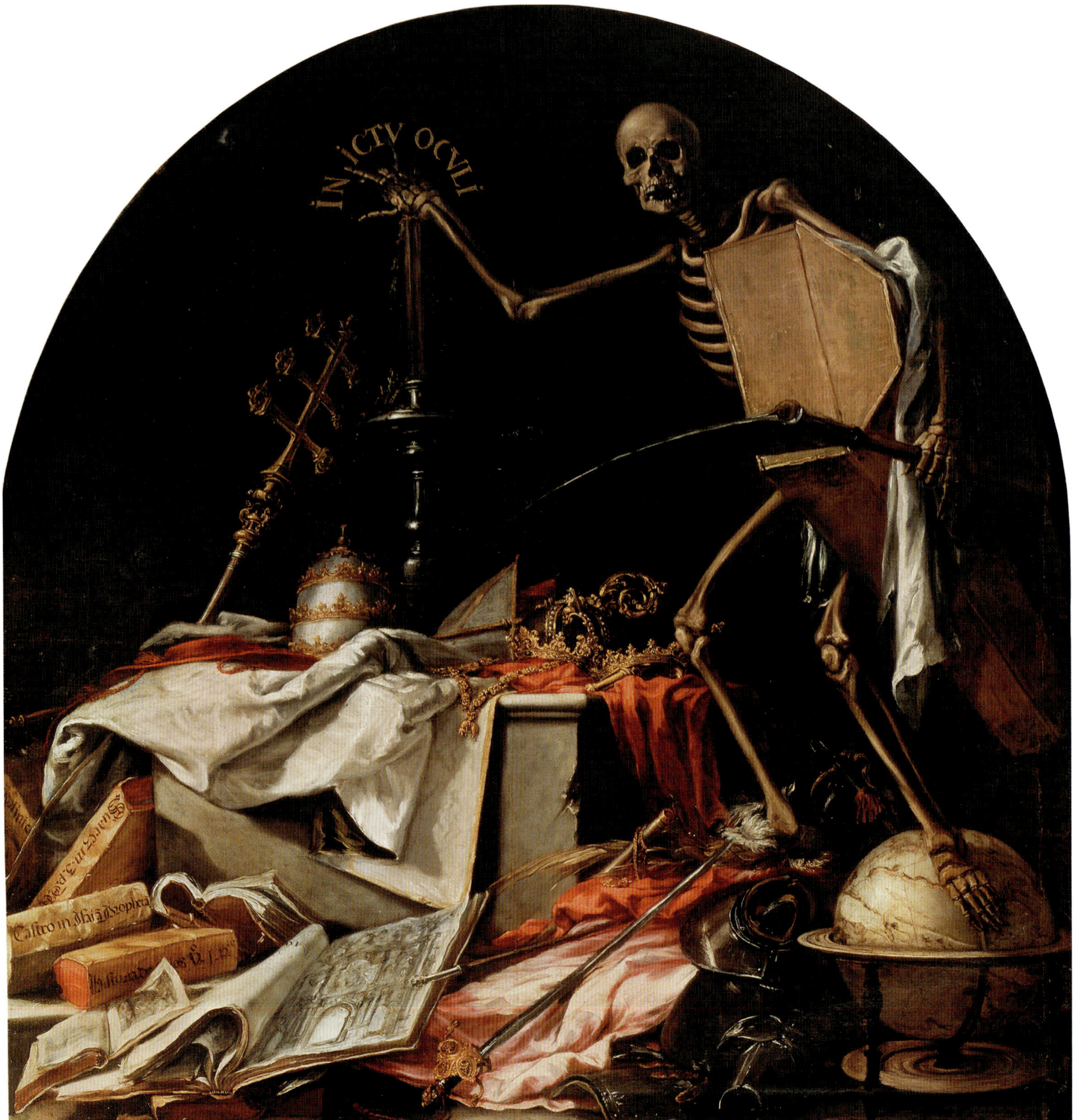

138 Juan de Valdés Leal, *In Ictu Oculi*, 1672, Hospital de la Caridad, Seville

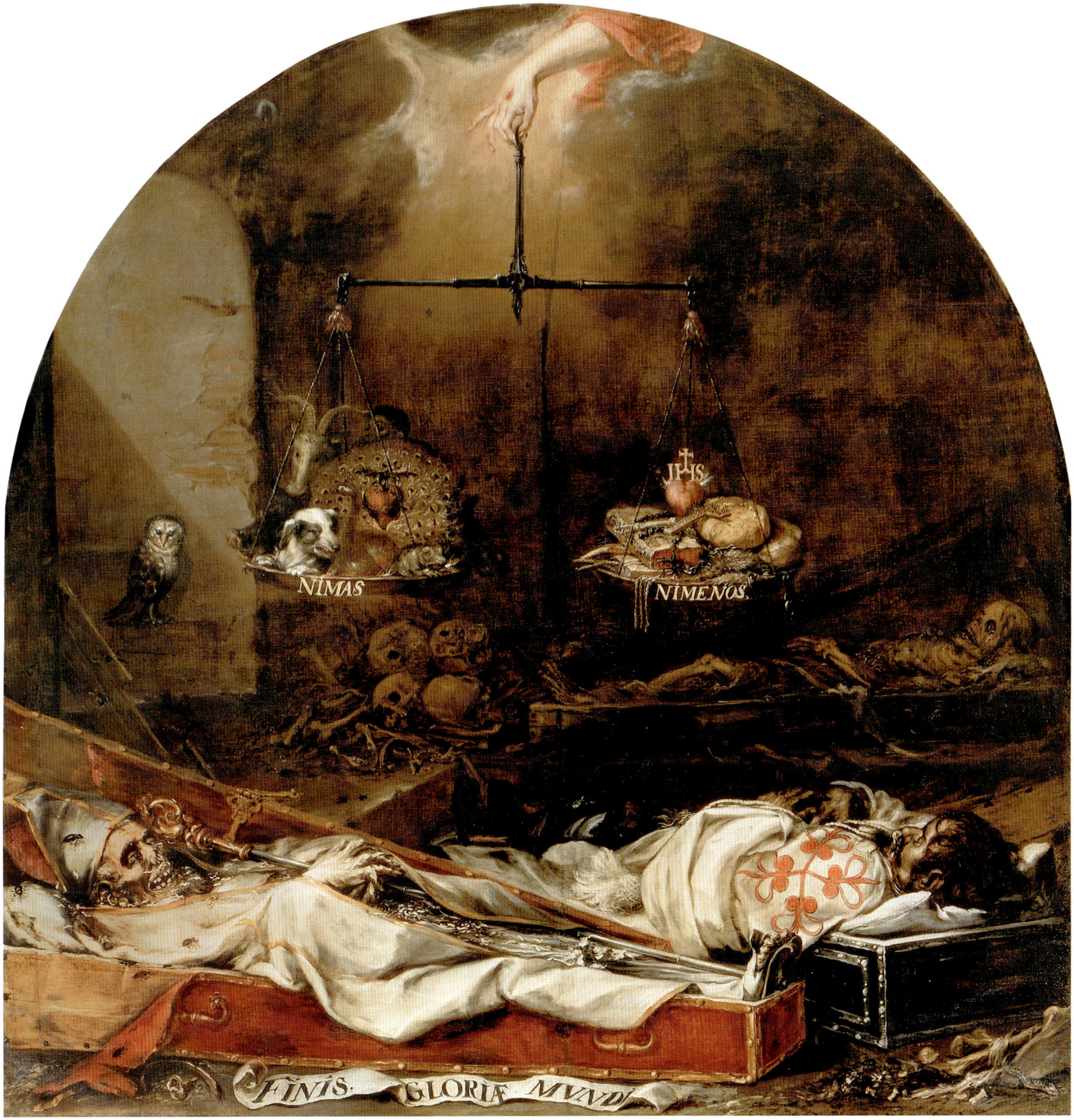

139 Juan de Valdés Leal, *Finis Gloriae Mundi*, 1672, Hospital de la Caridad, Seville

cants. Indeed, the canvas returned to favour later in the same century, after it had been restored to the Hospital in Seville and appraised by eyes newly attuned to Romantic art. Its ability to combine elevated grandeur with unsentimental realism was widely admired, helping to boost Murillo's reputation and gain him an esteem higher than he had ever enjoyed before.[19]

The human warmth suffusing *Saint Elizabeth of Hungary* becomes more pronounced still when set beside the two celebrated *vanitas* paintings executed for the Hospital. Mañara, who wanted an artist to deal with the transience of human life and glory, made a well-judged choice when he asked Valdés Leal to deal with these forbidding themes. For the inevitability of death and worldly decay could hardly have been presented in a more uncompromising manner. In the canvas inscribed *In Ictu Oculi* ('in the blink of an eye'; pl. 138), a skeleton clutching a scythe and holding a coffin under the bones of his left arm stretches out towards the tip of a candle. Judging by the three Latin words floating above it, he is about to snuff out the flame and consign the entire scene to terminal darkness. But for the moment, light still lingers on the rest of the image, enabling us to realise that an entire panorama of earthly achievements has already been reduced to ruin. With one foot placed on a globe, the Grim Reaper steps on the edge of this mouldering heap. Weapons, armour, the spoils of war and bound volumes filled with grand architectural designs are strewn across the picture. Above them rises a cracked plinth supporting the candlestick. Ecclesiastical attributes rest on the plinth, raised to a symbolically higher position than their secular equivalents below. But even they seem doomed to obliteration, and when the candle's flame is extinguished the blackness already surrounding this forlorn still life will close in on sacred and profane alike.[20]

As if this painting were not explicit enough, its companion proved even more remorseless (pl. 139). For Valdés Leal concentrates in *Finis Gloriae Mundi* on the bodies of the men whose worldly prowess was rendered so fleeting and insignificant in the other canvas. His teeth bared in a terrible mirthless smile, the most prominent corpse lies exposed in an open coffin. Although the attributes on his head and clasped in his hands identify him as an ecclesiastical dignitary, the high office he once held has not prevented him from succumbing to extensive decomposition. Bishops are as doomed as the rest of us to corporeal decay and the figure stretched out in the other prominent coffin will soon be rotting as well. Before long, in fact, both corpses can expect to find themselves in the same state as the skeleton lying in a more distant coffin, mercifully half-veiled by shadow. That spectre, in turn, could ultimately become part of the ignominious pile of bones and skulls detectable alongside.

It is a gruesome prospect, scarcely alleviated by the upper half of the painting where storm clouds part to disclose a hand holding scales in the balance. For unlike the similar scales held by Saint Michael in Rogier van der Weyden's Beaune altarpiece (see pl. 30), Valdés Leal does not incorporate a reassuring image of souls entering heaven. He keeps the viewer in suspense, showing merely a goat, dog and peacock on the left side of the scales as they are weighed against a book, an instrument and some religious beads on the right. Although the obvious conclusion might be that the latter group will eventually prevail, the word inscribed on it is ominous indeed. *Nimenos* ('No Less') it proclaims with Goyaesque bluntness, while the other end of the scales bears the equally terse message *Nimas* ('No More').

Unafraid of terrifying imagery, and usually at pains to avoid anything that flatters the eye, this passionate and almost feverish Seville-based painter produced here perhaps the most unnerving reminders of human mortality in Western art. Relentless in their emphasis on extinction, his *vanitas* pictures could never have offered their spectators the kind of rich sustenance that Murillo's cycle provided in such reassuring abundance. What, therefore, did Mañara hope to achieve by commissioning these visceral *memento mori* images and hanging them in the Hospital's church? It might be tempting to conclude that his faith was tinged with hysteria, and we certainly find ourselves recoiling from the horror that Valdés Leal defines with sombre yet fervent conviction. Well over two centuries later, in 1928, Georges Bataille decided to let the two canvases make an unexpected appearance in his pornographic *tour de force* called *Story of the Eye*, where he pointed out that in the picture of 'decomposing corpses . . . one of the eye sockets was being gnawed through by a rat'.[21]

In late seventeenth-century Seville, however, these single-minded canvases carried a rather different meaning. They confirmed what the inhabitants of that plague-ridden city already knew about the inevitability of death and its grotesque capacity to consume the flesh. Looking up at the paintings, the church's congregation would therefore have acknowledged their essential truthfulness, respecting Valdés Leal for stressing the utter vulnerability of even the grandest prelate. In this sense, he succeeded in mounting a powerful moral attack on the urge to aggrandise and pursue selfish ends. Since all these efforts are bound to terminate in dust, he implies, the citizens of Seville would be better advised to cast aside worldly delusions and concentrate instead on charitable enterprises – like the nurturing provided by the Caridad, where the abandoned and infirm could be assured of comfort, medical help and unbounded love.

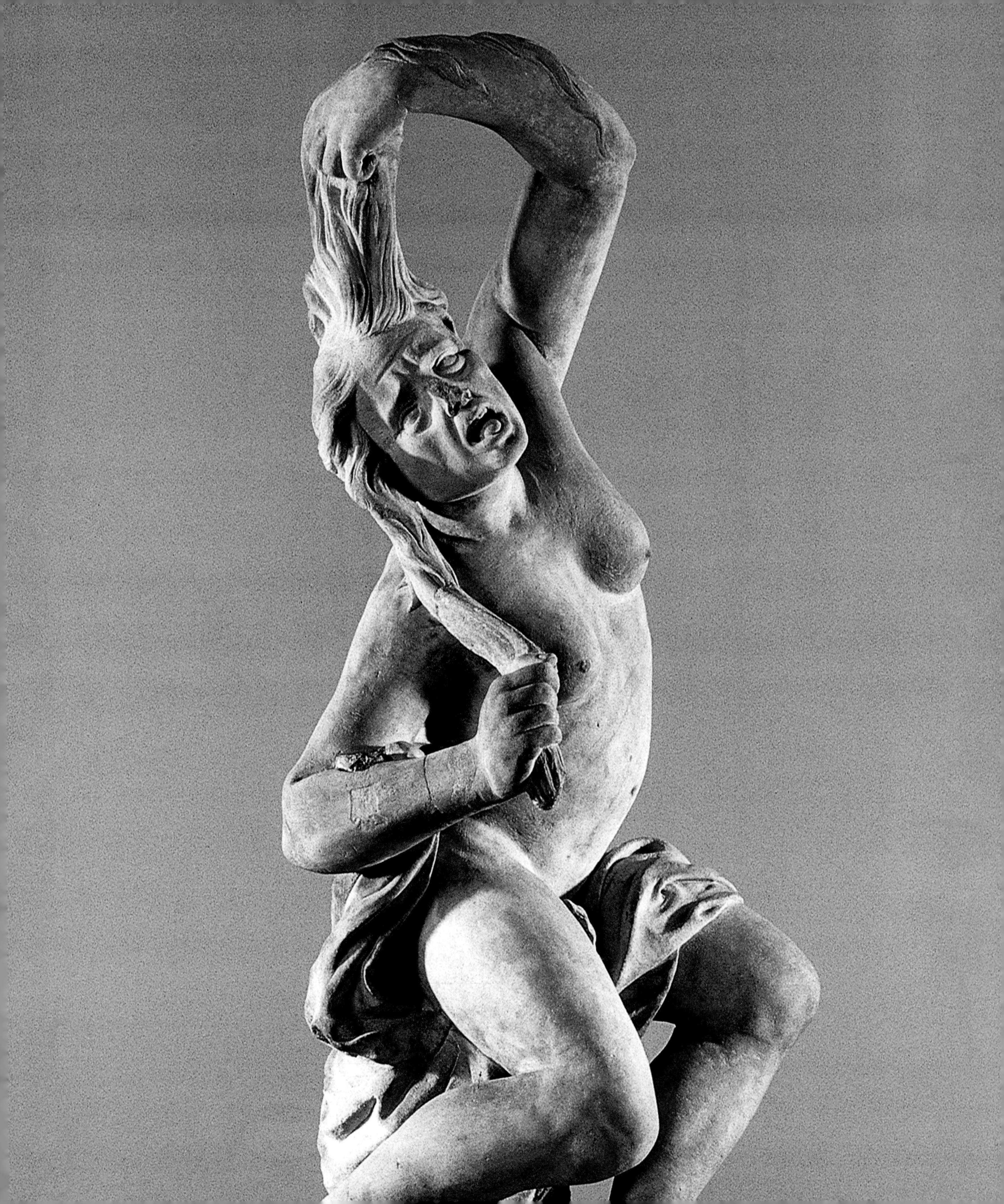

ELEVEN
FRENZY, BEDLAM AND 'THE CRIPPLES'

While so many painters in seventeenth-century Holland revolutionised the art of landscape, portraiture and still life, a few sculptors also dared to depict hospital inmates with a new and disturbing directness. The monumental carving of a woman from a madhouse, known only as *Frenzy*, once dominated the courtyard of the old Amsterdam lunatic asylum (pl. 140a). Attributed to Artus Quellinus the Elder, a major Flemish sculptor who was strongly influenced by Rubens, the crazed figure tugs at her hair with a raw, muscular vehemence that must have unsettled even the most seasoned madhouse visitor. The artist responsible for this forthright image clearly saw no point in disguising the effects of insanity, and may have wanted to arouse compassion for the plight of this possessed woman. Nevertheless, *Frenzy* looks hysterical to a fault when set against the carvings on the plinth where she sits, for its sides contain understated heads framed by the windows of their cells (pl. 140b). Realism here replaces melodramatic posturing and achieves a wholly disquieting intensity. Each inmate peers out with a pleading yet futile expression, determined to see and be seen while at the same time realising that any thoughts of escape are useless.

The quiet sympathy shown here for the plight of incoherent and isolated individuals is very remarkable, anticipating the exceptional understanding that Géricault would bring to a similar commission early in the nineteenth century (see pls 259–63). Moreover, the reticence of the plinth heads compares particularly well with the view of madness found on a stone tablet carved for the asylum at 's-Hertogenbosch (pl. 141). It was the first psychiatric hospital in the Netherlands, opened as early as 1442 with funding provided by Reinier van Arkel, whose generosity enabled the building of a safe house for six mentally ill men. Here, in an exclamatory and almost feverish sculpture installed on the madhouse facade, dishevelled faces grimace from windows like a demented chorus. In front of them, placed each side of a scroll bearing the inscription 'For six poor insane people', a pair of frowning figures lurch and gesticulate with alarming vigour. They look threatening enough, in their random movements, to give an alarmist vision of mental disturbance. Potential visitors might well have been discouraged from entering the asylum to discover the truth about madness for themselves.

Not that anyone was deterred from visiting the new Bethlem Hospital in London by two formidably stark carvings installed outside. When 'Bedlam', as it has often been nicknamed, was rebuilt on the south side of Moorfields in the latter half of the 1670s, it boasted the overwhelming grandeur of a palace (pl. 196). The first custom-designed British

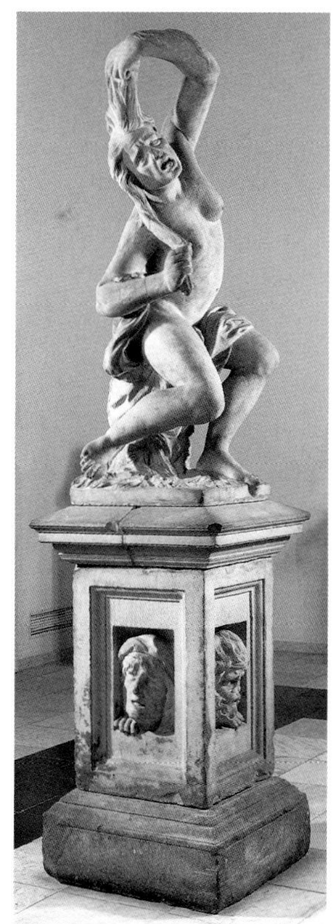

140a (*facing page*) and b (*above*) Artus Quellinus the Elder (attr.), *Frenzy*, 1650–1660, Rijksmuseum, Amsterdam

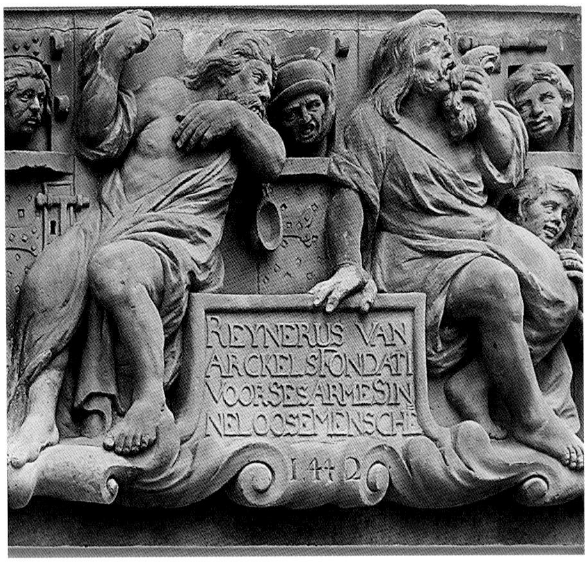

141 Anon., Faces on facade of Asylum at 's-Hertogenbosch, 1442

hospital for the insane, this resplendent showpiece was meant to impress. Its conspicuous monumentality bore out the truth of Thompson and Goldin's assertion that 'noble and bourgeois donors built for the sick poor in forms familiar to themselves', making it 'hard to distinguish a hospital from a gentleman's home'.[1] But the carvings of inmates commissioned from Caius Gabriel Cibber amounted to far more than extravagant ornamentation. They were radically unfamiliar, and would never have been seen in a stately mansion. Already much admired for his allegorical bas-relief at the base of The Monument near London Bridge, the Danish-born sculptor managed to provide the new Bethlem building with his finest surviving works. And these mighty images left no one indifferent to their raw, unsettling power (pl. 142).

Both figures, reclining on carved replicas of straw matting, occupied prominent positions on the ends of a broken pediment above the entrance gate's stone piers. As the official engraving of the Hospital makes clear, this gate was as imposing as the palatial edifice designed for the immense site by Robert Hooke, a friend and close collaborator of Christopher Wren. Cibber's carvings were perched about fourteen feet above the ground, yet their ample dimensions and expressive force combined to impress all those passing through the high walls on their way to the central pavilion beyond. They quickly became synonymous in the public's mind not only with 'Bedlam' but with the whole notion of madness itself. References to them abound in the art and literature of the following century, notably in Pope's description of 'Great Cibber's brazen brainless brothers' from *The Dunciad* and Hogarth's overt quotation in the 'Bedlam' scene from *A Rake's Progress* (see pl. 146) where the deranged and manacled Rake adopts a

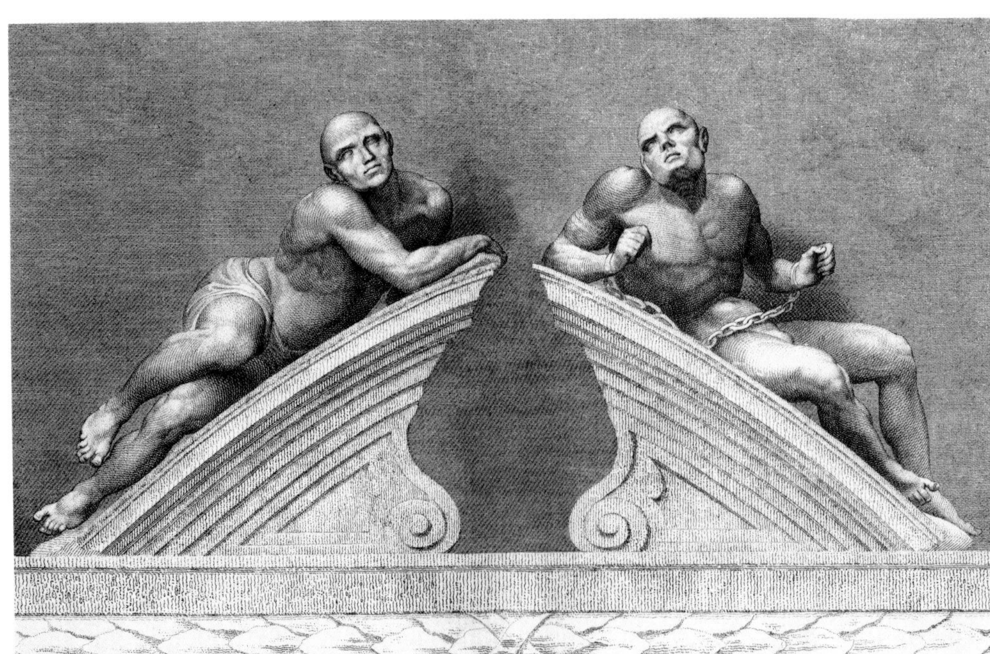

142 Caius Gabriel Cibber, Figures on Bethlem entrance gate, *c.*1676, engraving by W. Sharp after T. Stothard

pose frankly reminiscent of the statue on the right side of the Hospital gate.

Since Cibber's carvings are nowhere mentioned in the minutes of the new Bethlem building committee, we do not know who was responsible for choosing such an audacious subject. But the patron probably realised that precedents could be found in the Netherlands for the idea of embellishing asylums with images of the insane, and Cibber was cosmopolitan enough in his interests to be keenly aware of their existence (pls 140 and 141). Even so, he felt no need to rely on the frantic example set by Artus Quellinus the Elder, preferring instead to develop a grander and more imposing alternative based on his admiration for Italian sculpture. The debt he owes to the Medici tomb figures in San Lorenzo is obvious enough, and an enthusiastic member of the French Academy decided in 1772 that Cibber's figures 'may justly be compared to the noblest productions of Michael Angelo and his school'.[2] They also suggest, in their muscle-bound pathos, an awareness of the shackled bronze slaves who tug sorrowfully at their chains on Pietro Tacca's monument to the Grand Duke Ferdinand at Leghorn. The realism evident in Tacca's haunting figures may well have left its mark on the notable directness informing the 'Bedlam' carvings.

Cibber, who had studied in Rome before settling in London, seems to have fused this respect for veracity with an altogether more Baroque grandeur. As a student, he had plenty of opportunities to study the newly completed travertine *Fountain of the Four Rivers* in the Piazza Navona and his memory of Bernini's masterpiece clearly informed the four recumbent river-gods he made for a fountain in Soho Square, later sadly demolished. Bernini's figure of the *Rio della Plata*, with its raised left arm and thrown-back head, seems to have contributed to the statue on the right of the 'Bedlam' gate, although it is significant that Cibber stops well short of indulging in the expansive rhetoric favoured by Bernini. The task of personifying 'Raving and Melancholy Madness', as the carvings came to be known early in the nineteenth century, demanded an approach markedly more sober than Bernini's exuberant flourishes. The prevailing mood of these two immense Portland stone images is restrained and intensely pathetic, more akin to the downcast character of the manacled prisoners on either side of a statue personifying 'Amsterdam' over the entrance leading to that city's House of Correction.

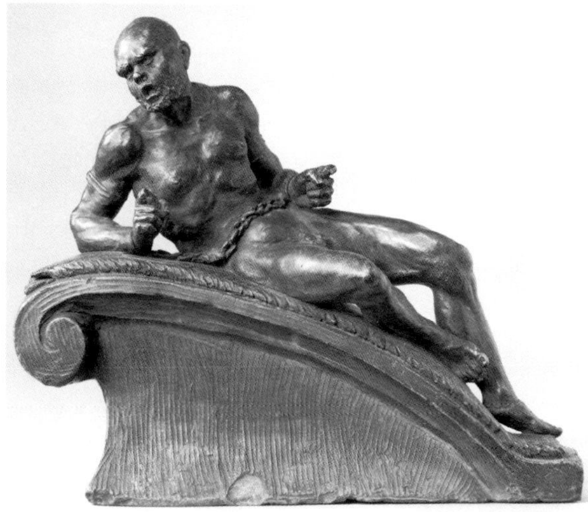

143 Caius Gabriel Cibber, Terracotta model for *Raving Madness*, *c.*1676, Staatliche Museen, Berlin

The two principal categories of mental disorder identified by contemporary authorities are represented by Cibber, and the figures' expressions differ accordingly. Christopher Smart mirrored this opinion very succinctly when he declared in 1751 that Cibber's representation of 'the two Species of Madness' could be defined thus: 'That on the Left is Melancholy, or sullen Madness; and the other downright Distraction.'[3] Despite the obvious con-

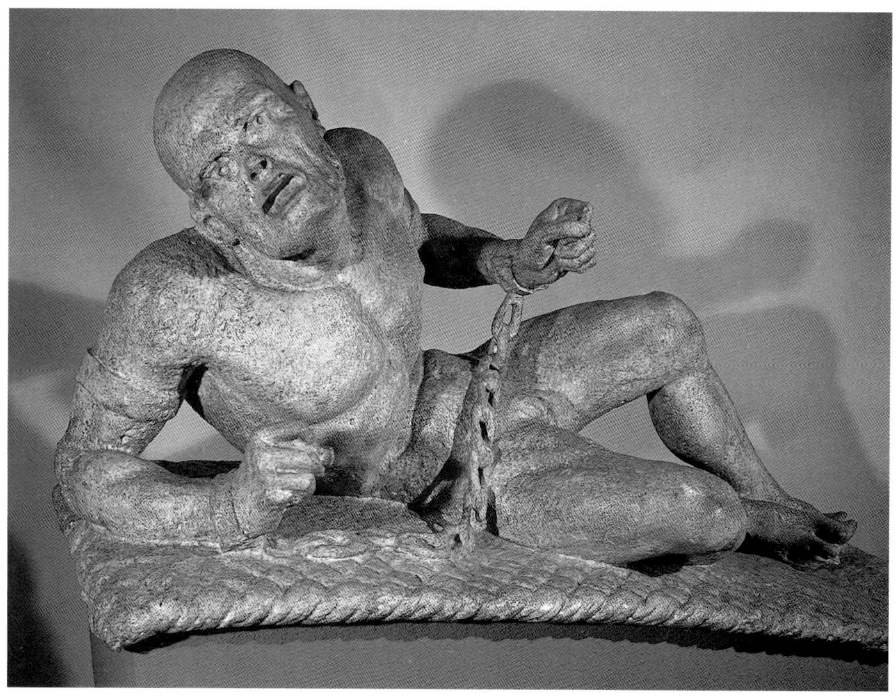

144 Caius Gabriel Cibber, *Raving Madness*, *c.*1676, Bethlem Royal Hospital, Kent

trast between the two figures, though, they are united by a profound sense of pathos. It has nothing to do with sensationalism or the desire to horrify. The chained statue on the right, who is the more exclamatory of the pair, opens his mouth to utter a cry (pl. 144). But the emotion he embodies is far closer to tragic despair than anything more aggressive or terrifying.

Cibber's terracotta model for the figure (pl. 143), revealing how carefully he related it to the form of the broken pediment below, has an authenticity that surely derives from studying inmates in the hospital itself. It is no accident that *'Raving Madness'* supposedly originated in Cibber's observation of Oliver Cromwell's unfortunate porter Daniel, who entered 'Bedlam' as a patient in 1656. His face, commemorated in an engraving, bears a resemblance to the statue, and the terracotta model has a directness and vivacity that could well derive from life. In the end Cibber decided, probably because he realised that the high position of the final figure demanded it, to lift the carving's left arm and push back the man's head to a more dramatic angle. This increase in tension and outspoken feeling would have been conveyed to the viewer below with greater effectiveness, and yet Cibber stops short of resorting to the frankly theatrical gesticulation that marred the Amsterdam *Frenzy* a quarter of a century before (see pl. 140). Instead, the melodramatic rending of hair has been replaced by an altogether more brooding alternative. *'Raving Madness'* may raise his fetters in the air, but he makes no real attempt to wrench them off his wrists. He knows, all too well, how firm his chains really are, and the cry he utters is an acknowledgement of helpless captivity. He no longer believes that someone might respond to the yell and set him free.

If Cibber's sympathy for this manacled victim of mental anguish cannot be doubted, his concern becomes even more clear in *'Melancholy Madness'* (pl. 145). Partially propping himself up on his matting, but in no sense motivated by any hope that his condition might change, the unfortunate man stares out at a world he will never again be able to inhabit. Although the new Bethlem Hospital was dedicated to 'the relief and cure of persons distracted',[4] Cibber's doomed inmate appears irrecoverably deranged. The extent of his predicament is conveyed not through theatrical bluster acting as the crazed outward manifestation of internal disorder, but by the lassitude afflicting his entire body. His legs bend abjectly as he realises that there is no point in raising himself above the bed. Here he reclines, massively powerful in build and yet incapable of applying all that Caliban-like strength to any coherent purpose. His mighty sinews have grown slack with disuse, rendered impotent and absurd by a mind that refuses to harness his physical potential any longer. All he can do is remain prone and abject. For Cibber's chisel has defined the forlorn face of a man divorced from any discerning awareness of the reality he was once able to identify. Worse still, his expression signifies utter emptiness, unrelieved even by a flicker of sentient recognition or the will to recover sanity. Dementia has set in for ever, and the sculptor's remarkable depth of understanding makes this statue the more impressive of the pair.

Precisely because they neither disguise nor exaggerate the conditions Cibber sought to define, these memorable carvings offered a corrective to the callous view of madness that made casual visitors throng the wards within 'Bedlam'. For a while, anybody who could afford a penny entrance charge gained admittance to the building. The frisson of

145 Caius Gabriel Cibber, *Melancholy Madness*, *c.*1676, Bethlem Royal Hospital, Kent

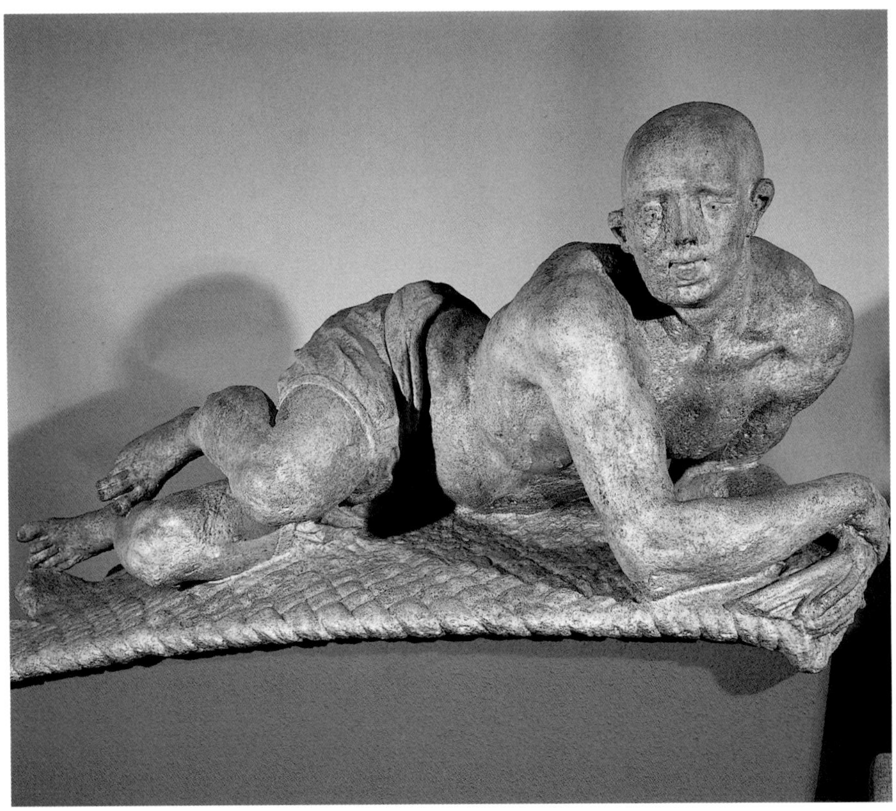

parading through its interior was regarded as an entertainment, like going to the zoo. Members of the inquisitive crowd encompassed 'everybody from gentlewomen going slumming to professional thieves who stole from the patients'.[5] Hogarth included a couple of idle society ladies smirking in his 'Bedlam' scene from *A Rake's Progress* (pl. 146). The presence of such lamentable voyeurs was bound to exacerbate the patients' unease. Most of them, after all, were incarcerated behind bars in spacious cells easily viewable from the visitors' corridor. One journalist reported in 1753 that he had witnessed 'a hundred spectators making sport of the miserable inhabitants, provoking them into furies of rage'.[6] And the pandemonium increased when other inmates began jangling chains or beating on the doors to support the protests of their beleaguered fellows.

Cibber's statues resisted this deplorable tendency to treat the insane as nothing more than a hilarious sideshow at the fair. Perturbed, helpless and embroiled in disorders of the brain so severe that they are deprived of all rational intelligence, his impotent figures are beyond mockery. How could anyone laugh at their suffering, when Cibber had gone out of his way to avoid all semblance of absurdity? No caricatured ideas about insanity can be discerned in these deeply troubled carvings. They were considered dignified enough to influence the new carved facade of Bart's Hospital in 1702, where reclining patients overtly reminiscent of Cibber's figures flank a commanding statue of their protective monarch. Until the early nineteenth century, both *'Raving Madness'* and its doleful partner continued to offer their onlookers a gravely compassionate vision of the alienation that mental disorder engenders in its victims.

The activities within 'Bedlam' eventually began to conform to the spirit in which Cibber had made the statues. By 1766 the Hospital had decided that the London crowd should no longer be allowed to turn its premises into a vulgar amusement, and just over twenty years later conditions had improved so much that a French observer described how 'the poor creatures there are not chained up in dark cellars, stretched on damp ground, nor reclining on cold paving stones . . . no bolts, no bars. The doors are open, their rooms wainscoted, and long airy corridors give them a chance of exercise. A cleanliness, hardly conceivable unless seen, reigns in this hospital.'[7] When Wordsworth wrote about his youthful London period in *The Prelude*, he ranked the experience of looking at Cibber's carvings very highly indeed, including them among

> Those other wonders different in kind,
> Though scarcely less illustrious in degree,
> The River proudly bridged, the giddy top
> And Whispering Gallery of St. Paul's, the
> Tombs
> Of Westminster, the Giants of Guildhall,
> Bedlam, and the two maniacs at its Gates.[8]

But attitudes towards 'madness' and its treatment were now changing so rapidly that, when the new Bethlem Hospital moved to Southwark in 1815, Cibber's statues were removed from open display. Hidden in the entrance hall, behind curtains only drawn aside on committee days and by special request, they were regarded as an embarrassing reminder of old attitudes towards the insane. Richard Dadd saw nothing wrong in using *'Raving Madness'* as the basis of his agonised watercolour in 1854 (see pl. 264). Two years later, though, the Hospital's surveyor Sydney Smirke dismissed them as 'the frightful figures', and declared that 'when the

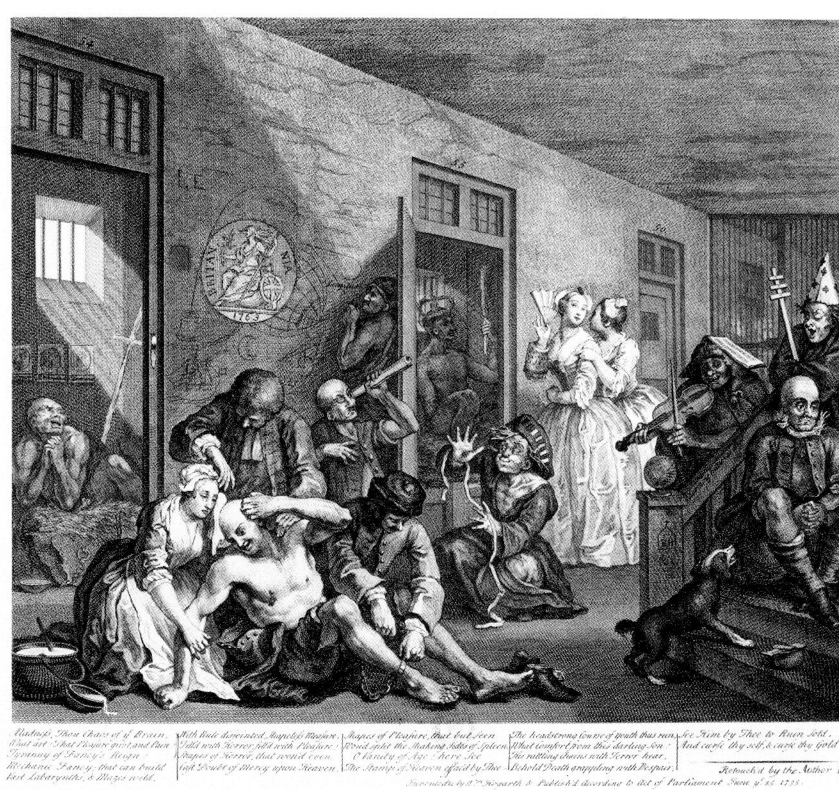

146 William Hogarth, 'Bedlam' Scene in *A Rake's Progress*, 1763, Guildhall Library and Art Gallery, London

Curtains in front of them were removed some years ago I thought it a measure of doubtful propriety and that it was the figures and not the Curtains which needed removal.'[9] The indignant Smirke soon put his disapproval into decisive action. In 1858 he ensured that the statues were taken off to the Victoria and Albert Museum, and remained banished from the Hospital for well over a century. Only now are they displayed with understandable pride in the Bethlem's own museum, where the archivist made perceptive amends for Smirke's condemnation by pointing out that 'Cibber, who must certainly have studied his subject from the life, showed more sensitivity to the full tragic despair of its extremes than has been appreciated even by his admirers: the name 'Melancholy' is a romantic misnomer for the deeply moving and disturbing image he has created.'[10] Victorian disdain has given way to contemporary admiration and Cibber's figures can once again be seen as a brave, haunting attempt to define the unfathomable tragedy of fractured minds.

The same words could hardly be applied to the five carvings made by Thomas Cartwright, the Saint Thomas's Hospital mason (pls 148–51). Sculpted for an entrance gateway designed by Nathaniel Hanwell, they are far more modest in their ambitions than Cibber's innovative and commanding figures. Cartwright lacked the grasp of powerfully expressive form displayed in the Bethlem statues, and the commission insisted that he place his four 'cripples' in the dominant context of royalty. Cibber's mesmeric carvings gained enormously from their isolation, marooned on the hospital gateway like outcasts enduring relentless social ostracism. Cartwright's patients, by contrast, were placed in deliberate subordination to the paternalistic presence of Edward VI, who refounded Saint Thomas's in 1551, eleven years after his father had decreed its closure during the Dissolution. In order to celebrate Edward's initiative, Cartwright was asked to carve him in full ceremonial regalia, sceptre in one hand and in the other a scroll that 'may be the charter presenting the Royal Hospitals to the City'.[11]

No pictorial record survives of the ornamental 'frontispiece' as it was first installed over the porch of the old Saint Thomas's building at Southwark. But an invaluable engraving does exist of the ensemble after it had been dismantled to make way for a larger entrance (pl. 147). Reassembled in the first court, to mark the passage through to the court beyond where the chapel and great hall were situated, it extolled the authority of the monarch by placing him in the most prominent niche beneath the hospital clock. He was also considerably larger than the 'cripples', who occupied subservient niches beneath him, and presided over the collegiate atmosphere of a building clearly reminiscent of a university or London's Inner Temple.

All the same, Cartwright's patients should not be underestimated. The presence of these anonymous figures in such an important site still represented a notable commitment on the part of the hospital's governors, who could so easily have restricted the 'frontispiece' either to the King alone or to regal and religious imagery in concert. Saint Thomas's placed great emphasis on Christian faith, after all: in every ward a charge to the patients was displayed in the eighteenth century, stressing that 'religion procures peace of mind, consolation under affliction, the prospect of God's blessing, through Christ, in this life, and the assurance of endless happiness and glory in the life to come'.[12]

Such sentiments reflected the fact that the Hospital's foundation had originated in the twelfth century as an *infirmarium* attached to the Priory of Saint Mary the Virgin in Southwark. Taking its name from the recently canonised Thomas Becket, the medieval hospital continued to care for the sick, poor travellers and the destitute aged. But Edward VI's Letters Patent of 1551 ushered in a new set of priorities. They referred to 'the miserable state of the sick and infirm poor men lying begging in the public streets and places of London and its suburbs'. Eighteen years later, the governors of London's four hospitals clarified this function still further. They issued a joint order

> for the Preventing of all Idle and Begging People, whether Men, Women, or Children, or other masterless Vagrants . . . to take the four Hospitals in London, by the sixteen Beadles belonging to the same, who had their several Standings and Walks in every Ward. Those that were Vagabonds and sturdy Beggars, they were to carry to *Bridewell.* Those that were aged, impotent, sick, sore, lame, or blind, to *St. Bartholomew's* or *St. Thomas's* Hospital. And all Children under the Age of sixteen to *Christ's* Hospital.[13]

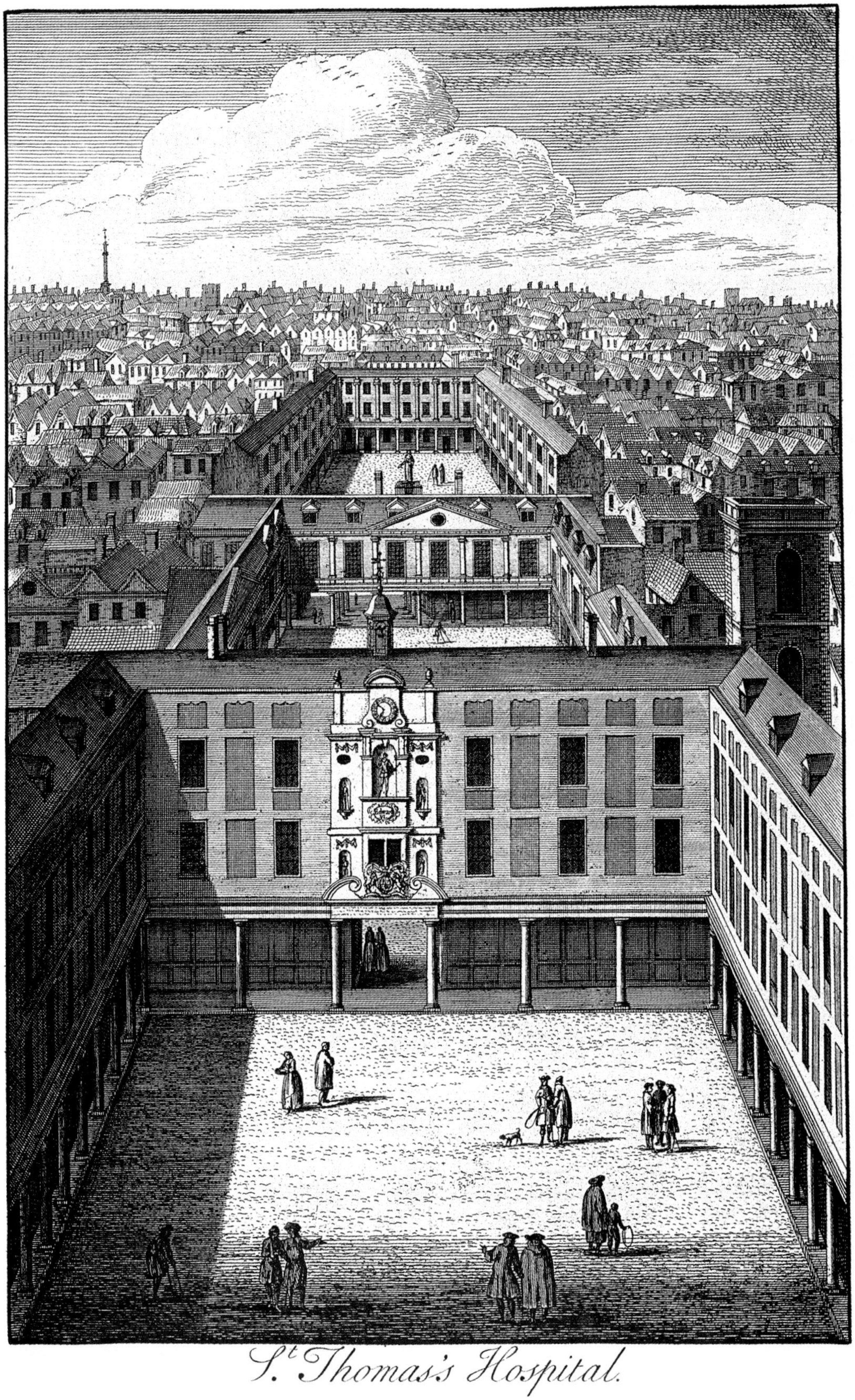

147 Thomas Cartwright, 'Cripples' ensemble reassembled in the first court of Saint Thomas's Hospital, London, engraving, 1739

148 (*top left*) Thomas Cartwright, *Youth with Wooden Leg*, 1681–1702, St Thomas's Hospital, London

149 (*top right*) Thomas Cartwright, *Young Woman with Arm in a Sling*, 1681–1702, St Thomas's Hospital, London

150 (*bottom left*) Thomas Cartwright, *Woman Resting on a Stick*, 1681–1702, St Thomas's Hospital, London

151 (*bottom right*) Thomas Cartwright, *Old Man Leaning on a Crutch*, 1681–1702, St Thomas's Hospital, London

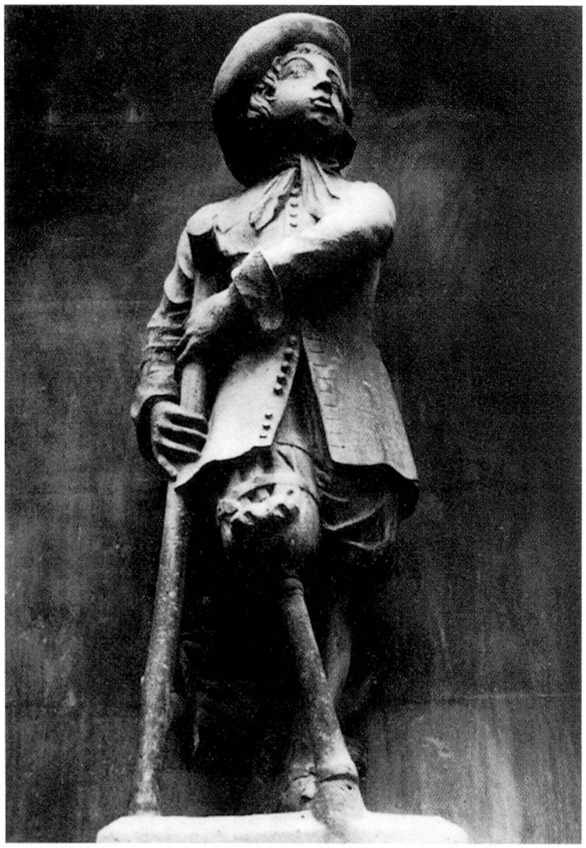

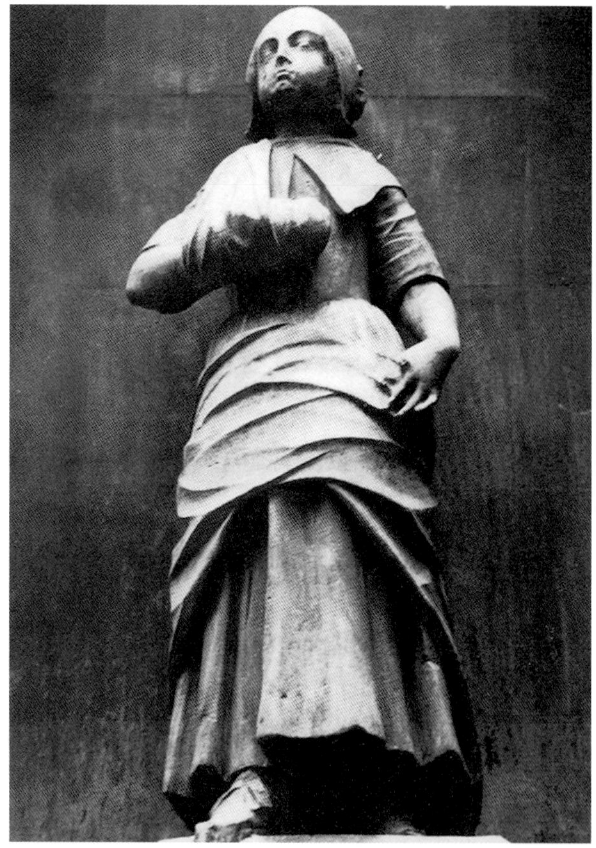

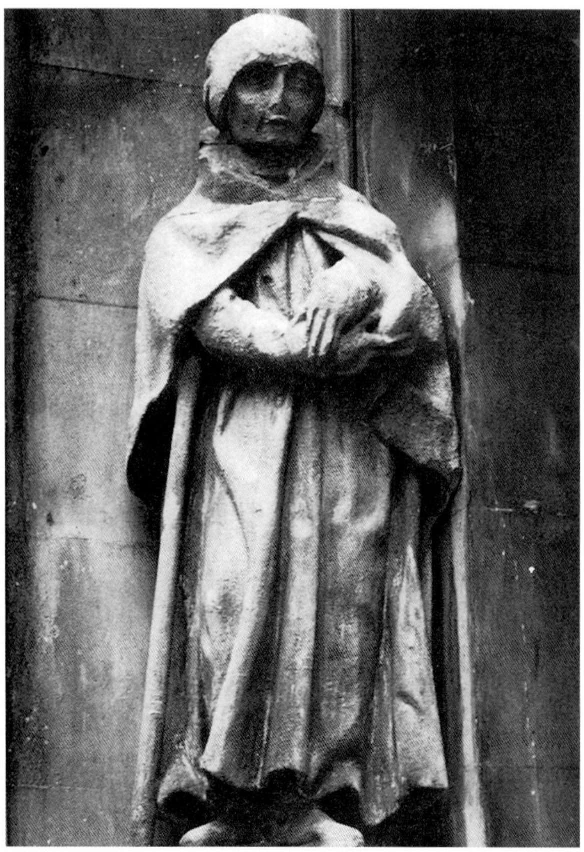

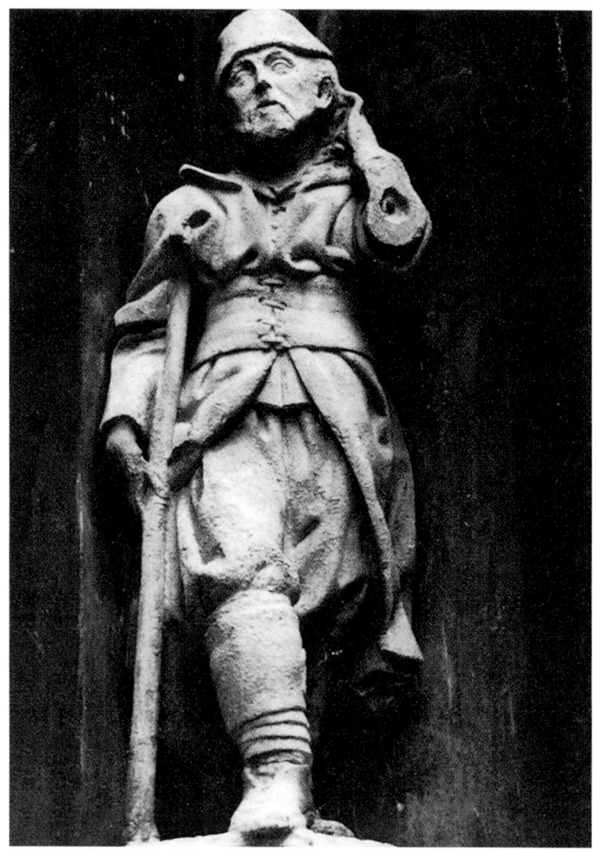

This, then, is the context in which to understand the reason why images of 'cripples' were installed over Saint Thomas's entrance rather than saints or angels. In post-Reformation England the Crown took over the church's role as the sponsor of hospitals and the wealthy citizens of London raised the funds to pay for a healthier environment. Hence the decision to place secular images of people drawn from the mass of 'aged, impotent, sick, sore, lame, or blind' in the niches of Saint Thomas's symbolic 'frontispiece'. Looked after by the omnipotent figure of the King, they quietly testified to the existence of deliberately varied ages of patient – an old man, a woman in middle age, a young woman and a youth – who had been taken off the streets and safely enclosed in an institution dedicated to their care.

Unlike Cartwright's statue of the monarch, a figure with a 'somewhat bloated and expressionless face'[14] who bears the inevitable hallmarks of a posthumous portrait, the 'cripple' carvings appear to be based on particular individuals. One historian of Saint Thomas's believed that 'the poor things who served as models for them were actual patients in the Hospital at Southwark',[15] and Cartwright's position as the mason of Saint Thomas's would certainly have given him ready access to the occupants of the wards. He made good use of the privilege, too. For all their obvious technical limitations, the statues he produced are distinguished by his willingness to stress the humanity of the 'cripples' rather than treating them merely as illustrations for a medical demonstration.

So direct was Cartwright's approach that the old man leaning on a crutch expresses the diffidence of someone who feels shy about posing for the mason (pl. 151). At a time when ordinary people were rarely singled out and portrayed in such a public manner, his reticence is understandable. But he holds his ground with calm dignity, his heavily bandaged leg prominently exposed so that no one could remain in any doubt about his ailment. The plight of the woman resting on a stick is, by contrast, less specific (pl. 150). A long dress hides the precise condition of her legs, and the hood enclosing her head like a helmet adds to the figure's enigmatic aura. All the same, her square-jawed face bears gaunt witness to the stoicism with which she handles her suffering, and her younger counterpart appears still more resilient in struggling to withstand adversity (pl. 149). The sling swathing her right arm does not prevent her from adopting a proud, erect posture. With her other arm falling gracefully down her side, where she hooks her thumb in the folds of an unusually full dress, she gazes out at the world with patience and fortitude.

So does the youth who is, perhaps, the most distinctive and memorable of the statues (pl. 148). Although encumbered with the gravest impediment of all, he refuses to let his wooden leg reduce him to the level of total inertia. Cartwright catches him at the very moment when he stretches an arm across to adjust his crutch, and this gesture implies considerable determination. But it appears vulnerable as well, the stance of someone who realises how vulnerable his amputated leg has made him. On the streets of London, before he was admitted to Saint Thomas's, such a boy would have found survival difficult. He might also have been subjected to mockery and humiliation by other vagrants, only too eager to scorn the 'spastic' in their midst. That is why the Hospital's decision to erect statues of 'cripples' was so salutary. It underlined the belief that nobody should be despised for labouring under grievous physical disability, and Cartwright's chisel did succeed in endowing his stoical, undaunted models with the dignity they deserved.

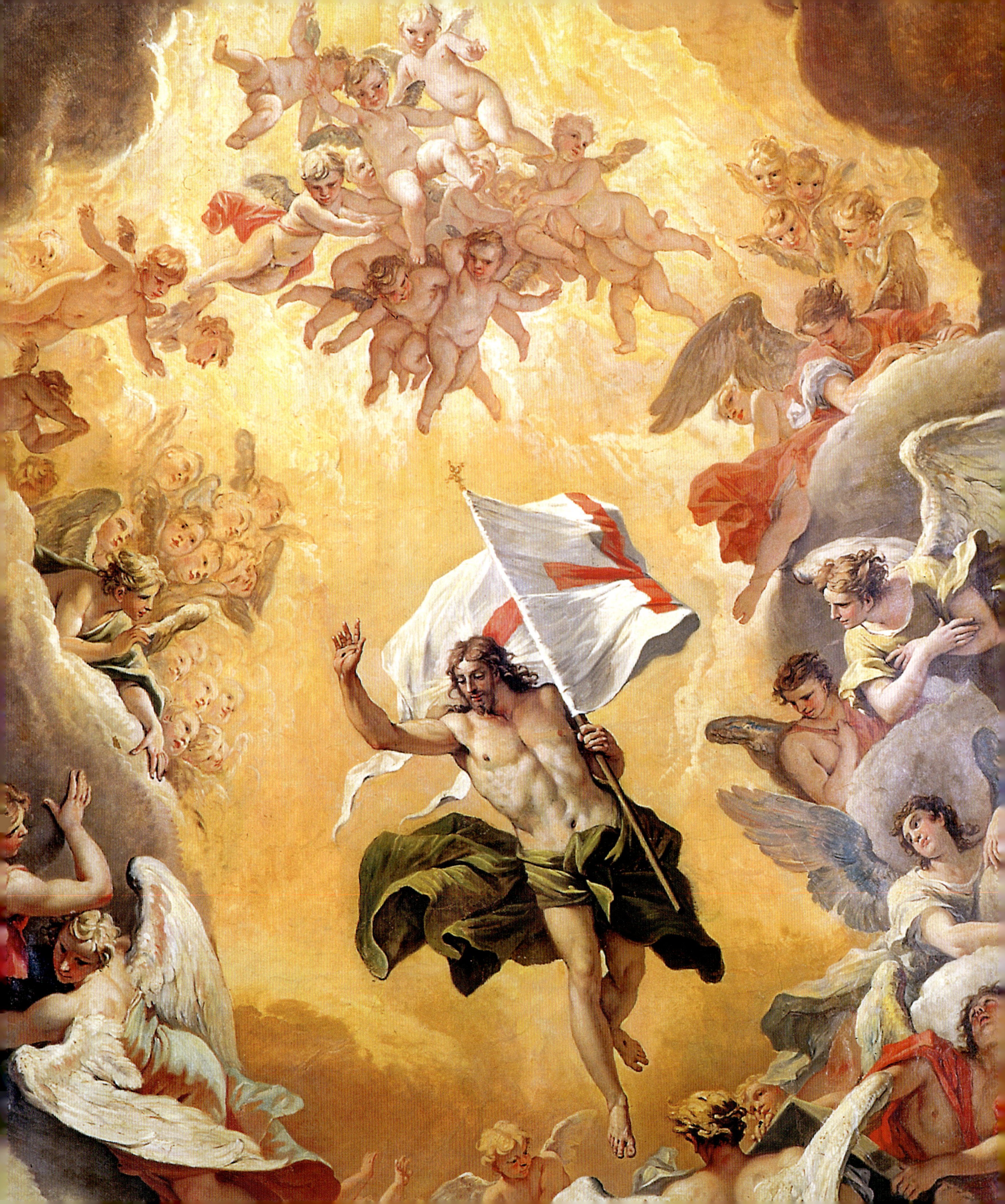

TWELVE
SHELTER FOR SOLDIERS

In seventeenth-century Paris, the most majestic new hospital made use of both painters and sculptors on a scale as yet undreamt-of in London. Founded by Louis XIV's royal decrees of January and April 1670, the vast architectural ensemble comprising the Hôtel des Invalides was intended to provide care and shelter for wounded, pensioned soldiers. Little time was lost in awarding the commission for the grandiloquent building to Libéral Bruant, who started work on the design in March 1671 and managed to lay the foundation stone eight months later. Although only three years elapsed before the first pensioners were allowed to move in, work on Bruant's design then became affected by his frequent absences. But the massive northern facade gradually rose from fields on the outskirts of Paris set aside for the king's ostentatious enterprise.

The ever-egocentric Louis made sure that Bruant's central pavilion, projecting from the rest of the immense frontage, took the form of a monumental arch with carved decorations glorifying the monarch's military prowess (pl. 153). Guillaume Coustou was responsible for installing, under a great curving band of stone festooned with trophies and a triumphant sun, the enormous bas-relief of the equestrian king riding between the figures of Justice and Prudence. This blatantly propagandist image rests on a plinth bearing the boast that 'Louis the Great in his royal munificence for his soldiers and with prudent foresight for eternity founded this edifice in the year 1675'. Not surprisingly, the bas-relief was destroyed by enraged Republicans during the Revolution. But Cartellier reinstated it once the monarchy had been restored, and the carving still retains its place today in a centrepiece whose high doorway is flanked by Coustou's flamboyant seated statues of Mars and Minerva. Backed by Bruant's mighty pilasters, against which they almost appear to rest, these extravagantly attired figures provide the building with a flourish it would not otherwise possess.

For Bruant's design is a stolid affair. As Anthony Blunt pointed out, it was the work of an architect who 'lacked entirely the sense of the spectacular',[1] and the Invalides would seem dull without the grimacing masks that surmount the ground-floor windows. The liveliest elements in this facade are, without doubt, the carved soldiers' breastplates and plumed helmets enclosing each of the twenty-four different dormer windows set into the high roof (pl. 154). With their faces gazing out from visors and plated arms extending down the side of each window, these fanciful additions introduce at times a macabre mood. One of the soldiers, whose face appears to be punctured by pockmarks, brandishes an empty armhole in a sling where his hand should

152 (*facing page*) Detail of pl. 165

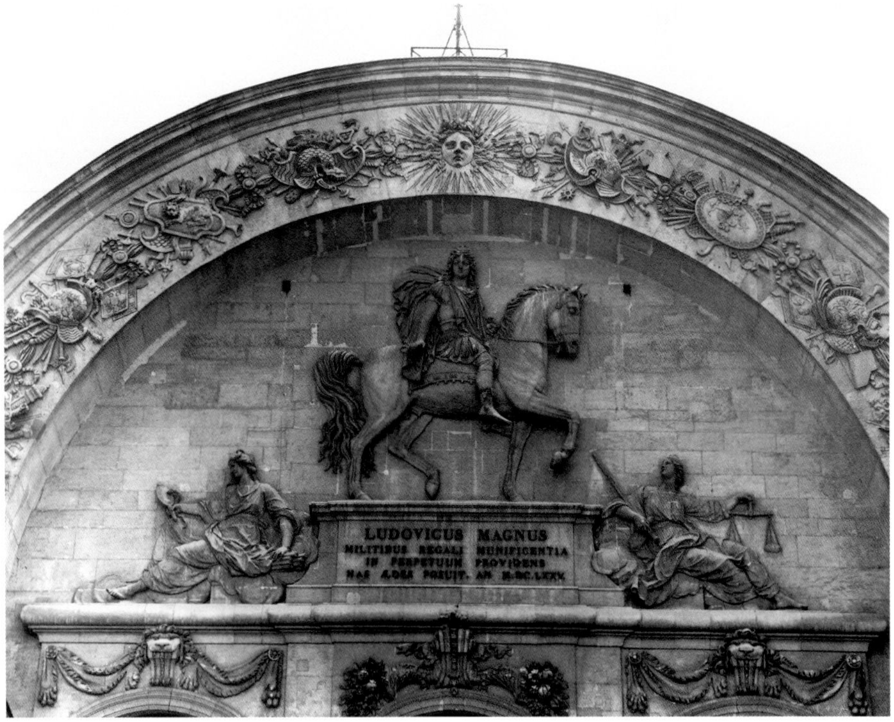

be. But these reminders of war's brutality, which may refer directly to the wounds suffered by some of the Hôtel's pensioned inhabitants, are rare. Their hints of pathos soon become outweighed by the drum-beating rhetoric elsewhere on the frontage, most extravagantly in the two fulsome bas-reliefs on the corner pavilions. Here the central breastplates are surrounded by the spoils of victorious campaigns. Cannons, winged standards, richly wrought shields and tasselled flags are all meant to evoke stirring memories of the Sun King's invincible career.

The brutal reality of military life, for many of the soldiers who had fought in Louis's incessant campaigns, was wholly removed from this bragging imperial rhetoric. Many of the wretched men admitted to the care of the Invalides had become beggars, and they must have felt hugely relieved to find that the Hôtel now offered them a permanent home. In order to qualify, applicants were required to prove that they had served in the army for at

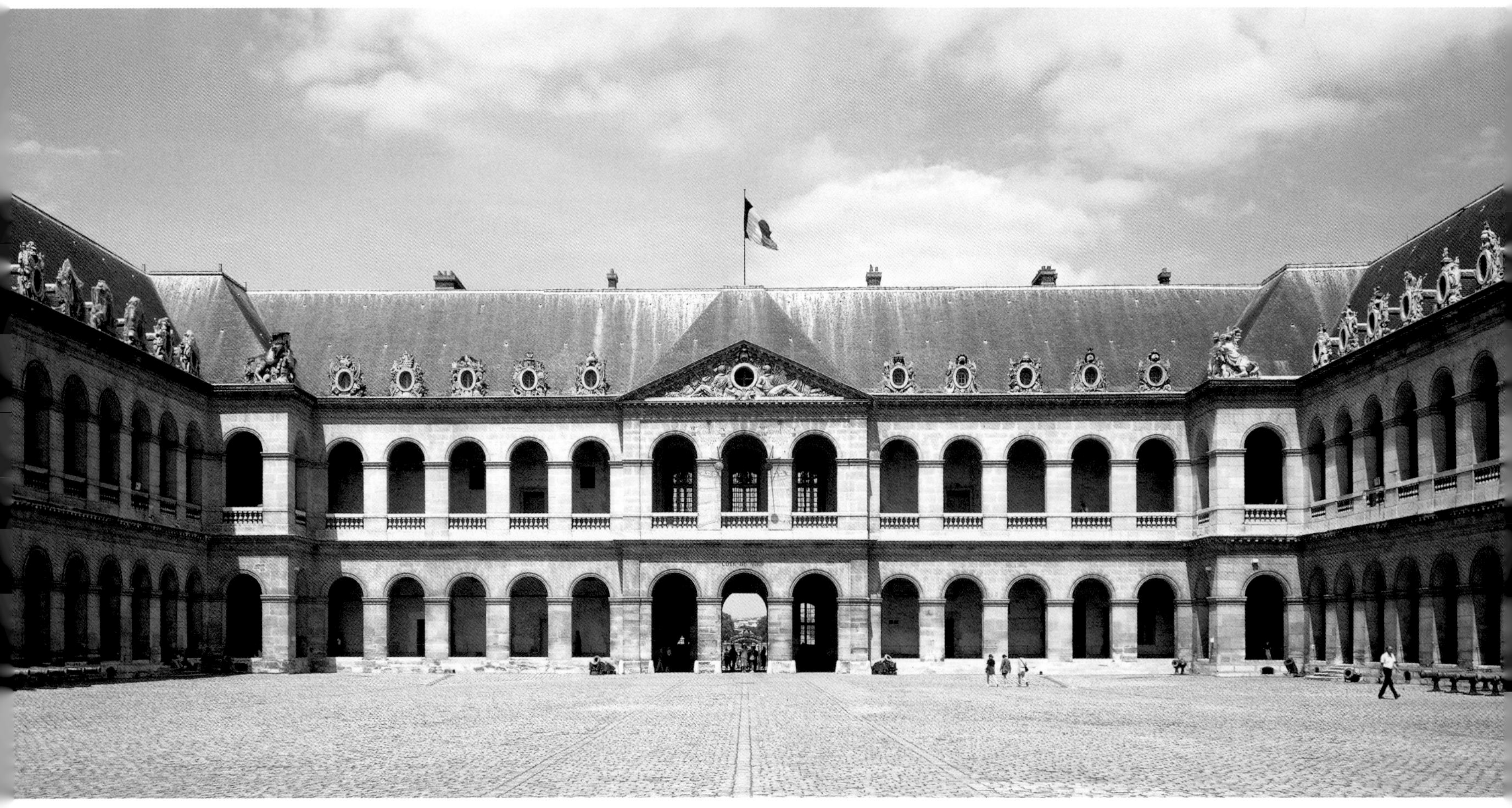

least a decade and that their careers had left them either crippled or disabled in some other way. The rule was strictly applied: Nicolas Apurillot, a seventy-year-old soldier nicknamed 'Grillot', was turned away in 1677 because 'he does not have the necessary service qualifications and is not crippled'.[2] When the accepted pensioners gained admittance, they found themselves subjected to a regulated existence with great emphasis placed on compulsory attendance at all religious services. Although they had been accustomed to discipline in their army days, many had since become so dissolute that the Invalides was forced to impose a strict regime. Drunkenness received stern punishment, for old age did not necessarily curb the soldiers' bibulous activities. The Hôtel registers singled out a notorious alcoholic lecher known as 'La Réjouissance', a sprightly sixty-three year-old who was 'always whoring, not only in the streets and shops, but even in houses'.[3] As a result, each pensioner was confined to half a pint of wine at meal-times, which might otherwise have degenerated into brawls.

Jacques Lepautre's engraving (pl. 155) shows the old soldiers dining at immensely long tables in one of the four grand dining-halls, with another table set aside in the centre of the room for 'water drinkers' whose wine rations had been banished altogether. The engraving also reveals the overwhelming magnificence of their surroundings. All the dining-halls were decorated with fulsome murals of Louis's victories, painted largely between 1678 and 1682 by Joseph Parrocel and Michel II Corneille. The contrast between the romanticised glory of these battle scenes, and the stoical stance adopted by the wooden-legged pensioner in the foreground of the engraving, is ironic indeed. Further back, Lepautre even includes the melancholy figure of a man whose legs have been reduced to stumps, forcing him to sit on the floor and move along with the aid of iron hand-clamps. But at least every effort was made to house the soldiers in surroundings that reflected wholehearted official appreciation of the gruesome sacrifices they had made.

Elsewhere in the Invalides, decoration was restricted to the uppermost levels of the building. Above the severity of the Hôtel's courtyard, where on the third floor many pensioners spent their days tapestry-weaving, illuminating hymn books or, on a more mundane level, shoemaking for the army, uninhibited carvings once again burst out on the edge of the roof. Sixty dormer windows are here surrounded by an array of sculptural caprices ostensibly derived from martial subjects but often indulging in heraldic images that involve an elephant, dog or ram. One window, reputedly depicting the arms of the Marquess of Louvois, plays on his name by crowning the decoration with a wolf's head peering cheekily through a flourish of reeds. These high spirits reach a crescendo at each corner of the court of honour, where groups of horses rear dramatically in the air (pl. 154). Their manes flare up with extraordinary abandon, as if to acknowledge both the danger and the exhilaration of the conflict they encounter on the battlefield.

From the ground floor of the Hôtel, the pensioners could gain access to their church where compulsory services were so often held. Built very hurriedly between 1676 and 1680, and dedicated to Saint Louis, the austere interior was enlivened by little other than the flags hung like trophies from the upper cornices. But Germain Pilon produced the organ-case, completing it by 1687;[4] and until 1873 an open way[5] behind the high altar linked Saint-Louis des Invalides with the outright architectural masterpiece of the entire Hôtel scheme, the Church of the Dome (pl. 156).

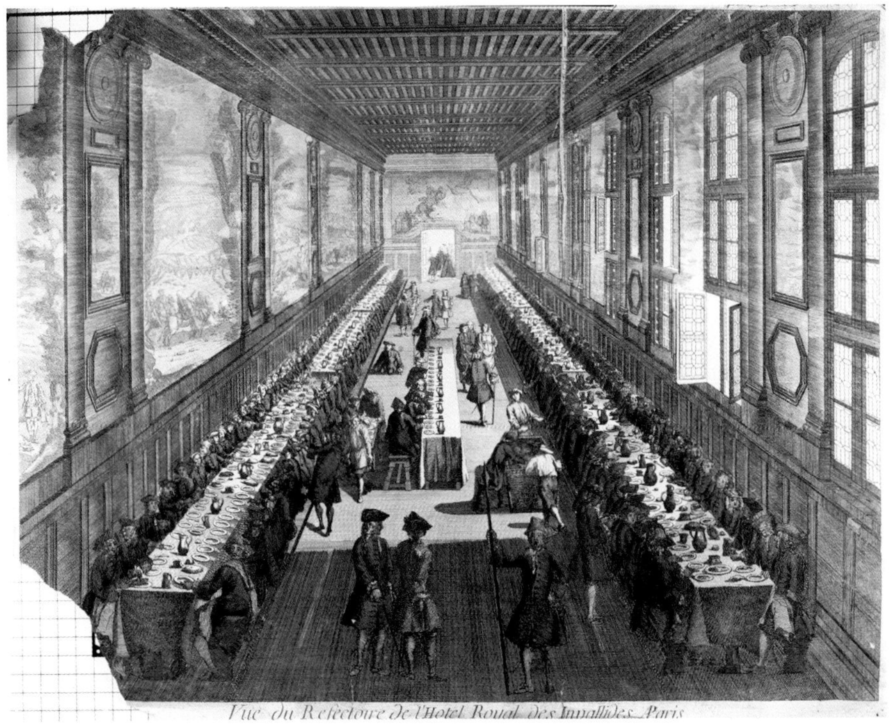

155 (*above*) Jacques Lepautre, *Old Soldiers Dining in Hôtel des Invalides*, 18th Century, Private Collection

153 (*facing page, top*) Guillaume Coustou, bas-relief of Louis XIV riding between Justice and Prudence, 1753, central pavilion of Hôtel des Invalides, Paris

154 (*facing page, bottom*) Carvings enclosing dormer windows, Cour d'honneur, Hôtel des Invalides, built 1671–1706, Paris

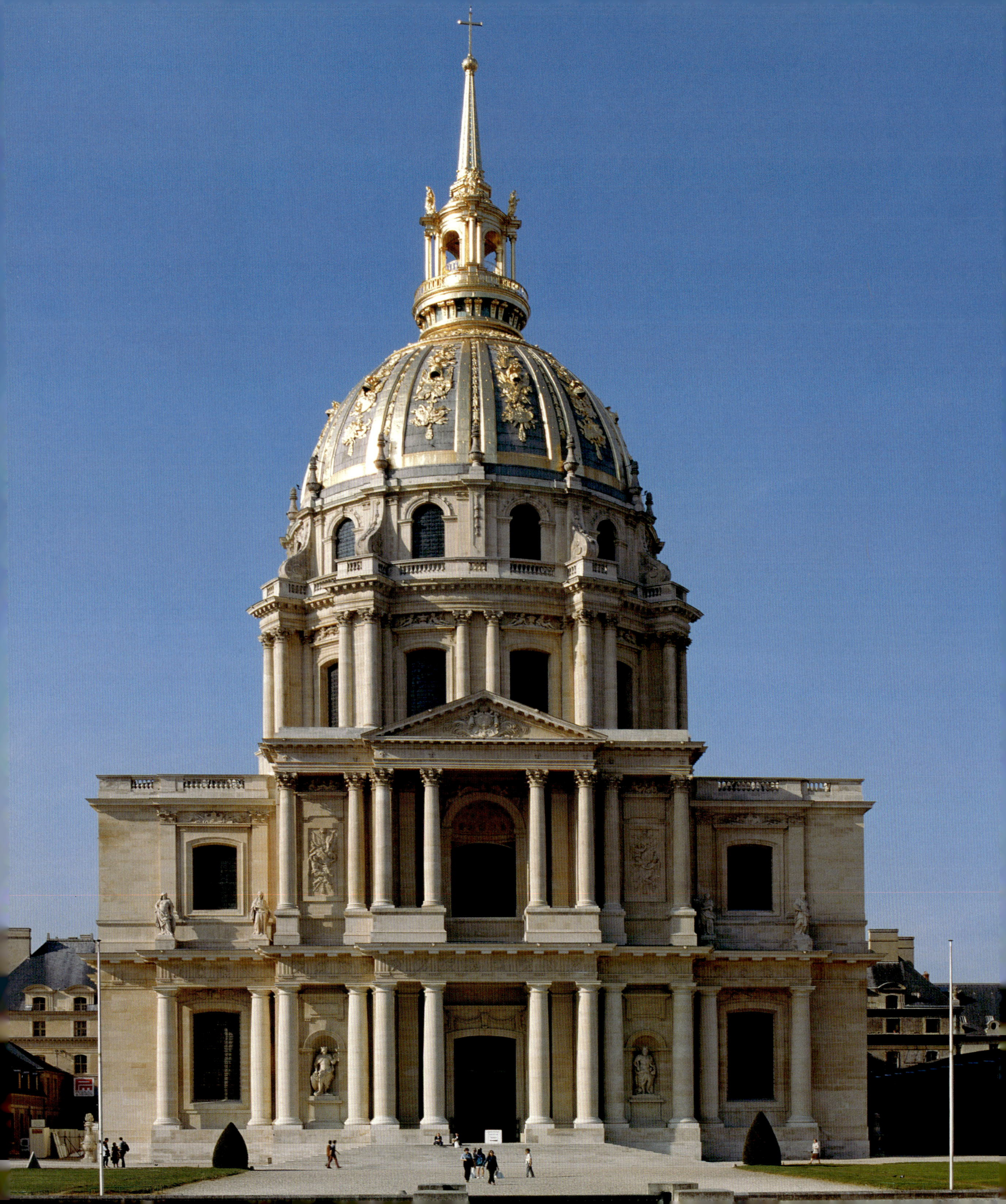

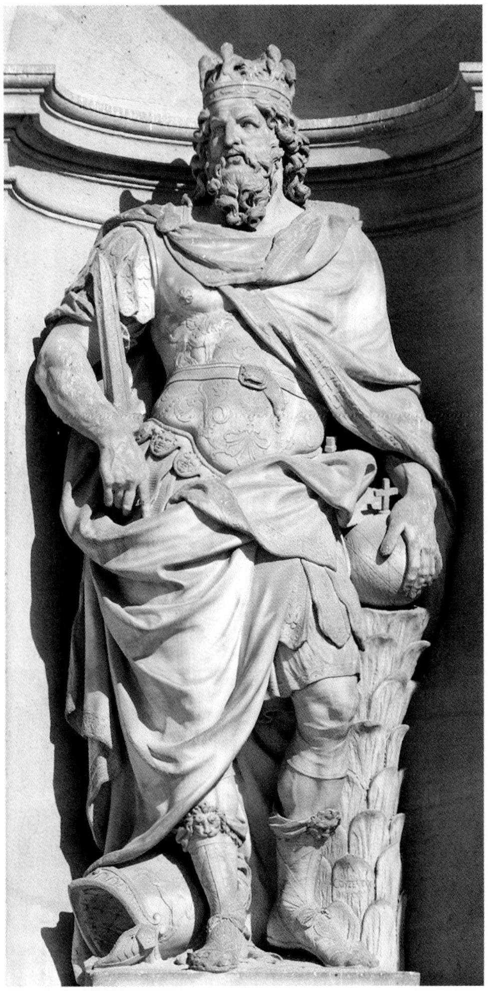 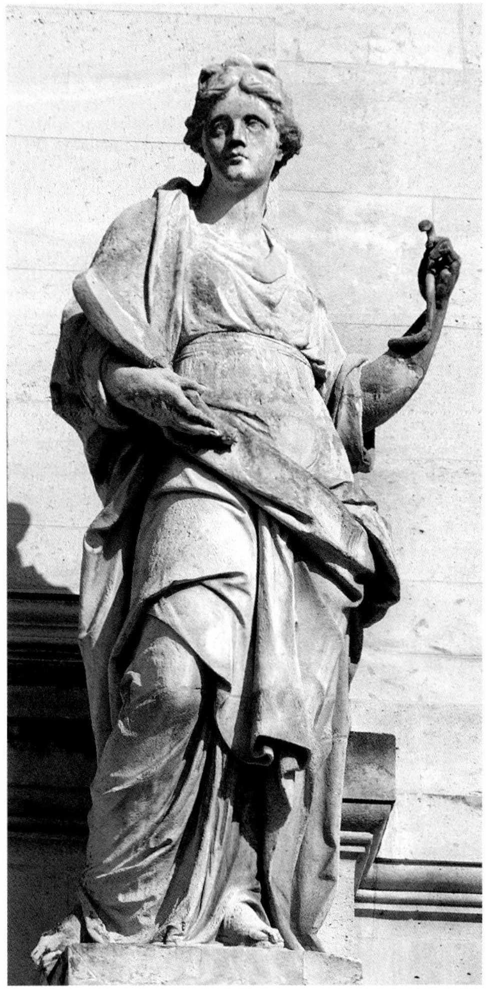 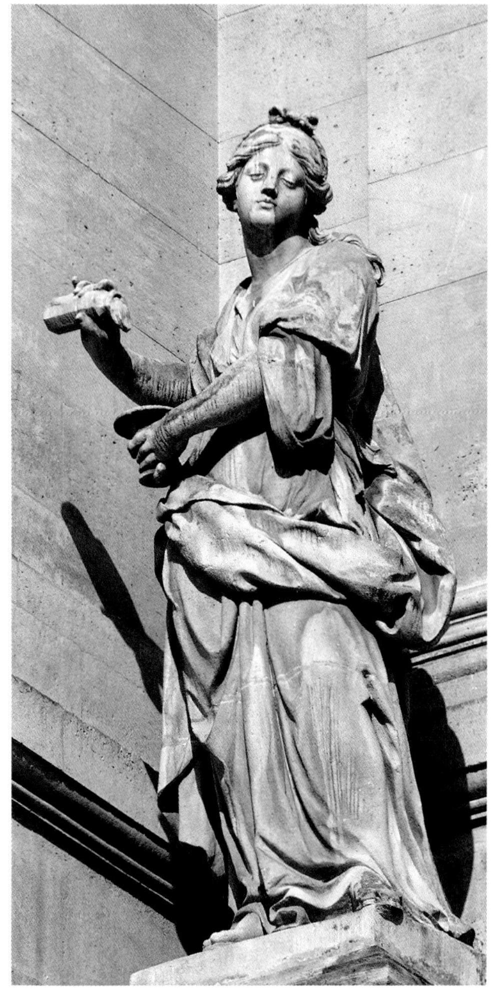

The idea of erecting this proud edifice behind the soldiers' church arose in the spring of 1676, when Louvois, then Under-Secretary of State for War and Superintendent of the Hôtel's buildings, contacted the thirty-year-old architect Jules Hardouin-Mansart. Dissatisfied with Bruant's progress on the Hôtel, Louvois commissioned his young protégé to design a building of such splendour that it would eventually come to be regarded as the Invalides' principal facade. Hardouin-Mansart started work on the project with a built-in advantage: since his great-uncle, François Mansart, had designed plans for the Bourbon chapel at Saint-Denis, he took over the blueprint and applied it to the new venture instead. After completing Saint-Louis des Invalides first, he began building the Church of the Dome in 1677 and continued for the next twenty-nine years. Lack of funds caused the delay in erecting the structure, and his ambitious proposal to complete it with a semicircular forecourt emulating Saint Peter's in Rome was never realised. But the church itself, capped by the superb dome, soon became recognised as one of Paris's most sublime buildings.

The importance of the role played by artists is announced at the very outset of a visit to the church. At either side of the main entrance, two monumental marble carvings occupy their niches with commanding authority: Coustou's statue of Saint Louis, on the left, represents the church's patron saint and (not by accident) the namesake of the king himself; while Coysevox's figure portrays Saint Charlemagne (pl. 157). The latter sculptor was also responsible for the four free-standing statues of *Prudence* (pl. 158), *Justice*, *Strength* and *Temperance* (pl. 159) above the Doric entablature. Their assurance lends the facade an enormous sense of poised elegance and it is a matter for intense regret

157 (*above, left*) Antoine Coysevox, *Charlemagne*, Church of the Dome, Hôtel des Invalides, Paris

158 (*above, centre*) Antoine Coysevox, *Prudence*, Church of the Dome, Hôtel des Invalides, Paris

159 (*above, right*) Antoine Coysevox, *Temperance*, Church of the Dome, Hôtel des Invalides, Paris

156 (*facing page*) Jules Hardouin-Mansart, Church of the Dome, completed 1706, Hôtel des Invalides, Paris

that the other thirty-four carvings in this sequence no longer remain *in situ*. Ascending as far as the lantern's summit, they once acted as an admirable sculptural complement to the intricate columnar interplay achieved by the architecture.

They are a great loss, and yet the elaborate paintings executed within the church still survive. Although their impact has since been impaired by the addition of Visconti's crypt for Napoleon, and by his no less intrusive high altar with its canopy supported by four wreathed marble columns, these sumptuous decorations must originally have arrested the attention of anyone exploring the building. The cupola of the first chapel on the right, Saint-Augustine, is emblazoned with paintings by Louis de Boullogne depicting the life of the saint to whom the chapel was dedicated. Other corner chapels in the sequence duly followed suit with equally competent, if unexceptional schemes, and the side entrance of each one bears a bas-relief representing an episode from Saint Louis's life.

The most prominent and expansive decorations were, however, reserved for the interior of the great dome itself. They commence in a relatively calm and restrained manner, with a low-relief carving of a guardian spirit embellishing each corner chapel entrance. But then monochrome sculpture gives way to heightened colour in the pendants above them, where Charles de la Fosse depicted the *Four Evangelists*. The act of writing does not prevent them from seeking divine inspiration by gazing and gesturing upwards, thereby directing attention towards the first cupola where Jean Jouvenet's twelve massive images of the Apostles[6] fill the tall, curving space allotted to them by Hardouin-Mansart's design. They form a majestic prelude to the circular painting executed by de la Fosse for the second cupola, lit by twelve semicircular openings invisible from within.

The subject chosen for this climactic image in the church was *Saint Louis offering his Sword to Christ after his Victory over the Infidels* (pl. 160). It was, no doubt, considered an appropriate theme for a building connected with the French army, but the painting is notable for de la Fosse's exclusion of any direct depiction of Louis's battles. The most overt references to his martial prowess are the shield and sword which he hands to Christ, a relaxed figure reclining on a cloud with a geniality far removed from any notion of omnipotent sternness. Illuminated by a blazing cloud behind him, he extends a finger to bless Louis for symbolically laying aside his weaponry. And as if to celebrate the cessation of conflict, the music-making angels who encircle the painting's rim strike up a joyful concert on harp, organ and flute. Like Noël Coypel's even more beatific paintings of the *Holy Trinity* and the *Assumption of the Virgin*, on the sanctuary's arched roof and the vault of the apse, the cupola decorations are dedicated to peace rather than aggression. They owe a debt to the exuberance of Correggio rather than the grim masters of battle painting, and reflect Louis XIV's new-found enthusiasm for religion. The invalids, well cared-for in an excellent infirmary, were required to attend religious services daily and found themselves described, somewhat disconcertingly, as 'heaven's militia'.[7]

Only on the outside of the dome, where twelve complex lead clusters of arms and trophies adorn the vault, are the priorities of soldiering asserted once more. They are, however, barely visible from ground level, where the viewer's attention finally comes to rest on the open-work lantern surmounted by a gilt obelisk and a cross. The priorities of religious faith are reasserted at the very apex of this masterly Jesuitic dome, which the gratified monarch finally inaugurated with all the members of his court in a splendid ceremony on 28 August 1706. Pierre Denis Martin recorded the scene in a panoramic canvas, including the throng of richly attired attendants around their monarch. But pride of place in the painting was reserved, quite rightly, for the pensioners' church beyond, a *pièce de résistance* gleaming with absolute serenity in the late summer sun.

Not long after work began on the Invalides, the decision was taken to erect in Kilmainham, County Dublin, a Royal Hospital to house three hundred army veterans who 'by reason of Age, Wounds, or other Infirmities, since their first coming into Our Army, are grown unfit to be any longer continued in Our Service'.[8] The idea of such a refuge, directly inspired by the Parisian precedent, was first mooted in the 1670s by the Earl of Granard and the Lord Lieutenant, the Earl of Essex. Charles II, ever competitive with Louis XIV, lost little time in consenting to a levy on Irish military pay as a means of funding the extensive enterprise. William Robinson, the Surveyor-General, was commissioned to design the building in Phoenix Park, and

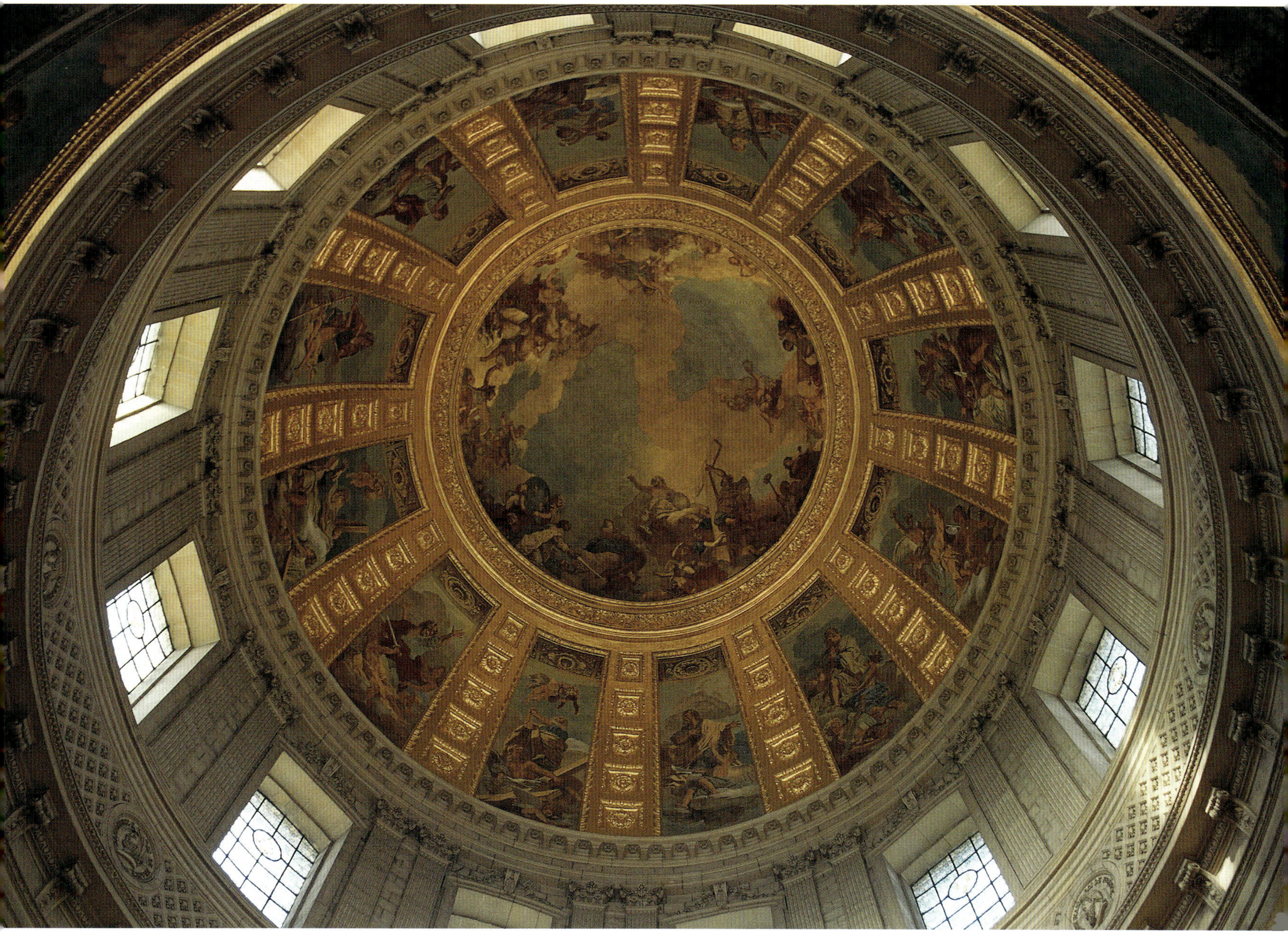

a site chosen where ruins still survived of the Priory of the Knights Hospitallers. The foundation stone was laid in 1680 by the Duke of Ormond and construction sufficiently advanced by spring 1684 for the Royal Hospital to receive its first residents. Along with a separate infirmary for sick and mad soldiers, the ensemble with landmark tower and steeple (pl. 161) ended up as the most distinguished building to be erected in seventeenth-century Ireland. And Robinson made sure that 'the hardy maimed veterans of our country's honour'[9] were housed in the country's first full-scale manifestation of classical architecture.

Writing a history of the Hospital in 1713, Thomas Wilson made clear that the Invalides had been the prime source of inspiration for the Kilmainham project.[10] The arcaded residential courtyard ranges, where the veterans could take exercise among '82 Lime Trees to be Planted Round the Quadrangle within the Hospital',[11] certainly echoed the Paris model. So did the five external tympana in the entrance arches (pl. 162), each carved in pine by a

160 Charles de la Fosse, *Saint Louis Offering his Sword to Christ*, Church of the Dome, Hôtel des Invalides, Paris

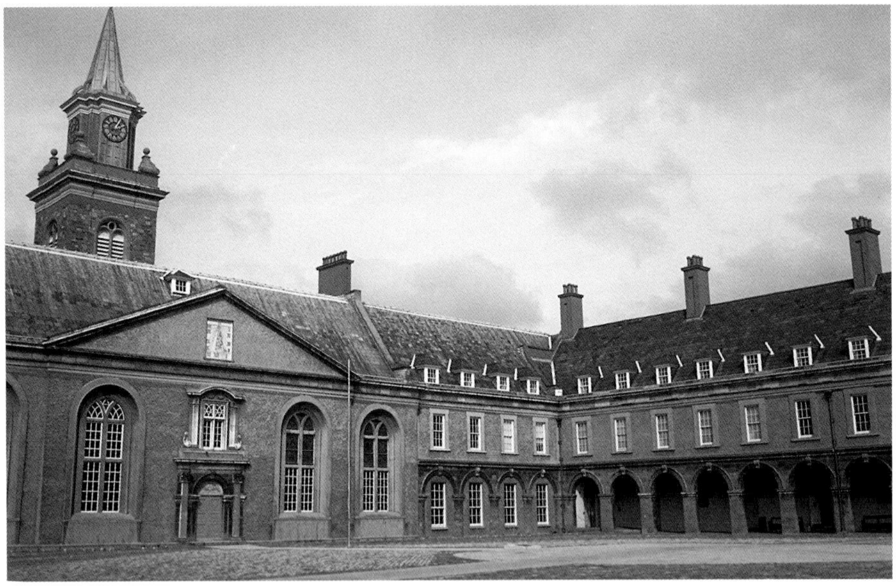

161 William Robinson, Royal Hospital (now Irish Museum of Modern Art), 1680–84, Kilmainham, Co. Dublin

162 James (or Jacques) Tabary, External tympana in the entrance arches, Kilmainham, Co. Dublin

sculptor impressive enough to substantiate Edward McParland's claim that the Hospital's 'carving is perhaps the finest ever to decorate an Irish building'.[12] Frustratingly, the lack of detailed accounts means that the sculptor's identity is uncertain. But he may have been the elusive James (or Jacques) Tabary,[13] who in 1682 was admitted as a freeman in Dublin and, five years later, is recorded at work on

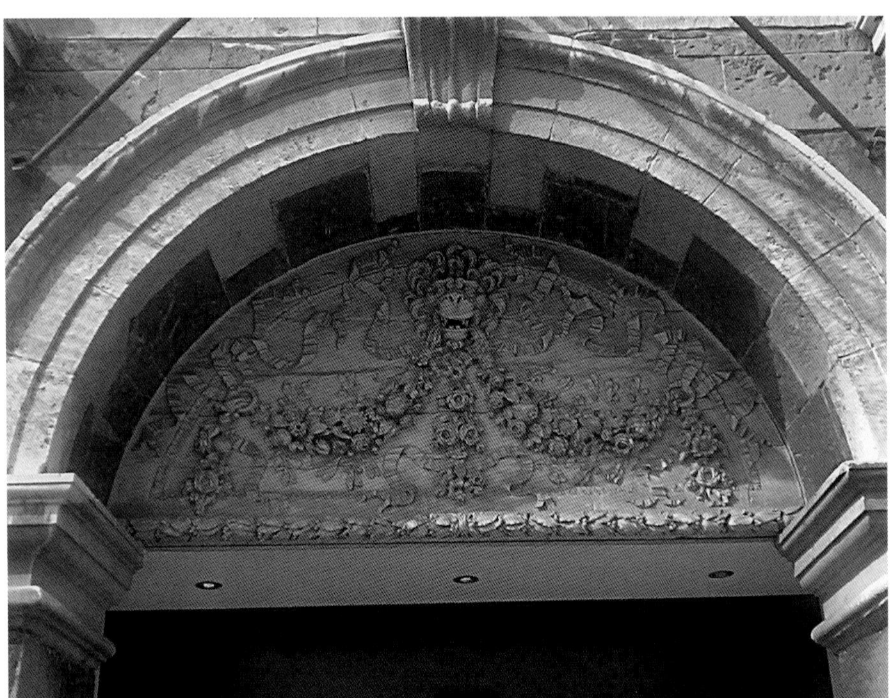

wood carvings in the east end of the Hospital's chapel. Executed with impressive skill, for a remarkable space which can be counted as the only Baroque interior in Ireland, Tabary's sprightly garlands, flowers and leaves have nevertheless been compromised by later alterations. Yet the external pine tympana retain all their original verve, assembling military trophies in celebratory Baroque clusters where helmets sprout animal heads and swords terminate in handles resembling birds with long, predatory beaks. They could have provided abundant fascination for the Hospital's occupants, thereby fulfilling the original charter where the sincere hope was expressed that 'such of the . . . Army, as hath faithfully served . . . in the Strength and Vigour of their Youth, may in the Weakness, and Disasters, that their Old Age, Wounds or other Misfortunes may bring them into, find a comfortable Retreat and a competent Maintenance therein.'[14]

Not to be outdone, London now decided to compete with Paris and Dublin.[15] The Royal Hospital, Chelsea (pl. 163), founded by Charles II in 1682 as a retreat for ailing and elderly army veterans, has a grandeur inspired by the Hôtel des Invalides. Charles was determined to emulate the French king's munificent gesture, thereby inaugurating a great era of hospital building in England. Until the sixteenth century, the state made no provision for old and injured soldiers, but by the time of the Civil War in 1642, pensions were being paid from national funds. Charles II's more ambitious aspirations are proclaimed at Chelsea not only by Christopher Wren's architecture but also by Grinling Gibbons's statue of Charles II presiding over the main Court (pl. 164). He looks like a Roman Emperor, and in his gilded condition the King must have appeared to his old soldiers as a gleaming saviour. Arrayed in their splendid scarlet coats and ceremonial tricorn hats, a modernised version of the service dress of the period, hundreds of army pensioners still live at the Royal Hospital. On Sunday mornings, their service in the chapel is dominated, on the semi-dome of its apse, by the colossal painting that provides a triumphant climax to Wren's interior (pl. 165).

To the chagrin of his ambitious British rivals, who bitterly resented the success of imported foreign artists, Sebastiano Ricci secured the prestigious chapel commission around 1714. It may have come, at the suggestion of the Duke of Shrewsbury, from George I. One historian has proposed that the

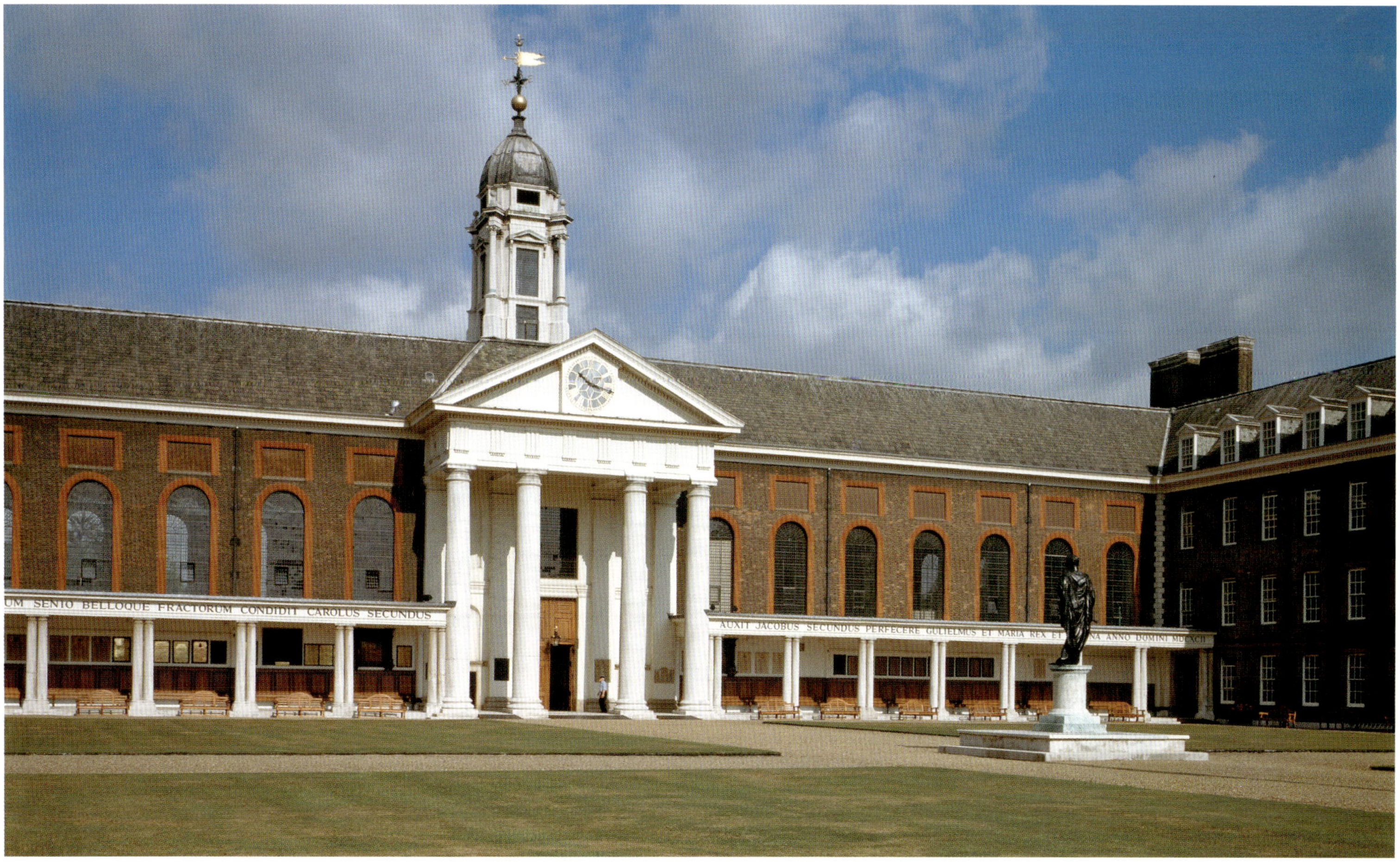
SENIO BELLOQUE FRACTORUM CONDIDIT CAROLUS SECUNDUS
AUXIT JACOBUS SECUNDUS PERFECERE GULIELMUS ET MARIA REX ET

Resurrection theme was chosen as a memorial to Queen Anne, who died in August 1714,[16] and it would indeed have been an appropriate subject for the decoration of a Royal Hospital chapel. The King may also have given this major commission to Ricci as a consolation prize, after he had been passed over in favour of Sir James Thornhill for the privileged task of decorating Wren's newly completed dome at Saint Paul's Cathedral. Patriotism dictated the choice of Thornhill, but George I was right to give the Italian invader an opportunity to excel himself on the grand scale in the Chelsea chapel. Ricci, brought over to England from Venice by his talented nephew Marco Ricci around 1709, was a skilful forerunner of Tiepolo. Indebted above all to Veronese, he is best known in England for the two large mythological compositions, *Diana and her Nymphs* and *The Triumph of Venus*, now hanging on the grand staircase of the Royal Academy's entrance hall in Burlington House. But the uneven Ricci surpassed himself on the apse at Chelsea. He

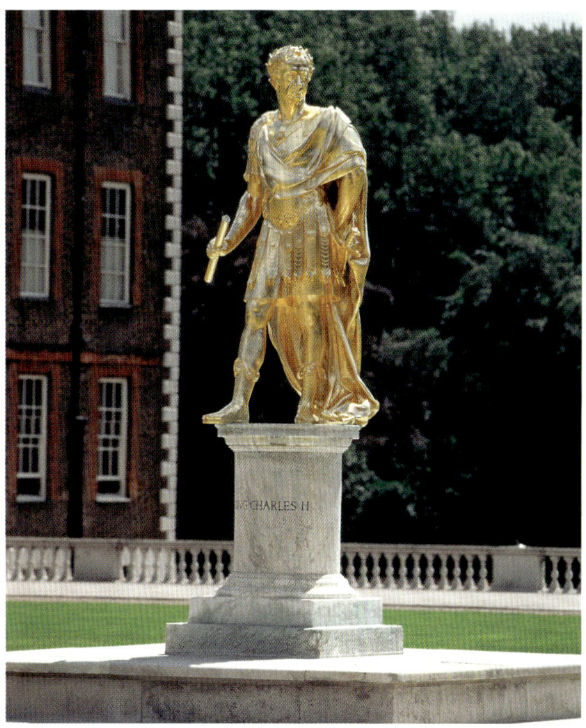

163 (*above*) Christopher Wren, Royal Hospital, Chelsea, 1682–91

164 (*left*) Grinling Gibbons, *Charles II* in the main court, 1676, Royal Hospital, Chelsea

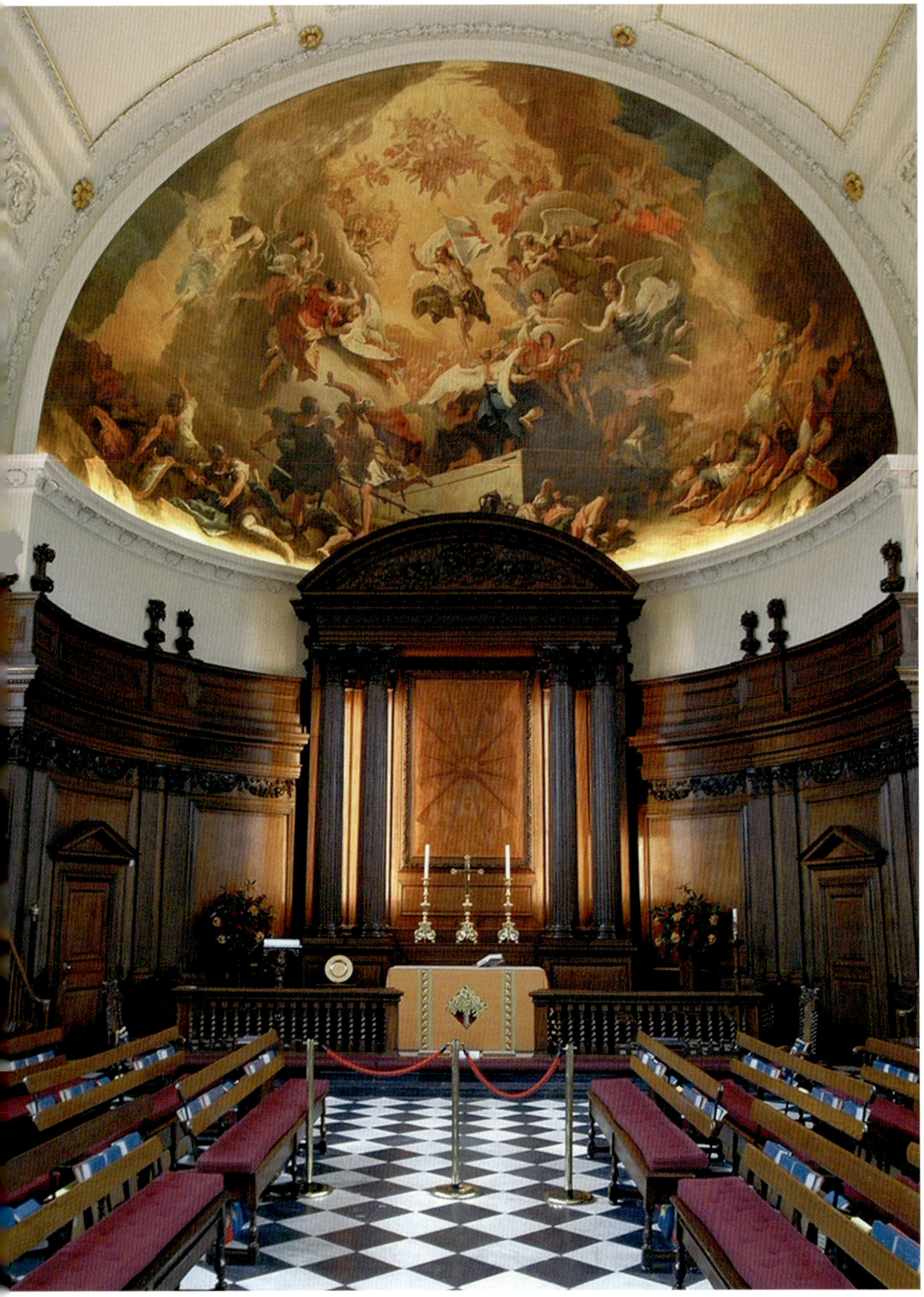

165 Sebastiano Ricci, *The Resurrection of Christ* at end of chapel, from 1714, Royal Hospital, Chelsea

gave the painting a Rococo panache vastly superior to the dull, heavy-handed decoration which Verrio and Henry Cooke had executed in the same hospital's Great Hall during the 1680s.

The verve and ambition of the *Resurrection* shows how much Ricci wanted to excel in this prominent metropolitan setting. Ellis Waterhouse describes it as Ricci's 'surviving masterpiece',[17] and two closely related, elaborate *bozzetti* reveal the thoughtfulness and painterly energy he expended on the project. The *bozzetto* now at Dulwich is a large and elaborately composed image, seizing on the dramatic instant when Christ is released by angels from his stone resting-place (pl. 166). Although partly reliant on Annibale Carracci's version in the Louvre, the grouping and lighting of Charles de la Fosse's semi-dome in the Versailles chapel,[18] and perhaps on a Veronese altarpiece now in Chelsea and Westminster Hospital Chapel (see pl. 409),[19] Ricci filled the painting with his own vivacity and flamboyant sense of theatre. Brandishing a triumphant banner with its symbolic red cross, Christ dominates the design. He scatters the soldiers in disarray, acknowledges the adoration of angels clustered so fervently around him and soars towards the brilliant source of divine light in the parted clouds above. The whole image seems complete enough but it was greatly enriched when Ricci, now possibly working in collaboration with his sprightly nephew Marco, addressed himself to the immense task of painting on the plaster of the chapel wall (pl. 165).

For the apse provided a generous expansion of the design at either side and Ricci knew precisely how to marry his decoration to the architectural space at his disposal. So the guards grow in number as they run, draw swords in a futile attempt to prevent the ascension, and gesticulate in terror at the cataclysmic shock of the event they witness. In the biblical source Ricci employed, Saint Matthew describes how the soldiers 'trembled and became like dead men'.[20] Ricci concentrates on their bewildered attempts to escape from the area around the tomb, which has increased in size and been given greater prominence than it possessed in the *bozzetti*. One figure, sprawled at the forefront of the painting, seems traumatised by fear and unable to move. Instead, he stares up at the four angels who have prised open the massively enlarged coffin lid with the aid of their exuberant wings.

Ricci vividly conveys the straining exertion involved in this enterprise and contrasts it with the altogether more abandoned choreography of the angels above, who converge in ecstasy on Christ (see pl. 152). Borne along by a current of air that makes his sage-green drapery billow and the white banners unfurl in extravagant undulations around his head, this regenerated deity seems, paradoxically, less dominant than he was in the *bozzetti*. Ricci has charged the outer areas of the design with so much vivacity and darting incident that they threaten to distract our gaze from the resurrecting figure himself. Yet Ricci compensates for this loss by drawing greater attention to the group of cherubs floating in such blissful profusion above Christ. The whole decoration has a Rococo *élan* and fluency that celebrates the sheer joyfulness of the revelation. Soon after completing the *Resurrection of Christ*, Ricci and his nephew felt so discouraged by the enmity of English artists that they abandoned London for Paris. But this ebullient image continued to offer the chapel's veteran congregation a vision of renewal, suffused in light and animated by the dynamism of an artist who had responded so energetically to the demands of the space he had been given.

The army pensioners cared for at the Royal Hospital were all old enough to be conscious of their mortality, none more so than William Hiseland (pl. 167). His sword-brandishing portrait, painted by George Alsop two years before Hiseland died at the prodigious age of 112, still hangs in the hospital museum at Chelsea bearing an inscription that describes how he sat for the painting 'in perfect health'. It serves as a suitably myth-making tribute to an indefatigable soldier who, having fought for Charles I at Edgehill, in Ireland and then under Marlborough at Flanders, ended up serving for more than eighty years in his country's forces.[21] As if to prove that his phenomenal longevity was accompanied by an equally remarkable sprightliness, he married when over a hundred years old. And Alsop's portrait stands as an affectionate tribute to the resilience of ex-servicemen who would often be regarded by the public as little more than beggars as the century proceeded. Pensioners like the redoubtable Hiseland would surely have been gratified to find, in the chapel where they worshipped,[22] an image of the liberated Christ offering hope to anyone who needed spiritual solace when confronted by the apparent finality of death.

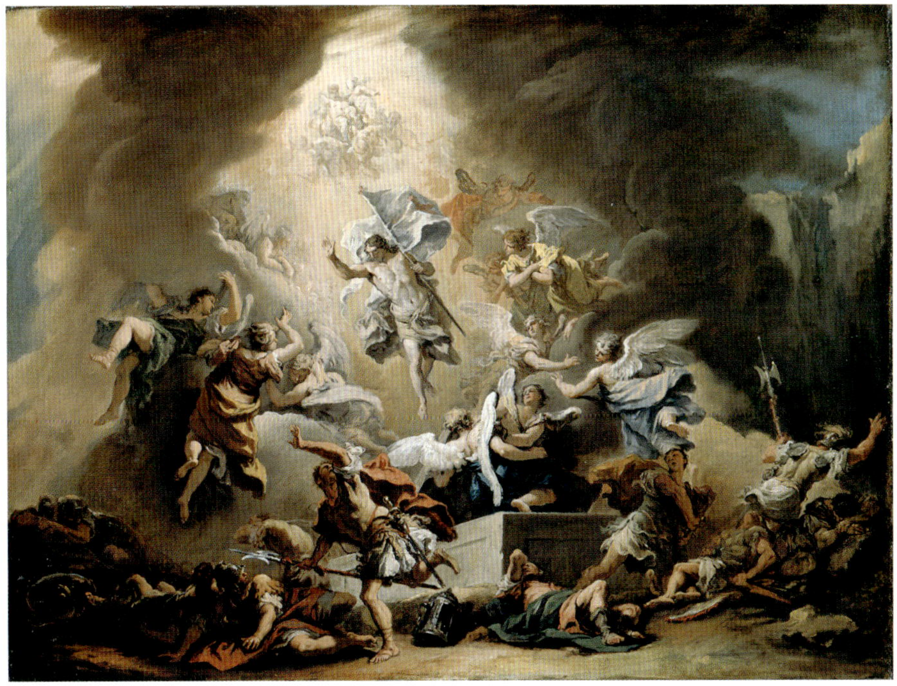

166 (*above*) Sebastiano Ricci, *Bozzetto for Resurrection of Christ*, 1714–16, Dulwich Picture Gallery, London

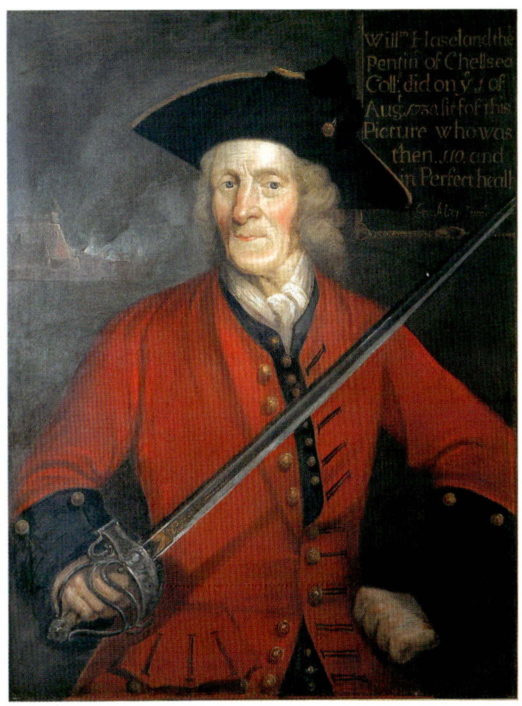
Pentin of Chellsea
Picture who was
then 110 and
in Perfect heal

167 (*left*) George Alsop, *William Hiseland,* 1730, Royal Hospital, Chelsea

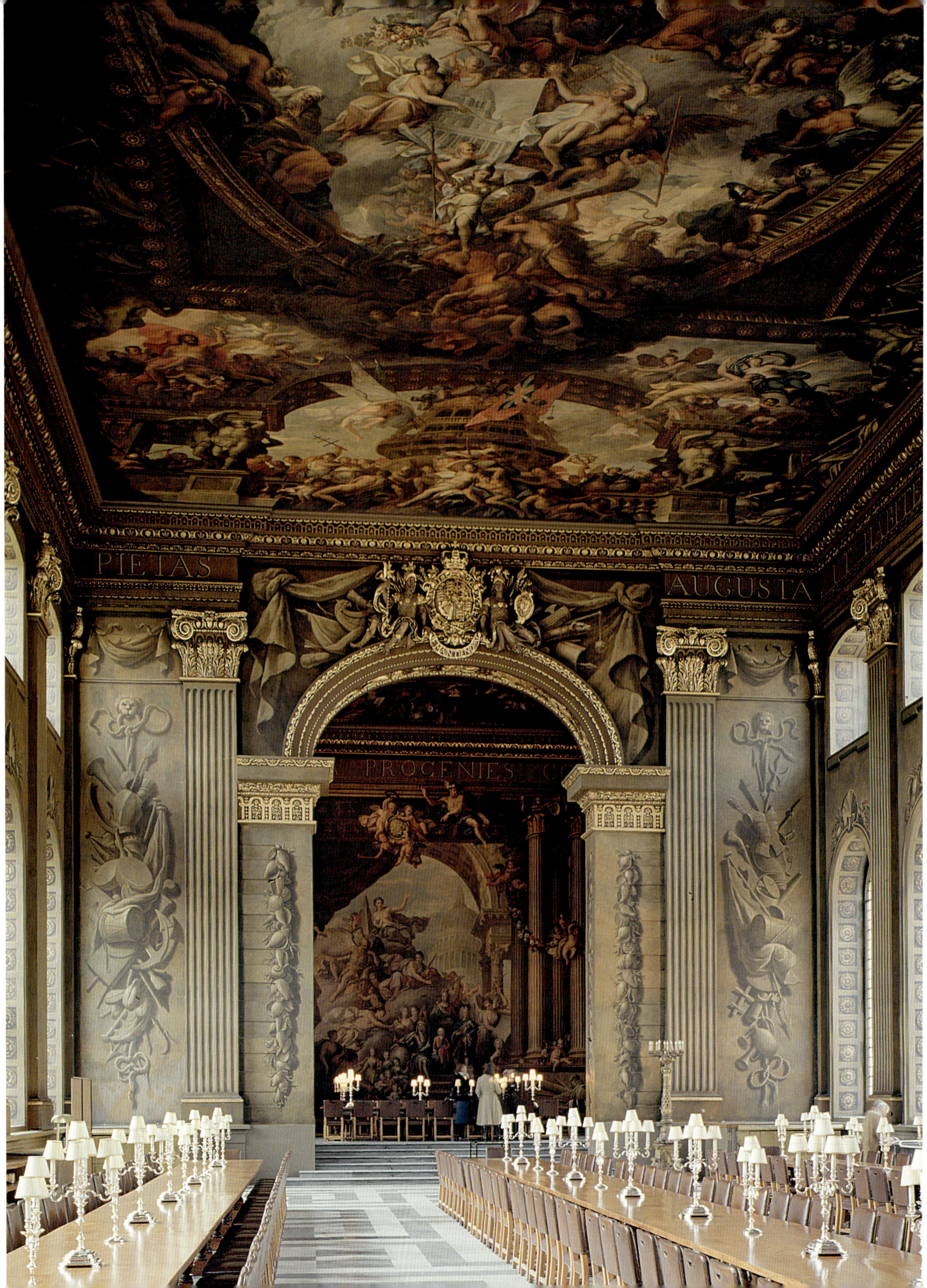
PIETAS
AUGUSTA
PROGENIES

THIRTEEN
SAVING THE SEAMEN

During the eighteenth century, London's determination to vie with Paris in the splendour of its hospitals produced a spate of building, either converting older premises or erecting handsome new structures for the purpose. The term 'hospital', which had previously encompassed so many disparate activities, now came to be regarded in the main as 'a place for the reception of the sick poor'.[1] Funded variously by the state, wealthy philanthropists and voluntary contributions, they often assumed such magnificent proportions that foreign visitors believed England's 'charitable foundations were more fitted, by their grandeur and extent, for the residence of kings; while her palaces, by their external appearance, seemed better calculated for the reception of the needy and unfortunate'.[2]

Nowhere was this waspish observation more spectacularly borne out than at Greenwich. Here the unfinished King Charles Building found itself developed with lavish panache as a hospital for old and disabled seamen, including provision for the 'Maintenance and Education of the Children of Seamen happening to be slain or disabled'.[3] Since William and Mary's joint succession to the British throne in 1688, war had been waged against Louis XIV in a sequence of naval battles that terminated when Admiral Russell inflicted a major defeat on the French army at La Hogue in 1692. Determined to mark the victory and honour the seamen who had made it possible, Mary decided that the King Charles Building (designed by John Webb in the 1660s as one wing of a proposed royal palace) should be completed in an even more resplendent style as a Royal Naval Hospital.

Although her early death intervened before the plan could be implemented, William ensured that his wife's scheme was carried through on the grandest conceivable scale. He asked Wren to design the new building, which stretched from the King's House by the water's edge up to Inigo Jones's celebrated Queen's House. Wren felt frustrated by William's insistence that the view of the Thames from the Jones building be preserved, but he managed to gain acceptance for the erection of massive twin domes on two projecting blocks named after William and his queen (pl. 170). With hindsight, they can be seen as forerunners of the even mightier dome he went on to erect over Saint Paul's Cathedral. But after laying the foundation stone of the Hospital in 1696, Wren left the elaboration of its design to Nicholas Hawksmoor,[4] who in 1698 became the Clerk of Works to the Greenwich Hospital and thereby directly responsible for the detailed creation of the most expensive, splendidly decorated part of the building: the Painted Hall (pl. 168).

168 (*facing page*)
Christopher Wren and Nicholas Hawksmoor, The Painted Hall, Royal Hospital for Seamen, now Old Royal Naval College, Greenwich

Working under only the most general direction from Wren, he set about producing an interior that eventually became the most swaggering manifestation of Baroque painted architecture to be found anywhere in Britain. Surmounted by a dome indebted to Michelangelo's design for the dome of Saint Peter's, the Painted Hall grew into a flamboyant demonstration of Hawksmoor's desire to achieve a convincing unity between architectural form and surface embellishment. He wanted the Hospital to 'equal in Strength, Beauty and Convenience'[5] the Invalides in Paris, and between 1696 and 1704 he presided over the construction of a Hall that offered immense opportunities to the painter capable of realising them with sufficient inventiveness and verve.

The artist who would undertake this titanic task had not yet been chosen, but by 1707 Hawksmoor had successfully overseen the completion of the decorative carvings he designed for the Hall. Robert Jones, later responsible for much of the carving at Castle Howard, supervised the execution of the gilded capitals running down either side of the Lower Hall. Derived from Serlio's *Third Book of Architecture*, they replaced the traditional acanthus leaf motif with wheat sheaves and give the interior they enhance a sense of harvest-like abundance. In a room intended to be the Hospital's dining-hall, such imagery was appropriate indeed. The former careers of the seamen were reflected in the carvings that Jones also executed, again from Hawksmoor's designs, over the arch leading to the Upper Hall, where Mars and Minerva sit at either side of William and Mary's arms (pl. 169). Mars, the god of war, symbolised the spirit of the naval engagements in which so many of the Hospital's inhabitants had fought, while the wisdom of Minerva was doubtless intended to counter his ferocity in times of peace. This balance between the rival demands of aggression and pacific sagacity would also run through the ceiling painting in the Lower Hall. For the underside of the same arch, by contrast, Jones carved highly Italianate personifications of the six northern signs of the Zodiac. Floating against a star-strewn sky, they link up with the Zodiac signs soon to be painted round the principal oval in the ceiling.

169 (*right*) Robert Jones, *Mars and Minerva*, *c*.1707, The Painted Hall, Royal Hospital for Seamen, now Old Royal Naval College, Greenwich

170 (*facing page*) Christopher Wren, exterior of the The Painted Hall, Royal Hospital for Seamen, now Old Royal Naval College, Greenwich

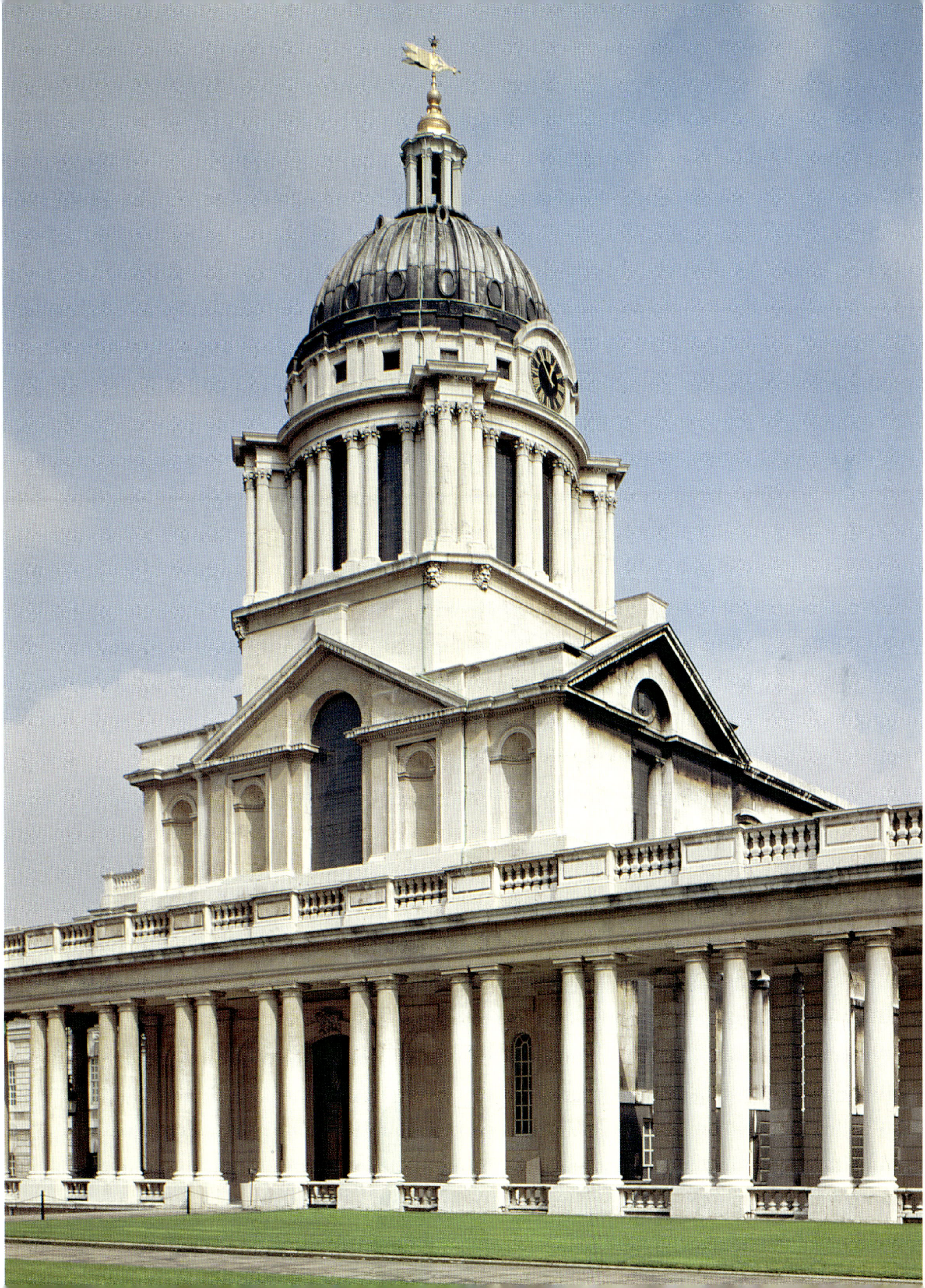

But who would be selected to carry out the painted decorations? Extensive enough to take its place in the noble tradition established in England by Rubens's great allegorical cycle for the ceiling of the Banqueting House in Whitehall, the Painted Hall provided surfaces that would tax the ability of even the most seasoned and ingenious artist. No one would have been surprised if the venture had been allotted to one of the foreign painters who earned considerable fortunes embellishing the walls, ceilings and staircases of grand institutions and private houses throughout the country. The commission could easily have gone to the skilful Laguerre, who had already collaborated with the equally admired Verrio on the decoration of Christ's Hospital in the 1680s. At Greenwich, however, the Governors turned to a less distinguished and relatively untried Englishman, James Thornhill. He owed a substantial debt to Laguerre, whom he succeeded at Chatsworth after the Frenchman had worked there, again with Verrio, on a number of important interior schemes. Although Verrio's blindness, followed by his death in 1707, ruled him out of consideration for the Greenwich project, the choice of Thornhill rather than his more illustrious continental competitors still came as a surprise. He secured the commission partly by encouraging a campaign of patriotic sentiment, which protested about the incessant awarding of great decorative ventures to foreign artists alone. The Hospital Governors perhaps also appreciated the fact that Thornhill the newcomer was cheaper than his esteemed rivals. Indeed, they later accounted for their unwillingness to pay him as much as he required by asserting that the Painted Hall 'was the first great work he ever undertook in England and served as an introduction to bring him into reputation'.[6]

Thornhill's energy and enthusiasm also played a significant part in obtaining the commission, for

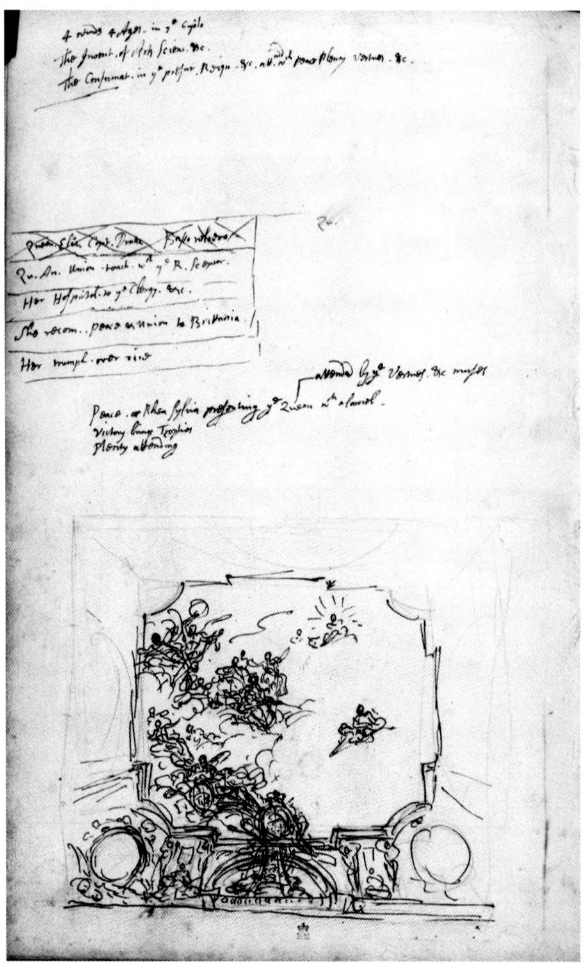

171a (*right*) James Thornhill, Preliminary drawing for the ceiling of the lower hall of the Painted Hall, Royal Hospital for Seamen, leaf from a sketchbook containing 149 leaves, 1699–1716, British Museum, London

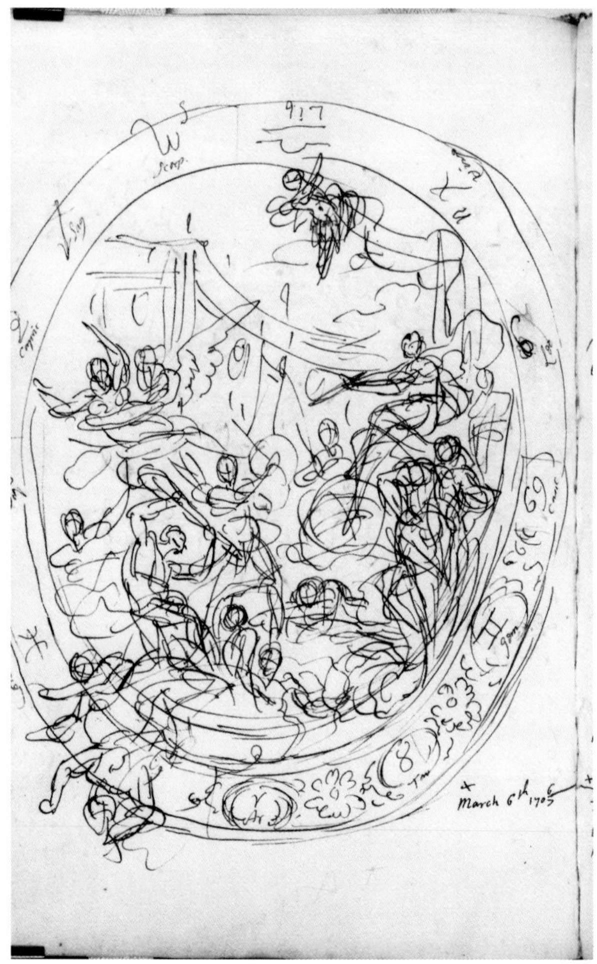

171b (*far right*) James Thornhill, Preliminary drawing for the central oval of the ceiling of the lower hall of the Painted Hall, Royal Hospital for Seamen, leaf from a sketchbook containing 149 leaves, 1699–1716, British Museum, London

the main ceiling of the Painted Hall turned out to be by far the most impressive work he ever executed. The vigorous confidence animating the final decoration of the Lower Hall is even more evident in his preliminary drawings for the scheme (pl. 171). Many of them rely on the expertise he had already gained as a designer of stage settings and elaborate decorations at Stoke Edith in Herefordshire. Carried out largely in crisp and rapid strokes of pen over pencil beginnings, the studies prove that he threw himself into the initial years of the Greenwich enterprise with commendable brio. The teeming allegory, which ended up containing almost two hundred figures, was intended to glorify William and Mary as the triumphant instigators of Peace and Liberty. Although the darting shorthand employed in Thornhill's sketches makes the elements of the complex design difficult to discern at this stage, the elaborately carved oval frame created the illusion that the ceiling, supported by eight slaves, had been pierced to open onto the canopy of heaven itself (see pl. 176).

Here the king and queen are enthroned, while above them Apollo drives the chariot of the sun in a blaze of light. Dressed in warlike armour, William rests a victorious foot on the dejected figure of Louis XIV, clutching a broken sword and swathed in a yellow tunic denoting fear and treachery. But the English monarch also receives an olive branch from Peace, and beneath him the fruits of armistice are glorified by the figure of Architecture pointing at the design for the Painted Hall itself. She thereby emphasised the 'unity of place' recommended by the theorists of history painting, while beside her the bearded Time supports the naked figure of Truth and exposes her to the full radiance of Apollo's rays. The Arts are victorious, their survival ensured by Pallas Athene and Hercules who, at the base of the main oval, club and spear the Vices out of heaven in a mass of writhing serpents.

172 James Thornhill, *Ship beneath arches carried on shoulders of Atlantes*, completed 1712, The Painted Hall, Royal Hospital for Seamen, now Old Royal Naval College, Greenwich

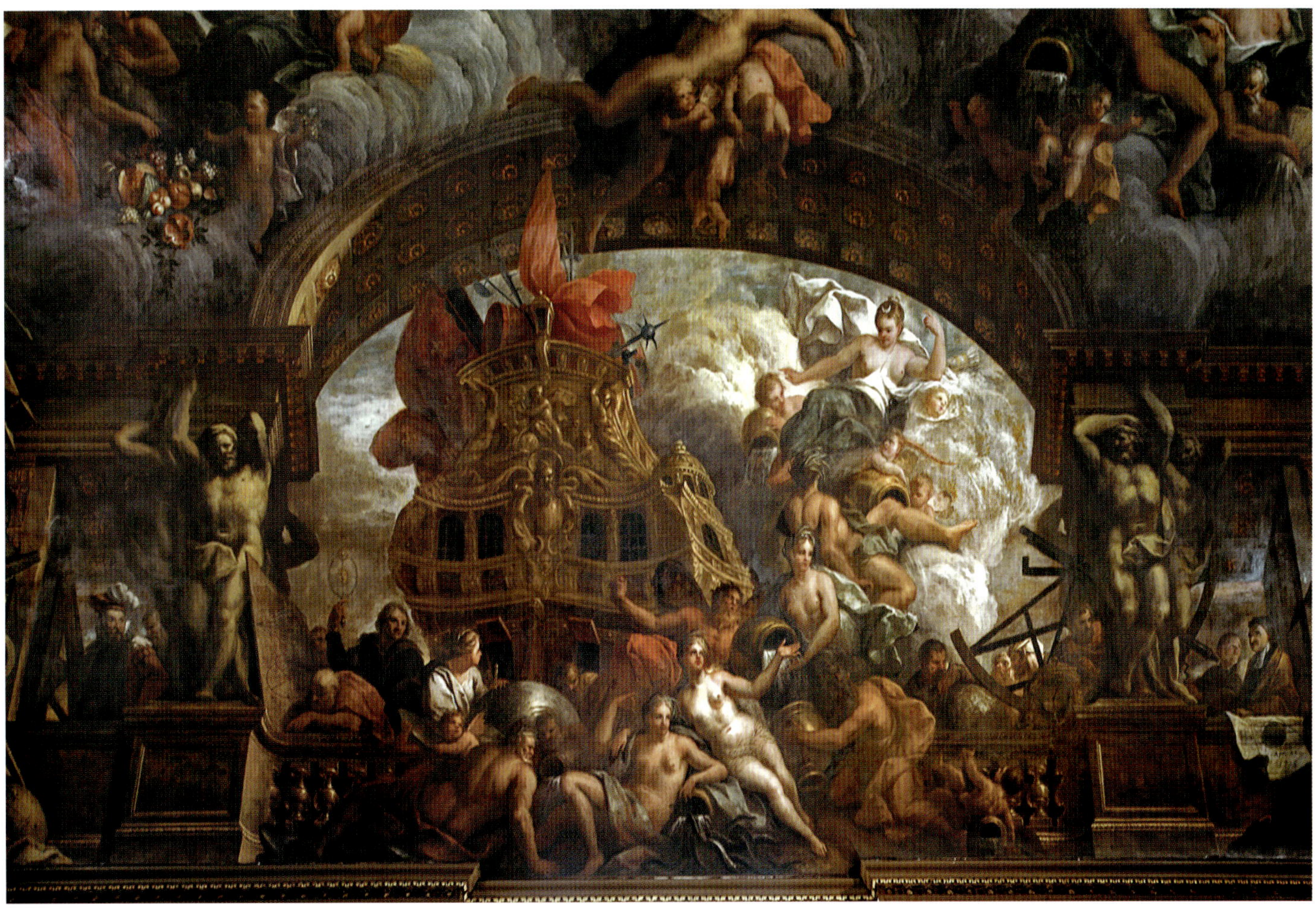

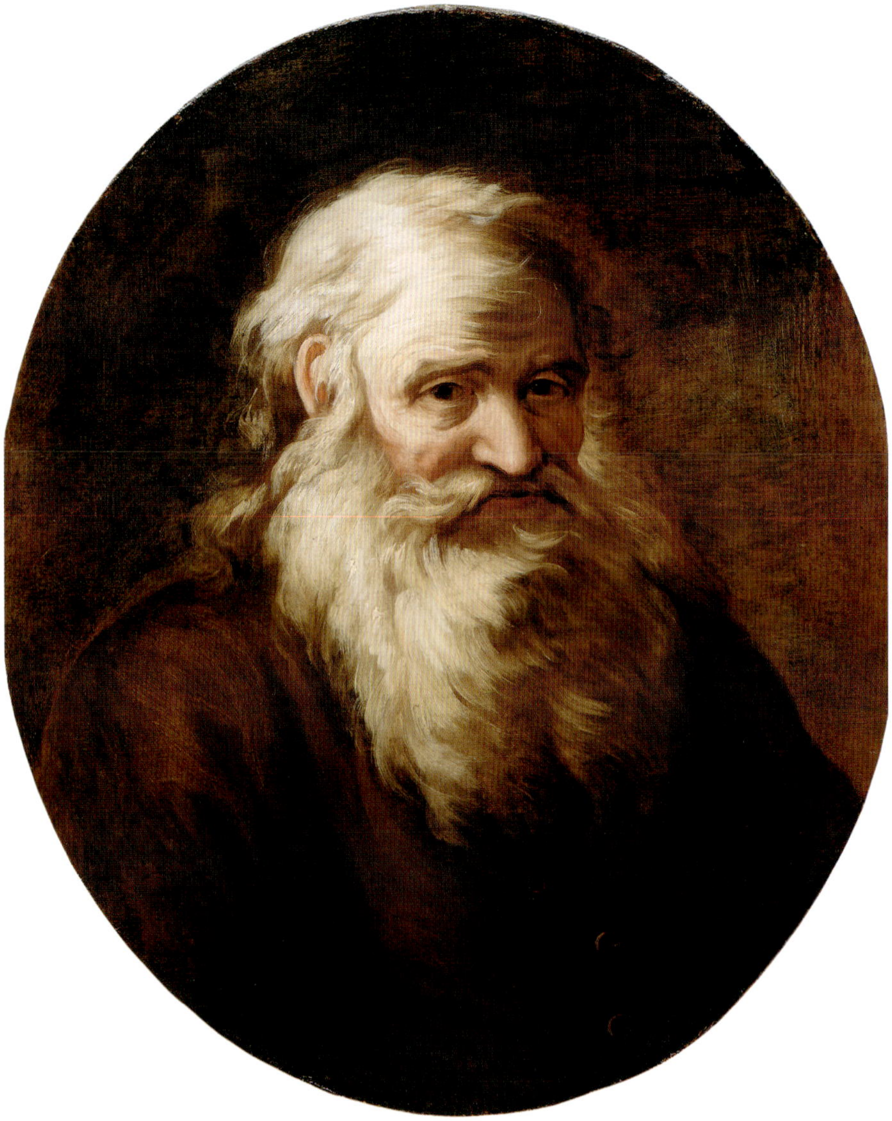

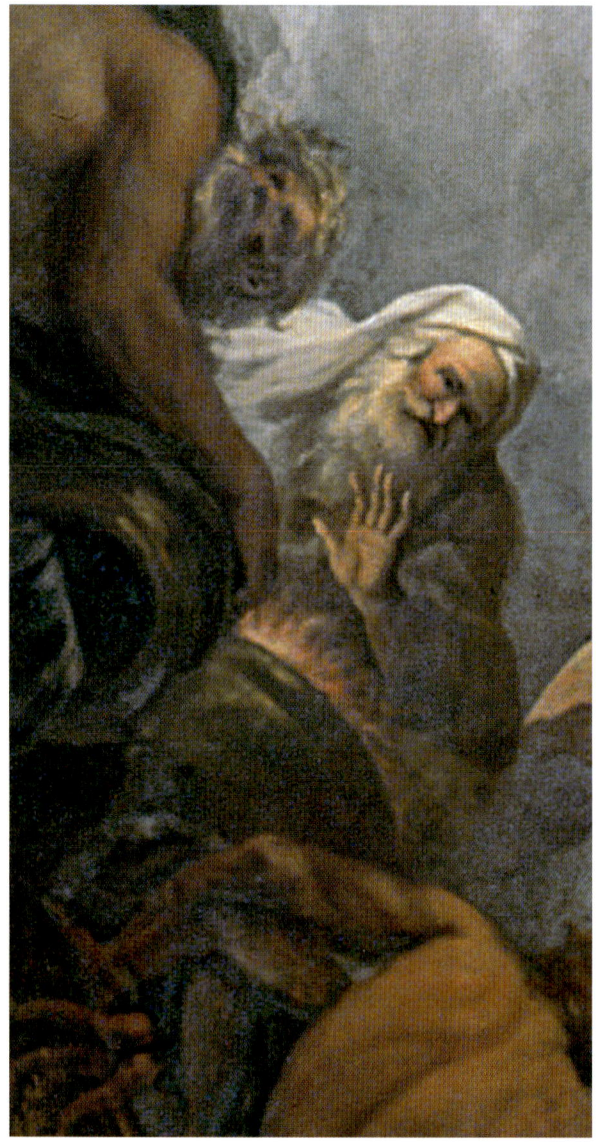

173 (*above left*) James Thornhill, Portrait of John Worley, National Maritime Museum, Greenwich, Greenwich Hospital Collection

174 (*above right*) James Thornhill, *Winter*, detail from the ceiling of the Painted Hall, completed 1712, Royal Hospital for Seamen, now Old Royal Naval College, Greenwich

The whole complex orchestration was so labyrinthine in its blend of mythology, Christian symbolism, modern history and Thornhill's own ideas that he eventually wrote a booklet expounding its meaning for spectators. But the preliminary studies won the qualified approval of the Governors in July 1707, when they 'ordered that as soon as the Scaffolding in the Hall is ready Mr. James Thornhill do proceed upon the painting thereof, by primeing it himself, or servants, and that he make such Alterations in his designe, in inserting what more he can relating to maritime affairs, till the same be approved by the Board'.[7] Later drawings demonstrate that Thornhill did his best to meet their criticism, and in the ceiling itself the maritime world is represented most effectively by the looming ships beneath feigned elliptical arches at both ends of the Lower Hall ceiling, each one carried on the sturdy shoulders of Atlantes (pl. 172). Laden with the spoils of battle and surrounded by rejoicing figures, the ships introduce a reference to the seafaring world that would undoubtedly have been welcomed by the men eating at their table below.

It still meant a great deal to naval families three centuries later, for Paul Nash's mother used Thornhill's ceiling as a means of instilling in her son some pride about her ancestors' long and distinguished professional commitment to the sea. 'In the Painted Hall at Greenwich', Nash recalled, 'I had been shown my great-grandfather's ship, the *Hebrus*, gaining a fierce victory over the French frigate, *L'Etoile*.'[8] The bulbous bulk of the fighting vessels helps to anchor Thornhill's airborne symbolism in a more readily approachable level of reality, and the maritime theme is continued round the oval frame in a frieze of cannons, drums, ropes, muskets and spars, all stone-coloured to act as a foil for the festive colours within the oval. Together with the figures representing British rivers at the east and west ends of the ceiling, they confirm the naval interests of the old men for whom the decoration was painted.

The pensioners would have been further delighted to identify, in the figure of Winter near the edge of the oval, a portrait of the ninety-six year-old John Worley (pl. 174). He was notorious among the inhabitants of the Hospital for inebriation and foul-mouthed behaviour. The Council Minutes record complaints that he had been 'very drunk in his ward . . . abusing his ward fellows and cursing and swearing saying that he was better than any in the house'. Advancing years had, it seems, failed to tame the habits Worley acquired during his seventy years' service at sea. But Thornhill's portrait of the veteran sea-dog, drawn in preparation for the painting of Winter, indicates that an attractive sense of humour might well have enlivened his weatherbeaten features (pl. 173). Moreover, Worley's miscreant ways are likely to have been cured by the stern punishment inflicted on him by the Council, who decreed that he was to be put in

> ye confining house for 4 days, and each meal to be exposed on ye elevated place in ye Hall and to lose this day's meals and to live on bread and water for a week and to wear ye badge for swearing, to lose a fortnight's allowance money and not to go out of ye Hospital for one month from ye date.[9]

A comparison between the final oil study for the central oval and the ceiling itself reveals how much Thornhill continued to improve his design as he worked on the scaffolding (pl. 175). The painted sketch is a sophisticated exercise, disclosing the extent of his reliance on Laguerre as he organises the clusters of monarchs, angels, deities and putti within the enormous oval. But unlike the bravura dynamism of the oil studies that Rubens made for his Whitehall ceiling, Thornhill's composition appears at this stage disappointingly timid and dutiful. The gusto of the preliminary ink drawings is not carried over into an image weighed down, no doubt, by its maker's conscientious attempt to give his elaborate subject a fully coherent form.

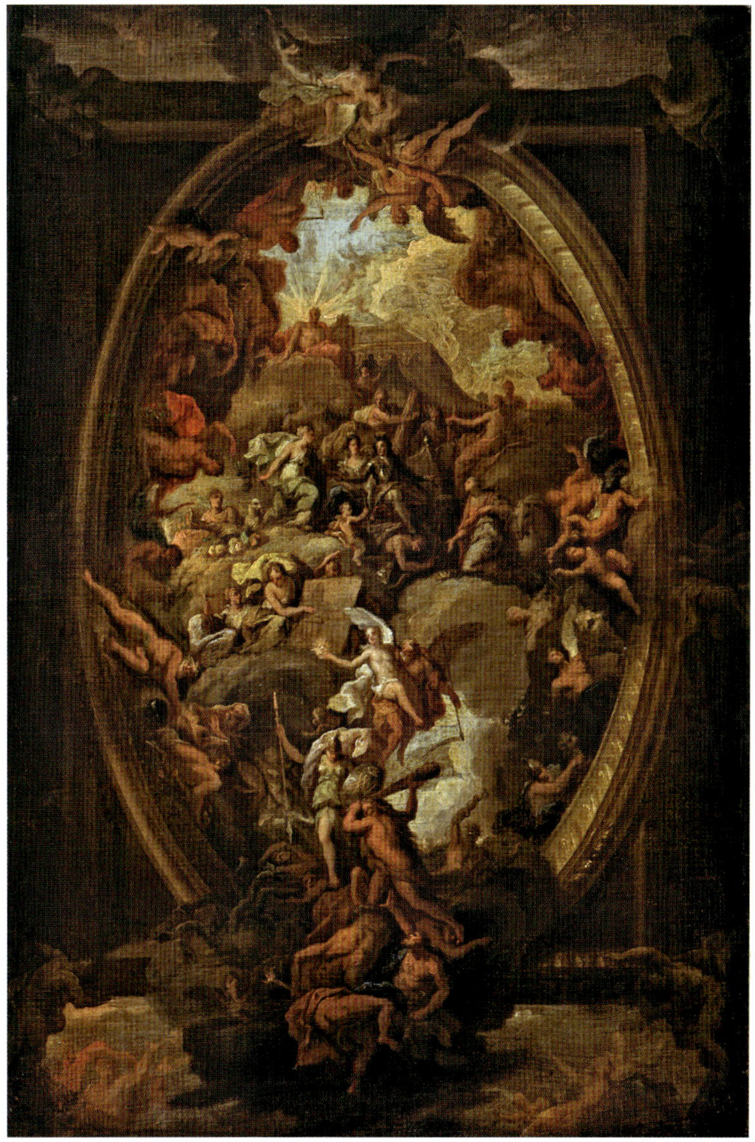

175 James Thornhill, Final oil study for central oval and ceiling of the Painted Hall, Royal Hospital for Seamen, *c.*1710, Victoria and Albert Museum, London

On the ceiling itself, though (pl. 176), Thornhill gave additional clarity and dramatic emphasis to the painted sketch's rather clotted profusion of figures and clouds. Apollo, who heads the moral hierarchy of the ceiling, adopts a far more dynamic stance as he raises a commanding arm in the air. The shafts of light exploding round him add

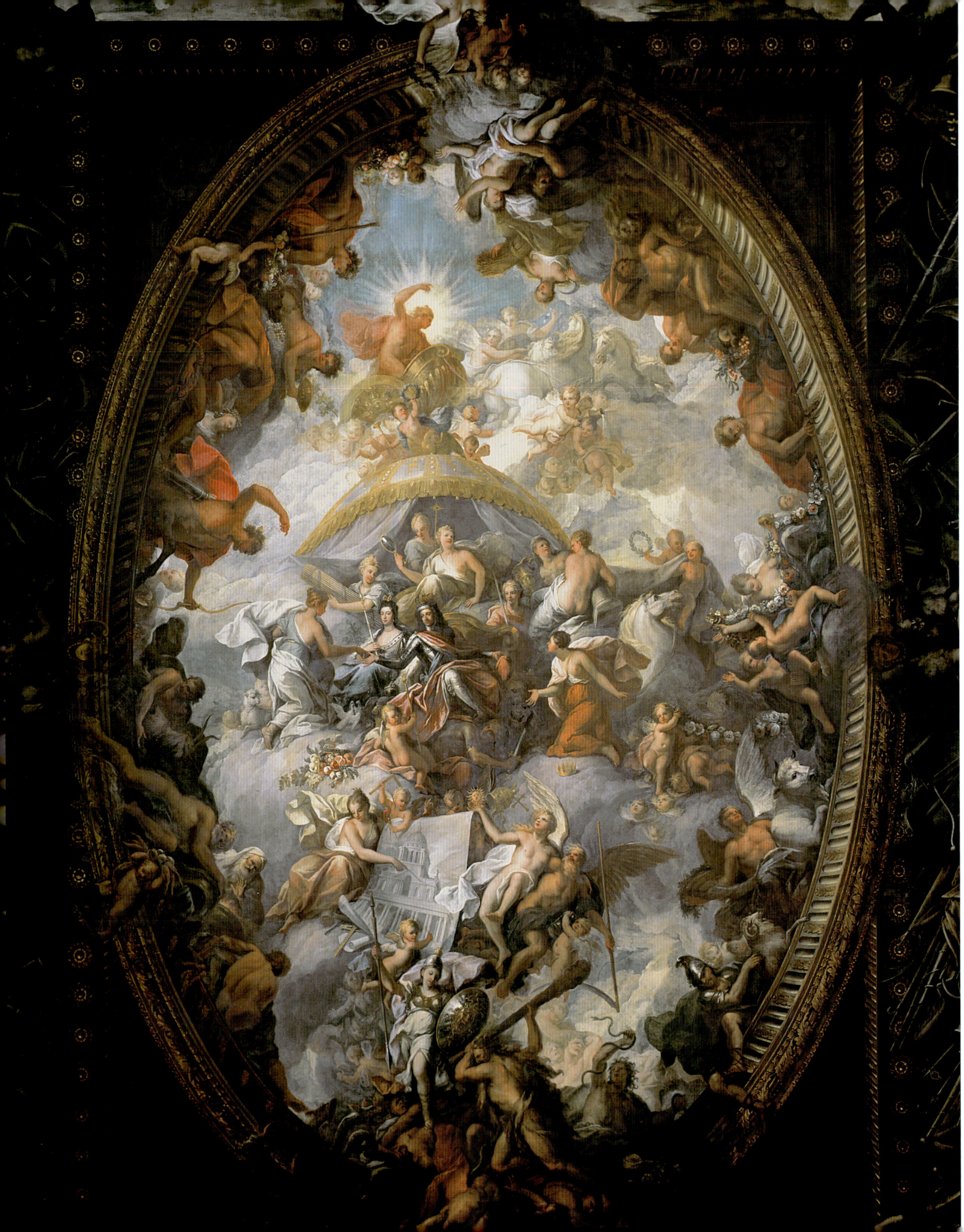

potency and his horses toss their manes energetically as they pound through the heavens. The tent is lowered from the position it occupied in the oil study, where it reared up behind Apollo and diminished his appearance. Now it serves clearly to separate the region inhabited by the charioteering god from the space below, where William and Mary reside. They have been moved slightly to one side so that Thornhill can place at the heart of his painting the red Athenian Cap of Liberty. This crucial change makes the entire ceiling less sturdily predictable. William, leaning now in a more lively diagonal position, hands the all-important cap to the figure of Europe, a kneeling woman who holds a rearing white horse by the rein. Thornhill's decision to give this particular area of the decoration additional emphasis was not prompted by compositional considerations alone. He was also reflecting Britain's exultation over the ultimate defeat of Louis XIV, for the Treaty at Utrecht was signed in March 1714 at a time when work on the ceiling reached its most intensive phase.

All over the painting of the Lower Hall, the somewhat indiscriminate activity depicted in the oil sketch is replaced by a more precisely ordered and articulated design. Look at the trumpeting figure of Fame who is scarcely noticeable at the top of the painted study. On the ceiling itself she is transformed into a far more purposeful creature, whose wings flare up dramatically as she blows her instrument and brandishes a laurel wreath like a weapon. For the organisation of this area, Thornhill appears to have relied on the precedent established by Andrea Pozzo's ceiling painting in the vast Jesuit church of Sant' Ignazio in Rome. The stance taken up by Thornhill's personification of the Wind, as he carries Fame along with a majestic hurling arm, looks like a reversal of the figure representing Europa in Pozzo's design. Compared with the soaring vertiginous disorientation that the Sant' Ignazio ceiling can induce in its viewers, Thornhill's heavenly oval is stable and harmonious indeed. But Pozzo did exert a palpable influence on the creation of the Painted Hall, for the architectural fantasies engraved in his book *Perspectiva pictorum et architectorum*, published in 1693, played a part in the design of the Greenwich building. Hawksmoor's assistant John James translated the book in an edition published in 1707, the same year that Thornhill embarked on his drawings for the Lower Hall. An 'approbation' of the book was signed not only by Hawksmoor, but by Wren and Vanbrugh as well.

Thornhill would have shared their enthusiasm, for he showed himself responsive to architecture throughout his career. Displayed most vividly by the drawings of buildings he made in his sketchbook during a tour of Belgium and Holland in 1711, this keen interest served him well at Greenwich Hospital. It helped to ensure that he reacted with sensitivity and assurance to the space Hawksmoor had provided, enhancing it with the illusionistic structure in his own painting rather than setting himself up in arrogant conflict with the rest of the interior. Thornhill's robust handling of its elements, and his ability to let them articulate the crowding figures they frame, is the main reason why the ceiling deserves to be regarded both as his masterpiece and as the climax of Baroque architectural painting in England. 'What is civilisation?' asked Kenneth Clark, before answering: 'A state of mind where it is thought desirable for a naval hospital to look like this and for the inmates to dine in a splendidly decorated hall.'[10]

The same level of achievement was not, unfortunately, sustained in the Upper Hall. Thornhill started work there in 1717, three years after the completion of his earlier *tour de force*, and the exuberant vitality of the Lower Hall had by now given way to a more stolid, decorous approach. A visit to France had convinced him that Charles Lebrun's decorations at Versailles were impressive enough to be emulated. Moreover, in his drawings for the walls of the Upper Hall Thornhill spends a great deal of time agonising over how best to deal with contemporary history in a style elevated enough to satisfy the demands of the grand manner. Although his own inclinations might have led him towards a greater degree of realism and faithful observation in his treatment of a subject like *George I landing at Greenwich in 1714*, his drawing for the scene listed the 'Objections yt will arise from yr plain representation of ye K. Landing . . . as it was in fact, & in ye modern way & dress'. Prominent among them were some substantial pitfalls: the landing had taken place in darkness, carried out by modest boats rather than majestic galleons, and the sober clothes worn by the king were not sufficiently 'worthy of him to be transmitted to Posterity'.[11] Thornhill opted for imaginative licence in order to overcome

176 (*facing page*) James Thornhill, Ceiling of the Painted Hall, completed 1712, Royal Hospital for Seamen, now Old Royal Naval College, Greenwich

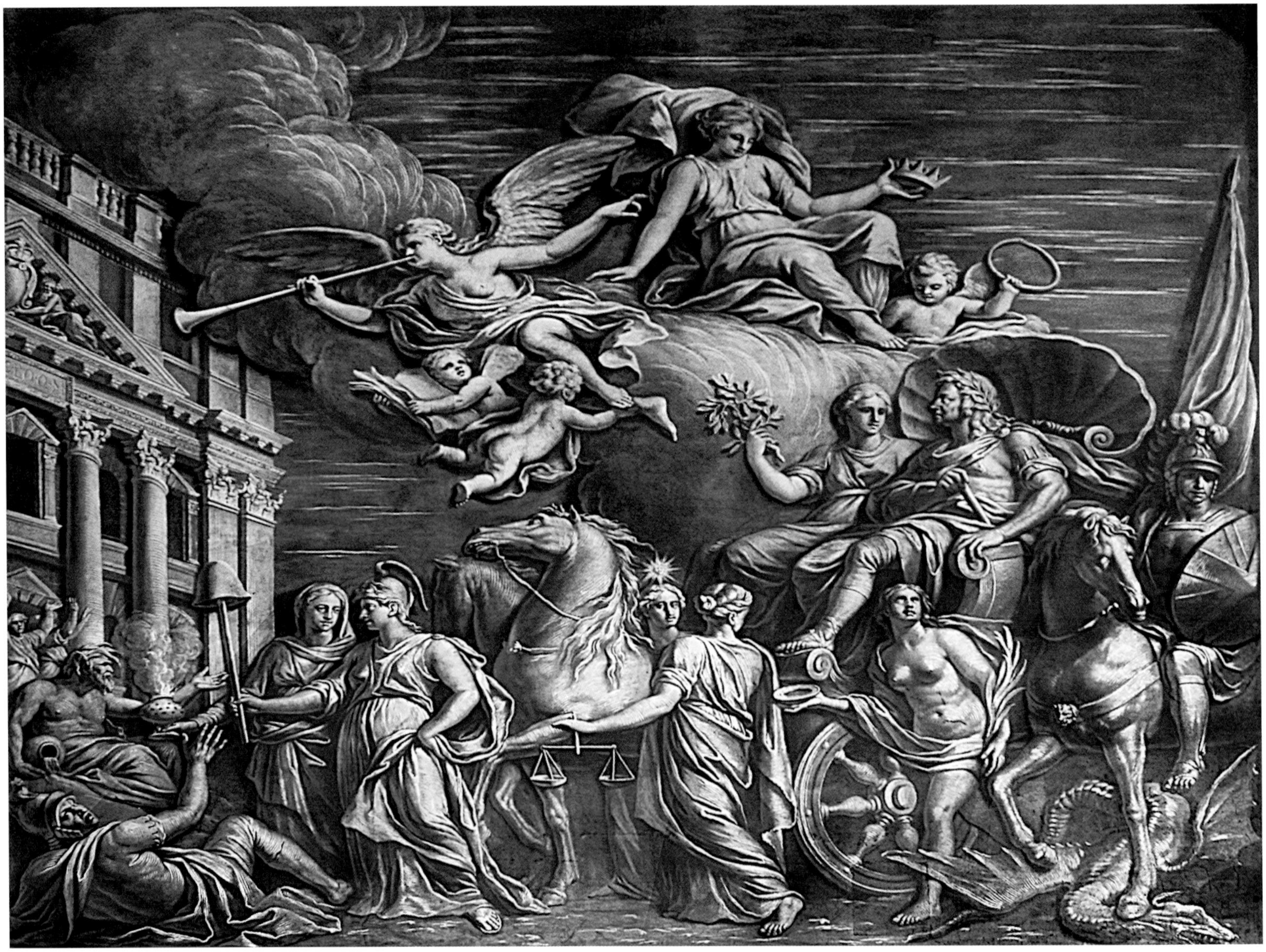

177 James Thornhill, *George I landing at Greenwich*, 1717–26, Upper Hall, Royal Hospital for Seamen, now Old Royal Naval College, Greenwich

these problems, even though he felt acutely divided in his loyalties when addressing the question of whether to depict the 'vast Crowd' who had attended the actual landing. 'To represent [it] would be ugly, & not to represent would be false', he wrote, torn between his desire to produce a suitably stirring image and his equally strong wish to respect historical truth.

In the end, the urge to enhance his artistic reputation by producing a graceful and dignified decoration triumphed over his leanings towards documentary fidelity. There was, ultimately, only one answer to the question of whether he should 'Take Liberty of an evening sky, & torches' in place of 'Night, wch to represent would be hard & ungracefull in Picture'. Besides, there were serious political considerations to be taken into account as well. Thornhill noted that 'the Real Nobles that were there, then, some of them are in disgrace now', so should he 'Make only 5 or 6 of ye Chief Nobles ye rest in ye crowd?' He must have known what the solution would be even as these questions were scribbled down beside his drawing, and in a subsequent study he plumps unashamedly for an allegorical composition. The revised design enabled Thornhill to include, alongside Father Thames and assorted Nymphs, an eagle surmounting the chariot – placed there, he admitted in the margin, not only

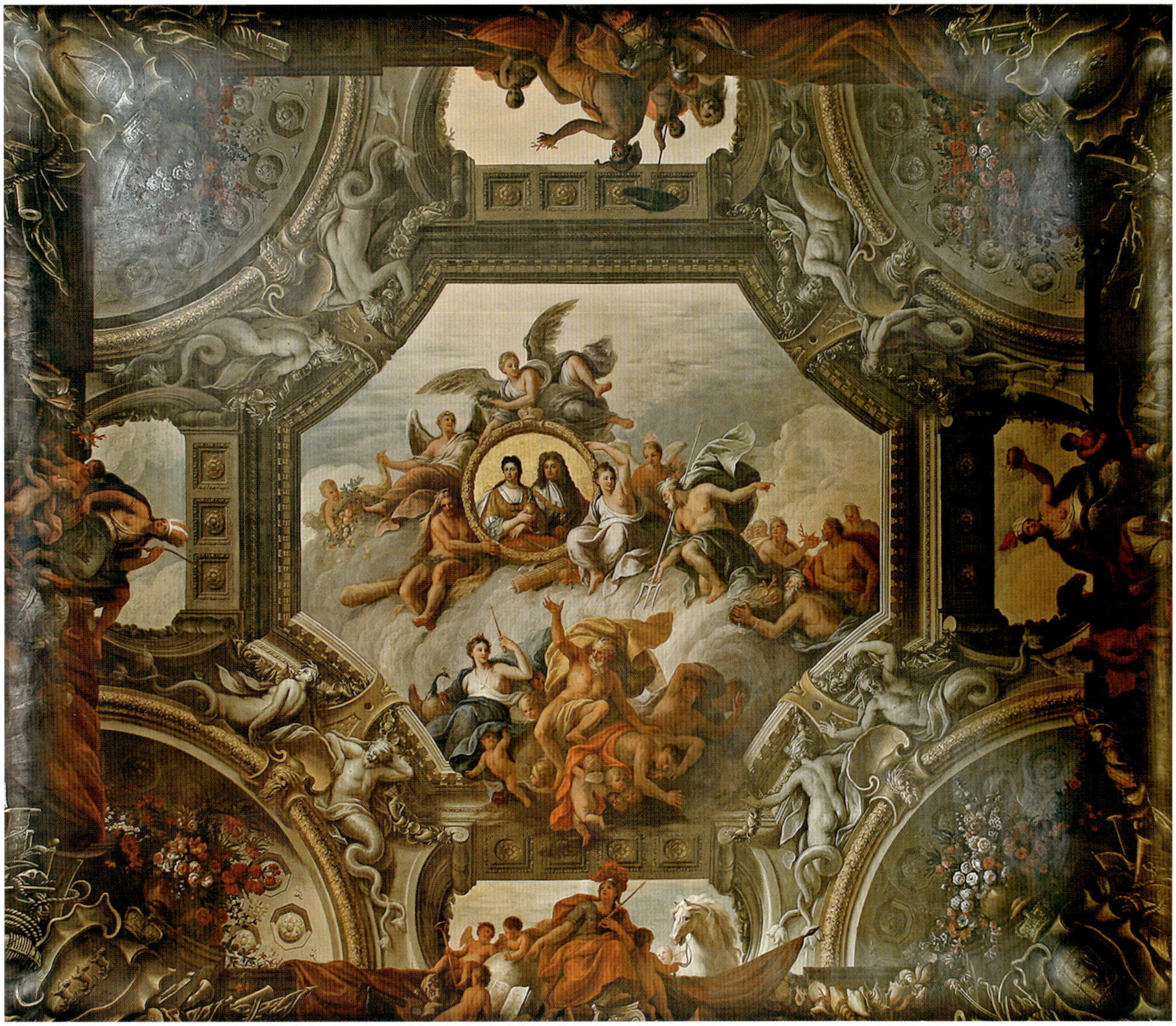

178 James Thornhill, Ceiling of Upper Hall, 1717–26, Royal Hospital for Seamen, now Old Royal Naval College, Greenwich

to 'shew the power of Jove' but also to give an airing to 'ye German Ensign'. Thus, as Charles Mitchell pointed out,[12] it would gratify supporters of the German succession without unduly antagonising viewers who felt little loyalty towards the new Hanoverian monarch. By debating all these considerations, Thornhill revealed himself as a cunning diplomat anxious to curry favour in as many quarters as possible – a propensity that would finally be rewarded with a knighthood in 1720, making him the first British-born artist to receive such an honour. But at least he had confronted the difficulties facing the painter of contemporary history with lucidity and frankness, entertaining the possibility of a more veracious approach before settling for the scene 'as it should have been then, rather than what it was'.[13]

The grisaille idiom used by Thornhill for his wall-painting of the scene, in order to emulate the stone carvings on Roman triumphal arches, accentuates the dullness that overcame him in the Upper Hall (see pl. 177). His other wall decoration there, showing William landing at Torbay to claim the throne, is equally bovine, and in the ceiling (pl. 178) he recovers only a semblance of the poise and vivacity evident in the Lower Hall. Perhaps Thornhill was bored, by now, with the prospect of dealing yet again with monarchs attended by Virtues, sea-gods

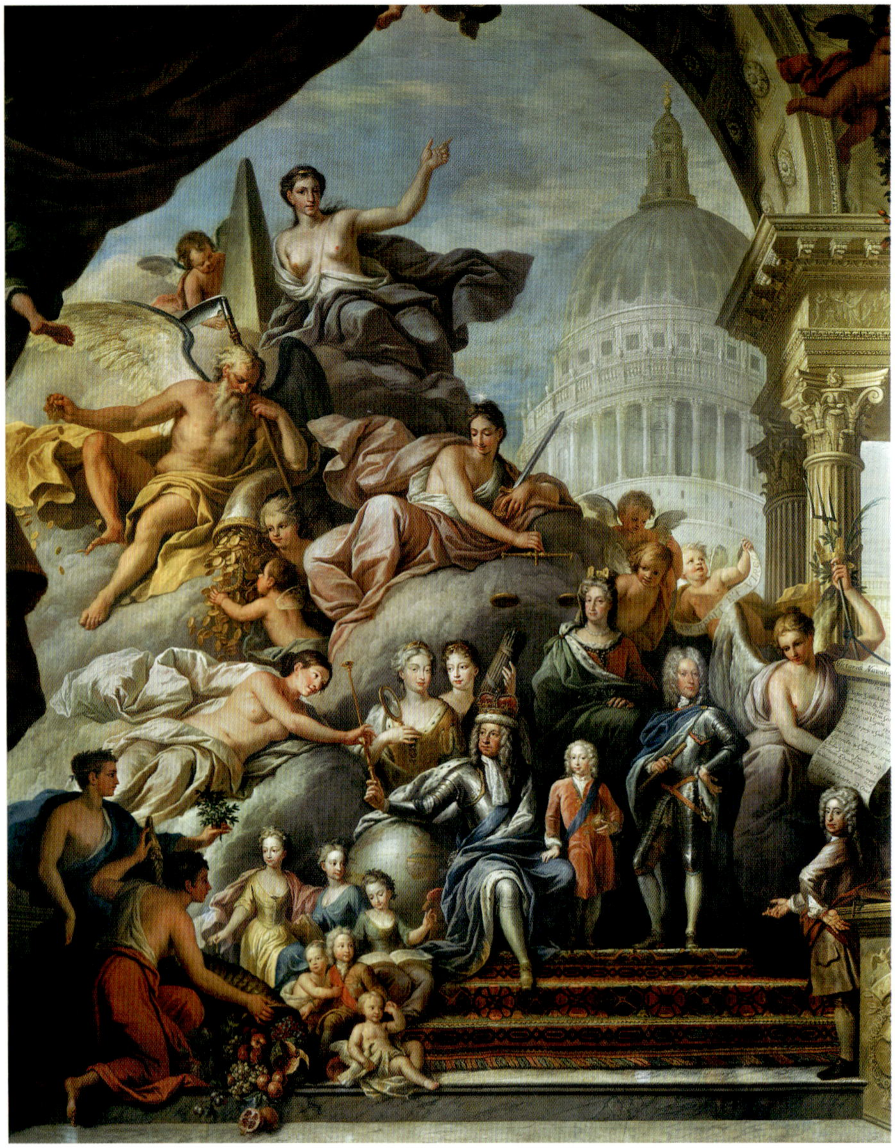

179 James Thornhill and Dietrich André, *The Return of the Golden Age*, 1717–26, Rear wall of the Upper Hall, Royal Hospital for Seamen, now Old Royal Naval College, Greenwich

and Victory. He tried hard to give Queen Anne and her husband Prince George of Denmark some dignity, as they reign over an imperialist ceiling with acclaim from figures representing Europe, Africa, Asia and America. He may even have enjoyed painting Asia's camel, Africa's lion and the Indian chief's regalia in which America is arrayed with such magnificence. But the ceiling as a whole pales in comparison with the oval decoration next door, and even the illusionistic window lacks the lightness of touch it needs to divert the eye.

Part of the trouble may have lain with Thornhill's increasing reliance on assistants as he laboured to complete the scheme by 1726. It had stretched over nearly twenty years of his by now faltering career and on the end wall of the Upper Hall he used the services of a Russian artist, Dietrich André, so extensively that the outcome is pictorially jarring (pl. 179). In this final painting, *The Return of the Golden Age*, where Fame sweeps back a curtain to disclose George I with his proliferating family attended by Peace, Time, Astraea the Star-maiden and other emblematic figures, André was entrusted with the important task of depicting the entire royal family. The manner he employs openly conflicts with Thornhill's handling of the upper section and André was even allowed to paint the portrait of Thornhill standing by a pillar at the right side of this highly theatrical tableau, where a backdrop of Saint Paul's proudly reminds viewers that he had painted some frescoes in the dome. André, who based the likeness on an early self-portrait drawn by Thornhill about thirty years before, shows his master gesturing towards the scene, with brushes, palette and mahlstick resting on the plinth beside him.

It was as if the increasingly unfashionable artist had turned his back on painting altogether, and after the completion of the Greenwich scheme Thornhill's career did indeed suffer an irreversible collapse. Hogarth, writing from his vantage-point as Thornhill's loyal son-in-law, tried to explain the heavy use of assistants in the Upper Hall by asserting later that 'the payment originally agreed upon for the work was so much reduced as made it not worth Sir James's while to finish the whole with his own more masterly hand'.[14] Robert Jones, who had received little acknowledgement for his sculptural decorations inside the Painted Hall, likewise suffered disappointment after he carved over fifty heads in Ketton stone for the exterior. They were supposed to be placed beneath the upper windows of the building's north and south sides but the lively images, ranging in subject from Galatea and Neptune to the inevitable British Lion, were never installed.[15]

In view of Thornhill's later decline, it is possible to detect a failure either of nerve or enthusiasm in his approach to this final chamber of the project. Unlike the Lower Hall, abounding in maritime references as robust as the great ship's stern exposing its hulk under one of Thornhill's feigned elliptical arches, the decorations in the Upper Hall bear scant relation to the lives and concerns of the Hospital's infirm and ageing seamen housed within its lofty allegorical pomp. Assembled below the proud announcement *Izam nova progenies caelo* ('Now a new race in heaven'), the pompous regal gathering on the west wall confirmed nothing except the triumph of the Protestant Succession in England. The only reference to maritime affairs was the figure of Naval Victory above Thornhill's portrait, holding a scroll where actions at sea dating back to the Armada are listed.

Just over half a century later, however, the Hospital authorities recovered their enthusiasm for commissioning ambitious and pertinent contributions from leading artists of the day. In 1779 the Chapel of Saint Peter and Saint Paul was gutted by a disastrous fire. Most of the distinguished interior designed by Wren and Ripley was destroyed but the Hospital decided to replace it with an even more sumptuous decorative scheme. Within a decade, services were resumed in a building transformed from the flamboyant Baroque dynamism of the nearby Painted Hall to the lightness and delicacy of 'Athenian' Stuart's Rococo idiom (pl. 180). In collaboration with William Newton, Stuart turned the old flat ceiling into a gently curving alternative, embellished with elaborate circular motifs and painted in colours pale enough to recall the pastel restraint of Wedgwood china. Although the interior is enriched with densely detailed plasterwork, much of it bearing maritime references like the dolphins intertwined with anchor and compass rose, there is no sense of decorative surfeit. Discretion rather than excess prevails, and throughout the chapel there is a consistent delight in skilful deception.

The panels containing apostles and evangelists between the upper windows on either side of the interior may resemble relief carvings, but they are in fact illusionistic paintings carried out with considerable technical virtuosity by the Italian specialist Biagio Rebecca. The massive Corinthian columns grouped in pairs at each end of the chapel are likewise made of *scagliola* (a blend of glue and plaster) in order to simulate marble. As for the cherubim supporting the altar and the roundels decorating the pulpit, they are made from a synthetic material called Coade stone (pl. 181). Benjamin West, soon to be elected the second President of the Royal Academy after Reynolds's death, designed these roundels, the most forceful of which depicts Saint Paul stretching out a dramatic arm towards Felix, the Roman governor of Judaea. Both Felix and his wife Drusilla trembled at the saint's fierce authority as he expounded the precepts of Christian doctrine, and the governor shrinks away from the assertiveness of the didactic index finger that Paul thrusts towards his face.

The virility of the roundels contrasts with the pacific mood of the four Coade stone statues designed by West for the niches of the chapel's entrance vestibule. Symbolising *Charity*, *Faith*, *Meekness* and *Hope*, they are the quintessence of gentleness.[16] But at the east end of the interior, Saint Paul's formidable tenacity was demonstrated on a truly colossal scale by the altar painting West installed there in 1789: *The Preservation of Saint*

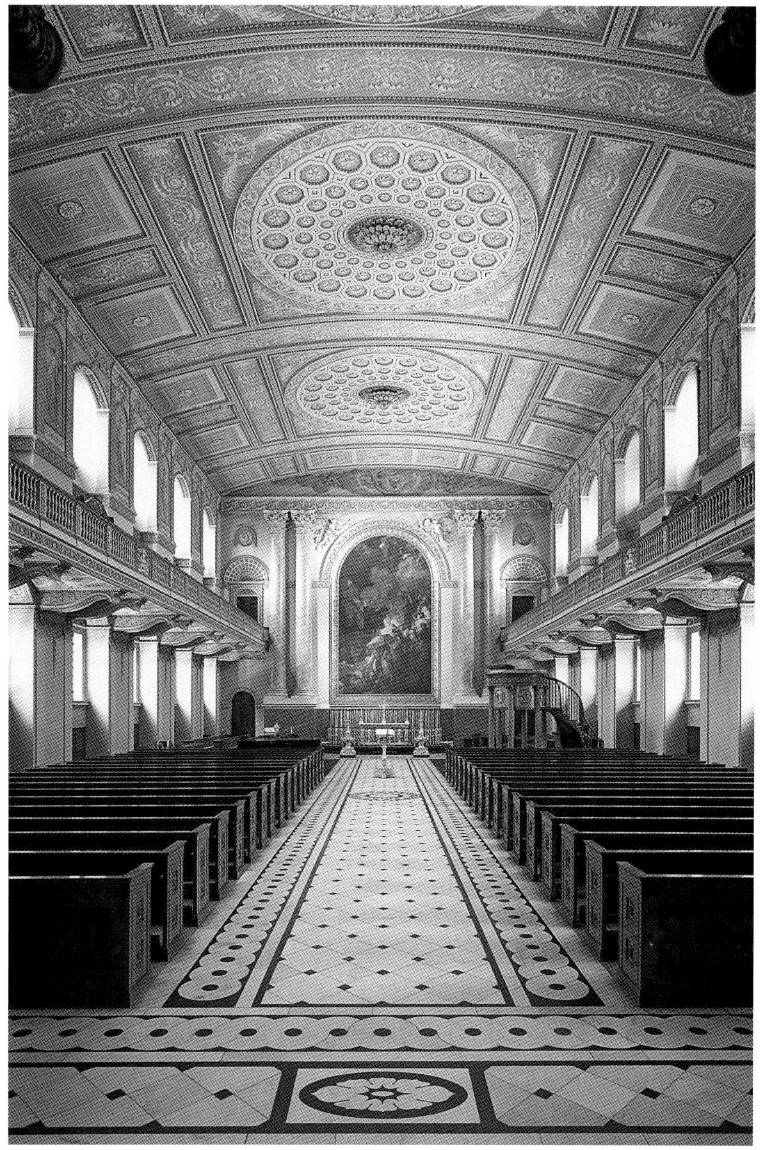

180 'Athenian' Stuart, interior of Chapel of Saint Peter and Saint Paul, 1779–89, Royal Hospital for Seamen, now Old Royal Naval College, Greenwich

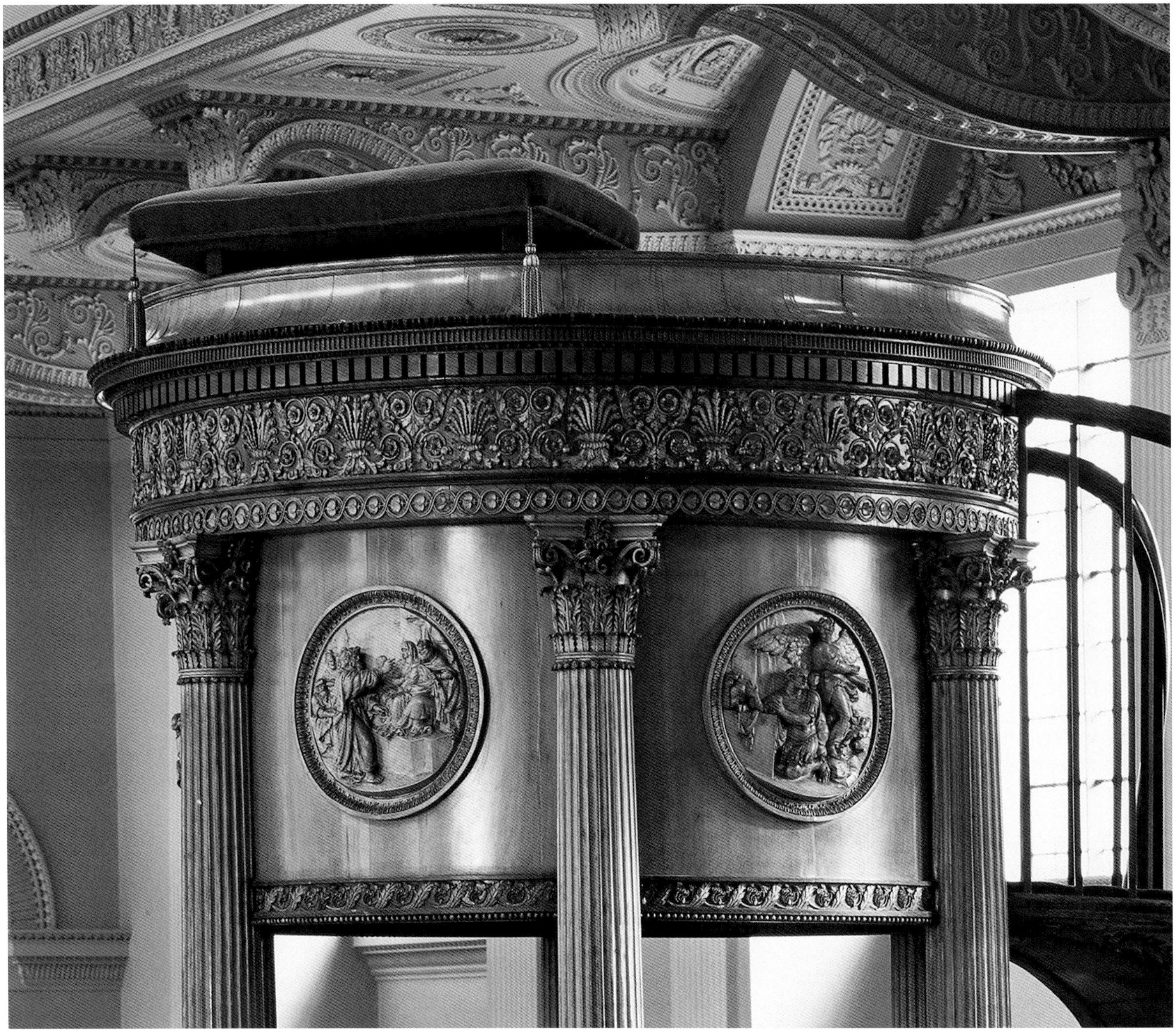

181 Benjamin West, Roundels decorating pulpit, 1789, Chapel of Saint Peter and Saint Paul, Royal Hospital for Seamen, now Old Royal Naval College, Greenwich

Paul after Shipwreck at Malta (pl. 182). Framed by Wren's imposing columns and, at the top, a pair of Coade stone angels, this dark and tumultuous canvas is calculatingly at variance with the lightness of Stuart's decorative scheme. It is difficult to discern the individual identity of many of the figures, clustered round a fire made for the storm-drenched company by the kind yet 'barbarous' people of Malta.[17] Perhaps West wanted to accentuate the superstition of the islanders by mantling them in deep nocturnal shadows, but his main reason for painting such pervasive gloom was surely to provide an arresting contrast with the flames. Bursting from the centre of the painting, they emblazon the people who throw up their arms in fear at the arrival of a snake. The Bible relates that when Paul had gathered a bundle of sticks, and laid them on the fire, there came a viper out of the heat, and fastened on his hand. And when the barbarians saw the venomous beast hang on his hand, they said among themselves, No doubt this man is a murderer, whom, though he hath escaped the sea, yet vengeance suffereth not to live.[18]

West concentrates on this moment of extreme suspense, when the islanders react with gesticulating dread while only Paul and the Roman soldiers he had befriended still retain their composure. The saint, his dark hair flying back from the wind of the fire, is about to drop the snake and disclose his unharmed hand to the islanders, who then conclude that he must be 'a god'. But in West's painting the crisis remains unresolved, and he makes sure that its tension is conveyed with a maximum amount of wonder.

The pensioners who congregated in the refurbished chapel could well have warmed to this large-scale dramatisation. It dealt, after all, with the survival of a storm, an experience familiar to many of them. The dangers confronting Saint Paul at sea and then by fire were likewise appropriate themes for ex-sailors, who had in many cases suffered grievous wounds in naval engagements.[19] However disfigured they may have been by these conflicts, the pensioners had at least returned alive, in some cases almost as miraculously as Paul when he shook the snake off his hand. So West's canvas, for all its vastness, bore intimately on their own concerns. Like the *Resurrection* mural executed by Sebastiano Ricci for the army pensioners of Chelsea Royal Hospital about seventy years before (see pl. 165), the Greenwich chapel sustained its worshippers at the century's end with a vision of survival, regeneration and hope.

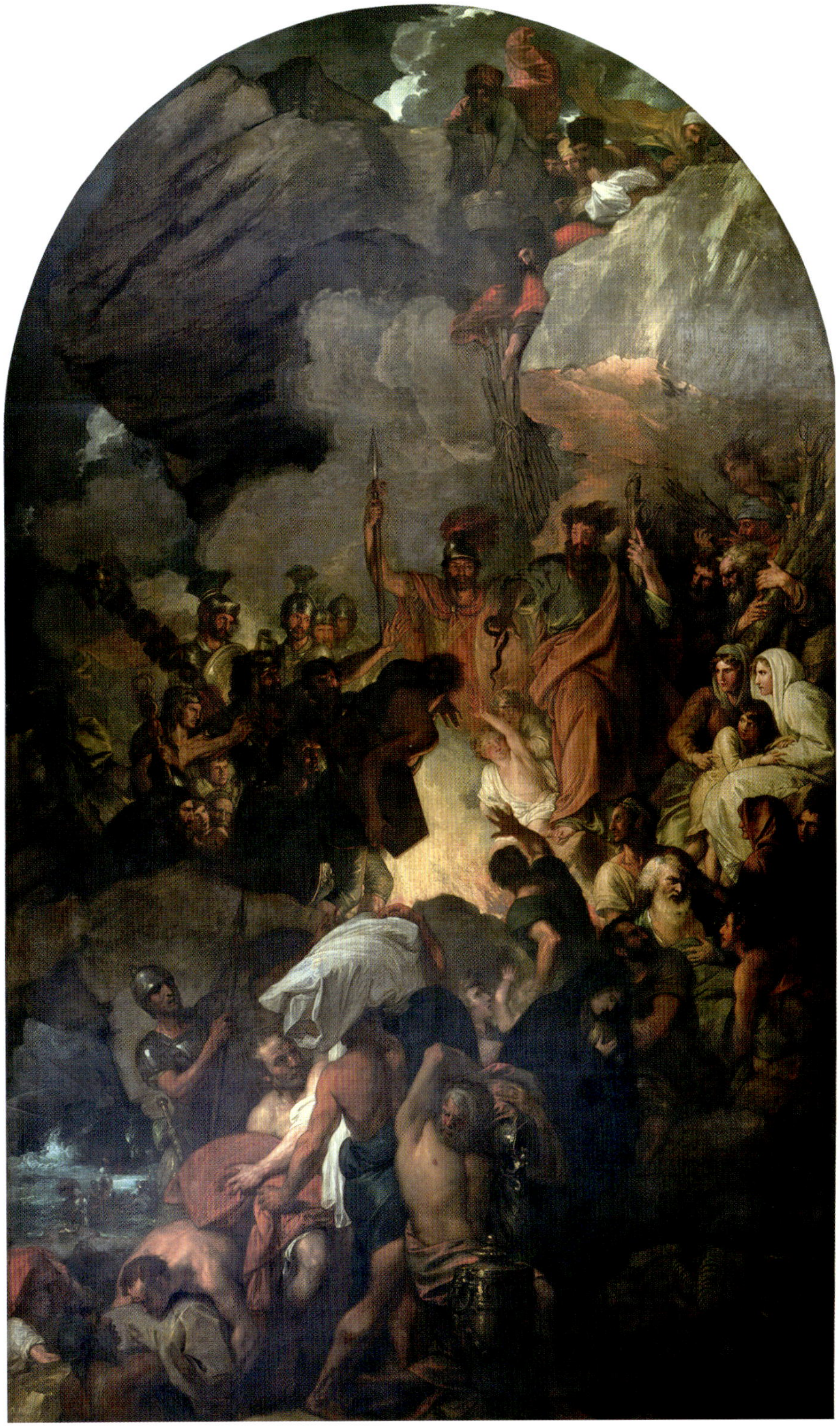

182 Benjamin West, *The Preservation of St Paul after Shipwreck at Malta*, 1789, altarpiece of Chapel of Saint Peter and Saint Paul, Royal Hospital for Seamen, now Old Royal Naval College, Greenwich

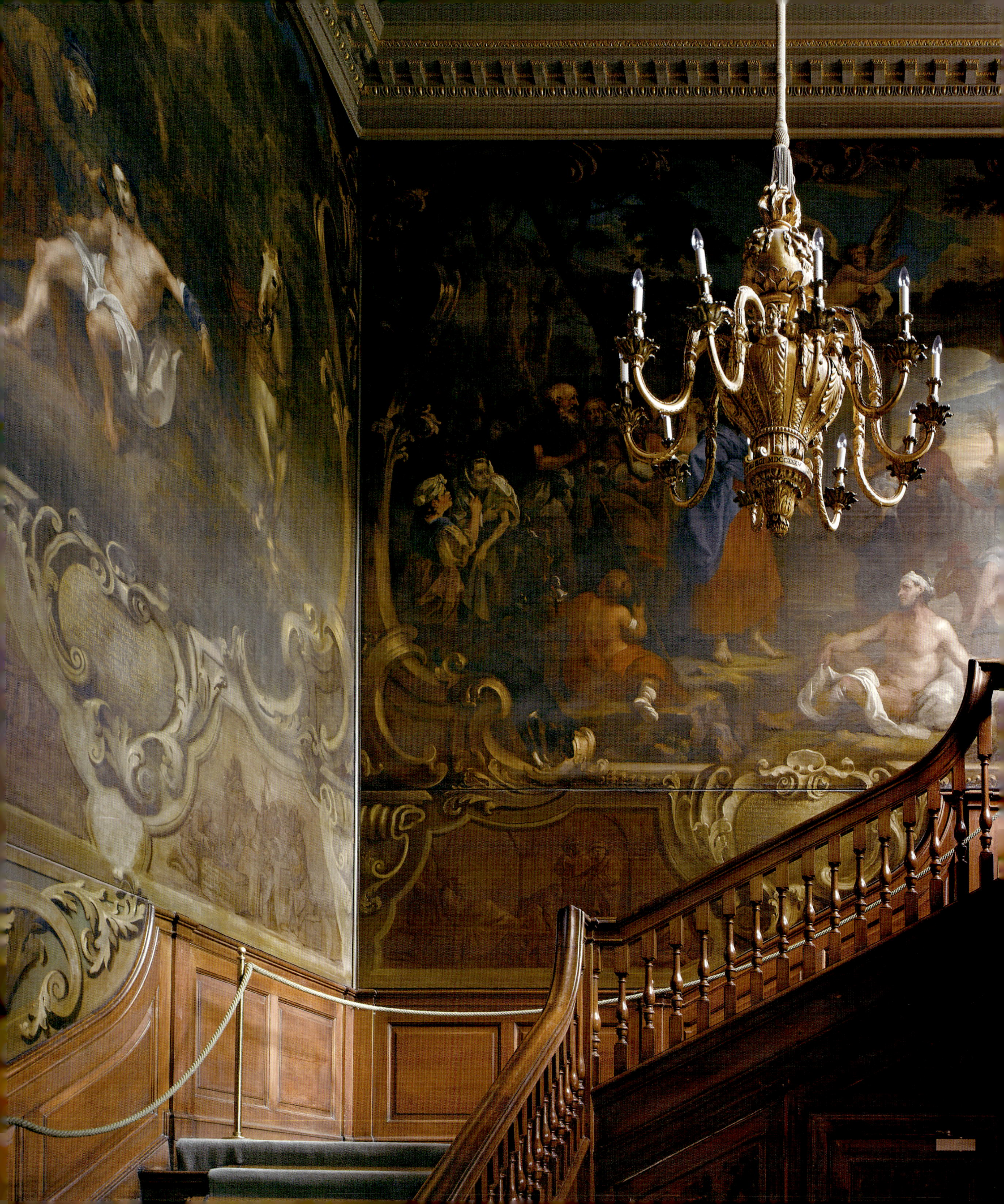

FOURTEEN
THE GOOD SAMARITAN AND CORAM'S FOUNDLINGS

Ever sceptical, and never afraid to assail mendacity in his art, William Hogarth regarded the medical profession with a particularly jaundiced eye. The greed and duplicity of doctors, no less than the ghoulish activities of surgeons, are lampooned with merciless wit and venom in many of his pictures (see pls. 210–11, 214). So Hogarth's willingness to spend an enormous amount of time on extensive painting schemes for major London hospitals, first at the ancient St Bartholomew's and then, with still greater commitment, at the newly established Foundling Hospital, may seem surprising. It discloses a quite different side of his work, far less familiar than the 'modern moral subjects' for which he is renowned.

His involvement can readily be explained, however. It stems in part from the friendships he enjoyed with two remarkable men: Thomas Coram, the Foundling's initiator, and John Freke, President of the College of Surgeons and a consultant at St Bartholomew's (Bart's). Hogarth's special affection for Bart's was quickened by the fact that he had been born in its neighbourhood, at St Bartholomew Close, Smithfield in 1697. His finest biographer, Jenny Uglow, observed that the 'elegant diamond' of Smithfield's marketplace had, like Hogarth's art, 'an in-built contradiction, ruled simultaneously by butchery and healing: by London's greatest meat market and one of London's greatest hospitals. Brick, flesh and blood'.[1] Moreover, his experience of growing up in the precincts of the Fleet Prison for debtors, where his father was incarcerated over a five-year period, left a profound mark on the work he subsequently produced. Ronald Paulson has argued that 'the problem of confinement, originating in childhood trauma, is discernible in almost every aspect of Hogarth's life and career: in his concern with institutions like St. Bartholomew's Hospital, with the establishment of the Foundling Hospital, and with the reform of prisons and madhouses.'[2]

All the same, the event that finally precipitated Hogarth into becoming an artist for Bart's had little to do with love of the locality or obsessive, subconscious motivations. It touched instead on his professional ambition to become a British painter in the grand manner, following in the tradition established with such enterprise by his father-in-law Thornhill at Greenwich (see pl. 176). Hogarth had no experience of tackling such a project, but he was incensed to hear that the Venetian history painter Jacopo Amigoni had almost secured the commission to paint elaborate wall decorations for the great staircase in Bart's new wing. Determined to put an end to foreign domination of important decorative schemes in Britain – a virtual monopoly

183 (*facing page*) James Gibbs, Staircase of administrative block at Bart's with Hogarth's *Pool of Bethesda* and *Good Samaritan*

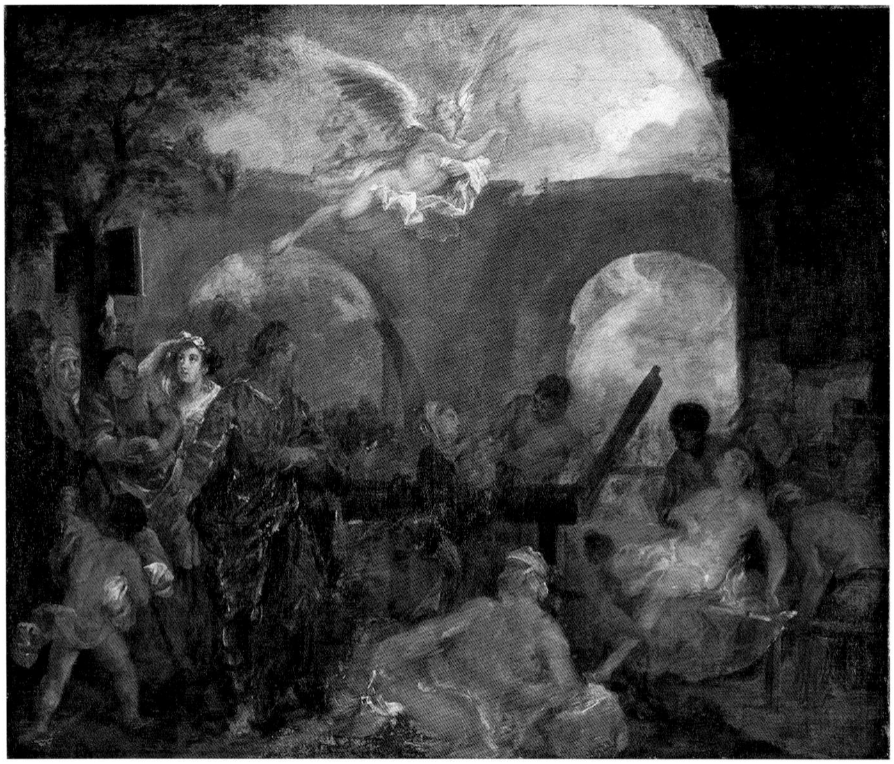

184 William Hogarth, Oil sketch for *The Pool of Bethesda*, *c.*1735, Manchester City Art Galleries

stretching back as far as Holbein and Rubens – Hogarth convinced himself that he could outdo Amigoni. Thornhill was about to die, a disappointed man who had been unable to crown his career with the further success he desired after Greenwich and the dome of Saint Paul's. So Hogarth, at the age of thirty-seven, felt even more strongly that the fallen baton should be picked up by the next generation of British painters. The Hospital he had known since boyhood seemed an ideal place to begin. Accordingly, he went to see the treasurer of Bart's, who was a friend, and brazenly offered to undertake the venture free of charge.

The offer was accepted, and in July 1734 it became sealed when Hogarth gained election to the hospital's governing board. But the task confronting him might easily have daunted an artist who had never before worked on a large scale in elaborate architectural surroundings. Bart's had recently decided to initiate a major rebuilding programme, transforming the inadequate medieval complex with its long, aisled ward and auxiliary cloisters into accommodation that took account of modern developments. Anxious to avoid the spread of either plague or fire, the hospital authorities commissioned James Gibbs, a governor since 1723, to design four separate ward blocks in a quadrangle. On the whole, though, this new ensemble was notable for its austerity rather than the exuberant embellishment enriching the Chelsea and Greenwich hospitals (see pls 163 and 170). Bryan Little observed of the Gibbs plan that 'the whole impression is not of luxury or of lavish expense, but above all of solid serviceability, and in the wards of a practical attention, given contemporary standards, to patients' needs'.[3]

The first building to be erected, though, was the most elaborate: a handsome administrative block distinguished by its two projecting 'pavilion' ends. Containing the treasurer's house, offices and a superb Great Hall ninety feet in length where the governors held their meetings, this was the wing housing Hogarth's staircase decorations (see pl. 183). One historian claimed that, since they occupied wall-space in a part of the building reserved for the Bart's board, 'it is most unlikely that patients ever saw these paintings'.[4] But in reality, as the inscription on the 'General Plan' of the Gibbs building reveals, the administrative block also housed 'a Room for admitting and discharging Patients and off of that another Room for the private Examination of them'.[5] These important areas of the Hospital adjoined the spectacular staircase with its ornamental plaster ceiling by John Baptist St Michele, so patients may have been able to look at Hogarth's prominently displayed canvases as they entered and departed from Bart's. In that sense, the paintings' subjects, described by the Governors as 'Characters (taken from Sacred History) wch. illustrate the Charity extended to the Poor Sick & Lame',[6] were well placed to leave inmates with a lasting visual impression of the hospital's priorities.

Hogarth's first painting, *The Pool of Bethesda*, was an idiosyncratic blend of satire and the sublime. Having recently completed his ambitious and uninhibited cycle *A Rake's Progress*, culminating in the madhouse scene with its quotation from Cibber's 'Bedlam' statues (see pl. 146), he was still in a mood to season the painting with macabre, even mordant incidents. But Hogarth also confessed that he 'entertained some hopes of succeeding in what the puffers in books call *the great style of History painting*', and other elements in the canvas adhere more firmly to the tradition honoured by Murillo in his version of the same subject (see pl. 133). These two disparate intentions do not fully cohere: the satirical side of the painting wars with its more elevated aim. Hogarth, however, did try very hard to make an original contribution to the iconography of Bethesda images, and it is fascinating to see how he prepared for the interpretation of a biblical text chosen, by the artist himself, as a theme appropriate to a Hospital for the poor.

His preliminary oil sketch for the *Pool of Bethesda* (pl. 184) is a crowded design, lacking the sense of spaciousness enjoyed by the final canvas. Brushed in very rapidly and lightly, the figures are unable to benefit from the ample foreground Hogarth develops in the finished painting. They also appear curiously indistinct in their characterisation. But the principal moral conflict between rich and poor is already confirmed as a key element in the design, and he had no intention of carrying the sketch's vagueness over to the decoration itself.

The existence of a careful chalk drawing for the semi-naked woman on the right of the composition (pl. 185) proves how thoroughly Hogarth prepared its principal figures. According to an inscription by Samuel Ireland, the drawing was executed 'in St. Martin's Lane', a reference to the 'Accademy for drawing from the life' which, as the engraver George Vertue recorded, began in St Martin's Lane under Hogarth's direction during the winter of 1735. This institution, now seen as the basis of the Royal Academy, encouraged the scrutiny of models assuming positions similar to the woman's stance in Hogarth's chalk study. So it may be that he executed the drawing at the class and then decided to incorporate the pose in his Bethesda painting.[7] Compared with the woman in the final canvas, the life model is altogether calmer and more dignified. She has none of the agitation afflicting the wealthy figure who so fussily implores her protector to secure an advantageous place in the pool. He orders the payment of an unscrupulous attendant, a rogue adept at receiving the bribe with one hand while brusquely pushing aside an impoverished woman and child with the other (pl. 186).

This aggressive episode, full of Hogarth's determination to show how ruthless the rich patients could be in their search for a cure, is typical of the *Pool of Bethesda*. Although the angel who troubled the pool's waters hovers overhead, resembling a figure in Thornhill's Sabine Room at Chatsworth,[8] this divine agent does nothing to quell the jostling that breaks out all over the uneasy painting. Behind Christ, a melancholy assortment of infirm people gesticulate and peer, amounting to a summary of the afflictions Hogarth may well have studied at first hand in the wards at Bart's. They include sufferers from blindness, anaemia, jaundice, inflammation of the breast, mental deficiency and hereditary syphilis.[9] It is a comprehensive array of ailments, vividly reflecting the diversity of patients found in many hospitals until the second half of the eighteenth century. Ivan Illich has described how, before then, 'the sick, the mad, the crippled, epileptics, incurables, foundlings and recent amputees of all ages and sexes were jumbled together'[10] in many

185 William Hogarth, Drawing of naked woman, 1735, The Royal Collection

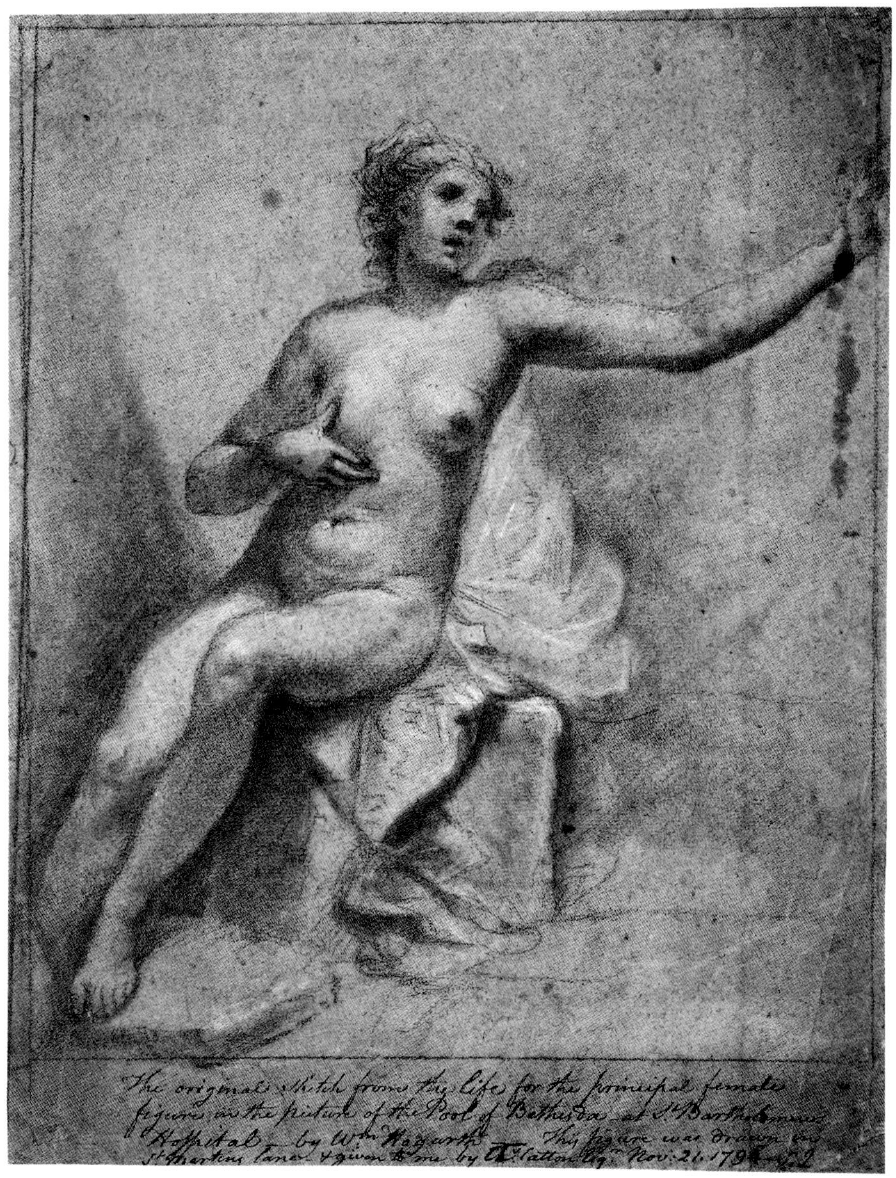

186 William Hogarth, *The Pool of Bethesda*, 1736, St Bartholomew's Hospital, London

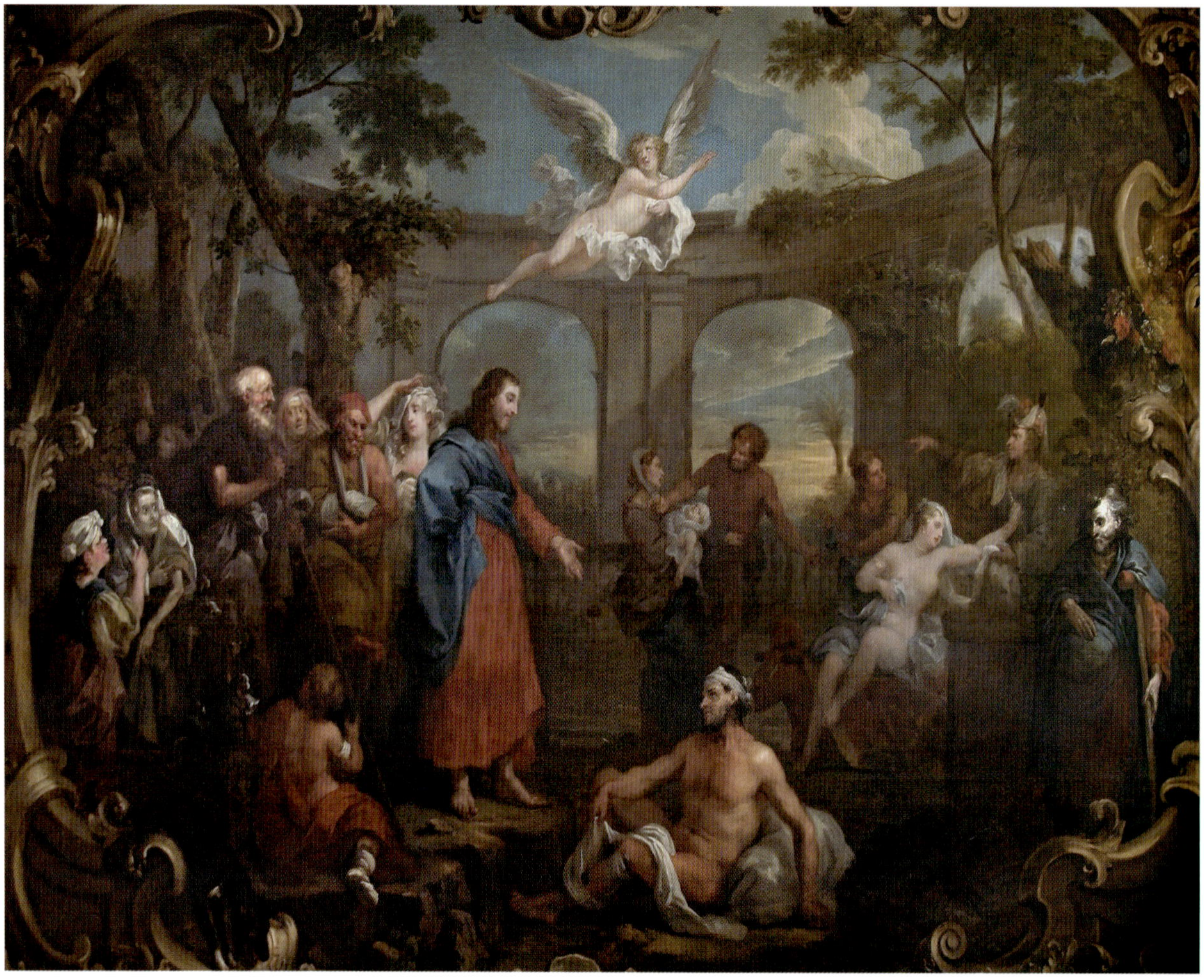

hospitals, and Hogarth's painting defines this gruesome clustering of unfortunates. Yet they are all beginning to realise that help might be obtained from Christ, who stands near the edge of a rock outcrop and extends a healing hand towards the paralysed man below.

Compared with Murillo, who created remarkable tension by focusing on the moment when the startled paralytic figure senses the first stirrings of life in his limbs (see pl. 133), Hogarth's version treats this central incident with surprising single-mindedness. The disabled man, who again recalls Cibber's 'Bedlam' statues (see pls 144–5), sits up and smiles as if the miracle were an entirely straightforward affair. His dramatic significance becomes the main focus of the painting, but it does not prevent us from exploring the subordinate groups, where Hogarth displays a racy vitality quite different from his depiction of the healing act. Here, away from the supposed centre of interest, he felt free to include among the heads a faithful likeness of Nell Robinson, a notorious prostitute with whom he had once been 'intimately acquainted'.[11] She possesses the energy and inventiveness animating all his finest work.

The companion painting, *The Good Samaritan* (pl. 187), presents a human act of charity to parallel its divine counterpart in the Bethesda canvas. Hogarth clearly intended the Samaritan composition as an extreme contrast to the earlier picture. Where the Bethesda image is replete with figures, and framed by monumental arches enclosing the entire scene, the Samaritan painting contains only a few people isolated in a wild and hostile landscape. The black dog who leans so cheekily over the edge of Bethesda's painted frame, and gazes down at anyone mounting the staircase, is replaced in the other picture by a wild-eyed hound who licks the

187 (*facing page*) William Hogarth, *The Good Samaritan*, 1737, St Bartholomew's Hospital, London

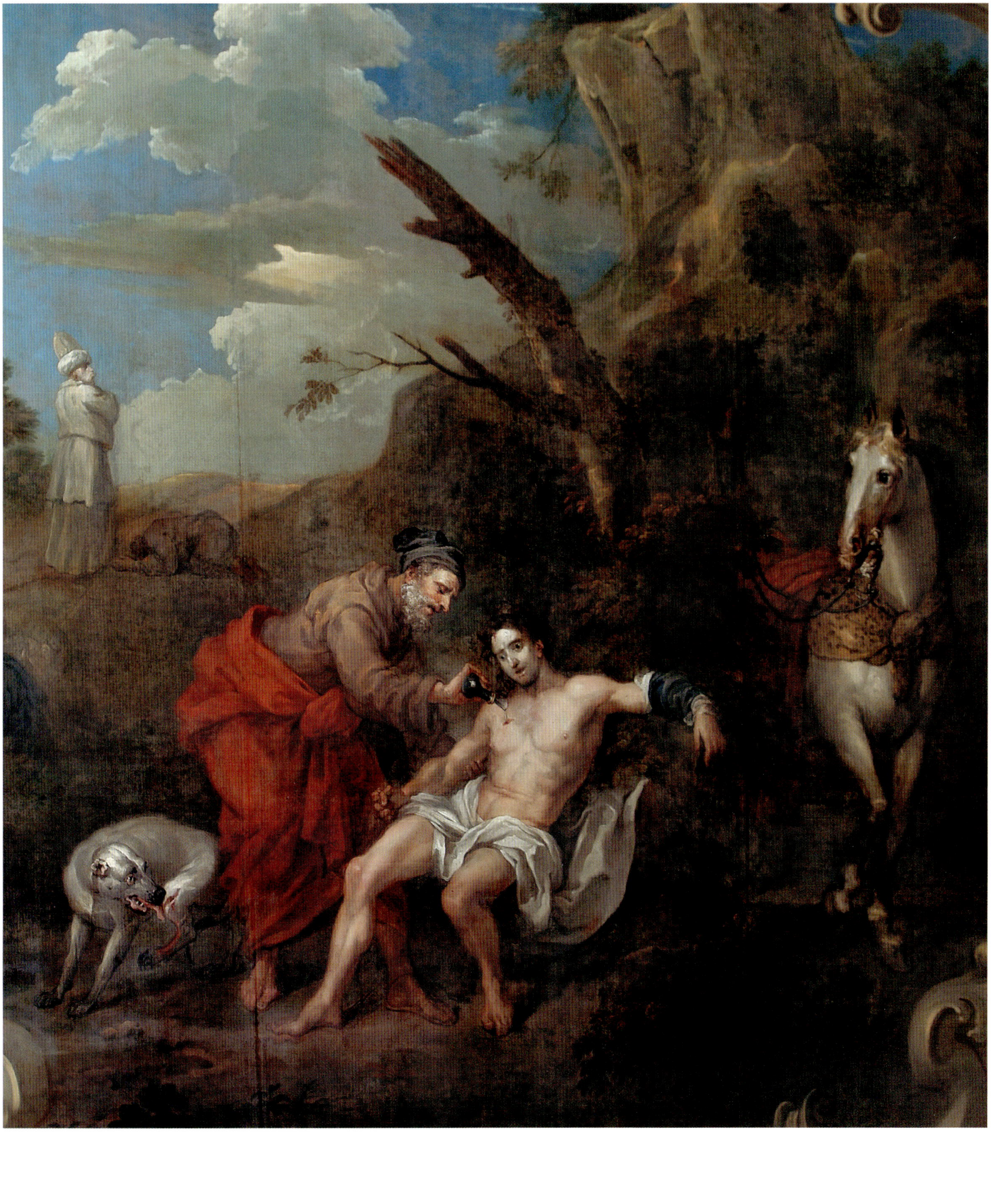

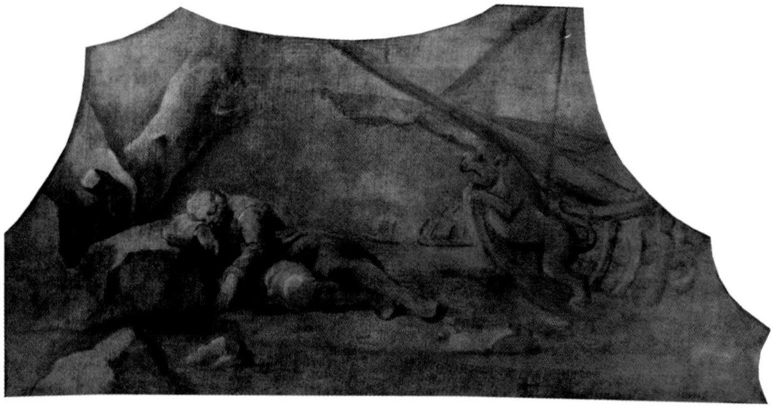

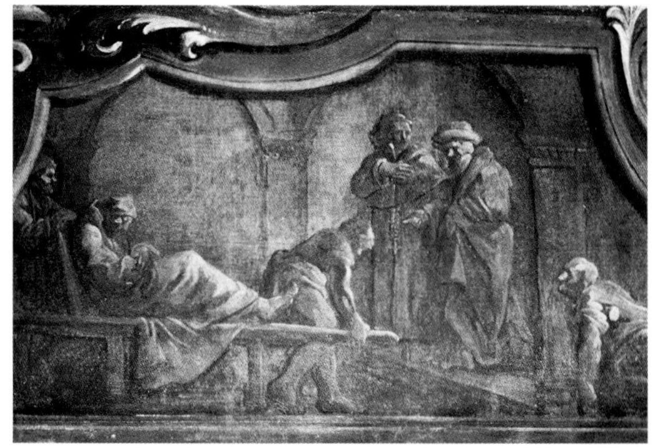

188a and b William Hogarth, Grisaille panels: *The History of Rahere*, 1736, St Bartholomew's Hospital, London

gash inflicted on his leg during a fight with his master's assailant. The difference between the two worlds is thoughtfully emphasised, and Hogarth afterwards boasted that the figures were seven feet high. But they appear ill at ease in the surrounding immensity. Emptiness is everywhere apparent, indicating that Hogarth was unwilling to activate the whole of his enormous picture surface with the predictable dexterity commanded by a more seasoned decorative artist. In this respect, he differs from Jean Restout whose monumental painting of the Good Samaritan was executed for the Hôpital de la Charité in Paris. For Restout shows no hesitation in allowing the two principal figures to dominate the canvas, focusing above all on the urgency and compassion of the Samaritan as he tends the traveller's injuries.

Hogarth, however, explores the relationship between Samaritan and victim with impressive sensitivity. Unlike the lavishly dressed figure in the distance, who walks away holding his haughty head aloft, the Samaritan lavishes anxious sympathy on the stricken man. Realising that the oil he pours into the wound will at first cause excruciating pain, the Samaritan tips the phial with conspicuous caution and delicacy. His little finger crooks itself carefully round the base of the container, as he tries hard to gauge the amount of liquid admitted to the gash. At the same time, he uses his other hand to hold the victim's arm. It is a compassionate gesture, for the injured man bunches the fist on that arm in order to cope with the agony. The feverish expression on his face shows how shocked and disorientated he feels, while the limpness of his left arm as it rests helplessly on the rock discloses the full extent of his exhaustion.

In the three *grisaille* panels beneath, Hogarth's spirited touch is a delight to the eye (pl. 188). He must have turned to them with enormous relief after the wearisome labour expended on the large paintings. The panels illustrate the history of Rahere, the founder of Bart's, who entertained his appreciative public with songs, stories, acrobatic feats and dancing bears. After becoming Henry I's favourite, he fell ill while returning from a pilgrimage to Rome and promised to start a hospital for the poor if he survived. Rahere kept his vow and in the finest *grisaille* Hogarth portrays him as the prior of the Augustinians who administered the institution during the medieval period. Hand outstretched in welcome, he greets a man bent with pain on a stretcher. The scene, summarised with great fluency and conciseness by Hogarth's confident brushmarks, contains in the figure of the cripple an outright homage to the Raphael Cartoons.[12] But the *grisaille* in its entirety remains an individual achievement, offering without any satirical excursions a sense of straightforward consolation for viewers who surely found it easier to scrutinise than the overwhelming paintings above.

The principal Bart's compositions did not lead Hogarth on to the commissions for grand decorative schemes he had hoped to obtain. His *Good Samaritan* achieved celebrity of a kind when it appeared in the cartouche of a splendid Rococo trade card for Dr James's fever powders around 1760. Even so, the staircase project never earned Hogarth the admiration he desired. 'Were there an inclination in England for encouraging historical pictures', he declared afterwards, 'such a first essay might prove the painting them more easily attainable than is generally imagined. But . . . religion, the great promoter of this style in other countries, rejected it in England.'[13] Ironically enough, a subsequent commission to paint a large altarpiece of the *Good Samaritan* for a private chapel at Cusworth Hall went to Francis Hayman, who relied on Hogarth's precedent established at Bart's for several elements in his painting. Over a century later, Richard Dadd followed Hogarth's example by producing a large *Samaritan* canvas for the staircase at Bethlem Hospital (see pl. 269). But for the moment, at least, Hogarth himself had to be content with helping Gibbs to frame the Hospital's redoubtable Henry VIII portrait, a school of Holbein full-length that they installed in the Great Hall with 'decent & respectfull Ornaments'.[14]

Even so, Hogarth did not wait too long before another, far more extensive and rewarding hospital venture gave him the opportunity to excel. It came from an unlikely quarter. Thomas Coram, the forthright sea captain whose greatest achievement was to establish the Foundling Hospital in 1739, had nothing to do with the medical establishment. Bluff, weatherbeaten and resolutely down to earth, he had earned wide admiration in his earlier career as a shipwright in colonial Boston and an authority on maritime trade. In 1735, three years after his appointment as a trustee for the settlement of Georgia, he was described by Horace Walpole as 'the honestest, the most disinterested, and the most knowing person about plantations I ever talked with'.[15] Since Walpole expressed these views in a letter to his father, who was then the de facto Prime Minister, Coram's reputation spread further. After his retirement from business, this hard-headed and single-minded character became increasingly preoccupied with a different cause. Prompted perhaps by childhood memories of the fate he had suffered after his own mother's death, when his father sent him off to sea at the age of eleven, the old captain decided to intervene on behalf of abandoned infants.

Coram was accustomed to walking between the City and his Rotherhithe home, often at night. He grew increasingly horrified by the sight of babies left to die on dung heaps in the street. Their plight had been a metropolitan scandal for many years. In 1713 the essayist Joseph Addison protested against London's unwillingness to make charitable provision for these pitiful children, pointing out that Paris, Rome, Madrid and Lisbon took their responsibilities far more seriously in this respect. But despite the passing of an Act in 1722, which brought about the building of workhouses where relief could be found, few of the infants admitted to these rudimentary institutions survived into adulthood. For seventeen years the doughty captain waged his campaign on behalf of abandoned children, while more and more poverty-ridden mothers were forced by the plummeting Poor Law to abandon babies whom they could not afford to support. He encountered formidable opposition, particularly from wealthy ladies who thought a foundling hospital would serve only to exacerbate lascivious behaviour. When he tried to deliver a petition to Princess Amelia at St James's Palace, her lady-in-waiting Lady Arabella Finch rebuffed him with 'very rough Words, and bid me begone.'[16] Unscrupulous journalists reinforced the attack by publishing lampoons like 'Joyful News to Batchelors and Maids', which claimed that Coram's plan was calculated 'To encourage the progress of vulgar Amours/The breeding of rogues and th'encreasing of Whores'.[17]

But Coram was undismayed. Once he had determined on a course of action, this obstinate man would not be deflected any more easily than a stubborn ship's captain bent on crossing the Atlantic as swiftly as possible. His friend Dr Brocklesby wrote of Coram that 'what he thought, he spoke, what he wished, he declared without hesitation, pursued without relaxation or disguise, and never considered obstacles any further than to discover means to surmount them'.[18] This singular tenacity enabled him, in July 1737, finally to present to George II and his Council a petition declaring itself written 'in behalf of great numbers of Helpless Infants daily exposed to Destruction'. The petition went on to ask the king for a Royal Charter to facilitate 'the Erecting and supporting an Hospital for the Reception, Maintenance and proper Education of such Cast of Children or Foundlings as may be brought to it'.[19]

More than two years passed before the endlessly optimistic Captain knew whether his proposal had received the assent he desired. But Coram was backed by powerful friends, including several dukes, almost a dozen earls and the most outstanding physician of the period, Dr Richard Mead. Their influence won the day and in November 1739 they gathered with other supporters at Somerset House for a ceremony where Coram received the Royal Charter 'for the Incorporation

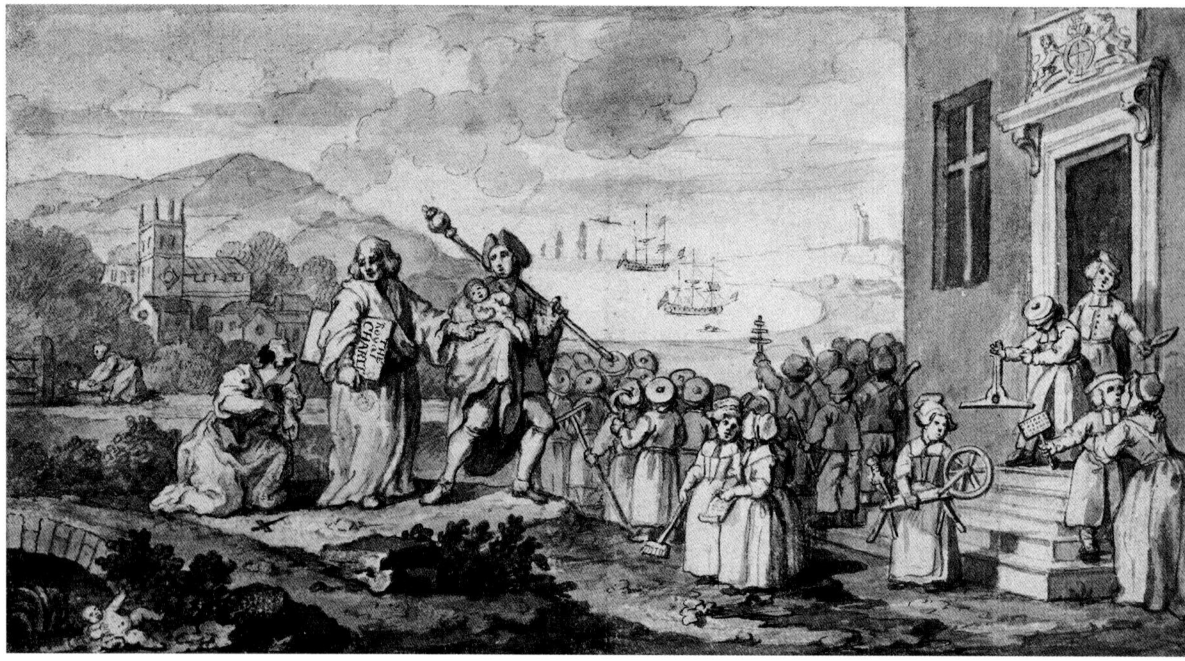

189 William Hogarth, *Heading to Subscription Roll*, 1739, Yale Center for British Art, Paul Mellon Collection

of the Foundling Hospital'. Among the assembled company was Hogarth, fired by the realisation that the obdurate Captain had committed himself to a humane concern with admirable resolve, level-headedness and lack of vanity. Here was a man Hogarth could respect without qualification, and he threw himself into the promotion of the Foundling's cause.

The aims behind it engaged his liberal and moral sympathies more deeply than Bart's had done. He approved of Coram's determination to implement child-care precepts well in advance of the time, not only providing for children in the Foundling home but acknowledging their need for family life, by providing a foster service. Hogarth's own wife Jane was one of the many foster-parents who became a part of the Coram Foundation's child-care service, and he did everything possible to place his art at the service of this compassionate endeavour. In the same year as the granting of the Royal Charter, he executed a heading to the Subscription Roll for the Hospital (pl. 189). It shows the kindly, silver-haired Coram assisting an officer with a baby while offering what comfort he can to its distraught mother. Reassuring her, he points towards a Foundling institution shown not in London but in an idealised rural location where the children are allowed to savour open fields and the distant prospect of a bay containing ships ocean-worthy enough to delight the Captain's heart. Although the reality proved considerably less idyllic, the Hospital was eventually erected in fifty-six acres of Bloomsbury fields with ample recreational space for the foundlings to enjoy. This lively subscription roll design, which adorned a document signifying that the Foundling authorities could now ask for contributions from potential benefactors, inaugurated Hogarth's work at the Hospital.

Only a few months later he followed it by donating a magnificent full-length painting of Coram that deserves to be ranked among the very finest of eighteenth-century European portraits (pl. 190). Such an image, grander by far than any other likeness Hogarth produced, fulfilled his ambitions to challenge the fashionable portraitists of the day. Just as his bulldog patriotism resented the near- monopoly exerted by foreign artists over decorative schemes in Britain, so he deplored the popularity among aristocratic sitters of a continental painter as mediocre as J. B. Van Loo. Hogarth recalled later that

> I exhorted the painters . . . to oppose him with spirit. But was answered, 'You talk! Why don't you do it yourself?' Provoked by this I set about this mighty portrait and found it no more difficult than I thought it. One day at the academy in St. Martin's Lane I put this question: 'If anyone now was to paint a portrait as well as Vandyke, would it be recognised and the person

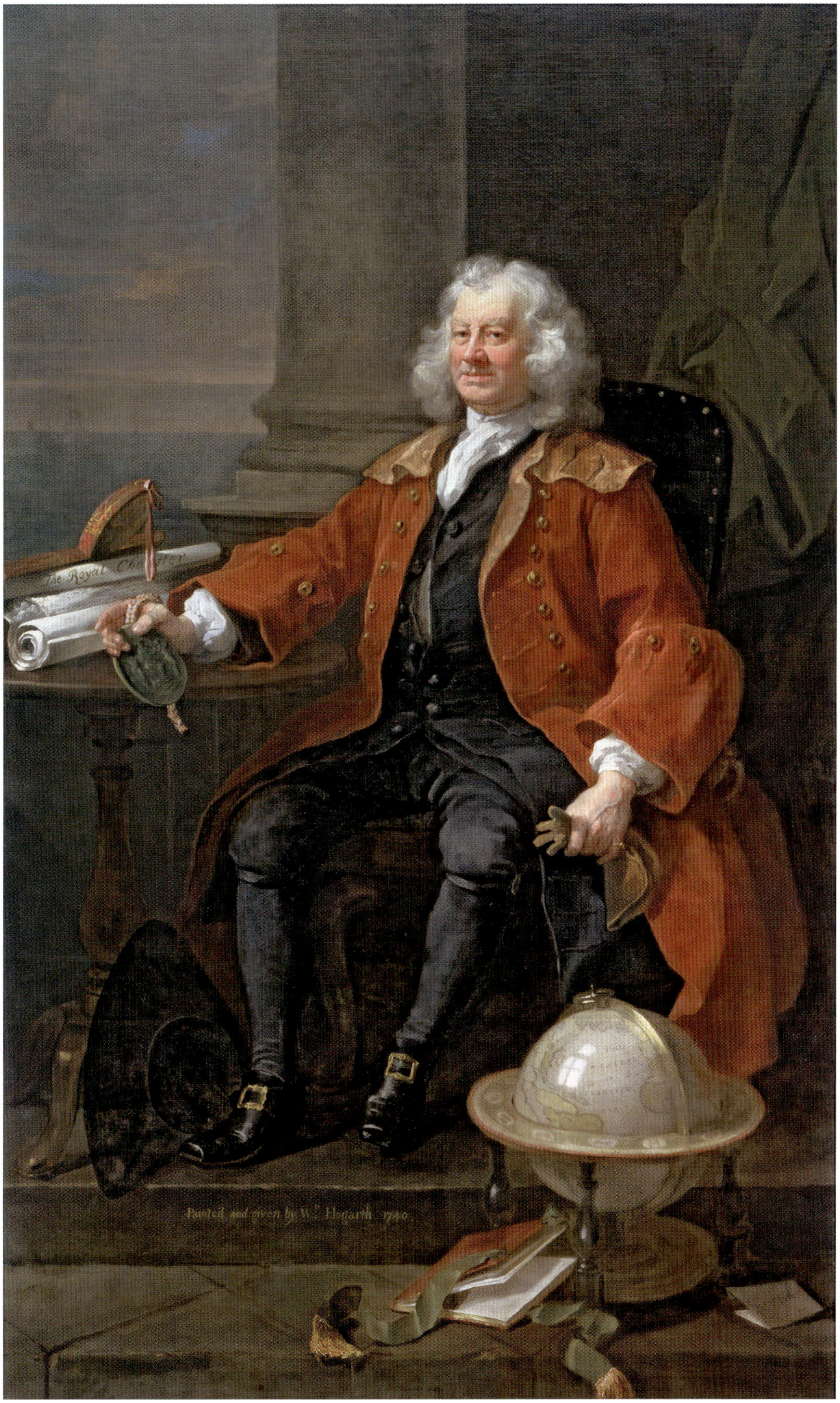

190 William Hogarth, *Captain Thomas Coram*, 1740, Foundling Museum, London

enjoy the benefit?' They knew I had said I believed I could. The answer was made by Mr. Ramsey and confirmed by the rest: 'Positively no' . . . Upon which I resolved, if I did the thing I would affirm it done.[20]

By presenting such robust and confident proof of his prowess to the Foundling Hospital, where he knew it would be seen by many influential visitors, Hogarth hoped to establish his reputation as a portraitist among those best able to commission further examples from him. 'Painted and given by Wm Hogarth 1740' runs the unusually elaborate inscription, easily visible on the step below Coram's feet. It reads like the verbal equivalent of a gauntlet flung at the feet of the portraitists he disliked – painters as ostentatious as Hyacinthe Rigaud, whose flamboyant likeness of the financier Samuel Bernard was a painting that Hogarth particularly wanted to reprove with his Coram portrait. It was a risky challenge to mount, for he could easily have made himself appear deluded. But the redoubtable painting of *Captain Thomas Coram* turned out to be a triumphant vindication of all his boasts, while at the same time subverting the empty poses and stylistic grandiloquence indulged in by so many of his fashionable rivals.

Although the mighty column and cascading drapery behind Coram are props deliberately borrowed from van Dyck's repertoire of theatrical effects, Hogarth does not employ them to bolster the esteem of a foppish, self-regarding grandee. Seated squarely and without pretension in a sturdy leather chair, the bluff sea captain makes no attempt to strike an imposing attitude. The parchment scroll of the hospital's Royal Charter is prominently displayed on the table beside him, and he clasps its seal with a firmness that implies his delight in obtaining at last the monarch's official blessing for his philanthropic venture. A plaque showing a Charity group hangs behind him, now scarcely visible yet clearly exposed in a mezzotint made by Nutter over half a century after the canvas was finished. None of these references is a form of personal aggrandisement, though. Hogarth and Coram have together ensured that the Foundling institution is celebrated here, and the sole personal mark of honour turns out to be a typically modest object: the three-cornered black hat leaning so informally against the leg of the Captain's desk. It symbolises the help he extended to London's hatters, who believed they were penalised in their Colonial trading. The only gift Coram would accept from them as sign of thanks was the hat, renewable free of charge whenever he wished.

Large yet plain, the hat is just as unadorned as the rest of the Captain's clothes. For his old-fashioned and almost homely rust-coloured coat has nothing to do with aristocratic finery, and no embellished ruffles can be found at the wrists of the old sailor's shirt. His linen is strong and simple, like the sturdy gold-buckled shoes with their blunt toe-caps. They are made for walking long distances rather than attending society soirées and Coram's seated position is restless enough to contain an unmistakeable promise of activity to come. His veined, coarse-knuckled left hand grasps a pair of gloves, as if to suggest that the Captain will soon put them on. A doer rather than a thinker, he appears ready at any instant to get up from the chair and hurry out in search of further benefactors for his Hospital.

The view of sea and ships beyond the pillar is redolent of a man whose horizons have never been bounded by the four walls of a room, and the globe isolated with such deliberation on a step of its own confirms the breadth of his outlook. Unlike the globes in comparable portraits of kings, soldiers or politicians, brazenly declaring the extent of imperial acquisitions throughout the world, Coram's is turned to focus on 'The Western or Atlantick Ocean'. This is the area he spent much of his maritime career sailing across, not subjugating in order to claim arrogant possession. Even the strip of America's east coast on the globe alludes to the efforts made by this devoutly religious man to establish Georgia as 'a charitable Colony', and the expression on his face has nothing to do with the haughty aggression of an empire-builder.

Kindly rather than ruthless, the ruddy sea-dog with his jutting chin smiles good-naturedly at the friend who paints him. The dark eyes remain surprisingly clear and intense for a man of seventy-two, and they have a shrewdness that enabled him to achieve his beneficent goal against formidable opposition. But they belong to a man of candour, not a master of duplicity: a robust and direct individual who would never let inhibiting codes of politeness prevent him from stating his case with refreshing independence. Spurning the modern periwig that excited Hogarth's derision in *The Company of Undertakers* (see pl. 212), he lets his own long, white curls descend like an untamed mane on shoulders wide enough to show the strength he still retains. His scalp is visible through the silver hair, and the portrait makes no attempt to pretend that Coram is anything other than an elderly man. But the sympathy between this old sitter and the equally outspoken, defiant artist who painted him gives the Captain an endearing liveliness. Happy to sit for a while until the picture is completed, Coram looks forward to the moment when he can relax, joke with Hogarth and give vent to the uproarious laughter that seems latent in his generous, immensely companionable face.

By using the conventions of the swaggering Van Dyck full-length to celebrate a man of modest social status, Hogarth here emancipated British portraiture with enormous brio and audacity. He never painted more confidently than in this ebullient canvas, and the fellow-feeling between sitter and artist surely contributed to the picture's irrepressible assurance. Hogarth must have identified with the Captain's success in taking on the established values of his day and winning the case for a more compassionate civilisation. If there is a hero to be found among the cornucopia of frauds, fools and sadists who pepper Hogarth's work, Coram must be the one. He is the very embodiment of the plain man who succeeds, despite daunting hostility from orthodox and snobbish opinion, in asserting a vigorous corrective to the prevailing order. The parallel with Hogarth's own attempts to replace contemporary artistic fashions with a more bracing alternative, rooted in trenchant observation of social reality, is clear enough. No wonder he needed scant prompting before grasping the opportunity to invest this epitome of stubborn, bloody-minded enterprise with as much nobility as grand-manner portraiture could provide. The dignity of the homespun seafarer from the everyday world is more convincing by far than the assumed loftiness in so many routine effigies of titled landowners and high-ranking officials.

The portrait was completed just in time. Only two months after it had been formally donated to the Foundling's Annual Court, 'for this Corporation to keep in memory of the said Mr. Coram's having solicited, and obtained His Majesty's Royal Charter for this Charity',[21] the Captain's wife died. After forty years of marriage, the effect on her husband was catastrophic. Unbalanced by grief, he allowed himself to decline into poverty and become, in the eyes of the Foundling's governors, merely interfering. He was, according to a report they received, expending most of his energies spreading scandalous rumours about the libidinous and deceitful behaviour of the Hospital's chief nurse. Coram alienated the sympathies of the governors so irrevocably that they refused to re-elect him as a member at the Foundling's general committee meeting in 1742. It was a tragic severance, barely ameliorated by the governors' decision in 1751 to let him be buried below the altar of the chapel in the Hospital's imposing building, near completion on the site where Coram's Fields can today be found.

However upset Hogarth may have been by the Captain's estrangement, he did not allow his own

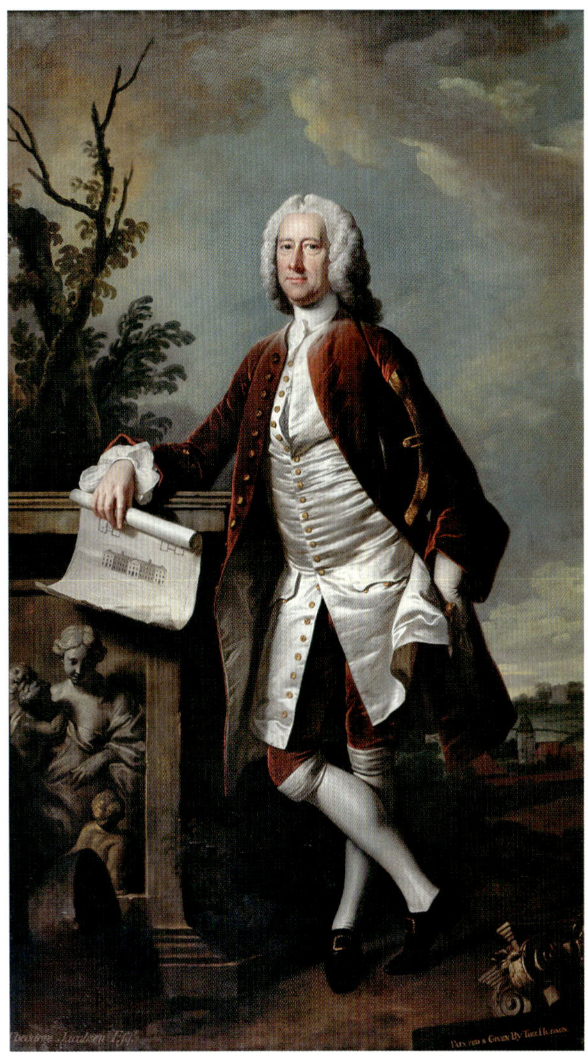

191 Thomas Hudson, *Theodore Jacobsen*, c.1742, Foundling Museum, London

involvement with the Foundling cause to slacken. He executed a half-length of Theodore Jacobsen, the architect of the hospital building. It lacks the grandeur of the full-length Jacobsen portrait painted for the Foundling by Thomas Hudson, showing the architect leaning on a plinth with a relief of Charity and holding Fourdrinier's engraving of the Hospital's plan and elevation (pl. 191). Although Jacobsen adopts what Ellis Waterhouse succinctly described as 'that foolish cross-legged style, which was to haunt British portraiture . . . for the next forty years',[22] Hudson overcame his usual dullness in this carefully wrought canvas. It does not possess the engaging humanity of Hogarth's picture, a direct image refusing to indulge in any unnecessary rhetoric. But Hudson succeeds in reflecting the character of a very practical man, a former City merchant of German descent who only became an amateur architect later in his career to satisfy his own substantial artistic and intellectual interests. Working free of charge, this Fellow of the Royal Society and the Society of Arts designed for the governors a severe three-sided structure (pl. 192), in accordance with the change in contemporary views about hospital architecture. By the middle of the eighteenth century, the unabashed splendour of buildings as palatial as the Greenwich Royal Hospital was regarded as inappropriate. 'Houses destined for the poor should have in them something of poverty' was the bleak opinion expressed by Marc-Antoine Laugier in his *Essai sur l'architecture* of 1755. He argued that 'hospitals should be solidly but simply built. There should be no building where sumptuousness runs contrary to propriety . . . Magnificence announces either superfluous funds in the foundation or very little economy in its administration.'[23]

It was a stern doctrine, and Hogarth seemed determined to disregard as vigorously as he could Laugier's chilling view that 'too much beauty in a house . . . will no longer attract the interest of the charitable'. In his capacity as a leading member of the Foundling's directing Court and its General Committee, he designed the red-trimmed uniform worn by the children and a shield that became incorporated in the Hospital's arms. But his commitment to the aims of the burgeoning institution, which housed six hundred foundlings by the time

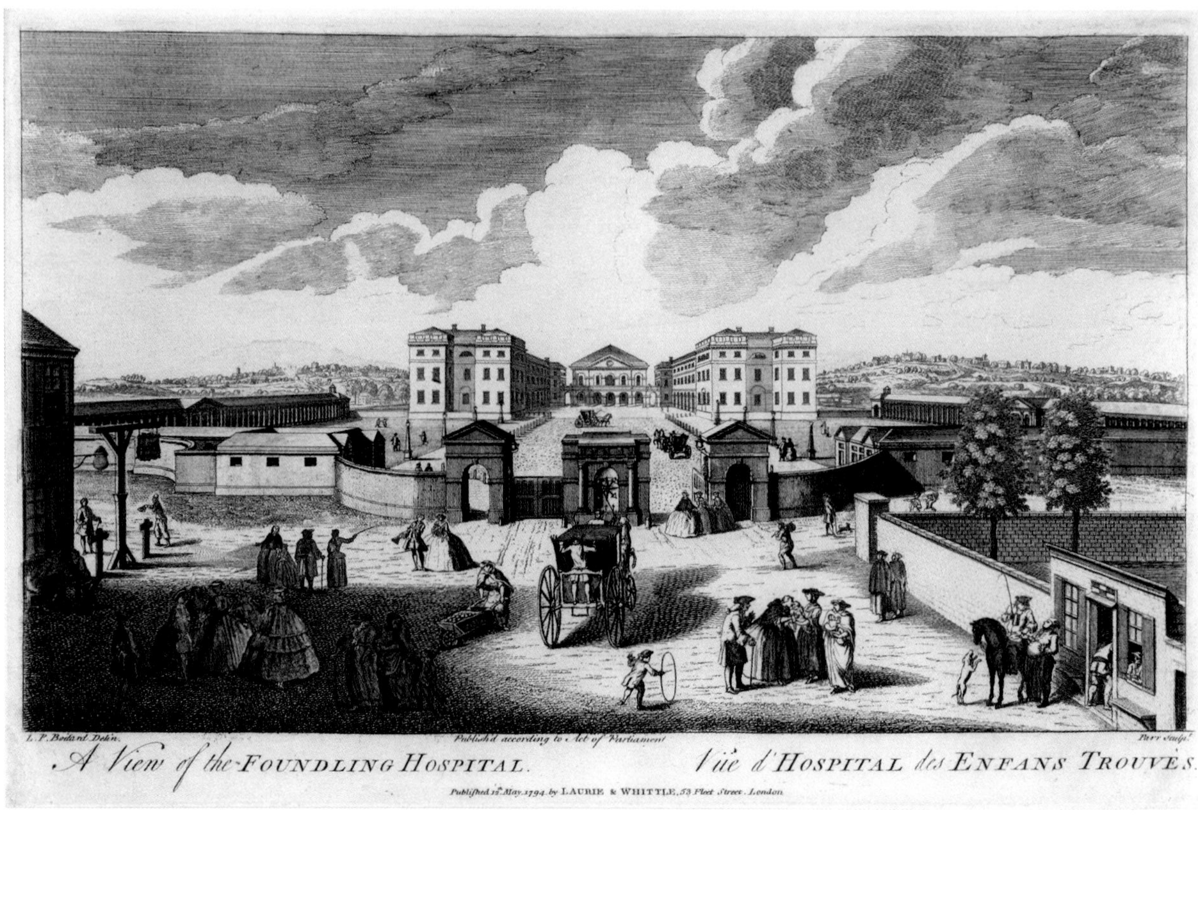

192 A view of Theodore Jacobsen's Foundling Hospital, originally published 1750, Foundling Museum, London

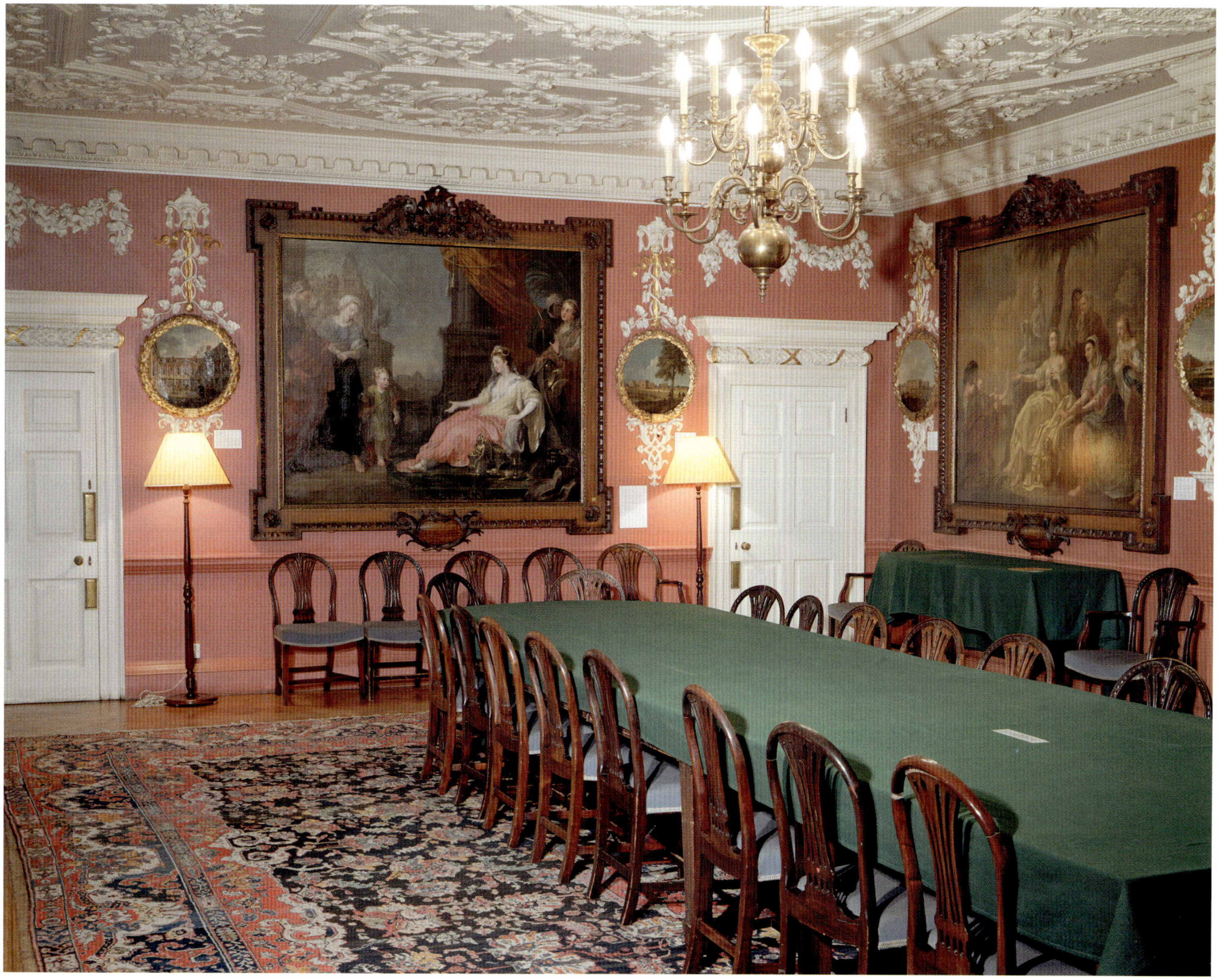

Jacobsen's building was finished in 1752, did not prevent him from presenting a special drawing to the London Hospital in 1744. Intended for the headpiece of a broadsheet appeal for subscriptions, and later used on attendance certificates as well,[24] the dignified design illustrated the Last Judgement text, 'In as much as ye have done it unto me'.[25] Hogarth's drawing indicated once again his instinctive support for institutions that offered genuine help to the sick and dispossessed, but he persisted in reserving his greatest generosity for the Foundling Hospital.

Even though the governors 'refused to apply any of the charitable contributions'[26] to the scheme he now devised, Hogarth went ahead with an ambitious proposal to decorate the Court Room in the new building's west wing. This resplendent chamber, intended for governors' meetings and embellished with an elaborate plasterwork ceiling by William Walton, was completed by October 1745 (pl. 193). Always on the lookout for public settings where British painters could execute decorations, Hogarth managed to persuade three fellow-artists to join him in producing large canvases, free of

193 Theodore Jacobsen and William Walton, Court Room of the original Foundling Hospital, London

194 Francis Hayman, *Finding of Moses in the Bulrushes*, 1746, Foundling Museum, London

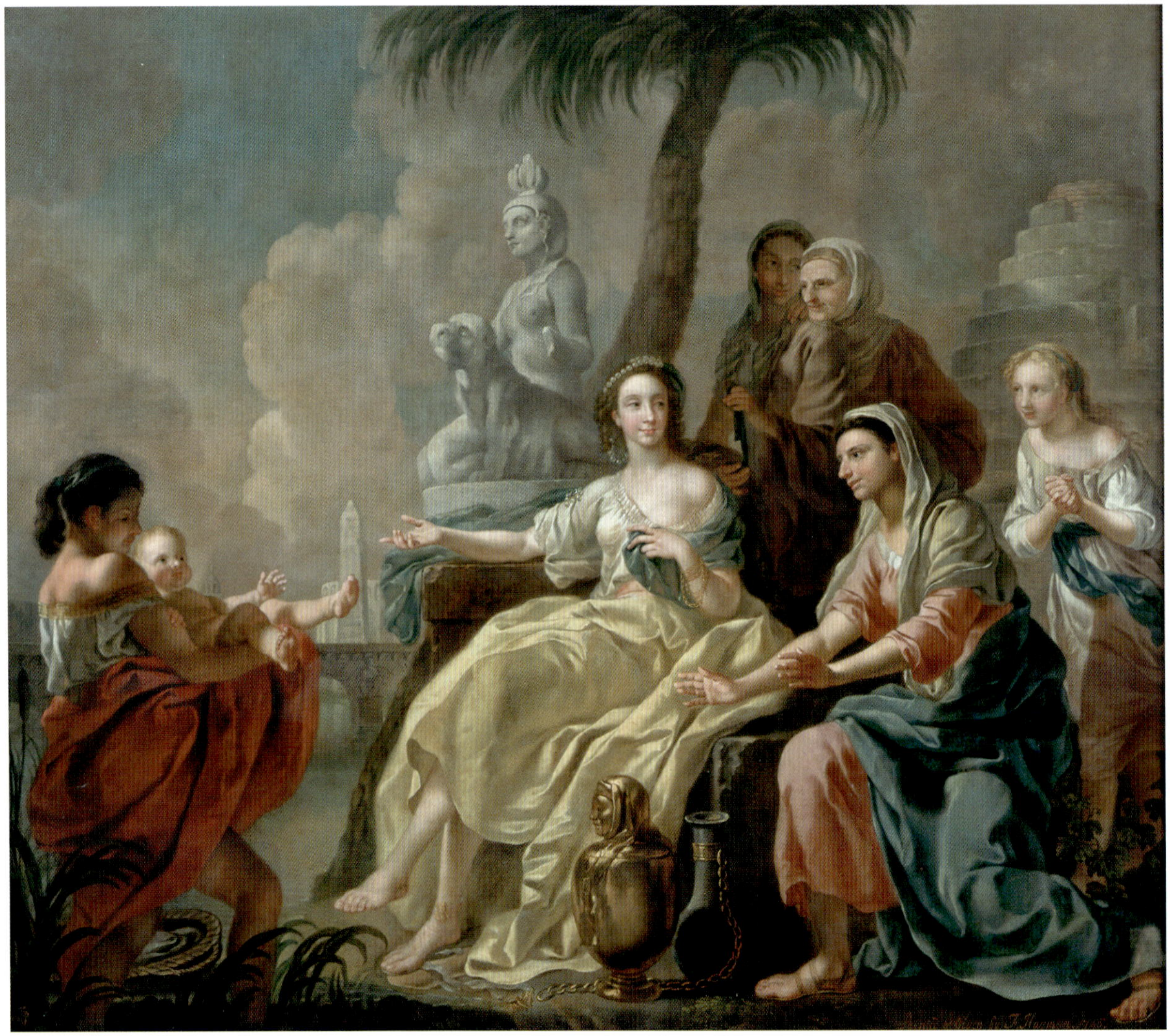

charge, for the Court Room's walls. John Brownlow, the Foundling's secretary and original historian, claimed that the pictures arose from the 'conjoint agreement' of the artists,[27] and all the canvases took their cue from the appropriate theme of young children rescued. Hogarth's subject was *Moses brought before Pharoah's Daughter*, Joseph Highmore tackled *Hagar and Ishmael*, James Wills depicted the *Little Children brought unto Christ* and Francis Hayman, the last of the four to complete a picture,[28] dealt with the *Finding of Moses in the Bulrushes*. But rather than deciding on the overall theme themselves, Hogarth and his friends probably followed the advice of Coram. For the Captain had presented the Hospital's first seal to its General Committee in 1739, explaining that the design he used there derived from 'the affair Mentioned in the Second of Exodus of Pharoah's daughter and her Maids finding Moses in the ark of Bulrushes which I thought would be very appropos for a hospital for foundlings, Moses being the first foundling we read of'.[29] Coram's partiality for the biblical story also resulted in a painting by Balthasar Nebot, where the founder of the Hospital is portrayed in front of his institution standing guard over a baby in a Moses basket beside him.

The iconography of the four main Court Room canvases may, therefore, have been Coram's last contribution to a foundation that had already ousted him from its membership. Hogarth was probably still inclined to take the advice of his old friend, and he must have arranged with Hayman for the two of them to depict consecutive episodes from the Exodus. Hayman dealt with the moment in Exodus 2:6, 7 when the baby Moses, having been hidden by his mother to prevent the Pharaoh's men from killing him, is discovered by the Pharaoh's daughter (pl. 194). She recognises that he is a Hebrew child but, instead of ordering his slaughter, 'had compassion on him' and arranged for 'a nurse of the Hebrew women' to look after him.[30] The nurse was, in fact, Moses' mother and, although Hayman places Pharaoh's daughter in the centre of the composition, its emotional focus lies with the woman whose baby has been temporarily restored to her.

Arms extended to receive the infant, she half-kneels as if overcome by the wonder of the occasion. Moses appears to recognise her, for his hand reaches towards the mother as he emerges from the river in the protective embrace of an affectionate 'maiden'. The whole canvas exudes a warmth of feeling matched by the colours Hayman employs. Serenity is accentuated by the carefully rendered Egyptian accessories, the fruit of scholarly research generated by the recently formed Egyptian Society. Brian Allen pointed out[31] that Hayman made full use of the authentic details of ancient Egypt published in 1743 by Dr Richard Pococke, whose *A Description of the East and Some Other Countries* illustrated plants and artefacts of the kind distributed with such deliberation in the foreground of this painting. They chime with the statue underneath the tree and the step-pyramid looming behind the monumental figures, each of whom possesses a Poussinesque restraint. Armed with knowledge of the biblical story, we can see that Hayman might have intended to give the picture a rather more poignant dimension as well. Although he swathes Pharaoh's daughter in a glowing yellow dress, and provides her with a regal smile, the fact remains that she occupies the sizeable gap between Moses and his mother. The two are not yet reunited, and Hayman knew that they would not remain with each other on a permanent basis. Hence, perhaps, Hayman's decision to choose the instant before the mother is able once again to grasp her baby. Pharaoh's daughter, seemingly the agent of recovery, signifies through the very forcefulness of her presence the role she will eventually play in parting Moses for ever from the woman who bore him.

The Bible does not describe how his mother felt when obliged, a few years later, to give her son to Pharaoh's daughter. The scene is tersely recounted in Exodus ('she brought him unto Pharaoh's daughter, and he became her son'), so Hogarth was obliged to imagine the scene without any significant help from his Old Testament source. Maybe the freedom he enjoyed here contributed to the gracefulness of the picture he produced (pl. 195). A more refined image than either of his earlier history paintings for Bart's (see pls 186–7), it concentrates on the dilemma confronting the little boy as he finds himself beckoned by the unfamiliar regal lady. Hogarth shows no complexity of emotion in the mother's face, possibly because he believed that she had long since resigned herself to the inevitability of this moment. Besides, he may also have decided that the tragic depiction of a bereft mother would have been too disturbing an image for the foundlings who contemplated his painting.

Yet there is nothing in the least comfortable about the relationship between the son and his would-be guardian. Although Pharaoh's daughter appears confident of her ability to reassure the child, and holds out a welcoming hand towards him, the gulf between them appears even more marked than the gap separating Moses from his mother in Hayman's canvas. Still reluctant to leave the shelter of maternal robes, he makes no attempt to reach out towards the proferred gesture. Instead, his hand dangles uncertainly in space and his expression reveals all the bewilderment of a small boy reluctant to leave the woman he loves. A sad and desperately lonely figure, caught between natural reluctance and the knowledge that Pharoah's daughter has promised to look after him, he personifies the profoundly wrenching experience undergone by many foundlings when their foster mothers returned them to the Hospital's care. The insight with which the boy's dilemma is interpreted marks this canvas out as the finest of the Court Room pictures, and George Vertue, the engraver and historian, reported that 'its Generally said and allowed that Hogarth's peece gives most strikeing satisfaction – & approbation'.[32]

The major Court Room canvases were applauded after their installation. Vertue related that they were 'by most people generally approvd & commended as works in history painting in a higher degree of merit than has heretofore been done by English Painters'.[33] The scheme was boosted by the addition of eight little roundels

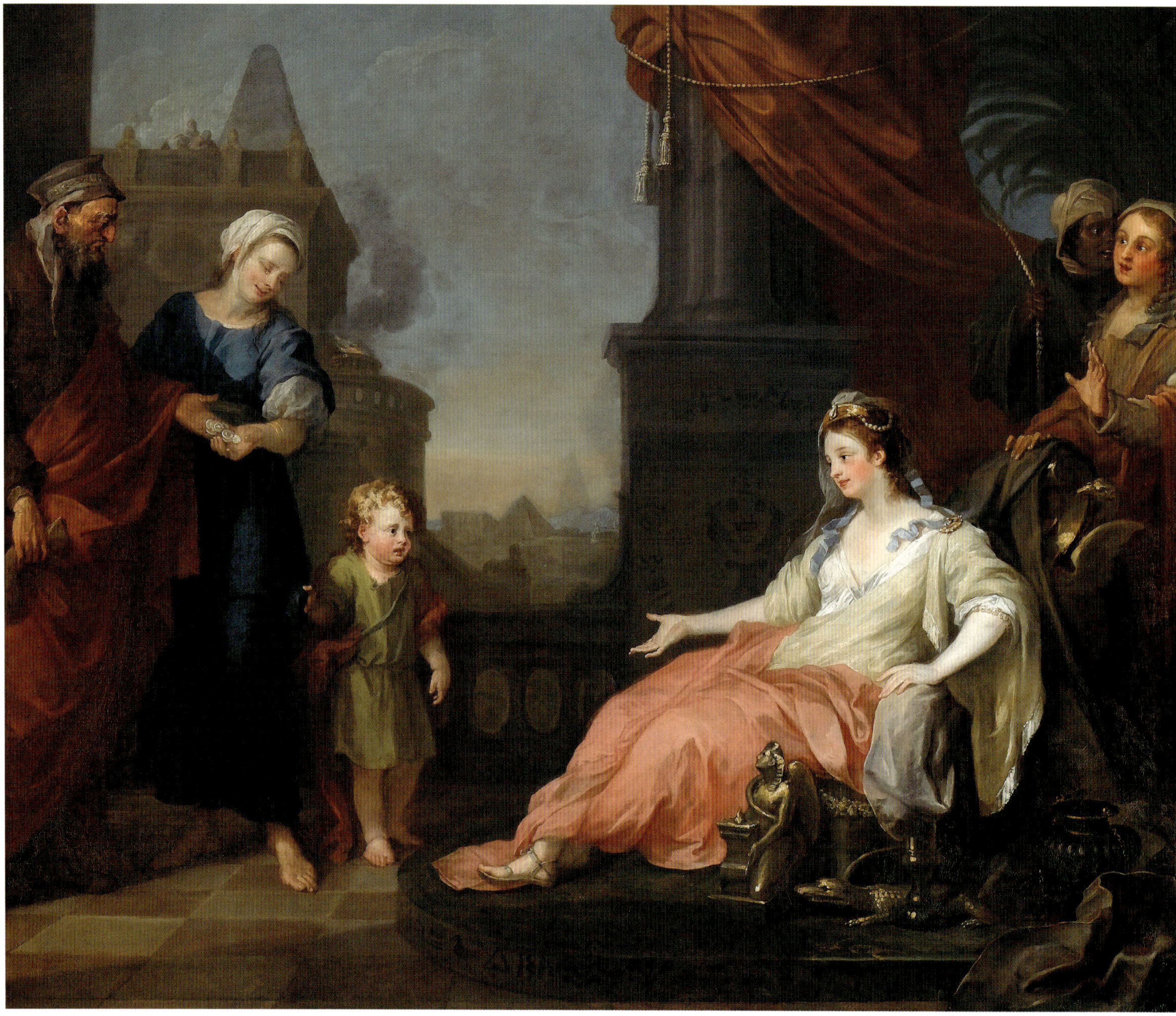

195 William Hogarth, *Moses brought before Pharaoh's Daughter*, 1746, Foundling Museum, London

depicting London's most important hospitals. Framed by delicate plaster scrollwork, they were installed between the big paintings to set the Foundling's aspirations firmly in the context of the city's other great medical institutions. Whether by accident or design, several of them offered fascinating pictorial evidence of works of art already adorning the hospital buildings. Although Gibbons's statue of Charles II cannot be discerned in Edward Haytley's Canaletto-like view of *Chelsea Hospital*, his painting of *Bethlem Hospital* (pl. 196) offers a clear and meticulous prospect of Cibber's colossal figures of the insane, surmounting the entrance gate and looming over the people passing by. Samuel Wale's roundel provides an intriguing view of *Christ's Hospital* founded by Henry VIII as a charity school for poor children, where the frontage is enhanced by prominent frescoes on its uppermost floor and an imposing statue in the niche below. His delicate painting of *Greenwich*

Hospital likewise provides a reminder of the splendour with which Wren and Hawksmoor endowed the home of Thornhill's masterpiece, while the same artist's view of *St Thomas's Hospital* shows Scheemaker's statue of Edward VI reigning over the courtyard of the new building completed in 1732 (pl. 197).

True to his predilections as an artist, Richard Wilson treats his roundels of *Saint George's Hospital* and Jacobsen's newly completed *Foundling Hospital* as landscapes rather than perspective views, thereby revealing how refreshing the buildings' surroundings must have been before the metropolis underwent its dramatic expansion during the Industrial Revolution (pl. 198). Together with the other roundels, Wilson's contributions amounted to an attractive survey of hospital architecture in the mid-eighteenth century. Their creation was doubtless spurred by Hogarth's ever-combative attitude towards foreign competitors, for he would have been pugnaciously aware of the new threat posed by Canaletto's arrival in London in 1746. The hospital views are, of course, far more modest than anything produced by the much-admired Venetian during his British sojourn, and they certainly did not prevent him from obtaining an abundance of covetable commissions; but they look delightful in the Court Room setting, even as they provide a lucid celebration of London's growing commitment to the care of its poor and old.

The most remarkable of all the roundels was donated in 1748 by Gainsborough, a precocious twenty-one year-old who responded to Hogarth's probable invitation[34] by painting a faithful yet strikingly individual view of *The Charterhouse* (pl. 199). If Hogarth's influence can be detected in Gainsborough's reliance on a powerful perspective thrust, as well as the idea of stressing the angle of a building, the young artist still feels at liberty to handle the subject in his own way. The Charterhouse gateway is placed in shadow, leaving Gainsborough free to emphasise the enticing atmosphere of the west walk of the cloister viewed from the Hospital's terrace on a warm and lazy afternoon. *The Charterhouse* is his sole surviving topographical canvas,[35] and he shows a countryman's impatience with the more dutiful aspects of urban view-painting. Ever attentive to the volatility of the English climate, he ensures that the building itself is subservient to the play of light as it animates the edges of leaves among the Dutch-influenced trees, strikes hard against the side of the chapel tower in the distance and plays among the soft clouds moving gently through the summer sky.

Gainsborough reserves the most evocative use of illumination for the path, however. The worn flagstones painted with such tactile sensuousness in the foreground of the roundel are suddenly emblazoned by the great bar of sun-glare flung across path and wall alike. Its richness is seductive enough to attract the two children playing at the edge of

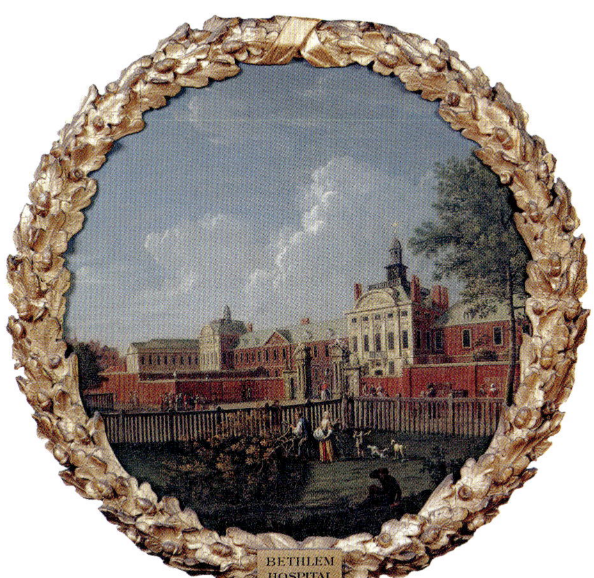

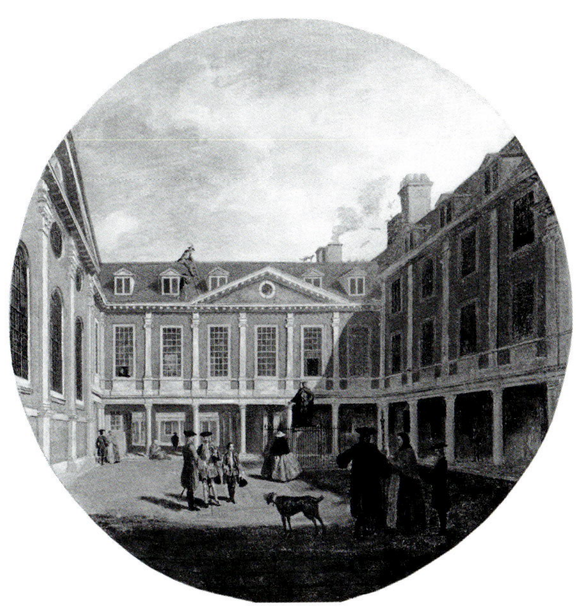

196 (*far left*) Edward Haytley, *Bethlem Hospital*, *c.*1747, Foundling Museum, London

197 (*left*) Samuel Wale, *St Thomas's Hospital*, *c.*1748, Foundling Museum, London

198 (*right*) Richard Wilson, *The Foundling Hospital*, *c.*1747, Foundling Museum, London

199 (*far right*) Thomas Gainsborough, *The Charterhouse*, *c.*1748, Foundling Museum, London

200 (*facing page, top*) Michael Rysbrack, *Charity*, 1745, Indianapolis Museum of Art, Gift of Mrs Albert J. Beveridge

201 (*facing page, bottom*) Michael Rysbrack, *Charity Children Engaged in Navigation and Husbandry*, 1745, Foundling Museum, London

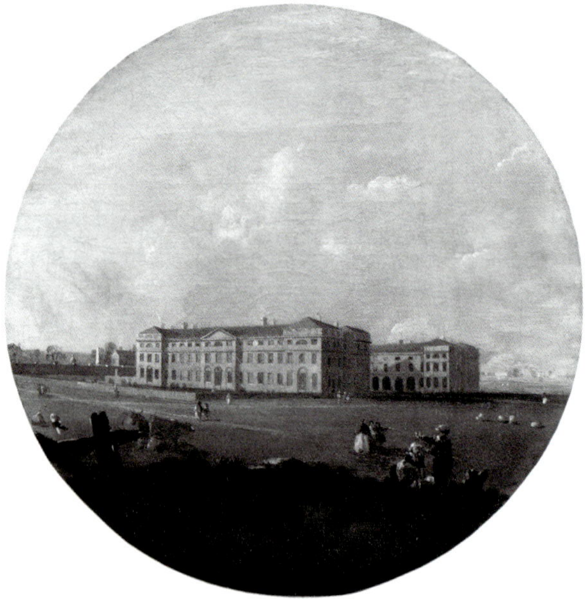

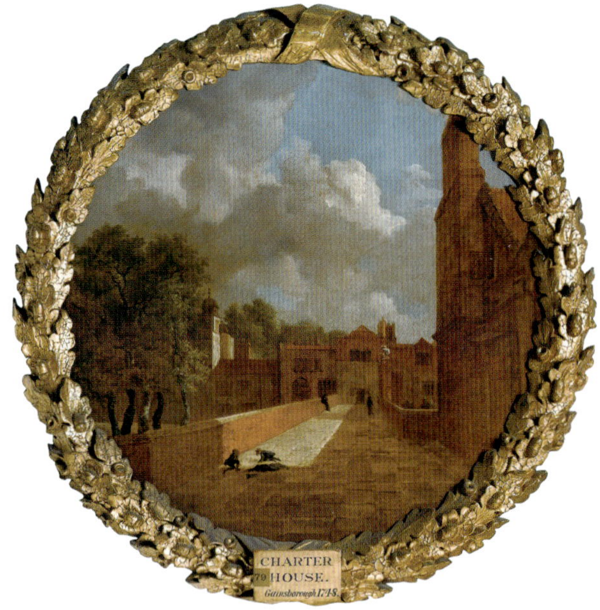

this outspoken lozenge of yellow and gold. Lost in their games, they are still able to revel in the heat it emanates. Further down the path, a silhouetted figure skirts the light while another gives himself up to its embrace and lolls against the wall. For all the roundel's ostensible purpose, as an accurate record of a building founded in 1611 as an educational and religious institution for the poor, it finally becomes a painting about childhood euphoria. Sufficiently young to recall his own boyhood memories of indolent summer holidays in Suffolk, Gainsborough was able to infuse this modest yet mesmerising roundel with the allure of an afternoon when the sun's potency promised to last for ever.

Only one sculpture was presented to the Court Room, but it proved a distinguished carving by Michael Rysbrack well able to enhance the interior. Since he was the first artist after Hogarth to be elected a governor of the Hospital,[36] Rysbrack must have been eager to donate a substantial example of his work. It took the form of a large marble relief over the fireplace, and he dealt with a subject once again close to Coram's heart: *Charity Children engaged in Navigation and Husbandry*. Rysbrack's sympathies were sufficiently stimulated by the theme of nurturing to make him execute a closely related terracotta statuette of Charity herself (pl. 200), a young woman feeding a baby at the breast while another infant tries to jump onto her lap. The whole group is instinct with movement either urgent or playful: the almost imploring eagerness of the little boy who attempts to leap upwards, one leg jutting at an exclamatory angle, is contrasted with the mischievous child round the other side ducking under the woman's protective drapery. Much of this engaging vivacity is carried over into Rysbrack's terracotta model for the mantelpiece. Vertue preferred it to the Foundling marble, although he considered the Court Room carving 'finely finisht and executed' when it was installed there in 1746. 'The Moddel of Clay of the same magnitude is admirably well done', he wrote, pointing out that 'wherein as the Materia is moleable, [it] still permitts the Artist to express his mind more Artfully & with greater freedom than on the laborious or durable marble.'[37]

The final Foundling relief is certainly a more restrained performance, deploying the precepts of classicism to arrange children, woman and animals in a chaste frieze across the entire width of the panel (pl. 201). Rysbrack was so enamoured of the inspiration to be derived from classical precedent that he did not even mind when an accident damaged his carving, for he explained to a patron that 'the Horn is broke . . . of ye Marble Basso Relievo at the Hospital, but it looks the more antique as Doctor Mead said of it'.[38] The infant in the terracotta sucking at Charity's breast now assumes a more discreet position on her arm, while the boy below no longer tugs quite so impetuously on her robes. Calmness prevails, and yet this serenity is entirely in keeping with the subject interpreted by Rysbrack. Nor does it prevent the boys on the left from applying themselves with some earnestness to 'coyling a cord' near a ship's anchor, while their female counterparts busy themselves with what Vertue described as 'huswifery and rural imployments milking the Cows &c'.[39]

Such pursuits accorded with the aims of an institution where many girls received a special apprenticeship for a life in domestic service. Yet the most Coram-like element in the carving is set at a jaunty angle to this harmonious blending of human and animal life. Beyond the tree, a ship's tilting stern can be glimpsed, a prophetic reference to the maritime service where most of the boy foundlings would be sent when they became old enough to leave the Hospital. In his poised and skilful way, Rysbrack implies that the education received by children at the institution was as natural and sustaining as the harvesting, milking and mothering which fills his relief with quiet yet fully absorbed activity.

As a reward for their generosity in donating these remarkable works to the Court Room, all the artists involved were elected governors. In December 1746, when Hogarth and Rysbrack were present, a formal meeting declared that the other painters who had produced canvases for the decorative scheme could now be admitted to the select ranks. They would have regarded their election as an honour and a reward well worth having, for the Royal Academy with its system of providing artists with much-coveted titles did not yet exist. As well as enhancing their social status, the Court Room project gave them a valuable opportunity to display their abilities before a large audience. In April 1747 Vertue recorded that an 'Entertainment, or publick dinner' was held at the Hospital for 'the Governors and other Gentlemen that had inclination – about 170 persons great benefactions then givens towards the hospital'.[40]

So the dividends flowed both ways. While funds were raised for the Foundling's future, the Court Room decorations were admired by an influential public. The Hospital became even more renowned as an enlightened centre for the arts when Handel offered his services. On May Day 1750 *The Messiah* was performed there to mark the dedication of the

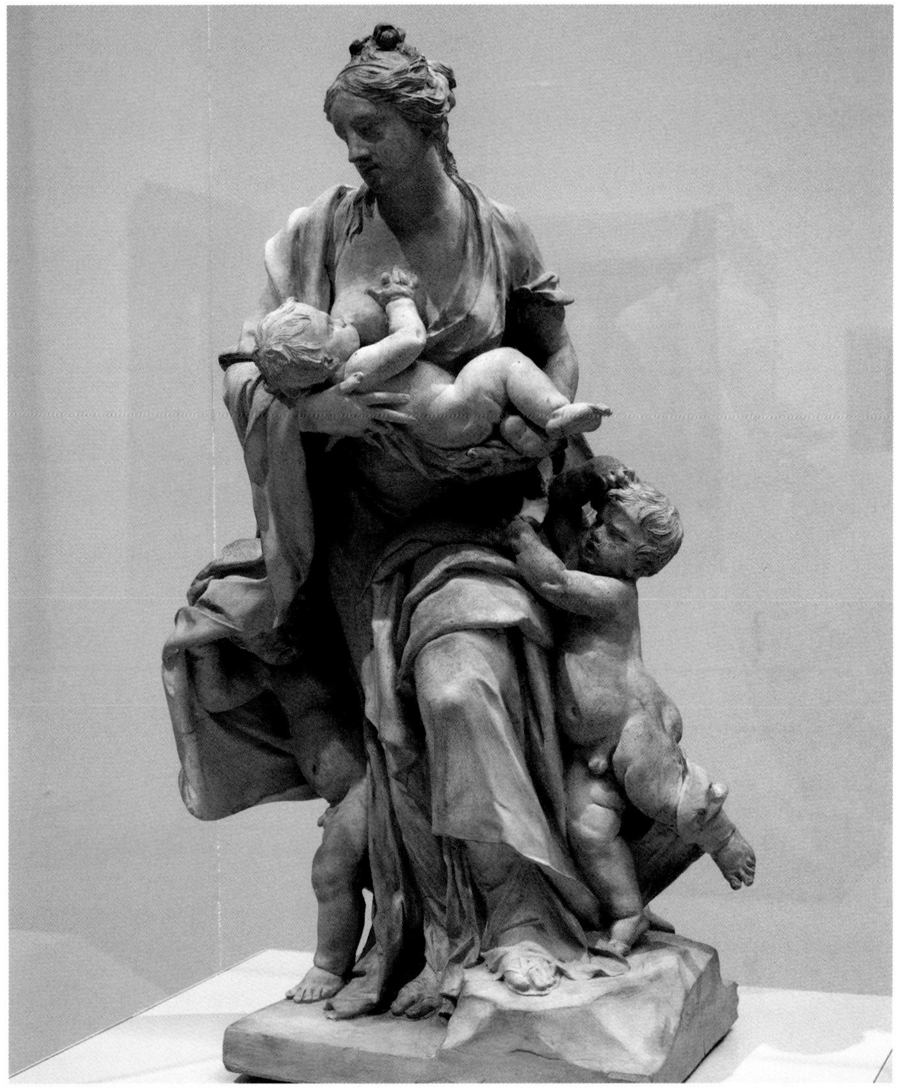

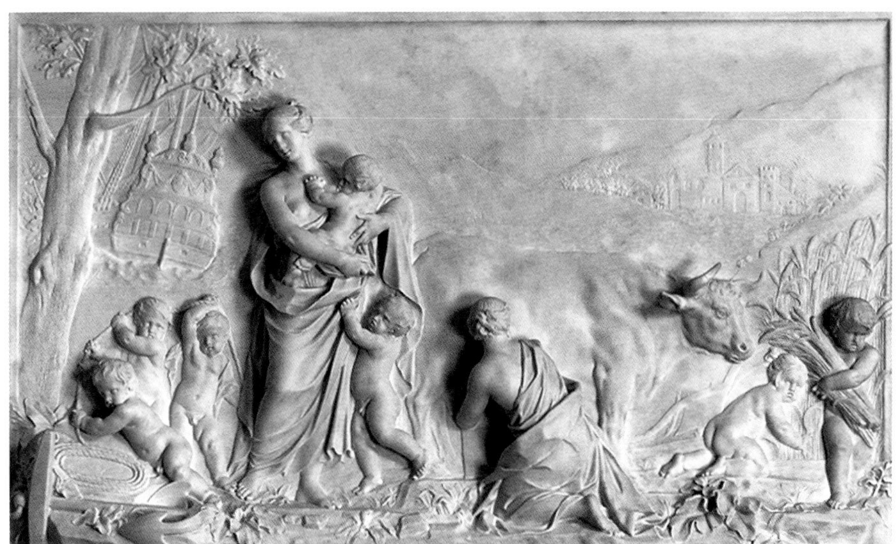

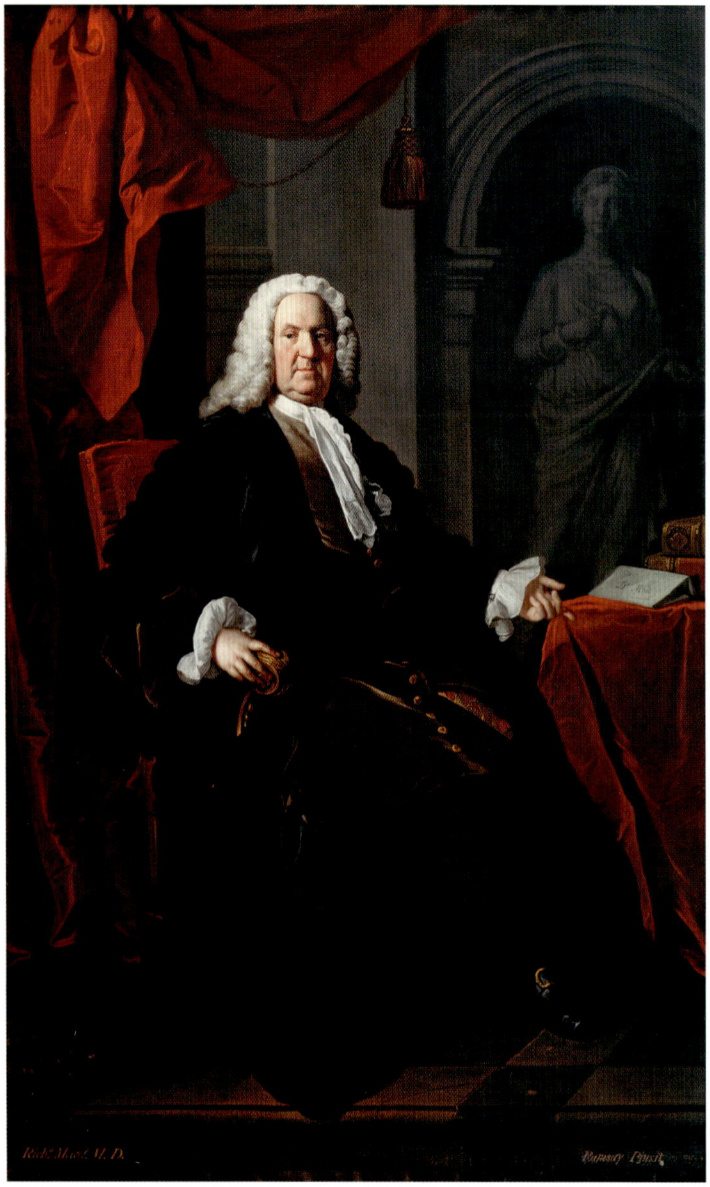

202 Allan Ramsay, *Dr Richard Mead*, 1747, Foundling Museum, London

organ, and Handel went on to enliven the grand formal opening on 16 April 1753 with his *Music for the Royal Fireworks*, selections from the oratorio *Solomon* and other works, among them his specially composed Foundling Hospital anthem, *Blessed are the Poor*. Handel continued to superintend annual performances there for several years, raising enormous sums for the institution. When he died in 1759, the Hospital inherited a fair copy of the score and all parts of the *Messiah*. By then, the Foundling was so esteemed that it had an important effect on the social position occupied by artists in Britain. The painters made a habit of holding annual feasts at the Foundling, generally on Saint Luke's Day, replacing the earlier gathering in taverns. Their works on view in the Court Room helped to convince them that regular exhibitions of contemporary art would be of inestimable value. Hogarth's enterprising experiment at the Hospital thereby paved the way for annual exhibitions at the Society of Arts and, eventually, the establishing of the Royal Academy itself.

At these feasts the cause of Coram's institution was not forgotten. The Hospital's Minute Books reveal that the annual dinner was preceded by a committee meeting 'to consider of what further Ornaments may be added to this Hospital without any expense to the Charity'. Among the early and most remarkable fruits of this continuing commitment was Allan Ramsay's full-length portrait of *Dr Richard Mead* (pl. 202). A leading physician and antiquarian, whose art collection and library were housed in rooms specially designed by James Gibbs,[41] Mead had been among the first members of the medical establishment to support Coram's visionary plan. Ramsay, by then acquiring a substantial reputation as a portraitist in London, did full justice to the doctor's *gravitas*. By instinct more a painter of women than men, he made an exceptional effort with this monumental image. Aware of the need to measure up to the exacting standards set by Hogarth's *Coram* seven years before (see pl. 190), and determined no doubt to produce a more profound interpretation of character than Hudson had managed with his portrait of Jacobsen (see pl. 191), Ramsay surpassed himself in the Mead portrait.

The learned doctor inhabits his seat with a more weighty assurance than Coram. Nor is there any suggestion that Mead is about to leave his chair, for he occupies it as securely as the antique statue inhabits her ample niche behind him. Gesturing with innate authority towards a document on the nearby table, he gazes out from the canvas like a man well used to commanding the respect of his profession. Even so, there is nothing unduly pompous about this imperturbable figure. If Ramsay had yet to master the tenderness and subtle delicacy that he would develop after his second visit to Italy in the mid-1750s, the masculinity of his earlier style suits Mead admirably. The doctor's jowelled face is constructed with forceful assurance. Ramsay's grasp of large pictorial masses, which

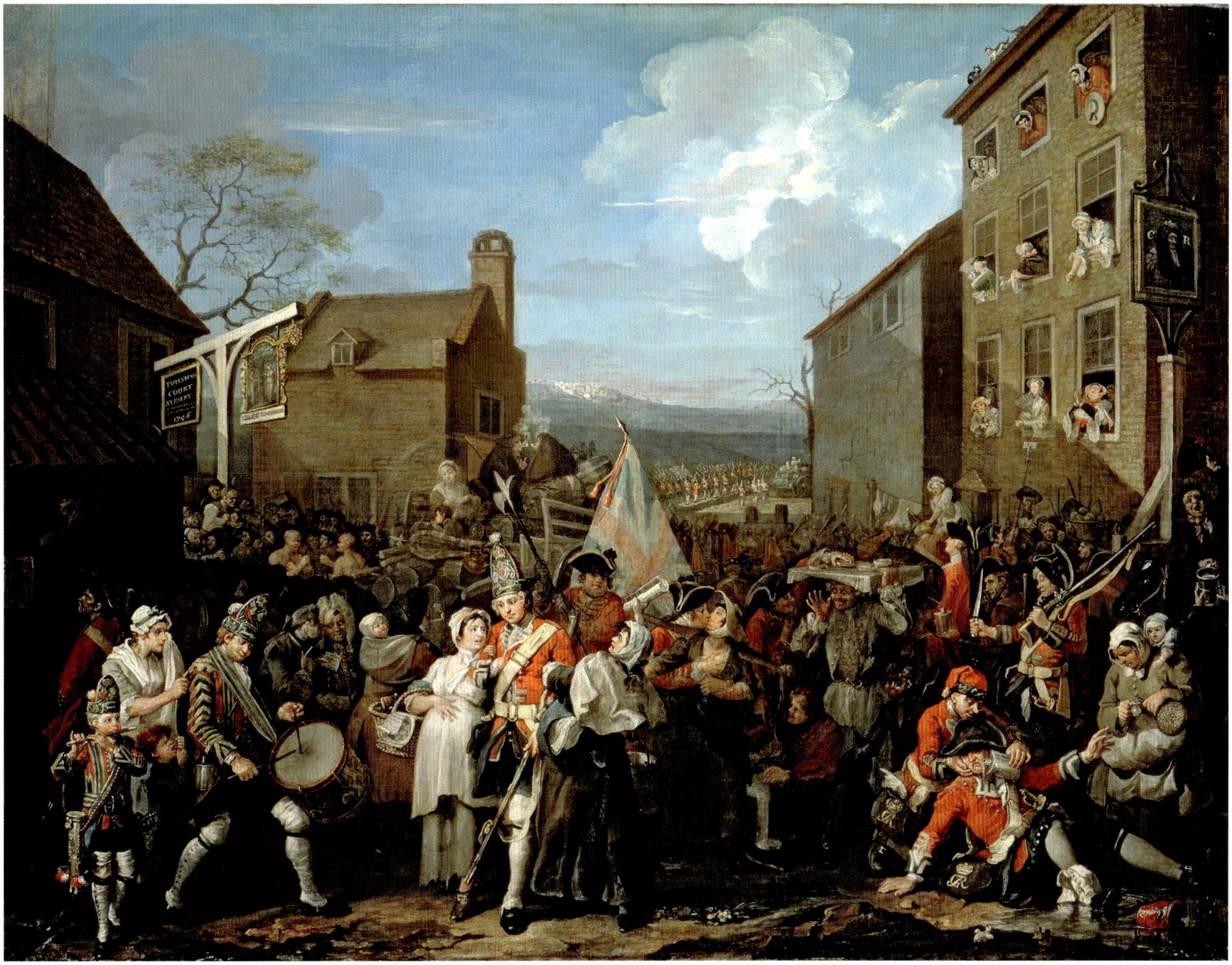

203 William Hogarth, *The March to Finchley*, 1749–50, Foundling Museum, London

anticipates Reynolds's later pursuit of the grand manner in portraiture, does not prevent him from paying proper attention to the psychological complexity of his sitter. Unlike some of the picture's subordinate areas, where a drapery painter helped him[42] with the execution, the features are handled in an incisive and vigorous manner. Ramsay's fondness for preliminary modelling in deep red, which gives the face's shadows a vermilion vitality, helps to prevent Mead's countenance from becoming somnolent. The wart beside the doctor's right nostril is not forgotten, and neither are the frown-marks creasing the skin between his redoubtable eyebrows.

This is a man who might well be capable of an intimidating anger, and yet Ramsay also succeeds in suggesting the level-headed sanity of a practitioner who had opposed the contemporary notion that plague was caused by 'a corruption of the air'.[43] Mead sensibly proposed that, while 'a corrupted State of Air is without doubt necessary to give these Contagious Atoms their full Force', it was evident 'that *Infection* is not received from the Air itself, however predisposed, without the Concurrence of something emitted from Infected Persons'.[44] Arguments as sound as this earned Mead respect throughout Europe. When Watteau came to

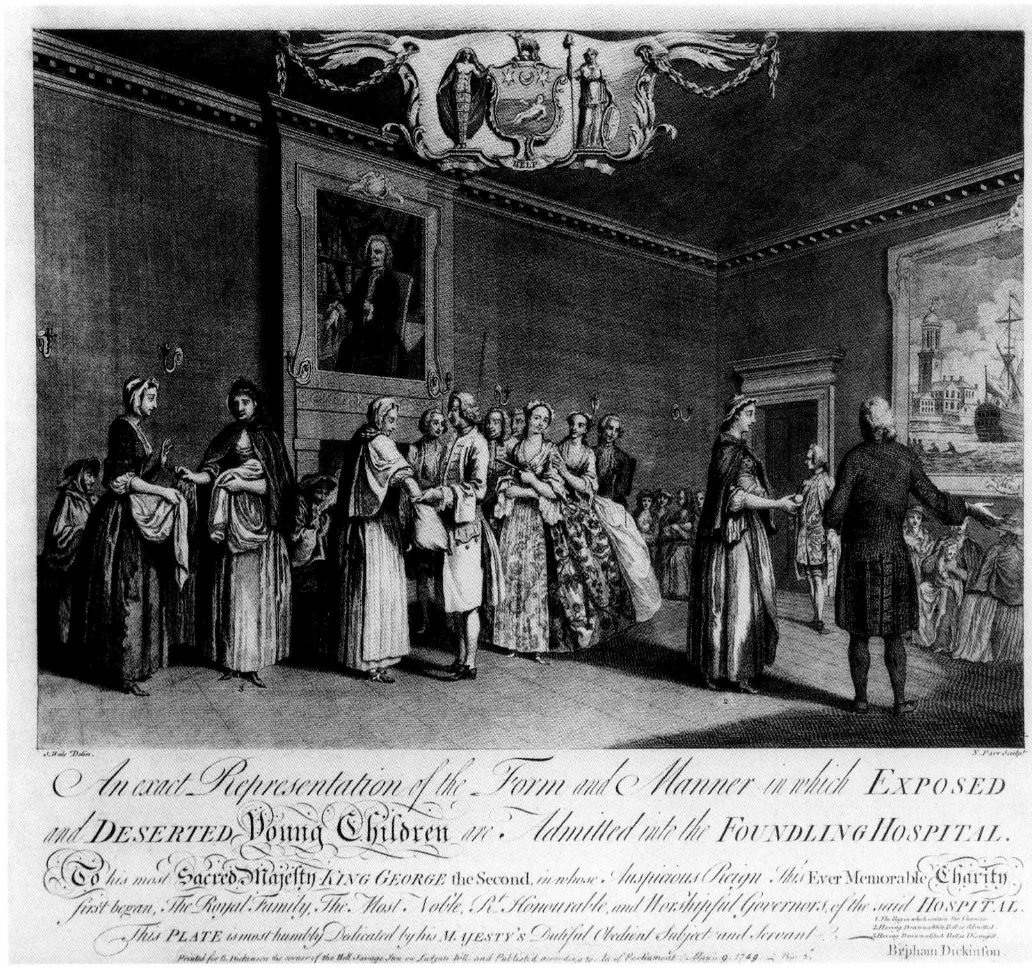
An exact Representation of the Form and Manner in which EXPOSED
and DESERTED Young Children are Admitted into the FOUNDLING HOSPITAL.
To his most Sacred Majesty KING GEORGE the Second, in whose Auspicious Reign this Ever Memorable Charity
first began, The Royal Family, The Most Noble, Rt Honourable, and Worshipful Governors of the said HOSPITAL.
This PLATE is most humbly Dedicated by his MAJESTY's Dutiful Obedient Subject and Servant
HELP

204 After Samuel Wale, *Admission of Foundlings*, engraving by N. Parr, published 9 May 1749, Foundling Museum, London

London in 1719, he met Mead and probably sought treatment for tuberculosis. Watteau painted two pictures for Mead, a discerning collector whose sensibility is well-defined in the Foundling portrait. Here, Ramsay defined the very pulse of the doctor's intellect in a painting that wholly fulfilled Jonathan Richardson's call for the portraitist to 'understand mankind, and enter into their characters, and express their minds as well as their faces'.[45]

The Foundling collection did not stop with Ramsay's presentation of the Mead portrait. In 1750, it received an unexpected windfall. Hogarth decided to dispose of his Rabelaisian painting *The March to Finchley* by offering it as a prize in a lottery of two thousand tickets, each of which was distributed with a subscription for the engraved version of the picture (pl. 203). Having originally intended to dedicate the picture to George II, he was incensed by the king's disapproval of the rumbustious canvas. The monarch's reaction was predictable. For Hogarth shows some of the English guards, in a dissolute and tipsy state, staggering off to join orderly troops defending London against the forces of the Young Pretender. The satire was so bawdy and literally unbuttoned that it prompted George II to utter the celebrated cry: 'I hate bainting and boetry too. Does the fellow mean to laugh at my guards?'[46] Hogarth took his revenge by dedicating the print to the King of Prussia, an encourager of the arts and sciences. He also gave the unsold 157 lottery tickets to the Foundling and the winning number ensured that the Hospital acquired this splendidly irreverent example of Hogarth's work.

Beyond the Court Room, paintings occupy prominent positions on the walls in Samuel Wale's print of 1749 (pl. 204) where the poignant admission of foundlings is taking place within the Hospital. Like Hogarth's picture, the children were chosen by lottery and their mothers are accompa-

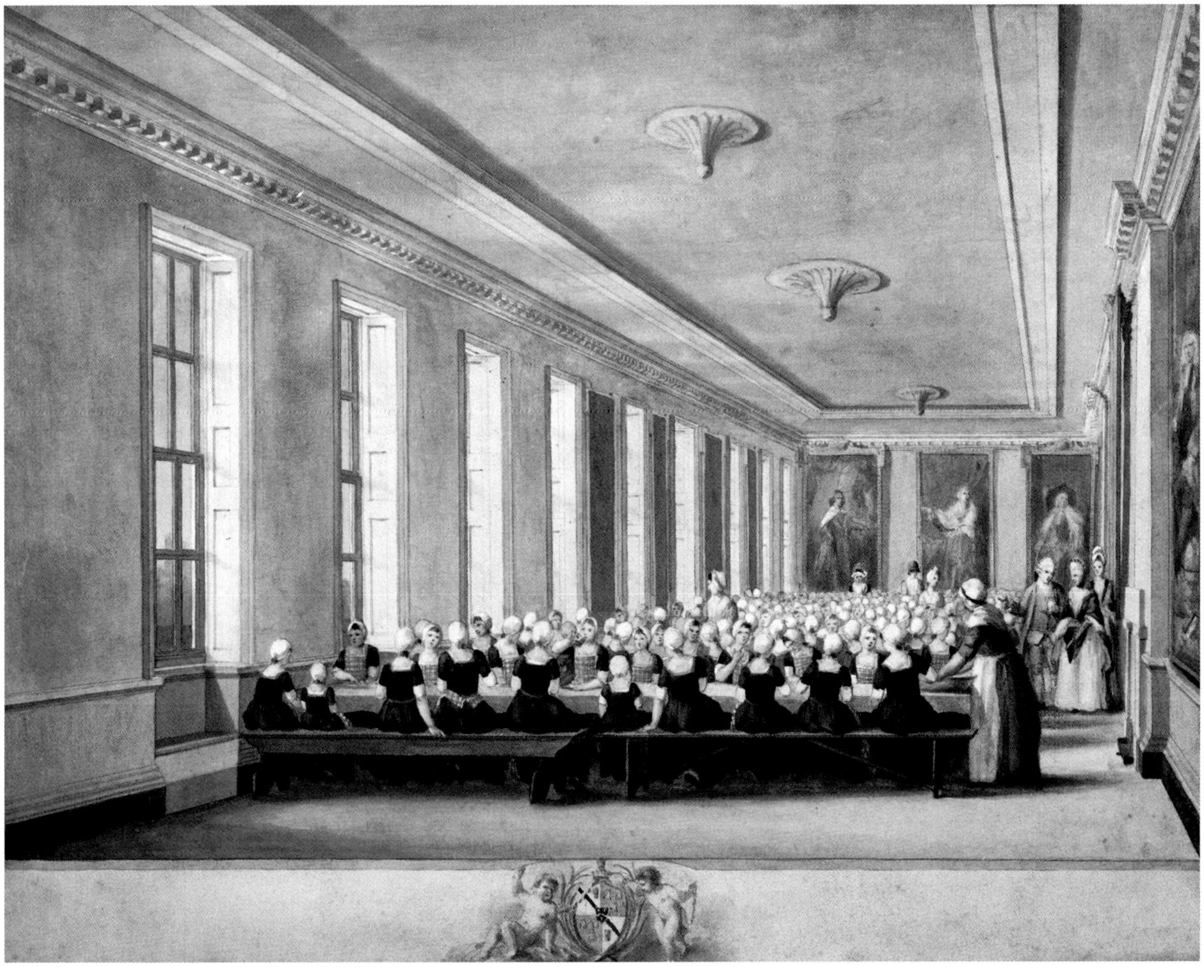

205 John Sanders, *The Girls' Dining Room at the Foundling Hospital*, 1773, Foundling Museum, London

nied by several petitioning ladies as well as representatives of the governors. The place where the *March to Finchley* hung is unrecorded, but just as Coram would have wished, many of the boys went on to become sailors and their Dining Room at the Hospital was dominated by an enormous canvas by Charles Brooking. He donated *A Flagship before the Wind and Other Vessels* to the Foundling in 1754, possibly after some prompting by his barrister patron Taylor White who served as the Hospital's Treasurer for twenty-seven years. It is the grandest and most elaborate work by the finest British marine painter of the period and, along with its lost companion piece by Peter Monamy, would have given the boys assembled for their meals an enticing vision of maritime existence.

The Foundling's collection was not confined to all-male areas of the building. John Sanders's watercolour, executed with a diligence matching the disciplined behaviour he depicts, proves that the Girls' Dining Room was lined with the Hospital's full-length portraits (pl. 205). While the neatly uniformed foundlings sit at their long refectory tables, supervised by staff and gazed at by wealthy visitors contemplating a donation, Hogarth's great *Coram* canvas can be seen presiding over them from the wall on the right. The children may not have been granted many opportunities to look at the paintings in the Court Room, but they could see this superb likeness of their founder casting a genial gaze over the orderly, protected life he had done so much to bestow on them.

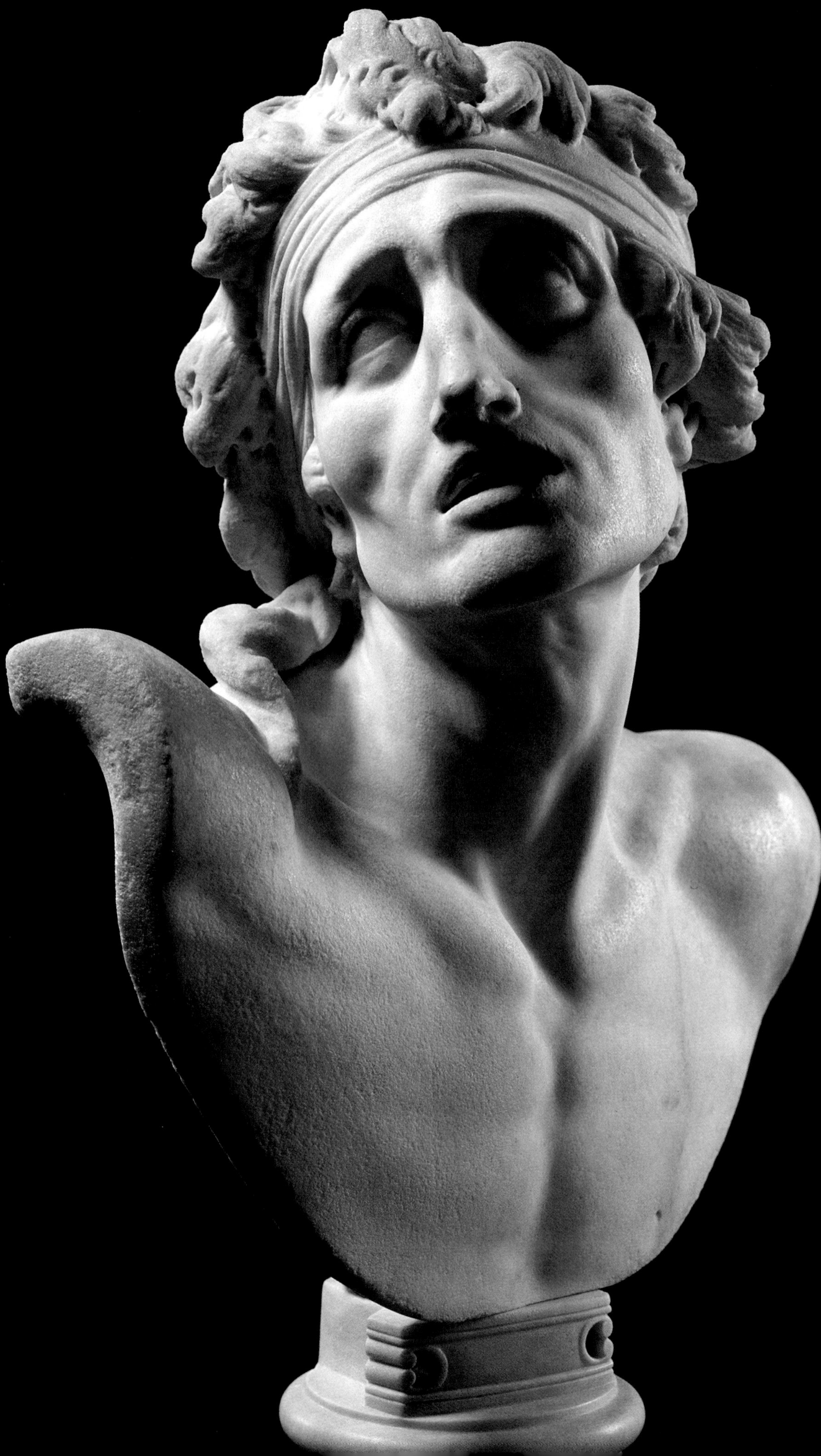

FIFTEEN
BENEFACTORS, DOCTORS AND QUACKS

As the building of new British hospitals proceeded apace, a fashion grew for acquiring portraits of the philanthropists who founded them. In London alone, no fewer than five hospitals were established between 1720 and 1745: Guy's, Westminster, the London, St George's and the Middlesex. The portraits they commissioned were, however, preceded at least two decades earlier by a full-length marble statue of Sir Robert Clayton, executed for St Thomas's by Grinling Gibbons (pl. 208). A former Lord Mayor and staunch Whig politician, Clayton became President of the Hospital in 1692 and spent the next fifteen years keeping its finances in order. He also gave a substantial amount of his wealth for the erection of a new wing, Clayton Court. One of St Thomas's historians has confessed that 'Sir Robert does not appeal to me very much. I like neither his face nor his record.'[1] But the all-powerful Board of Governors respected him enough to present Clayton's statue to the Hospital six years before his death. A sub-committee was established for the purpose, and in June 1701 it reported that the members

> had agreed with Mr. Grinling Gibbons to cutt the said Statue in the best Statue Marble and to set the same up in the Middle of the lower Quadrangle of this Hosp'll upon a Pedestall of the same Sort of Marble by Christmas next, For which he is to have £50 in hand – and £150 more as soon as the Work is finished.[2]

Gibbons had previously executed a gilded[3] statue of Charles II, arranged and posed in an imperial Roman manner, which still stands glistening in the Figure Court of Chelsea Royal Hospital (see pl. 164). It possesses a formidable dignity, and St Thomas's doubtless hoped that the same sculptor would perform a comparable act of ennoblement for this new Clayton commission. Gibbons did not disappoint them. The outcome was an imposing effigy in mayoral robes displaying the profusely bewigged Sir Robert, parchment scroll in hand, as a lofty dispenser of 'bountiful' benefaction. A fulsome testimony on the pedestal, which bears cherubs holding a coat of arms, testifies to his generosity and declares that the statue was erected to 'preserve his Memory after Death'. One of only four known works by Gibbons in marble, it lacks the lightness and virtuosity of his finest wood carvings. But the Clayton statue remains a formidable personification of the philanthropy which, spurred on by the burgeoning preoccupation with scientific enquiry in general, invested much munificence in the building of hospitals.

For more than a hundred and fifty years Gibbons's statue stood undamaged behind protective railings in the third square of St Thomas's,

206 (*facing page*) John Bacon the Elder, *Sickness*, 1778, Royal Academy, London

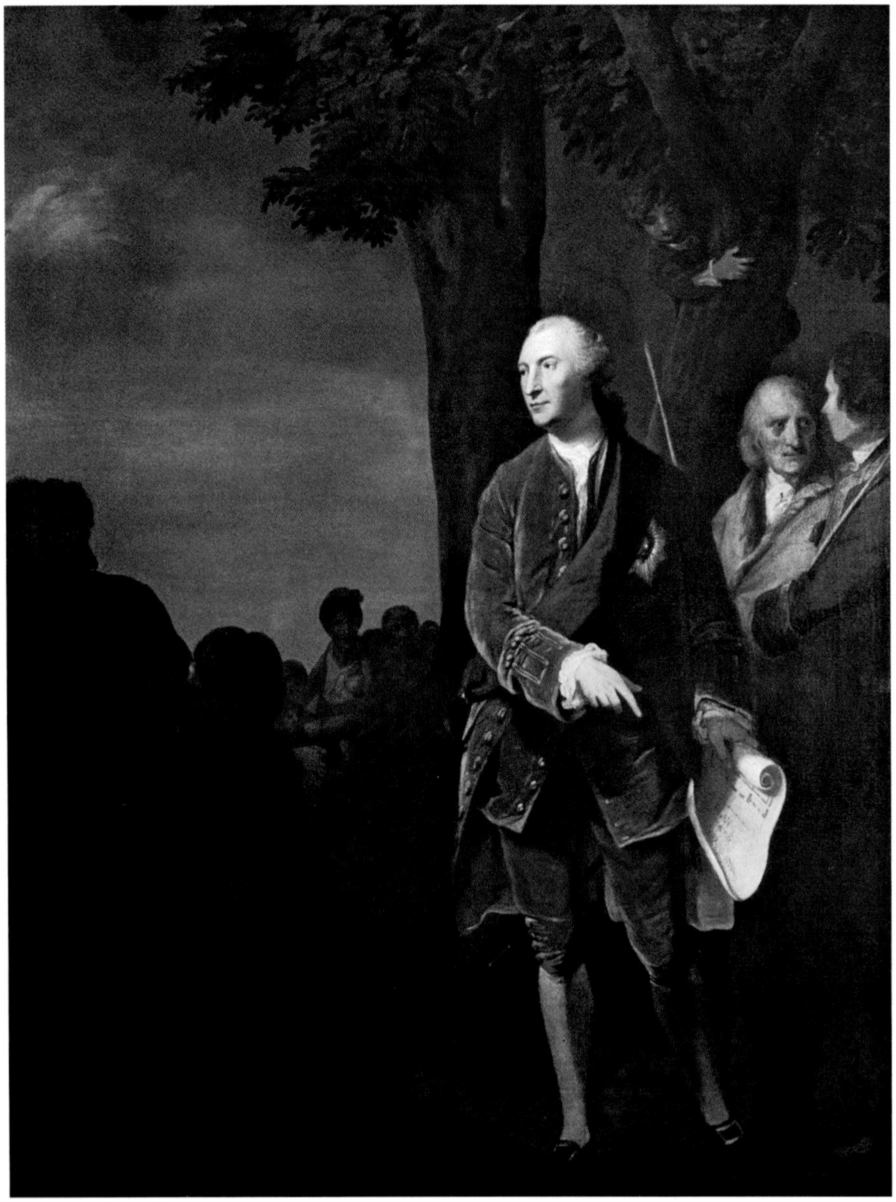

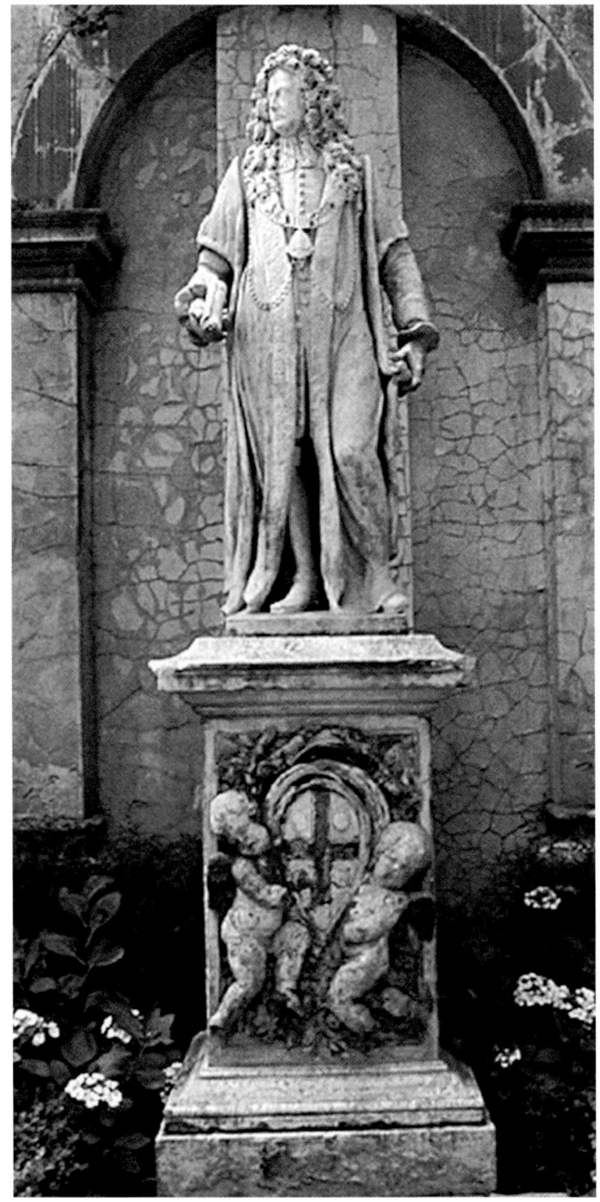

207 (*above left*) Robert Edge Pine, *Hugh Percy, Earl [later First Duke] of Northumberland*, 1768, UCLH NHS Foundation Trust

208 (*above right*) Grinling Gibbons, *Sir Robert Clayton*, 1702, St Thomas's Hospital, London

which became known as Clayton Square. Yet the clause in his will directing that the figure be preserved from any 'Spoyle or hurt save only by time' did not shield it after the Hospital moved to Surrey Gardens in 1864. As a temporary measure, the sculpture was unwisely installed next to a tavern frequented by medical students, one of whom decided after a convivial evening to climb Sir Robert as a dare. Clayton's right hand broke off, and about sixty years later a similar incident led to the severing of his other hand. Happily they were both restored, so Gibbons's statue continued to stand at St Thomas's as a distinguished precursor of the portraits commissioned by younger London hospitals for their walls.

In 1761 Middlesex Hospital invited Robert Edge Pine to execute the most grandiloquent of all these benefactor images: Hugh, the First Duke of Northumberland, laying the building's foundation stone in 1755 (pl. 207). Secure in the conviction that he was the handsomest man in the country, the Duke adopts a self-consciously statuesque pose while pointing to the plan of the Hospital building clasped in his other hand. He does not demean himself with the business of manhandling the stone, a task left to an anonymous assistant in a shadowy area of the foreground. But the artist, who presented the canvas to the Middlesex in 1768, shows more interest in the white-haired man behind the posturing Duke. The most lively passage in the portrait is reserved for the boy looking down mischievously at the whole pompous ceremony from the safety of a tree.

By this time St Thomas's, not to be outdone, had used a bequest of 500 guineas from its treasurer to commission from Peter Scheemakers another effigy of Edward VI, doubtless to stress the Hospital's regal origins (see pl. 197). The result, a more imposing image than Cartwright's earlier modest carving for the same hospital, was placed in the second or administrative court of the building, thenceforth known as Edward Square. Here Scheemakers breaks away from his previous, confining dependence on classical precedent in the handling of draperies. Although he bases the head and garments on a painting of Edward attributed to Holbein,[4] Scheemakers shows great confidence in composing arm gestures redolent of calm, relaxed authority. Edward's left hand rests confidently on his hip, while the great curving folds of his cloak proclaim a new spirit of independence on the sculptor's part. No wonder George Vertue declared that 'the attitude of the Statue and graceful disposition of the limbs is judiciously done and merits great applause'.[5]

Even so, the most original portrait of a London hospital benefactor is the *Monument to Thomas Guy*, carved in pictorial relief by John Bacon in 1779 (pl. 209). Here the founder is seen, not isolated and remote on a plinth like Scheemakers's earlier statue of Guy, but gravely involved with the plight of a haggard man who needs help. Far from being absorbed in contemplating his own fame, Guy stares down at the ailing figure and grasps his right wrist. The two men, one elaborately attired and the other semi-naked, gaze at each other. Guy smiles at the anguished man, whose draperies swirl dramatically around his back as if in response to the assistance he is receiving. Although on the edge of emaciation, he attempts to push his right leg against the jutting ledge. He wants to get up, and in this respect the deeply religious Bacon must have wanted his sculpture to stir memories of Christ's miraculous action at the Pool of Bethesda (see pls 133 and 186). However, the building behind is a hospital courtyard and Guy points towards its portico confident in the knowledge that medical assistance will always be available there. Beneath his hand, two orderlies can be seen carrying another man into the building on a stretcher. So even if Guy's life-sized effigy dominates, the plight of patients is the true subject of this impressive relief. Bacon felt sufficiently satisfied with *Sickness*, (see pl. 206) a powerful marble study for the seated figure's anguished head,[6] that he donated it to the Royal Academy as his Diploma work in 1778.

Within the hospitals, however, disappointingly little thought was given to embellishment of any kind. A revealing 'prospect of one of the wards' at

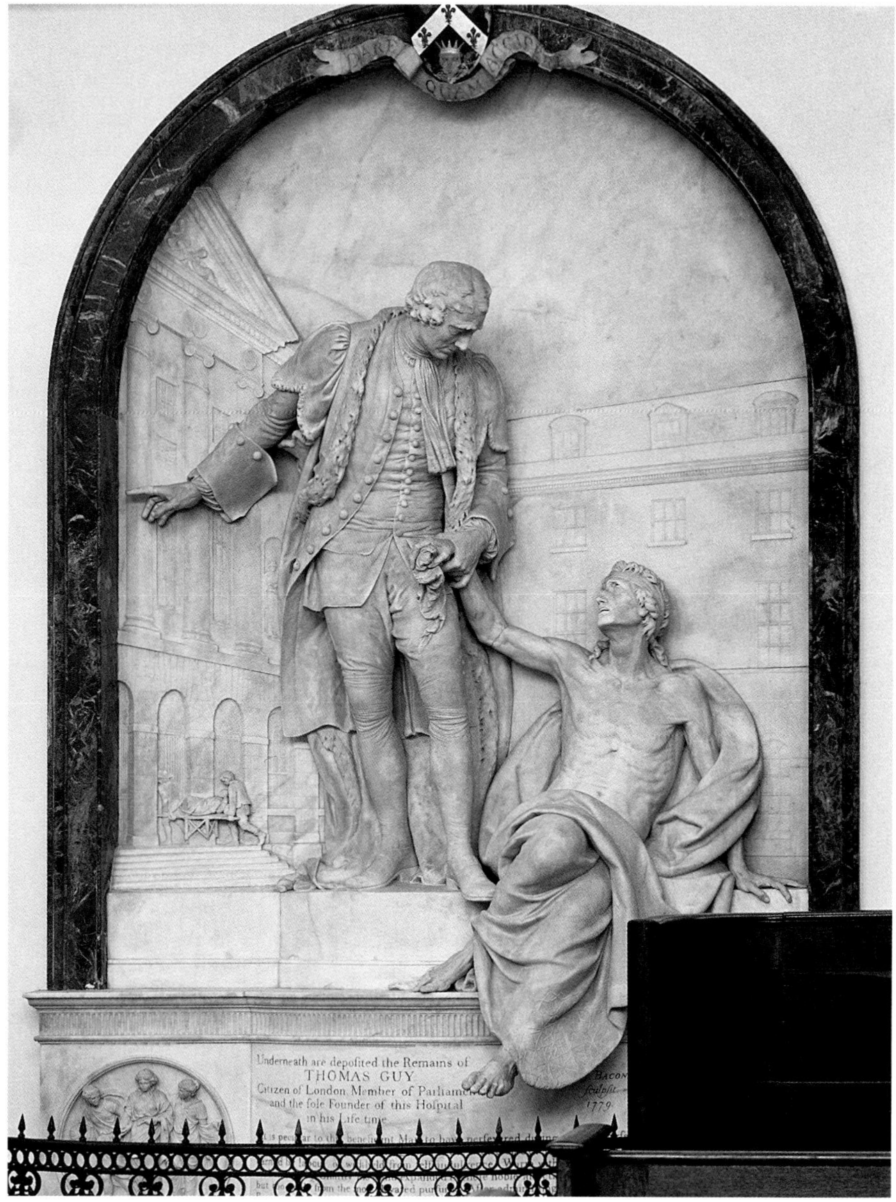

209 John Bacon the Elder, Monument to Thomas Guy, 1779, Guy's Hospital, London

Guy's, produced in the year when the building opened, testifies to their spartan bleakness. Nothing is displayed on the walls to alleviate the rectilinear bareness of the patients' cubicles and the stark, forbidding character of the room helps to explain why wealthy citizens still preferred to be nursed at home. The exteriors of the new London hospitals may have been lavish but the level of medical achievement inside was still rudimentary. Their charitable status reflected the fact that they were regarded as the preserve of the poor and, except for smallpox inoculation, disappointingly few major discoveries furthered medical expertise during this period. 'Operations were performed without the benefit of antiseptics or anaesthetics, frequently by trainee surgeons', wrote Celina Fox, pointing out that

> nurses were untrained and badly paid. Hospitals even discouraged the admission of chronic or highly infectious cases, for which nothing could be done. It is no accident that Hogarth's moral cycles are littered with Londoners going about their lives bearing the marks of disease; those suffering from the effects of sexual, alcoholic or gastronomic excess remained at large. The concept of personal and public hygiene barely existed.[7]

Even when operations were carried out in the relative safety of a doctor's surgery, they usually turned out to be acutely painful affairs. In Antwerp, Joseph Horemans the Elder painted just such an event, diligently depicting the range of surgical and pharmaceutical equipment stacked on the neat shelves of the surgeon's house. Despite the plentiful evidence of order and expertise, nothing can prevent the patient from suffering. Supervised by the white-wigged surgeon, his younger apprentice makes an incision in the unfortunate man's side. Blood spurts freely onto his shirt and he cries out in an agony unrelieved by any of the analgesics we take for granted today. As if in sympathy with his suffering, the seated woman who may be his wife or mother turns away from the spectacle, her mouth likewise open in protest. Even the dog starts and swings his head, alarmed by the sounds of distress echoing through the room.

As one might expect, Hogarth took an eagerly satirical view of the medical profession. He made merciless comic capital out of the fatuous surgeons and physicians who believed an illiterate woman called Mrs Tofts when she claimed to have given birth to seventeen rabbits. Soon afterwards, he portrayed two notorious quacks, Dr Misaubon and Dr Rock, squabbling over the effectiveness of their rival remedies for venereal disease while the patient herself expires in utter wretchedness.

Just over a decade later he was even more indignant, giving savage vent to his disgust in a drawing of an operation scene (pl. 210). Situated in the 'cutting room' of a hospital,[8] it dramatises the full horror of a leg cauterisation in progress. Once again the physician is seen staring at a urine bottle rather than offering any support or sympathy to his charge. He may even be as inebriated as the servant who has collapsed on the floor in front of him. Taking his inspiration from an incident that supposedly occurred at Queen Caroline's deathbed,[9] Hogarth shows the semi-conscious woman letting her candle ignite the doctor's full-curled wig. The same accident would reappear, more than a decade afterwards, in Laurence Sterne's *Tristram Shandy*, but Hogarth ensures that it seems paltry when set beside the agony of the heavily bandaged patient. For the surgeon, dressed in over-sleeves to prevent blood and pus spattering his frock coat, has pulled the wounded leg out of the sheet and applied a burning cauteriser. Steam rises from the scorched flesh, so the patient's suffering must be intense, but no one bothers to extend a comforting hand. The surgeon's assistant is lost in contemplation of his implements and he thrusts an elegantly stockinged leg forward with posturing vanity.

210 William Hogarth, *Operation Scene*, c.1745, Pierpoint Morgan Library Department of Drawings and Prints

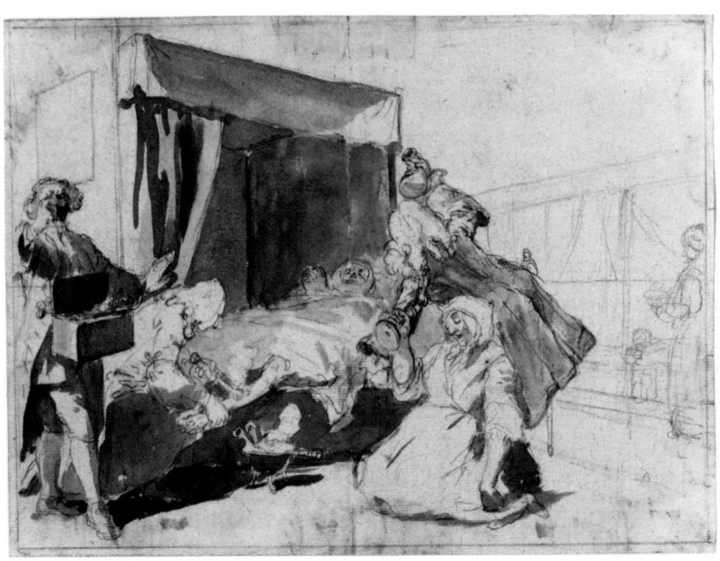

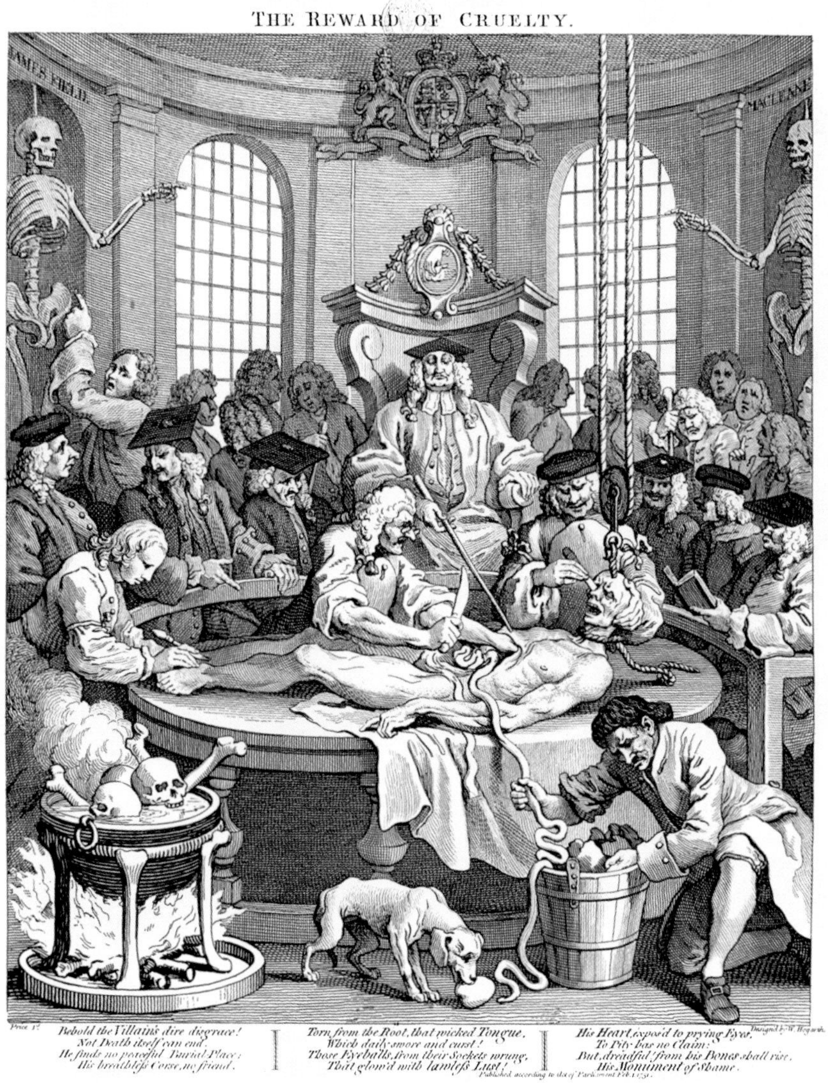
THE REWARD OF CRUELTY.
Behold the Villain's dire disgrace!
Not Death itself can end.
He finds no peaceful Burial Place;
His breathless Corse, no friend.
Torn from the Root, that wicked Tongue,
Which daily swore and curst!
Those Eyeballs, from their Sockets wrung,
That glow'd with lawless Lust!
His Heart, expos'd to prying Eyes,
To Pity has no Claim:
But, dreadful! from his Bones shall rise,
His Monument of Shame.

211 William Hogarth, *The Reward of Cruelty*, plate IV from *The Four Stages of Cruelty*, 1751, Guildhall Library and Art Gallery, London

Hogarth's contempt for medical practices reached its powerful zenith a few years later with the publication of *The Four Stages of Cruelty*. He set the last and most excoriating of these images in an operating theatre, where the corpse of sadistic Tom Nero receives its gruesome comeuppance at the surgeon's hands (pl. 211). Presided over by the callous indifference of physicians observing the proceedings, Nero's body is subjected to the most humiliating dissection imaginable. While a young assistant makes incisions in his feet and another butcher-like figure gouges his eye socket, the grotesquely haggard senior surgeon carves into his bowels, pulling out an extended length of intestine that trails down ignominiously into a bucket. The carelessness of the man assigned to the cleaning up of Nero's waste means that a dog is permitted to gnaw at his remains. Hogarth saw this ultimate degradation as a suitable fate for a man who had been guilty of terrible cruelty against animals. He came to believe that the publication of *The Four Stages of Cruelty* had 'checked the diabolical spirit of barbarity, which, I am sorry to say was once so prevalent in this country'.[10] The final print in this outspoken sequence could also be regarded as an assault on the cold-blooded brutality and indifference of the surgeons. They were widely held to have deprived the criminals whose bodies they dissected of decent religious burials, not to mention the chance of life after death. Public disapproval also centred on the ruthless opportunism of body-snatchers, who capitalised on the growing demand

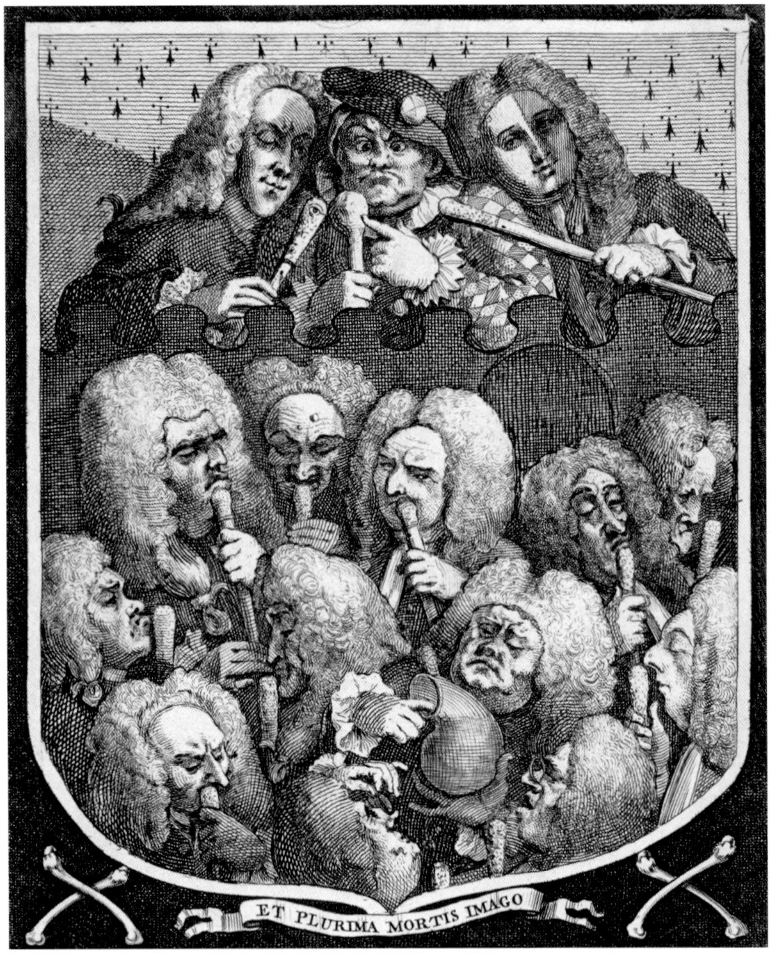

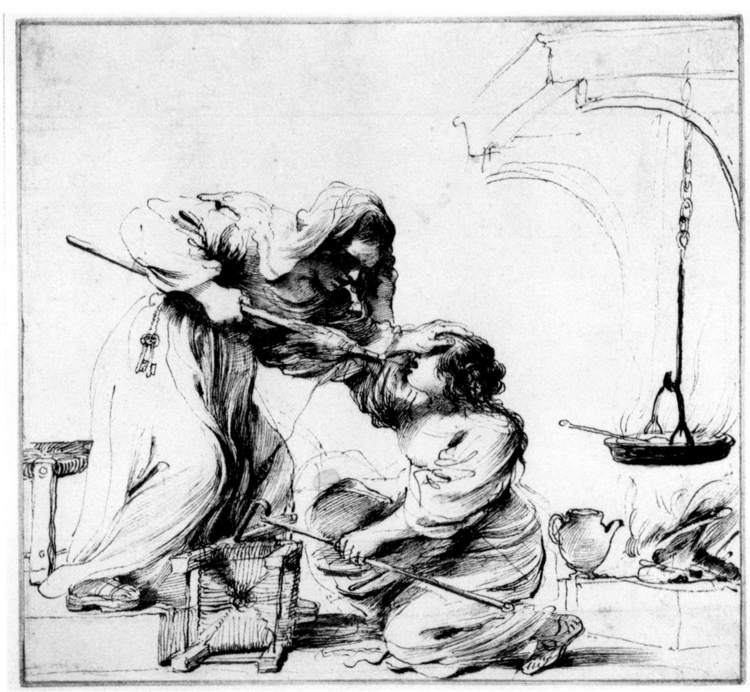

for corpses among a medical profession eager to augment the number of bodies officially allowed for the performing of anatomies. *The Reward of Cruelty* suggests that Hogarth shared this general antipathy towards the ghoulish activities of surgical practitioners.

In view of his strongly expressed condemnation, it may seem inconsistent of Hogarth to devote so much energy to carrying out extensive paintings for major London hospitals, at Bart's and then the Foundling institution (see pls 186–7, 190–95). But the undoubted sincerity of Hogarth's involvement with Bart's did not prevent him from issuing, in the same year that he completed the staircase decorations, another unfettered assault on the dignity of physicians. This time it was a print called *The Company of Undertakers*, pithily advertised as 'Quacks in Consultation' (pl. 212). Here the medical profession is mocked for pomposity, addiction to cane heads, donnish secrecy and a fetishistic preoccupation with periwigs. Surrounded by emblems of death, the conspiratorial grotesques filling most of the composition with their gargoyle-like features are surmounted by a trio of notorious charlatans. Mrs Mapp, the cross-eyed bone-setter, is sandwiched between John Taylor the oculist, dubbed by Dr Johnson as 'an instance how far impudence would carry ignorance', and a pill-pusher called Joshua 'Spot' Ward, whom Hogarth had already pilloried in the death scene of the *Harlot's Progress*.[11] His scorn for such dangerous imposters knew no bounds, and yet his condemnation was rooted in precise observation. One eighteenth-century writer insisted that 'the physicians in Hogarth's prints are not caricatures. The full dress with the sword and great tye-wig, and the hat under the arm, and the doctors in consultation, each smelling to a gold-headed cane . . . are pictures of real life in his time'.[12]

By the early 1740s, Hogarth's commitment to the Foundling Hospital did not lessen the venom in his depiction of the medical profession's more disreputable members. The third canvas in his masterpiece of 'comic history-painting', *Marriage à la Mode*, deals with a visit to the quack doctor (pl. 214). It is a gruesome indictment of dubious curative practices. Brought by her ruthless aristocratic lover to the quack's broken-down room, a frightened young girl hopes to find a remedy for the venereal disease which the viscount has given her.

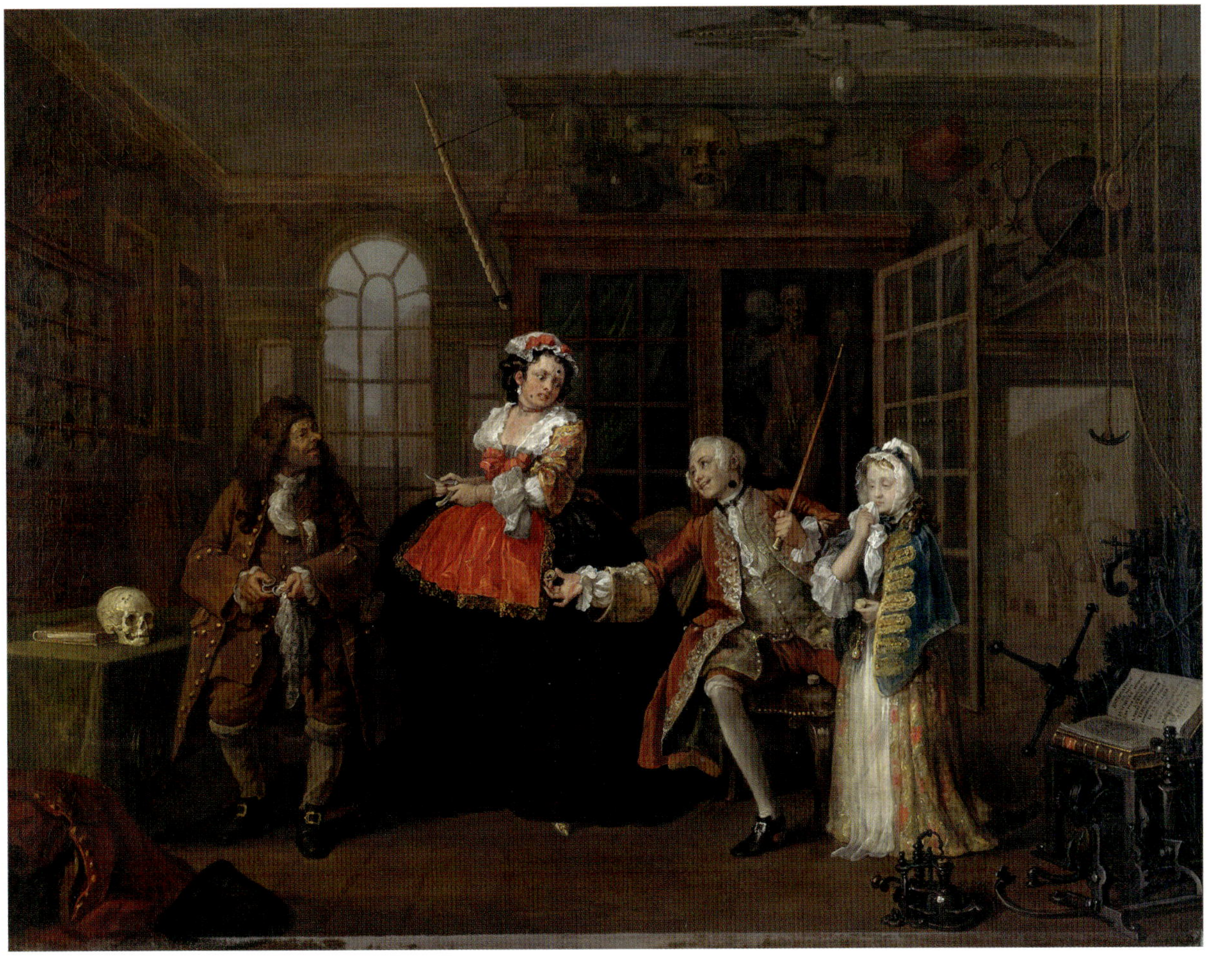

214 (*left*) William Hogarth, *Marriage à la Mode: Visit to the Quack Doctor*, c.1743–5, National Gallery, London

212 (*facing page, top*) William Hogarth, *The Company of Undertakers*, 1736, Guildhall Library and Art Gallery, London

213 (*facing page, bottom*) Guercino, *Woman Pulling Out a Girl's Tooth [The Enraged Housewife]*, early 1620s, The Ashmolean Museum, Oxford

But any hope she harbours must be dashed by a survey of her wretched surroundings. The hole in the ceiling, the stuffed crocodile and the sinister shoulder- straightening machine are more suited to a chamber of horrors than a doctor's surgery, and fear leads to disgust in the cupboard where a skeleton makes an amorous advance on an anatomical figure. The quack himself, the same Dr Misaubon whom Hogarth had already attacked in the *Harlot's Progress*, looks dirty and unscrupulous beside the table bearing a diseased skull. And the woman next to him, probably identifiable as Betsy Careless the brothel keeper, does nothing to counter his air of irredeemable seediness, deception and greed.

After Hogarth's death in 1764, other artists continued to explore the most grotesque aspects of medical care. The idea was by no means new: at one stage early in the 1620s Guercino had devoted his formidable skills as a draughtsman to defining the moment when a woman pulls out a girl's tooth (pl. 213). Holding her young companion steady with one hand, the woman prepares to yank with the other. The girl is so distressed that she clutches the woman's hair, and still holds an implement for hooking the pan over the nearby kitchen fire. Guercino ensures that the flames and smoke add to the sense of alarm, but he also succeeds in conveying the trust between both participants in this gruesome drama. The girl trusts the woman, who seems to be acting in a responsible and compassionate manner.

She could hardly be further removed from the cackling sadism with which popular dentistry was explored in the next century, when a number of relentless pictures were painted by the itinerant schoolmaster John Collier. Known also as Tim Bobbin, he specialised in a macabre panel painting of a dentist pushing his leg against a patient's chin.[13] With both hands, he tugs on the thread round his victim's tooth. While the patient's face

215 John Collier, *Laughter and Experiment*, from *Human Passions Delineated*, 1773

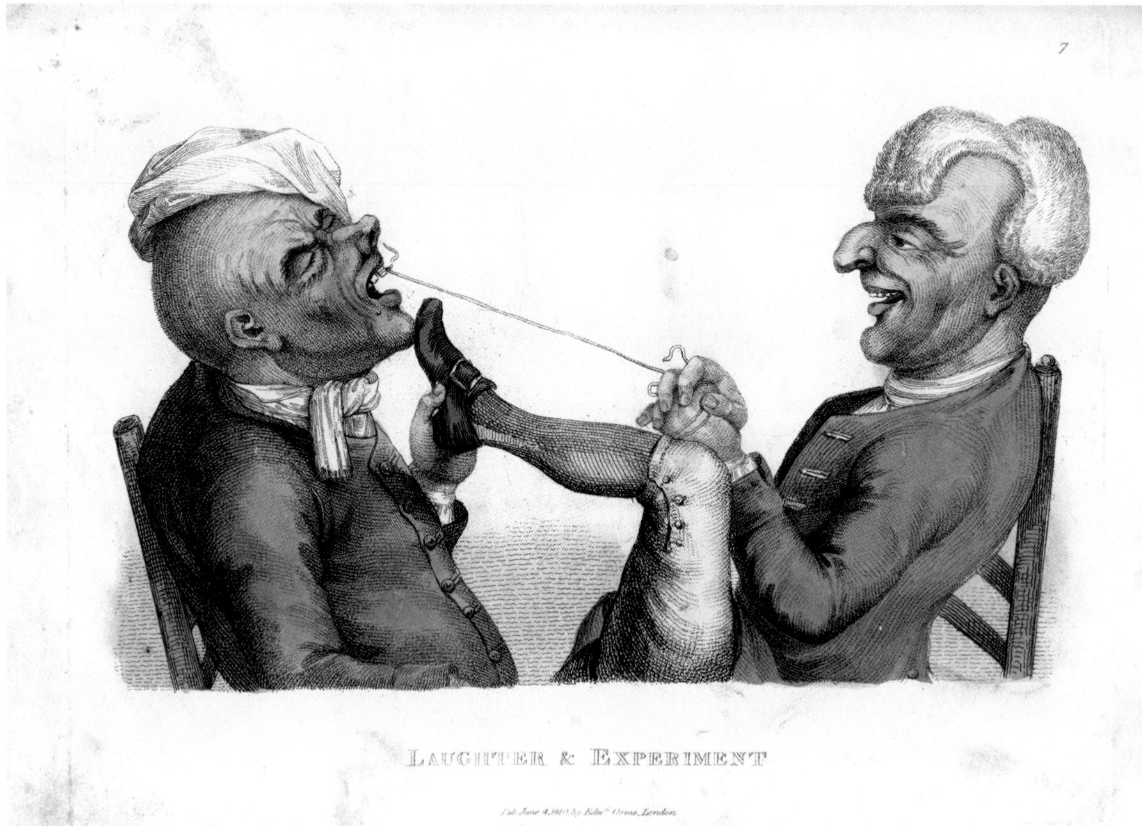

216 John Hamilton Mortimer, *Doctors Dissecting*, *c.*1770–79, Yale University Historical Library, New Haven

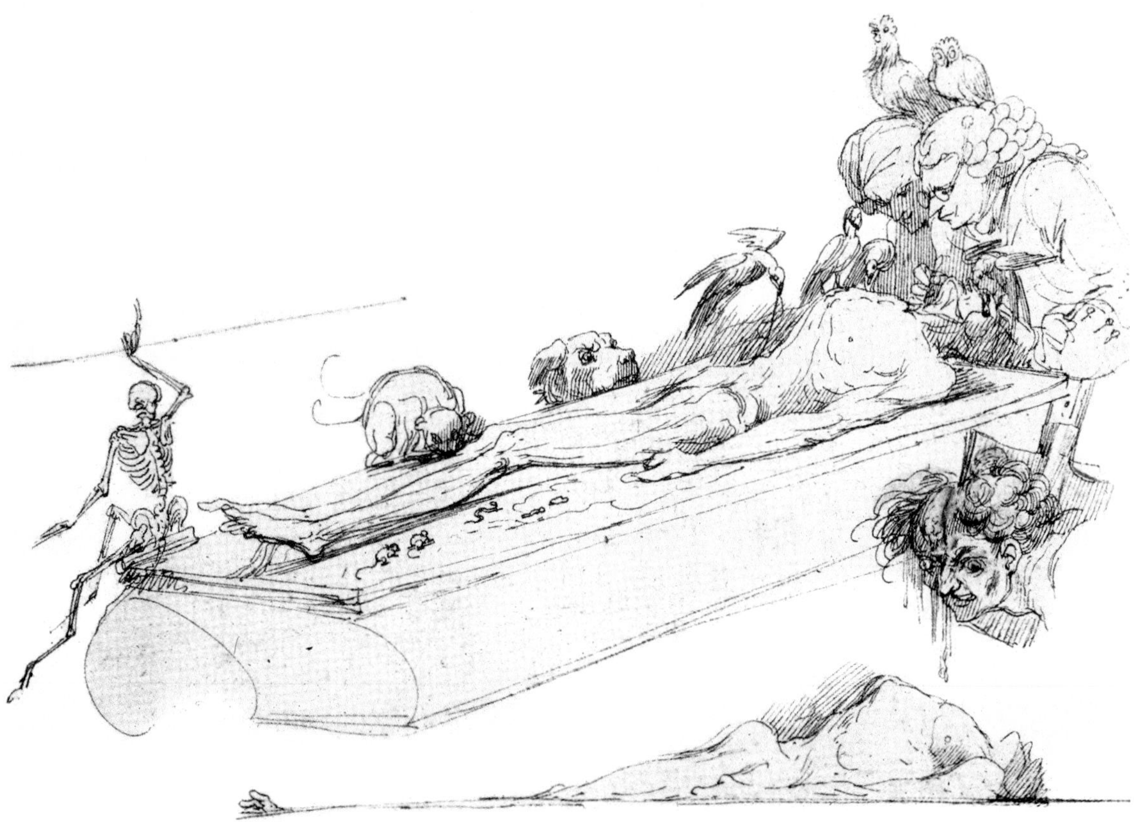

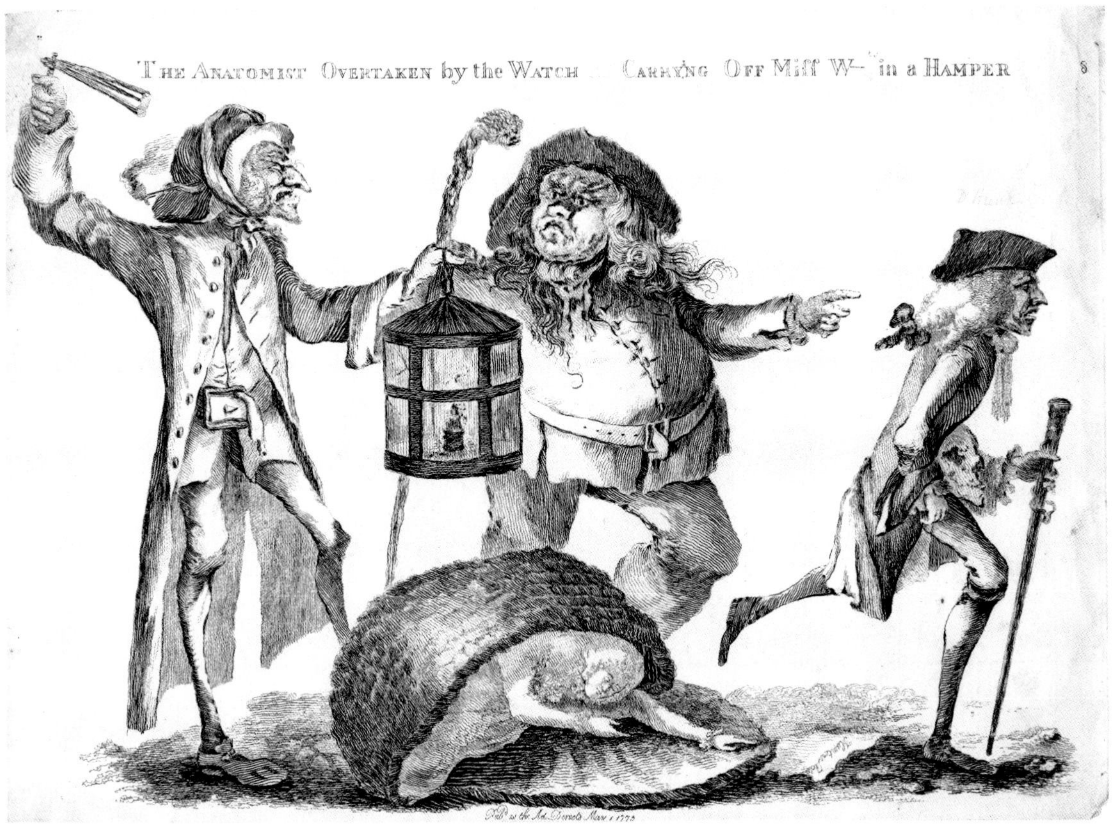

217 Anon., *The Anatomist Overtaken by the Watch in Carrying off Miss W—tts in a Hamper*, 1773, British Museum, London

twists in unimaginable agony, the dentist leers with vulpine relish. Collier called the same scene *Laughter and Experiment* when he published an engraved version in his 1773 book of verse and cartoons called *Human Passions Delineated*, where the English professions were all mercilessly satirised (pl. 215). The accompanying verse described how

> A packthread strong he tied in haste
> On tooth that sore did wring:
> He pull'd, the patient follow'd fast,
> Like Towzer in a string.
> He miss'd at first, but try'd again,
> Then clapp'd his foot o'th chin;
> He pull'd – the patient roared with pain,
> And hideously did grin.[14]

On the whole, though, artists reserved their greatest vilification for surgical subjects. John Hamilton Mortimer drew a particularly repellent pen study of *Doctors Dissecting* (pl. 216). The surgeons bending with such manic zeal over the corpse are scarcely less predatory than the assortment of birds perched on their periwigs and pecking at the body's chest. Lower down, a dog and cat lurk impatiently for any morsel they can grab, while two mice and a worm advance towards the dead man's attenuated legs. It is a grisly scene, made still more repugnant by the miniature skeleton gesturing with perverse delight at the end of the slab.

Mortimer's disgust was undoubtedly magnified by the knowledge that illegal body-snatching for dissection was reaching the proportions of an epidemic. A popular print published in the 1770s revealed the macabre spectacle of *The Anatomist Overtaken by the Watch in Carrying off Miss W–tts in a Hamper* (pl. 217). The paper dropped on the ground bears the inscription 'Hunter's Lectures', a topical reference to the brilliant surgeon John Hunter and his brother William, whose 'museum' in Windmill Street housed the anatomical collections now displayed at the Hunterian Museum in Glasgow. However, the hapless Miss W–tts, whose body tumbles pitifully from its ignominious hamper, may well have been exhumed by the Resurrectionists who operated in graveyards with such ruthless disrespect.

Her figure probably provided Thomas Rowlandson with the starting point for the dead woman

218 (*right*) Thomas Rowlandson, *The Dissection*, *c.*1775–80, The Huntington Library, Art Collections and Botanical Gardens, San Marino, California

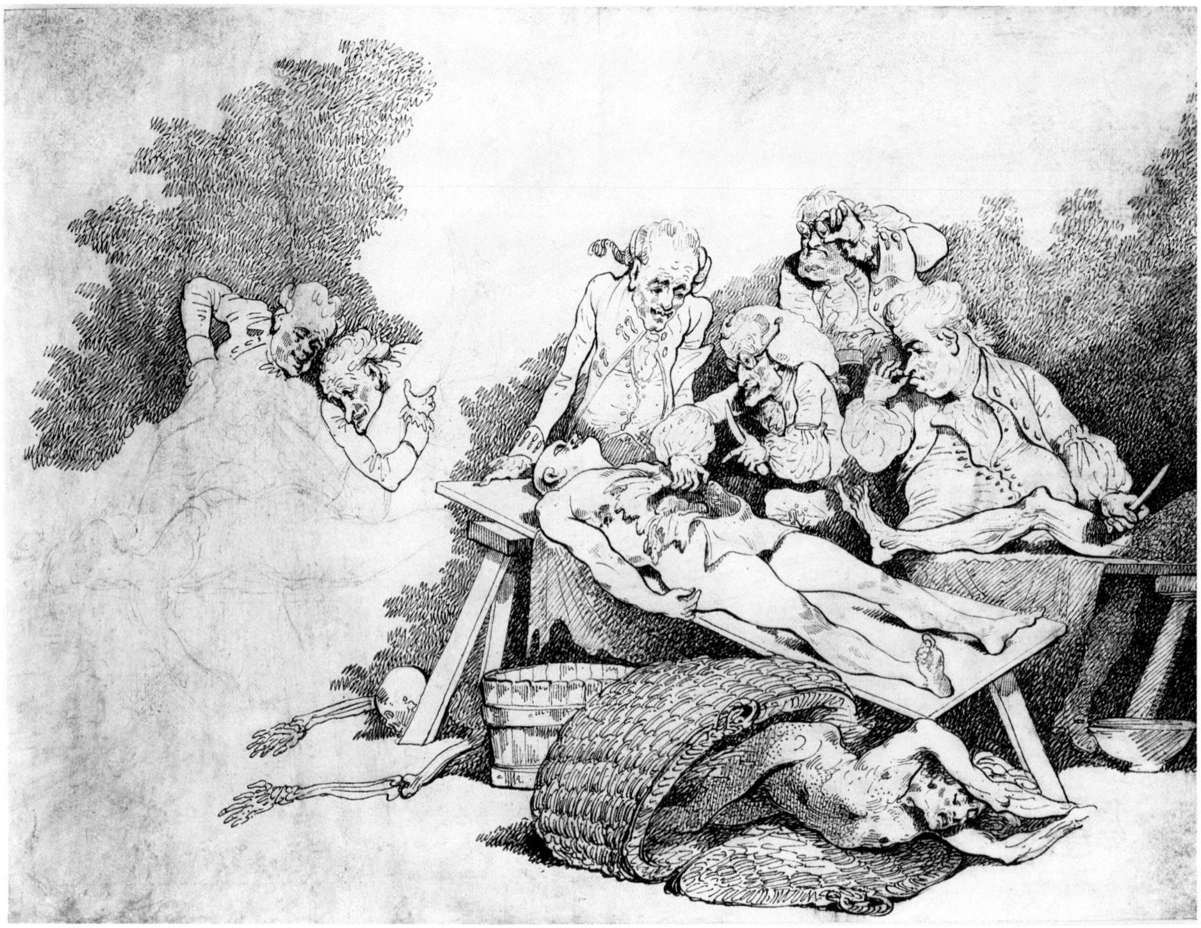

219 (*facing page, top*) Edward Pierce, *Baldwin Hamey Jnr*, 1675, Royal College of Physicians, London

220 (*facing page, bottom*) William Hoare, *Dr Oliver and Mr Peirce Examining Patients*, *c.*1742, Royal National Hospital for Rheumatic Diseases, Bath

who has plummeted from a similar basket in his drawing of *The Dissection* (pl. 218). An early work, which reveals the full extent of his admiration for Mortimer,[15] this trenchant satire is a more boisterous affair than *Doctors Dissecting*. The table bearing the corpse is collapsing under his weight and the gaggle of anatomists display a repellent vitality as they peer and grin over the gaping incision. One of them, turning irresponsibly away from the body he should be working on, takes a pinch of snuff as an antidote to the cadaver's stench. The most disturbing area of the drawing can be found in an unfinished passage, however. Here Rowlandson's pen-nib, as precise and wounding in its way as a surgeon's scalpel, wirily defines the two gloating doctors. Yet the object of their salacious attentions has been left, perhaps deliberately, as a mass of pencil lines. Only a detailed scrutiny discloses that a naked woman lies there, with one leg held up in the air by an anatomist anxious to see her genitals. Maybe delicacy forbade even the uninhibited Rowlandson from developing this incident with greater clarity.

Even so, the revulsion aroused by such practices did not prevent several leading artists from accepting commissions to portray distinguished physicians of the day. After the multi-talented mason, carver, architect and sculptor Edward Pierce had produced a large bust of Baldwin Hamey Junior back in 1675 (pl. 219), British hospitals and the Royal College of Physicians accumulated an impressive number of images dignifying the medical profession. The finest of them amount to a great deal more than officially sanctioned flattery. Dr Hamey may boast a flamboyant Restoration hat and long curls falling over elaborately attired shoulders, but the frowning face belongs to a man haunted by his professional responsibilities. An air of seasoned assurance goes hand in hand, here, with compassion and a melancholy awareness of life's frailty. Hamey looks the very opposite of a charlatan interested only in fleecing his patients without a thought for their future well-being. Pierce's ability to respond to the doctor's *gravitas* led Margaret Whinney to conclude that he was 'the best portrait sculptor of the century in England; it is sad that either his other activities or lack of commissions prevented him from doing more in this field'.[16]

Pierce's pupil Richard Crutcher carved an elaborate funerary sculpture of St Thomas's benefactor Sir Robert Clayton and his wife at Bletchingley, Surrey, in 1705. Soon afterwards the Hospital supported so generously by Clayton acquired Jonathan Richardson's painting of its most celebrated surgeon of the period, William Cheselden. But British portraiture's involvement with physicians only reached a stronger sense of engagement after the artist William Hoare moved to Bath in 1738. Hoare's ability combined with his first-hand knowledge of Italy to earn him rapid approval among wealthy Bath patrons eager for their portraits. At the same time he became fascinated by the treatment of rheumatism at the newly created Bath General Hospital (now the Royal National Hospital for Rheumatic Diseases). From the moment it was founded in 1738, Hoare served as a Councillor at the Hospital and for the next twenty years 'he took his duties as Governor and Visitor very seriously'.[17] Around 1742 he decided to publicise the pioneering work of the Bath General by embarking on a large, deeply felt painting, *Dr Oliver and Mr Peirce Examining Patients* (pl. 220).

Like Hogarth and the other artists associated with the Foundling venture in London, Hoare eventually presented this remarkable canvas to the Hospital he supported. But unlike the Foundling's painters, who avoided direct representations of the activities within the institution, he decided to show two distinguished medical men at work in their consulting room. Dr William Oliver, portrayed in profile making notes at the table, had played an important role fund-raising for the Bath General, where he served as the Governor and one of its chief physicians between 1740 and 1761. His colleague Jeremy Peirce, a senior surgeon at the Hospital, turns to Oliver while holding the extended hand of a man suffering from 'wrist drop'. Heralding the sympathetic gesture adopted by Thomas Guy in John Bacon's carving (see pl. 209), Peirce's fingers carefully probe his patient's bone-structure while he tries to define the nature of the ailment. Both he and Oliver have already examined the boy

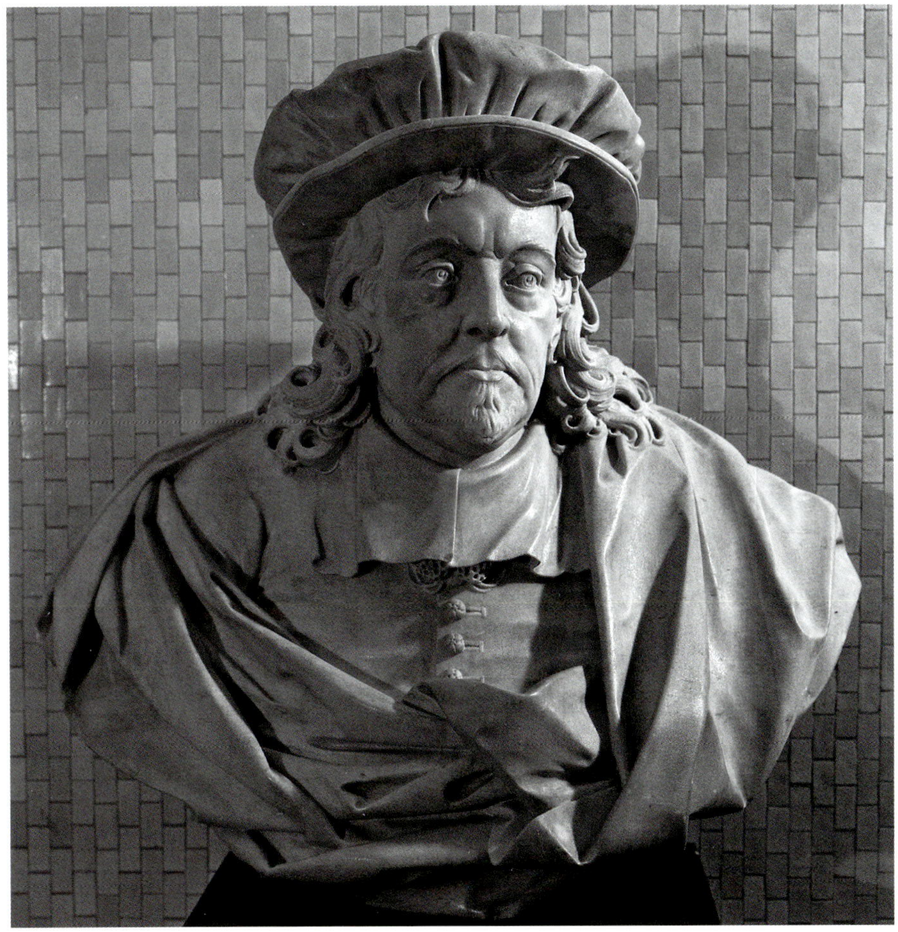

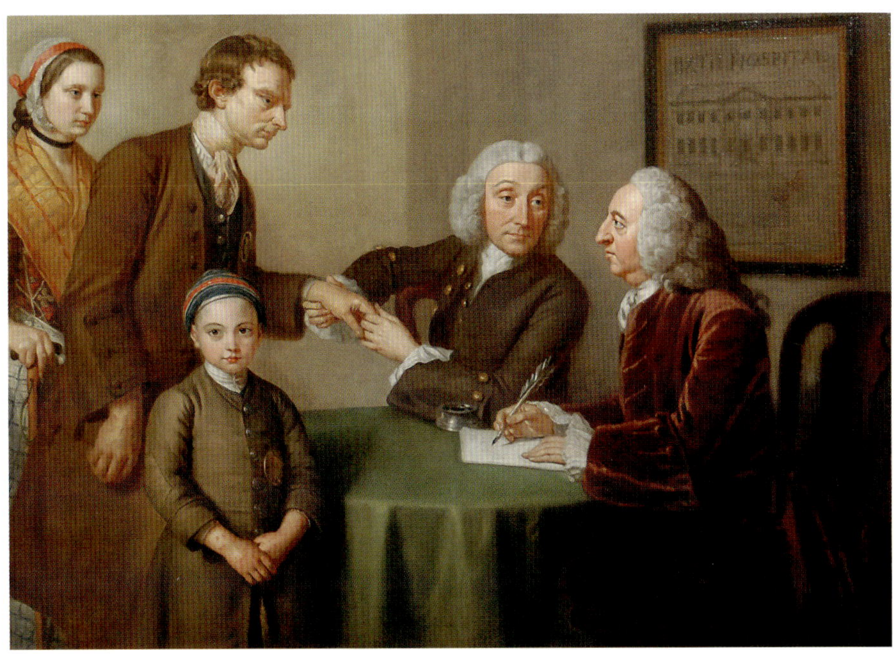

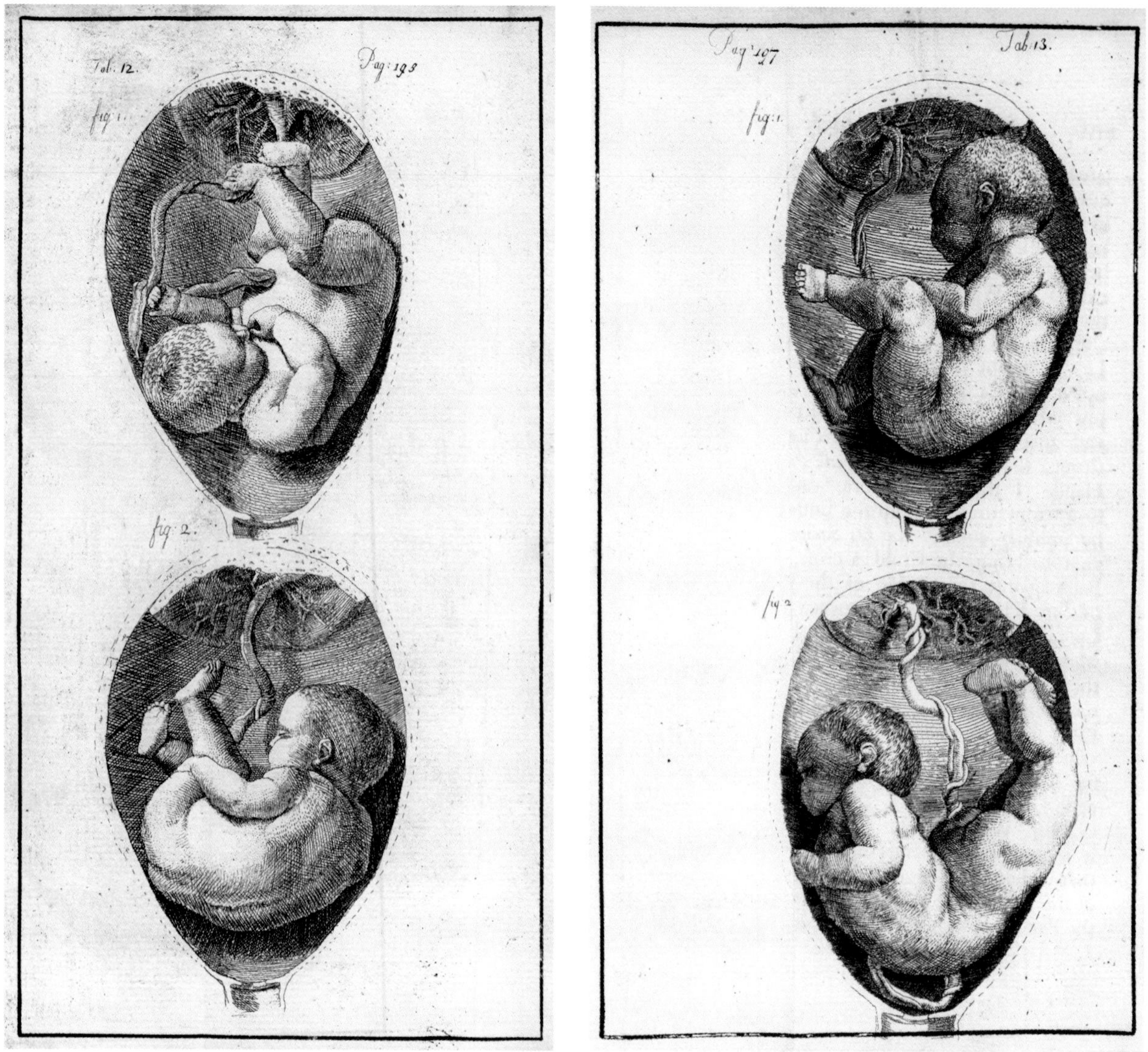

221a and b (*right*) George Stubbs, images from John Burton's *Essay towards a Complete New System of Midwifery*, 1751

222 (*facing page*) Louis-François Roubiliac, *Dr John Belchier*, Hunterian Museum at the Royal College of Surgeons of England

in the foreground, who is clearly afflicted by a serious skin disease and wears a brass badge identifying his ward and bed number, which gave him free admission to the Corporation Baths. The plan framed on the wall behind displays John Wood's classical frontage of the Hospital's new building and the entire painting celebrates, in a restrained and thoughtful manner, the growth of dedicated medical expertise in Bath. Hoare ensured that the trio of patients represented the three main types of illness treated by the Hospital: rheumatism, 'leprosy' and paralysis. After exhibiting the canvas at the Society of Artists in 1762, he gave it to Bath General. And in 1780, the elderly Hoare demonstrated his continuing commitment by donating to the Hospital a painted portrait of its Treasurer, Daniel Danvers, who had recently died after nearly twenty years of service. The Committee of Governors, who thanked Hoare for 'his valuable present', also asked him to 'make the Hospital a present of his own [portrait]',[18] probably the early pastel still preserved in its collection, as testimony to the warm relationship between Bath General and its devoted artist.

Soon after Hoare painted his remarkable portrait of Oliver and Peirce, the young George Stubbs moved from his family's Liverpool home to start working as a portrait painter in York, where he stayed for about eight years. He was soon involved in studying and teaching anatomy with the surgeon Charles Atkinson at York Hospital. According to Ozias Humphry, who wrote a memoir of Stubbs based on conversations with him, anatomy had begun to fascinate the artist at the age of eight. Stimulated by a Dr Holt, who lent the boy bones and other material, he made drawings. The fascination returned in York, where Atkinson found Stubbs his first cadaver. He started dissecting animals and humans, while Atkinson gave him lessons in anatomy. Stubbs made friends with a number of Liverpudlians belonging to Jacobite and Roman Catholic circles centred on York Hospital. He learned so much that, within a few years, the hospital's students attended anatomical lectures delivered by Stubbs.

And he also came into fruitful contact with Dr John Burton, York Hospital's founder, who wrote *Essay towards a Complete New System of Midwifery* and asked Stubbs to illustrate it with eighteen etched plates. Humphry maintained that Stubbs robustly insisted on making the dissections for them himself (pl. 221). He even enlisted the help of his hospital students when taking, from a graveyard, the corpse of a woman who had died in childbirth. Such activities earned him 'a vile reputation' in York: one writer recalled that 'to dissect the human body was also his diligent pursuit, inasmuch that (as I have heard a relative of his declare) to procure subjects for his improvement, Mr Stubbs has, an hundred times, run into such adventures as might subject anyone with less honourable motives to the greatest severity of the law'.[19] Perhaps Stubbs's awareness of the risks he was taking in his anatomical obsessions was one of the reasons why he withheld his name from *Essay towards a Complete New System of Midwifery*. Like hospitals and surgeons, he had to guard against the disrepute so easily associated with this kind of pioneering research. He may also have wanted to distance himself from the notoriety of Dr Burton, who provided Sterne with satirical inspiration for the male midwife Dr Slop in *Tristram Shandy*. Burton's preface launched an attack on Dr William Smellie, an outstanding surgeon in the field of midwifery who 'was about to publish my Improvements with some other Work of his own; this put upon me the Thoughts of publishing them myself'.[20] But Burton's scholarly book was poorly received when published in 1751, and Smellie's landmark *Treatise on the Theory and Practice of Midwifery*, the first volume of which appeared only a year later, was applauded by its reviewers.

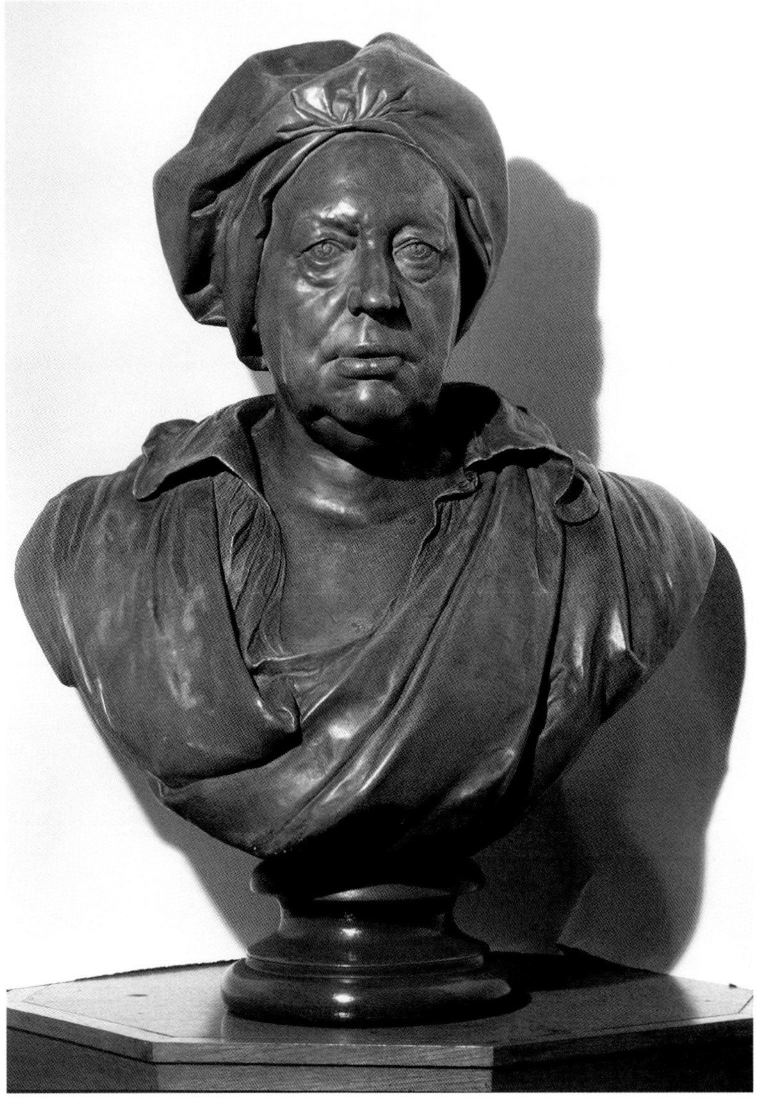

The expansion of medical knowledge during the eighteenth century is reflected in the increasing gravity of the finest physicians' portraits. Louis-François Roubiliac, the most brilliant of the sculptors working in England at that time, carved a notably solemn bust of *Dr John Belchier* (pl. 222). The elderly surgeon, simply dressed in an open-necked shirt, stares forward with unusual intensity. Far from basking in his social status, he seems absorbed in contemplating the meaning of an incessant professional struggle to save his patients from death. Roubiliac made no attempt to hide the scar running down from Belchier's left eye towards his mouth. The line evokes the incisions made by the doctor in the operating theatre, while the sense of tension is accentuated by the slight parting of the surgeon's lips.

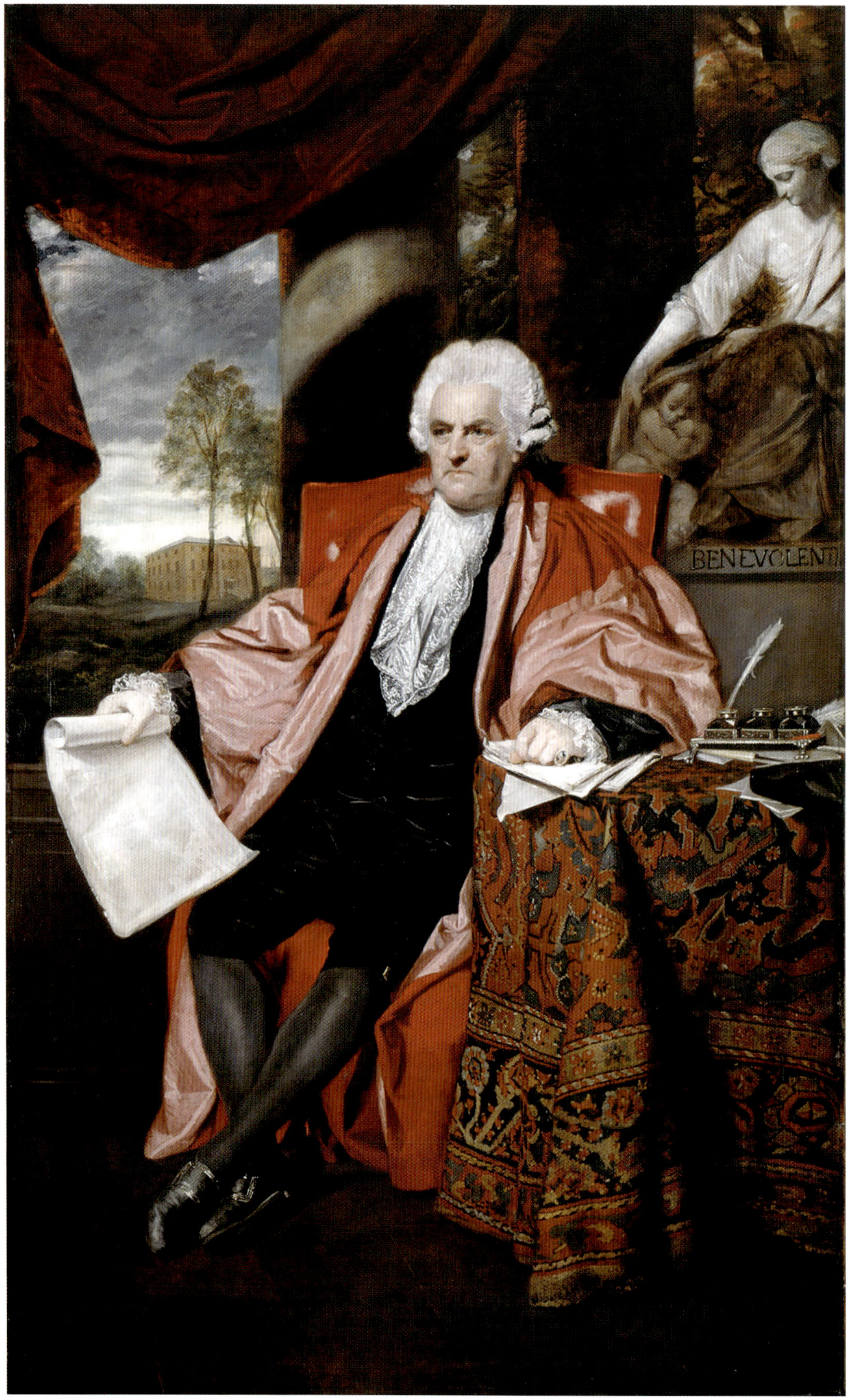

223 Joshua Reynolds, *Dr John Ash*, 1787, Birmingham Museums and Art Galleries

By no means all doctors' portraits in this period possess the insights conveyed by Roubiliac. Compared with the profundity of his Belchier bust, Joshua Reynolds's three-quarter-length study of *Percival Pott* lacks distinction. Painted in 1784 for presentation to Bart's, where it was displayed in the Great Hall near the staircase adorned with Hogarth's wall-decorations (see pl. 183), it fails to communicate the vigorous grasp of character shown in Reynolds's subsequent painting of *Dr John Ash*, portraying a widely respected Birmingham physician who had been instrumental in founding and planning the city's General Hospital (pl. 223). Although he had earlier been prey to periods of mental disorder, Ash was a man of impressive intellectual achievement. The General Hospital venerated him and, after his departure for a fellowship of the London College of Physicians in 1787, the Governors decided to 'perpetuate his presence in Birmingham by means of portraiture'.[21] Possibly acquainted with the Pott painting at Bart's, they invited Reynolds to produce a portrait that turned out to be one of his most successful, magnificent and incisive late full-lengths.

Progress on the commission might have been quickened by a growing rapport between sitter and artist. They were exactly the same age, sixty-five, and after the portrait was completed Reynolds attended on at least three occasions evening sessions of the Eumalian Club, a 'convivial learned society'[22] founded by Ash himself. He bestowed the Greek name for an ash tree on his club, whose members gathered at the Blenheim Tavern in Bond Street. Here Reynolds would have felt at home, since several close friends including Boswell and Richard Payne Knight were among its members. He certainly provided Birmingham General Hospital with a very complete and sympathetic portrait, showing Ash resplendent in his Doctor of Medicine gown, lace cravat and an elegant suit of black velvet. The physician displays the Hospital's ground-plan with understandable satisfaction, while the building itself appears in the tree-framed distance.

Compared with Hogarth's Coram (see pl. 190), whose general position is echoed in this painting, Ash is a grave and imposing figure formally attired in a powdered wig. Yet his kindly eyes flash with the same glinting vivacity to be found in the diamond-studded ring on his little finger. Behind him, the principles governing his professional life are embodied in a classical statue of *Benevolentia*, a woman who extends her mantle over a vulnerable child even more protectively than Rysbrack's *Charity* had done at the Foundling Hospital twenty years before (see pl. 201). The modern critic Roger Fry, fascinated by Reynolds's *Discourses* since his student days at Cambridge,[23] was immensely impressed and excited when he encountered *Dr John Ash* in an exhibition at the Royal Academy. Writing in *The Athenaeum* in 1906, he declared that 'it is one of those splendid compositions, at once simple and rich, which show Reynolds had acquired a greater command of artistic resource, and used it with a more unerring taste, than any other British painter. This is worthy of Titian or Rubens, and scarcely another portrait painter can lay claim to have given so much pictorial splendour to the subject.'[24]

The most remarkable alliance between art and doctors in eighteenth-century Britain centred, however, on the Hunter brothers. William, the elder of the two, was an eminent Scottish surgeon, anatomist, obstetrician and collector. In 1746 he became surgeon-*accoucheur* to the Middlesex Hospital and then sealed his immense reputation by establishing a lecture theatre, dissecting room and museum at his London house in Great Windmill Street. The anatomy school was revolutionary for England: it promised hands-on anatomy, a corpse for every student. Hunter's distinguished career was crowned by his appointment as Professor of Anatomy at the Royal Academy in 1768. There he behaved with great generosity towards an Irish model called George White, whom Reynolds had discovered laying down paving stones in the street. After Reynolds had clothed, fed and painted him, White was introduced 'as a subject for the students of the Royal Academy to paint from'. When Hunter saw him there, he thought

> Old George the finest muscular subject that he had ever seen, and, in consequence, had him, during the course of his lectures, at his Theatre, in order, by comparison, to elucidate the 'superficial' anatomy of the human system. The benevolence of the Doctor induced him to do more, for he took him into his house where he resided some time; but I have understood that the irregularity of Old George, his inmate, who had been

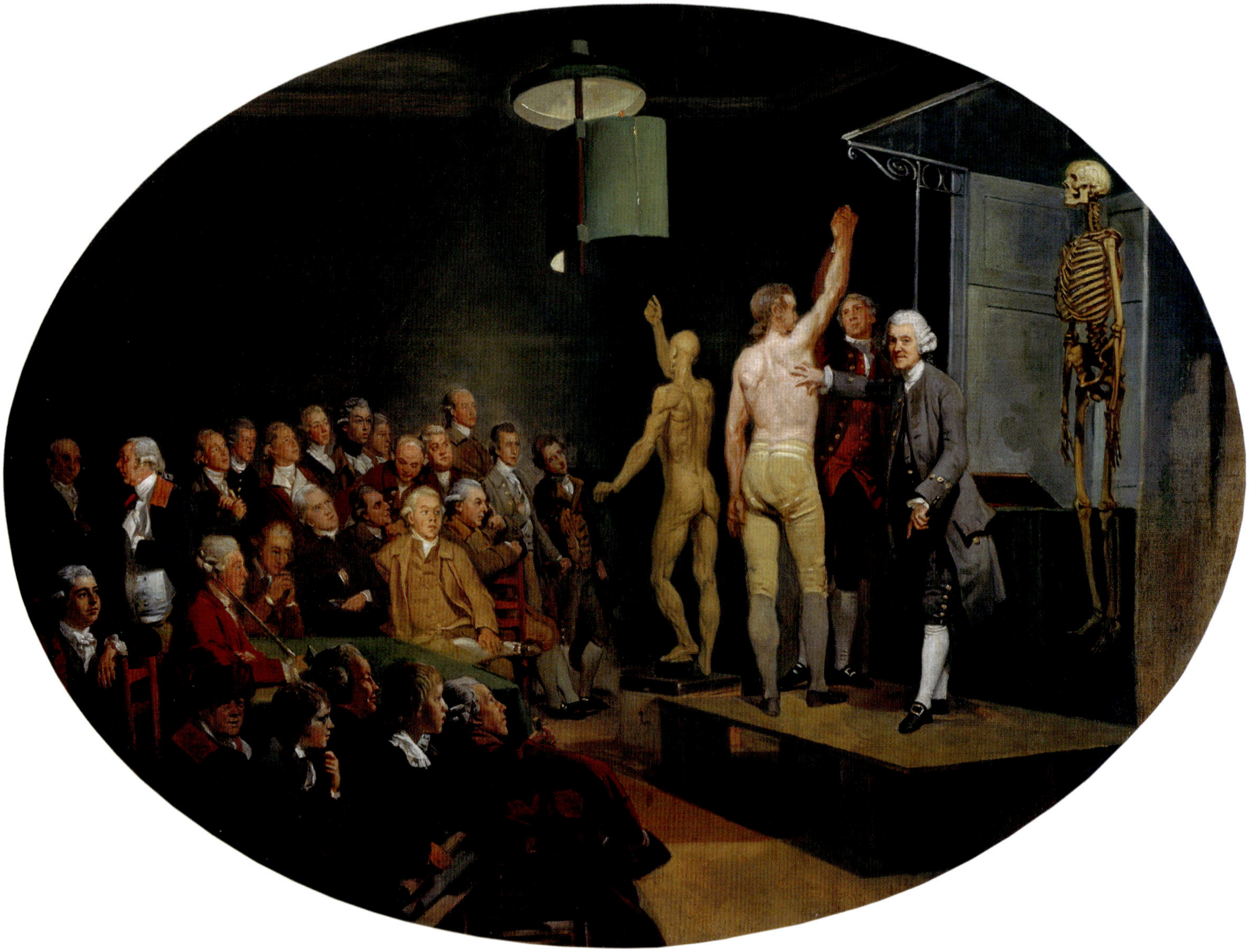

224 Johan Zoffany, *Doctor William Hunter' teaching Anatomy at the Royal Academy*, c.1772, Royal College of Physicians, London

used to a dissolute course of life, induced his patron at last to part with him, though I think he received an allowance both from him, Sir Joshua, and others, that rendered his old age comfortable.[25]

Hunter's lectures were especially popular with students, and around 1772 Johan Zoffany painted a dramatic demonstration he gave at Somerset House before a spellbound audience (pl. 224). With a skeleton hanging in a wooden cubicle behind him, Hunter stands on a platform and smiles as he arranges his live model in a pose echoing the plaster *écorché* figure on the left. Reynolds, seated in the centre, holds his ear trumpet and listens eagerly while Hunter demonstrates the formation of the muscles. On other occasions, though, the attraction of Hunter's lectures lay in his willingness to use not only live models, but also the corpses of hanged criminals. One day, during a dissection at Surgeons' Hall, he examined a corpse and decided that the musculature was so impressive that it should be preserved. So the corpse was transported to the Royal Academy schools, where the sculptor Agostino Carlini agreed to make a cast. The dead man had been a smuggler, and Carlini posed him as the Dying Gladiator. This cast was esteemed enough to stay on display at the Academy for

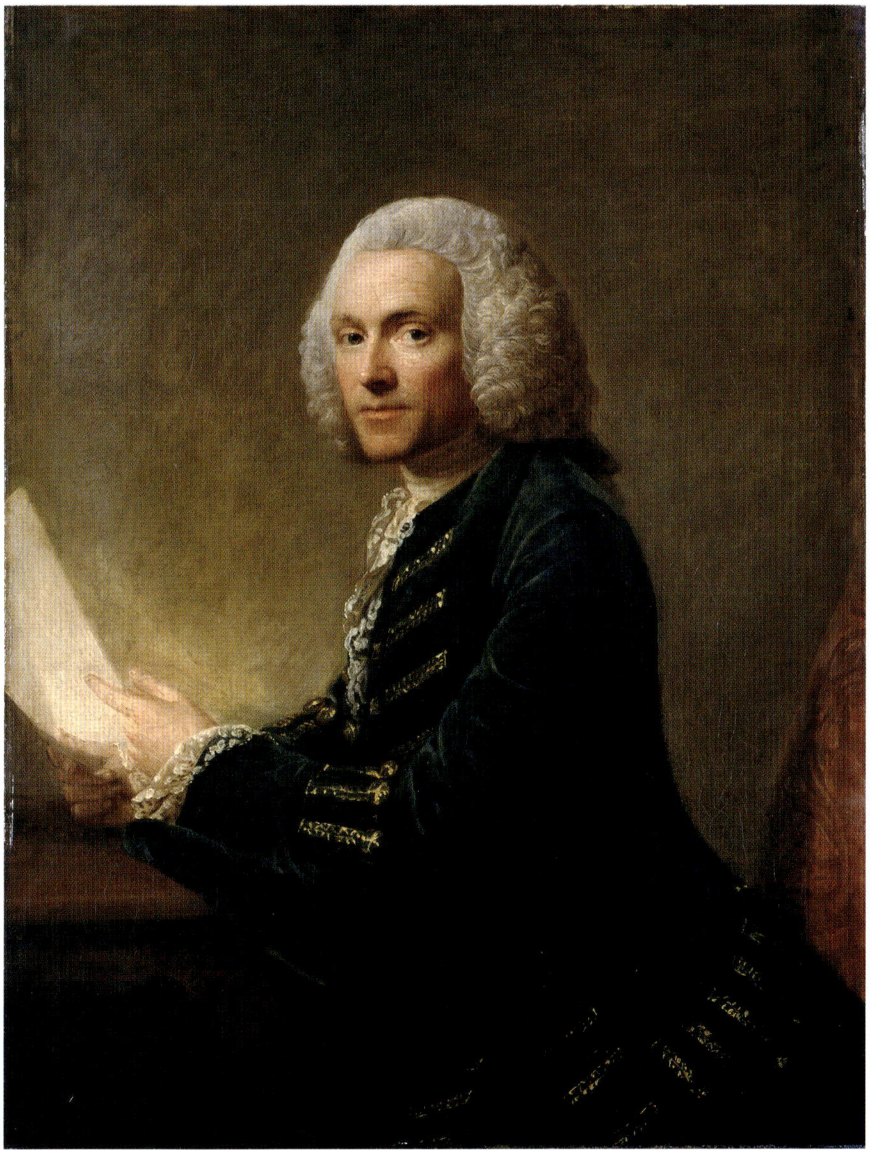

225 Allan Ramsay, *William Hunter*, *c*.1764–5, Hunterian Museum and Art Gallery, Glasgow

decades and successive generations of students referred to him by the affectionate nickname 'Smugglerius'.

Reynolds painted a posthumous portrait of Hunter in 1787, where the sitter is shown pausing at his work-desk, looking up and smiling in a remarkably open, friendly way.[26] His charm may well have helped him to gain the confidence of patients who valued discretion. Probably an abortionist, as well as a trusted male midwife to Queen Charlotte and many other titled ladies, he also saved several mothers of dead babies from the gallows; his *Uncertainty of Signs of Murder in Bastard Children* is regarded as a landmark in the history of forensic medicine. Hunter's discernment as a collector was demonstrated when he chose Allan Ramsay as his portraitist (pl. 202). This gentle half-length image, showing Hunter pointing at a sheet of paper in his right hand, can be ranked among Ramsay's most free, subtle and sympathetic paintings. The sitter looks impeccable in his powdered wig and deep blue coat slashed with gold trimmings, but his intent gaze indicates the importance Hunter attached to the act of painting. Although the portrait probably commemorates his appointment in 1764 as Physician Extraordinary to Queen Charlotte, no pompous ostentation mars this understated canvas.

It is easy to imagine Hunter relishing the opportunity to converse with Ramsay, who may have drawn his sitter's attention to the merits of Chardin.[27] At any rate, Hunter acquired three outstanding early works by Chardin for his collection, paying £8 for *Lady taking Tea* and also purchasing a pair of smaller, no less superlative images of melancholy servants, *The Scullery Maid* and *The Cellar Boy*. He also commissioned George Stubbs to execute paintings of a moose, a nylghau, an antelope and cavies. Some of Hunter's acquisitions have turned out to be misattributed: he bought a panoramic landscape by de Koninck in the belief that it was a Rembrandt. Nevertheless, the oil study of *The Entombment of Christ* is a genuine Rembrandt and the Reynolds portrait of Hunter's patient Lady Maynard is an excellent example of the artist's work. Hunter spent so much of his fortune on paintings, coins, souvenirs from Captain Cook's voyages and thousands of books and manuscripts that his younger brother John described him as 'in the strictest sense a miser'. Yet he was much loved by patients and students alike, and public-spirited enough to leave the entire collection, with funds for a special building, to his *alma mater*. Hence the creation of the Hunterian Museum at Glasgow University, where everything from superb paintings to unsettling anatomical specimens can be viewed to this day.

John Hunter, often described as 'the father of modern surgery',[28] performed his first human dissection at the age of twenty in his brother's anatomy school. There John spent twelve years, dissecting more than two thousand bodies to supply William with 'preparations' (preserved body parts) as proofs of his theories. To complete this toughening-up process, John also served on the front line looking after the British army during the Seven Years War. William Blake satirised him as the anatomist 'Jack Tearguts', but the truth is that Hunter's research transformed understanding of anatomy, dentistry, embryology, transplantation and much else besides. He regarded operating only as a last resort and his proposal that every life form possesses an innate capacity for malformation and deviation from nature was instrumental in leading Darwin to his theory of evolution. No wonder St George's Hospital venerated him so much that it commissioned a memorial bust by Alfred Gilbert in 1893 (see pl. 312).

Like his brother, John Hunter amassed a prodigious collection of more than thirteen thousand anatomical, pathological, botanical and zoological specimens at his home in Leicester Square. The Resurrectionists, or 'Sack 'Em Up Men', would deliver corpses from London's cemeteries to his back door. Hogarth would not have approved but when Hunter's collection was opened to the public in 1788, it demonstrated the interrelatedness of all life on earth. Seventy years before Darwin published *On the Origin of Species*, Hunter insisted on displaying monkey and human skulls together in a sequence. He told visitors that 'our first parents, Adam and Eve, were indisputably black'. The immense cost of acquiring all the specimens left him with huge debts and half of the collection was destroyed by Nazi bombs in 1941, but the rest is still preserved at London's Hunterian Museum in Lincoln's Inn Fields.[29]

As a brilliant Enlightenment figure, Hunter knew several of the leading painters of his time. He commissioned Stubbs to paint him images of a rhinoceros, a yak, a baboon and a macaque monkey. Both Gainsborough and Reynolds became his patients and since they were artists he treated them without payment, as he did medical colleagues and the poor. When Gainsborough was dying from a growth in his neck, Hunter looked after him. The Royal Academy announced, too optimistically, that 'from Mr Hunter's skill it is hoped that ten days or a fortnight may restore [Gainsborough] to the practice of that science of which he is so distinguished an ornament'.[30] In reality, as Gainsborough himself admitted, the growth had been remorselessly enlarging for three years. 'What this painful swelling in my Neck will turn out, I am at a loss at present to guess', he wrote in April 1788. 'Mr John Hunter found it nothing but a swell'd Gland, and has been most comfortable in persuading me that it will disperse by the continued application of a Sea:water poultice'.[31] Gainsborough's trust in his doctor was complete: he insisted a month later that 'I shall not on any account interfere in what Mr Hunter is about'.[32] But by August the cancer had killed him.

Four years afterwards, Hunter found himself professionally concerned with the death of Reynolds as well. He had been painted by Sir Joshua in 1786, seated at his desk with skeletal illustrations in a book opened beside him (pl. 226).

Hunter looks grave: he seems to be implying that his own head will soon resemble the skulls displayed with such disconcerting prominence on the page nearby. The human bones on the wall above add to the suspicion that this painting is, above all, a *memento mori*. Reynolds reworked it in 1789, after illness had altered Hunter's face. The two men were neighbours and Reynolds declared that, if he had been a surgeon rather than a painter, 'he should not have been obscure, for as fame was allways his desire he would have study'd physick and at least have attemted if not realy made the greatest physician in the world'.[33] After Reynolds died in 1792, Hunter was called in to perform the melancholy task of a post-mortem. Then, within only a year, the ominous prophecy hinted at in Reynolds's portrait of the surgeon with his skeletal specimens was fulfilled with Hunter's own death.

No amount of friendship between artists and doctors, however, could prevent the British public from regarding physicians with instinctive alarm. Human life expectancy, about thirty-seven years in the eighteenth century, had improved little in the previous two millennia. This was a period when, as George Orwell pointed out

> medical science had grown bolder than before without being any more successful [and] the whole business of doctoring was looked on with horror and dread by ordinary people. Surgery, in particular, was believed to be no more than a peculiarly gruesome form of sadism, and dissection . . . was confused with necromancy . . . When you consider what an operation without anaesthetics must have been like, what it notoriously *was* like, it is difficult not to suspect the motives of people who would undertake such things. For these bloody horrors which the students so eagerly looked forward to ('A magnificent sight if Slasher does it!') were admittedly more or less useless: the patient who did not die of shock usually died of gangrene, a result which was taken for granted.[34]

Suspicion and outright contempt continued to bedevil the medical profession's relationship with the public as the eighteenth century came to a close. Even an innovation as beneficent as Dr Edward Jenner's revolutionary smallpox vaccine was condemned in some quarters, and the satirists seized on its origins with venomous relish. Jenner had begun experimenting with cow-pox in 1796 and, after great difficulty finding subjects willing to be inoculated, started testing a vaccine three years later. News of the discovery spread swiftly, provoking a rash of vaccination prints. Only one declared itself in favour of Jenner's great breakthrough,[35] and far more typical was James Gillray's outrageously uninhibited *The Cow-Pock — or — the Wonderful Effects of the New Inoculation!* (pl. 227). Set in the Smallpox and Inoculation Hospital established by Jenner at St Pancras in London, the print marked the publication of the news that Parliament had granted him £10,000 for his research. Gillray was unimpressed, and he gave the Hospital no credit for

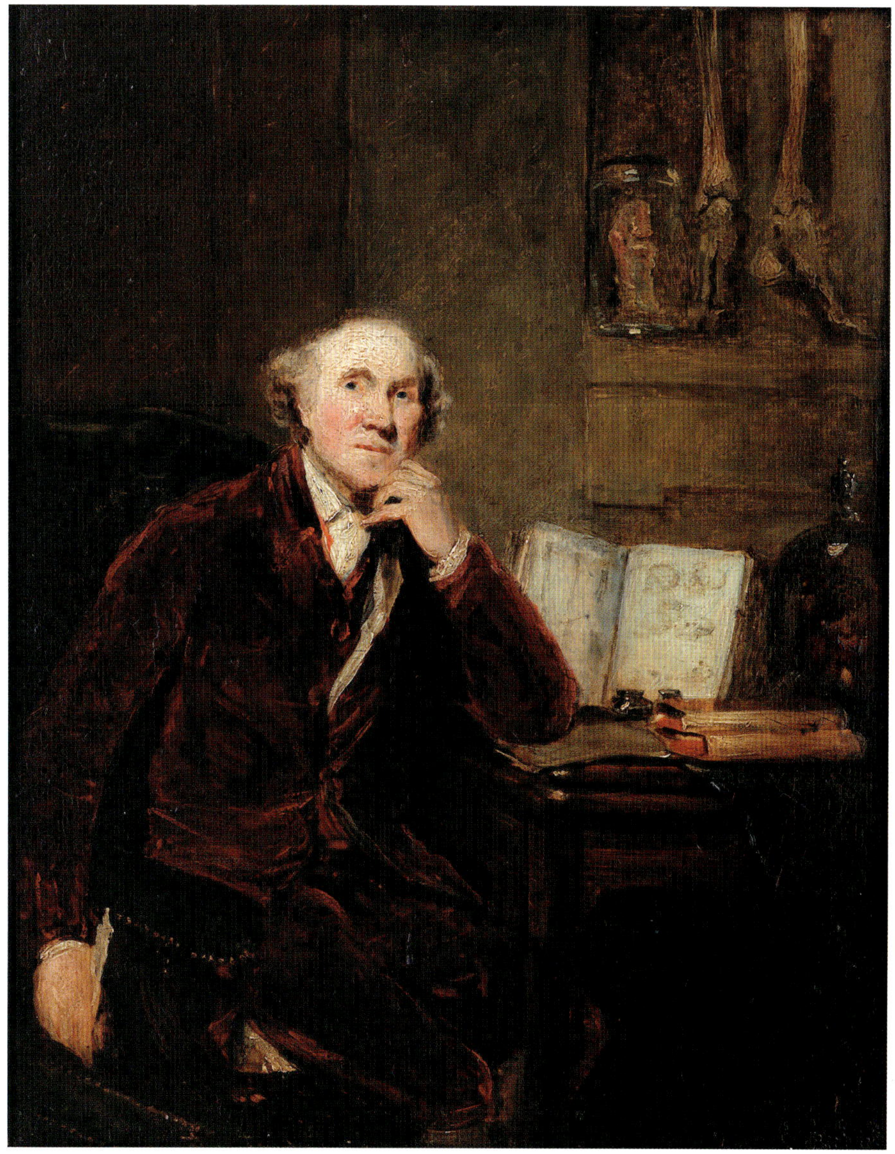

226 Joshua Reynolds, *John Hunter*, 1786–9, Private Collection

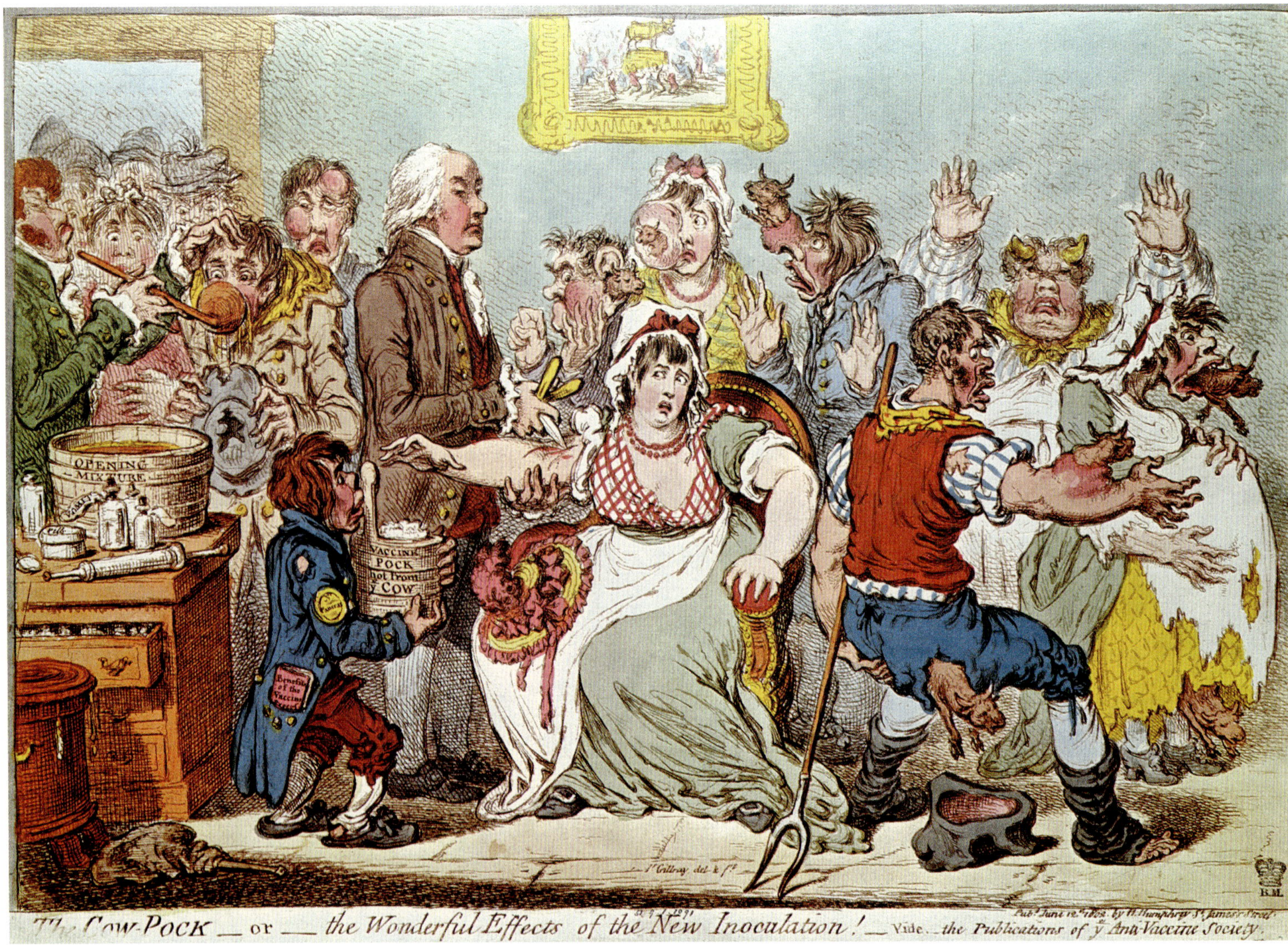

227 James Gillray, *The Cow-Pock — or — the Wonderful Effects of the New Inoculation!*, published by H. Humphrey, 1802

instituting free vaccination for the poor. In his bilious view, Jenner was the perpetrator of a horrifying confidence trick which only the most gullible members of society would be foolish enough to accept.[36] All the dupes crowd eagerly through the Hospital doorway, staring with crazed anticipation at the ladle filled with 'Opening Mixture' which a haughty assistant is cramming into the mouth of a hapless wretch. Dr Jenner stands next to him, coolly carving into the arm of a woman who shudders as his blade draws blood. Her outstretched hand hovers over the vaccine bucket, labelled 'Pock hot from ye Cow', held by a ragged assistant whose jacket badge suggests that he is a charity schoolboy of the district. The woman's attention is concentrated, understandably enough, on the doctor's knife. But if her eyes turned the other way, she would realise that the vaccine had a variety of instantaneous and grotesque results.

Gillray defines these calamities with shameless gusto. A wild-eyed farmhand stares incredulously at his bloodstained forearm, where a miniature cow emerges from the skin. Another cow charges out of his right buttock and patients leaving the Hospital reel from a barrage of similar inflictions. Cows eject themselves from the mouth, nose, ear and cheek of people who witness the eruptions with panic and disgust. Perhaps the most distressed of all the victims is an obese lady whose arms are raised in abject terror as yellow horns sprout from her head. Gillray's command of line makes each of these macabre deformations nastily believable. His manic inventiveness may well have taken as its springboard the information in a recent study of 1795, *Morbid Poisons*, which revealed that 'when the cow pox is communicated to the human, it produces, besides ulceration in the hand, a considerable tumour of the arm, with symptomatic fever, both of which gradually subside'.[37] Far from subsiding, Jenner's vaccine here threatens to transform its recipients into animals. Gillray damns the patients still further by equating them with the Israelites who worship the idolatrous golden calf in the painting displayed on the Hospital wall. Clamorous, surreal and laced with hysteria, *The Cow-Pock* shows how even the most enlightened of medical advances could be greeted with fearful derision.

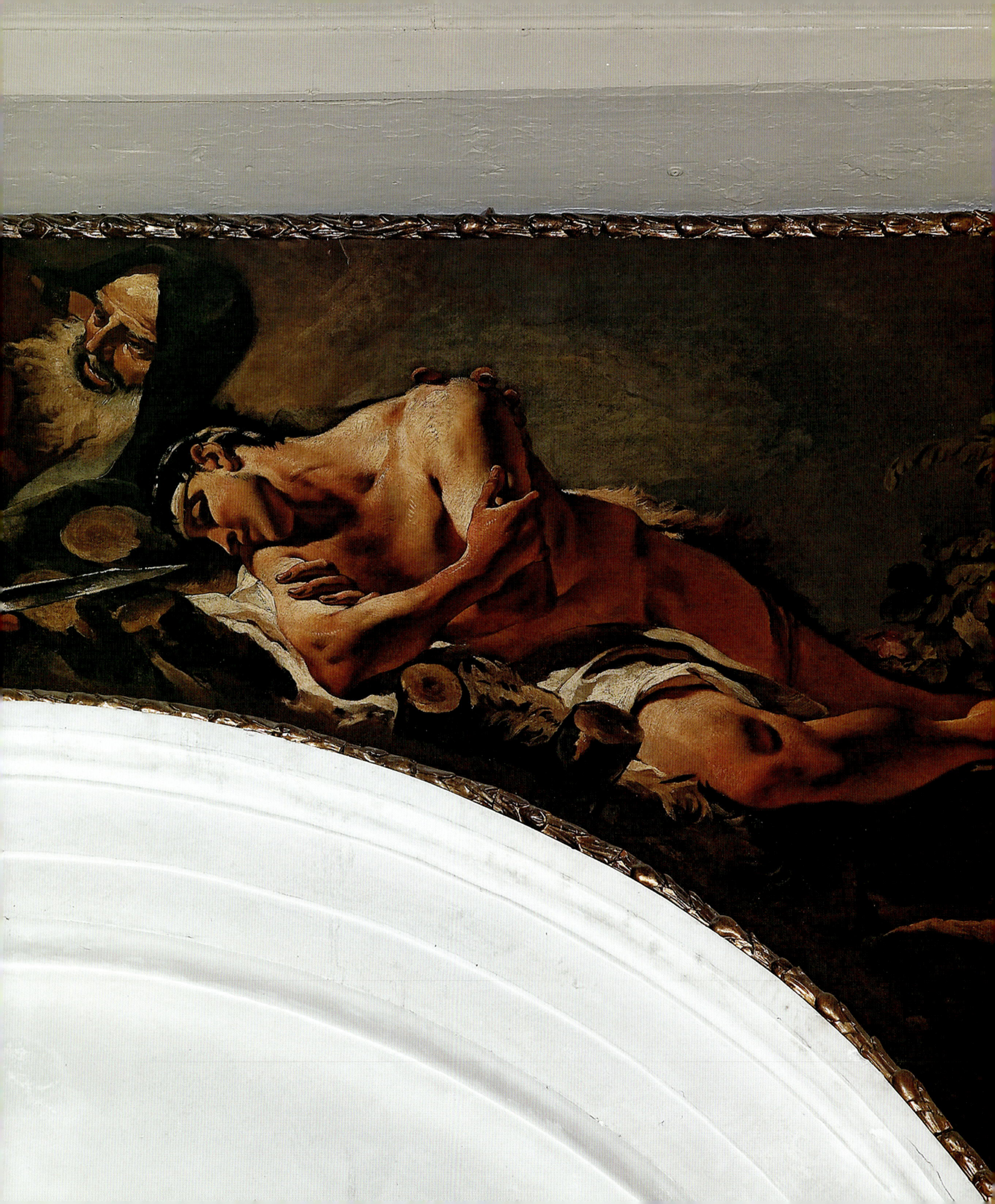

SIXTEEN
ENFANTS-TROUVÉS, LYING-IN AND MUSIC-MAKING

The facade of the Ospedaletto church in Venice, where Tiepolo produced his first surviving painting for a public setting, contains nothing to suggest that it was built for an orphanage. Baldassare Longhena, who designed this bizarre frontage in the early 1660s, loaded it with an abundance of grotesque carved apparitions (pl. 229). They leer down at anyone pausing to survey the church from the *calle* in front, a passageway so narrow that it forces the spectator into a disconcertingly close relationship with the bulk of the building ahead. Longhena was bent on flouting all the Venetians' preconceptions about classical propriety and his outsize imagery still manages to disturb today. With Baroque effrontery, he permitted a macabre giant to stick out his tongue at passers-by, who feel assailed by equally flagrant aggressors wherever they look. The grossly built *telamones* seem determined, not simply to support the church's entablature, but to threaten and crush with their ogre-like physiques. Contorted lion masks convey a similar truculence, so it is a relief to pass through this fusillage of brazen sculptural exaggeration and penetrate the dark interior of Santa Maria dei Derelitti.

When the young Tiepolo received his commission for the church, just before 1720, a considerable array of large-scale canvases were already installed there. Several *seicento* artists of merit had contributed to the nave's embellishment, among them Johann Carl Loth, Pietro Liberi and Ermanno Stroiffi, whose *modello* for his altarpiece of the *Madonna and Child with SS John the Baptist, Francis and James the Great* has a tender simplicity in handling and sentiment alike (pl. 230).[1] Tiepolo did not share the advantage enjoyed by Stroiffi and the other painters, who were able to brandish their abilities on the grand scale in prominent sites. But his precocious image overcame its awkward shape and high location with outstanding verve, easily outshining all the canvases by different artists installed in similar positions above the altars.[2]

Tiepolo, who was supposed to have been nineteen when he produced the Ospedaletto painting, owed this crucial early commission to the influence exerted by his teacher, Gregorio Lazzarini. The older man carried out a painting of the *Pool of Bethesda* in the same church, directly underneath Tiepolo's contribution. While lacking the psychological insight and compassion of Murillo's Bethesda canvas in the Hospital de la Caridad (see pl. 133), not to mention the satirical gusto of Hogarth's response to the subject (see pl. 186), Lazzarini's version is still an accomplished work, borrowing from Veronese in order to arrive at a stolid yet sincere and well organised treatment of a subject suited to the Ospedaletto's context.

228 (*facing page*) Detail of pl. 231

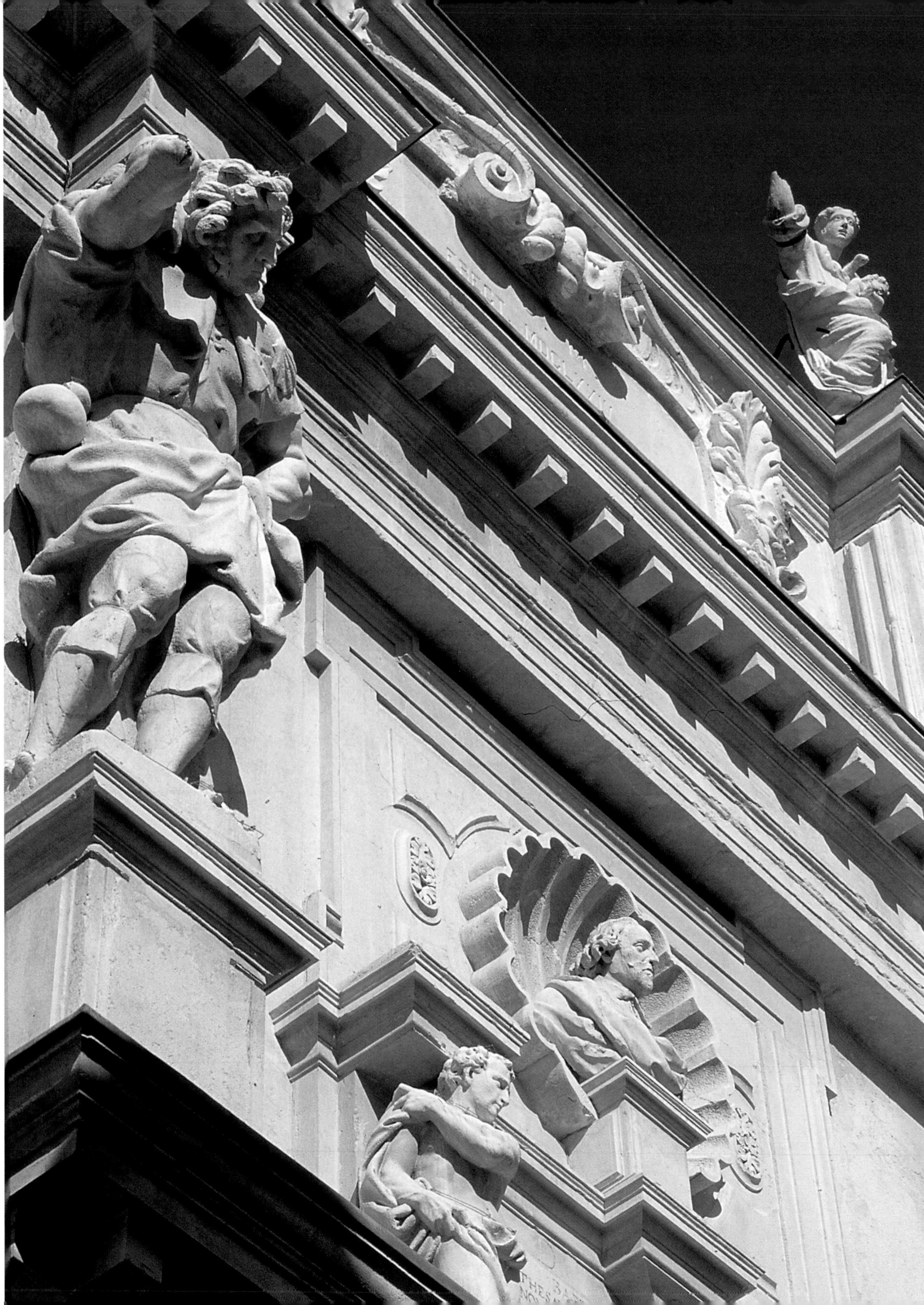

It cannot, however, compete with the conspicuous flair and dramatic inventiveness of Tiepolo's *Sacrifice of Isaac* (pl. 231). In his 1732 *Life of Lazzarini*, Vincenzo da Canal described how the youthful prodigy 'abandoned his master's painstaking manner, inasmuch as, all spirit and fire, he adopted one resolute and rapid'.[3] Both adjectives apply well to the image Tiepolo produced for the Ospedaletto, but they should not be taken to imply that he gave his theme only the swiftest consideration. He was, after all, obliged to struggle with the constraints of an unusually taxing arched space. This did not prevent him producing a strikingly original interpretation of his well-worn biblical material. Michael Levey pointed out that 'the deep curve of the canvas serves to suggest the top of the mountain on which both Abraham and Isaac recline'.[4] Tiepolo thereby turned this problematic picture-space to his own advantage, heightening the sense of vertiginous danger that confronts the hapless son.

The logs abandoned by Isaac jut violently from the ground beneath him like the elements in a sinister funeral pyre, and Abraham's sharp-pointed knife is shown perilously close to the youth's flesh. A second away from thrusting the blade into his beloved son, whose shoulder he clutches with desperate resolution, the hooded patriarch has the

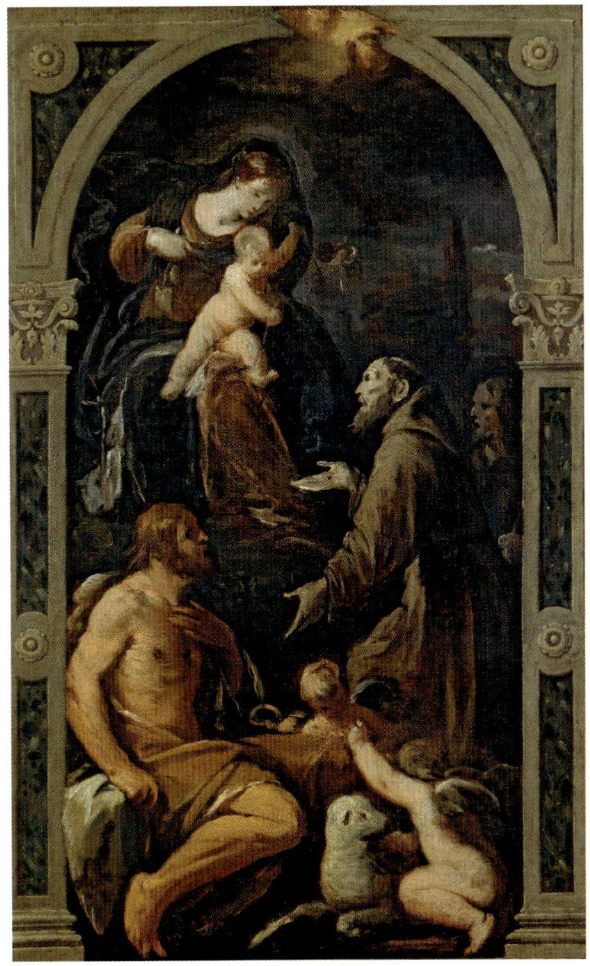

230 (*left*) Ermanno Stroiffi, Modello for altarpiece in Ospedaletto Church, *c.*1662, Ashmolean Museum, Oxford

231 (*below*) Giovanni Battista Tiepolo, *Sacrifice of Isaac*, 1716, Ospedaletto Church, Venice

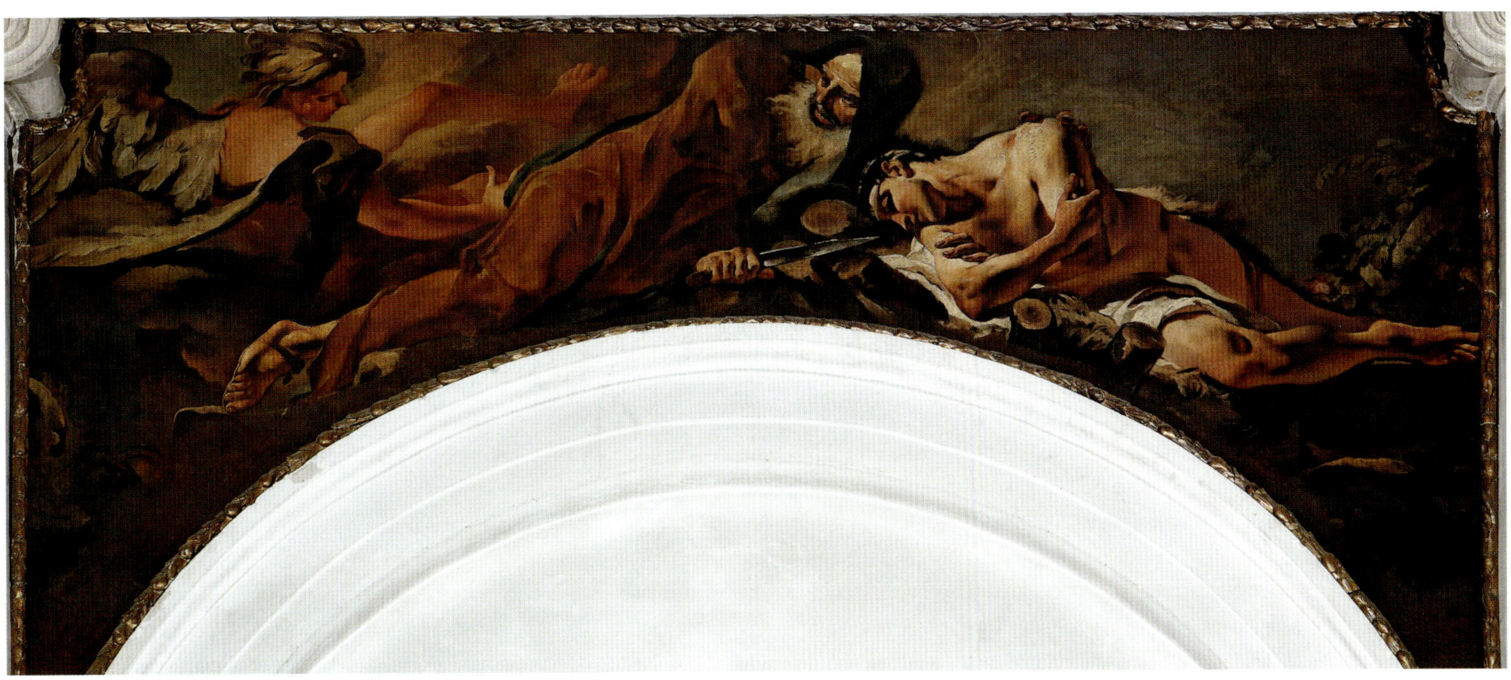

229 (*facing page*) Baldassare Longhena, Facade of Ospedaletto Church, Venice, 1660–74

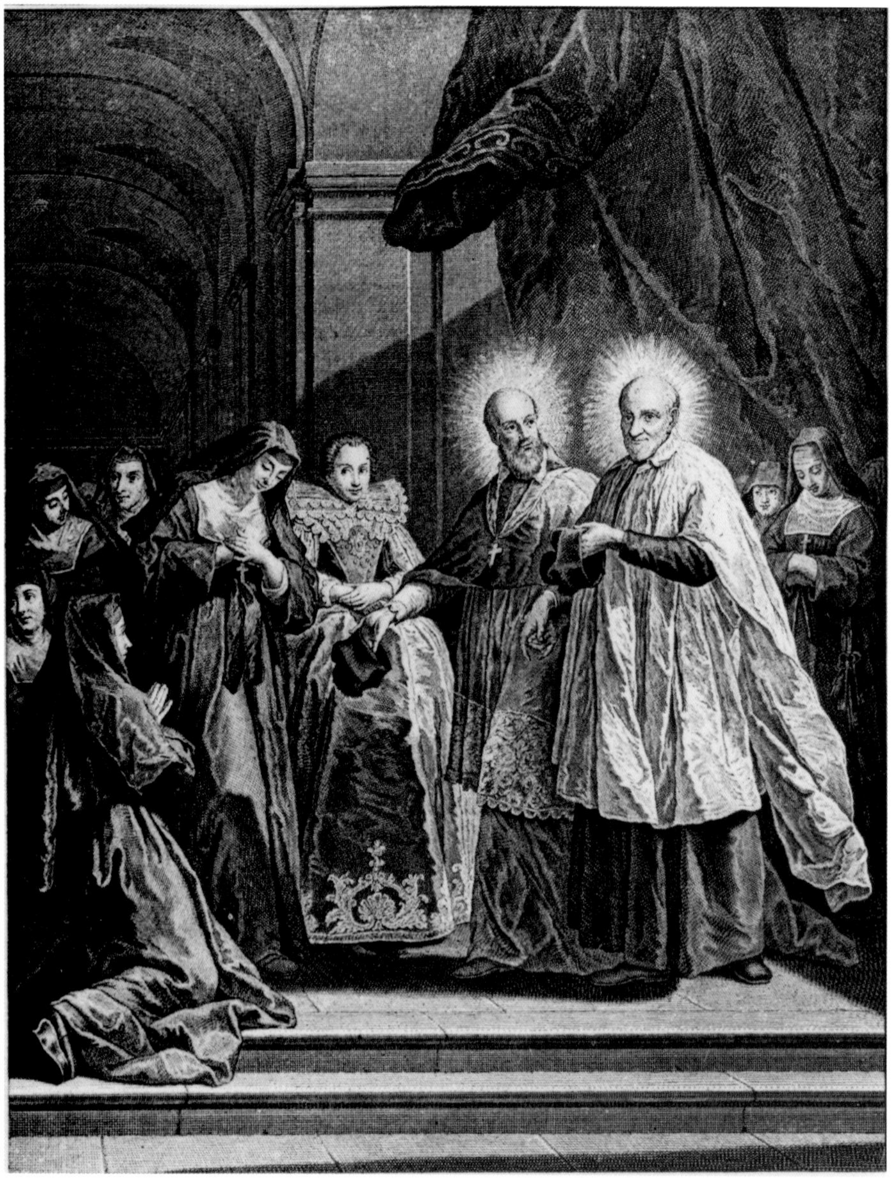

232 Jean Restout, *St Vincent de Paul with St Francois de Sales*, Hôpital de Saint-Lazare

hunched appearance of a man grievously ashamed of the sacrifice he is required to carry out. Although Tiepolo may have been forced by the space to make Abraham lean on the mountain, his pose is eloquent of an old man so distressed that his legs are no longer able to support him. There he lies, half stricken and half determined to obey the word of God. Almost as much of a victim as the son he is about to kill, he swings his head round with an understandable air of furtive guilt as the angel appears. The suddenness of the winged figure's advent is forcefully conveyed. Since Tiepolo had no room to include a more conventionally positioned angel, he once again capitalised on acute spatial limitations by portraying the messenger as a brusquely intrusive presence, reversing into the picture with upflung legs caught up in the slipstream created by his own velocity. This brilliant foreshortening stresses the extreme urgency of his quest, and Abraham gives a start as he registers the explosive intervention of God's emissary. He has not yet had time to realise the true, joyful significance of the angel's action and neither has Isaac.

Tiepolo handles the youth with equally superb insight (see pl. 228). Although he crosses his arms to protect his body from attack, Isaac simultaneously submits to his father's command. With head resting on shoulder in eerie mimicry of death, he appears to accept the inevitability of his fate. But this strangely peaceful figure could equally well have gone into a swoon, brought on by a terrified realisation of the doom about to overwhelm him. The ambiguity of Isaac's stance is movingly expressed and Tiepolo deploys an already consummate command of illumination and shadow to enhance the beauty of the son's body. Stretched out on the mountain with an almost supine deference, he personifies the athletic gracefulness of youth. His life therefore seems still more precious than it would normally have been, and the saving of it an act that acknowledges the unique value of an individual's being. Perhaps the context of the Ospedaletto affected Tiepolo's imaginative approach to the commission, encouraging him to stress in this powerfully felt painting the immeasurable sanctity of human existence.

The Venetians' concern for the welfare of foundlings was echoed by the tireless Saint Vincent de Paul in France. During the previous century his crusading emphasis on the need for pastoral care had been enormously influential, transforming the priorities of the French church and leading to the establishment of orphanages throughout the country. His beatification in 1729 prompted the Prêtres de la Maison, the congregation he had founded over a hundred years before, to celebrate the occasion by commissioning an elaborate cycle of paintings for their church. The Prêtres, who became known as the Lazaristes after they occupied the Hôpital de Saint-Lazare, did not stint over the implementation of their ambitious scheme. During the early 1730s eleven vast canvases were installed in the church, several by prominent artists of the day. The entire sequence gained even greater attention after engravings were made of them in 1737, to mark Vincent's formal admission to sainthood. He thereafter enjoyed the status of a national religious hero and the Lazaristes paintings disclosed the full extent of his multifarious activities. Jean-Baptiste Féret's canvas revealed how Saint Vincent anticipated the concerns of the Invalides by exhorting his supporters to look after soldiers wounded in battle, while Frère André emphasised his compassion for the poor in a painting of the saint preaching to a congregation afflicted by severe hardship.

Jean Restout, who had recently established his reputation as an eloquent religious painter with his dramatic yet restrained painting *The Death of Saint Scholastica*,[5] made perhaps the most memorable contribution to the scheme. His picture of Saint Vincent preaching to galley-slaves now survives only as an engraving but Restout's other canvas, *Saint Vincent de Paul with Saint François de Sales* (pl. 232), is preserved well enough to show how he responded with vivid actuality to the challenge of defining a man he had never met. Restout's sense of historical propriety, later instrumental in helping him to pursue an outstanding professional career culminating in the directorship of the Academie, is apparent throughout the picture. Every attempt has been made to arrive at a faithful representation of the clothes worn by the saints and the Dames de la Visitation, to whom Saint Vincent is being presented as an almoner by Saint François.

Although Restout's zeal for authenticity of costume reaches its height in the elaborate attire worn by Sainte Jeanne de Chantel, her brocaded stiffness looks somewhat uneasy in the centre of the composition. It contrasts unfavourably with the more supple movements of the nuns themselves, who react with gracious, flowing rhythms to the advent of Saint Vincent. He returns their cordial reception with a quirky geniality of his own, which shows how far Restout tried to go beyond a stereotyped image of his protagonist. Vincent here resembles a flesh-and-blood Frenchman rather than a remote archetype of piety. The glow of a nimbus round his head does not unduly detract from Restout's candid portrayal of a humane, smiling individual, who has no desire to aggrandise himself with ostentatious robes. Nor did Restout indulge in any of the rhetorical gestures that another, more flamboyant painter of the period might have wanted to brandish. Saint Vincent's innate humility is further conveyed by the understated colours deployed throughout the painting, its quiet harmony derived from subtle variations on the theme of white and grey.

Louis Galloche, another of the artists at the Saint-Lazare church, devoted his canvas to Saint Vincent instituting the Hôpital des Enfants-Trouvés. Then, nearly twenty years later, the same Hôpital consecrated a new chapel where a superlative marriage of painting and architecture was achieved. Although the structure of the building seemed straightforward, the interior was transformed into a delightful *tour de force* of illusionistic decoration. It was subsequently destroyed but not before Fessard published an engraving that showed just how thoroughgoing, resourceful and inventive the scheme had really been.

Germain Boffrand, the chapel's architect and one of the administrators of the Hôpital des Enfant-Trouvés, was responsible for proposing that the interior should be painted with scenes from the Nativity and the Adoration of Kings and Shepherds. He presumably hoped to imply that even children born in the least propitious of circumstances deserved cherishing, just as the infant Christ had been honoured in his cattle-shed. It was an inspired choice of subject, and a pamphlet printed to coincide with the chapel's opening in 1751 explained that Boffrand also hoped, like Hogarth at Bart's and the Foundling Hospital, to demonstrate how well French artists could handle architectural spaces if they were presented with the chance to decorate them.

The confidence with which Boffrand advanced this claim was well founded, for he had brought about an enchanting alliance of painting and architecture at the Hôtel de Soubise in Paris more than a decade before. There, on the walls of the Salon de la Princesse refurbished for the Prince de Rohan, he had arrived at a fusion of his own spirited design and Charles-Joseph Natoire's paintings. The canvases, depicting the story of Psyche, are exquisitely attuned to the rhythms, colours and light-hearted architectural play so evident in the rest of this delightful oval room. And Boffrand doubtless hoped that, with Natoire again by his side, the Enfant-Trouvés project could be as memorable.

Judging by the engraving that records the appearance of the chapel interior, his ambitions

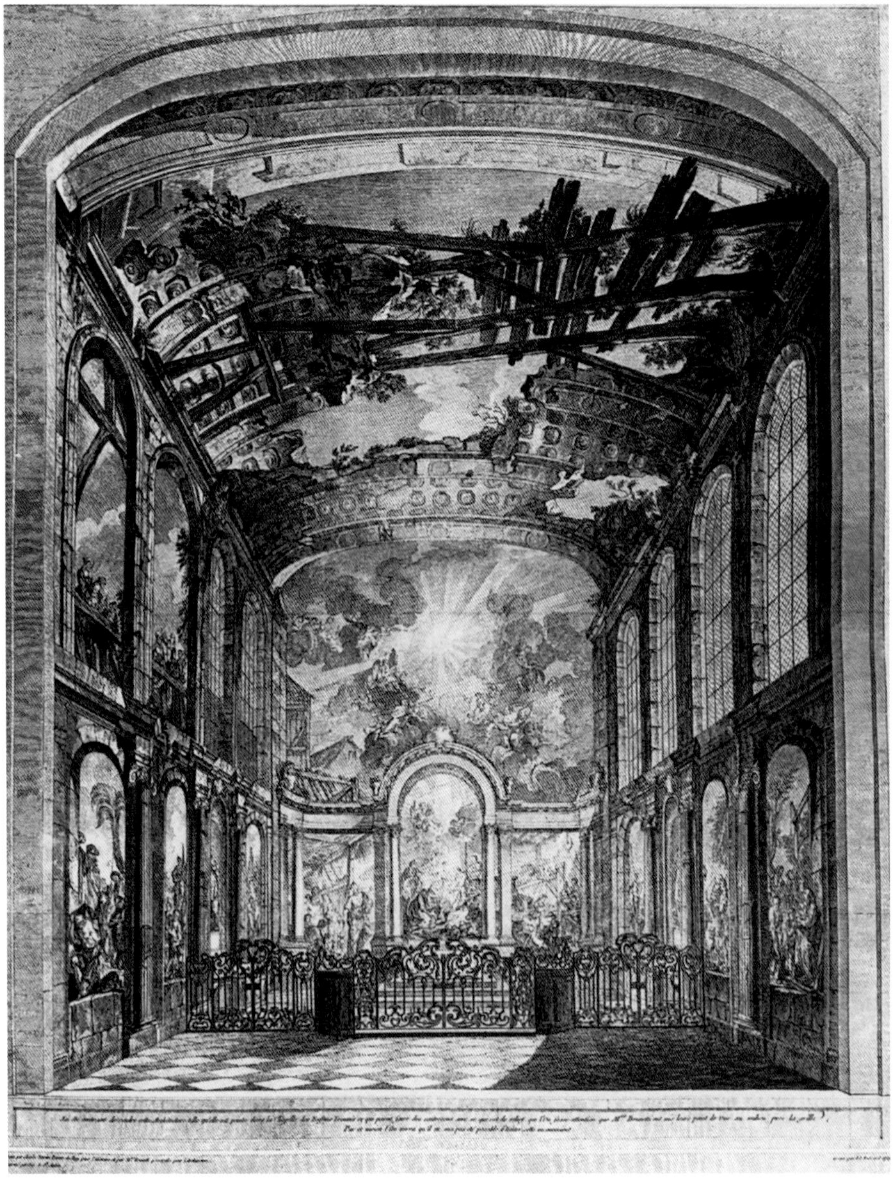

233 Etienne Fessard, Engraving of Chapel with wall paintings by Charles-Joesph Natoire, completed 1751 for the Hôpital des Enfant-Trouvés

were handsomely fulfilled (pl. 233). The architecture itself does not look as inventive as the Salon de la Princesse, but its simplicity is quite deliberate. It becomes the shell within which Natoire, assisted by the illusionistic skills of the Italian specialists Gaetano and Paolo Antonio Brunetti, produced a brilliantly deceptive painted environment more complete by far than the oval room at the Hôtel de Soubise. Indeed, the engraving indicates that their interior deserves to be ranked among the finest mural decorations in eighteenth-century Europe. With the Brunettis' cunning and expert help, a beguiling fictive architecture was painted on the walls of the chapel. Visitors entering the space found themselves in an immense classical ruin, its roof broken so severely that nothing more than a rudimentary network of wooden trusses remained in several places. They hang there precariously, ready at any instant to split, dislodge themselves and plummet to the floor. Weeds and other vegetation sprout from the fragments of coffered ceiling that still adhere to their original location, and they look equally doomed to collapse. Already the sky can be seen in large areas, and its prominence must have increased the feeling of vulnerability, of a barn-like space open to whatever damage storms were capable of inflicting.

Far from being merely a whimsical caprice, the riven ceiling could have been intended as a metaphor to underline the hardship undergone by so many of the children in the Hôpital. The roof's precarious state may even symbolise the danger that threatened them at infancy: if they had shelter at all, it was just as liable to fall in and crush them as the rickety beams and coffering so cleverly simulated on the ceiling of the Enfants-Trouvés chapel. Boffrand and Natoire did not, however, want their interior simply to reflect the most hazardous aspects of a foundling's life. They aimed, in the rest of this deftly manipulated environment, at an affirmation. Lit by four tall plain-glass windows on the first floor of the right wall, the murals offered a far more heartening view of babyhood. Below the windows, a row of ample panels gave the advancing shepherds a festive and processional air, as if to acknowledge the importance of the event in the most heightened manner imaginable. On the opposite wall this triumphant mood was reinforced by the panels depicting the journey of the Kings, travelling through an exotic landscape punctuated by Tiepolesque palm trees. Visitors, accompanied at either side of the chapel by these representatives of humanity at its humblest and most exalted, could therefore walk towards the altar like first-hand observers of the Nativity themselves.

The cumulative rhythm created by the wall panels must have been compelling, as it drove worshippers onwards until the choir was reached. There, beyond the convoluted ironwork screen, *grisaille* figures of Vincent de Paul and Genevieve, the chapel's two patron saints, joined the adoring throng from their vantages in niches bordering the altar. They both resembled statues, presumably in order to differentiate them from the level of reality inhabited by the shepherds and kings. However, the three panels on the lower half of the altar wall represented the Adoration of the Magi in a blaze of uninhibited colour once again. The stable where they honour the infant was as dilapidated as the broken architecture simulated on the chapel roof. All the same, Natoire countered the wretchedness of the baby's surroundings with a joyful, heart-warming interpretation of the Nativity. The altar-piece in the centre rose into an arched top, its greater height accentuating the heavenly dimension of this central scene. Above, an ecstatic Glory opened out to cover the width of the end wall, filling the vastness with a soaring, visionary painting where cloud-borne angels laud the holy birth among shafts of flaring sunlight.

The most moving aspect of this remarkable decoration, though, was located away from the impressive pictorial climax over the altar. On the wall leading up to the choir, above the panels where the Kings processed with such flamboyant zest, Natoire and the Brunettis painted a rustic balustrade across two panels. Behind it the figures of nuns and children were shown, staring down in wonder towards the miraculous event (pl. 234). Since they were placed directly opposite the first-floor windows that provided illumination for the entire chapel, this Veronese-like cluster of excited witnesses would have been clearly visible to anyone surveying the interior. Their presence there, in a prominent position so near the source of awe, demonstrated the Hôpital's clear commitment to its staff and foundlings alike. All the painted decoration in this chapel was dedicated to involving worshippers more completely in the implications of Christ's birth, and the decision to depict orphans within the illusionistic scheme must have fortified the real orphans enormously when they gazed around, in wonder, at this captivating celebration of hope for humanity as a whole.

Over in Ireland, a similar sense of awe and excitement was generated by the chapel of Dublin's radical Lying-in Hospital, designed by Richard Castle just before he died in 1751. Also known as the Rotunda because of the assembly room next to it, this pioneering building became the first maternity hospital to be erected anywhere in Britain. Its founder, Bartholomew Mosse, was as determined and ambitious as Captain Coram. Intended for poor

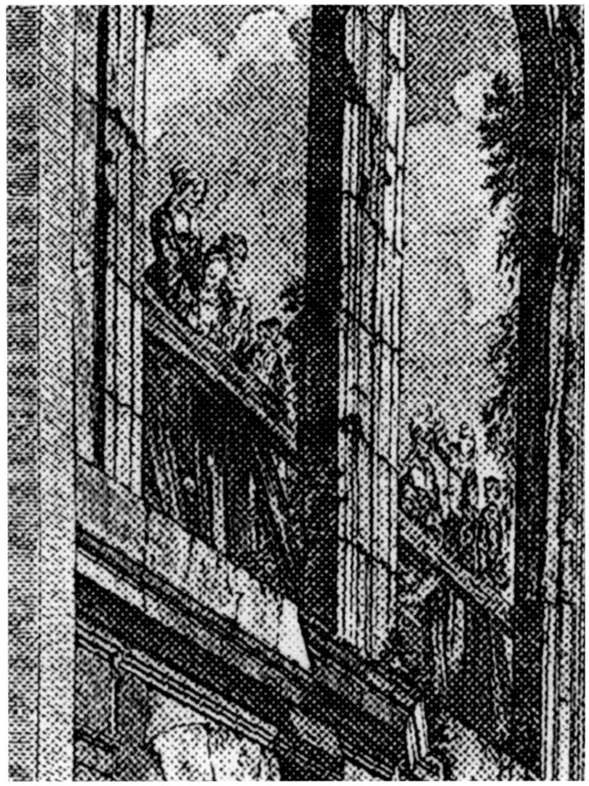

234 Detail of pl. 233

pregnant women, the Lying-in Hospital occupied a site in a remote, north-eastern area of the city. But Castle designed a grand neo-Palladian structure, with colonnaded quadrants leading from the central block. It was set in four acres of garden that played a key role in the replanning of Dublin during the late eighteenth century (pl. 235). According to Mrs Delany, the garden became the city's equivalent of the fashionable pleasure-centres at 'Vauxhall and Ranalagh.'[6] No less than six hundred elms were planted there by Robert Stevenson and the gardens opened to the public with great acclaim in 1749.

Eight years later the Lying-in Hospital was completed by the architect John Ensor, who faithfully adhered to Richard Castle's original plans. If Mosse's hopes had been more than fulfilled by the fashionable success of the gardens, he was frustrated in his plan to instal two monumental statues by John van Nost, 'to be Brunz'd in Gold',[7] on the building's end pavilions. Inside the Hospital, however, the chapel became a place of uninhibited Rococo delight. The first patients discovered, after making their way through the Palladian entrance hall with its imposing columns and pilasters, that the staircase hall was lavishly

235 (*right*) Richard Castle, Lying-in Hospital, Dublin, 1751–7

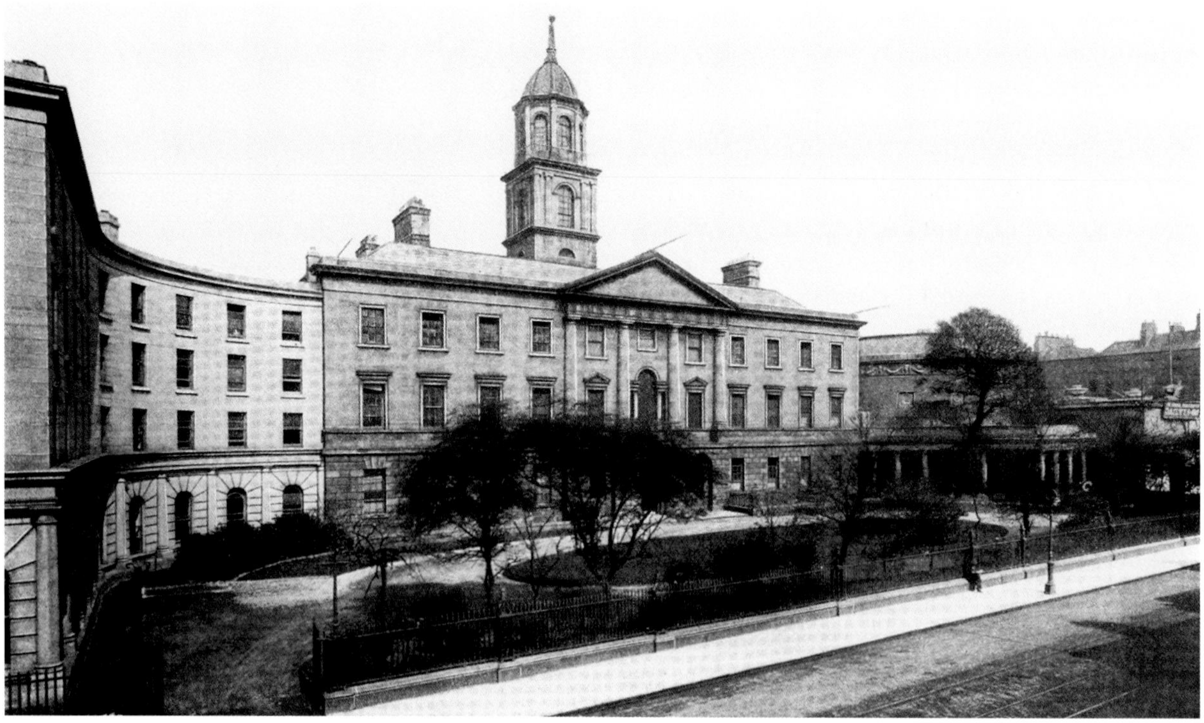

236 (*below left*) Bartholomew Cramillion, Ceiling Stuccowork, 1755, in Lying-in Hospital, Dublin

237 (*below right*) Bartholomew Cramillion, East Wall stuccowork, 1757, in Lying-in Hospital, Dublin

embellished with stucco and wrought iron. Yet nothing could have prepared them for the astonishing *coup de théâtre* in the chapel, adorned with what Edward McParland has described as 'the finest stuccowork in the country' (pl. 236).[8] Executed with great panache by Bartholomew Cramillion, an elusive plasterworker who left no clear evidence of any achievements elsewhere, it

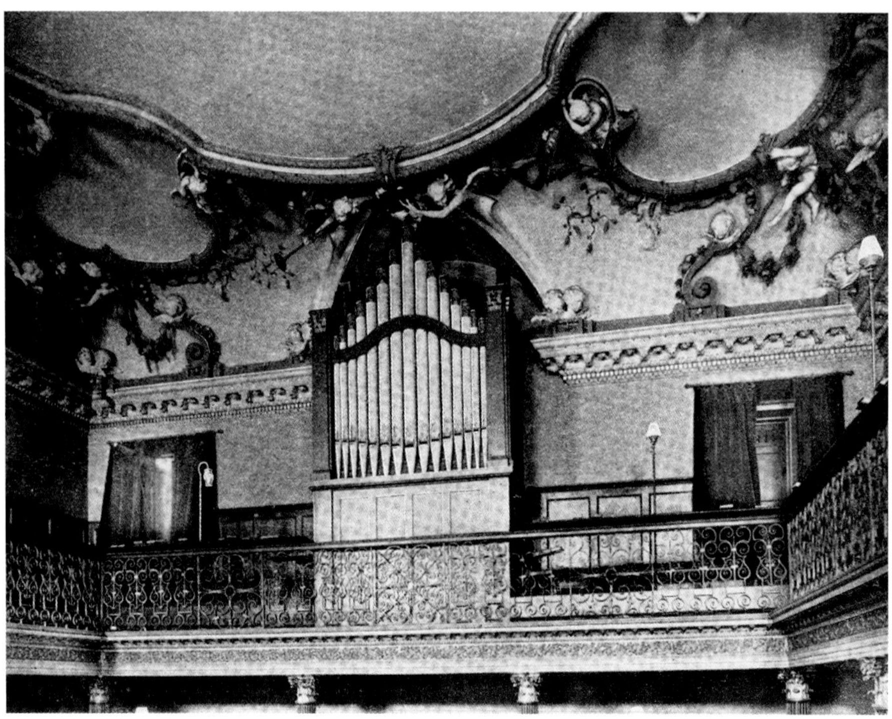

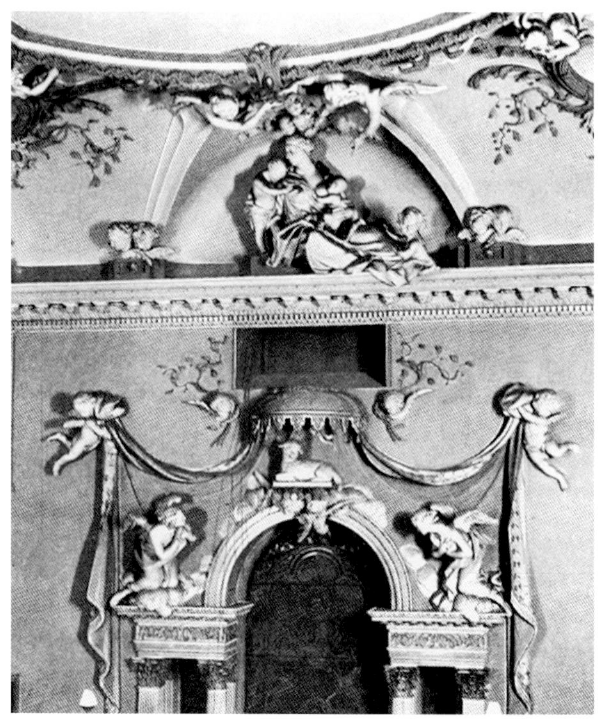

turned the ceiling and east wall into a lyrical display of airborne energy and love.

Mosse never succeeded in commissioning the ceiling paintings he discussed with Giovanni Battista Cipriani, but the chapel decorations are a triumph. He ensured that twenty thousand leaves of gold were used for 'Gilding the Corinthian Collumns & Pillasters the Capitals & Bases & the Whole Entablature',[9] while Cramillion was probably given considerable creative licence in the execution of his sprightly stucco figures. When the chapel was formally opened, the indignant preacher asked: 'why such Grandeur? Relieve these poor Objects, tis Right, but why in a Palace?'[10] Mosse knew, however, that the resplendent, double-height interior would attract fashionable donors and he wanted Dublin society to feel beguiled there by 'sacred Oratorios'.[11] He had already organised a fund-raising performance of Handel's *Hester* in 1746 and music played a remunerative part in adding to 'the Yearly Income of the Hospital'[12] for many decades.

In this respect, the Lying-in may well have taken its inspiration from London's Foundling venture, where fund-raising chapel concerts were likewise regularly staged. The two Hospitals shared the same president, the Duke of Bedford, and the iconography of Cramillion's stuccowork displays an emphasis on children that echoes Coram's most abiding concerns. All round the ceiling buoyant babies can be detected, holding garlands of flowers even richer than Tabary's wood carvings in the chapel at Kilmainham (see pl. 162). The international standard of excellence achieved at the Royal Hospital was inspirational throughout eighteenth-century Dublin, and nowhere more delightfully than in Cramillion's masterpiece. Ecstatic infants and angels are interwoven with undulating swags and sprays across this supremely festive ceiling. Above the east wall, they gather round a niche where a seated mother clasps her contented offspring. Directly below, winged putti draw a curtain behind adoring angels who flank the Lamb of God (pl. 237). The Hospital's impoverished pregnant patients would all have been gratified to discover, beneath the Lamb, two robust babies lodged at the apex of the window illuminating the rest of this spellbinding interior.

Music-making was even more important in the new Venetian church of the ancient Santa Maria della Visitazione, called the Pietà (pl. 238). As its compassionate name suggests, it was an institution originally dedicated to the care of orphans. An inscription can still be found near the church, spelling out the grave consequences that awaited any parents who handed over their children to the foundation without genuine economic duress. Once the orphans had been admitted, they were looked after well and trained to sing in an excellent choir. The Pietà was held to be foremost among the conservatoires attached to the four Venetian Ospedali, and Antonio Vivaldi had been instrumental in creating its reputation. He wrote for the female orphans, providing them with concertos, masses and oratorios that helped a great deal to enhance the Pietà's fame as a first-class centre for music-making. Singing under Vivaldi's direction for the best part of half a century, between 1703 and 1745, the foundling girls enchanted observers with their ability and appearance alike. Writing in his *Lettres familières sur l'Italie*, the Président des Brosses could not decide which he appreciated more ardently – the choir's musical expertise or the attractiveness of the beautiful young orchestra leader with her flower-garlanded hair.

As if determined to take his cue from the choir's inspiration, Giorgio Massari seems to have designed the new church with a musical stimulus firmly in his mind. The interior of the Pietà, completed in 1750 after five years' construction, looks more like a concert auditorium than a full-blown ecclesiastical environment (pl. 239) and performances are regularly held there to this day. The cool discipline that informs Massari's handling of the space acts as an ideal architectural counterpart to the stringent elegance of Vivaldi's music. A similar desire for rigour led the Pietà's governors to decide that they did not want their building painted as comprehensively as the Chapelle des Enfants-Trouvés in Paris (see pl. 233). When they approached Tiepolo around 1753, he was invited to produce frescoes only for the principal vault and two smaller spaces. The rest of the ceiling would remain unadorned and the canvases commissioned from other artists were restricted to the four altars at the curved corners of the oval interior – apart, of course, from the culminating high altarpiece which occupied a recessed space of its own. Piazzetta, who had been admired by the youthful Tiepolo and connected with him in the decoration of previous Venetian churches, was supposed to provide the high altar with a painting of *The Visitation*, but he

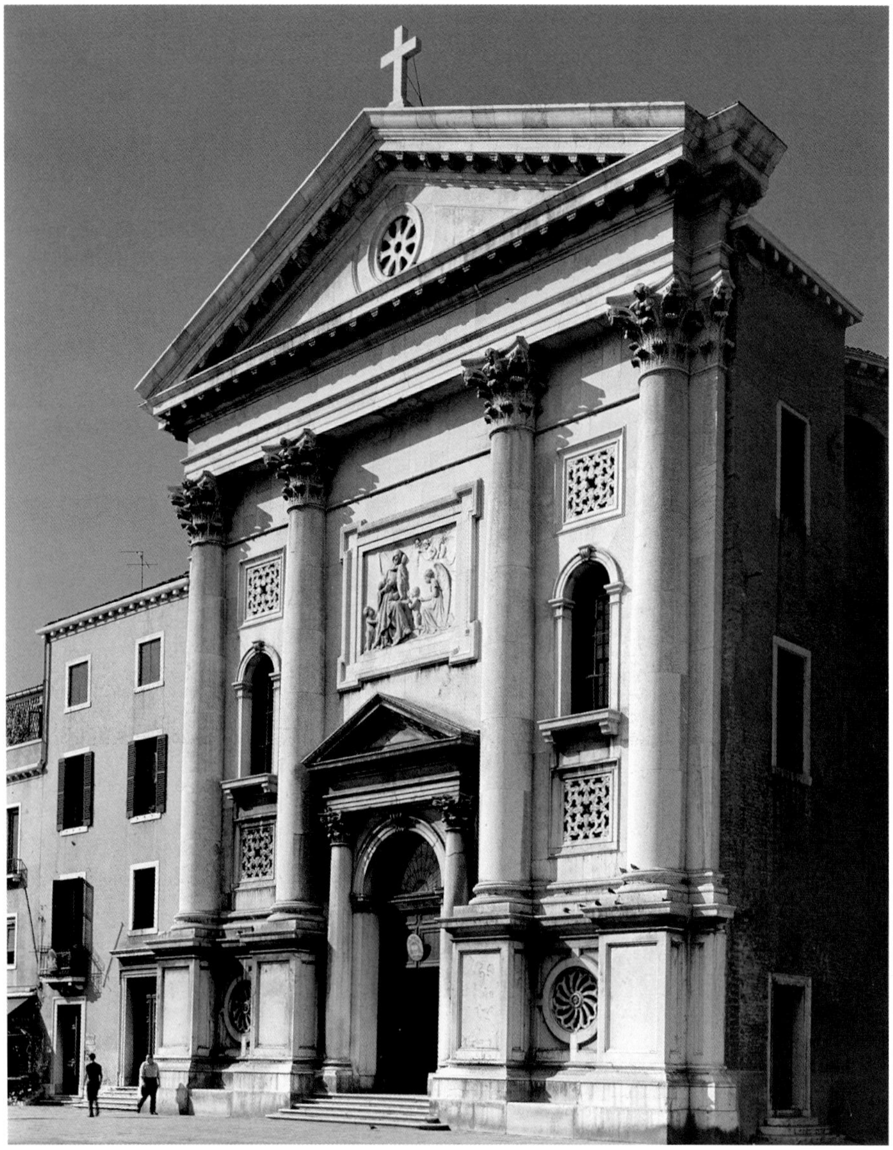

238 (*above*) Giorgio Massari, Facade of the Church of Santa Maria della Pietà, 1745–50, Venice

239 (*facing page*) Giorgio Massari, Interior of the Church of Santa Maria della Pietà, 1745–50, Venice

died before its completion. His pupil Giuseppe Angeli had to finish the canvas as well as executing an altarpiece of his own for a corner altar donated by Doge Francesco Loredan. The opposite altarpiece, depicting a miracle performed by Saint Spiridon, was also painted by another artist who had studied under Piazzetta, Domenico Maggiotto. They are both respectable paintings and satisfyingly attuned to the architectural character of the interior they embellish. But, as Hugh Honour has observed, these corner altarpieces 'by minor masters of the *settecento* seem tame indeed'[13] compared with the pyrotechnics displayed on the surfaces where Tiepolo's frescoes hold sway.

The restraint governing this pale interior provides a discreet foil for his supremely spirited contributions, even if they start quietly enough above the high altar with a grisaille wall-roundel where King David is visited by an angel. Nearby, the ceiling carries a fresco of *Faith, Hope and Charity*, (pl. 240) a theme whose relevance to the aims of the Pietà orphanage was clear enough. Tiepolo here appears to be stressing the importance of nurturing an independent outlook among the foundlings, for the child supported by Charity insists on standing proudly erect. Surely based on the artist's own scrutiny of a particular model, this alert offspring is depicted with conviction and seems eminently capable of playing a part, when the time comes, in the musical activities of the Pietà foundation.

Quite understandably, Tiepolo reserved his most prodigious powers of invention for the great oval in the high ceiling of the church's main interior (pl. 241). Antonio Morassi supposed that the Pietà's songs 're-echoed through the mind of the artist when he was thinking out the composition of the fresco',[14] and the painting indeed contains plentiful references to the orphans' musical prowess. The two swaying balconies that erupt at the base and apex of the oval provide a context for the ethereal proceedings above, where the Triumph of Faith is personified by the *Coronation of the Virgin*. Performers throng the balcony areas, peering down at the congregation while brandishing their instruments in a spirit of infectious gusto. They inhabit the lofty perches with insouciance, dangling their limbs over the side or leaning back almost cheekily as they perform on violin, organ and lute.

The sheer exuberance of music-making produces, at times, an intoxicated mood. Halfway round the oval's left side, where the balcony dwindles to a slender curve, a trumpeter is represented only by an insolent leg resting on the edge. This holiday mood is sustained at the top of the fresco as well. An uninhibited cellist, her draperies hitched up to the thigh, straddles the balcony while playing with vigorous aplomb. Nearby, a group of girl singers clustered behind their score perform so wholeheartedly that an angel seems to be flapping his wings in ecstatic appreciation of their voices.

While all this rippling, darting and tumbling activity plays around the perimeter of Tiepolo's oval, celebrating the Pietà's renowned concerts with all the fervency at his disposal, a far more

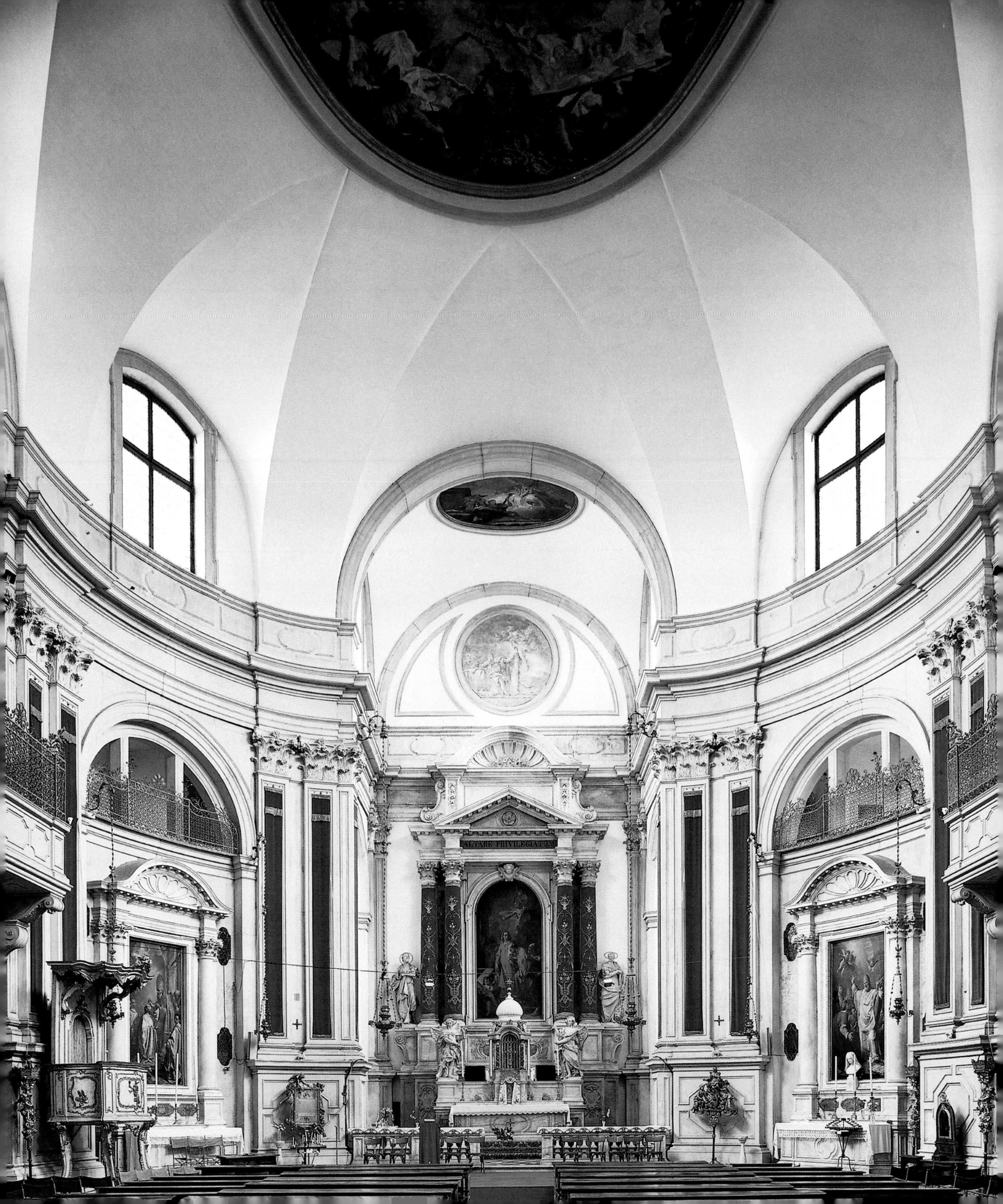
ALTARE PRIVILEGIATUM

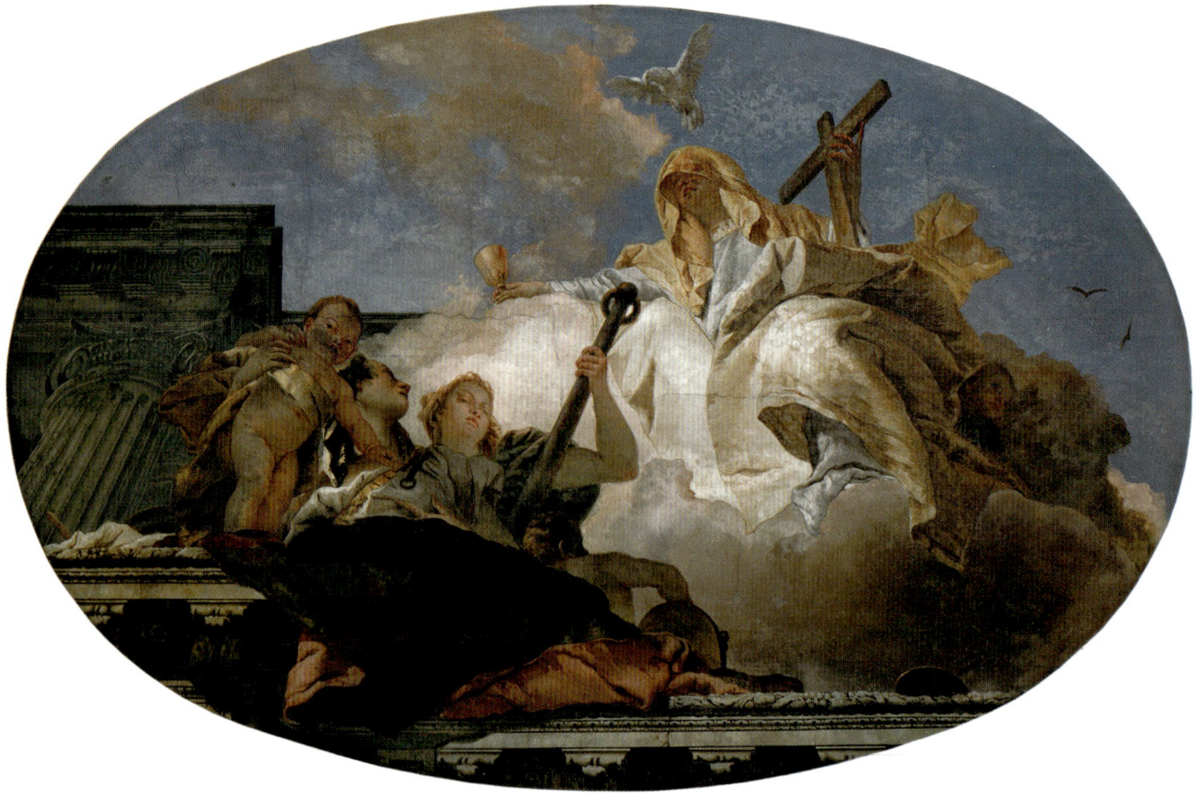

240 Giovanni Battista Tiepolo, *Faith, Hope and Charity*, 1754, Church of Santa Maria della Pietà, Venice

transcendent event takes place above. It is no less giddily exhilarating. Surrounded by a proliferation of angels, who dive over each other in their eagerness to honour and support her swaying body, the Virgin balances precariously on the side of the globe. Without the help of her boisterous attendants, and the clouds that buttress the group even more reassuringly, she might have been in danger of falling. Poise triumphs, however; and the Virgin's ample shawl seems to be billowing around her head, as if impelled by an irresistible rush of movement towards God the Father. Drastically foreshortened, so that his body is half-obscured in the plethora of beating wings and expansive clouds around him, the bearded patriarch is nevertheless able to exert an imperious hold over the Virgin.

The crown he holds aloft, near the blazing form of a dove transfigured by beams of light, appears to be pulling her up from the globe towards a mystical union in the heavens. Christ, grasping his cross at one side, honours the overriding power of this ascendance by gesturing in the crown's direction as well. Even so, Tiepolo ensures that the jostling excitement centring on the Virgin's progress does not lead to a sense of intolerable congestion. The upper half of the frescoed oval, whose complete form felicitously echoes Massari's plan for the church, is given over to a limpid sky largely devoid of figures. Here, in the light-saturated empyrean, the rapturous activities of music-making and crowning are both dissolved in a region of radiance alone.

With this sublime ceiling, which according to Pietro Gradenigo was 'made visible'[15] in August 1755, Tiepolo brought his prolonged sequence of Venetian religious frescoes to an exalted conclusion. His benevolence towards the Pietà was demonstrated a couple of years later by his generous loan to the governors. Although it must have helped them in their struggle to pay for the church, Massari's initial proposal to flank the church with the Hospital's two wings was never realised.[16]

Financial constraints did not, however, prevent a similar institution elsewhere in Venice from commissioning another distinguished decorative scheme twenty years later. The Ospedaletto, where the young Tiepolo had worked in the church with

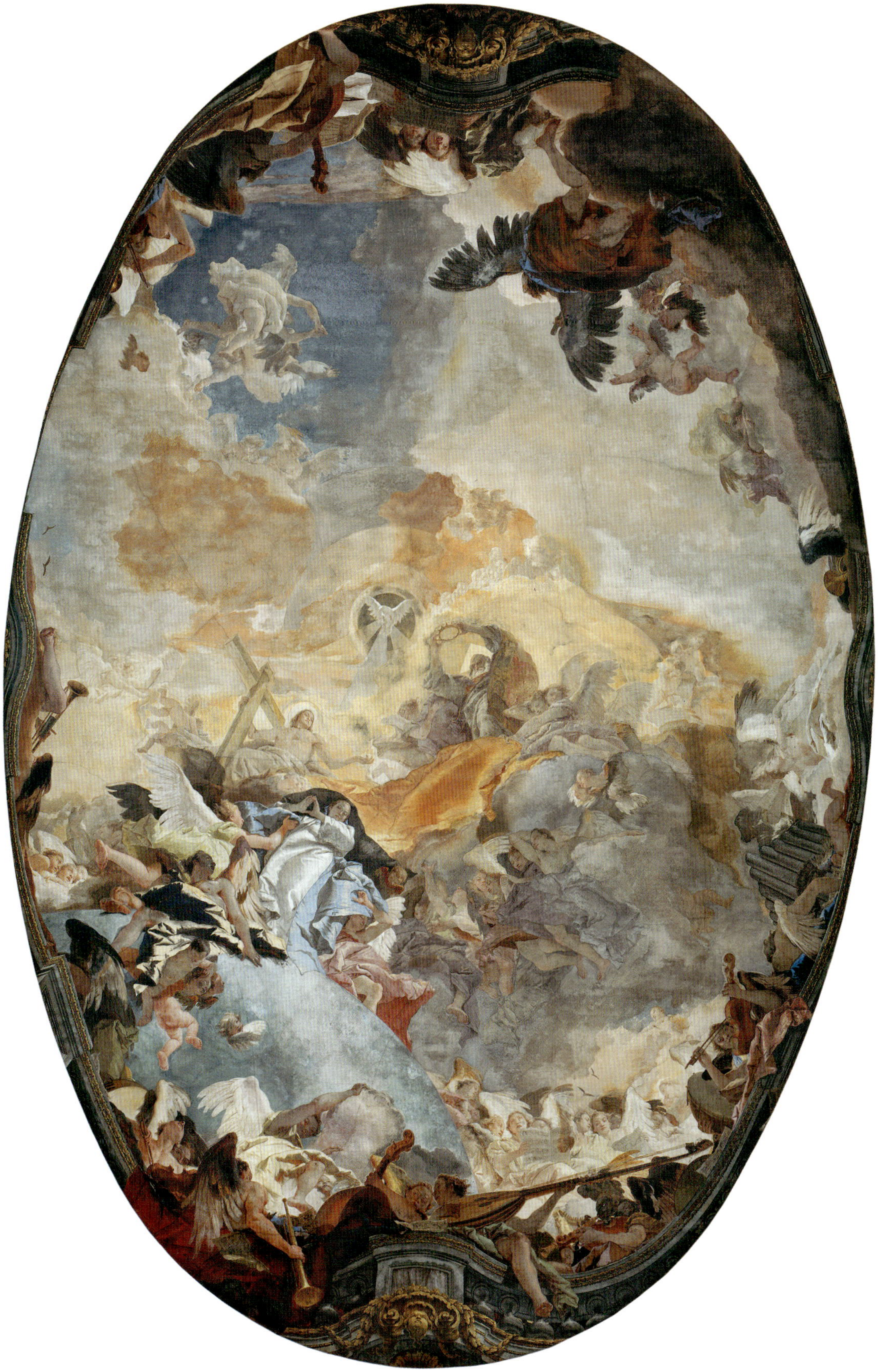

241 Giovanni Battista Tiepolo, *Coronation of the Virgin*, 1754–5, Church of Santa Maria della Pietà, Venice

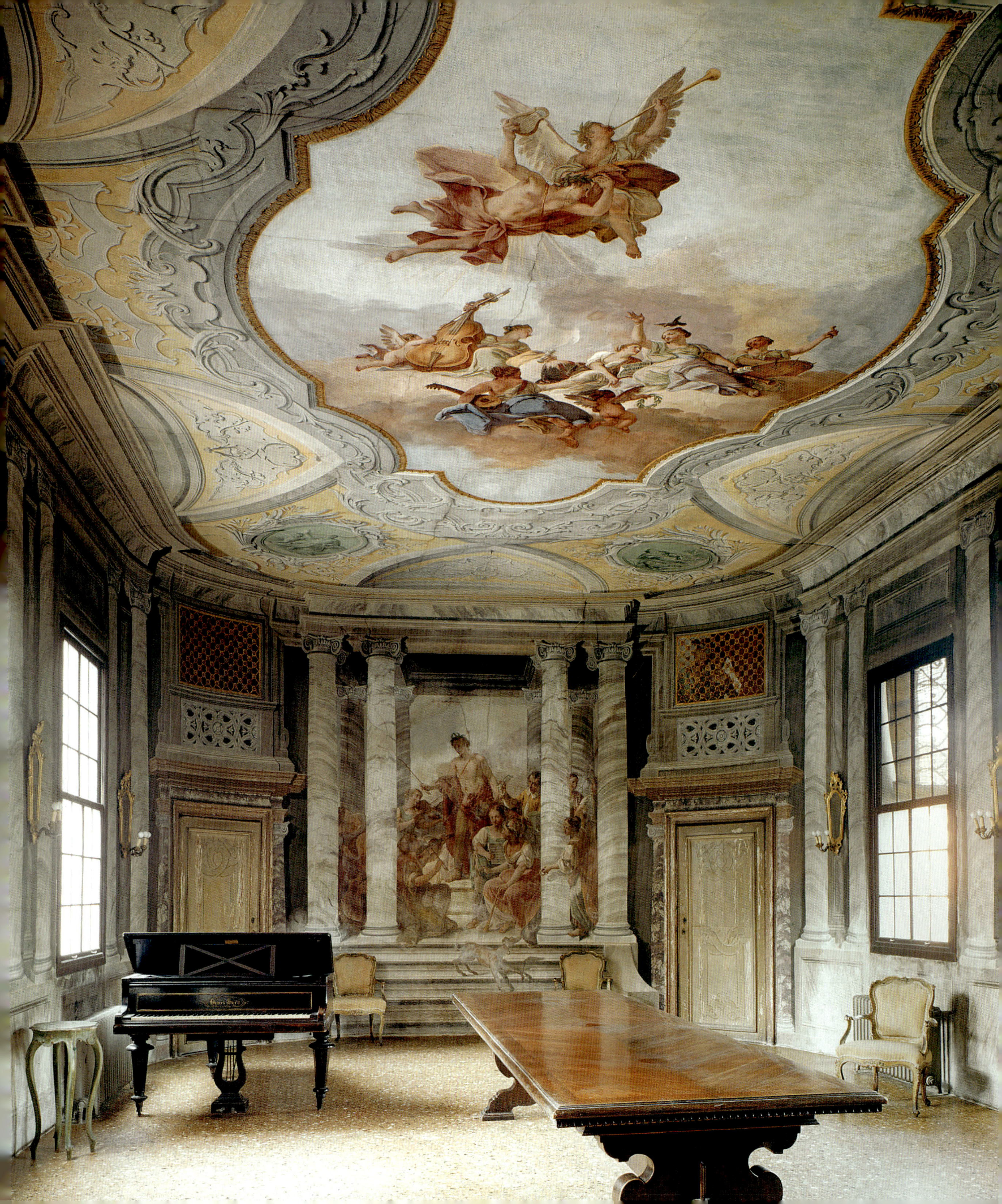

such brilliance at the beginning of his career (see pl. 231), likewise boasted a renowned conservatoire. Indeed, the Président des Brosses, who enthusiastically compared the girl choirs in all four of the Ospedali with the singing of angels, believed that Anna Maria at the Ospedaletto was among the finest violinists in Italy. As for Rousseau, he confessed that 'I cannot imagine anything so voluptuous, so touching as this music' and rapturously described how 'every Sunday . . . during Vespers, motets are performed with full orchestra, composed and conducted by the most famous Italian masters, executed in the latticed galleries by young girls only, all under twenty years of age.'[17]

Realising no doubt that their church was now replete with altarpieces and other images, the Ospedaletto governors turned in 1776 to the creation of a sublime music room (pl. 242). It became one of the most delightful manifestations of *settecento* decoration in Venice, and was an ideal setting for the celebrated concerts performed there by the children of the institution. Agostino Mengozzi-Colonna was commissioned to produce the *trompe l'oeil* architectural setting that gives the Sala della Musica so much of its light-hearted charm. Benefiting from the immense experience gained by his father when collaborating on similar projects with Tiepolo, he painted double columns between the windows. They established a perfect airy avenue leading the eye to the fresco on the end wall. There, under a Palladian-style portico that gives the double columns an even more persuasive reality than before, an allegory of music was painted by Tiepolo's pupil Jacopo Guarana (pl. 243).

Since the simulated architecture in this scene chimes so well with the rest of the Sala della Musica and the fresco extends downwards as far as the floor, Guarana's gossamer fantasy appears to be an extension of the oval room. It invites the viewer to enter an ideal region, where the sensuous, pink-robed Apollo conducts equally alluring female music-makers with an expression of blithe concentration. His performers, assembled round the plinth where he stands, play on their violins from the score of the aria 'Combatteremo insieme', written by the Maestro Pasquale Anfossi. He helps the proceedings along behind the women, partly obscured by a column and yet clearly an integral part of the company.[18]

While this spirited concert runs its course, other figures introduce a more humorous mood. The dog who casts such a persuasive, albeit cartoon-like shadow on the illusionistic steps threatens to disrupt the harmony of the players above. In an attempt to lead him away from the performers, a woman emerges from behind a pillar and holds out a doughnut to the animal. He pauses, attracted by the proferred reward for good behaviour; and Guarana allows the reverberations of this witty episode to continue over the door at the right of the fresco. There, half-hidden by a grille painted in collaboration with Mengozzi-Colonna, two conspiratorial women spy smilingly down on the antics below.

Their droll presence is so subtly handled that they only become apparent after careful scrutiny. Guarana knew, however, that the audiences attending concerts at the Sala della Musica would have plenty of time to scrutinise his work and enjoy discovering its playful felicities as the performance continued. The whole ingenious treatment of this end wall shows how blithely Guarana and Mengozzi-Colonna entered into the spirit of the context. Just as Veronese had not hesitated to spice even his most ambitious and carefully orchestrated scenes with profane, even irreverent details, so the wall fresco in the music room blends gracious allegory with everyday comedy in a delightful manner.

A more decorous approach is adopted on the ceiling, where four side ovals accompany a large central representation of the *Triumph of Music*. Concert instruments are again in evidence, floating weightlessly on clouds that support a cluster of female figures with equal ease. Two angels hover over them, blowing a trumpet and plucking a lyre respectively. They address themselves to their tasks with dedication, while the birds above appear to be closing in a union made all the more harmonious by the music they can hear. For all its demonstration of joy, though, the *Triumph of Music* lacks the sly fusion of solemnity and comedy in the Apollo fresco. The principal group of women seems conceived in a more dutiful mood, as if Guarana knew that most viewers' attention would be focused, not on the ceiling but on the wall ahead.

So it was there, against the lightest of cloudless Venetian skies, that his masterpiece was painted, providing the girls' choir with an irresistible picto-

242 (*facing page*) Agostino Mengozzi-Colonna, and Jacopo Guarana, Music Room, Ospedaletto, Venice, 1776

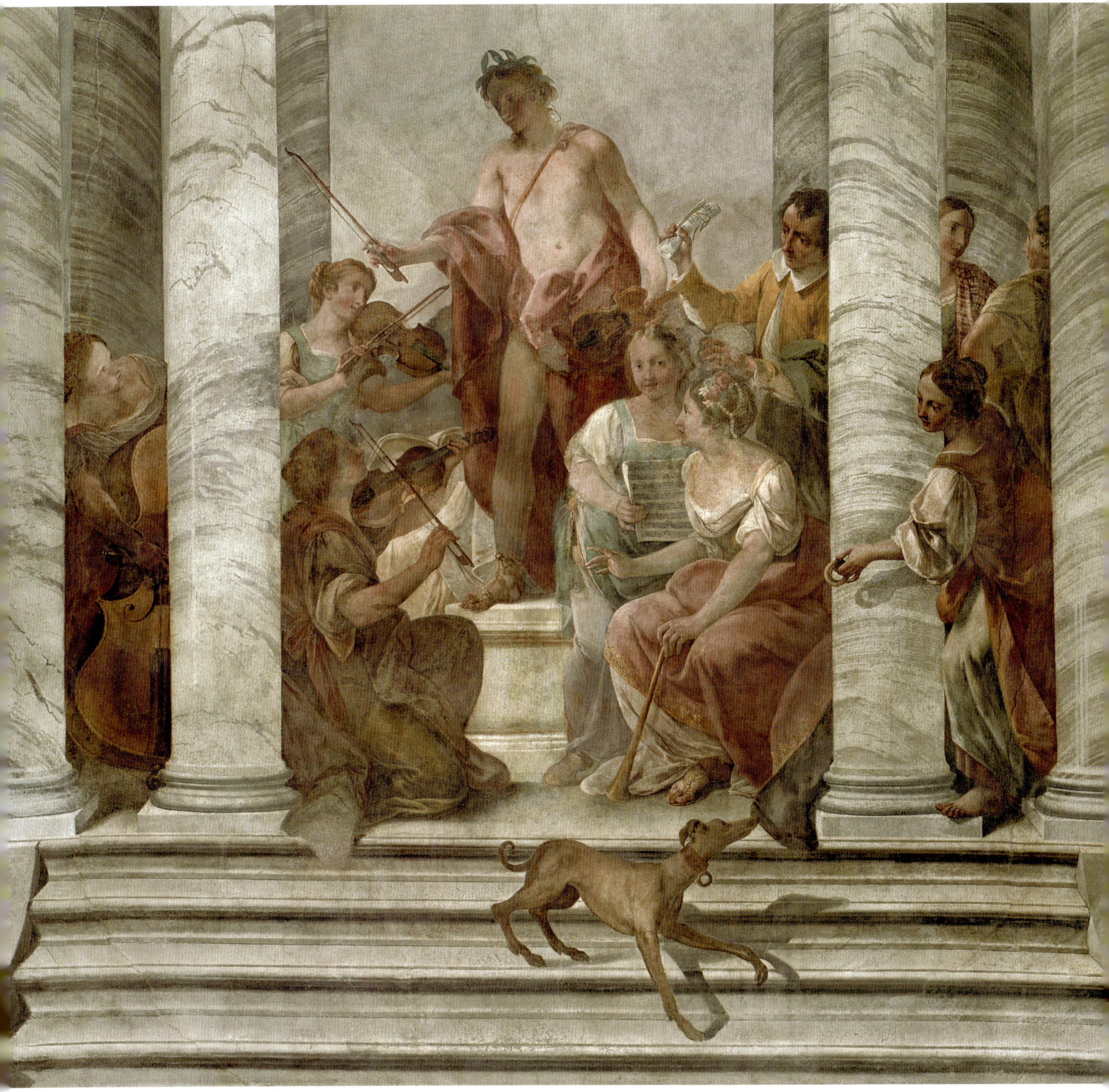

rial accompaniment. Little known and for a long time poorly preserved, the Apollo fresco and Mengozzi-Colonna's deceptive setting add up to a spirited illusionistic interior. It acts as a worthy coda to the great sequence of related fresco schemes carried out in Venice for very different patrons over the preceding two centuries. With hindsight, Guarana's fresco can now be seen as one of the final manifestations of a playful era, about to be abruptly replaced by a far more troubled and revolutionary alternative.

243 (*facing page*) Jacopo Guarana, *Allegory of Music*, 1776, Music Room, Ospedaletto, Venice

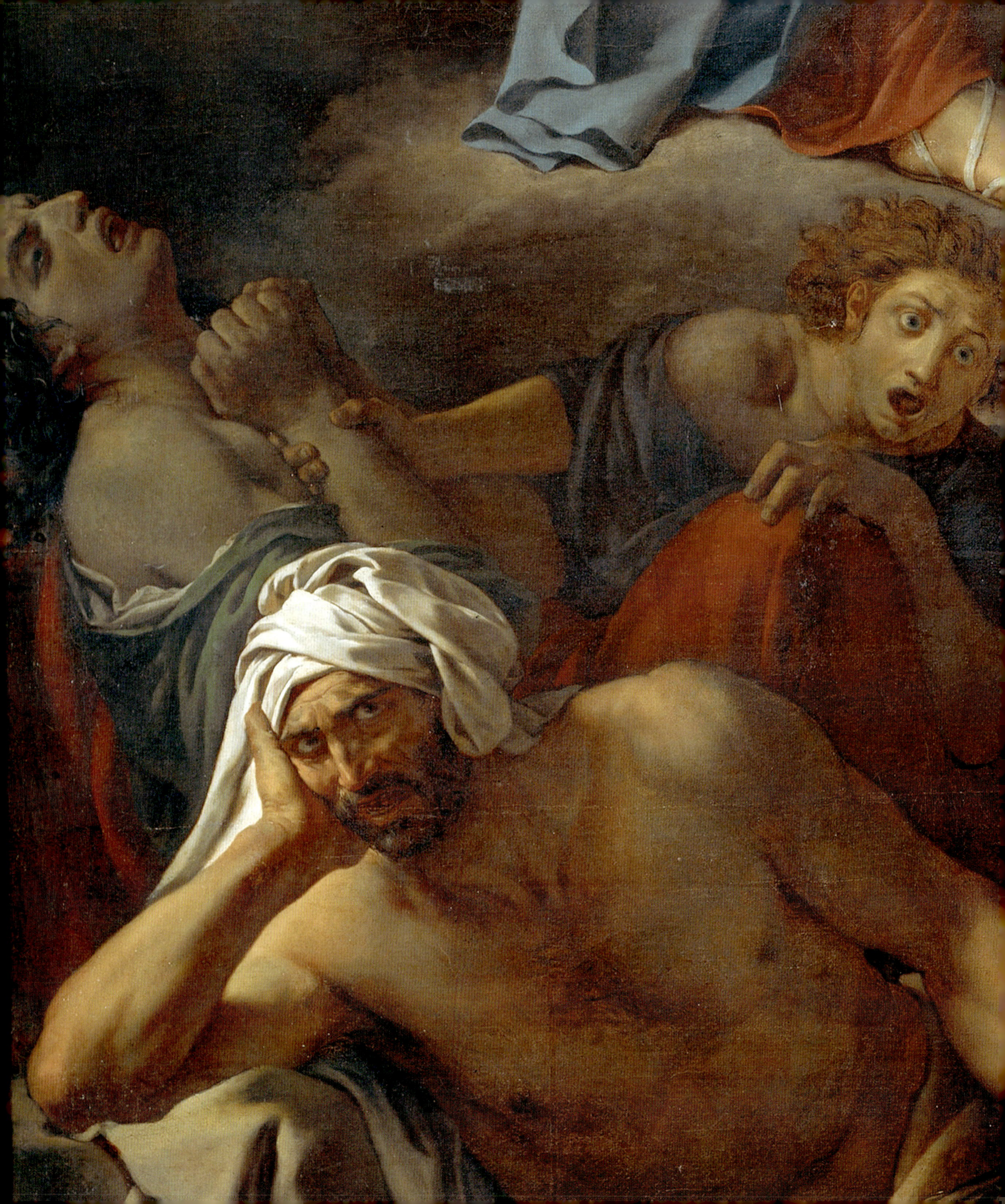

SEVENTEEN
PESTILENCE AND THE PHYSIOGNOMY OF MADNESS

Jacques-Louis David, one of the most zealous proponents of a disturbing new post-Rococo era, responded with typical directness when he received his first major commission from the Office of the Marseilles Health Service. He started work on the project in the autumn of 1779, only three years after the Sala della Musica was completed in Venice (see pl. 242). But the difference in attitude between his stark painting and Guarana's genial caprice is symptomatic of the profound, convulsive changes then galvanising European culture. The subject of the commission, assigned to the ambitious young David by his former teacher Joseph-Marie Vien, was far more gruesome than the light-hearted theme animating the interior of the Ospedaletto's music room. The Department of Health wanted a large painting of *Saint Roch imploring the Intercession of the Virgin for Victims of the Plague*, as an altarpiece in the Chapelle du Lazaret, the plague hospital's chapel.

It was intended to commemorate the terrible epidemic of pestilence that decimated the population of Marseilles back in 1720, and David's preliminary sketch discloses his impetuous willingness to heighten the dramatic significance of the scene. A rarity in his oeuvre, this small study (pl. 245) arrives at the fundamental elements he would deploy in the eventual painting; but the Caravaggesque lighting stresses the urgency of the saint's pleading intervention and, most important of all, the tragic isolation of the ailing figure who sprawls across the foreground. Utterly removed from the idealised Virgin behind him, this brooding victim is ensnared in suffering. In order to convey the brutal reality of the plague's onslaught, David stresses the man's agony and even seems to entertain the possibility that the gracious woman beyond might never penetrate his hellish reality. If the altarpiece had pursued these ideas to their logical conclusion, it could have been in danger of implying that Christian faith was powerless to combat the ravages of such a fearsome epidemic. But the final painting (pl. 246), completed in 1780 and greatly admired by visitors to David's Rome studio, pulls back from such a potentially heretical confrontation. The disparity between Virgin and victim is lessened here, in a canvas that brings the three principal performers into a greater degree of pictorial unity. But if the contrast announced in the study has been softened, David still ensures that the altarpiece is fired by a memorable intensity of feeling.

A comparison with Tiepolo's great Este Cathedral altarpiece of 1759, which deals with a similar theme, is enlightening (pl. 247). With considerable frankness, Tiepolo emphasised the horror of the

244 (*facing page*) Detail of pl. 246

245 (*right*) Jacques-Louis David, Study for *Saint Roch imploring the Intercession of the Virgin for the Victims of Plague*, *c.*1779, Musée Magnin, Dijon

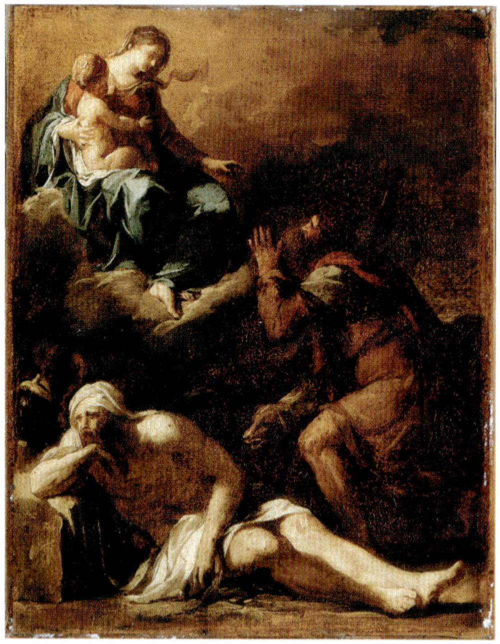

246 (*below*) Jacques-Louis David, *Saint Roch imploring the Intercession of the Virgin for Victims of the Plague*, 1780, Musée des Beaux-Arts - Palais Longchamp, Marseilles

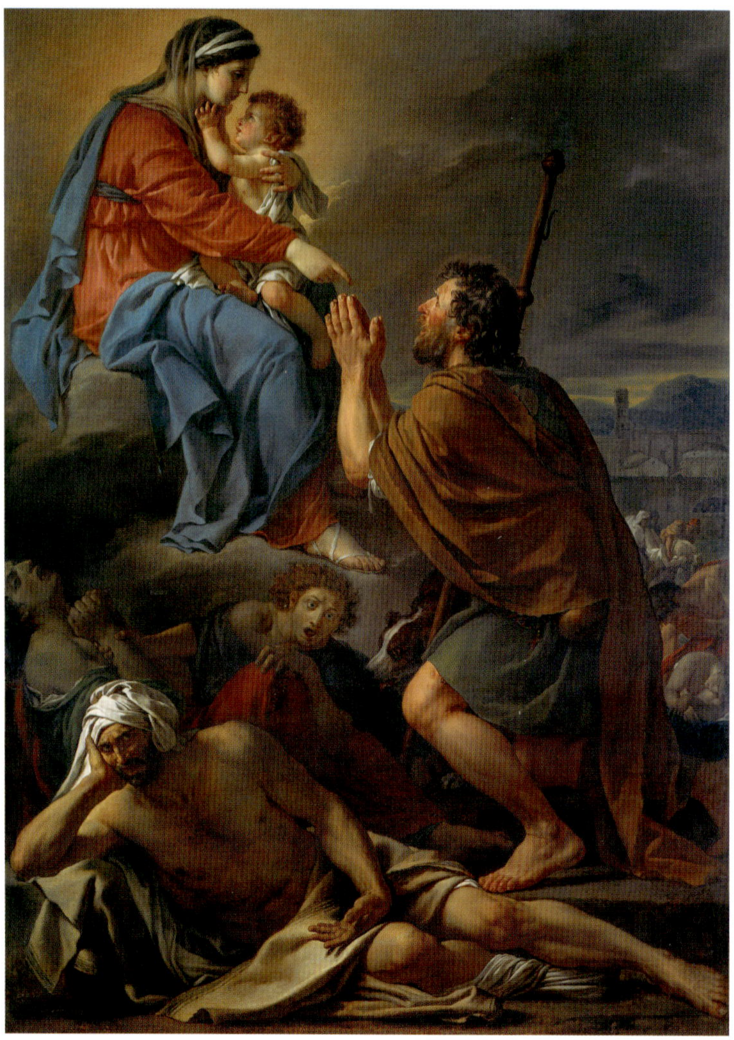

plague in Este by showing a woman holding her nose to stave off the stench of the corpses. He also reinforced the epidemic's pathos in a prominent area of the design, where a weeping child clutches at the mother's blanched body in a futile attempt to revive her. David may have been aware of Tiepolo's powerful precedent, for he includes a group of distant mourners whose straining poses, as they carry a dead figure to burial, echo a similar group in the Este altarpiece. But in every other respect, he diverges from Tiepolo's *tour de force* – replacing the dynamic airborne deity with a more earthbound alternative, giving the interceding saint a more active role and insisting that the full reality of plague-ridden humanity occupies a far more inescapable place in his painting.

Although David's conception of the Virgin is indebted to Guercino and the Bolognese tradition, she is given a quite singular, statuesque presence in the hospital canvas. Lacking the ability of Tiepolo's flying God to move his awesome authority through the heavens, she nevertheless embodies distinct virtues of her own. For one thing, the Virgin is prepared to listen to the entreaties of her own child, who turns to her and pleads the plague-victims' case with an earnest charm that no mother could resist. For another, her proximity to the scene of suffering implies a willingness to become wholly involved with the epidemic. Rather than remaining at a distance, like the deity at whom Tiepolo's Saint Tecla gazes with no hope of contact, David's Virgin places herself daringly near the infected city.

Although clouds surround and protect her, the finger she points at Saint Roch almost touches him. Whereas Saint Tecla's praying hands point to the ground, he pushes up his stubby, clasped fingers with the eagerness of a man almost expecting to catch the Virgin's beneficence like drops of holy water. David defines Saint Roch's half-stumbling eagerness, showing a man who ignores the sinister sore above his knee as he bends in pleading anticipation before the potential source of help. Despite his evident weariness, which prompts him to lean heavily on a stout pilgrim's staff, the saint's body is charged with the hope that his fervent prayers will be granted.

Nevertheless, David insists on presenting the dilemma of the victims with a quite uncompromising forcefulness. Tiepolo occupied the very forefront of his altarpiece with a shadowy region, where a coffin-like form floats near the archway of a bridge. Yet the entire foreground of the Chapelle du Lazaret painting is occupied by the ailing man who, Antoine Schnapper argued, remains 'entirely detached from the miraculous scene behind him' (see pl. 244).[1] Unlike the principal victim in Tiepolo's painting, whose lifeless head is turned away from the spectator, this agonised man stares outwards, as if determined to confront us with the full reality of his plight. David strengthens this direct appeal by adding another anguished head beyond, holding the arm of a woman contorted with pain as he calls out of the canvas for our help. Both he and the dog staring in horror nearby seem just as oblivious of the Virgin as the bearded man beyond Saint Roch, bending over a dying woman and holding his nose (like one of the observers in Tiepolo's picture), to counter the stench of putrefaction. Yet neither of these figures in David's painting carries the moral weight of the recumbent man before them. He cannot be avoided. Although his head and pose derive from Poussin and Lebrun respectively, as Philip Conisbee pointed out,[2] David transformed his sources by turning them to innovatory account.

For this obstinate figure, who props his head on hand and glares brazenly at us, carries an accusatory charge. His mighty musculature has not prevented him from succumbing to a disease of terrifying potency, and he lies helpless on the ground like a great stricken tree felled by a storm. All the same, David gives him enough reserves of willpower to direct his eyes away from the Virgin, with her promise of imminent succour, and towards an unsettling confrontation with the misery of his own death. The victim's angry expression, as he opens his mouth in a cry of pain and protest, forces us to ask why such grotesque suffering is permitted in a world over which the holy family supposedly presides.

If the haunting, obstinate face of David's plague victim still has the capacity to disturb, so too does the mesmeric sequence of heads by Franz Xaver Messerschmidt. Made around the same period as the Marseilles altarpiece, but without the stimulus of a commission, they were the product of his self-imposed isolation in remote Pressburg (Bratislava). These images have occupied a marginal place in art history ever since they were displayed at the Vienna Burgerspital (or Citizens' Hospital) in 1793, a decade after Messerschmidt's death. It was the first time they had been placed on public view and the clinical setting provided by the Burgerspital encouraged a medical interpretation of these strange, unsettling presences. Their individual titles, along with the collective name 'Character-heads', were given to them on this occasion. The authority responsible for organising the exhibition has gone unrecorded, but an effort was clearly made to account for Messerschmidt's aberrant work by locating it within late eighteenth-century ideas about the physiognomy of madness.

Joseph II of Austria and the physician Gerard van Swieten were both prominently involved in reforming the treatment of insanity, and Messerschmidt was well placed to know about their initiatives. He had established his reputation in 1760 with bronze portraits of the Emperor and his wife,

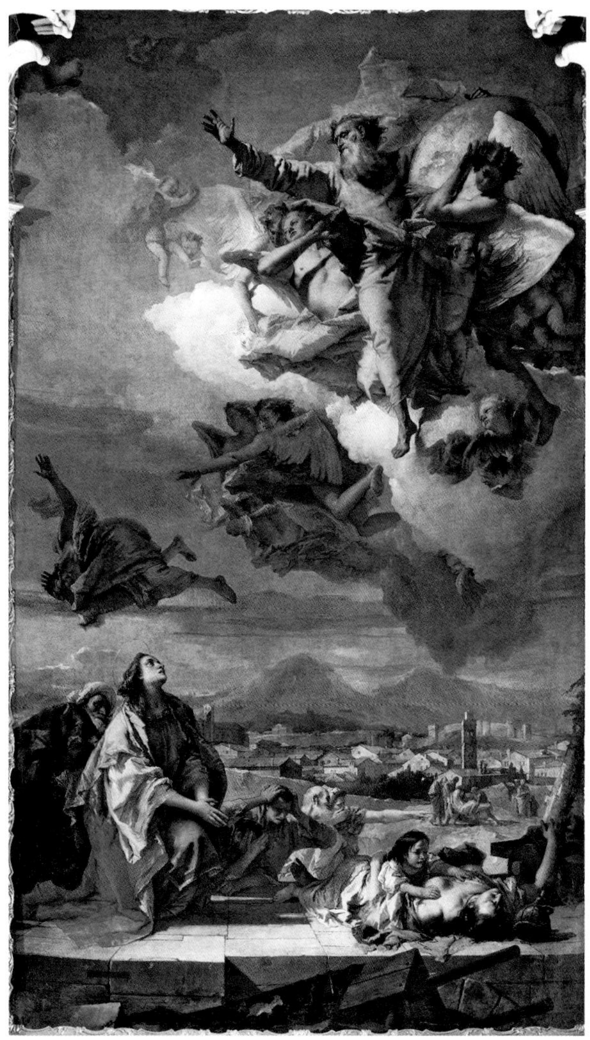

247 Giovanni Battista Tiepolo, *Saint Tecla interceding for the plague-stricken Este*, 1759, Altarpiece for Este Cathedral

248 (*right*) Franz Xaver Messerschmidt, *The Yawner*, after 1770, Szepm, veszeti Muzeum, Budapest

249 (*far right*) Franz Xaver Messerschmidt, *A Seriously Wounded Man in Agony*, after 1770, Galerie im Belvedere, Vienna

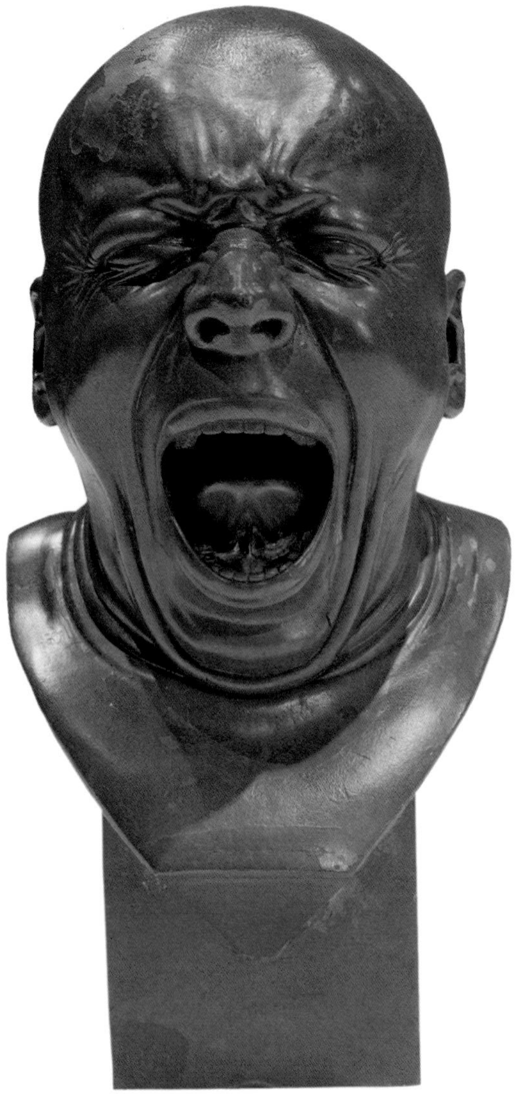

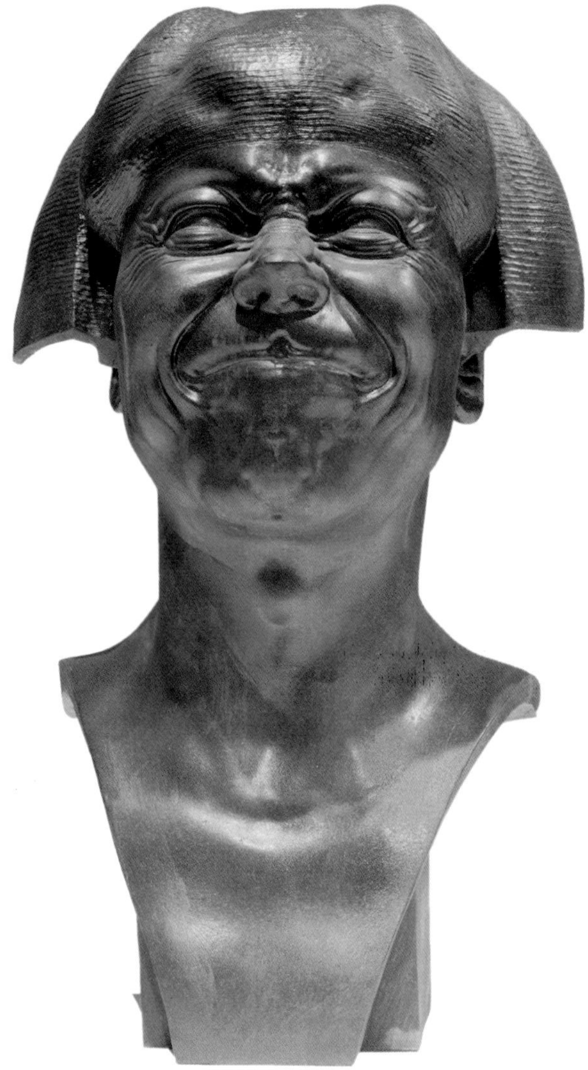

and two busts of van Swieten survive from Messerschmidt's hand.[3] So the hospital exhibition may well have been intended to imply that the mysterious heads, without any parallel in contemporary European art, were intended as illustrations of the pseudo-scientific systems of Lavater and Lichtenberg, or Lebrun's physiognomic treatise widely followed by artists after his schematic images of *Expressions* were published in plentiful editions from 1696 onwards.

However understandable this attempt to make sense of Messerschmidt's 'Character-heads' may have been, it ended up locating them too far outside the sculptural context. They became hereafter associated with psychiatric enquiry rather than art, and rumours about their maker's supposed mental illness only reinforced the interpretation. Tantalisingly little is recorded about the breakdown he was supposed to have suffered, but it is known that Messerschmidt underwent a crisis which destroyed his promising career as a conventional, if skilful, Baroque portraitist. Having been promised the Viennese Academy's Professorship of Sculpture at a precocious age, he was then disqualified on the grounds of 'mental instability'. Premature retirement swiftly followed and, after refusing a pension, the ostracised sculptor met further rejection when he applied for employment at the Munich court.

By that time, in 1775, the series of 'Character-heads' had already commenced. Their startling

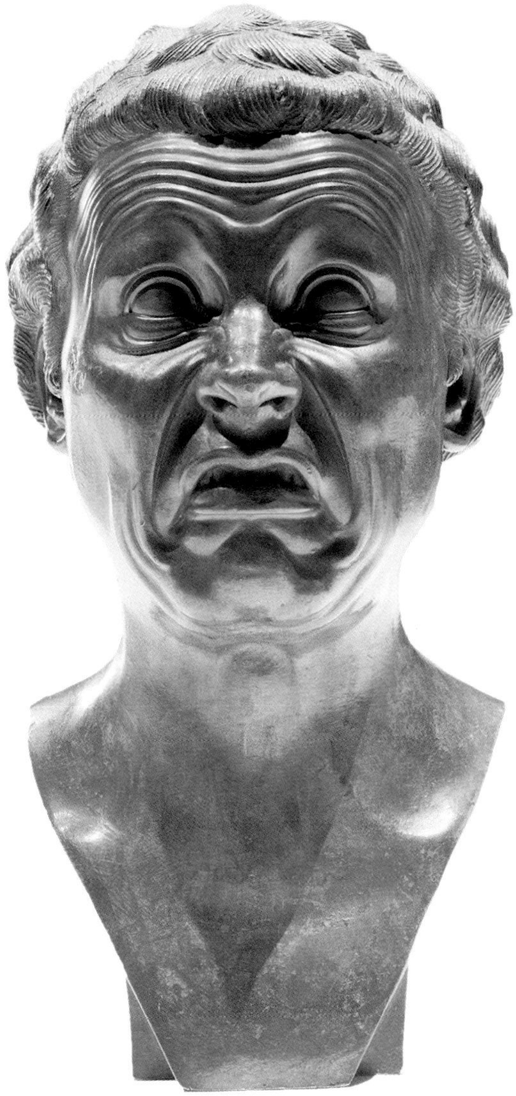

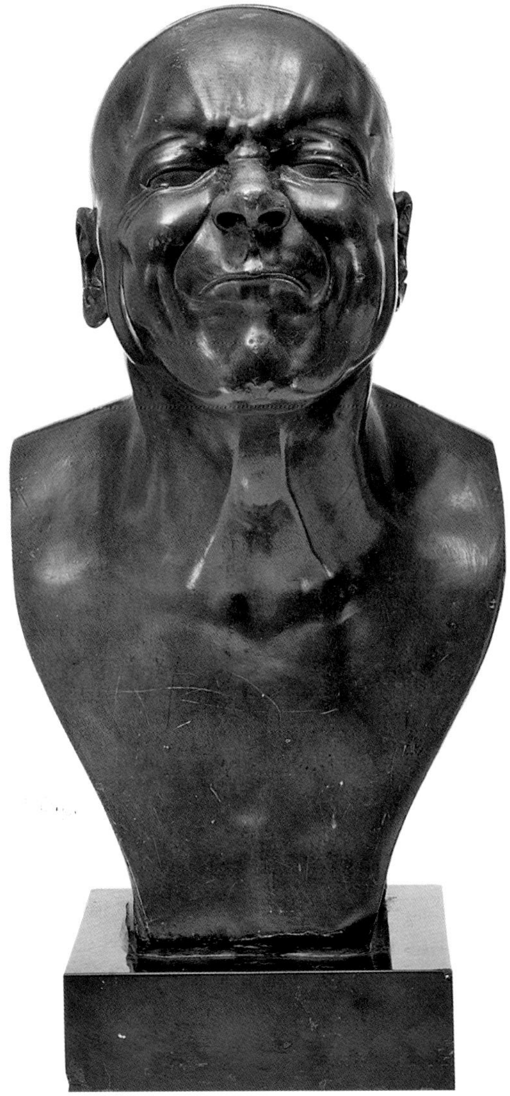

250 (*far left*) Franz Xaver Messerschmidt, *A Childish Weeper*, after 1770, Szepm, veszeti Muzeum, Budapest

251 (*left*) Franz Xaver Messerschmidt, *The Strong Smell*, after 1770, Victoria & Albert Museum, London

intensity of expression would have been regarded as outlandish in regal circles and his subsequent retreat to the loneliness of Pressburg was probably inevitable. Shunned by former colleagues and cut off from the metropolitan world he once knew, Messerschmidt pursued his disconcerting obsession in spartan, poverty-ridden surroundings. Friedrich Nicolai, whose account of a meeting with the recluse furnishes the only detailed information about his final years, records that 'his entire domestic effects consisted of a bed, a flute, a tobacco-pipe, a ewer, and an ancient Italian book on the Proportions of the Human Figure'.[4] Nicolai was sensible enough to treat this hermit with the utmost sympathy and respect, recognising that 'my good Messerschmidt' was a sculptor of immense seriousness and originality. Rather than dismissing him as a madman, and thereby forgoing any attempt to understand the reason why he concentrated on such unclassifiable aims, Nicolai tried hard to obtain an explanation from the recluse himself.

Messerschmidt made clear that 'it was spirits that so affrighted and tormented him, especially at night', while during the day he was plagued by incessant pains in the abdomen, thighs and other parts of his body. 'Since his vanity deluded him that he had made novel and unheard-of discoveries concerning the proportions and their effects', wrote Nicolai, 'he fancied the Spirit of Proportion envied him for approaching so near perfection in the knowledge of proportions, and that this motivated it to cause him the pain.' So a bizarre battle began, whereby Messerschmidt pinched himself in the painful areas while contorting his face in the mirror. He became convinced that 'power over the spirit' could be attained, and believed that as many as sixty-four heads could be produced to fit his system by illustrating 'these grimacing proportions'. Nicolai watched him at work on the sixty-first, marvelling at the sight of a sculptor who would 'look upon the glass continually, and, with the greatest accuracy would pull the face he required'.

The astounded visitor can hardly be blamed for concluding that the entire ritual was irredeemably deluded, but Nicolai still remained perceptive enough to recognise the prodigious amount of skill, intelligence and discipline it required, and the quality of the heads provoked his admiration. Nevertheless he decided that Messerschmidt had been 'misled by a blighted imagination and by insane hypotheses.'[5] As late as 1932 Ernst Kris declared that the sculptor was a victim of schizophrenic psychosis.[6] Kris presented this diagnostic interpretation with such ingenuity that Messerschmidt continued to be regarded as a lunatic oddity for decades afterwards. Only with the publication of Margaret and Rudolf Wittkower's *Born under Saturn* in 1963 was an alternative interpretation proposed, and an unprejudiced examination of the heads suggests that their book was right to escape from a confining preoccupation with lunacy alone.[7]

252 Henry Fuseli, *Scene in the Hospital of S. Spirito in Rome*, 1772, British Museum, London

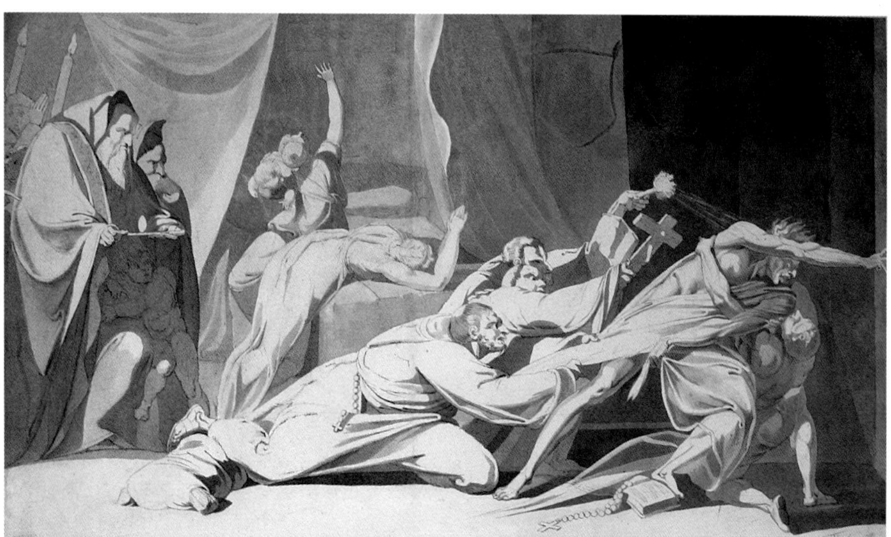

For however deluded Messerschmidt may have been, the images he produced are remarkable above all for their analytical rigour and, paradoxically, a sense of poise. On one level, *The Yawner* may present an alarming vision of a man opening his mouth in a Munch-like scream (pl. 248), but this zinc face is modelled with a lucidity and control far removed from hopeless mental incoherence. Spurning his former Baroque fluidity in favour of a less ostentatious manner, Messerschmidt stiffened each head with stern classical discipline. Several, most notably *The Gentle Peaceful Sleep*, could hardly be more serene in their unruffled resolution. Moreover, images as distorted as *An Arch-Villain* or *A Seriously Wounded Man in Agony* turn out, on prolonged inspection, to be very clear and faithful studies of specific facial poses (pl. 249). The peculiar power of Messerschmidt's most outspoken heads stems, in fact, from the contrast between their manic expressions and the calm precision of his handling. He was quite capable of carrying out more conventional portrait commissions while producing the 'Character-heads', and there is nothing agitated or hysterical about the careful, precise, almost matter-of-fact definition of these snarling, leering, pouting, wincing and frowning visages.[8]

Some of them, like *The Constipation Sufferer* and *A Childish Weeper*, seem to reflect an impish humour on Messerschmidt's part, as if he delighted in his capacity to reveal humanity in all its fallible absurdity (pl. 250). Indeed, the most ferocious of his heads often arise from a keen awareness of the human comedy. The man in lead who cranes his neck forward, and twists his features into an expression of seemingly unbearable stress, is saddled with the satirical title *The Strong Smell* (pl. 251). Even if Messerschmidt himself might have wished to give it a less knockabout name, the fact remains that a distinct strain of subversive wit runs through the entire collection. It indicates a hitherto unsuspected layer of meaning in his work, closely bound up with a discerning awareness of the manifold links between 'normality' and 'lunacy' in the human mind.

In this respect, the powerful exhibition of his heads at the Citizens' Hospital in Vienna marked the appearance in European sculpture of an artist who, despite his possible derangement, was resolved to deal with mental disorder in an entirely new, lucid and ordered way. Although the Burgerspital show limited contemporary understanding of Messerschmidt's achievement as an artist, it may therefore have contributed to the enlightened fascination with 'madness' that bore early pictorial fruit in the work of a few outstanding painters.

Around 1772, Henry Fuseli produced an alarming pen and wash drawing (pl. 252). It was engraved and reproduced in the first English edition of an influential three-volume treatise on *Physiognomy* by the theologian Caspar Lavater, whom Fuseli had befriended as a young man in Zurich.[9] They shared radical beliefs and, after publishing a fiery political pamphlet, had been forced to leave Switzerland. Fuseli probably made this drawing while training as an artist in Rome: its shallow, frieze-like design reflects his passion for the antique. Yet, while professing neo-classical ideals, he could not prevent his turbulent imaginative life from having far more in common with emergent Romanticism. The frenzied energy of the three lunging monks, who strive to restrain a patient with wild hair, possess a nightmarish intensity. Although one of the trio brandishes a cross, performing last rites on the resisting hospital occupant, success eludes him. Hysteria seems to have broken out on the bed behind, where two more figures gesticulate, writhe and collapse. Terrified, a naked child reels back from them and hides in the shadowy robes of heavily bearded elders advancing on the bed. They stare aghast, as if powerless to prevent the insanity from reducing the entire hospital to a state of permanent chaos.

An inscription beneath the engraved version of Fuseli's drawing claims that he had observed these deranged people at first hand in a Rome hospital. Soon after its publication in Lavater's *Physiognomy* in 1792, this profoundly unsettling print may have been seen by Francisco de Goya. Recovering in Cadiz from a serious illness that left him partially paralysed and permanently deaf, he spent his convalescence painting twelve small '*Caprichos*' on tin plate. They were, for him, a decisive breakthrough, leading to the darker, more personal and painful of his later paintings. Juliet Wilson-Bareau has emphasised the cardinal importance of 'these completely independent works, perhaps the first that he painted entirely to please himself rather than in response to a commission or a friend's request'.[10] Like Fuseli, Goya became increasingly preoccupied with violence and nightmarish images, focusing in his case on fire, shipwreck and murderous theft. Yet the most powerful of these turbulent small paintings shows a *Yard with Lunatics* (pl. 253) and the struggling figures in the centre may have been inspired by their manic predecessors in Fuseli's drawing.

Goya, however, transforms his source so completely that he creates a different world: Fuseli's melodramatic stage-set has given way to a far more unsettling and believable place. Declaring that it 'shows a yard with lunatics, and two naked figures

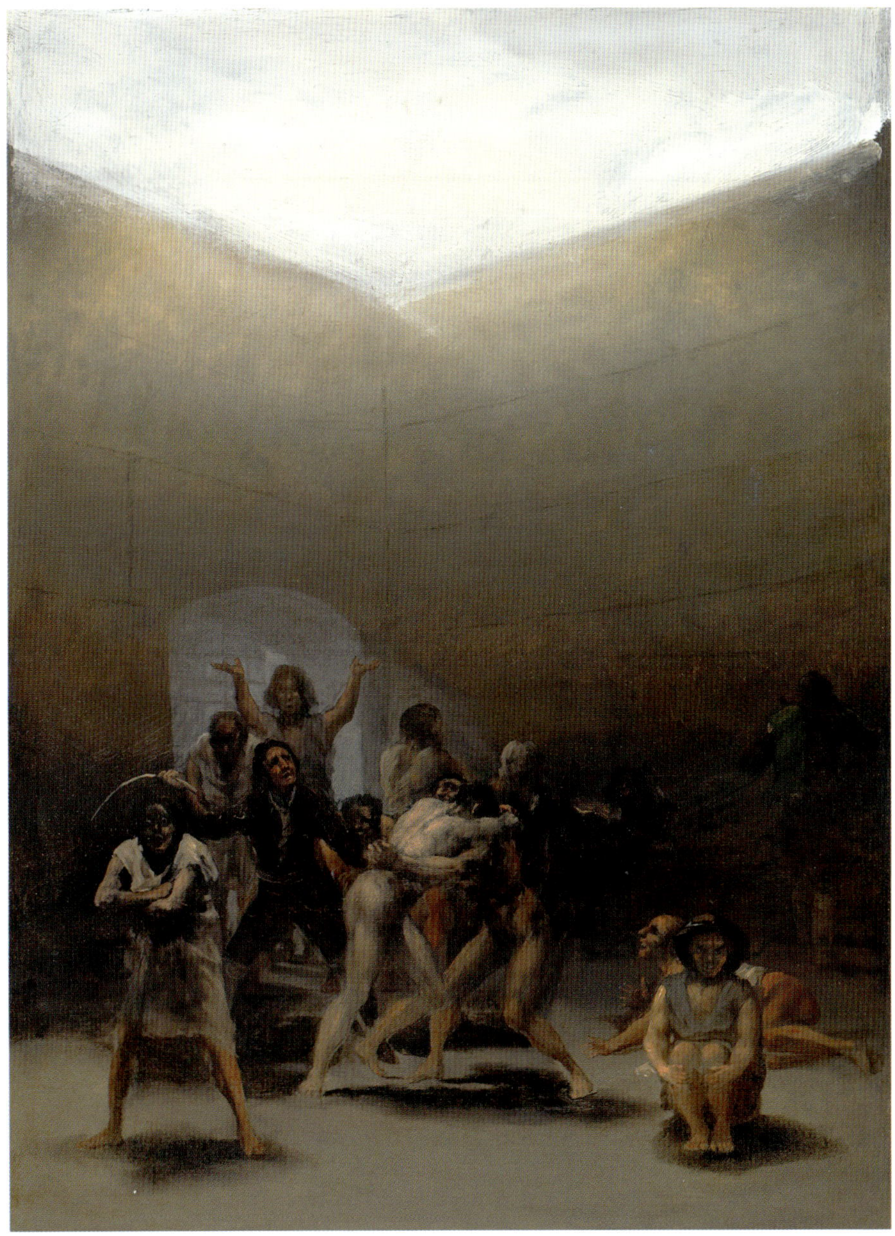

253 Francisco de Goya, *Yard with Lunatics*, 1794, Algur H. Meadows Collection, Meadows Museum, Southern Methodist University, Dallas, MM67.01

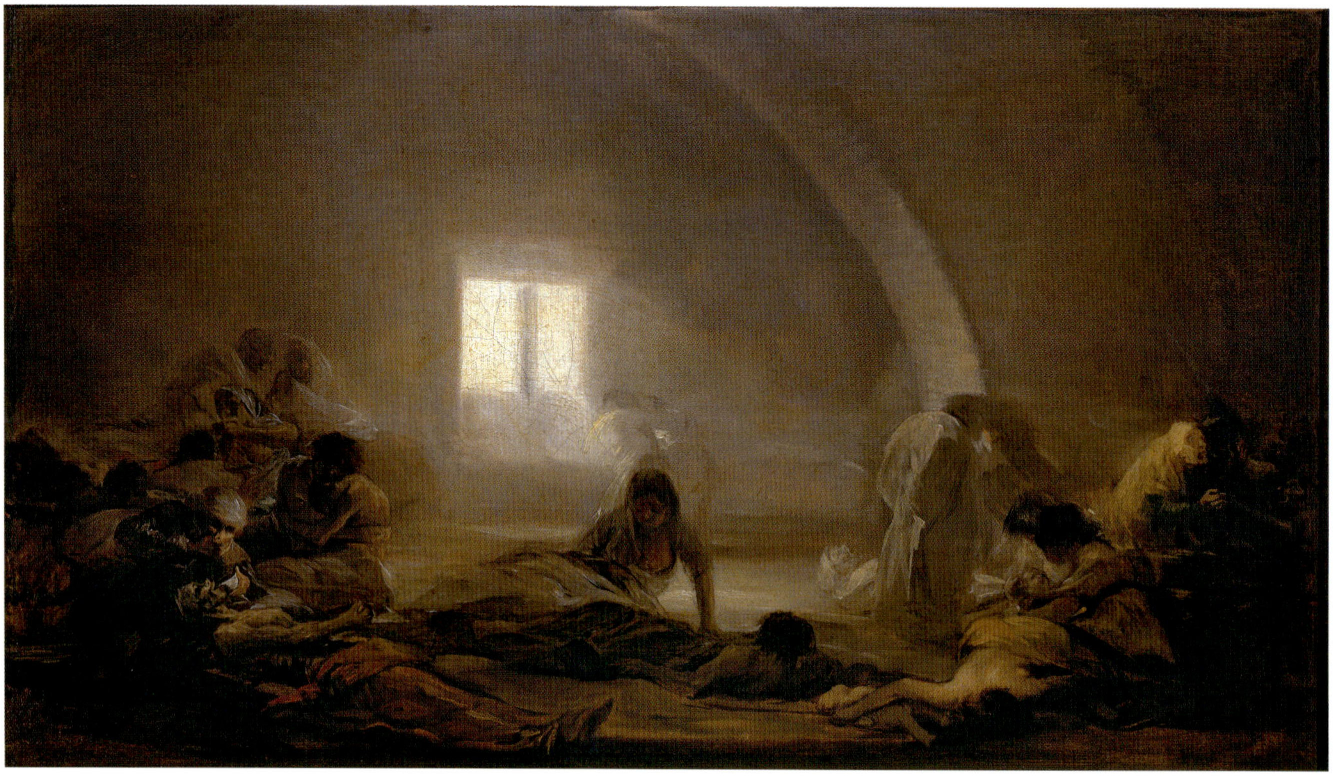

254 Francisco de Goya, *A Plague Hospital*, 1808–10, Private Collection

fighting', Goya explained that 'the keeper beats them, and others in sacks'. He also asserted, less reliably, that 'it is a scene I once saw in Saragossa',[11] a claim questioned by several historians, who conclude that 'Goya's painting and description are pure fantasy, based on a precedent which had struck his imagination'.[12] Whatever the truth may be, *Yard with Lunatics* looks authentic enough to have been painted by an eyewitness. Stranded in the grim austerity of an exercise compound open to the sky, the inmates grimace, gaze wild-eyed and bare their teeth while two naked men struggle in the centre. A frowning, open-mouthed custodian lashes them. But it is not clear whether he aims at restraining or exciting them to further combat. Nobody else incarcerated in this shadowy chamber seems to care. Although one long-haired 'lunatic' raises his arms, he appears locked in his own mind rather than reacting to the fight. Others turn their heads to the wall, as if overcome by terminal depression or the deafness that Goya himself now suffered. As for the two figures at the front, one seated in a hunched position and the other standing with his legs apart in seeming shock, they both stare out at the viewer. But they make no attempt to communicate, and Goya makes us feel uncomfortably like voyeurs who have stumbled on a scene we have no right to scrutinise.

A few years later, when he painted *A Plague Hospital*, the sense of tragedy is so overwhelming that we feel almost incapable of confronting it at all (pl. 254). This time, no open sky can be discerned at the top of the image. Goya takes us deep inside a round-arched room reminiscent of the oppressive, paranoid architecture in Piranesi's *Prisons* engravings. It is strewn with the bodies of the dying and the dead. Some lie sprawled, with gaping mouths and arms outflung, beyond all assistance; but one silhouetted and emaciated form, prone at the heart of the foreground, still manages to raise his head. Perhaps he is looking at the woman beside him, propped up on one arm and gazing dejectedly down. She is succumbing to the pestilence, and does not even possess the energy of the skeletal figure on the far right who lifts up her head to scream in the blackness. Nearby, a young mother leans over a baby whose anguished face seems caught in the plague's final stage. She will not leave her offspring, and the same selfless devotion motivates the older woman on the left who pours liquid into the mouth of the man stretched out below her.

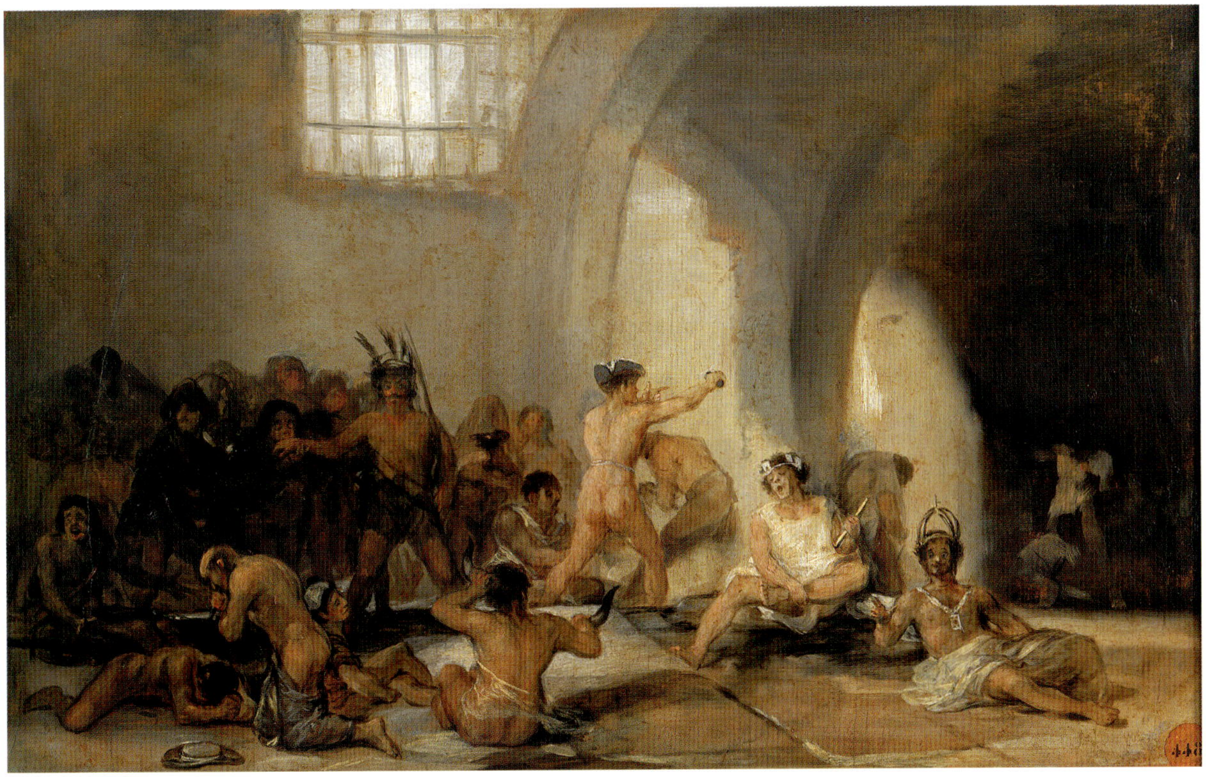

255 Francisco de Goya, *The Madhouse*, 1815–19, Museo de la Real Academia de Bellas Artes de San Fernando, Madrid

Goya's economical brushmarks define his haggard, bony torso and skull-like face. The stench of his decaying body is so repugnant that the woman holds her nose, struggling not to vomit. She must realise that prolonged contact with such a pestilential smell can only result in her own death as well. But the urge to minister overcomes her fear, and the couple behind have abandoned caution to end up locked in a mortal embrace. Goya defines their love as convincingly as he conveys despair elsewhere in the painting, yet the overall mood of this harrowing image is summed up in the blurred, flickering brushstrokes. They dart across the doomed hospital with restless sensitivity, applied with such deftness that everyone seems about to melt in the light. This feeling of transience reaches its height in the distance, where two figures clutch one another as they seem to stumble towards the window. Goya's handling makes their indistinct forms hover on the edge of dissolution, almost engulfed by the obliterating whiteness of the luminosity beyond.

Since his illness in 1792–3, Goya had led an almost schizophrenic existence as an artist. While successfully pursuing his privileged career as the Court Painter, executing church decorations and portraits of the royal family, aristocrats, ministers and officials, he also insisted on exploring the obsessive and often unnerving world of his private imagination. Nobody knows precisely when *A Plague Hospital* was painted but it belongs to a powerful series of eight paintings probably bought from the artist by Don Juan de Salas, an art collector in Mallorca. His daughter was married to the 3rd Marquess of La Romana, and the entire sequence of canvases still belongs to their family. Believed to have been executed between 1798 and 1810, these *'Caprichos' of the Marquess of La Romana* possess manifold links with Goya's celebrated 'Collection of Prints on Fanciful Themes', published in 1799 and soon known simply as *Los Caprichos*. Nothing, however, could be less fanciful than *A Plague Hospital*, which may at its deepest level reflect Goya's continuing anxieties about the state of his own health. An urge to ruminate on life and death runs through all the *'Caprichos' of the Marquess of La Romana*, with their remorseless concentration on bandits attacking, raping and murdering women, as well as a particularly brutal, traumatic image of *Shooting in a Military Camp*.

256 Francisco de Goya, *Self-Portrait with his Doctor Arrieta*, 1820, Institute of Arts, Minneapolis

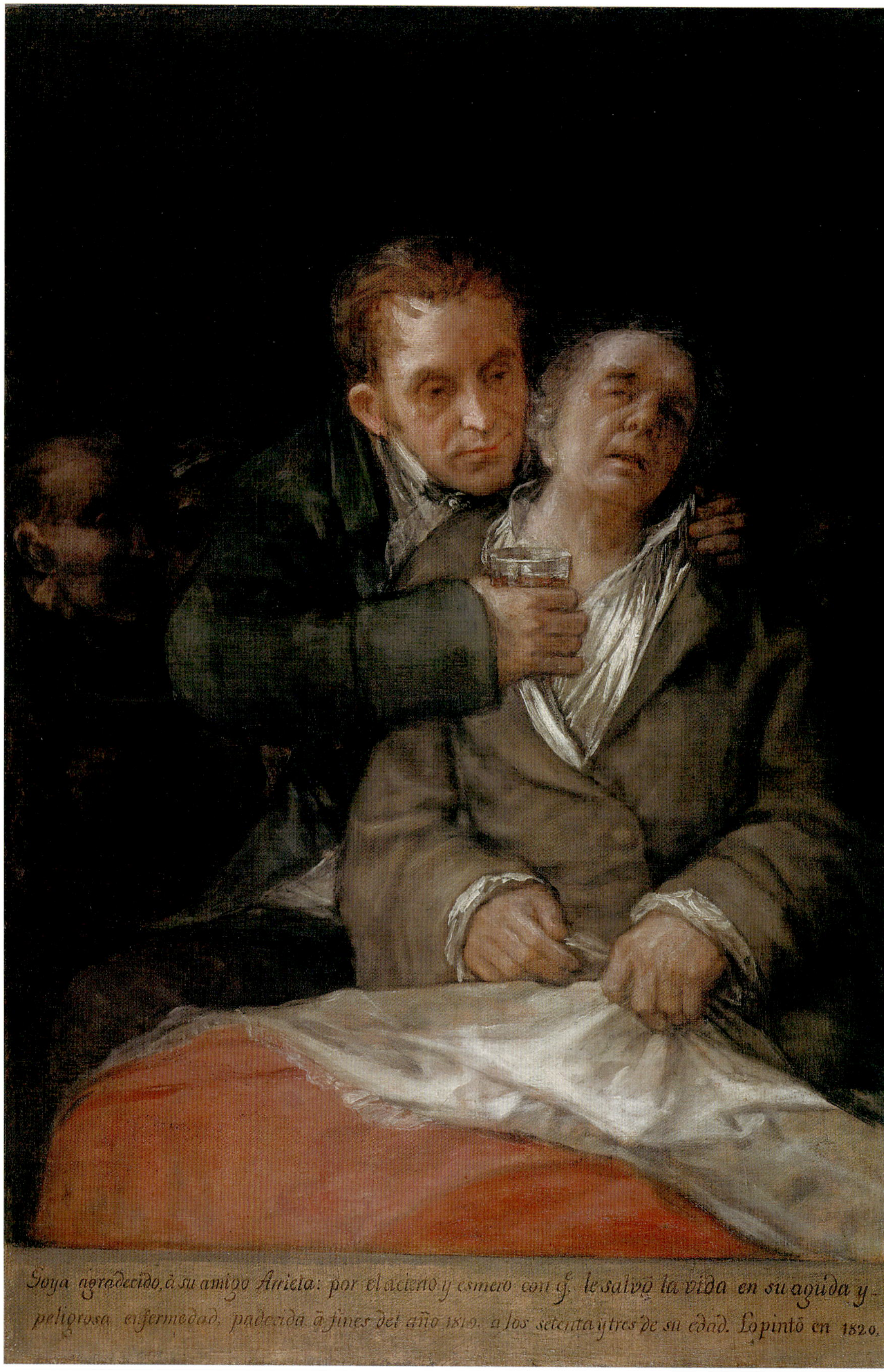

No wonder these dark and haunted canvases have often been mistakenly linked with Spain's later War of Independence. They prefigure the work Goya made in response to the uprising against the French invaders in 1808, and his later *Madhouse* painting reflects his mood of bitter disillusion following Fernando VII's return to the Spanish throne in 1814. After an anxious period when Goya found himself in danger of being branded a traitor, and threatened by a summons from the Inquisition to account for two 'obscene' paintings of a Maja, he was finally acquitted. However, the fear and despair remained, for Fernando soon reasserted his old bullying and tyrannical ways. Hence the savagely satirical *Madhouse*, one of four '*Caprichos*' panels bequeathed by the French sympathiser Don Manuel García de la Prada to the Royal Academy of San Fernando in 1836 (pl. 255). Painted at some point between 1815 and 1819, when Goya had increasing reason to mourn the passing of the brief liberalism engendered by the Regency in Madrid, it signals a return to the mood of the paintings he had produced while recovering from his near-fatal illness some twenty years before.

This time, however, he made no claims that *Madhouse* was based on a scene witnessed in Saragossa. Unlike *Yard with Lunatics* (see pl. 253), this new panel is filled with figures openly symbolising the folly of those who seek to dominate humanity. Sitting in a round-arched room reminiscent of the doomed chamber in *A Plague Hospital*, an inmate poses as a monarch. Clutching a sceptre with one hand and his own bare leg with the other, he opens his mouth in an idiotic yell. Nobody pays any attention to him, least of all the risible figure on the right who sprawls on the floor. Wearing a papal tiara on his head and a glistening chain and pendant round his neck, he raises his hand to bless; but no one kneels to receive his benediction, and the 'pontiff' ends up looking merely absurd. So does the would-be savage chieftain, even though his extended arm is rewarded with a kiss by a black-cowled woman. Both he, the military commander and the murderer are mocked by Goya as embodiments of posturing futility, in a room lit well enough to reveal the utter emptiness of their antics. Goya even allows us to see what is happening in the distant shadows on the far right, where his free, summarising brushmarks define a standing nude and a figure crouched directly below. Engaged either in a cruelly humiliating ritual or a joyless sexual act, they convey the abject nullity of an institution where the occupants are able to indulge their fantasies unchecked by attendants of any kind. At least in *Yard with Lunatics* a keeper could be detected, albeit one addicted to beating his charges with savage energy. But now, in *Madhouse*, no warders attempt to supervise or prevent the patients from inflicting arbitary violence on each other.

Hence, no doubt, the immense gratitude felt by the ageing Goya to the doctor who managed to cure him when, in the winter of 1819, he fell victim to another serious and potentially mortal ailment. He painted a heartfelt tribute to Don Eugenio García Arrieta (pl. 256), a much admired doctor who probably left Spain soon after treating Goya in order, very courageously, to study the bubonic plague in Africa. The exact nature of Goya's complaint is not recorded but the *Self-Portrait with his Doctor Arrieta* movingly communicates his dependence on the medicine and human sympathy he received. Unlike Frida Kahlo, who would hail her doctor in a painting where the artist is seen alone in her studio (see pl. 395), Goya showed the two men together.

Propped up in bed, while his head lolls in agony, Goya is seen struggling to endure what the novelist Anita Brookner has described as 'an extremity of suffering, the structure of his face and body disintegrating beneath the gravity of his pain, his expression both naked and disbelieving'.[13] But he finds himself supported by a man quite willing to court infection by holding his patient with remarkable intimacy. One of Arrieta's steadfast hands closes round the medicine while the other rests reassuringly on Goya's slumped shoulder. The proximity of their two heads, the one so desperate and the other so consoling, implies that Arrieta's help was as much psychogical as physical. Although the liquid in the proferred glass may well have brought genuine relief, the doctor's close and steadfast dedication to Goya's welfare doubtless proved decisive as well. The solemnity with which this dramatic moment is presented in the canvas gives the act of providing the medicine a sacramental significance. Death, in this intensely moving canvas, seems very near. It could easily be imagined as a painting where Arrieta administers the physician's equivalent of the last rites to his expiring patient.

Before succumbing to this illness Goya had in fact completed, free of charge,[14] a vast *Last Communion of Saint Joseph Calasanctius* for the chapel of the Esculeas Pías de San Antón in Madrid. The priest places the wafer in the saint's open mouth with as much care and compassion as Arrieta displays. Yet the devout congregation praying with such solicitude behind Saint Joseph are replaced, in the self-portrait with Arrieta, by more shadowy and sinister faces who belong to a darker region of Goya's imagination. Soon to embark on the so-called 'black paintings', where disease, madness and senility were explored with a vehemence quite unprecedented even in his own work, Goya was probably invaded by these ominous spectres during his ailment. Here they appear to be lurking, in grim and implacable expectation of the artist's demise. But Arrieta's brave, purposeful intervention holds them off and Goya's canvas ends up as an arresting affirmation which, the inscription explains, was painted 'in gratitude, for his friend Arrieta: for the care and attention with which he saved his life in his acute and dangerous illness, suffered at the end of the year 1819 when aged 73. He painted it in 1820.'[15]

Self-Portrait with his Doctor Arrieta was intended essentially as a personal offering of thanks from one man to his devoted physician. In a wider sense, though, it happened to be painted at an extraordinary moment in European art when a prominent French doctor befriended another outstanding painter and encouraged him to study the patients under his care. Dr Etienne-Jean Georget, a pioneer researcher into insanity who worked at the Salpêtrière women's asylum in Paris, may have met Theodore Géricault after the artist's breakdown in the late autumn of 1819. The two men seem to have recognised a kinship between them, for Lorenz Eitner has argued that 'Georget resembled Géricault in the passionate intensity of his temperament, in his excessive sensitivity, and his self-destructive habits of work.'[16] They would, in fact, both die at a tragically young age within a few years of befriending each other. By the time Géricault began work on his extraordinary portraits of the insane, probably between 1819 and the early 1820s,[17] Georget may have realised that the young painter would soon succumb to a terminal illness. The doctor certainly knew, from personal experience of the most painful kind, what it was to suffer from an ailment he described as 'the horrors of hypochondria of the third degree' – a malady to which 'poets, men of letters, scholars, philosophers, and artists'[18] could be particularly prone. Perhaps, therefore, Georget encouraged Géricault to paint his patients because he knew that the artist would bring to them an exceptional degree of insight and understanding.

Several historians proposed that the portraits were undertaken as a form of therapy, prescribed by a doctor anxious about Géricault's state of mind,[19] but it is more likely that Georget commissioned the paintings in order to supply himself with illustrations for his lectures and writings. Whatever the truth may be, the doctor was allied with a school of psychiatric research which had recently identified a type of madness called 'monomania'. One of the five principal forms of insanity categorised at the time, it served to describe obsessive delusions that appeared deceptively logical in their grasp of reality. Georget's teacher, Jean-Etienne-Dominique Esquirol, believed that patients suffering from monomania were especially rewarding to study because their affliction had been shaped by 'the dominant ideas, the prevailing errors, the general beliefs, right or wrong, that constitute the life of society'.[20] Esquirol concluded that research in asylums would therefore lead to a comprehensive understanding of the history of the age; and he also believed that the physiognomy of patients yielded fascinating insights into the nature of their complaints. He had himself commissioned more than two hundred drawings of the insane to prove his point, and in 1818 the British psychiatrist Sir Alexander Morison (see pl. 266) was amazed to find on a visit to Esquirol that 'he has near 200 plaster of Paris casts of the faces of insane persons and 600 skulls'.[21]

Georget began studying with Esquirol at this time, but he soon developed a materialist theory of neurological injury that carried with it little interest in speculation about the physiognomy of madness. He may have invited Géricault to execute the portraits for Esquirol's benefit rather than his own, although Georget certainly became interested in the defence of insane criminals whose monomania had led to prosecution. All five of the portraits that survive from Géricault's original sequence of ten depict patients suffering from afflictions likely to make them commit a crime: addictive gambling, hopeless kleptomania, delusions of military rank, compulsive kidnapping and obsessive envy. Georget, who owned all the portraits until his death in 1828, probably dictated the form of the whole scheme to Géricault. He must also have been instrumental in helping the artist to locate the patients, not all of whom could be found among the women housed at the Salpêtrière. The men portrayed in the series were housed at Charenton or Bicêtre, asylums where Géricault would have been granted permission to study them under close supervision by guards ready, at any moment, to protect him from the possibility of sudden, violent assault.

Considerable courage was required to carry out such an unnerving assignment, but Géricault had already proved himself capable of studying subjects that most artists would prefer never to contemplate. A few years before, while preparing himself for his monumental painting *The Raft of the Medusa*, he had visited the Beaujon Hospital to scrutinise human illness. Although his biographer Charles Clément maintained that Géricault's 'ardent scrutiny' missed nothing, 'from the first seizure to the final agony',[22] he showed special interest in the bodily remains presented to him by hospital students. The severed heads and dissected limbs he arranged in his studio form, perhaps, the most disquieting still life in the history of Western painting (pls 257–8).

They are, nevertheless, also characterised by a curious serenity, enabling him to stress the intimacy between an amputated arm and the feet with which it is intertwined. The harrowing theme of his *Raft* canvas, strewn with the dead and dying bodies of people who resorted to cannibalism during their desperate fight for survival, helps to explain why Géricault transformed his studio into a temporary

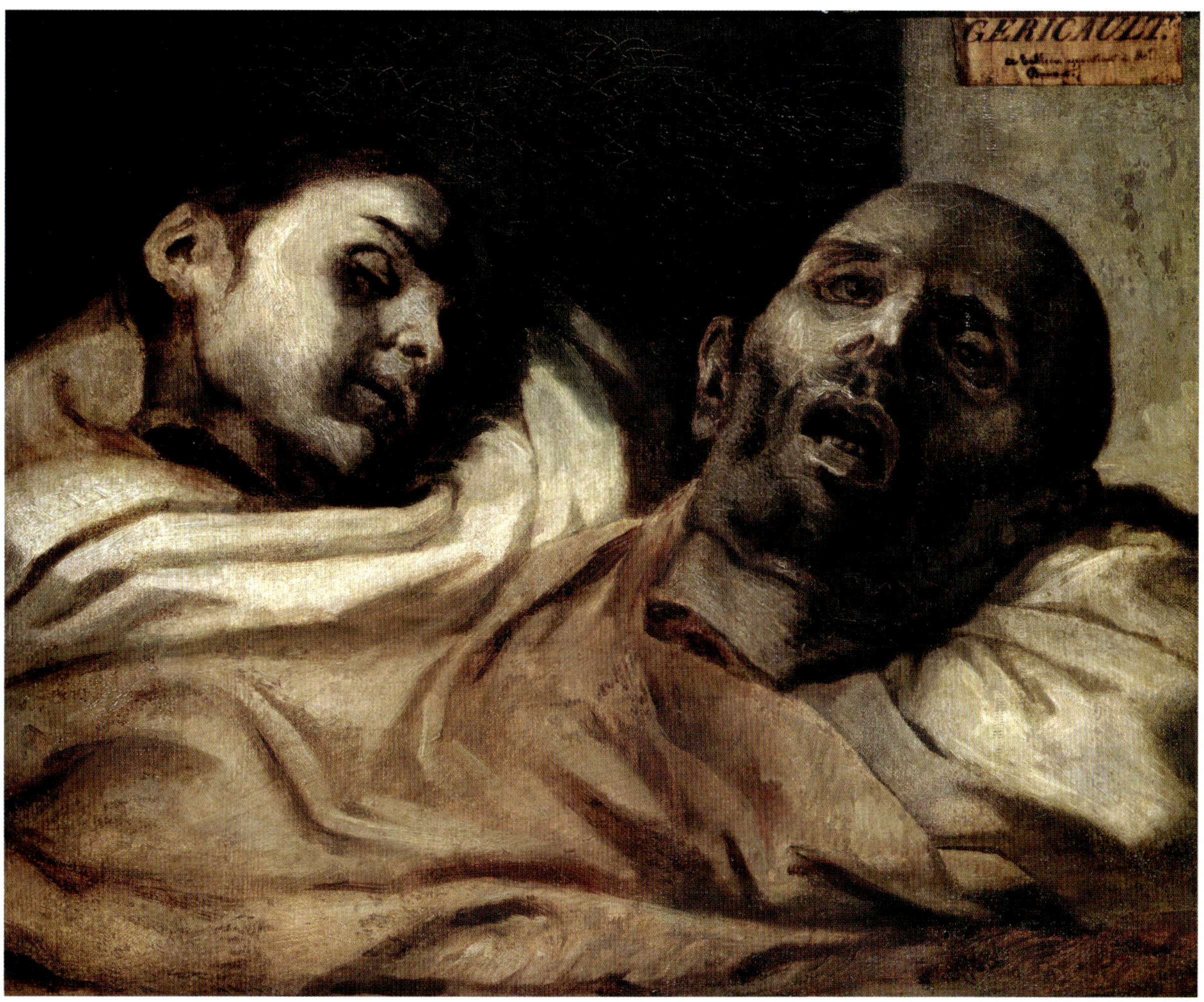

257 Theodore Géricault, *Severed Heads*, study for *The Raft of the Medusa*, *c.*1819, Musée des Beaux-Arts, Rouen

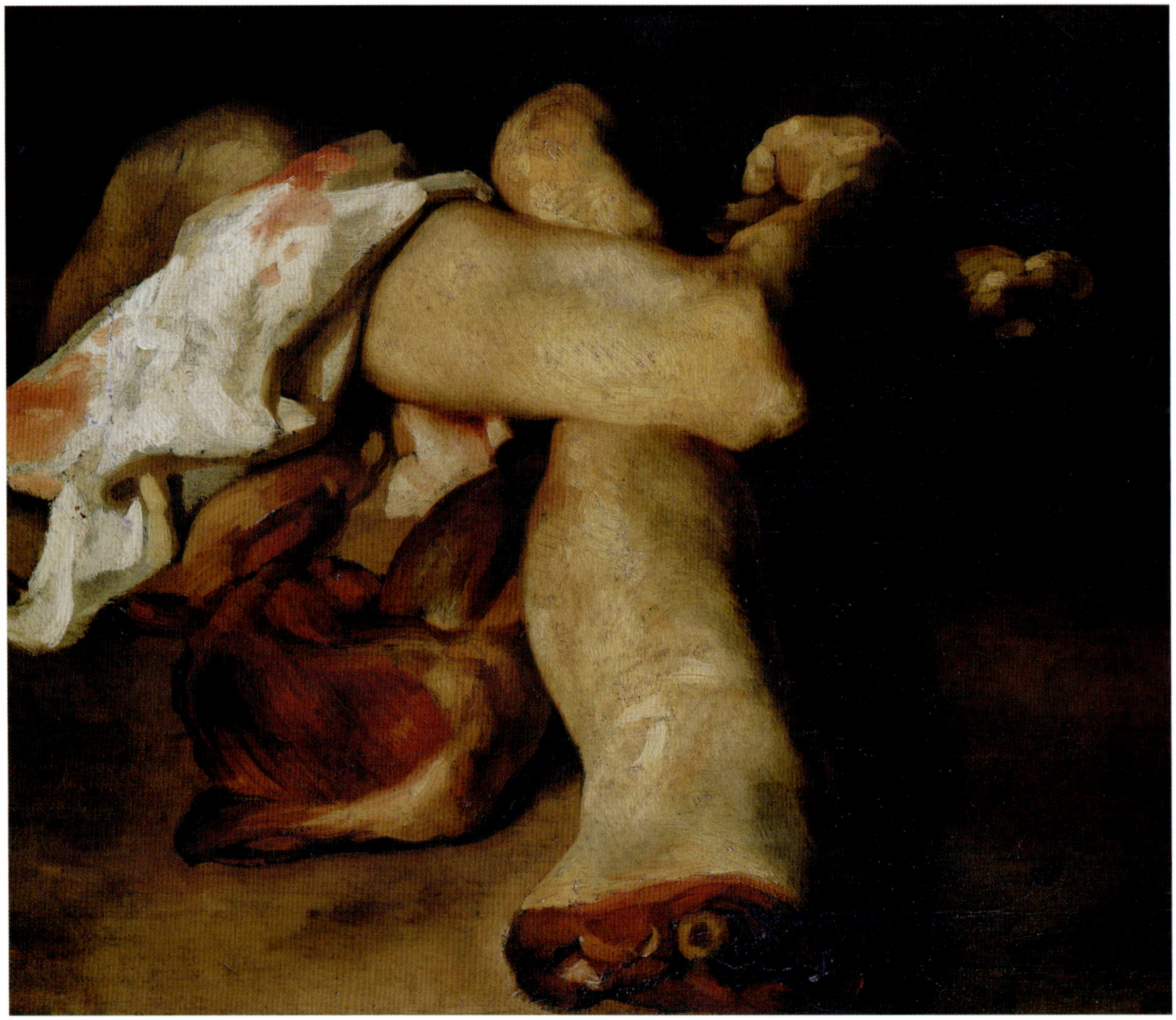

258 Theodore Géricault, *Dissected Limbs*, *c*.1818–19, Musée des Beaux-Arts, Rouen

charnel-house. It does not, however, wholly account for his determination to immerse himself in the most chilling manifestations of mortality. The oil studies of amputated fragments from the Beaujon Hospital played no direct part in his final painting: they stand as fully achieved images in their own right, the remarkably controlled and open-minded outcome of a preoccupation with human extinction that only degenerated into morbidity at the end of his life.

This open-mindedness remains a central strength of the five surviving 'monomania' portraits. Compared with the macabre exaggeration that earlier artists like Quellinus had invested in their images of frenzied lunacy (see pl. 140), Géricault approaches his deranged sitters with quiet, intimate perception. He treats them all like fellow humans rather than seeing them as the bestial puppets who squat, crawl and struggle in Goya's little painting of *Yard with Lunatics* (see pl. 253). Although Goya himself told a friend that his picture was based on personal observation of 'a scene I once saw in Saragossa', he stayed at a firm remove. The screaming and gesticulating wretches trapped within the dark, claustrophobic compound are beyond Goya's reach, in every sense of the word. He dramatised their degradation, whereas Géricault initiates an entirely different response to the phenomenon of madness.

No crazed gestures are here permitted to distract attention from his close concentration on heads alone, looming out of the otherwise pervasive darkness of their cells. By painting them with the same sympathetic attention found in his portraits of sane

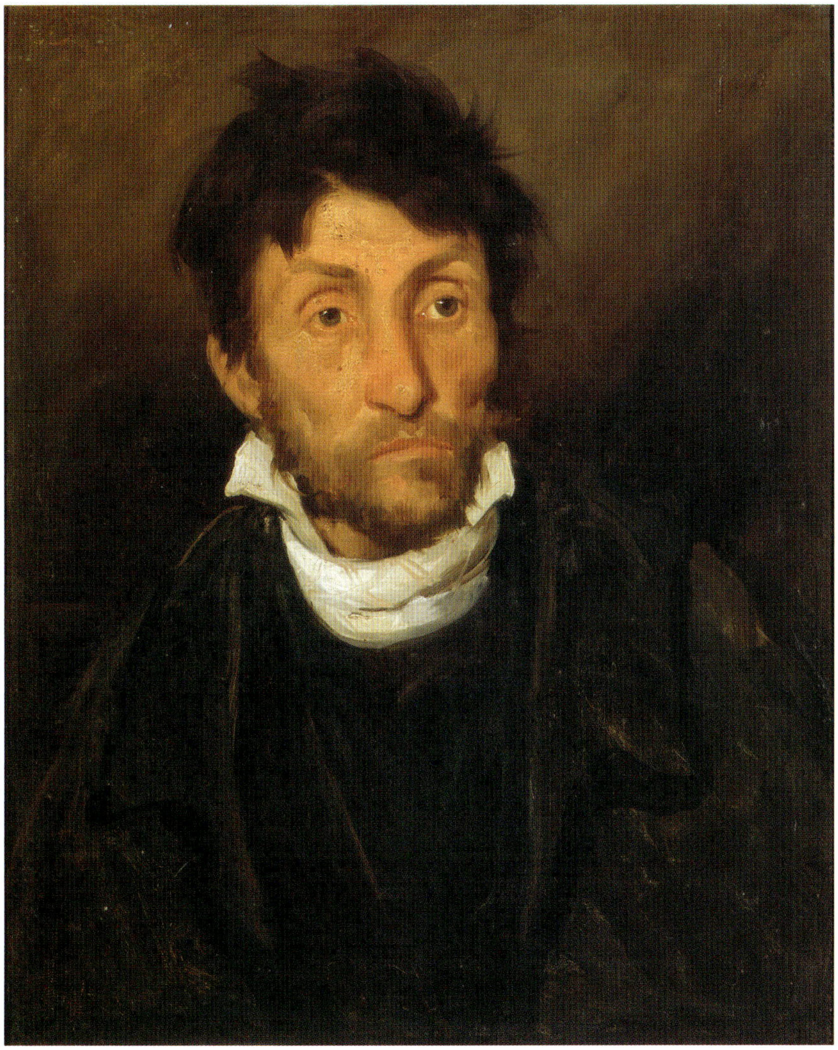

259 Theodore Géricault, *Kleptomoniac*, 1822, Museum voor Schone Kunsten, Ghent

people, he revolutionised the depiction of lunatics and implied that they deserved to be seen not as freaks, fit only to illustrate a case history of irredeemable derangement, but as sad and alienated human individuals. Just as Velázquez had charged his portraits of dwarfs with an engaging dignity that entirely overrode their physical deficiencies, so Géricault gave his monomaniac subjects a depth of insight which portraitists normally reserved for relations, friends and other sitters with whom they enjoyed a special affinity.

The kleptomaniac who posed for the artist in an asylum had no prior claim on Géricault's affections, yet the painting he produced is alive with an instinctive sympathy (pl. 259). Without knowing that the man laboured under this affliction, we would not immediately think of him as 'mad' at all. Instead of regarding the kleptomaniac as a specimen, a generalised embodiment of a medical condition, Géricault paints him with a directness unfettered by preconceptions of any kind. Although his hair is slightly dishevelled, and he wears the somewhat dazed expression of a man who remains baffled by existence, there are no signs here of the melodramatic symptoms that a less understanding artist might have been tempted to portray.[23]

A similar refusal to indulge in exaggerated poses marks the portrait of the man suffering from delusions of military rank (pl. 260). He could even be mistaken for a genuine old soldier, proudly displaying the cap he had worn as a uniform during his career in the armed forces. Géricault realises how convinced his sitter really is of the military

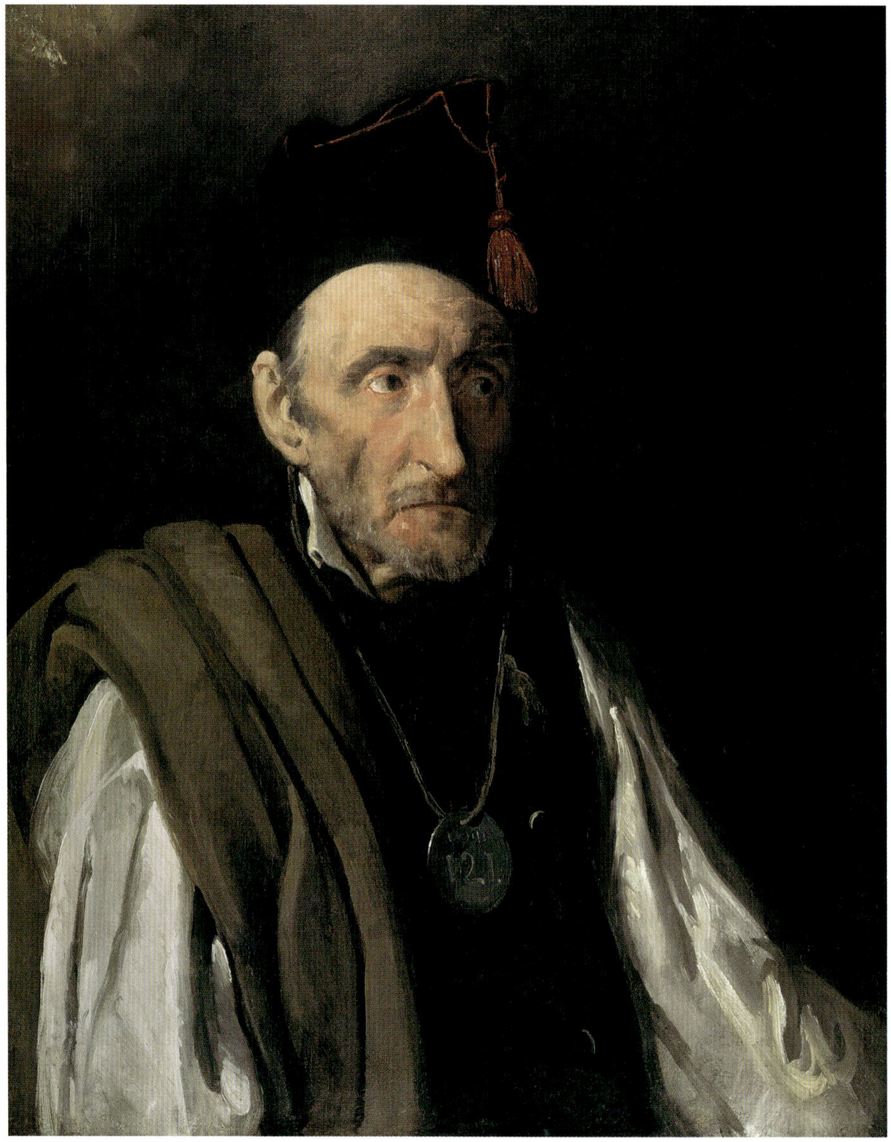

260 Theodore Géricault, *Man suffering from Delusions of Military Rank*, *c* 1819–22, Collection Oskar Reinhart 'Am Römerholz', Winterthur

status he assumes. The cap is not, for this hapless fantasist, a prop to be used in a charade. Rather is it a vital adjunct of his daily life, a means of bolstering and even defining his defective sense of self. Far from mocking the man's delusion, Géricault takes it seriously. There may be something absurd, or at the very least pathetic, about the tassel dangling in a bedraggled and listless fashion from the peak of the cap, but it is not presented here as a matter for scorn. Only in the direction of his sitter's eyes does the artist reveal a haunted disquiet, suggesting that no amount of borrowed military grandeur can ultimately prevent the man from sensing his fundamental insecurity. He looks wary and defensive, as if expecting to come under attack at any instant from an unnameable adversary. Fearing assault may well be an integral part of his condition, the inevitable corollary of his delusion. And Géricault succeeds in eliciting pity for the vulnerability of this acutely isolated patient.

The *Portrait of a Kidnapper* displays a rather more alert and positive subject (pl. 261). His cap, rather than solemnly projecting a soldierly persona, is tipped at a more jaunty angle on the sitter's head. His beard is fuller than the wispy, grey-flecked growth on the military man's chin, and he stares out of the picture with restless energy. Georget might have concluded that the kidnapper's expression disclosed his inner urge to snatch, bear away and imprison a victim, but Géricault refrains from pro-

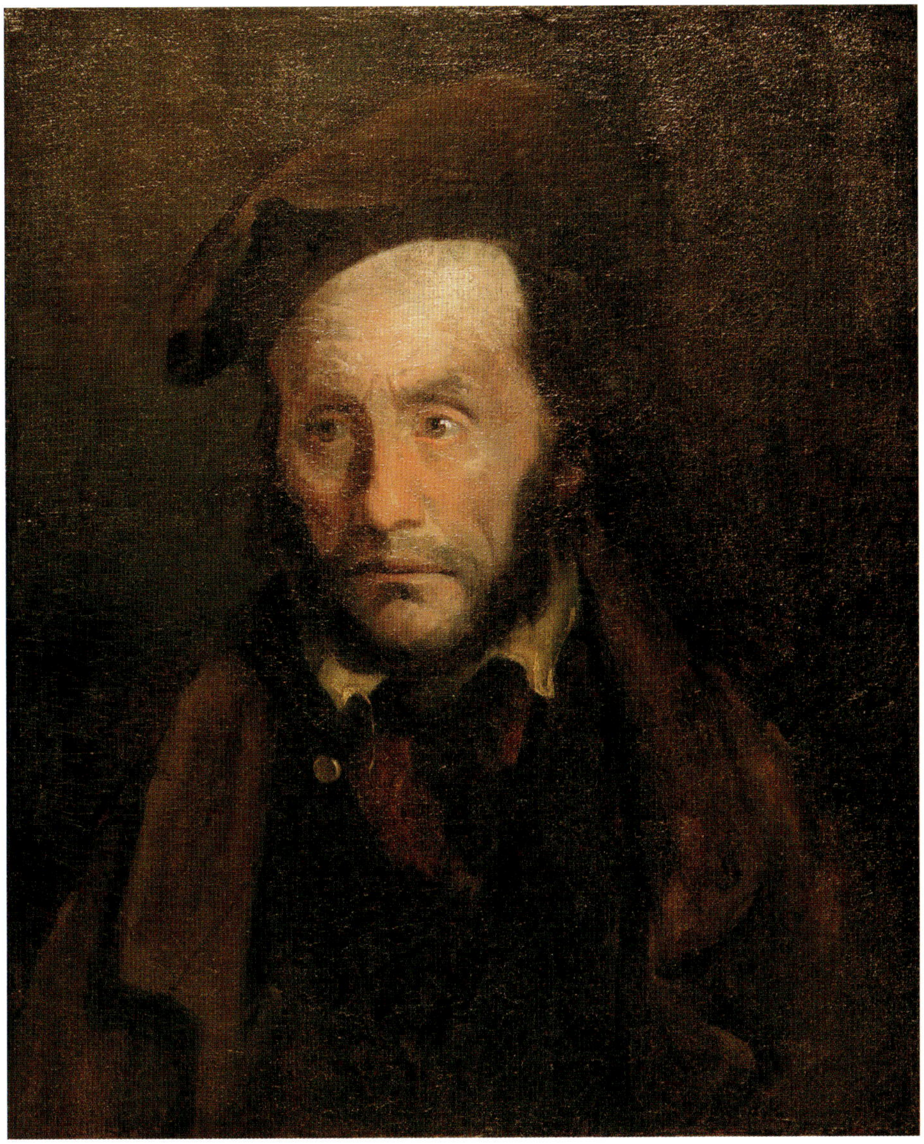

261 Theodore Géricault, *Portrait of a Kidnapper*, 1822–3, The James Philip Grey Collection, Museum of Fine Arts, Springfield, Mass.

ducing an image that could be identified in any facile or predictable way with such a compulsion. There is nothing repellent or overtly violent about this figure. If his mottled skin signifies that his health is less than robust, he can hardly be said to exude symptoms of a diseased mind. Géricault does, however, give him a strange certitude around the eyes. Unlike the man suffering from military mania, he gazes at the world with the steadiness of someone unwilling to be deflected from the *idée fixe* holding him in its thrall.

No such unwavering force can be discerned in the portrait of the woman addicted to gambling (pl. 262). Sallow to the point of bloodlessness, and hunched in a position enabling her to look up only with difficulty, she is the most abject of the five patients. Perhaps her physical stoop helps to account for her mania, providing the old woman with a mental excitement that releases her, albeit momentarily, from the bodily constraints she endures. The trembling eagerness of her expression confirms such a hypothesis. She looks up expectantly, ready to believe that something momentous might happen to compensate her for the severe limitations of life in an asylum. The crutch jutting from her cloak suggests that she might be disabled by the deformation giving her head its awkward, craning rigidity. But the gambler refuses to be entirely crushed by her chronic disabilities. The prospect of transforming her existence with a spec-

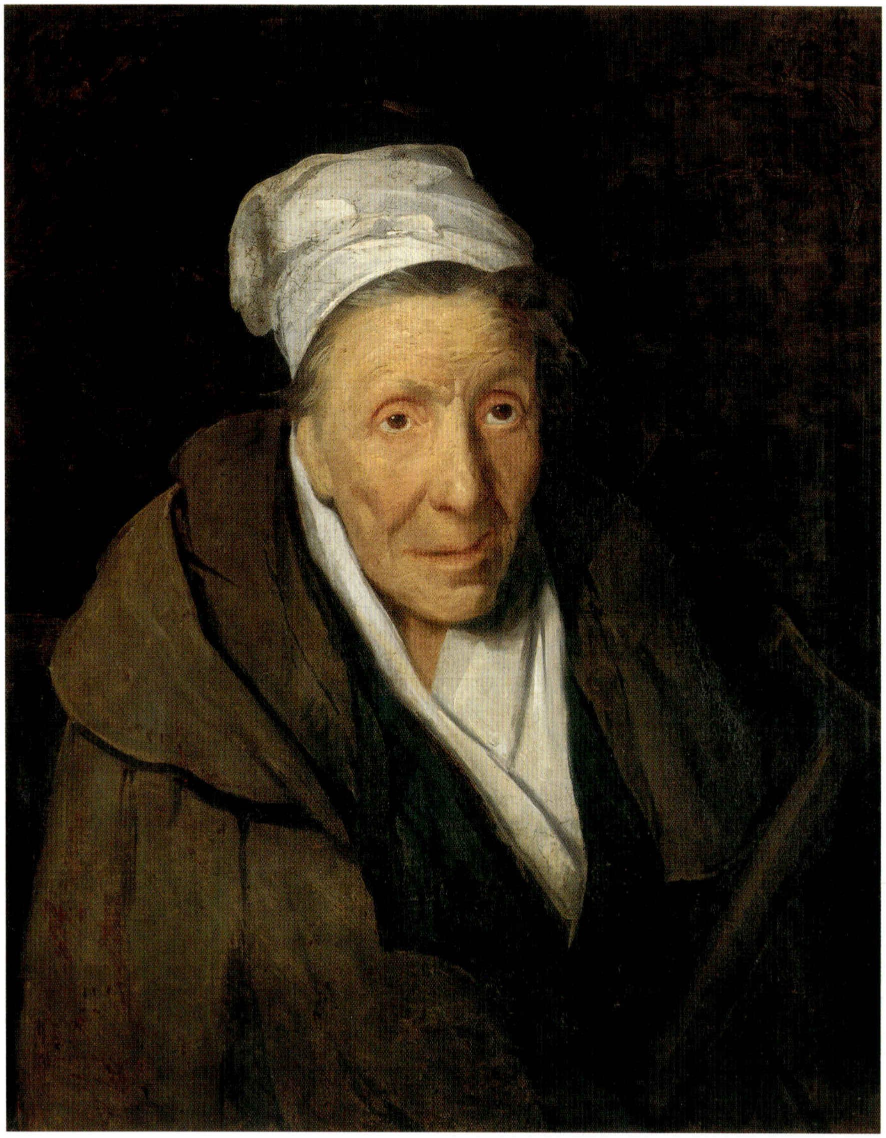

262 Theodore Géricault, *Woman addicted to Gambling*, 1819–24, Musée du Louvre, Paris

tacular, extravagantly risky venture still exerts a mesmeric hold over her mind. And Géricault seizes on this stubborn strain of hope in his arresting portrait.

The other painting of a woman, this time suffering from obsessive envy, is the most openly disturbed image (pl. 263). Impressed by his sitter's frowning concentration, which seems powerful enough this time to counter the infirmities of age, Géricault injects a greater animation into his study of this fierce inmate. Her years in the Salpêtrière have not dulled the overweening emotion she feels. Menacing and almost predatory, the woman bears down on the object of her incisive gaze as if nothing else mattered. Géricault defines the creases and veins in her forehead, the red rims of her bloodshot eyes, and the harsh lines stretching from nostrils to lips, with greater precision than in the other portraits.

These distinguishing features have a rasping potency here, and he accentuates them still further by letting her bonnet explode from the sides of her head. Even the folds in her mantle are emphatically handled with urgent sweeps of the brush. They appear as vengeful as the four long strings of the bonnet, hanging down over her russet scarf like tentacles ready to twine themselves round the victim she wants to destroy. It is a compelling examination of a mania fuelled by boundless anger, and yet Géricault resists even here the temptation to lapse into theatricality. Excited neither by disapproval nor the urge to sensationalise, he retains the objectivity that enables him to understand this enraged woman rather than condemn her out of hand.[23]

By painting these unfortunate patients with such subtlety and restraint, Géricault must have hoped to support the medical efforts of Georget and his colleagues. Having undergone a nervous collapse himself, he was predisposed to approach monomania with unusual sympathy and a desire to assist the search for effective therapy. Behind the probing intimacy of the 'insane' portraits lies an implicit conviction that lunatics are by no means as incurable as society in general imagined. The great achievement of these five canvases rests in his ability to reach an intense rapport with each sitter, and at the same time temper it with a realistic awareness of the uncontrollable passions distorting their perceptions of the world.

Géricault knew enough about mental illness to appreciate how frightening its aberrations could be. A vivid idea of his extreme volatility is conveyed by Charles Cockerell, who befriended the troubled artist during his stay in London. After admiring Géricault's 'deep feeling of pity, the pathetique, at the same time vigour, fire and animation of his works', Cockerell wrote with concern in his diary about more alarming extremes in the painter's own wildly oscillating behaviour patterns: 'Lying torpid days and weeks then rising to violent exertions. Riding tearing driving exposing himself to heat cold violence of all sorts.'[24] At the same time, Géricault was able to study psychology and expression with as much realism as the Scottish rationalists John and Charles Bell, whose illustrated studies of

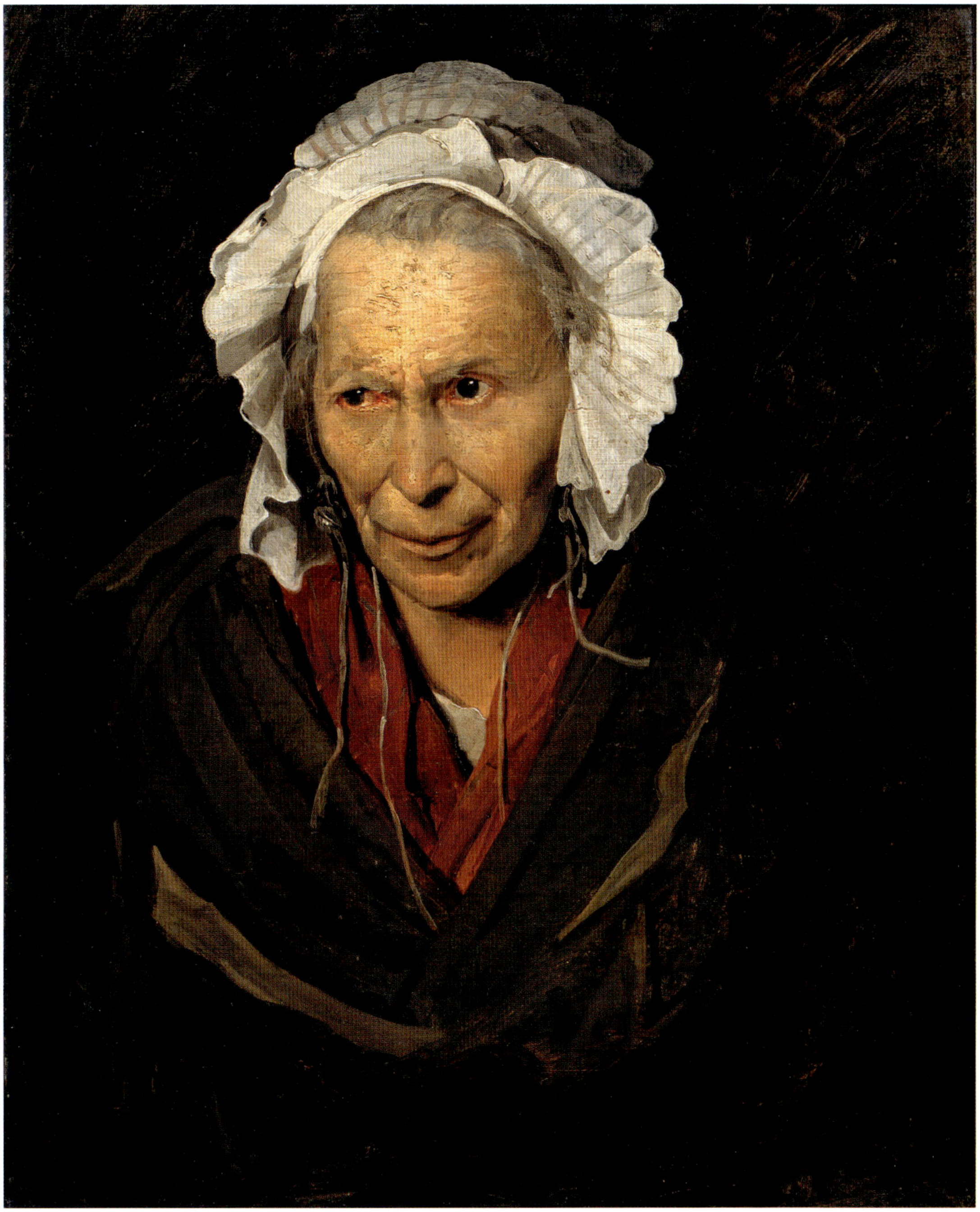

263 Theodore Géricault, *Woman suffering from Obsessive Envy*, 1822, Musée des Beaux-Arts, Lyon

the anatomy of expression attracted Géricault's attention before his London sojourn.[25]

Nevertheless, none of his portraits underestimates the malevolent power of madness. He never attempted to present it as a harmless phenomenon. Rather did he arrive, in his profoundly original *Monomania* portraits, at a masterly balance between compassion and frankness. Disturbing, poignant and utterly clear-sighted, these honest studies executed with such deft authority in the gloom of asylums herald a turning point in Western society's attitude towards demented humanity.

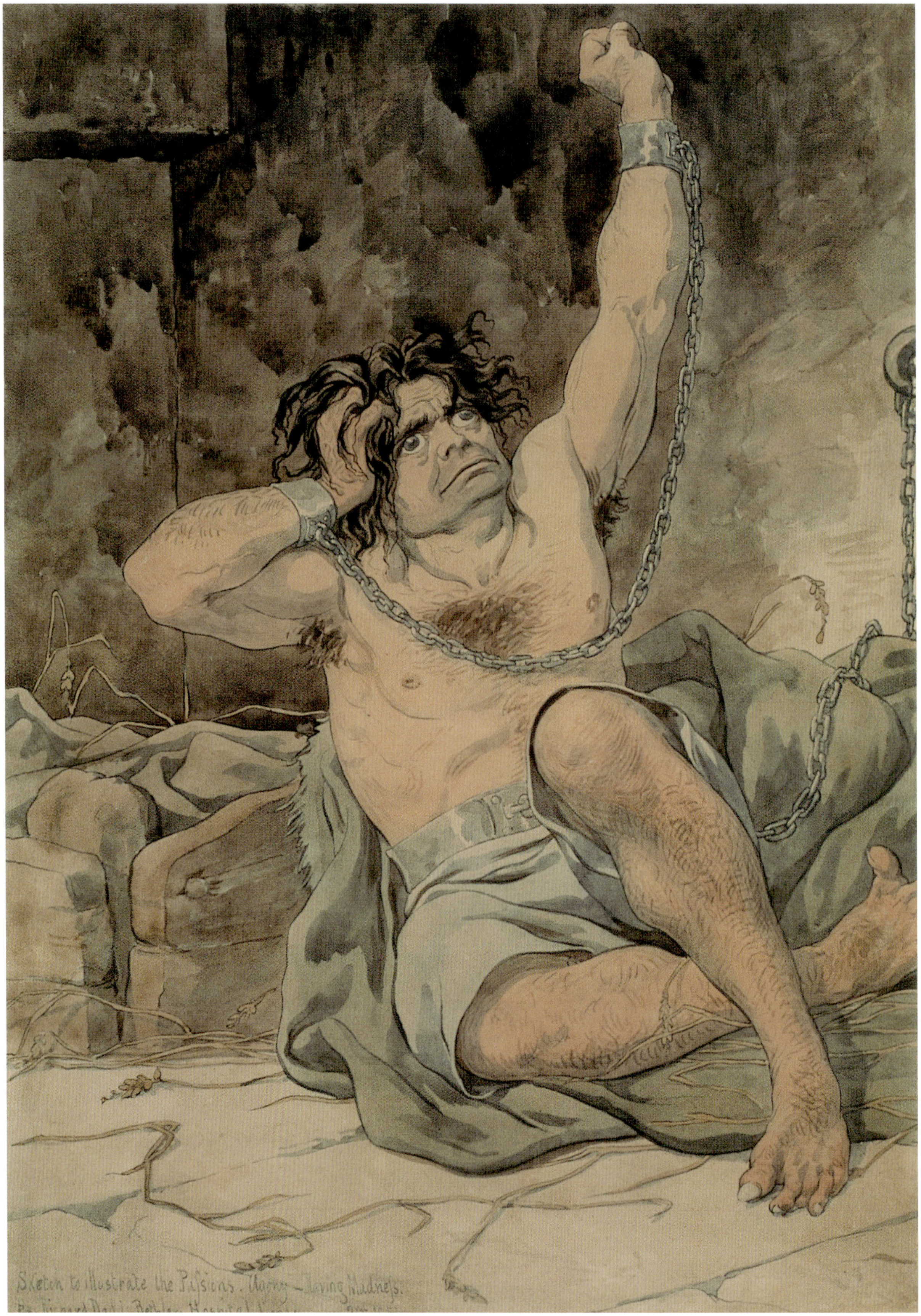

264 Richard Dadd, *Sketch to Illustrate the Passions. Agony – Raving Madness*, 1854, Bethlem Royal Hospital Museum, Kent

EIGHTEEN
'CLASSED AMONG THE DEAD'

Before long, Géricault's uncompromising images of monomania gave way to a more sentimental alternative. Sir Alexander Morison, sincerely believing that he was following in the steps of Esquirol, published a *Physiognomy of Mental Diseases* in 1843, profusely illustrated with lithographic portraits of the insane. In an understandable desire to escape from the stereotypical image of madness, Morison ensured that all the pictures dressed the patients up in impeccably respectable clothes, as well as smoothing away any hint of disfiguring neurosis from their equable faces. It was a well-meaning travesty of the truth, but soon after Morison published his findings he came into fortuitous contact with the work of an artist who, although permanently confined to asylums, continued to produce coherent and astonishingly powerful work for many years.

He first came across Richard Dadd in 1844, when the deranged painter, then aged twenty-seven, was sent to the criminal lunatic department of Bethlem Hospital. Having killed his father with a spring knife, in a notorious and premeditated incident during a walk in Cobham Park, Dadd was never again able to pursue the promising professional career that had begun to flower before insanity claimed his mind. Although Bethlem was much improved since Hogarth's day, when the public's freedom to 'view the lunatics' was a national pastime (see pl. 146), Dadd's existence there was circumscribed. He may have been freed from the strait-waistcoat confining his movements in prison directly after the murder was committed, but life in the criminal department offered little stimulus for a man of Dadd's unusual imaginative powers.

The gallery housing him in the daytime was a stark structure, about thirty metres long and chronically overcrowded. From the highly educated to the illiterate, inmates suffering from all kinds of derangement were herded together in this single space and expected to cope with each other's company at all times. The macabre atmosphere was reinforced, unintentionally, by the creation of areas separated from the main gallery by iron rods. These confined spaces gave access to the sleeping rooms next door. But the result, according to one visitor in 1857, was to create cages 'more like those which enclose the fiercer carnivora at the Zoological Gardens than anything we have elsewhere seen employed for the detention of afflicted humanity'.[1] This was the grim institution where J.M.W. Turner's mother Mary had been sent by her family just after Christmas 1800, disordered in her senses and possibly afflicted by a violent form of schizophrenia. Thereafter, Turner seems never to have talked about her, and reacted angrily if anyone else even mentioned her name. In such a forbidding context, Dadd's future must have appeared bleak and admirers of his early landscapes and fairy pictures feared that the *Art Union* was right when it gloomily referred, in 1843, to 'the late Richard Dadd. Alas! we must so preface the name of a youth of genius that promised to do honour to the world; for, although the grave has not actually closed over him, he must be classed among the dead.'[2]

Bethlem's patients were, however, encouraged to occupy themselves with reading, chess and handicrafts. Dadd would certainly have been assisted in his stubborn efforts to resume painting as soon as he revealed signs of wanting to take up his brushes once more. Dr Edward Thomas Monro, the physician supervising him, had inherited from his celebrated father Dr Thomas Monro a distinguished collection of watercolours produced by Girtin, Turner and other members of the 'Monro School'. He probably urged Dadd to start working again; and Sir Alexander Morison, the other visiting physician, would have done likewise. In his diary for 1844 Morison made a tantalisingly brief note that 'Mr. Gow brought drawing of Nolan dementia . . . says Dadd is an extraordinary artist.'[3]

It was, no doubt, the first time that Morison learned of Dadd's outstanding abilities, and Gow was well placed to assess them. An artist himself, he executed many drawings of Bethlem inmates for works on the physiognomy of madness and became one of the few visitors Dadd received in his early years at the asylum. Having known Dadd before insanity overtook him, Gow was embarrassed enough to try avoiding an encounter as he passed 'through the ward, with a portfolio under his arm'. But Dadd noticed Gow and brought him to a halt with the peremptory enquiry: 'What brings you here; have you killed anybody?' The two men then entered into a prolonged and detailed debate about the drawings of the patients in Gow's portfolio. Dadd commented that 'those fellows look mad, every one of them'.[4]

When he tried to depict an insane man himself, however, the outcome demonstrates that Dadd had little interest in studying his fellow inmates (see pl. 264). The watercolour belongs to a series produced in 1854 and inscribed with the title *Sketch to Illustrate the Passions. Agony – Raving Madness.* Far from relying on the appearance of the men around him at Bethlem, he reverted to a more traditional image of the manacled lunatic seated semi-naked in a straw-littered cell. It referred to the asylum's grim past rather than its more enlightened present. The pronounced sculptural character of the deranged figure suggests that Dadd also remembered the brooding power of Cibber's *Raving Madness* carving (see pl. 144), executed for the gatepost of the previous Bethlem building nearly two centuries before. Like Cibber's statue, Dadd's lunatic does not appear to be struggling to liberate himself from the chains. His exclamatory arms seem to protest against the inner agony he endures, and one hand presses despairingly against his brain as if to combat the unruly voices besieging him there. Compared with the forces conspiring to undermine his sanity, the manacles are a minor irritant. It is reasonable to assume that Dadd, while making no attempt to produce a recognisable self-portrait, has dramatised the mental pressure and disturbance that at times became so unbearable within his own beleaguered head.

For much of his life, he did nevertheless find merciful solace in his art. A photograph taken at Bethlem around 1856 shows him working with apparent contentment on one of his greatest paintings, *Contradiction: Oberon and Titania* (pl. 265). The thin brush held so delicately between his thumb and index finger testifies to the meticulousness with which he was able to work, loading each millimetre of his picture surface with an abundance of miscroscopic details. Although the proliferating minutiae are the result of an obsessive concern that may be symptomatic of his insanity, they also prove that Dadd possessed an exceptionally sharp eye and a firm hand. The amount of work he produced during his forty long years in asylums bears eloquent witness to an overriding spiritual need. However depressing his outward circumstances and inner turmoil may alike have become, he held on to his imaginative vision as tenaciously as the victim of a shipwreck grasping the flotsam that sustains his existence in the turbulent sea. Patricia Allderidge, a former Archivist to the present-day Bethlem Royal Hospital, believed that 'Dadd survived as a person throughout these terrible years because he survived as a painter. Never, on the evidence of his work, did he draw or paint merely to pass the time, and there can be little doubt that for the rest of his life he lived and worked as a dedicated artist, who had never abandoned his profession.'[5]

Sir Alexander Morison was more than ready to acknowledge and assist Dadd's dedication. His interest in the artist continued long after his retirement from Bethlem in 1853. Three years later he sent Dadd £5 for several drawings. The proposed transaction incurred the disapproval of the Bethlem authorities, for the Treasurer returned the money to Morison with the apologetic yet firm explanation that 'we must not allow any more of Dadd's drawings to leave the hospital. So long as they remain in hands such as yours no objection can be made but it is possible they may at some future time find their way into the market, a result which might lead to much inconvenience.'[6]

In 1852, however, Dadd had sealed his relationship with Morison by painting an arresting portrait of the seventy-three year-old physician (pl. 266). Doubtless a commission, the painting arrives at a disconcerting amalgam of naturalistic fidelity and visionary strangeness. The obsessive detail seems at first to ally the picture with the work of other Victorian artists who filled their images with an abundance of piercingly observed pictorial information. Morison is positioned in front of his seaside estate at Anchorfield on the Firth of Forth by Newhaven, and Dadd depicts both the house and its maritime setting with a veracity that might suggest he had visited the locale to study it on the spot. In reality, of course, he was never allowed out of the asylum and relied on a sketch provided by Morison's daughter Anne. Similarly, the two fisherwomen, whose diminutive proportions contrast so eerily with the physician's elongated bulk, were probably taken from the famous calotype studies of Newhaven fisherfolk by D. O. Hill and Robert Adamson. Dadd had painted similar figures on previous occasions, most notably in a large oil called *The Fish Market by the Sea*, but here they assume an oddly dream-like appearance, standing with unexplained and almost proprietorial dignity between the sitter and his home.

Although their statuesque presence ought to ameliorate Morison's isolation, they are so detached that his acute loneliness is intensified. The elderly physician lived for another fourteen years after Dadd painted him, yet he stares out of the picture with the gaunt anxiety of a man ruminating on his own mortality. The top hat held in one of his hands adds to the funereal mood, and no sign of family or friends softens the starkness of a figure who stands before us with stiff Calvinist formality. The opposite of the country gentlemen who recline at their ease in so many traditional British portraits, Morison appears to derive no pleasure from his idyllic surroundings. Rather does he gaze, with unconcealed disquiet sliced deeply into his haunted features, towards the man who painted him with such precision. His furrowed face may even reflect a sorrowful empathy with the plight endured by Dadd. In this respect, the painting ends up as a tribute to a physician's pioneering compassion for the mental anguish of the patient in his care.

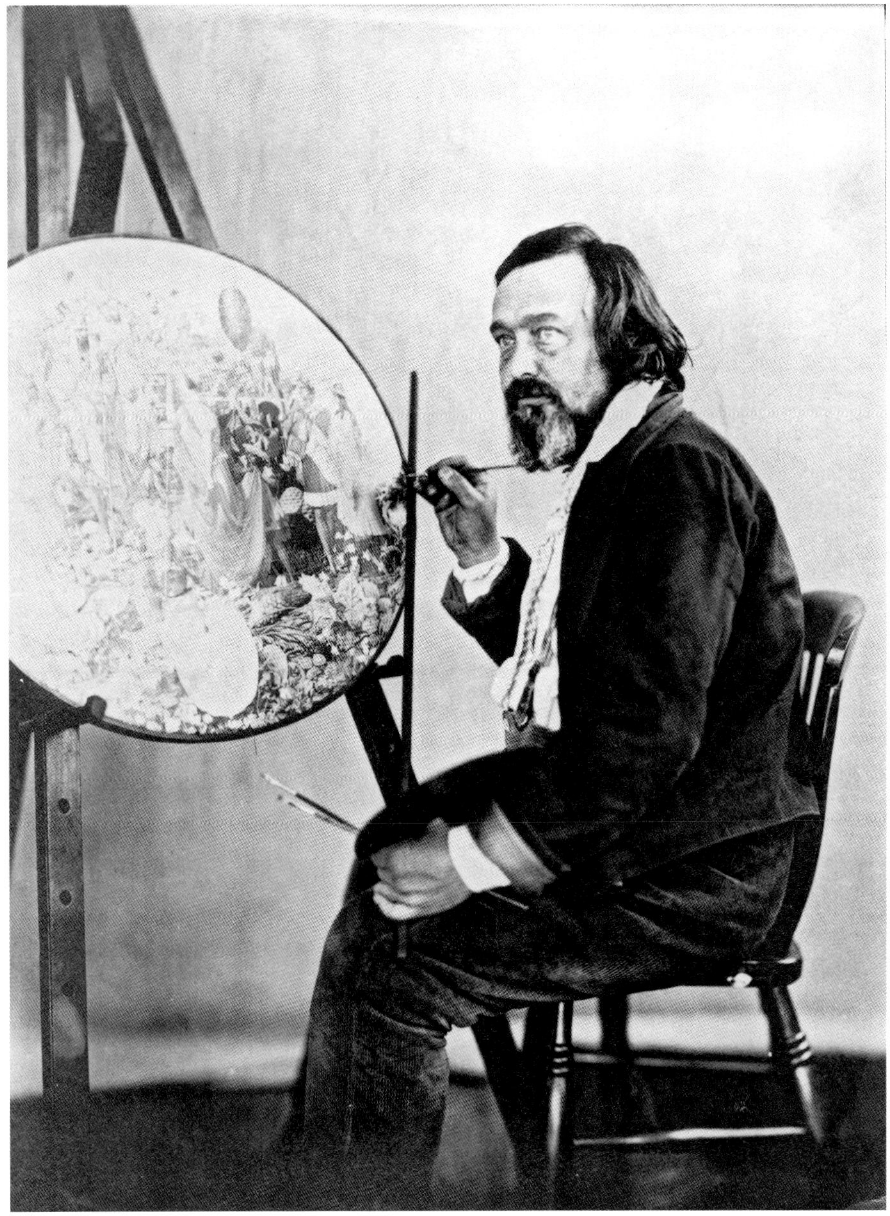

265 Henry Hering, Photograph of Richard Dadd around 1856, Bethlem Royal Hospital Museum, Kent

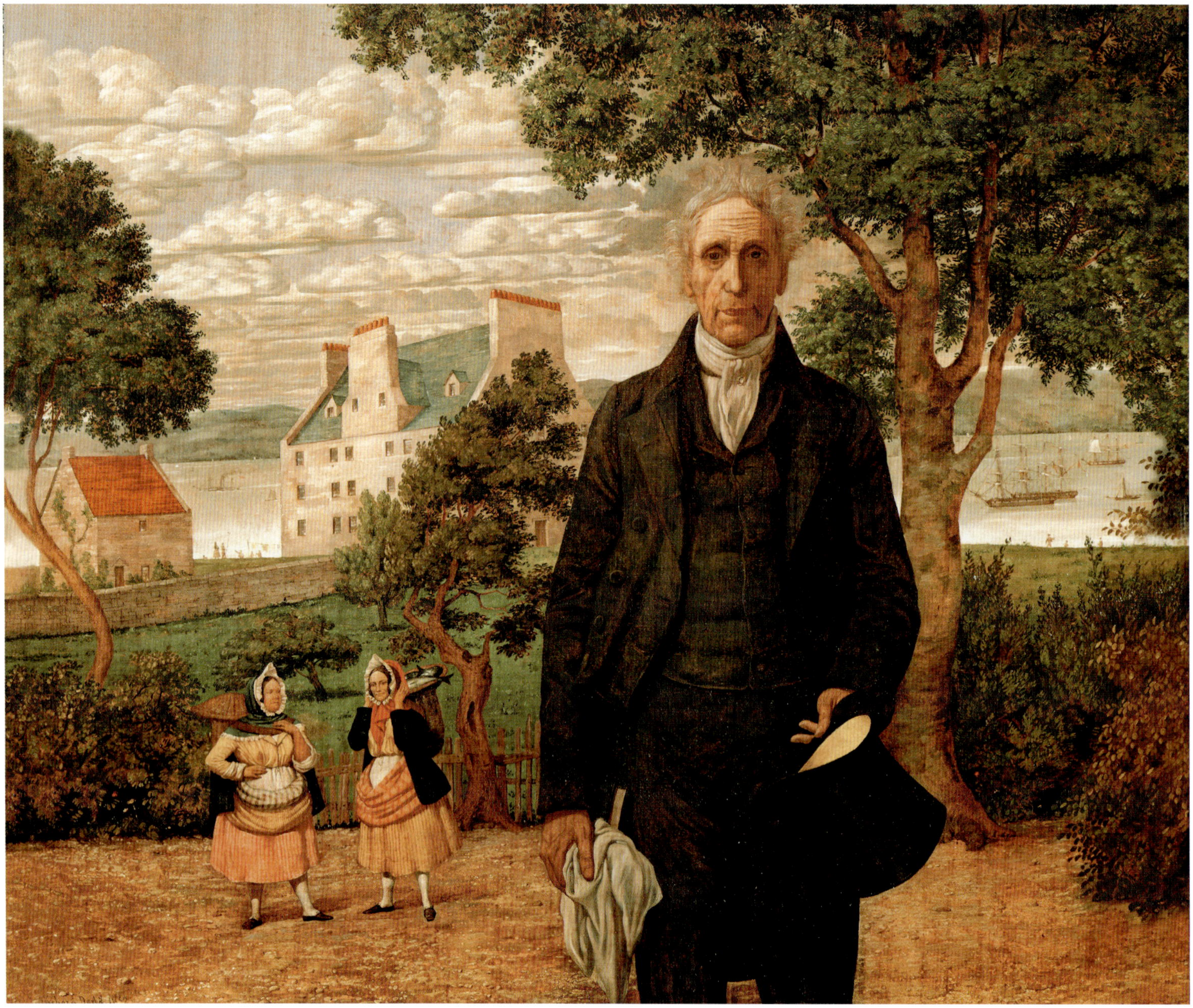

266 Richard Dadd, *Sir Alexander Morison*, 1852, Scottish National Portrait Gallery, Edinburgh

The handkerchief gripped by Morison's right hand reappears, the following year, in another remarkable portrait (pl. 267). Its sitter has been identified, albeit tentatively, as William Charles Hood, an energetic young man responsible for revolutionising the treatment of Bethlem's patients. In 1852, around the time when Dadd's output significantly increased, Hood was appointed as the first resident physician superintendent. He devoted himself full-time to the inmates, giving them more attention than the sometimes neglectful visiting physicians had hitherto provided. Before long, the galleries at Bethlem were transformed. The windows enlarged by Hood, no less than the birdcages, paintings and hanging plants he introduced to the formerly austere spaces, countered the grimness of the ward illustrated in an engraving of the period.

Dadd must have savoured the change, even if Hood and his new steward George Henry Haydon

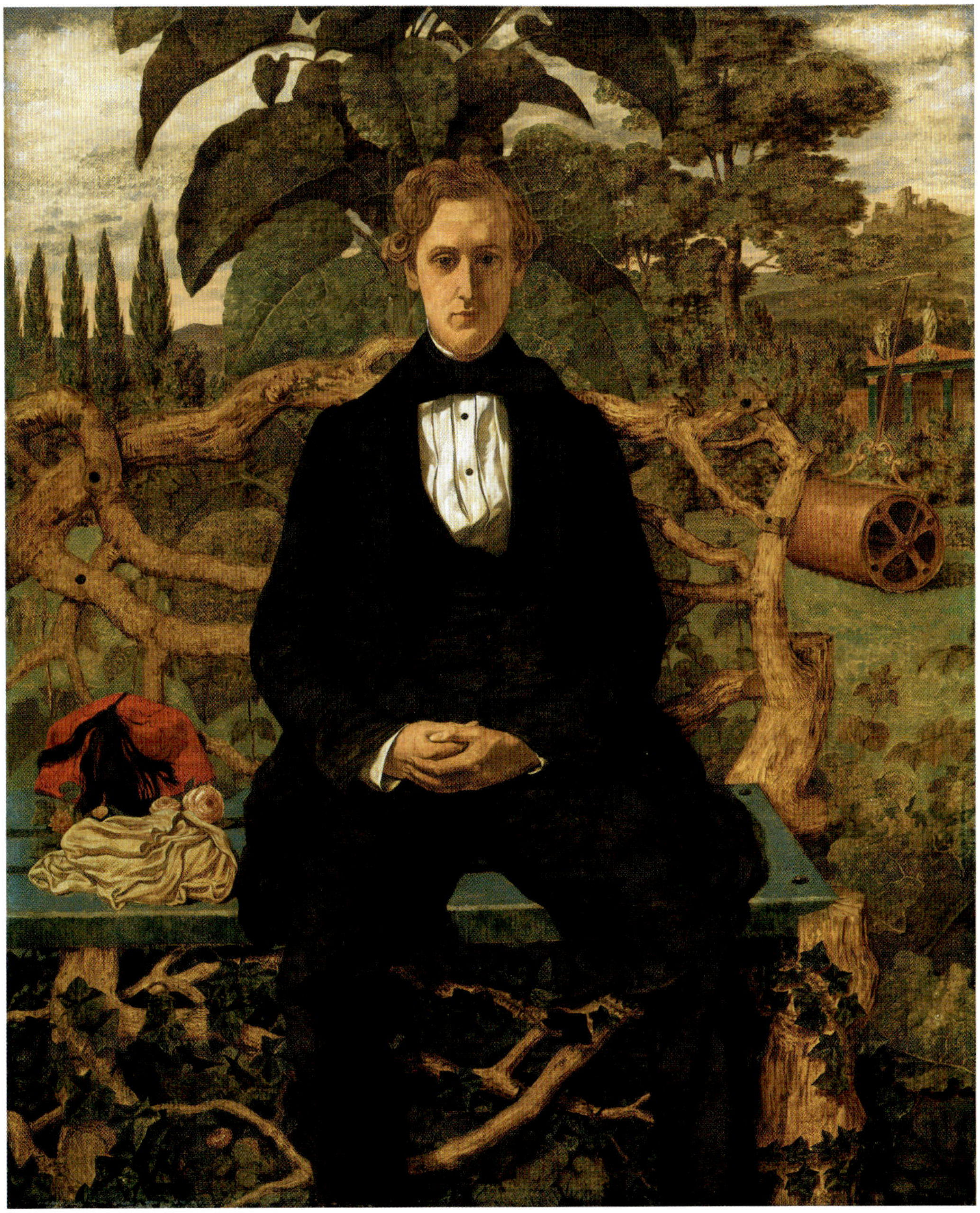

267 Richard Dadd, *Portrait of a Young Man* (William Charles Hood?), 1853, Tate, London

(another possible candidate as the sitter) found that their zeal was somewhat thwarted by the congested and architecturally gruesome criminal department where Dadd was housed. He benefited from Hood's company, for the enlightened doctor recorded in his case-notes of 1854 that Dadd was, at his most lucid, 'a very sensible and agreable companion, and shews in conversation, a mind once well educated and thoroughly informed in all the particulars of his profession in which he still shines'.[7] Hood's enthusiasm for his patient's work was sincere enough for him to amass more than thirty of Dadd's pictures in his own collection,[8] among them *Contradiction: Oberon and Titania*, triumphantly completed after four years' intensive work.[9]

Whether or not Hood is depicted in the *Portrait of a Young Man*, it commemorates a notable sympathy between sitter and artist. There is little, here, of the tension pervading Morison's portrait. Instead of standing with erect propriety in a landscape that seems strangely detached from the sitter, the man rests on a sturdy garden seat and wears a meditative expression. A handkerchief lies on the blue seat beside him, no longer clutched with the fervency displayed by Morison. The fez next to it, reminiscent of that worn by Dadd himself on his early journey to the Middle East, gives an exotic warmth to the picture, as do the enormous leaves of the sunflower sprouting behind the sitter's head, lending the image an expansiveness that the rest of the landscape does nothing to dispel. For the countryside beyond is burgeoning with the growth of high summer, its richness no doubt reinforced by the yearning memories of an artist whose life outdoors had not always been exclusively limited to a bare exercise yard. Drawing on nostalgic recollection and material in his sketchbooks, Dadd paints the kind of garden that accords most closely with his own fantasies of the setting he would have liked to inhabit. From the line of vigorous poplars to the fat garden roller idling on the freshly-cut lawn, everything seems to exude pastoral contentment. The castle on the distant hilltop, a thoroughly romantic motif also included in several of his previous imaginary landscapes, confirms that Dadd is indulging in unashamed wish-fulfilment about a world he could no longer experience.

The sobriety of the man seated in this horticultural paradise contrasts with his hedonistic context. He maintains a sense of professional composure, and his dark clothes make no concession to the luminosity around him. If signs of Dadd's instability are anywhere to be detected in this otherwise beguiling picture, they lie in the strange disparity between man and nature. He looks altogether too correct and prim for such a place, and an element of English repression has perhaps been allowed to shape Dadd's interpretation of his personality. The sitter almost appears to be refusing, in a puritanical way, to savour the delights of the location. He clasps his hands together with a resolution that implies a desire to avoid direct contact with the plant textures and dewdrops painted so enticingly among the growth around him. The meticulous attention Dadd pays to the branches writhing in the back of the garden seat adds to the suspicion of incipient unease, as does the ivy that chokes the area behind his legs with its clinging force. Yet these elements should not be exaggerated. Their hints of another, more disconcerting mood are outweighed by a prevailing air of satisfaction, both with the natural order Dadd longed to enjoy and with the sympathetic attitude of a young man who regarded him as a gifted human being rather than a lunatic beyond assistance.

Commissioned portraits of physicians apart, most of Dadd's time at Bethlem was taken up with watercolours seemingly executed for his own satisfaction alone. Relying on the resources of his prodigious inventiveness, he made little attempt to portray fellow-patients or to depict the condition of insanity with the explicitness that marks his image of *Raving Madness* (see pl. 264). An exception can be found in the powerful and exquisitely refined watercolour inscribed 'Sketch of an idea for Crazy Jane', which may have been based on a male inmate posing for the purpose (pl. 268). Dadd's choice of the word 'sketch' does no justice to the deliberation expended on this poignant work, where he took as his starting point the ballad 'Poor Crazy Jane' and its melancholy tale of a meeting between an itinerant, deranged girl and a passer-by who is horrified by her distress:

> Why fair maid in every feature
> Are such signs of fear expressed!
> Can a wandering wretched creature,
> With such horror fill thy breast.

After Crazy Jane explains that her lover's cruel desertion precipitated the madness she now endures, the ballad arrives at a disconsolate conclusion:

> Now forlorn and broken hearted
> And with frenzied thoughts beset,
> On that spot where last we parted,
> On that spot where first we met
> Still I sing my lovelorn ditty
> Still I slowly pace the plain,
> While each passer by in pity
> Cries God help thee Crazy Jane.

The ballad offers an uncompromising picture of the damage that irreparable feelings of betrayal and loss can inflict on a young mind. Dadd's *Crazy Jane* is fired by his readiness to respond to her tragic predicament. Garlanded with an Ophelia-like assortment of wild flowers and leaves festooning her bedraggled hair, the forlorn girl stretches upwards with a determination that implies a desire to escape from her misery. The feeling of resolve is

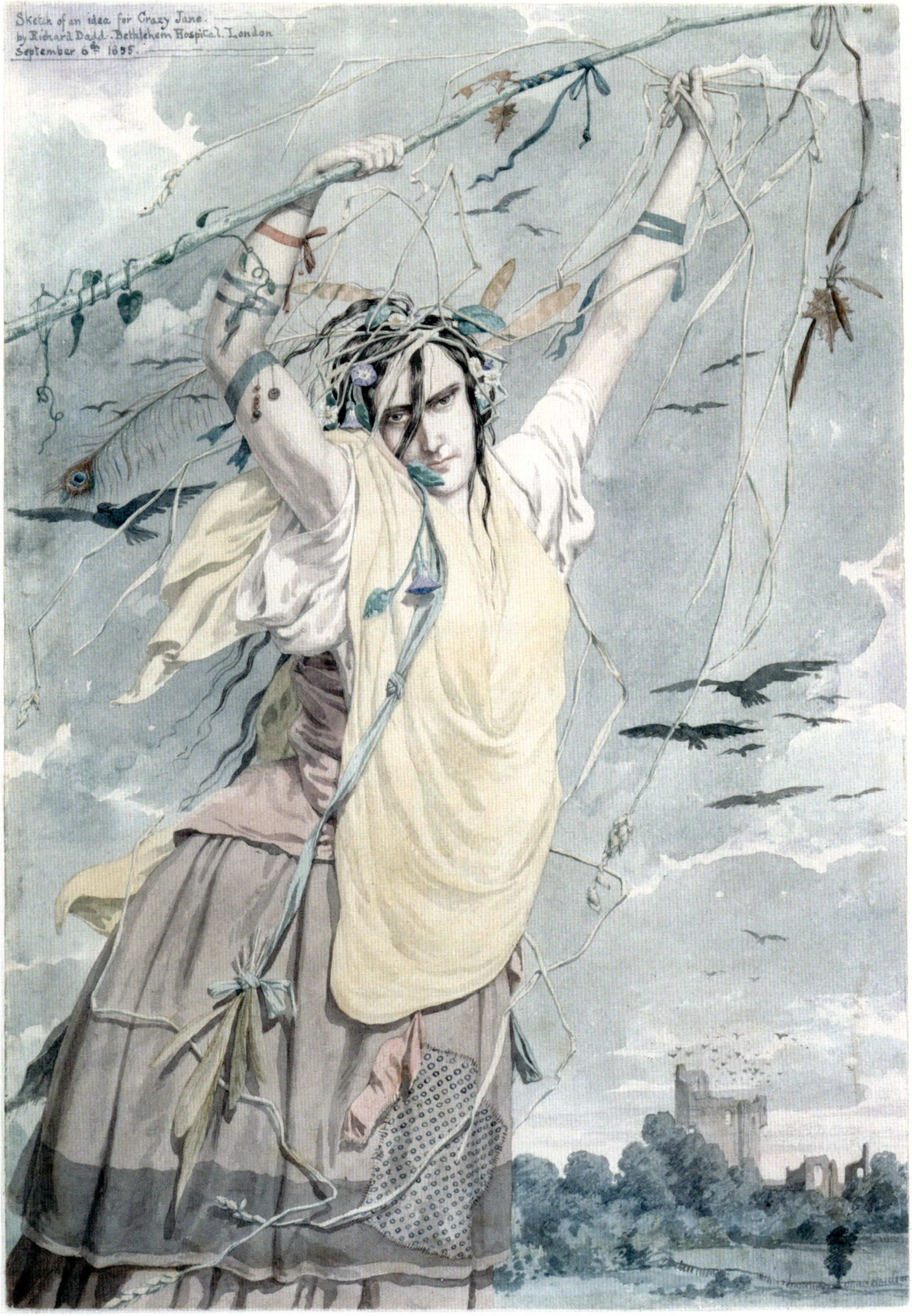

268 Richard Dadd, *Sketch of an Idea for Crazy Jane*, 1855, Bethlem Royal Hospital Museum, Kent

strengthened by Jane's stern expression, for Dadd has spurned the temptation to give her features a predictably 'lunatic' appearance. He knew, from personal experience as much as observation of other sufferers, that the condition of madness did not automatically manifest itself in facial distortions. The model who posed for the picture may well have looked deceptively composed, and Jane takes on the coherent air of someone calmly convinced that her behaviour is quite rational.

Her action, however, is marked above all by futility. Try though Jane might to reach out in a yearning diagonal towards the freedom of the sky, she cannot transcend her earthbound limits. The branch she wields like a makeshift javelin should, ideally, assist these efforts to divest herself of mortal sorrow. But the bulk of her skirt, painted in more leaden colours than the pale lemon drapery flung across her shoulders, weighs heavily on Jane's slender body and frustrates her fantasies of flight. Her right arm, which should be aiming the would-be projectile upwards with single-minded vigour, seems to acknowledge the uselessness of her endeavour. For Jane's hand is bent over the branch, in a position that signifies dangling rather than throwing, and her inability to soar is confirmed by the leaves, ribbons and convolvulus hanging down as well. The broken ears of wheat reveal the full extent of her ineffectiveness as they droop from the uppermost end of the branch, while Jane is helpless to prevent the trailing straws grasped by her left hand plummeting almost the entire length of the picture. Their limpness makes a nonsense of the supposedly triumphant thrust of the girl's left arm. She is condemned to confront her plight in a landscape uninhabited by anything except an appropriately ruined castle, and the raven-like birds flapping towards Jane's alienated form appear to be anticipating her imminent collapse.

The finely judged precision with which Dadd defines this figure shows how much discernment and control he was able to exert over his art. Its clarity contrasts, eerily yet effectively, with the dishevelled wildness of the poor girl in his picture, but the image of madness presented by *Crazy Jane* is cheerless enough. It suggests that she will forever be trapped within her torment, and Dadd would by now have reached similar conclusions about his own state of mind. Although he retained formidable powers of intellect and rallied to a certain extent after the murderous fit that confined him to the asylum in the first place, he knew that his crime would oblige the authorities to keep him incarcerated for life. Moreover, he was still prey to sudden rages and inexplicable assaults on his companions, driven as he thought by the dominant influence of the Egyptian god Osiris and other spirits. Dadd never freed himself from the terrible delusions behind his father's murder: one visitor described in 1877 how the sixty-year-old artist remained at the mercy of 'thick-coming horrors and portentous visions – meditative, gloomy, abstracted'.[10]

By this time, however, he had executed a large-scale painting that presented a more optimistic vision of the curative process. This canvas, about three metres wide, hung on the Bethlem staircase for many years (pl. 269). Its unusual size indicates that Dadd produced it specifically for that site, and in location and subject alike it suggests his awareness of Hogarth's decoration for the Great Staircase at Bart's (see pl. 183). For Dadd painted *The Good Samaritan* in a frieze-like design, presenting the wounded man and his helper at the very forefront of the picture. The photograph of this lost painting is sadly indistinct but enough can be discerned to ascertain that Dadd concentrated on an affirmative moment in the biblical story. He could have shown the victim at his most abandoned, newly injured with the Samaritan still a great distance away. Instead, he chose to follow Hogarth's precedent and depict the time when, having been propped against a rock and already swathed in a bandage above his right elbow, the man lies back gratefully while the Samaritan binds his other arm. Unlike Hogarth's painting, where the afflicted figure is gashed yet alert and able to retain a seated position, Dadd's canvas emphasises the seriousness of the wounds. With eyes shut and legs stretched inert across the ground, the victim is scarcely conscious in the Bethlem version. Yet Dadd has given him a shaggy, heavily muscled physique, suggesting that he may be capable of making a complete recovery. Furthermore, most of the shallow picture-space is filled with the reassuring forms of both the Samaritan and a donkey waiting patiently for the ministrations to finish.

Although the surviving photograph hardly facilitates a confident assessment of *The Good Samaritan*, Dadd appears to have adopted a distinctly different manner here. Knowing that the result

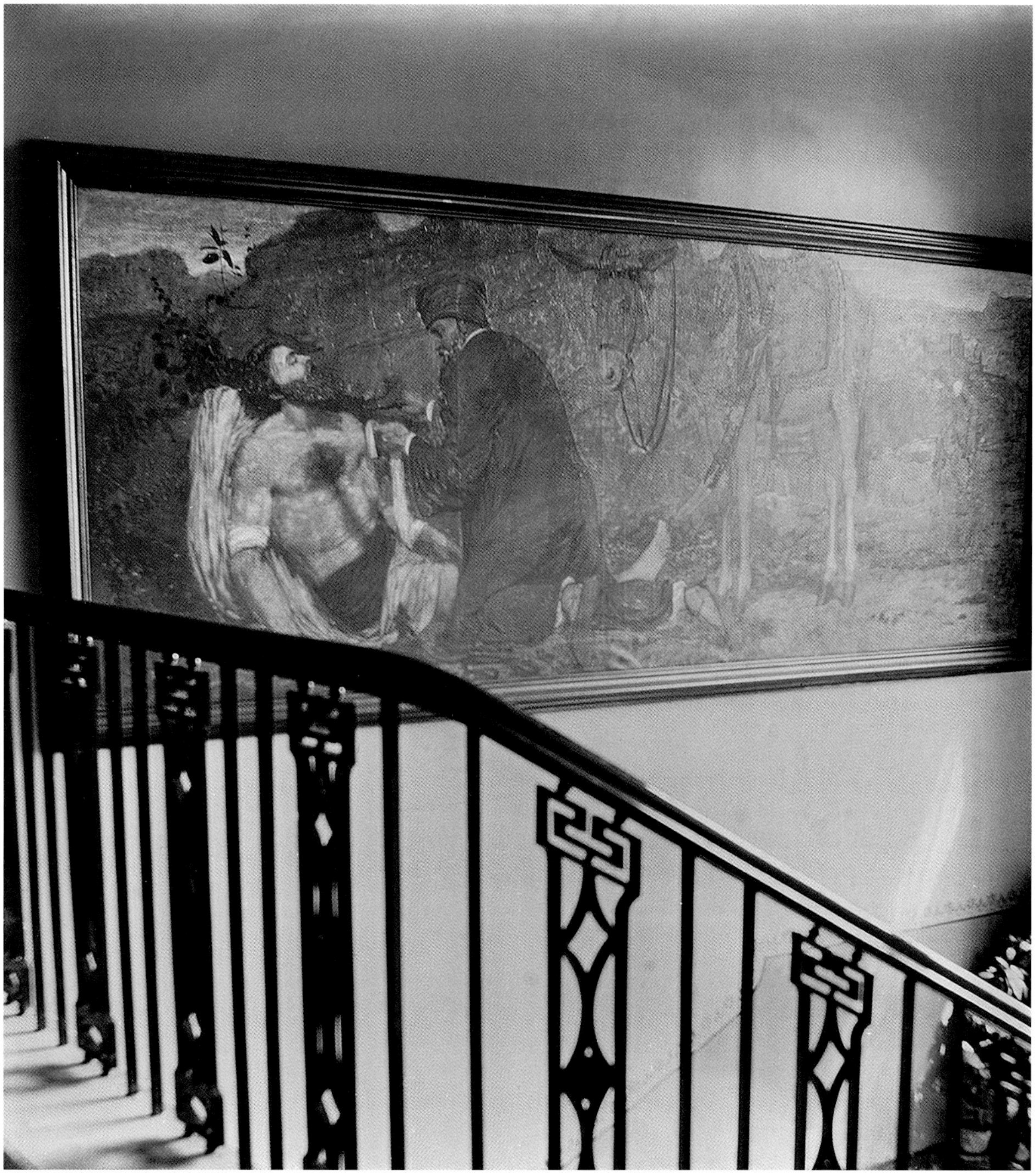

269 Richard Dadd, *The Good Samaritan* on Bethlem staircase, *c.*1859, Bethlem Royal Hospital Museum, Kent

would be seen by everyone at Bethlem, he employed a more monumental and straightforward form-language – presumably in an attempt to produce an image accessible to even the most visually illiterate onlooker. One observer noted that the decoration, in place by 1859, was 'a vigorous though unfinished painting',[11] and indeed it seems to have lacked the obsessive quality of Dadd's smaller, more private and personal works. William Michael Rossetti, who visited him and was perhaps adversely affected in his judgement by the 'undercurrent of sullenness' he detected in Dadd's attitude to him, considered that *The Good Samaritan* was an unexceptional work, 'with no trace of the impressive talent demonstrated by Dadd before madness claimed him.'[12]

270 Richard Dadd, *The Fairy Feller's Master-Stroke*, 1855–64, Tate, London

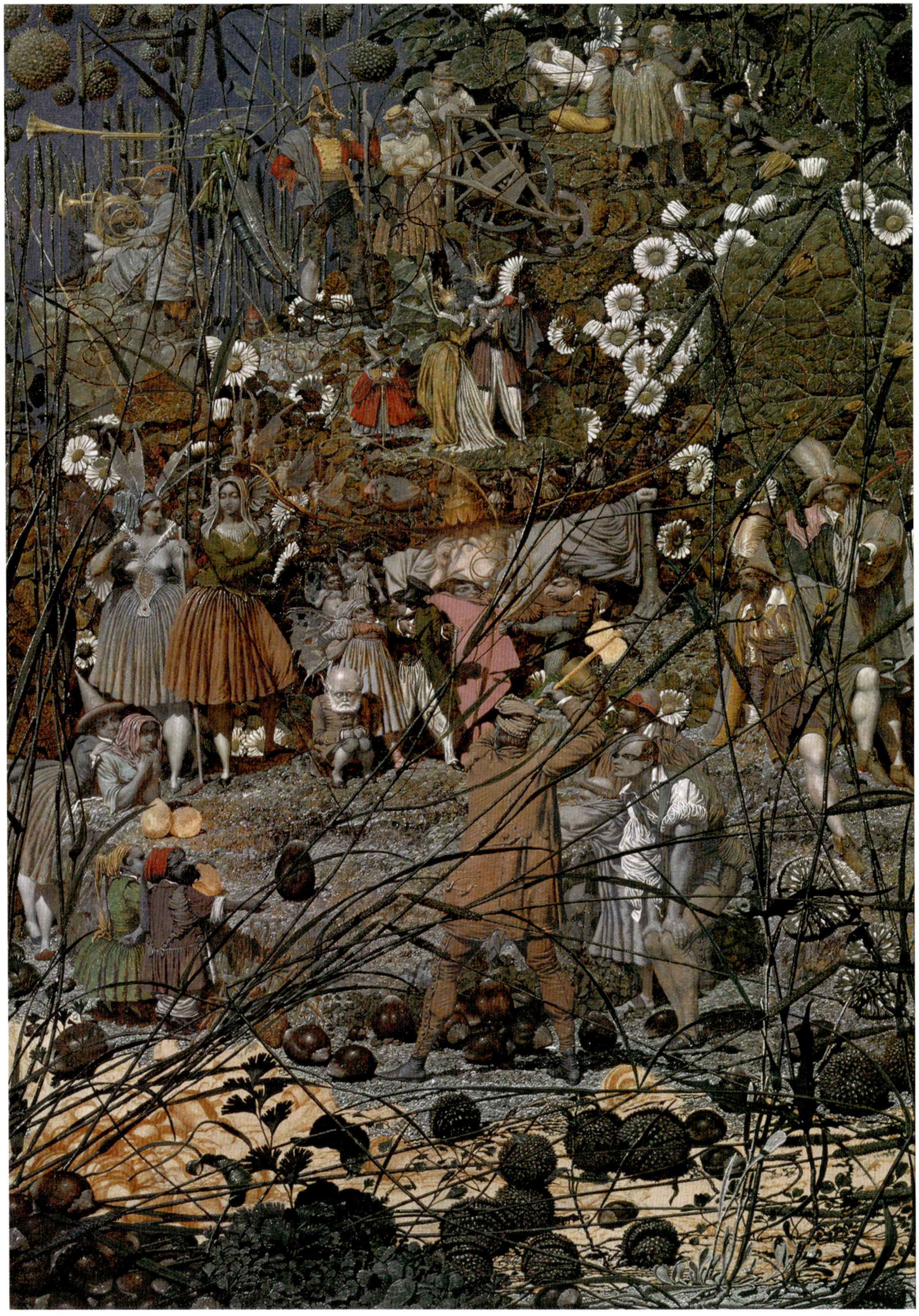

Whatever its shortcomings, the painting was clearly an ambitious and sincere attempt to provide the hospital with a grand statement about humanity's readiness to help and comfort the afflicted. The fact that Dadd procured a canvas large enough to suit this prominent public space, and was encouraged to make a painting for the pleasure of Bethlem's staff, inmates and visitors alike, says a great deal about the faith that Hood and Haydon had in his abilities. They gave the picture a substantial frame, enough to imply that it deserved a permanent place in the institution. And the two men surely took justifiable pride in the installation of a work proving that a so-called 'insane' patient could, with sufficient help from sympathetic staff, produce a wholly coherent pictorial testament to the humane principles behind the transformation of Bethlem's *modus operandi* in the 1850s.

The extent of Dadd's gratitude to his friends can be gauged by his willingness, possibly between 1855 and 1864, to paint for Haydon *The Fairy Feller's Master-Stroke*,[13] the most trance-like of all his works (pl. 270). It is also, in terms of the brutal crime committed by the artist, the most unnerving. As the title indicates, its central tension is focused on the leather-clad fairy woodman, who lifts up his axe to split open a hazelnut as large as a human skull. Although his face is turned away from view, this bucolic executioner could be a portrait of the artist as murderer. Dadd's father, who was an apothecary, is probably included at the top of the painting, in a group of figures representing the children's fortune-telling game 'soldier, sailor, tinker, tailor, ploughboy, apothecary, thief'. Everybody in this fanatically detailed canvas belongs to what Dadd described, in his bizarre poem purporting to explain the painting, as 'A Fairy band'.[14] He also claimed that work could only begin on the picture once his mind had been cleared of all conscious intention:

> I thought nought on nought – a shift
> As good perhaps as thinking hard. . .
> Indefinite almost unseen
> Lay vacant entities of chance,
> Lent forms unto my careless glance
> Without intent, pure fancy 't'is I mean.

Perhaps this act of emptying his imagination enabled him to deal, albeit indirectly, with his own tragic downfall. When Dadd knifed his father to death in Cobham Park, he was certainly not surrounded by the large cast of 'Fays, gnomes, and elves and suchlike' who have assembled here to stare at the fairy-feller. But they all seem fascinated by his raised axe, and determined to witness the fateful striking of the hazelnut. Through the diagonal lines of the timothy grasses sweeping across the picture-surface, their faces can be discerned, whether leering, squinting, goggling or peering. The cross-eyed, gnome-like figure squatting on the ground just above the fairy-feller is, according to Dadd, a critic whose 'business is to teach to do./ Do it himself? Oh! no! tis you.' The group clustered round him include a couple of eavesdropping elves and, theatrically arrayed in a pink cloak, a politician 'with senatorial pipe . . . /To hear him talk, Lord! how 't'would make you laugh.' But this diminutive gaggle is overshadowed by the monumental pair of maidservants on the left, one holding a broom and the other a mirror. They are the most openly erotic figures ever painted by Dadd, who clearly relished the girl with ample breasts threatening to burst through her bodice. He must have envied the 'satyr' peering lasciviously under the skirts of the other maid, for Dadd's poem dwells enviously on this gleeful voyeur:

> His right to look,
> I care not to dispute. . .
> All are not saints on earth below. . .
> Or are shut out from natures game.

Yet the most potent observer is the white-bearded patriarch, whose 'triple crown of subtle might' probably identifies him as the Pope. During a trip to Rome in 1843, Dadd saw the pontiff at a public appearance and afterwards admitted to his doctors that he was 'overcome by an urge to attack him, only refraining, because he was so well protected'.[15] This sense of awe is carried over into Dadd's painting, for he explained that in his canvas the Pope's right hand is raised not to bless everyone but to issue an order to the fairy-feller: 'Except I tell you when, strike if you dare.' Hence, perhaps, the curiously frozen pose of the leather-clad axeman. Seemingly unable to strike without permission from the holy father, he may also be mesmerised by the bizarre calligraphic swirls round the Pope's crown. Dadd devoted one of the most bizarre passages in his poem to this hypnotic spectacle:

Turn to the Patriarch & behold
Long pendents from his crown are rolled,
In winding figures circle round
The grass and such upon the mound,
They represent vagary wild
And mental aberration styled.

There can be little doubt that Dadd was meditating on his own breakdown in this mysterious, claustrophobic painting. The figures all appear ensnared in a wild and overgrown setting where, as Dadd wrote in his poem, they seem in thrall to a bewitching sense

Of power a potent spell to loose
Which binds the better slave to worse
Swindles soul, body, goods & purse
T'unlock the secret cells of dark abyss
The power which never doth its victim miss.

Ultimately, though, Dadd could not bear to confront the full, distressing reality of his crime in this haunted picture. In order to prevent viewers from concluding that *The Fairy Feller's Master-Stroke* is above all a confessional image, obsessed by the violence implicit in the raising of the axe, he concluded his long, rambling poem with an eloquent disclaimer:

But whether it be or be not so
You can afford to let this go
For nought as nothing it explains
And nothing from nothing nothing gains.

The vehemence of this extraordinary final line suggests that Dadd must have felt relieved to turn away from such alarmingly personal concerns and focus on a new environment. So far as his hospital surroundings were concerned, the execution of the *Good Samaritan* gave him the confidence and ambition to undertake an extensive series of wall-paintings for the building where he was moved in the summer of 1864. All the criminal patients of Bethlem were transferred to the new and more spacious Broadmoor asylum at that time, and the change must have been revelatory. For Broadmoor Hospital, set in the wooded Berkshire countryside, offered its inmates an open rear terrace more heartening by far than the brickbound exercise yard at Bethlem. The move did not prevent Dadd from continuing to produce his small, visionary watercolours in the same fervent spirit as before. It did, nevertheless, inaugurate a period of intensive experiment.

Most of his energies at Broadmoor were focused on the decoration not just of a staircase but of entire interiors. Like the *Good Samaritan*, most failed to survive the hospital's move in 1930. Until then, though, the building's inhabitants were able to savour Dadd's work on a truly spectacular scale, for a report in *The World* declared in 1877 that 'he has adorned and beautified the asylum-walls'. The writer did not, unfortunately, specify all the rooms containing these images, which would have constituted a compelling alternative to the traditional framed picture seen decorating a day-room for male patients in a contemporary illustration. Yet it is clear that the theatre at Broadmoor had become the particular focus of Dadd's activities. The murals, according to *The World*, 'were lavished [with] decoration of a curiously florid kind, quaint arabesques, and lines painted in a medley of vivid colours'.[16]

They sound, from this tantalisingly brief account, more idiosyncratic and uninhibited than the relatively sober *Good Samaritan*. Prompted no doubt by the dramatic purposes to which the room was devoted, Dadd cast reticence aside when he undertook the transformation of the Broadmoor Theatre. The loss of these murals can only be deplored, for they constituted his most sustained attempt to animate an architectural space. Congenial new surroundings, combined with encouragement from the superintendent Dr William Orange, spurred him into experimenting with new materials and contributing to the embellishment of the stage itself. Dadd painted an elaborate drop-curtain for which a detailed watercolour sketch still exists (pl. 271). It seems placid enough, with a golden galley burnishing the foreground and a richly foliated hill reflecting perhaps the inspiration of the Berkshire landscape. Yet nothing as spectacular as this mountainous terrain could be found in the vicinity of Broadmoor. The rock rises to a giddy height, culminating in the elegant temple structure that presides like a lighthouse over the Mediterranean scene. Set in an unspecified past, the 'sketch' allowed Dadd to give rein to his love of a full-blown romantic landscape, where dignified architecture close at hand is juxtaposed with mountainous terrain beyond and a spectacularly tall bridge spanning the vertiginous depths of a ravine.

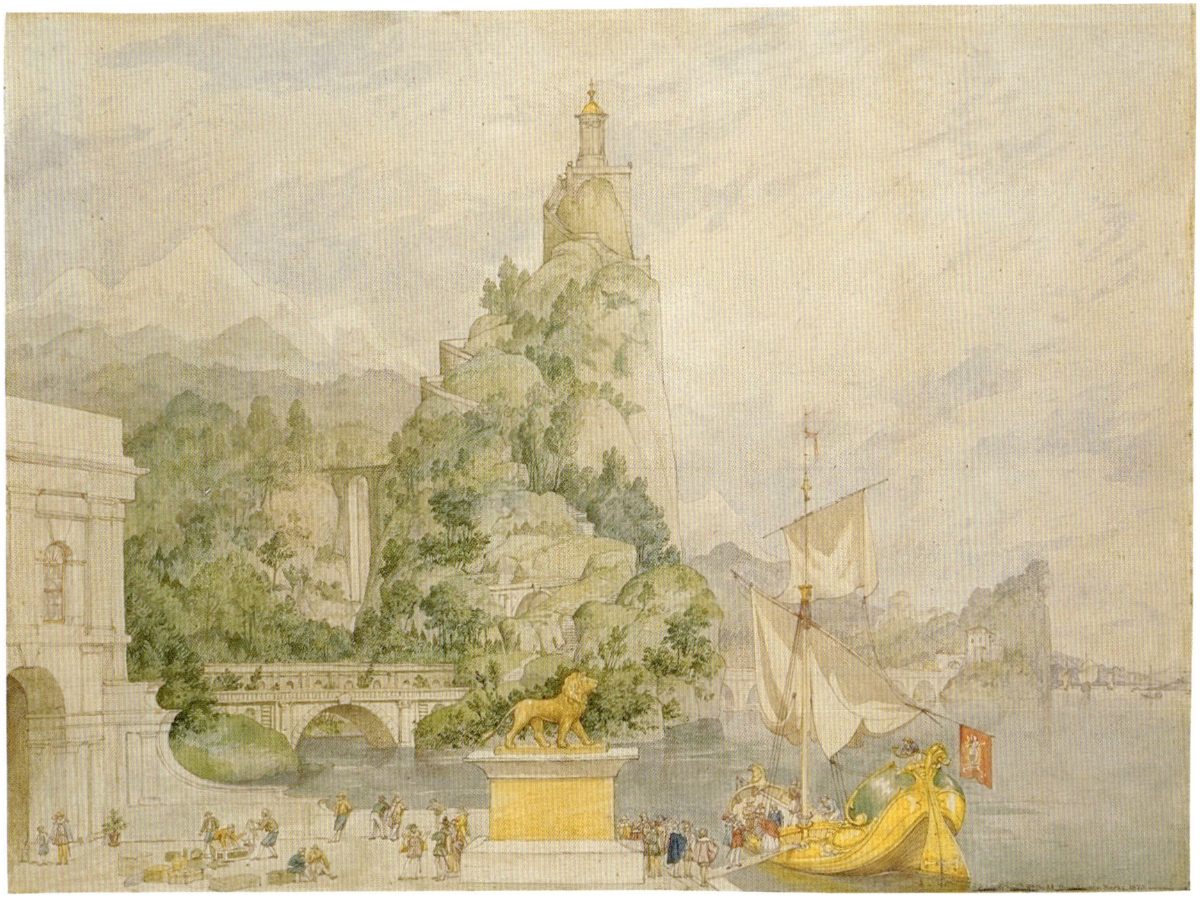

271 Richard Dadd, *Design for the Broadmoor Stage Drop-Curtain*, 1873, Victoria and Albert Museum, London

When he executed the drop-curtain itself, though, this warm and enchanting caprice underwent a turbulent metamorphosis. The disturbed side of Dadd's fantasy, so disarmingly suppressed in the 'sketch', was released now with overwhelming force. 'The drop-scene is a masterpiece', declared *The World* in 1877,

> and exhibits all the lurid imaginative power that might be looked for from a 'mind o'erthrown'. It represents the temple of Fame; an elegant Greek edifice standing on a single peak, which soars high into the clouds of a wild and stormy sky. Crowds press onwards and upwards by a series of winding stairs and platforms, but upon the crag-summit there is foothold for but one at a time; and he who outstrips his fellows at first and wins the ascent is in danger of being overtaken, displaced, and hurled down the sheer straight precipice into the angry waves of a tumultuous sea. In the foreground is a wide terrace, paved with marble – it might be The Piazzetta of Venice – which is the starting-point for all who climb. It is crowded with figures – some eager, some apathetic, some pointing with feelings of envy or contempt to those who are already on the rise, while new arrivals are making the shore in triremes and galleys under oar and sail. In all this work – meritorious, nay, painfully excellent – there is but one fault – no single figure is perfectly drawn. Some detail is wrong – arm, leg, hand, head.[17]

It reads as if Dadd charged his drop-curtain with an unfettered apprehension of life as an essentially perilous undertaking. At the risk of over-interpreting a design that may have taken a theatrical text as its starting point, it could even have contained a very personal allegory of Dadd's own tragic experience: a young artist who, at the precise moment when he had succeeded in scaling the heights of professional success, was himself 'hurled down' into

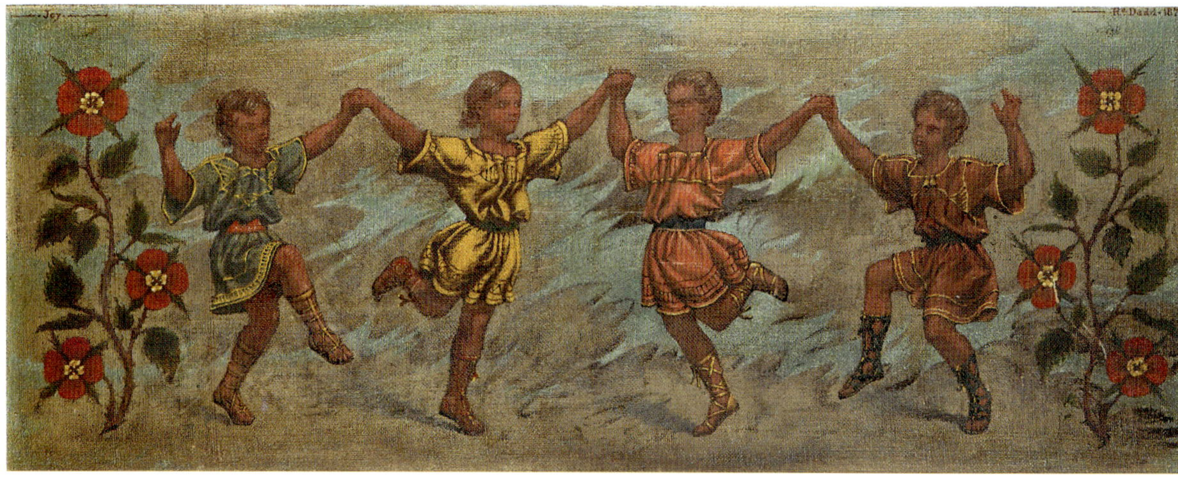

272 Richard Dadd, *Panel from Broadmoor Stage: Joy*, 1874, Bethlem Royal Hospital Museum, Kent

the 'angry waves' of mental dislocation and despair. Nevertheless, Dadd did not treat the decoration of the Broadmoor stage simply as an opportunity to expose his inner conflicts. He also painted six panels for the front of the stage, which survive to demonstrate his capacity for playfulness and delight.

Remembering perhaps the hundred untraced panels he had produced as a precocious student for Lord Foley's house at 26 Grosvenor Square in London, inspired by Byron's *Manfred* and Tasso's *Jerusalem Delivered*, Dadd adopted the same frieze arrangement in each design. One panel called *Joy* (pl. 272) shows children dancing with a pleasure that their neo-classical draperies do little to dampen, and in *Love* they display loyal affection with calm, statuesque dignity. Since three of the panels depict *Avarice*, *Grief* and *Hatred*, Dadd's darker impulses might be expected to erupt in them; but order prevails in all three, along with a clear conviction that the children are consistently engaged in theatrical rituals rather than anything more sinister. Even in *Hatred*, where two of them clash swords with stylised deliberation, their movements have been choreographed into balletic elegance. The only panel to hint at unease is *Folly*, where the diminutive figures advance on each other and disguise their true selves with bearded masks (pl. 273). Perhaps the disparity between the players' innocent expressions and the frowning, almost grotesque features of the masks mirrors a fascination on Dadd's part with the theme of double identities.

The blitheness exuded by the participants in these painted *divertissements*, which owe a great deal to Dadd's memories of studying Pompeiian

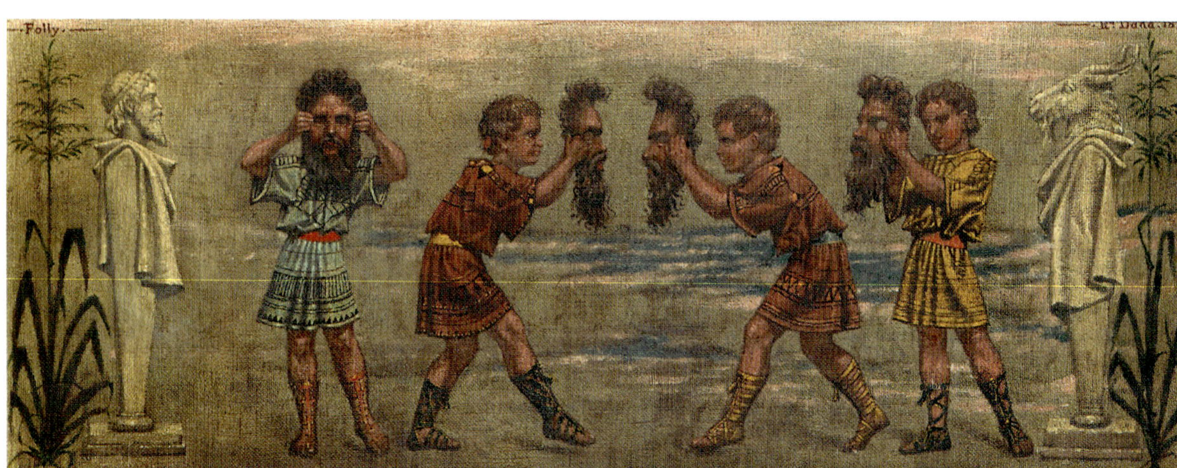

273 Richard Dadd, *Panel from Broadmoor Stage: Folly*, 1874, Bethlem Royal Hospital Museum, Kent

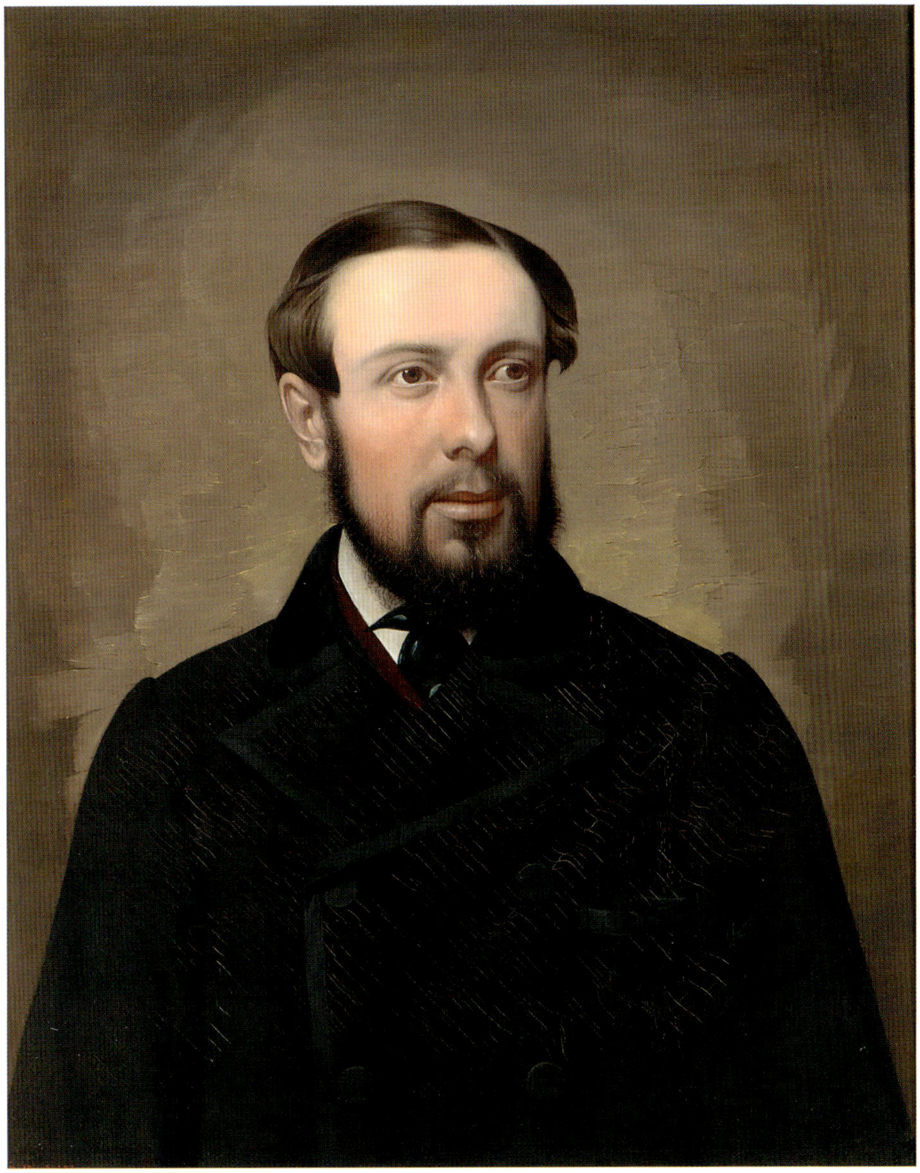

274 Richard Dadd, *Portrait of a Broadmoor Office (Dr Orange?)*, 1875, Bethlem Royal Hospital Museum, Kent

friezes representing playful cupids, gains much of its conviction from his ability to study real children at Broadmoor. Dr Orange, who became the institution's widely admired Superintendent in 1870, was enlightened enough to allow Dadd access to his own house at the hospital (pl. 274). Early in the 1880s, after the completion of the theatre decorations, Orange commissioned Dadd to paint a large fresco on the hall wall. Since Orange's son Hugh watched Dadd working on the project during his school holidays, the artist might well have enjoyed refreshing contact with an observant and intelligent boy after the long years when company was restricted to adults alone. For his part, Hugh Orange never forgot the experience, and many years later he recalled that the fresco's

> subject (chosen I believe out of compliment to my mother whose name was Florence) was a large figure of Flora, bearing flowers and fruits, – It was full of detail, some critics thought it was too full of detail. I am no art critic, but I admired the work, and am sorry to have recently learned from Dr Hopgood that it had been effaced by one of his predecessors, in the course, I expect, of some structural alterations.

Hugh also remembered that Dadd was 'accompanied by an attendant' while he worked on the fresco

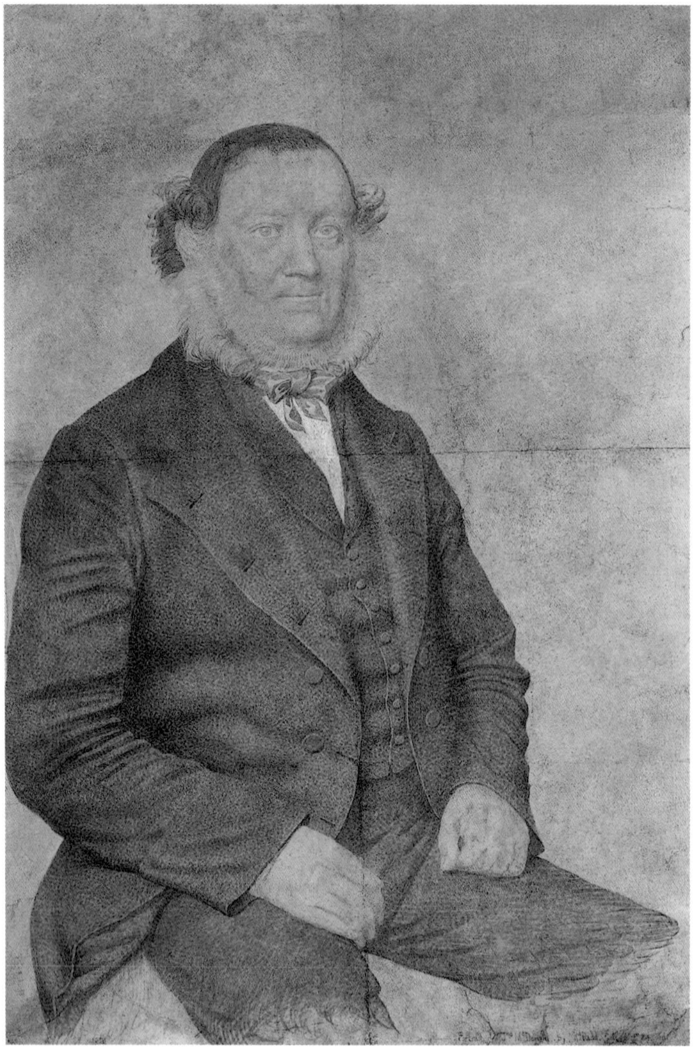

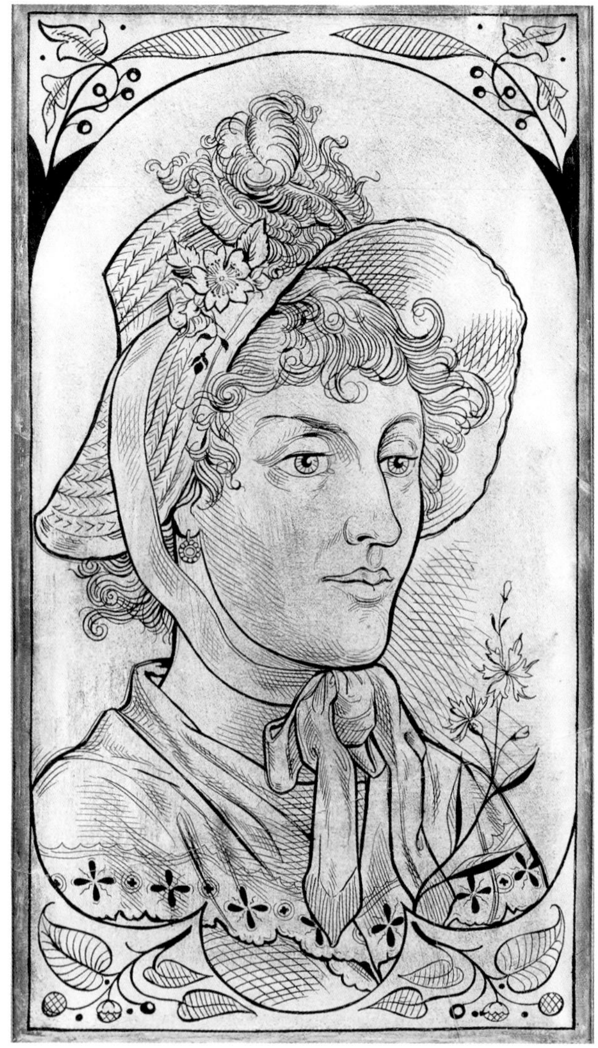

275 (*above left*) Richard Dadd, *John McDonald*, *c*.1857–64, Bethlem Royal Hospital Museum, Kent

276 (*above right*) Richard Dadd, *Female Head*, after 1864, Bethlem Royal Hospital Museum, Kent

and that he was 'a man of mild and dignified appearance, evidently absorbed in his work and taking pleasure in it'.[18]

By this time Dadd was in his mid-sixties and only a few years away from death. Advancing years did not repress his appetite for work and his Broadmoor activities show increasing versatility. While continuing to produce watercolours of great delicacy and dream-like poise, he painted a surprisingly naturalistic portrait of his latest patron. The Orange oval is quickened by a vivid grasp of individual features and seems inspired by genuine affection. Fortunate in his physicians, Dadd repaid the debt as best he could by applying his talents to every aspect of the environment at Broadmoor. As well as his extensive mural schemes, he appears to have decorated chairs with painted designs and even embarked on a large sequence of panel images scraped through a white ground on glass. Possibly intended as a set of small windows for the theatre or a day-room, they are reminiscent of traditional playing-card forms in their representation of a troubadour, a turnkey, a jester and other figures redolent of the medieval period. Only one panel, a close-up portrait of a bonneted young lady, depicts a contemporary face (pl. 276), and Dadd here deploys a tender sentiment that probably characterised the Christmas decorations he is also supposed to have produced.

Ready to turn his hand to diagrams and illustrations for lectures and entertainments as well, he eventually made himself an indispensable part of Broadmoor life. Recently discovered evidence from the Bethlem archives proves that John

McDonald, whose watercolour portrait Dadd painted in 1874 in his most diligent, stippled technique (pl. 275), was an attendant at the hospital from 1855 until 1876. He worked in the main department rather than the criminal lunatic section, and Dadd invests the blue-eyed, extravagantly bearded official with an almost photographic realism.[19] For all his Victorian formality, McDonald seems open, equable and responsive to the artist. Both staff and patients at Broadmoor were constantly entertained by Dadd's puckish ability to sit down and in just 'a few hours . . . produce a host of humorous cartoons, comical street figures'.[20] Yet these spirited activities were brought to an end when he became terminally ill with consumption: soon after New Year's Day 1886 he died. His sister confessed herself 'truly thankful to know him at rest, it is less grief to me, than it was to think of him in the changed condition in which he has lived for many years past, his life has been to me a living death'.[21]

While her emotions are wholly understandable, the 'living death' did generate a body of work that gave forceful yet pellucid expression to the resilience of Dadd's fecund imagination. He managed to share this inner intensity in a positive way with the other inhabitants of the hospitals housing him. One perceptive visitor was right to claim in 1877 that

> art is thus his mistress still . . . it is to his beloved brush that he clings, and wields continuously, with that enthusiasm and unwearying ardour the true painter alone can know. Many works will live after him, the product of these thirty-odd years of absolute seclusion – melancholy monuments of a genius so early shipwrecked, but which never went actually to ruin.[22]

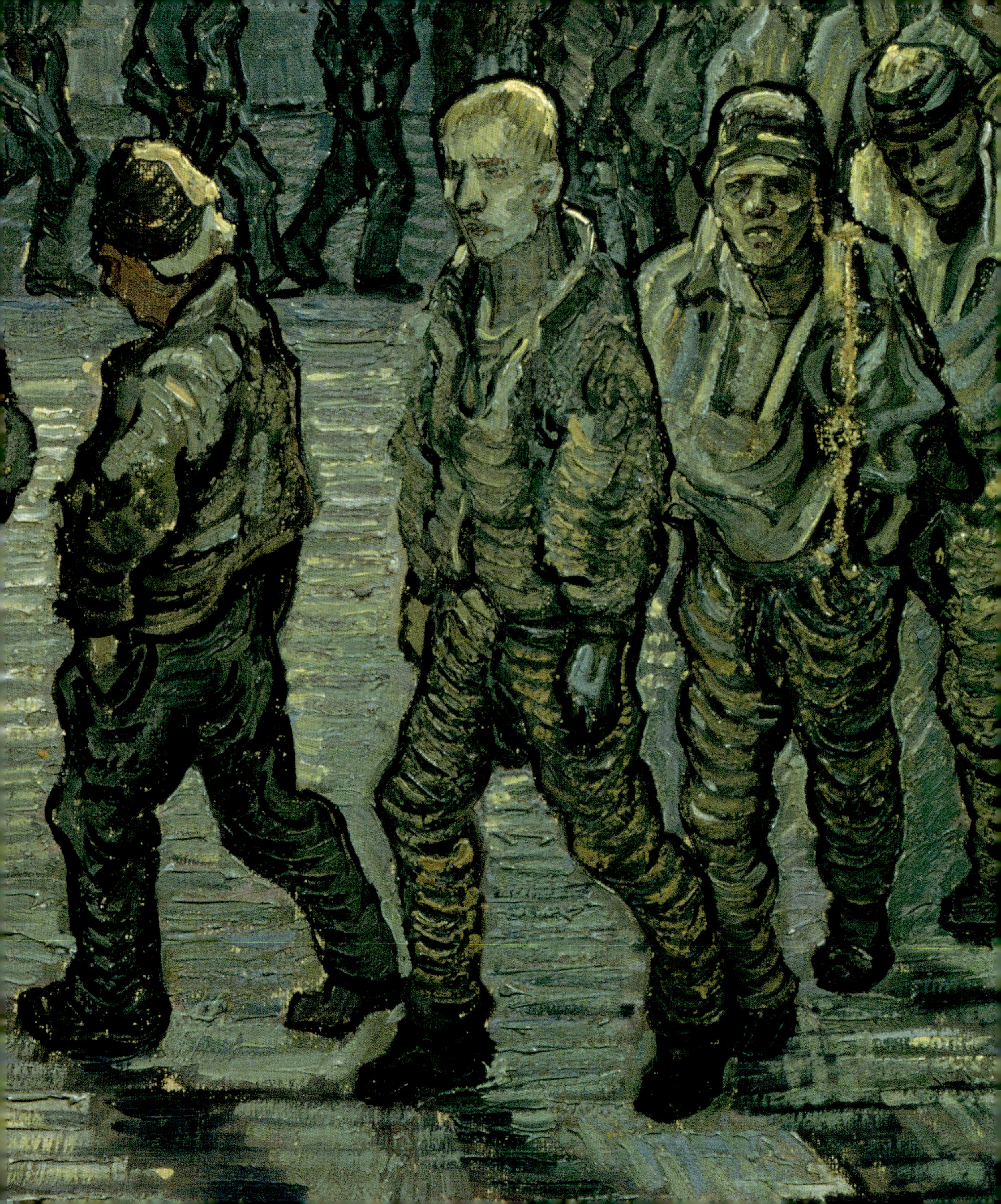

NINETEEN
'ACUTE MENTAL DERANGEMENT'

In May 1889, Vincent van Gogh was admitted to a mental home near the village of Saint-Rémy-en-Provence. The attending physician, Dr Théophile Peyron, recorded on the certificate of entry that his patient, aged thirty-six, had been 'stricken by acute mental derangement, with hallucinations of his sight and hearing, which led him to mutilate himself by cutting off his ear'.[1] The affliction was terrible enough to make van Gogh remain, quite voluntarily, in the Saint-Paul-de-Mausole asylum for an entire year. The illness did not, however, prevent him from pursuing his art with a remarkable sense of discipline, concentration, audacity and impassioned commitment.

Van Gogh was determined to recover from his catastrophe, even though he knew it had destroyed all the idealistic hopes that inspired his move from Paris to the South of France. He had hoped, in Arles, to establish a co-operative community of artists. Fired by the strong light and heightened colours of Provence, he persuaded Paul Gauguin to join him. The two men had become close friends in the 1880s, sharing many ideas about the need for drastic renewal in art. They both admired the clean-cut energy of Japanese prints, and in 1888 Gauguin journeyed south to live with van Gogh in the so-called Yellow House he rented there. For a while, everything went well. Van Gogh saw Gauguin's arrival as a triumphant first step towards realising his dream of an artists' society, revolutionising European painting in a 'Studio of the Tropics'. However, he was too restless, argumentative and unpredictable to preside in tranquillity over a peaceful community of like-minded innovators. Before long, he and Gauguin began fierily disagreeing about the future course of art, and van Gogh admitted that their debates were electric.[2]

At the centre of these seismic rows lay a fundamental divergence. Van Gogh wanted to retain a direct, nourishing connection with the natural world. He continued to cherish the work of great Dutch landscape painters from the past like Meyndert Hobbema and Jacob van Ruisdael. Gauguin, by contrast, was bent on liberating modern painting from what he saw as a disabling reliance on nature. Fascinated by non-Western art, he aimed at a more abstract style where bold outlines, flat colour-fields and harmonious rhythms predominated. As a result, van Gogh and Gauguin were set on an aesthetic collision-course. The tension between them grew unbearable when poor weather obliged the two artists to work irritatingly near each other, feeling increasingly fractious within the cramped confines of the Yellow House.

Giving way to paranoia, van Gogh became convinced that Gauguin would renounce him alto-

277 (*facing page*) Detail of pl. 294

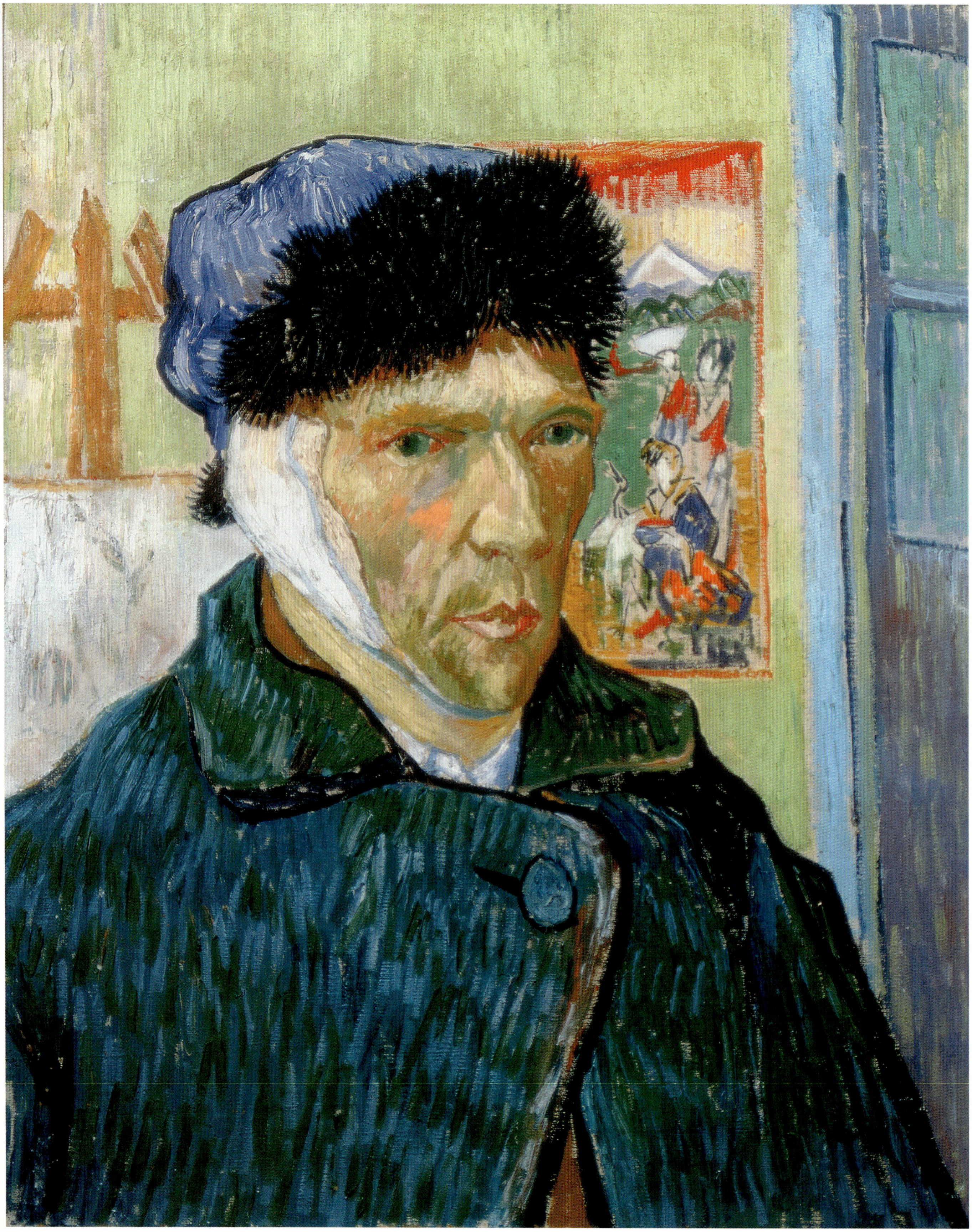

gether and leave Arles for good. In despair, the Dutchman resorted to reckless self-mutilation. After threatening Gauguin with an open razor in the street, he retreated indoors and sliced off part of his left ear instead. Having sealed this curious sacrificial offering in an envelope, he delivered it to the local brothel. The girl who opened the envelope fainted, causing a commotion. But somehow, van Gogh's old friend Roulin the postman led the heavily bleeding artist back to his house. He was admitted to the local Arles hospital, the Hôtel Dieu, while Gauguin turned his back on the torment and escaped to Paris. The idealistic alliance was over, leaving van Gogh incarcerated and inconsolable.

In less than a month, he had benefited so much from the kindness and sympathy of Dr Félix Rey, the resident surgeon at the hospital, that recovery seemed to have been achieved. By early January 1889 he was ready to go back home with Roulin, whose devoted family had cleared up the blood-smeared Yellow House. Soon van Gogh was ready to embark on some portraits, including a confessional painting of his gaunt, bandaged face juxtaposed, hauntingly, with a Japanese print where robed courtesans flaunt themselves against the idyllic backdrop of Mount Fujiyama (pl. 278). But he could not continue to live alone for long. Van Gogh, fortified by medicine, hoped that his mind would never again succumb to what he described as moods of 'indescribable mental anguish when the veil of time and inevitability seemed for the twinkling of an eye to be parted'.[3] Yet the hallucinations returned. He became paranoid again, suspecting that everybody was out to poison him. Passers-by found themselves shouted at on the street and he provoked tumult in local cafés. By early February van Gogh was forced to re-enter the hospital and recover from this second attack. Within a week or two, he was permitted to go home again, but many of his neighbours signed a petition to the mayor, describing him as a public danger who should be confined. After van Gogh lost control once more, pushing open his windows to scream at the people he thought were staring in at him, the mayor decreed that he must return to the Hôtel Dieu.

This time, the protesting painter was locked up in a prison-like room for weeks on end. Van Gogh equated it with his hatred of big cities, remembering that when he saw Paris for the first time, 'I felt above all the dreary misery, which one cannot wave away, as little as one can wave away the tainted air in a hospital, however clean it may be kept.' He lapsed into sullen, shocked silence, broken only when the Protestant pastor Dr Frédéric Salles visited him and made clear that van Gogh had been unfairly treated. 'The neighbours', he wrote to Vincent's brother Theo, 'have roused a tumult about nothing. His first foolish act had made them interpret unfavourably every singularity of the poor young man.'[4] Responding to Dr Salles's concern, van Gogh finally spoke. 'If the police had prevented the children and grown-ups from crowding round my house and climbing the windows as if I were a curious animal', he said, 'I should have controlled myself and done no harm to anyone.'[5]

Staring out of his hospital window, he found that the advent of spring blossom roused his desire to paint. His door was unlocked and a visit from the sympathetic young artist Paul Signac reinforced the urge to resume work. With Signac, he brought back from his house brushes, canvases and paints to the hospital. The mood of optimism was backed by Dr Rey, who told Signac that if van Gogh could lead 'a very methodical life, eating and drinking normally and at regular hours, he will have every chance of avoiding a repetition of these terrible crises'.[6] Such hopes proved unfounded, but for the moment the wounded, frightened artist managed to overcome his despair and produce a few forthright images of his surroundings. One canvas, of the hospital dormitory (pl. 279), provides a robust and relatively faithful view of the bed-lined ward, curtains drawn back while the patients huddle round the stove to read, smoke or gaze disconsolately at the floorboards rushing in giddy recession towards the distant wall. The claustrophobia, made more disturbing by the brutal form of the stove-pipe cutting its way through the composition, mirrors van Gogh's anxious condition tersely enough.

While most of his fellow inmates resigned themselves to a life of lassitude, he remained feverishly active. In the courtyard of the hospital, he painted a view showing how some patients could pause on the yellow-pillared balcony and survey the garden below (pl. 280). Since a nun is the only figure walking among the flowerbeds, they were probably out of bounds to everyone except the staff. Even

278 (*facing page*) Vincent Van Gogh, *Self-portrait with Bandaged Ear*, 1889, Courtauld Institute Galleries, London

279 Vincent Van Gogh, *Hospital dormitory at the Hôtel Dieu, Arles*, 1889, Oskar Reinhart Collection, Winterthur

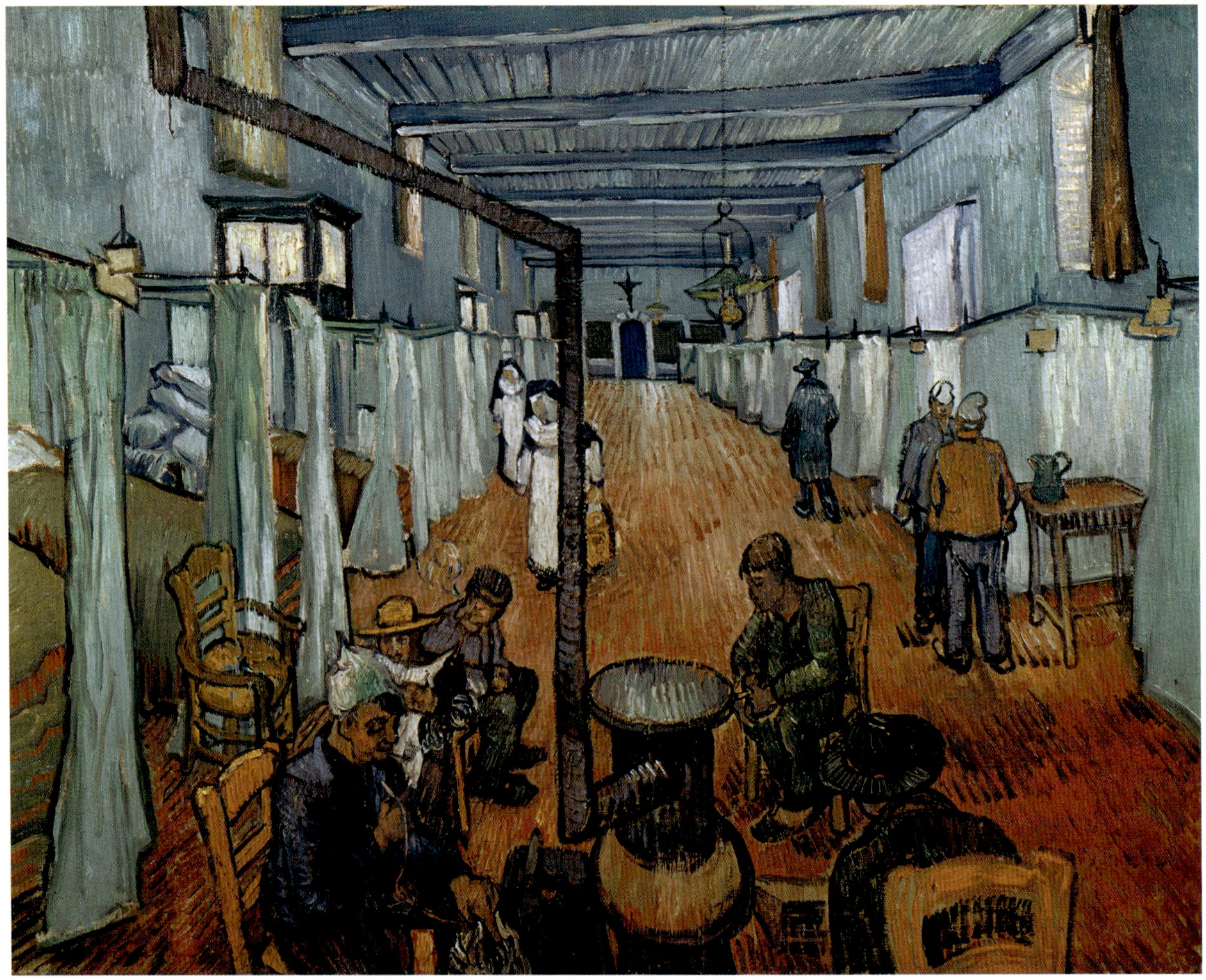

so, van Gogh enjoyed scrutinising the foliage surmounting the small trees' crooked trunks, and tracing the geometry of the paths as they converged on a central pool where goldfish flash their bright scales beneath the turquoise water.

At a slightly later stage in the spring, when the garden had begun to bear a rather more exotic crop of blooms, he carried out a large and exuberant drawing of the courtyard in vigorous strokes of pencil, reed pen and brown ink (pl. 281). By this time the pool was surrounded by vegetation so thick that it threatens to hide the goldfish from view. The assurance with which van Gogh defines this complex array of plants and flowers suggests that he relished the pictorial challenge they presented to him. Far from using his art as an outlet for his most agonised emotions, he succeeded in subjecting himself to the rigorous discipline of keen-eyed observation. The outcome is at the opposite remove from the images so often produced by psychiatric patients, with their agonised concentration on inner turbulence alone.

Vincent trained his art resolutely outwards, asking Dr Rey to pose for a small portrait that reveals a considerable rapport with his sitter (pl. 282). The doctor appears to regard his portrayer with kindness, and there is no hint in Rey's open, fresh-faced expression that van Gogh saw him as a remote or threatening personification of medical authority. Only the agitation of the patterned wallpaper behind the doctor's head hints at a less genial order of feeling. Here, orange arabesques dance on a green ground punctuated by scarlet splashes redolent of blood. They testify, ominously, to the assertion of a more restless and alarming mood, and whatever hopes van Gogh may have harboured about Rey's ability to understand his art were soon cruelly confounded.

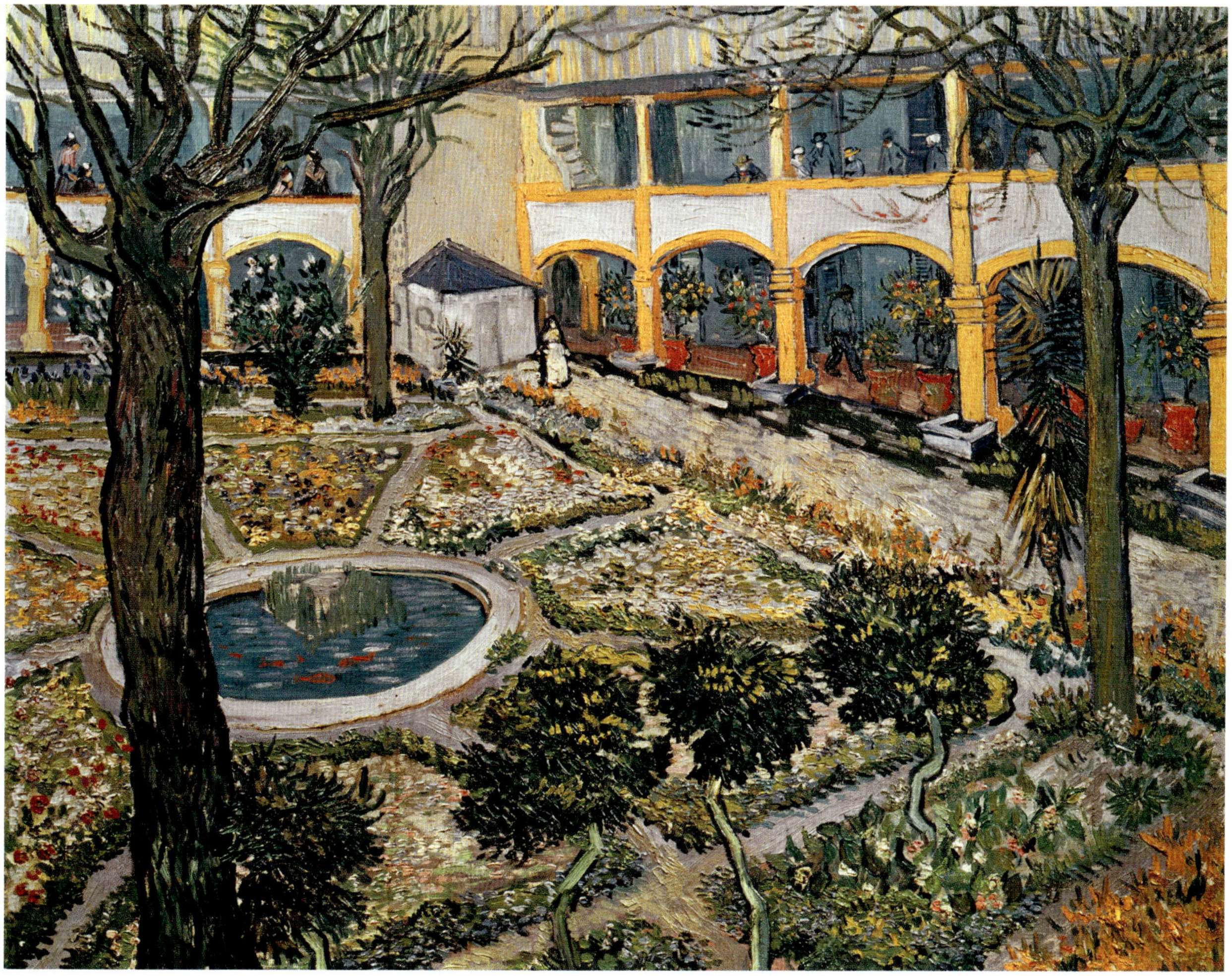

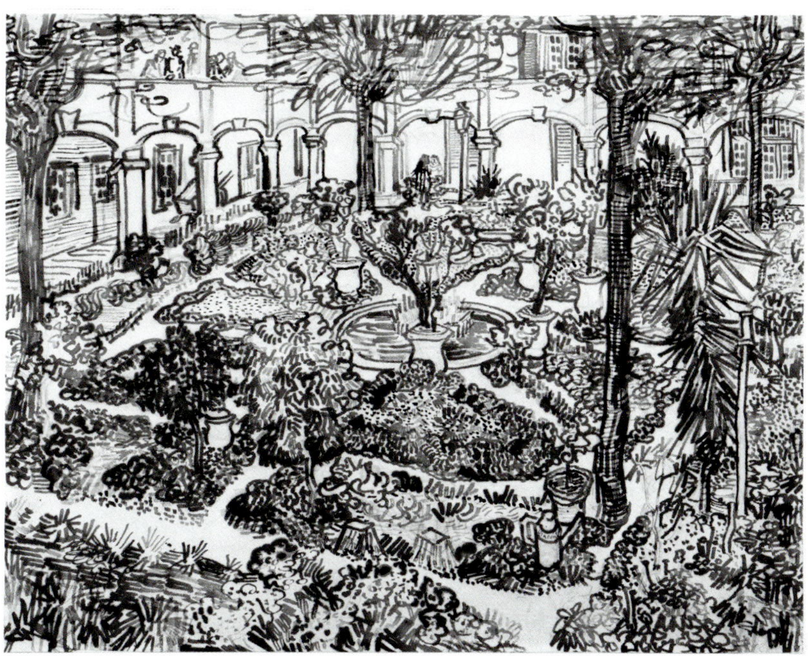

280 (*above*) Vincent Van Gogh, *Garden courtyard of the Hôtel Dieu*, 1889, Oskar Reinhart Collection, Winterthur

281 (*left*) Vincent Van Gogh, *Drawing of the Hospital Courtyard*, 1889, Vincent van Gogh Museum, Amsterdam

282 (*facing page*) Vincent Van Gogh, *Portrait of Dr Félix Rey*, 1889, Pushkin State Museum of Fine Arts, Moscow

With characteristic generosity, Vincent wanted to give the paintings he had executed at the hospital to either the doctor[7] or the hospital itself, probably as a thank-offering for the help he had received there. But his admirable gesture was treated with contempt. Rey's portrait was used for a while to close a gap in his hen-house. 'When I saw that he outlined my head entirely in green', Rey recalled later,

> that he painted my hair and my moustache – I really did not have red hair – in a blazing red on a biting green background, I was simply horrified. What should I do with this present? Nor did I know what to do with other paintings, *The Hospital Garden* and *Dormitory in the Hospital*, that were also presented to me. I offered them to the Administrator of Hospitals, who happened to be visiting, but he would have no part of them and passed them on to the secretary of the clinic. You see, this gentleman is himself a painter . . . Unfortunately, van Gogh's paintings did not find favour with him either. This gentleman called them 'dirty obscenities' and presented them, now for the fourth time, to the druggist.[8]

Vincent did not stay long enough at the hospital to hear about this hostile treatment of his donations. Salles accompanied him to the Yellow House, where they took down all the paintings, packed them up and cleared away the furnishings as well. The whole melancholy operation made him feel that he had failed his faithful brother Theo, who had done much to encourage and finance the move to the South of France. 'I thought how you had given me all these things with such brotherly love', he wrote to Theo, 'and how you had kept me all these years, and then for me to have to tell you this wretched ending to it all – oh, I can't tell you what I felt!' Yet he realised that there was no alternative to a stoical admission of defeat. 'I've tried to found a studio in the south', he wrote. 'My satisfaction must be in that. I can't face the isolation any more.' Van Gogh admitted that after his third attack 'it isn't at all easy to begin life again, for a lot of despair remains inside me'. Returning to his former life seemed out of the question: 'my head is not steady enough to work at stretch by myself as I did before. And I dare not risk making any more public scenes.'[9] Hence his willingness to tell Salles, with alarming honesty, that 'I'm not fit to govern myself and my affairs'.

Realising how desperate van Gogh felt, Salles searched for a place where a greater degree of psychiatric care might be found. He settled for the old monastery of St Paul, newly converted into an asylum. The journey from Arles to Saint-Rémy would not be too arduous, and the mental home's director Dr Peyron told Salles that the artist could be looked after there for a hundred francs a month. The negotiations nearly collapsed when Peyron announced that van Gogh would not be permitted to paint outside the asylum. Vincent was distraught, threatening to join the Foreign Legion if he could only find somewhere to paint without paying for the privilege. His gloom intensified when heavy spring rains flooded the basement in Arles where his paintings from the Yellow House were stacked. However, after Theo told him that the Foreign Legion was nothing but *un pis aller*, and promised to persuade Peyron to let him work in the open air, van Gogh relented. 'I should like to be shut up for a while', he confessed, 'as much for my peace of mind as for others.'[10]

On 8 May, he left Arles with Salles and travelled to the Saint-Rémy asylum. Here, Theo believed, he would receive specialist help in surroundings more conducive to his recovery. At any rate, such a hope was fostered by the asylum's brochure. Its fulsome text claimed that the building, with its graceful medieval chapel and single-storey quarters for patients, was 'better designed than most for service of the sick'. Moreover, its site on the northern slope of a hill in the Alpine chain was considered eminently salubrious: 'Air, light, space, large and beautiful trees, drinkable waters – fresh, abundant, of good quality, originating from the mountains – and sufficient remoteness from all large population centres: such are the principal justifications for the learned founder's choice of location.' Above all, though, the asylum was founded in the conviction that 'the cruelty with which we once treated the mentally ill has been replaced by humane understanding . . . It is no longer the *illness* which the doctor has to treat, but, rather, the sick *person*, for whom the complex treatment varies according to the diverse circumstances which led to the illness.'[11] These precepts, echoing the new ideas informing Richard Dadd's treatment at Bethlem and Broadmoor, promised well for helping van Gogh to regain his composure.

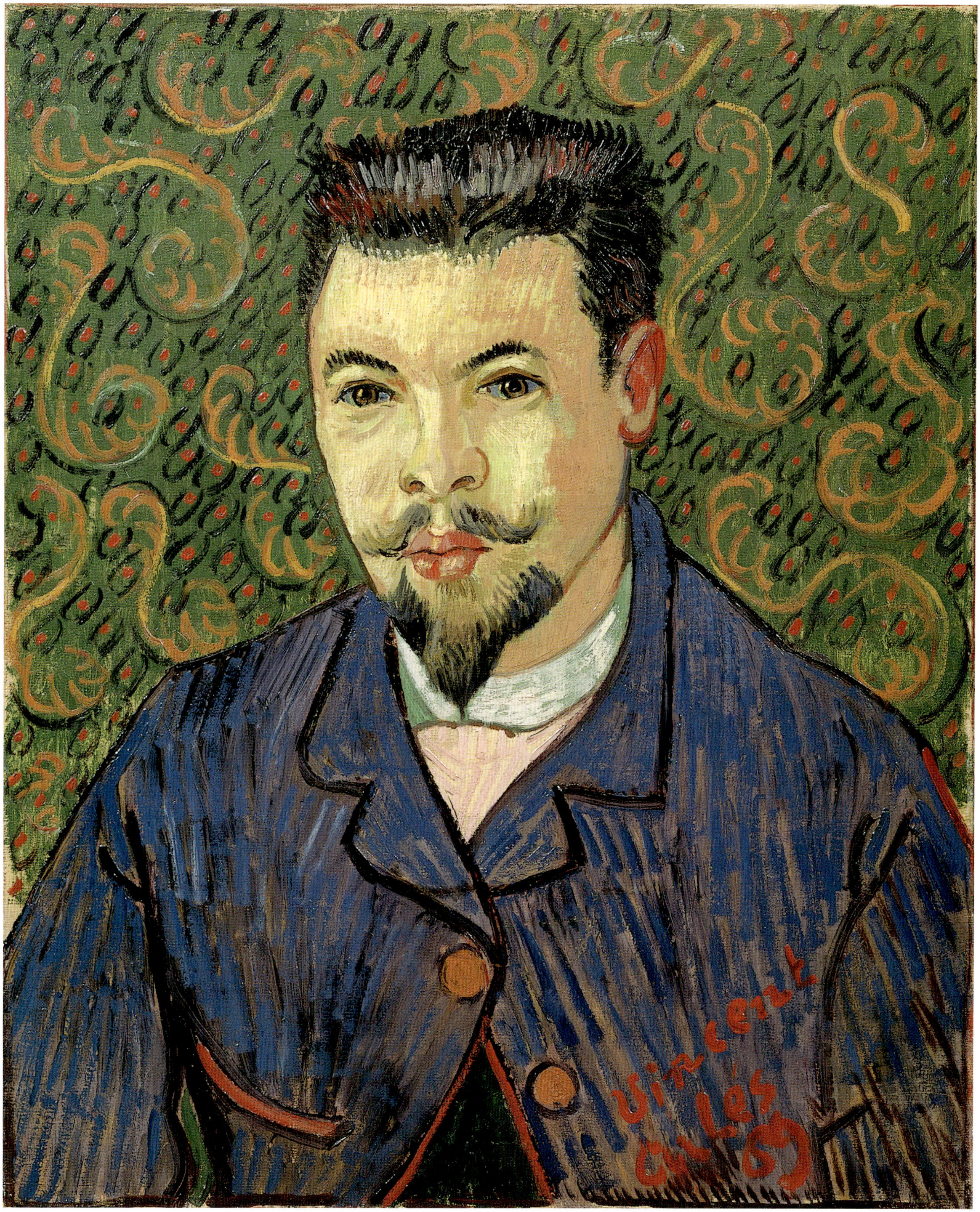
Vincent
Arles
89

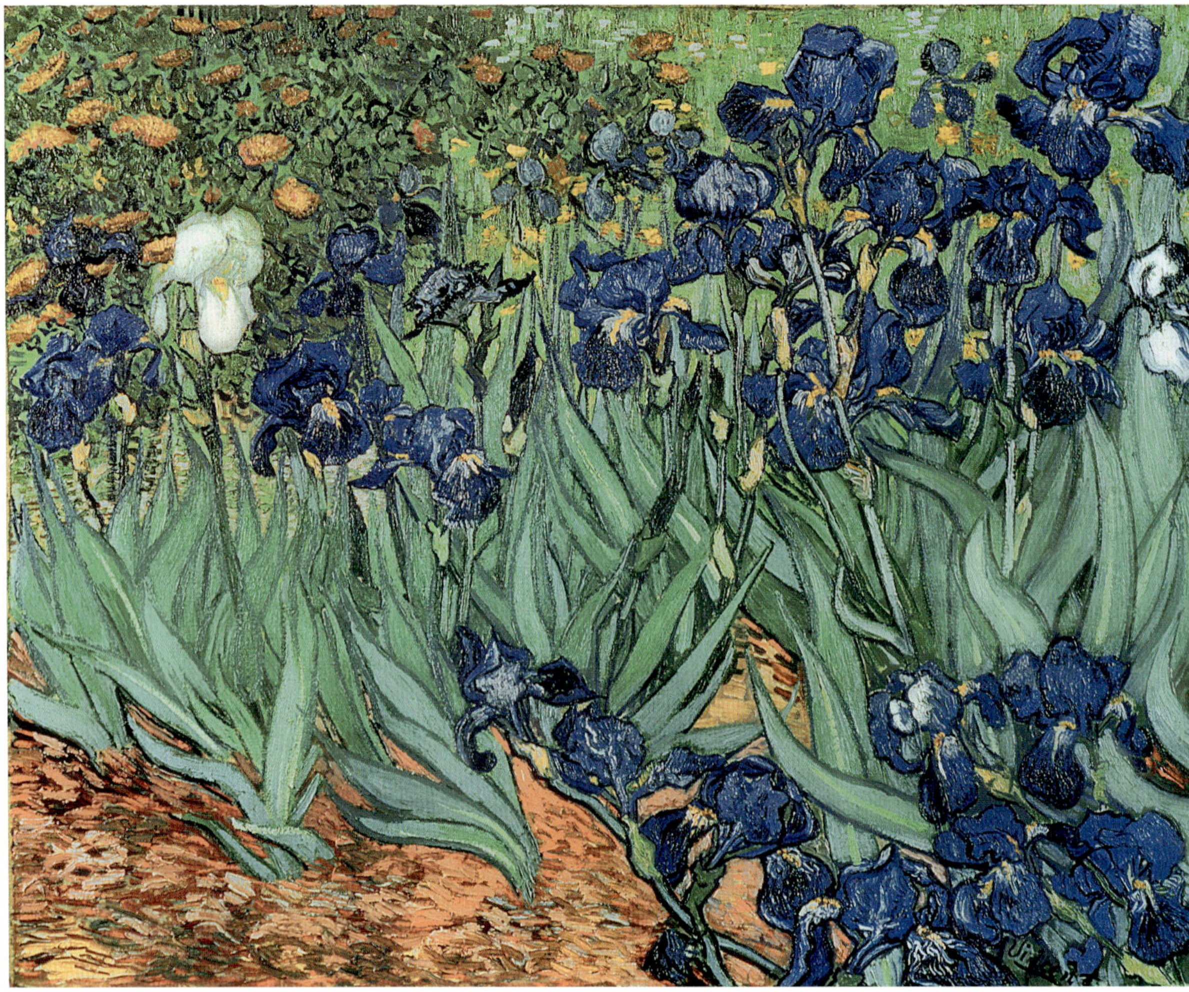

283 Vincent Van Gogh, *Irises*, 1889, J. Paul Getty Museum, Los Angeles

Although Dr Peyron came to the hesitant conclusion that Vincent was suffering from 'a state of epilepsy', and warned Theo that 'if this should be confirmed one should be concerned about the future',[12] he was encouraged by his patient's initial progress. After recurrent painful nightmares during the first few days, van Gogh's sleep improved along with his appetite. Towards the end of May, Peyron was able to report that 'he spends the whole day drawing in the park here, but as I find him entirely tranquil, I have promised to let him go out in order to find serenity outside this establishment.'[13] There can be little doubt that van Gogh gained therapeutic release from his ability to resume working. Despite his distress, he seemed adept at discovering continual inspiration in whatever surroundings confronted him. A few weeks earlier, near the end of his stay in Arles, he had bravely asserted that 'if I had to stay for good in an asylum, I should make up my mind to it and I think I could find subjects for painting there as well.'[14] The prophecy was borne out to spectacular effect at Saint-Rémy, where he painted many of his most satisfying and eloquent canvases.

Within a week of arriving at the asylum he was hard at work on two paintings of the garden,[15] one of which turned into the superlative *Irises* (pl. 283). At first sight it appears festive, revelling in the piercing clarity of the violet-blue flowers as they thrust and wave with an exuberance worthy of a Hokusai print. After a while, though, more disturbing elements demand attention. The irises and their blaring green leaves fill the canvas with insistent movement, as if jostling for room in the confined picture space. They crowd round the solitary white flower in their midst, provoking the suspicion that Vincent equated their clamorous behaviour with the more disturbed patients confined inside the asylum's walls. He was probably unaware of the parallel himself, on a conscious level at least, categorising *Irises* among the paintings that were 'more studies from nature than subjects for pictures'.[16] Even so, aggressive symbolism was detected in the image when Theo sent it for exhibition at the Salon des Indépendants later that year. Writing in *La Vogue*, the perceptive Félix Fénéon declared that 'the "Irises" violently slash their petals upon sword-like leaves'.[17]

A similar ambiguity can be detected in some of van Gogh's powerful pen and ink drawings of the asylum garden. One in particular, a study of an ivy-smothered tree related to a lost painting,[18] stresses the extremity of the curve in the trunk scything through the composition (pl. 284). Fiery pen-strokes accentuate both the possible collapse of the tree and the forcefulness of the ivy, clinging to the bark like an especially tenacious cancer. Van Gogh himself had linked ivy with malignant growth in human bodies when writing from Arles. The drawing derives much of its tensile strength from an implicit conflict between the sagging yet defiant trunk and the plant attached unshakeably to its surface.

All the same, he claimed that a similar image of ivy-covered trees 'represents the eternal nests of greenery for lovers',[19] and it would be a great mistake to regard these garden drawings as unrelievedly tragic in meaning. One of the finest, *Fountain in the Garden of the Asylum*, rejoices in the almost sexual ejaculation of water from the nozzle at the centre of the pool (pl. 285). It spurts up in a thin jet that contrasts, in its rigidity, with the wayward lurching of the gnarled trees ranged around the fountain at intoxicated angles. Release is likewise apparent in another drawing of the garden, where the imprisoning fence and urgent swaying of flame-like trees give way, further up, to a liberating expanse of untroubled sky.

A far more enclosed and oppressive mood is, however, generated by a trio of freely handled views of the asylum's interior. Ronald Pickvance has proposed that these three chalk and gouache studies, all the same size, might have been envisaged as a triptych.[20] They certainly seem to represent a concerted attempt to convey three different aspects of van Gogh's life at the asylum. His view of the vestibule (pl. 286a) includes a framed painting and a portfolio, both propped up near the entrance as if ready for an expedition outside. The doors are

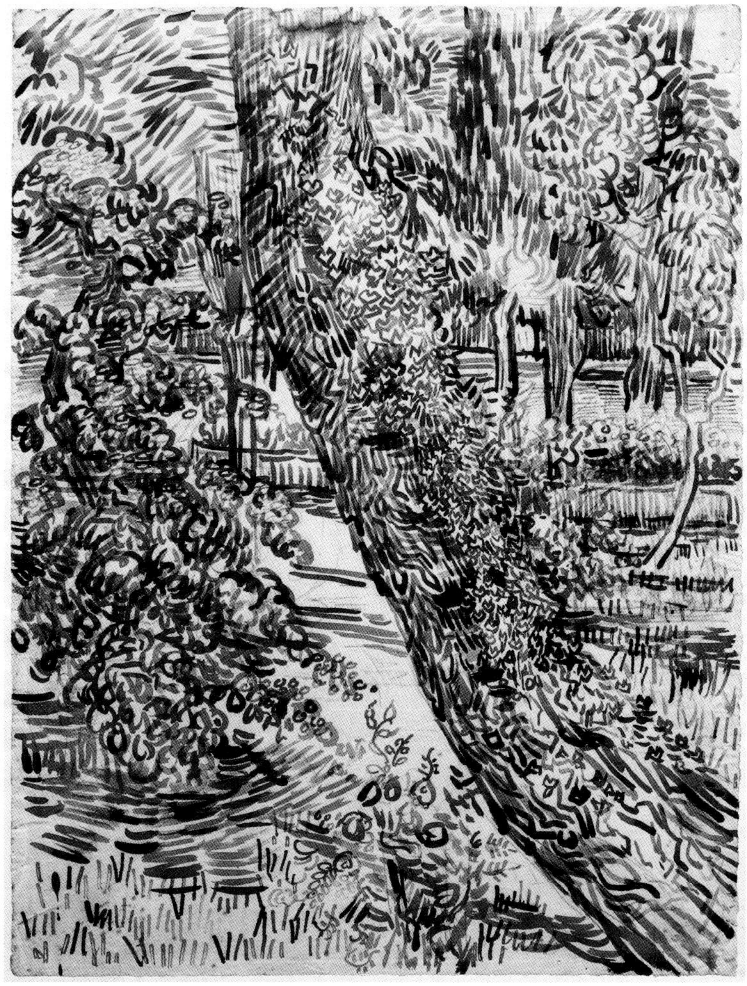

284 (*above*) Vincent Van Gogh, Drawing of ivy-covered tree in asylum garden, 1889, Vincen Van Gogh Museum, Amsterdam

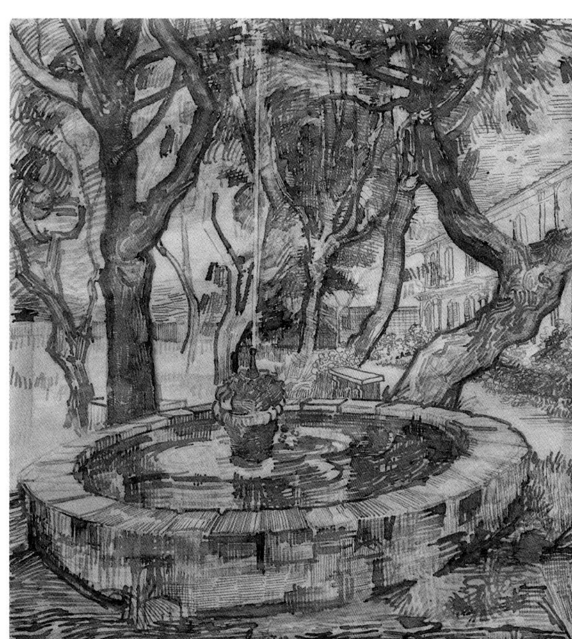

285 (*left*) Vincent Van Gogh, *Fountain in the Garden of the Asylum*, 1889, Vincen Van Gogh Museum, Amsterdam

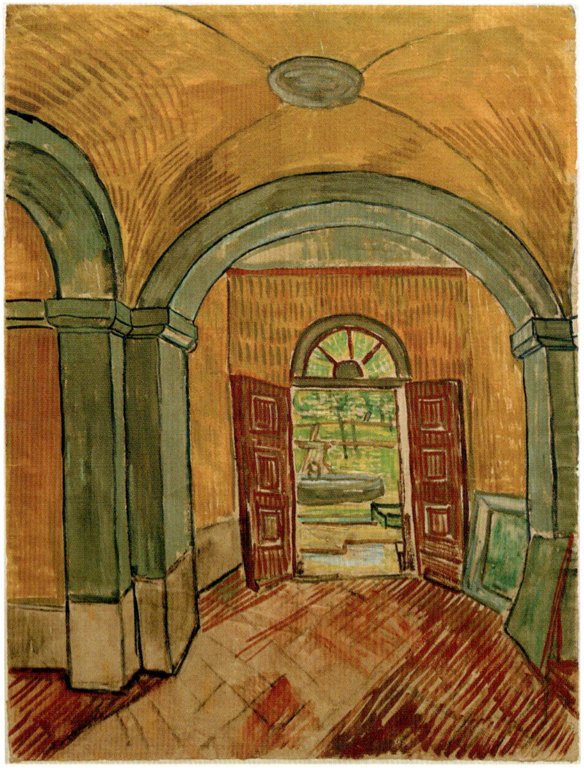

286a Vincent Van Gogh, *Three Studies of the Asylum: Vestibule of the Asylum*, 1889, Vincent van Gogh Museum, Amsterdam

open, giving onto the sunlit garden where he produced so many exhilarating studies. But the vestibule picture is dominated by the architecture of the asylum's interior, handled with an insistence that stresses its overbearing presence. The archways press down on the space, determined to emphasise their containing force on the man who paints them.

This sense of imprisonment becomes more apparent in the view of an asylum corridor (pl. 286b). Apart from the overhead pressure exerted by the archways, whose forms gain in constricting power through their repetition, the picture leads into a tunnel-like space that grows increasingly irksome as the perspective recedes. The air of desolation is reinforced by the institutional barrenness so evident here, devoid of decoration and inhabited only by a solitary patient. He turns away from the corridor, as though anxious to escape from its Kafkaesque atmosphere. Perhaps van Gogh's response to this macabre interior was affected by his awareness that, as he informed Theo, 'there is someone here who has been shouting and talking like me *all the time* for a fortnight; he thinks he hears voices and words in the echoes of the corridors, probably because the nerves of the ear are diseased and too sensitive'.[21]

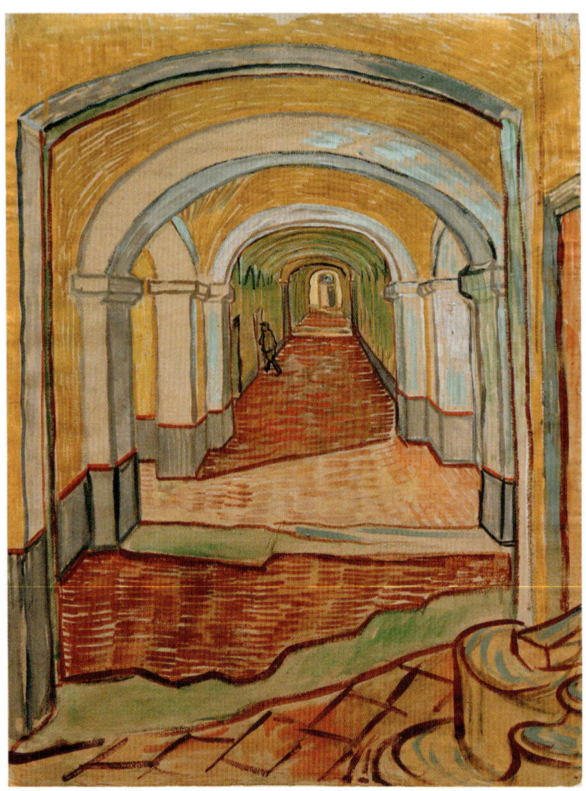

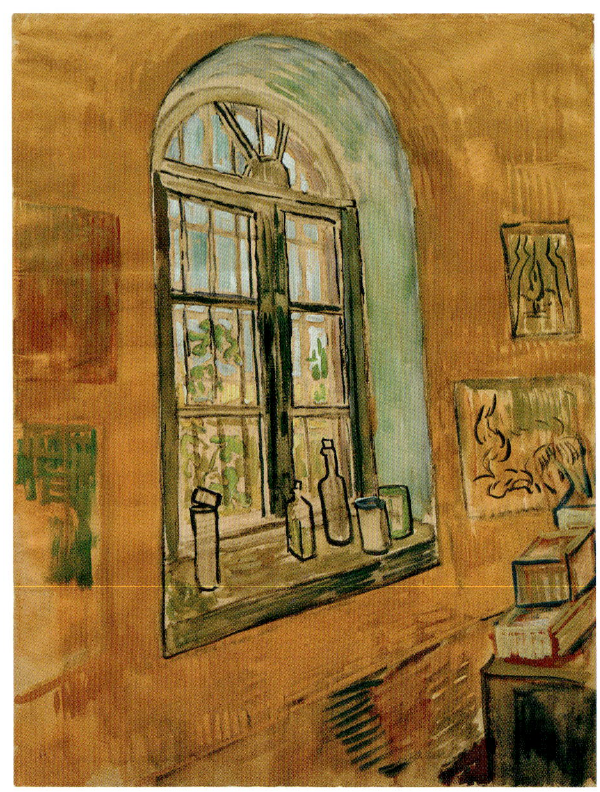

286b (*right*) Vincent Van Gogh, *Three Studies of the Asylum: Corridor of the Asylum*, 1889, Bequest of Abby Aldrich Rockefeller, Metropolitan Museum of Art, New York

286c (*far right*) Vincent Van Gogh, *Three Studies of the Asylum: Window in Vincent's Studio*, 1889, Vincent van Gogh Museum, Amsterdam

At least van Gogh was able to humanise this prevailing drabness in his own studio, the subject of the third image in the putative triptych (pl. 286c). He explained to Theo that, 'as there are more than thirty empty rooms' at the asylum, he had been given 'one to work in'. He lost little time in hanging on its walls his unframed works, four of which can be seen in this gouache. Two seem to contain whirling forms derived from his work in the garden. His decision to devote much of the gouache to the window indicates that he wanted to meditate on the poignant difference between the enclosed room and the sun-dappled world outside. The bars of the window are painted with particular forcefulness, as if to accentuate their prison-like structure; but the pictures displayed nearby prove that the asylum permitted him to transform the room with blazing affirmations of his ability to continue painting, despite his inner turmoil. He longed, like Dadd before him, to animate the whole asylum with his art, telling Theo that 'it would be splendid to hold an exhibition in, all the empty rooms, the large corridors'.[22] The asylum's rules must have forbidden such an ambitious project, not to mention the inevitable disapproval of staff and patients ready to bridle at the raw radicalism of van Gogh's work. But if the opportunity had been granted, he would have transformed the building into an arena for his prolific, ever increasing output.

He was irrepressible as an artist for much of his long stay in the asylum. Towards the end of May 1889 he described his excitement over the view from his bedroom, where 'through the iron-barred window I see a square field of wheat in an enclosure, a perspective like van Goyen, above which I see the morning sun rising in all its glory'.[23] Soon after Dr Peyron allowed him to work in the field, he began an extended sequence of views which amount, in their entirety, to the finest series of paintings he produced at Saint-Rémy.

The first canvas, *Mountainous Landscape behind the Asylum* (pl. 287), is one of the most outspoken in its desire to use nature as a metaphor for his own emotional condition. The turbulence of the wheat, heaving in its enclosure like an angry sea, surely reflects van Gogh's view of his plight within the institution's walls. He described the painting to Theo on 9 June, explaining that the foreground contained 'a field of wheat ruined and hurled to the

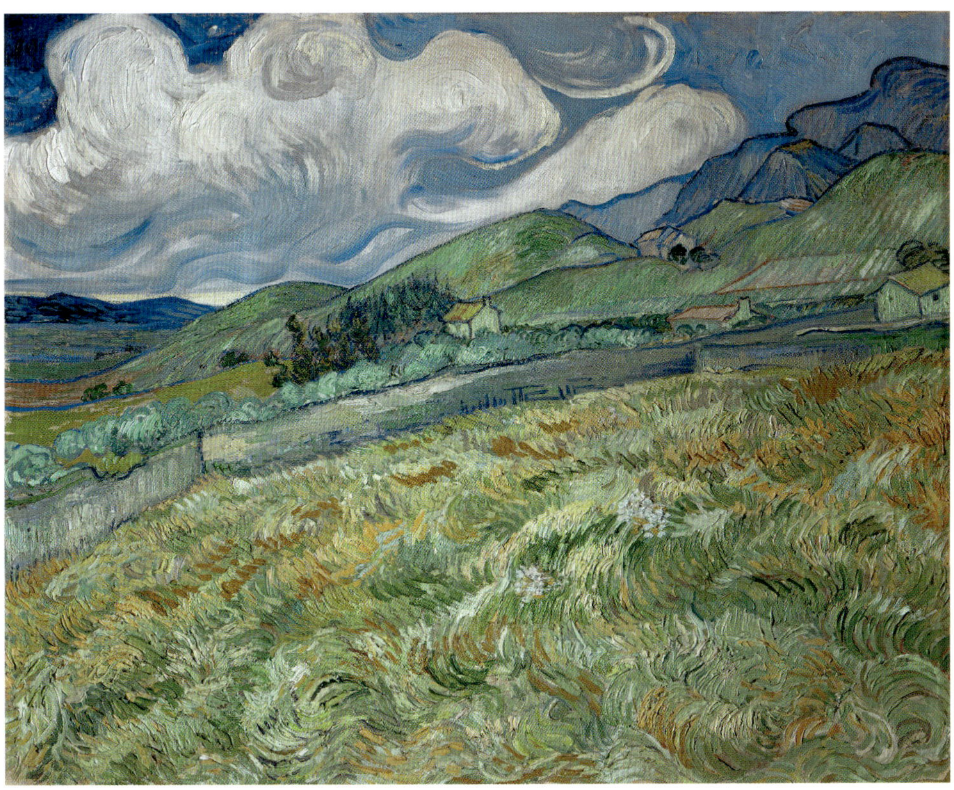

287 Vincent Van Gogh, *Mountainous Landscape Behind the Asylum*, 1889, Ny Carlsberg Glyptothek, Copenhagen

288 Vincent Van Gogh, *The Reaper*, 1889, Vincent van Gogh Museum, Amsterdam

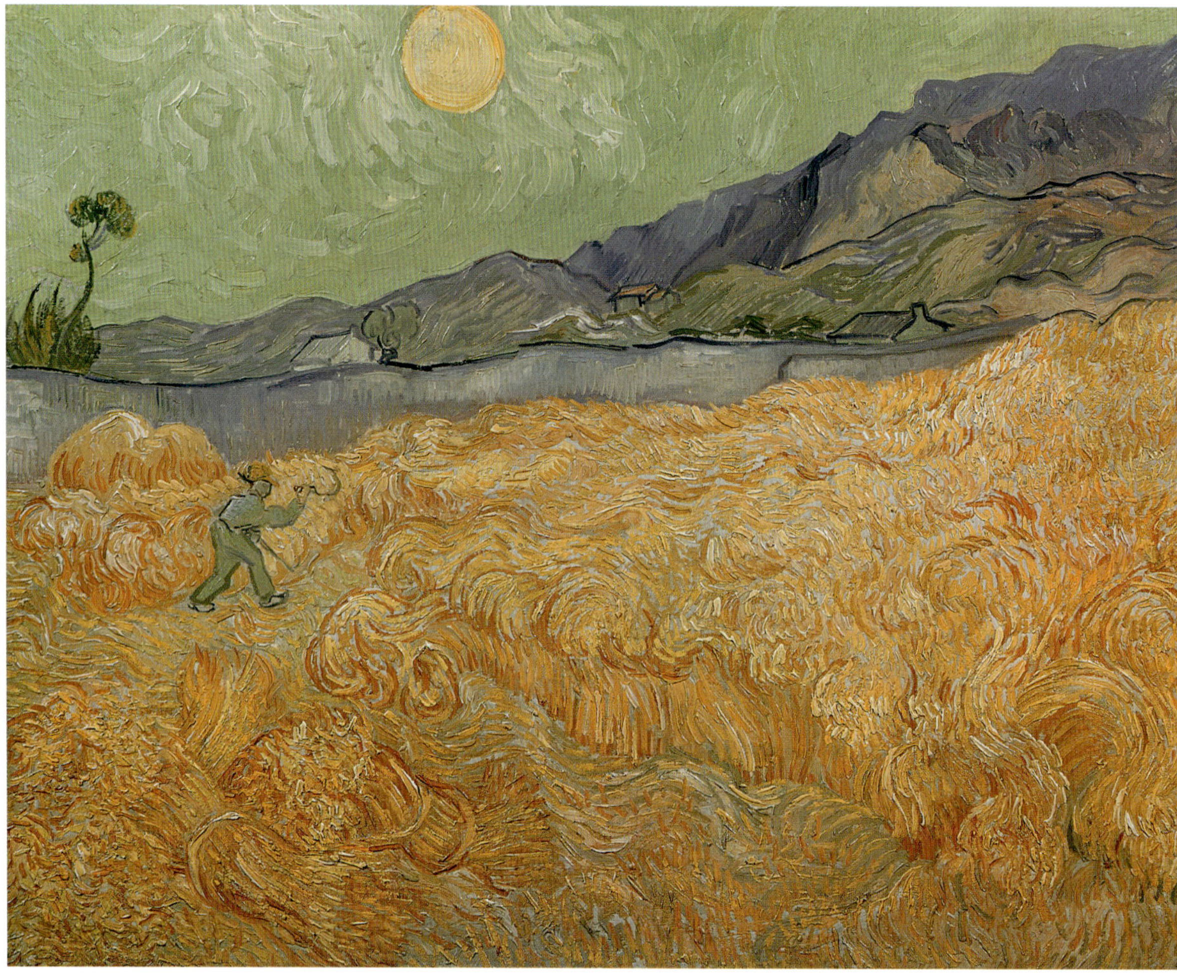

ground after a storm'.[24] Van Gogh may well have been correct in identifying the cause of the tumult as a natural one, for his art was rooted in precise and, according to his own lights, faithful observation. But he must have been conscious of the fact that he, too, was trying to recover his shattered composure 'after a storm', and subsequent canvases in the wheat-field sequence continued to refer to the extreme vulnerability of his emotional state.

Towards the end of June, for example, he started work on a painting called *The Reaper* (pl. 288) and brought it to virtual completion before suffering a serious breakdown for several weeks. The choice of theme may reflect an awareness that mental crisis was imminent, for when van Gogh resumed work on the 'terribly thickly painted' picture early in September, he told Theo that 'I see in this reaper – a vague figure fighting like the devil in the midst of the heat to get to the end of his task – I see in him the image of death, in the sense that humanity might be the wheat he is reaping.'[25] This toiling peasant could embody van Gogh's realisation that he was engaged in a struggle against mental illness to complete his task as an artist. The unusual amount of impasto helps to reinforce the formidable extent of the harvest-work confronting the isolated figure. Van Gogh's letter makes clear that he was also dwelling on the destructive outcome of the reaper's activity – as if each new painting brought him nearer to extinction. Yet he insisted that 'there's nothing sad in this death, it goes its way in broad daylight with a sun flooding everything with a light of pure gold'.[26]

As the year advanced van Gogh became aware of the new life preparing to grow once again the following spring. After completing an overcast picture called *Rain*, where the wheat field is slashed by the lancing diagonals of a heavy downfall, he

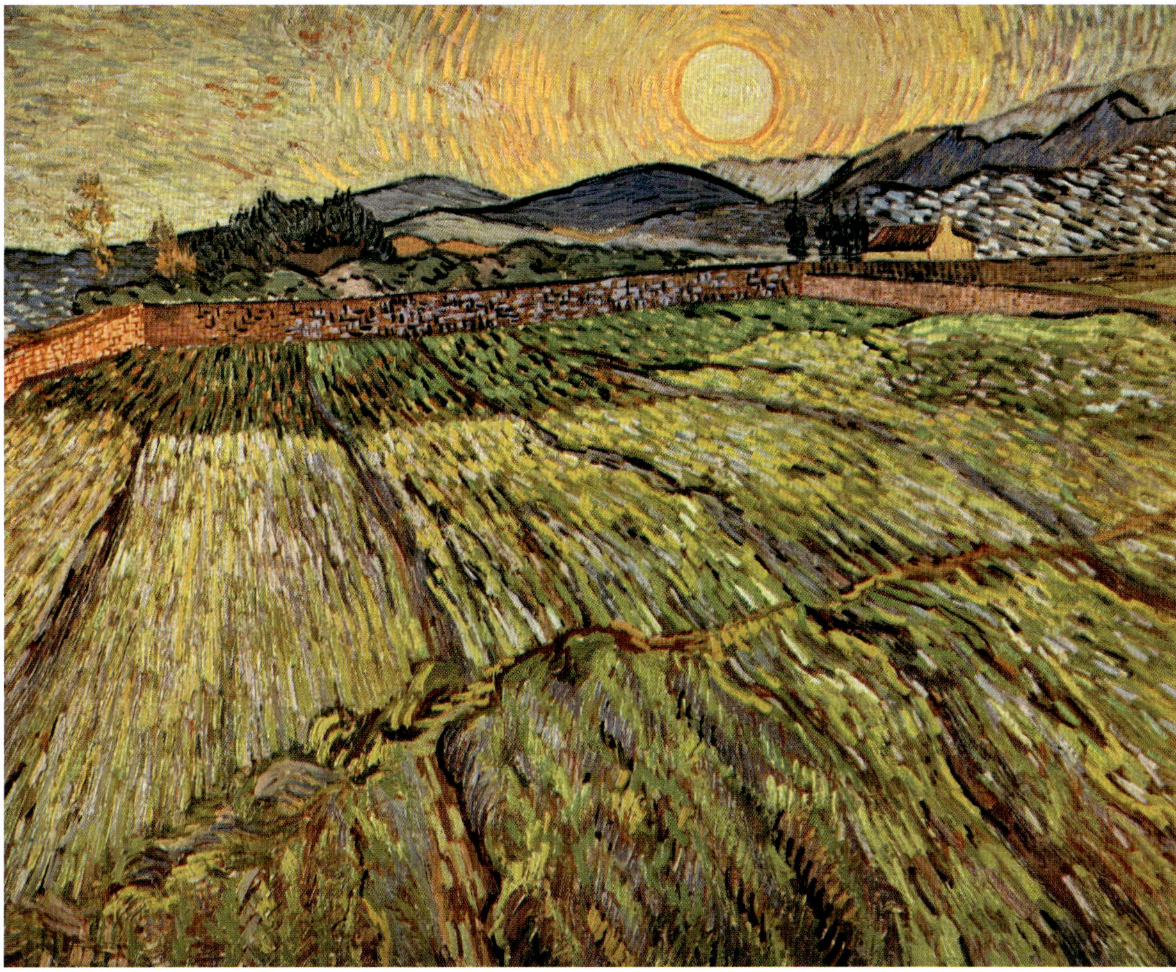

289 Vincent Van Gogh, *Wheat Field with Rising Sun*, 1889, Private Collection

started work in November on a painting that brought the whole field series to a magisterial conclusion. *Wheat Field with Rising Sun* (pl. 289) was produced specifically for a major Les XX exhibition in Brussels. Using a thinner technique that replaced impasto with a handling more alive to the nuances of atmosphere, he defined the hurtling rhythm of the furrows as they rush in undulations towards the distant wall. The effect is affirmative and van Gogh maintained that 'it is the result of the quiet, secluded life that I am leading, and I am all the better for it. Fundamentally I am not so violent as all that, and at last I *myself* feel calmer.'[27] Indeed, he aimed in this superbly vibrant picture at inducing in its viewers a serenity comparable with the most peaceful of religious compositions: 'It is not necessary to portray the characters of the Sermon on the Mount in order to produce a consoling and gentle motif.'[28]

Implicit in this remark is van Gogh's belief that his art could have a healing effect. So he must have wondered whether the other asylum patients could benefit from seeing his work on their walls. He certainly continued the policy initiated at Arles with the portrait of Dr Rey, deciding this time to paint a study of Trabuc, the head attendant at Saint-Rémy, and once again giving it to the sitter (pl. 290). Just as Dadd had portrayed the staff caring for him (see pls 266–7), so van Gogh tried to express the gratitude he felt towards a man whose presence he valued. Writing to Theo, he explained that Trabuc 'was at the hospital at Marseilles through two periods of cholera; altogether he is a man who has seen an enormous amount of suffering and death, and there is a sort of contemplative calm in his face'.[29] The attendant frowns as he poses for the artist, staring with an alertness that belies his age. It led van Gogh to describe how

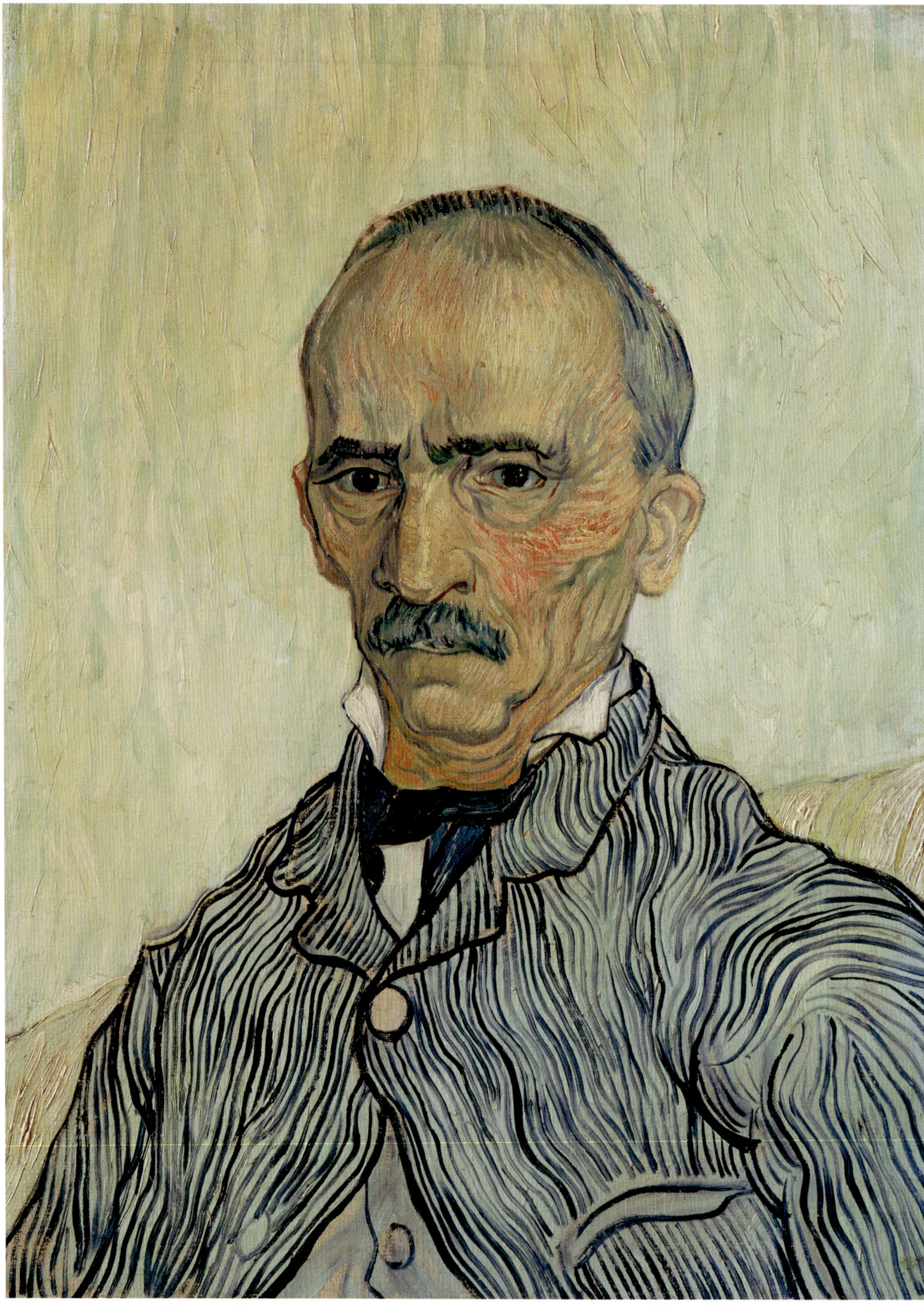

'he has something military in his small quick black eyes'.[30] Vincent appreciated the concern that Trabuc felt for his patient, even though the painting presents a stern individual whose demeanour is reinforced by the harsh lines running through his jacket like the grain in very rough wood. The no-nonsense Madame Trabuc, who likewise became the subject of a portrait that van Gogh presented to her,[31] even tried to minimise the significance of his troubles. 'I have talked to her sometimes when I was doing some olive trees behind their little house', he told Theo, 'and she told me then that she did not believe that I was ill.'[32]

However much he might have liked to agree with Madame Trabuc's diagnosis, van Gogh was unable to conceal the seriousness of the ailment from himself. In one mood he transformed a view of *Hospital at Saint-Rémy* (pl. 291) into an ecstatic image, rejoicing in the vigour of trunks and foliage as they soared above the buildings. 'I tried to reconstruct the thing as it might have been', he explained, 'simplifying and accentuating the haughty, unchanging character of the pines and cedar clumps against the blue.'[33] Yet the element of agitation in this dynamic picture soon developed into outright anxiety. *A Corner of the Asylum Garden* (pl. 292) discloses this darker mood, and in a fascinating letter to his painter friend Emile Bernard he revealed how he hoped the landscape would convey the predicament confronting the asylum's inmates. After describing how the pine trees reared up beside 'some deflowered rose bushes', standing out 'against an evening sky with violet stripes on a yellow ground', he concentrated on the painting's principal symbol:

> Now the nearest tree is an enormous trunk, struck by lightning and sawed off. But one side branch shoots up very high and lets fall an avalanche of dark green pine needles. This sombre giant – like a defeated proud man – contrasts, when considered in the nature of a living creature, with the pale smile of a last rose on the fading bush in front of him.

Then, after discussing the other colours he had deployed in his sullen and bilious canvas, van Gogh went on to declare that

> this combination of red ochre, of green gloomed over by grey, the black streaks surrounding the contours, produces something of the sensation of anguish, called 'noir-rouge', from which certain of my companions in misfortune frequently suffer. Moreover, the motif of the great tree struck by lightning, the sickly green-pink smile of the last flower of autumn serve to confirm this impression . . . One can try to give an impression of anguish without aiming straight at the historic Garden of Gethsemane.[34]

A clearer indication of van Gogh's aims in this haunting picture could hardly be imagined. While it would be wrong to conclude that every picture

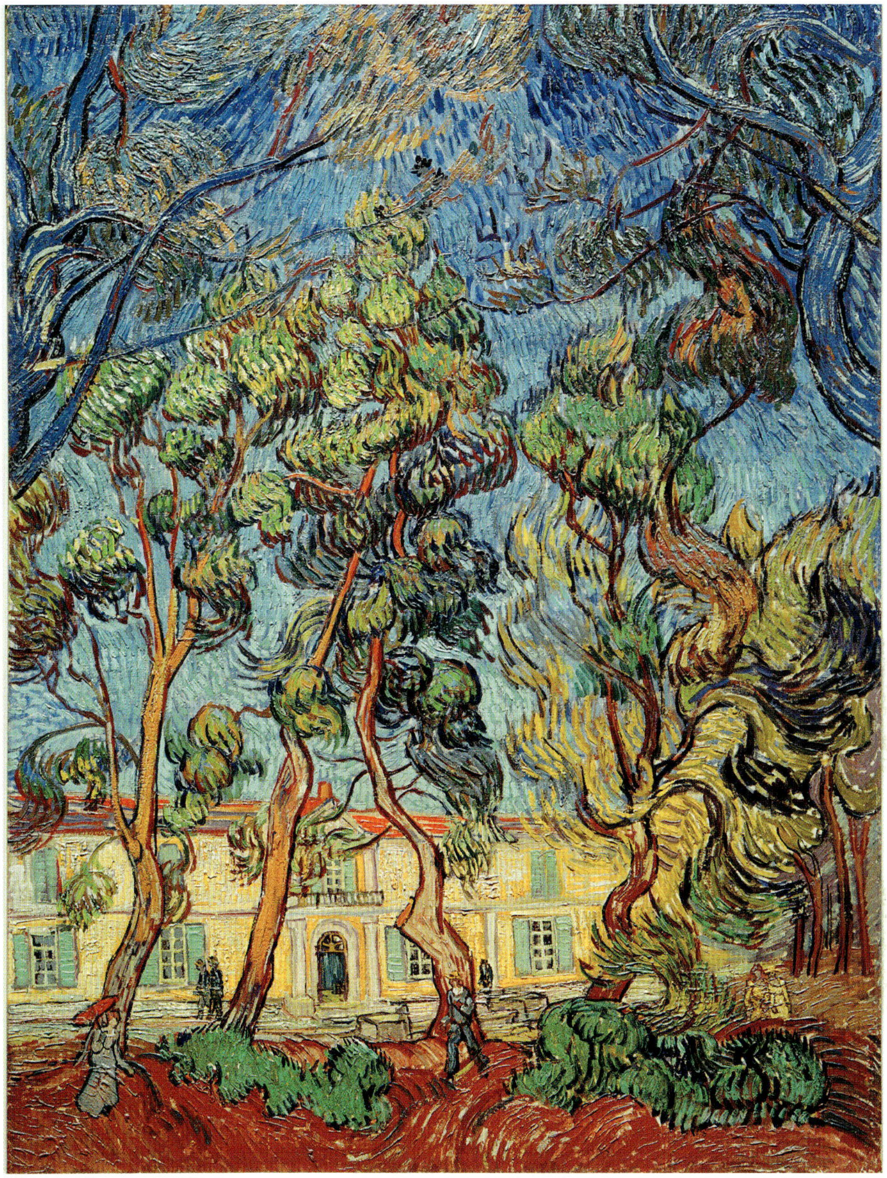

291 (*above*) Vincent Van Gogh, *Hospital at Saint-Rémy*, 1889, The Armand Hammer Collection, Armand Hammer Museum of Art, Los Angeles

290 (*facing page*) Vincent Van Gogh, *Portrait of Trabuc*, 1889, Kunstmuseum Solothurn, Switzerland

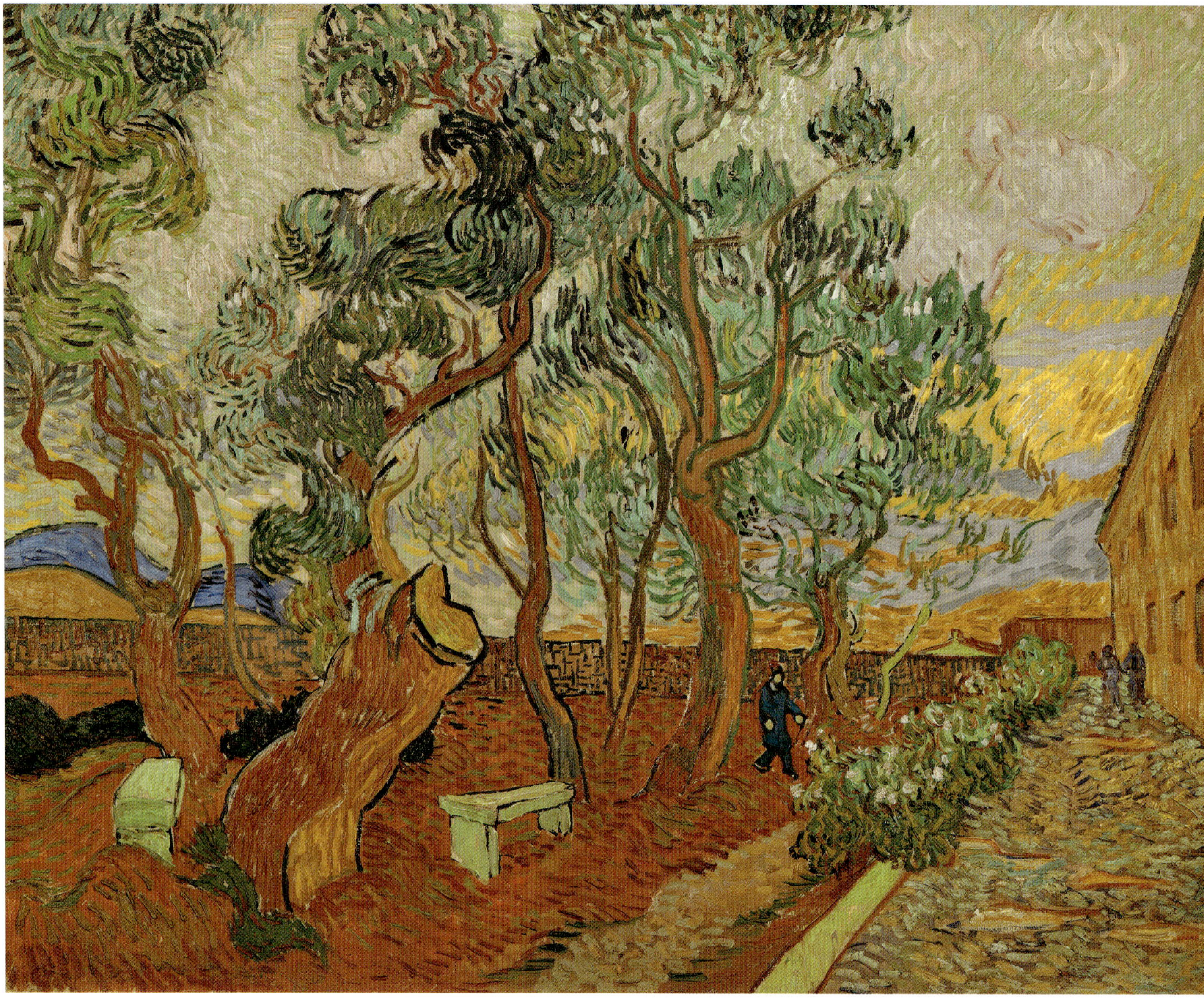

292 Vincent Van Gogh, *A Corner of the Asylum Garden*, 1889, Museum Folkwang, Essen

he painted at the asylum bore so directly on his own plight, certain images take on intense autobiographical significance. Among the most melancholy is a painting called *The Prison Courtyard*, begun only a few days after he was stricken with one of his periodic attacks (pl. 294). Like several other pictures executed during his confinement at Saint-Rémy, it was copied from a print sent by the devoted Theo. In this case, Gustave Doré's dour view of prisoners exercising at Newgate in London (pl. 293) provided the starting point. Van Gogh remained faithful to the composition in most respects; but the acid colours envenoming the picture are his invention, and he magnifies the claustrophobia of the yard by stressing the harshly scored brickwork as it extends high above the prisoners. No hint of sky is permitted to alleviate these relentless walls, and the birds included by Doré in the upper reaches of his woodcut have been banished from view. The four windows set brutishly into the wall are either blocked or barred, frustrating any escape. Vincent's treatment of the foreground paving-stones is equally remorseless, enlarged from Doré's original and slashed with strokes of thick, blue-green pigment. They act as metaphors for the

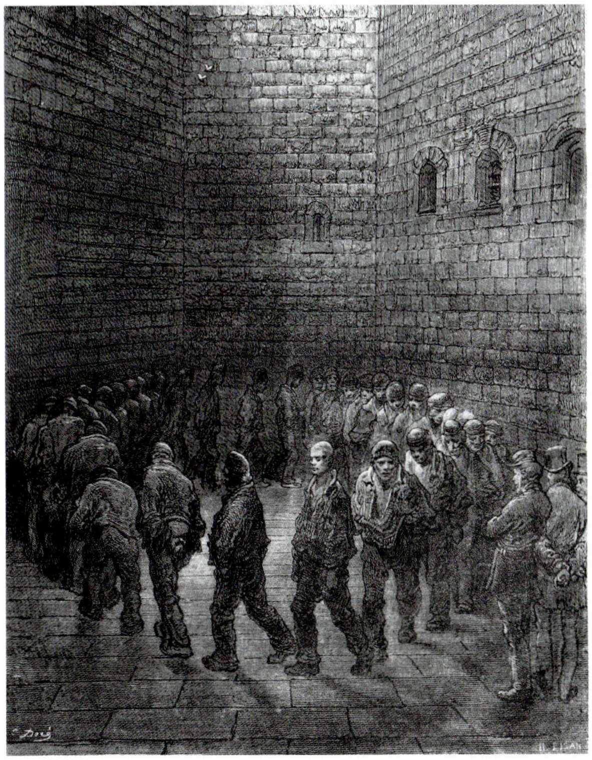

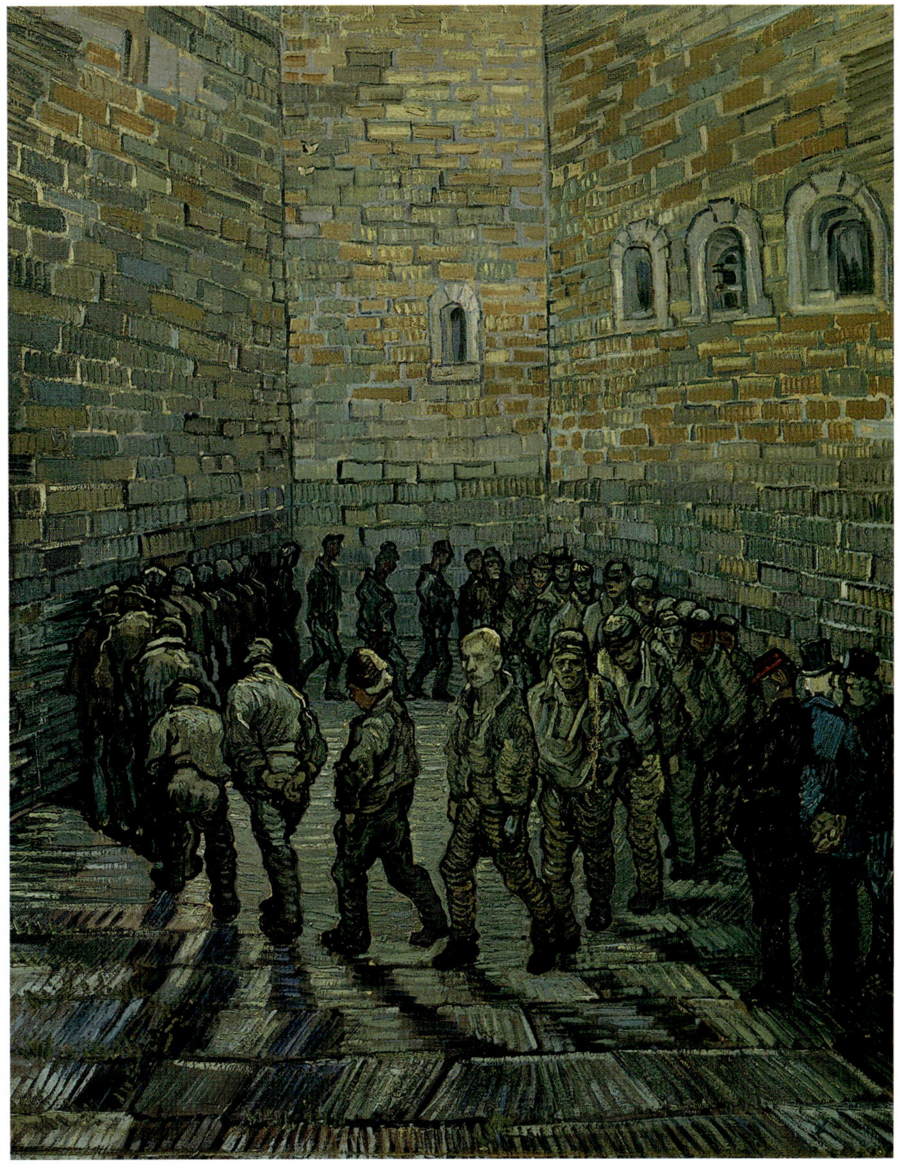

flagellating emotions experienced by the figures in this gruesome arena.

Van Gogh disclosed his painfully personal reason for choosing the prison subject by turning the most prominent of the exercisers into a self-portrait (see pl. 277). His close-cropped hair and blanched features belong to a man of sorrows, confined not by walls and warders but by a terror of his own inner malaise. Although he attended the Saint-Rémy asylum out of his own volition, and was able to wander beyond the building's limits for much of the time, this grim painting indicates that he felt as trapped by his illness as the gaunt felons serving their sentences by plodding round the dank and infernal courtyard.

By this time, any hopes that van Gogh may once have nurtured about achieving a full recovery at Saint-Rémy were gone. During the first few months of his stay, he rallied from the initial shock of other inmates yelling and screaming in nearby rooms, at night as well as in the day. He started talking to them, though they were incapable of coherent replies. As he reported to his sister, 'though there are some seriously ill here, the fear of madness that I felt has already largely disappeared. Although one is always hearing howls and cries like beasts in a zoo, the people here understand each other very well and help each other when they fall into a fit.' Despite Theo's protests, he resigned himself to the probability that

> I shall stay here for a long time. I've never been so quiet as here and in the hospital at Arles, and at last I can paint a little. The small mountains, grey or blue, are very near here with very, very green fields and pines at their feet. I shall count myself very fortunate if I can work enough to earn my living – I'm very worried when I think that I've made so many drawings and paintings without a sale.[35]

293 (*above left*) Gustave Doré, *Prisoners exercising at Newgate*, 1872, Bibliothèque Nationale, Paris

294 (*above right*) Vincent Van Gogh, *The Prison Courtyard*, 1890, Pushkin Museum of Fine Art, Moscow

Yet he never succeeded in selling more than one canvas, to a collector in Brussels just before his thirty-seventh birthday. Dr Peyron's early optimism, prompting him in July to let van Gogh pay a visit to Arles, did not prove well founded. Soon afterwards, the artist suffered a gruelling attack while at work in the foothills near the asylum. The onset of a mistral, blowing a half-finished painting off its perch, seems to have precipitated his collapse. A protracted fit of yelling left his throat acutely painful for days, and he attempted suicide by gulping down his own paints. Nightmares and hallucinations dogged van Gogh. They made him realise how wrong Dr Rey had been to suggest that simply leading a more regular life would release him from mental illness altogether. His opinion of the staff at Saint-Rémy darkened. Dr Peyron seemed to have neither the time nor the patience to attend to him properly, while most of the sisters viewed his art with alarm and disapproval. When Epiphane, the sympathetic head sister, proposed displaying his work in their living-room, they dismissed the idea with outraged hostility. In their eyes, he was allowed far too much freedom at the asylum, and should not have been encouraged to produce his barbaric paintings at all.

Hiding away in his room, where he struggled to cope with this alienation by working harder than ever on self-portraits filled with an unbearable sense of strain, van Gogh felt tormented. 'If one could resign oneself to suffering and death, surrender one's will and love and self!' he wrote. 'But I love to paint, to meet people, to see nature.' The severity of his attack in the foothills left him doubting if he could continue much longer, and he fell back on the thought that his experiments might at least provide the seed for artists in the future. 'I believe that my work will be carried on', he declared.

> Not directly perhaps, but after all I'm not the only one to have faith in the truth. And if someone carries on the work, what do I matter? People are like the corn; both are ground between millstones to make bread. Happiness or unhappiness, what is the difference if one looks to the result? Both are necessary, both useful. Death, life, all is relative.[36]

Increasingly obsessed by the prospect of his own death, van Gogh could not even be helped by the further trips he made to Arles, at Christmas and again in late January 1890. Renewed contact with his former life unsettled him so much that he succumbed to more attacks. The news that his old friend Madame Ginoux was assailed by depression prompted him to write her a devastatingly honest letter. 'I assure you that last year the fear of suffering a relapse almost prevented me from being cured, so little did I wish to begin again', he wrote.

> I very often said to myself that I'd rather there was no more of it and that it should all be over. However, we are not the masters of our own fate and it seems to be a question of learning to want to live again even while suffering. Ah, I feel myself to be so cowardly about this. Even with my health coming back, I still fear.[37]

He had good reason to be despondent: successive attacks left him unable to write or work properly. Dr Peyron ruled out any further trips to Arles and in April van Gogh at last announced to Theo that his period in the asylum should now be terminated. 'The society of the other invalids influenced me so badly', he revealed, 'that finally I could think of nothing.'[38]

His sense of regret was intense. He could not bear the thought of leaving the South with all its fertile inspiration and going instead to live with Camille Pissarro's old friend Dr Gachet, an avid collector of Impressionist art. Auvers-sur-Oise, where Gachet had a house, was only an hour outside Paris and van Gogh knew he would miss the powerful, sensual stimulus of Provence. 'I can scarcely bear to leave the Midi', he told Theo. 'This morning I saw the country again after the rain – it was so fresh, and the flowers . . !'[39] Just before departing, he painted 'a field of grass with dandelions in full sunlight'.[40] The energy derived from this experience may well have inspired him to react defiantly when Theo, ever anxious, proposed coming down to Saint-Rémy and keeping him company on the long retreat north. 'I am not dangerous', van Gogh protested to his sister. 'I've been a patient for a year or more, I've never done harm to anyone – is it just that I should be accompanied like a wild beast? Anyway, I'm so cut up to be leaving in this way that I shall be far too upset to go mad in the train.'[41]

He was right: the journey on the night train in May 1890 proved mercifully uneventful, and he then managed to paint some of his most outstanding images under Dr Gachet's care in Auvers. Nevertheless, this burst of productivity could not be sustained. Just over two months after he left Saint-Rémy, van Gogh went out into the summer fields and clumsily shot himself in the stomach with a revolver. His arduous attempts to recover mental stability with medical help had all failed, and he died two days later. On his deathbed, when the distraught Theo asked him why he had decided to commit suicide, van Gogh only managed to reply with another, equally anguished question: 'Who would imagine that life could be so sad?'[42]

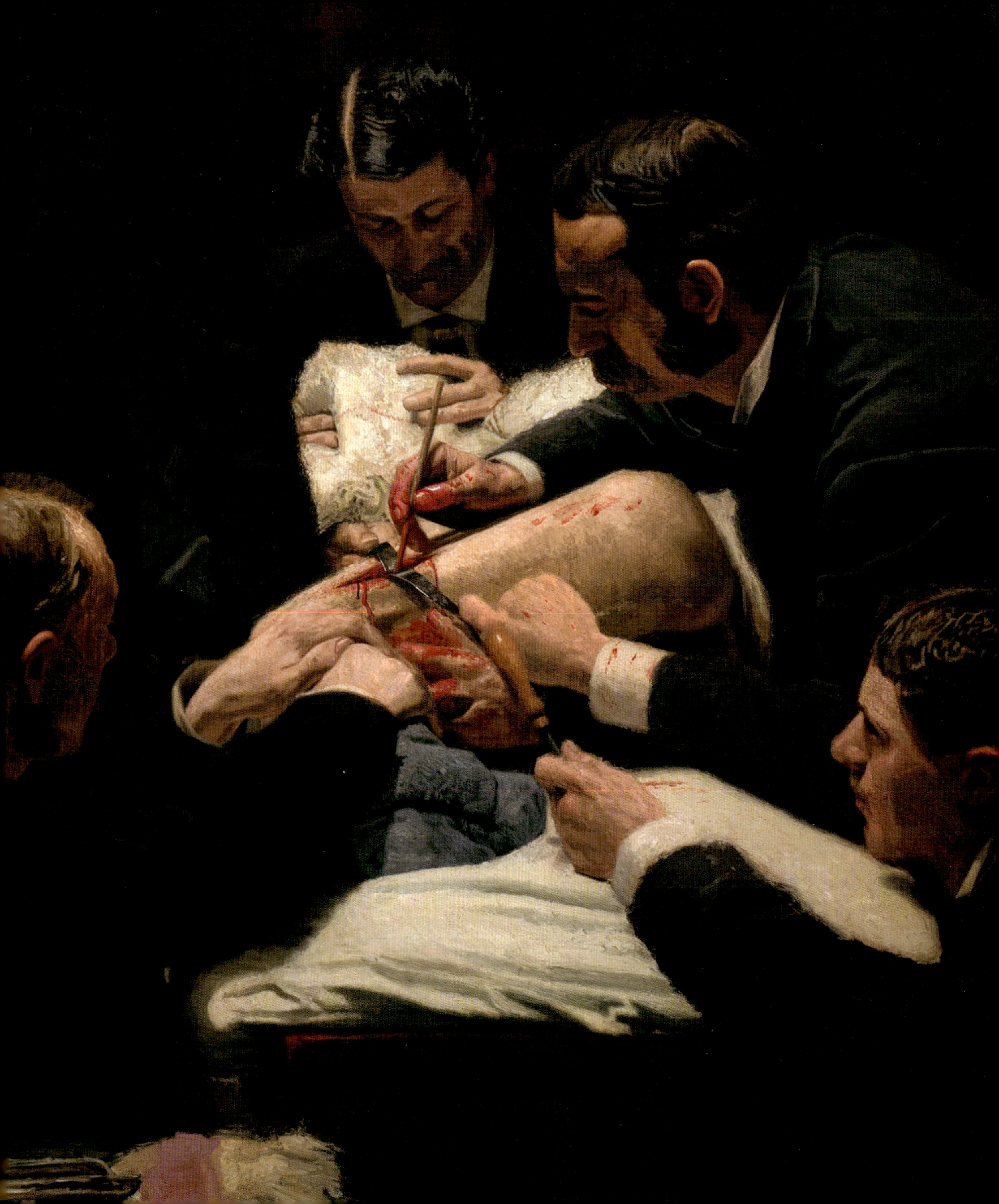

TWENTY
VICTORIAN VALUES

It is ironic that Richard Dadd's intense unofficial activity at Bethlem and Broadmoor coincided with a period when artists in Britain were rarely called upon to enhance general hospitals. The fate of a vast painting called *The Triumph of the Duke of Wellington* by James Ward, presented to the Chelsea Royal Hospital by the British Institution in 1820, is symptomatic of the prevailing lack of interest. Even though the substantial sum of a thousand guineas had been lavished on the canvas, which extended no less than thirty-five feet (10.5 metres) in width, it was not displayed at the Hospital for several years. Then, perhaps hoping that an image of Wellington's triumph might elicit an enthusiastic response from the occupants, the Hospital authorities hung it over the gallery in the Great Hall – with the aid of some folding. This experiment did not, however, prove successful. The unwieldy painting, which showed the Duke riding triumphantly in a chariot through a war-devastated landscape with serpents on the ground and a hydra-headed monster tumbling from the sky, was eventually consigned to the storeroom. Then, in 1879, it suffered the ultimate indignity and was returned to Ward's son. Only the oil sketch (pl. 296) for the unwanted canvas, far more manageable in size, remains in the Hospital today as a reminder of the whole farcical and humiliating episode.

Even the apotheosis of Florence Nightingale failed to generate a demand in hospitals for portraits of the heroic nurse. During the Crimean War she became a national icon, and Jerry Barrett gained enormous popularity through engravings of his epic canvas *The Mission of Mercy: Florence Nightingale receiving the Wounded at Scutari, 1856*. Having established a wide reputation with his earlier hospital painting of *Victoria and Albert visiting the Crimean Wounded*, where the monarch tours a British ward filled with blanched and cruelly injured patients unable even to acknowledge her presence, Barrett journeyed to Scutari in 1856 and made on-the-spot sketches. His final *Mission of Mercy* painting (pl. 297), completed two years later, shows the cool and dignified Nightingale standing beneath a window in the Barrack Hospital where Barrett himself looks down on the scene.[1] Sick and wounded soldiers are making their way through the gateway from a rudimentary landing-stage on the Bosphorus. In the distance, the gardens of the Seraglio and the Mosque of Hagia Sophia are visible, reminding viewers that Scutari was a suburb of Constantinople. Yet the focus of the painting rests with Nightingale, who adopts a Christ-like attitude above the soldier on a stretcher extending his arm in her direction. Memories are stirred of the Pool of Bethesda (see

295 (*facing page*) Detail of pl. 305

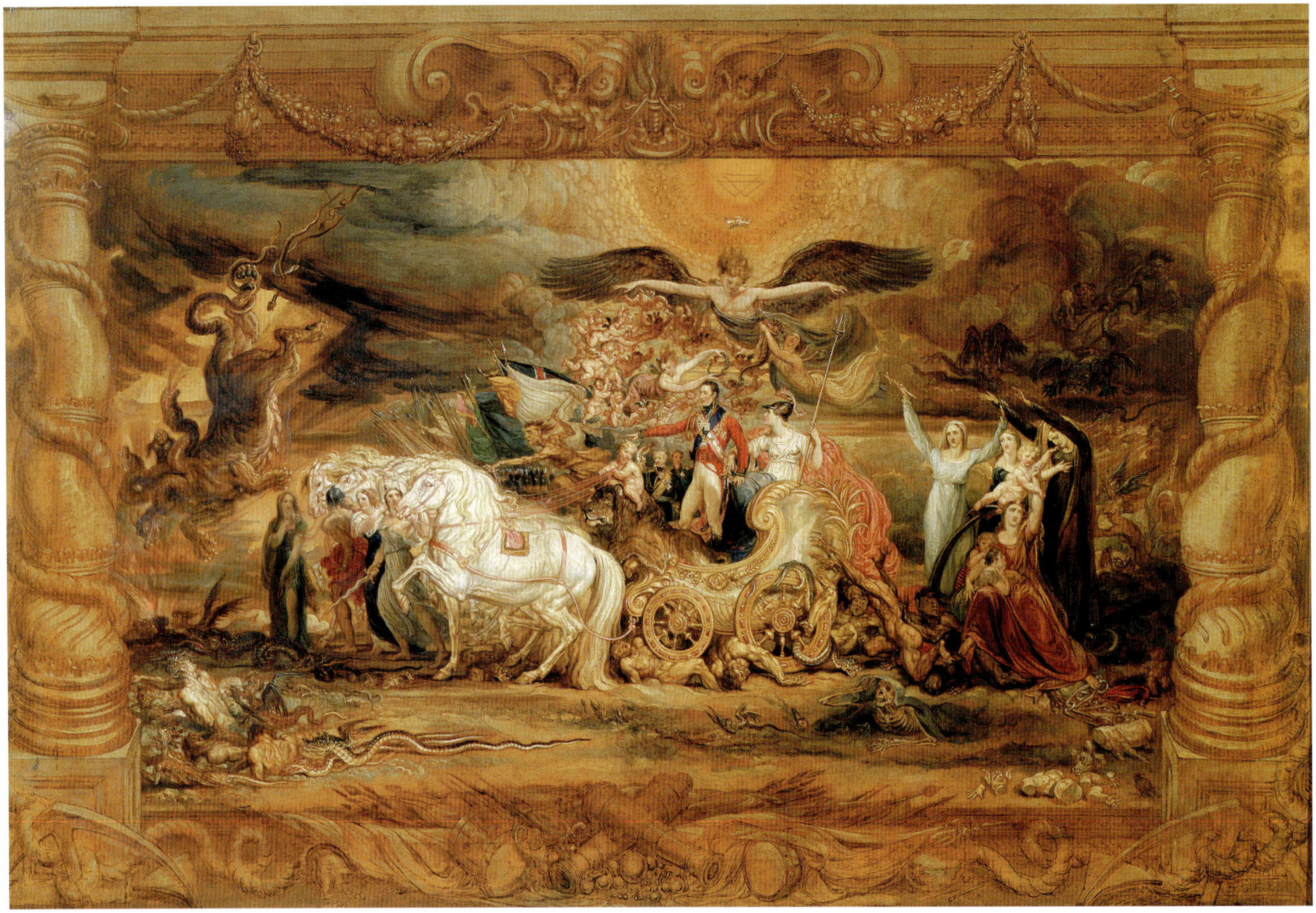

296 James Ward, Oil sketch for *The Triumph of the Duke of Wellington*, 1820, Royal Hospital, Chelsea

pls 133 and 186) and Barrett undoubtedly saw Nightingale as a secular saviour.

Such an image, stressing the saintly courage and competence of the woman who had struggled to overcome pestilential conditions at the notorious Barrack Hospital, still did not lead medical bodies to procure similarly elevated paintings for their institutions in their charge. Nightingale did her best to discourage them, too. She granted Sir John Steell only two sittings for his iconic bust and declared that she harboured moral objections to having her likeness taken in any form: 'I do not wish to be remembered when I am gone'.[2]

No hospital would have dreamed of commissioning a portrait of Mary Seacole, the other woman who gained an impressive reputation for looking after troops in the Crimean War. She first began caring for British officers in her native Jamaica, having been trained in herbal medicine. But Seacole's subsequent attempt in England to volunteer her services as a nurse in Nightingale's contingent was rejected by the British government, probably on racial grounds. Undaunted, she set out for Balaclava at her own expense in the mid-1850s. There, her ramshackle boarding-house called the 'British Hotel' quickly became legendary in army circles. Seacole held surgeries for countless soldiers suffering from intestinal diseases, giving them remedies made from boiled pomegranate skins. She also made regular visits to the battlefield, administering food and drink as well as nursing the wounded and dying. Her bravery, warmth and stamina were widely admired, not only in the Crimea but also in Britain where newspapers often reported on her medical feats and unfailing hospitality.[3] Yet after the war she returned to England

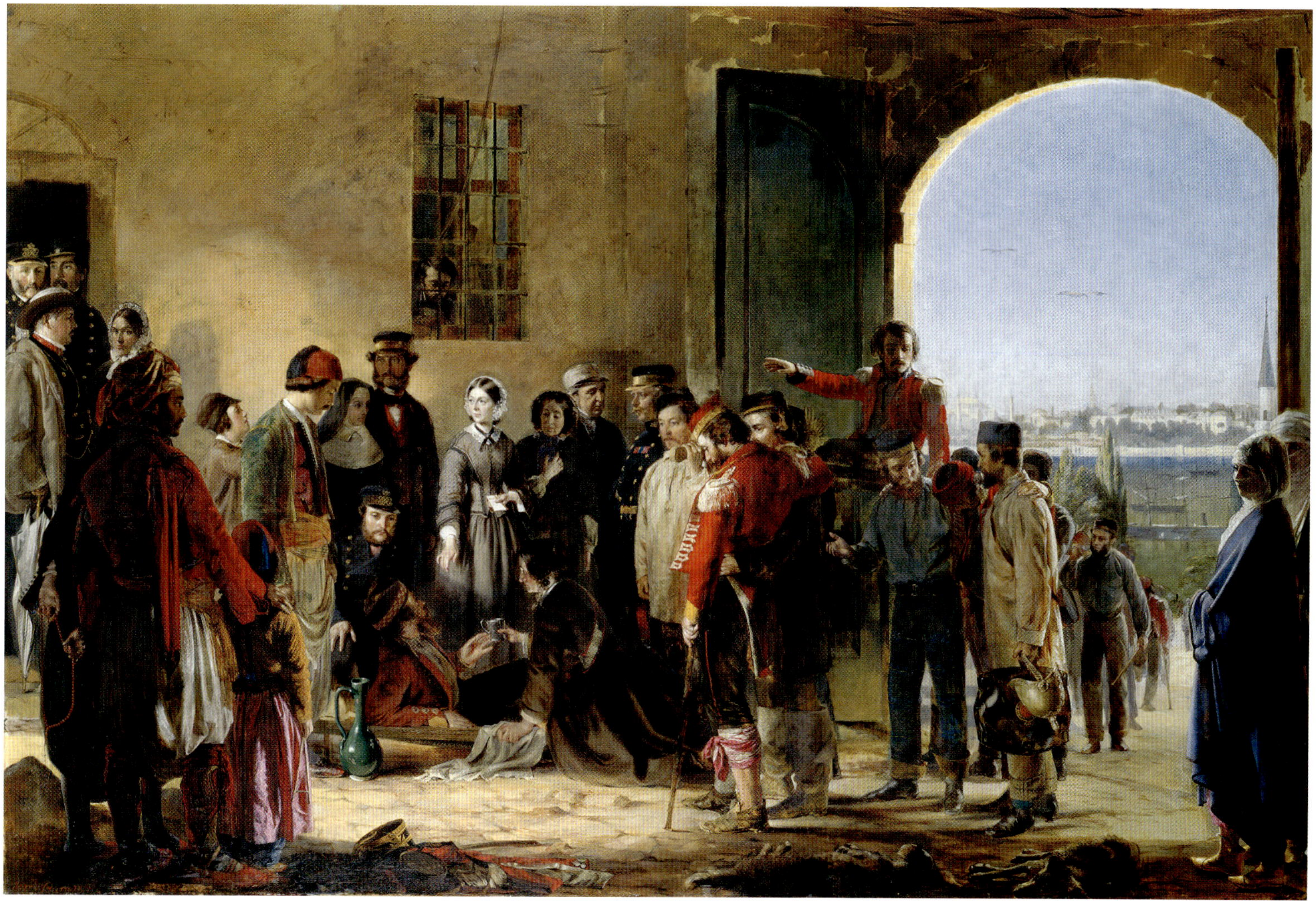

297 Jerry Barrett, *The Mission of Mercy – Florence Nightingale receiving the Wounded at Scutari*, 1858, National Portrait Gallery, London

destitute. Queen Victoria, who lauded Nightingale, never bothered to meet the woman who became known to troops throughout the Crimea as 'Mother Seacole'. Her habit of selling alcohol in Balaclava was frowned on, and Nightingale once sharply remarked that 'anyone who employs Mrs Seacole will introduce much kindness – also much drunkenness and improper conduct wherever she is'.[4] Helen Rappaport, a leading Seacole scholar, has explained that Nightingale 'was trying to establish nursing as a profession for middle-class women, and she could not be associated with a freewheeler and maverick like Mary'.[5] The only known painting of Seacole is a recently discovered oil portrait by the obscure London artist Albert Charles Challen, who produced a freely handled image of the tough, resolute Jamaican displaying her medals – the French Legion of Honour, the Turkish Medjidie and the British Crimean medal – with defiant pride (pl. 298).

Only in exceptional circumstances were artists given opportunities to produce anything other than portraits of resident physicians for Victorian hospitals. When William Calder Marshall produced a grand full-length figure of *Dr Jenner* in 1858, it was installed in Kensington Gardens rather than a medical institution. Its heroic dignity is far removed from Gillray's delirious satire of Jenner in the *Cow-Pock* more than half a century earlier (see pl. 227). Even so, the seated physician looks somewhat lost in this outdoor setting. No wonder the *London Review* complained that 'the statue of Jenner is not a bad one, but it is entirely out of place. Surely a more appropriate site could be found for the commemoration of one of the benefactors of the human race'.[7]

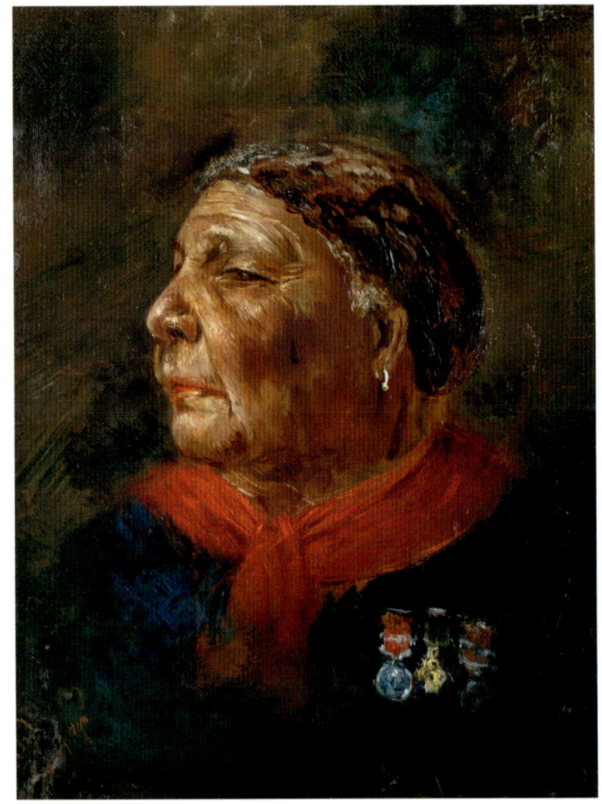

298 Albert Charles Challen, *Mary Seacole*, 1869, National Portrait Gallery, London

Emma Brownlow's work for the Coram Hospital, by contrast, owed everything to her personal connections with the institution. In 1858, when Barrett completed his panoramic *Nightingale* canvas and Calder Marshall's *Jenner* was unveiled, Brownlow began her uneven yet fascinating sequence of paintings for the Coram. She was lucky: her father John, who had himself been a foundling, was the hospital's Secretary and instrumental in securing benefactors' funding for the enterprise.[8] Moreover, she had been brought up in the Coram building. Although not a foundling, she was therefore predisposed to treat the hospital's activities with special sympathy and understanding. Both qualities are well to the fore in the earliest and best of her Coram canvases, *The Foundling restored to its Mother* (pl. 299). Set in the Secretary's room at the hospital, this diligent and compassionate painting depicts John Brownlow presiding with geniality over the reconciliation he has helped to bring about. The original receipt for the child lies on the floor, symbolically discarded by a woman anxious to reclaim her small daughter. Emma Brownlow emphasises the gulf between them by ensuring that a sizeable distance separates the two figures – the child standing uncertainly with her Foundling nurse, and the mother stretching out eager yet apprehensive hands to her long-lost girl. A box of toys has been opened, ready for use. But the moment of uncertainty shown here stresses the painfulness of reunion as well as its joy.

Since several pictures from the Coram collection are displayed prominently behind, Brownlow might be suspected of drawing a parallel between their subjects and the drama enacted in front of the Secretary's desk. No particular significance can be attached to the inclusion of the portraits of Shakespeare and Jonson, the tapestry of Salome after Guido Reni and a detail from a painting of *Elijah raising the Son of the Widow of Zarephath*, attributed to Giovanni Lanfranco. The main canvas on the wall, however, is Hogarth's *March to Finchley* (see pl. 203), where dissolute soldiers reluctantly struggle free from the women with whom they have been carousing. Brownlow could, perhaps, be using the Hogarth painting to indicate how babies might be born from such casual liaisons, and afterwards consigned to the Foundling Hospital. She had certainly showed a preoccupation with the fate of abandoned children in earlier paintings like *The Foundling Girl* or *The Orphan*,[9] and Pamela Gerrish Nunn suggested that growing up in the hospital 'encouraged a social conscience in the young woman'.[10]

A childhood spent in the Coram premises also furnished Brownlow with an insider's grasp of how the institution worked. Her next painting for the Foundling Hospital, *The Christening* (pl. 300), concentrates on the scene in the chapel dominated, appropriately, by Benjamin West's large canvas *Christ presenting a Little Child*. Since many of the applicant mothers were domestic servants, who had been made pregnant by the young men of the household, they found it easiest to present their unwanted offspring on Saturdays. The christening took place on the following day, observed in Brownlow's painting by two gentlemen standing at a discreet distance from the proceedings. While older foundling girls carry in the babies, each one neatly swathed in fresh linen, the Coram's morning preacher, the Reverend J.W. Gleadell, gives the infant he carries a new name. Brownlow invests the picture with well-observed warmth. The girls, conscious no doubt that they were once as forlorn as

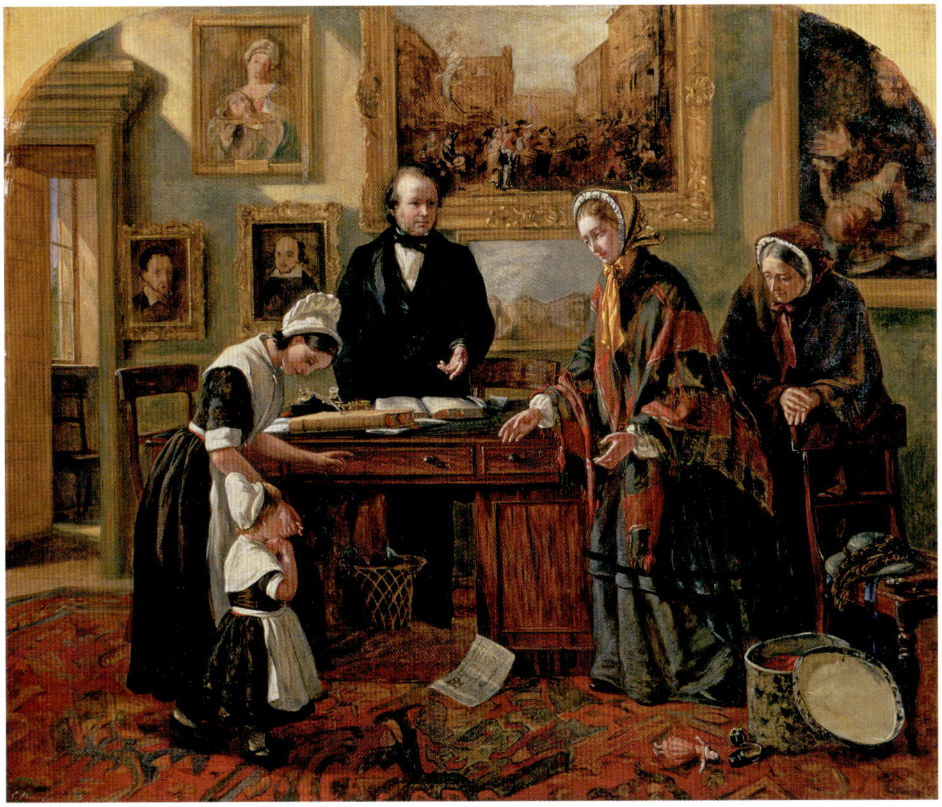

299 Emma Brownlow, *The Foundling Restored to its Mother*, 1858, The Foundling Museum, London

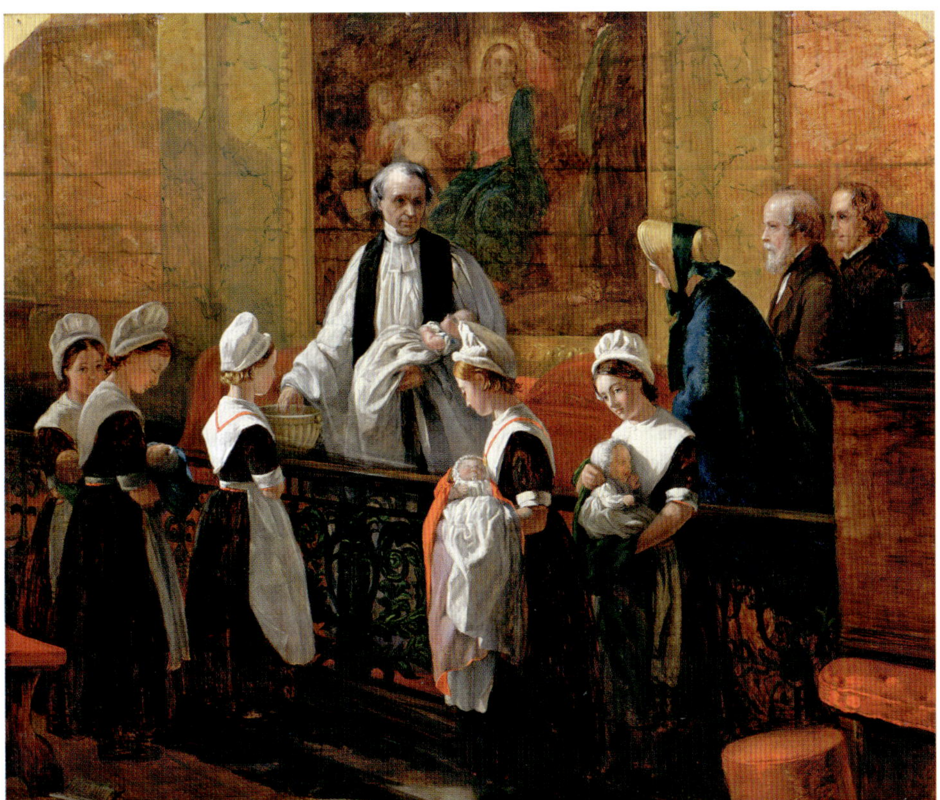

300 Emma Brownlow, *The Christening*, 1863, The Foundling Museum, London

the babies in their arms, cradle their charges with tender devotion. As for Gleadell, he watches the procession with a mixture of quiet benevolence and sadness.

Charles Dickens, whose house in Doughty Street was a short walk from the hospital, found himself much affected by the melancholy fate of the orphans he studied from his rented pew in the Coram chapel. He allowed the full strength of his reaction to be expressed in *Little Dorrit*, when Mrs Meagles visits the chapel and describes how,

> when I saw all those children ranged tier above tier, and appealing from the father none of them has ever known on earth, to the great Father of all of us in Heaven, I thought, does any wretched mother ever come here, and look among these young faces, wondering which is the poor child she brought into this forlorn world, never through all its life to know her love, her kiss, her face, her voice, even name![11]

Compared with Dickens's shameless outpouring, Brownlow is notable for her restraint. Even her third Coram canvas *The Sick Room* (pl. 301), a subject that could easily have led her into cloying, tearful excess, remains subdued. First-hand knowledge of medical care at the hospital probably prevented her from indulging in emotional overkill. The patient, rather than suffering a piteous death according to the most heart-wrenching traditions of Victorian fiction, seems relieved to see Dr Thomas Wormald, the Surgeon and Governor. With practised intimacy, he sits on the bed and takes the child's pulse while other foundlings are allowed to gaze at the proceedings and even play on the floor with dolls. It amounts, no doubt, to a rosy improvement on the reality of life in hospital sick-bays, but the Coram was regarded as an admirably humane place in the nineteenth century.

Brownlow's fourth painting demonstrates her willingness to reveal the sterner side of the Coram's activities as well. Painted a decade after her first canvas in the series, and showing considerable signs of compositional awkwardness, *Taking Leave* (pl. 302) depicts the solemn moment when two foundlings bid farewell to their guardians. The formality of the ceremony has a stiffness that contrasts poignantly with the familial atmosphere of the *Sick Room*. Here, the children seem inhibited by the unbending behaviour of their elders, the most senior of whom gazes at them from his chair with a disconcerting expression of furrowed concern. He does not appear to view their future optimistically. Instead, the sadness of imminent departure is allowed to prevail, and Brownlow's decision to include on the wall Hogarth's *Moses brought before Pharaoh's Daughter* (see pl. 195) intensifies the sense of foreboding. That painting focused on the figure of the boy, deeply upset at leaving his mother and alarmed at the prospect of approaching a new life. Perhaps Brownlow wanted, with commendable thoughtfulness, to let Hogarth highlight the hidden emotional implications of the leave-taking in the room itself.

By this time, the Foundling Hospital was enough of a celebrated national institution to be made the subject of a widely reproduced painting. Exhibited at the Royal Academy in 1863, Edward Matthew Ward's *Hogarth's Studio, 1739: Holiday Visit of Foundlings to view the Portrait of Captain Coram* presents an idyllic view of orphans and painter alike. The cherubic children, dressed in immaculately laundered pinafores, exude a cheerfulness and ruddy health which prettify historical reality with unapologetic zeal. Ward's coyness reaches its apogee behind the Coram portrait, where the old captain gleefully hides in order to eavesdrop on the foundlings' joyful response. It is a preposterous conceit, testifying above all to the Victorians' limitless capacity for sentimentality of the most arch and calculating kind. But the picture also shows how Ward and contemporaries like William Mulready venerated the precedent set by Hogarth. When the painting was displayed at the Academy, Ward accompanied it with a quotation from a recently published essay by George Augustus Sala, who stressed Coram's saintliness.[12] Reviews of the picture likewise emphasised its faultless morality, exclaiming over the 'natural and healthy tone of feeling' and concluding that an engraving of the painting would arouse responses 'both pleasurable and wholesome'.[13]

Where the embellishment of hospitals was concerned, the Victorian preoccupation with unimpeachable respectability came to a formidable climax in June 1871, when the new St Thomas's building was unveiled on its Albert Embankment site opposite the Houses of Parliament. Dignity was of the essence when Queen Victoria herself, standing on a dais in the Central Hall, declared the

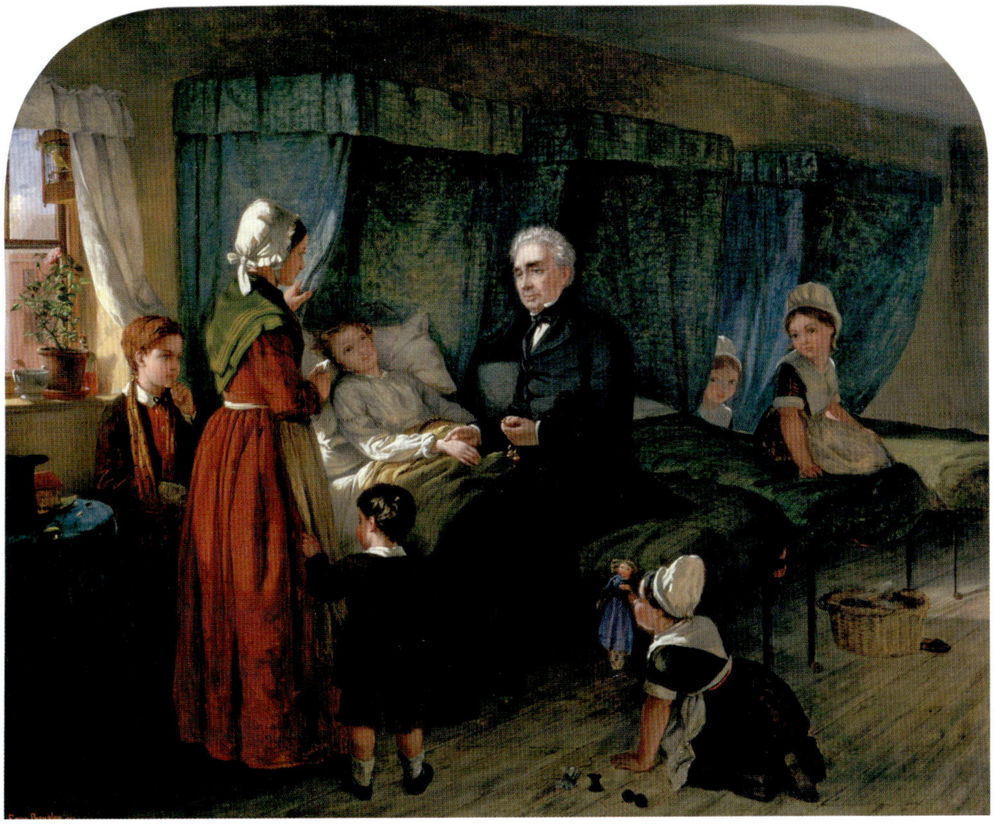

301 Emma Brownlow, *The Sick Room*, 1864, The Foundling Museum, London

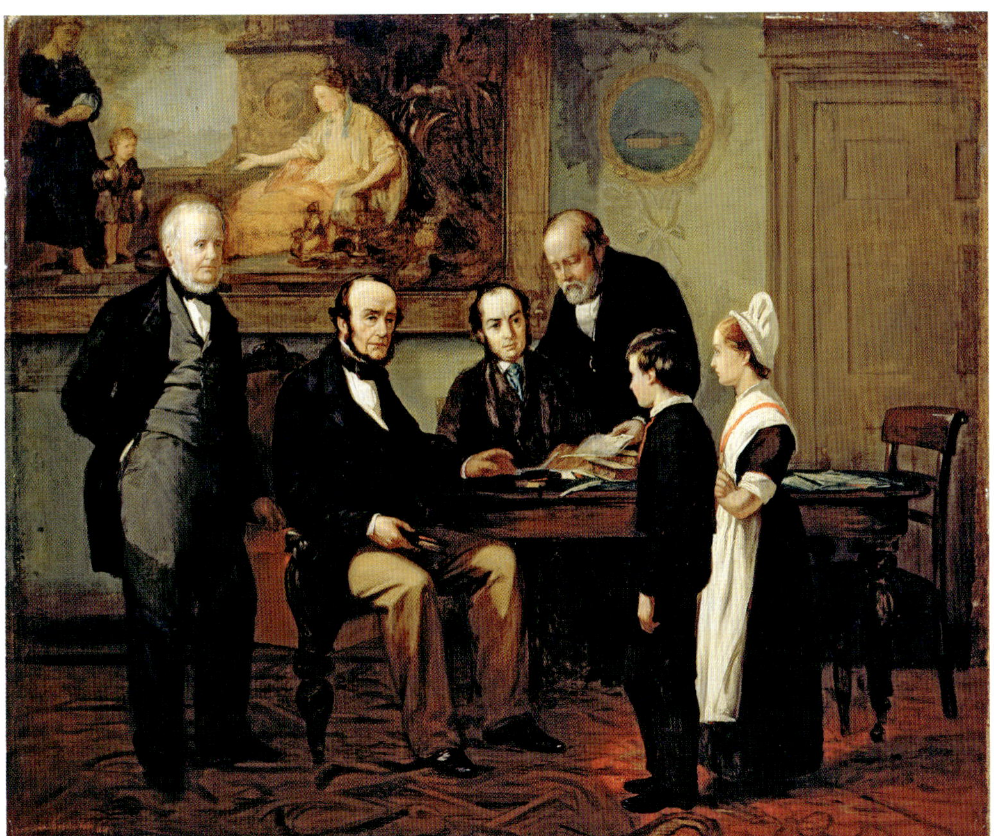

302 Emma Brownlow, *Taking Leave*, 1868, The Foundling Museum, London

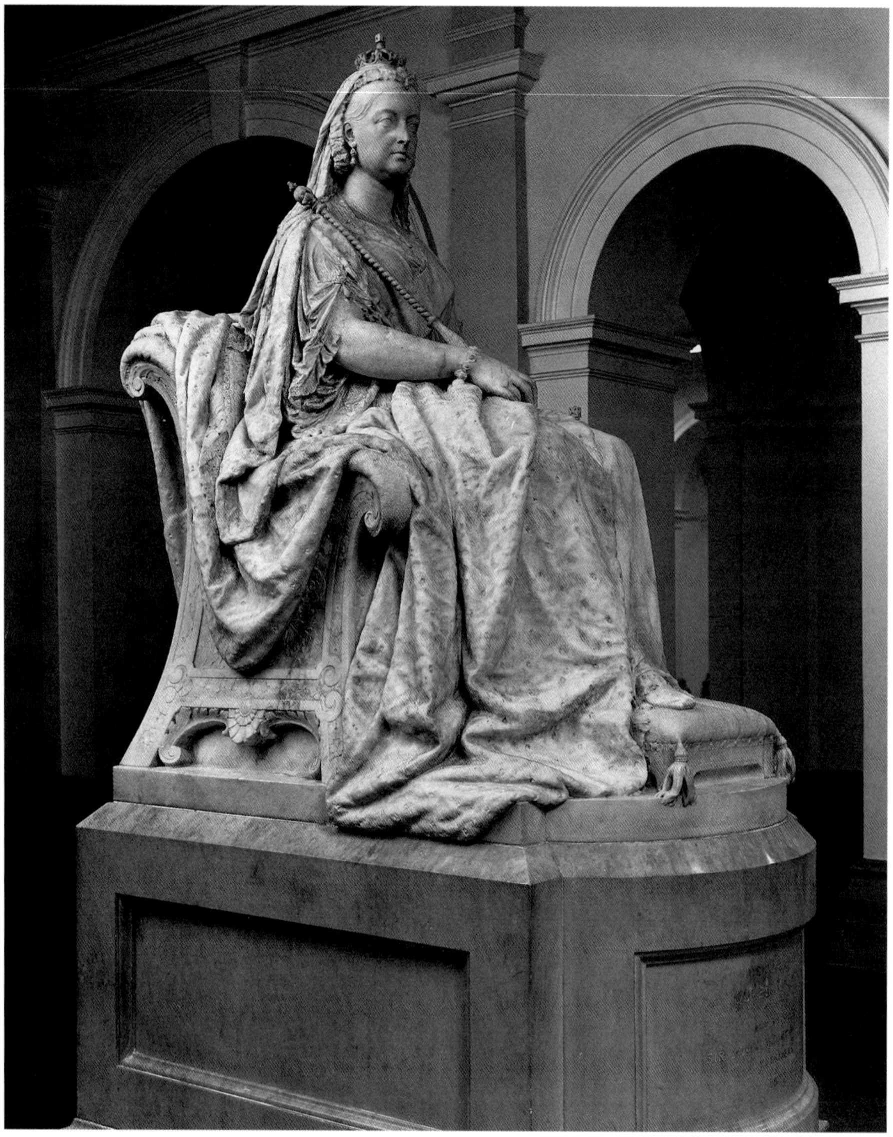

303 Matthew Noble, Statue of Queen Victoria, *c*.1871, St Thomas's Hospital, London

hospital open. To commemorate the event, Noble's immense marble statue of the enthroned monarch (pl. 303) was installed soon afterwards, a gift from the President Sir John Musgrove. For many years, this somnolent effigy loomed over the Hall as a crowning confirmation of medicine's hallowed place in the hierarchy of Victorian values.

Its presence there doubtless inspired the creation of the double row of St. Thomas's worthies, grave marble busts memorialising the hospital's most distinguished members of staff. Although one of them is a copy of Roubiliac's earlier portrait of Sir Richard Mead,[14] most of these bewhiskered countenances depict nineteenth-century physicians. Even today they give the Central Hall an overwhelming air of mournful authority. One of the hospital's historians proudly described it as 'our Valhalla'.[15] Here is Sir John Simon, known as the 'Apostle of Sanitation' for his seminal contribution to public health in London, and nearby we find the nervous diseases specialist Dr John Syer Bristowe, whose textbook on medicine became a standard work. Assessed as sculpture, these busts are competent and unremarkable, the partial exception being Sir Francis Chantrey's bust of Henry Cline, donated by his admiring students. However, the busts manage to make even the least memorable of men appear imposing. Samuel Solly, for instance, was a surgeon without special merit, and yet his curled side whiskers combine with a Roman toga to give him an immensely dignified aura. Sir William MacCormac's professional record likewise suggests that he did little to deserve the immortality bestowed on him here, for his dresser admitted: 'I cannot look back upon him as a really first-class surgeon; while as a lecturer and teacher he was very poor indeed'.[16] Overall the busts confirm Francis Turner Palgrave's withering assertion that 'the present time will probably be looked on in future years as the *nadir* of English sculpture'. His scorn knew no bounds:

> More money than ever, it is credibly stated, is now in the course of expenditure upon marble-chipping and smoothing . . . And yet, in fact, we all know, and sadly have to confess it, – nobody believes in or cares for English sculpture, except the prosperous few who fall thus within range of the genial shower which, if it cannot transmute ignorance into artistic skill, performs at least the more tangible metamorphosis by which bronze refines into gold, and bank-notes freely form themselves upon the surface of the marble.[17]

To discover more impressive and personal Victorian portraits of medical specialists, one has to look elsewhere. In 1864, when Palgrave unleashed his critical venom on Henry Weekes's 'inaccurate and tasteless' statue of Dr Hunter, George Frederick Watts received a memorable commission for a physician's portrait (pl. 304). It came from William Bowman, whose precocious prowess in the treatment of eye complaints had led to his appointment as a full surgeon in the Royal London Ophthalmic Hospital at Moorfields. Bowman, an enthusiastic and discerning art collector, had already commissioned Watts to produce a self-portrait and a study of Tennyson. Since Watts's painting of Bowman is the same size as his own self-portrait, the two paintings can be seen as a pair. Watts depicts himself heavily bearded in a broad black hat, gazing out somewhat defensively and clasping his hands with nervous rigidity, but he portrays Bowman as a more relaxed individual, leaning back informally over a chair with hands folded in a calm, composed manner. The mutton-chop whiskers and flowing silver hair are painted with notable vivacity, and Bowman's remarkably dark, intent eyes testify to the clarity of his own vision.

Watts had suffered ocular problems and consulted Bowman,[18] whose expertise often brought him into contact with artists worried about their eyesight. In this painting, Bowman could be listening to Watts as the artist compares the demands of ophthalmology with the importance of close, focused scrutiny in portraiture. But the image testifies above all to friendship rather than the formality of a doctor–patient relationship. Barbara Bryant has observed that *William Bowman* 'also showed a new direction for male portraiture in suggesting mood and meaning beyond mere likeness'.[19] It won widespread approval when exhibited at the Royal Academy in 1865. Several reviewers commended its Titianesque qualities, while *The Times* declared that 'Mr. Watts's portrait of Mr. Bowman, the oculist, best satisfies the true requirements of a portrait. It interests without one's knowing the person painted.'[20]

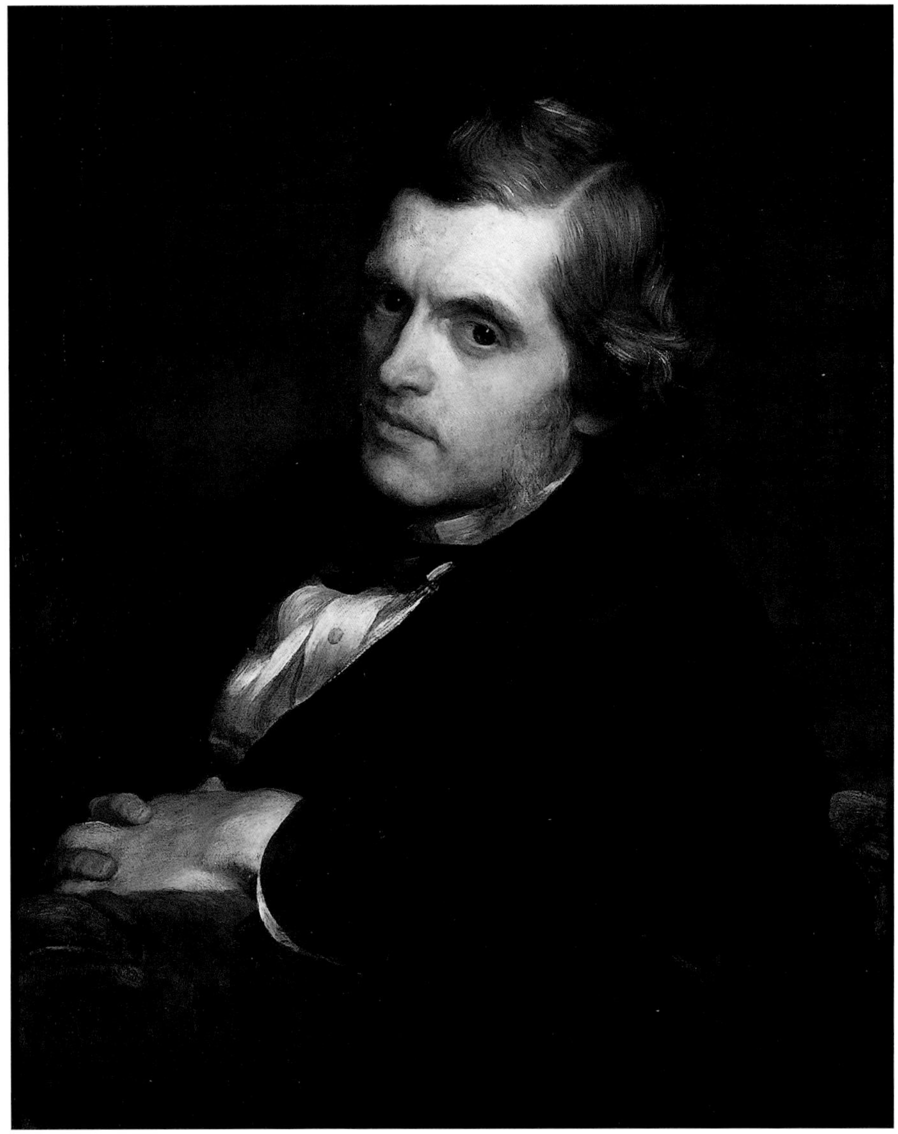

304 George Frederick Watts, *William Bowman*, 1864, Private Collection

To find a truly outstanding painting of a physician in this period, however, we must leave Britain and travel to Philadelphia. There Thomas Eakins spent most of 1875 executing an ambitious and profound portrait of Dr Samuel D. Gross, surgeon and teacher at Jefferson Medical College. Rather than showing him posed as an isolated figure inside the artist's studio, Eakins decided to place Gross in the context of surgery's dramatic role as a health-giver. Even in the preliminary oil sketch, a swiftly handled affair where Gross's head looms out of the surrounding darkness, he is placed next to surgical colleagues and a body prone on a table. Eakins received no commission for this large, complex canvas: he initiated it himself and Marc Simpson has emphasised that, as with Eakins's paintings of athletes, *The Gross Clinic* 'was a new type of subject, virtually unknown in American art and with few precedents even in the European tradition'.[21]

Conscious no doubt of Rembrandt's two great paintings of anatomy lessons (see pls 114 and 116), Eakins emulates his Dutch precedents by investing the subject with an intensely meditative gravity. Unlike Tulp and Deyman, though, Dr Gross is conducting a remedial operation on an anaesthetised patient (pl. 305). Light falls on the thigh of a young figure, probably identifiable as a charity case, who is suffering from osteomyelitis.[22] The incision, to remove a segment of diseased bone and thereby retain the limb, is depicted with unprecedented realism. The blanched vulnerability of the patient's flesh is conveyed without any flinching by

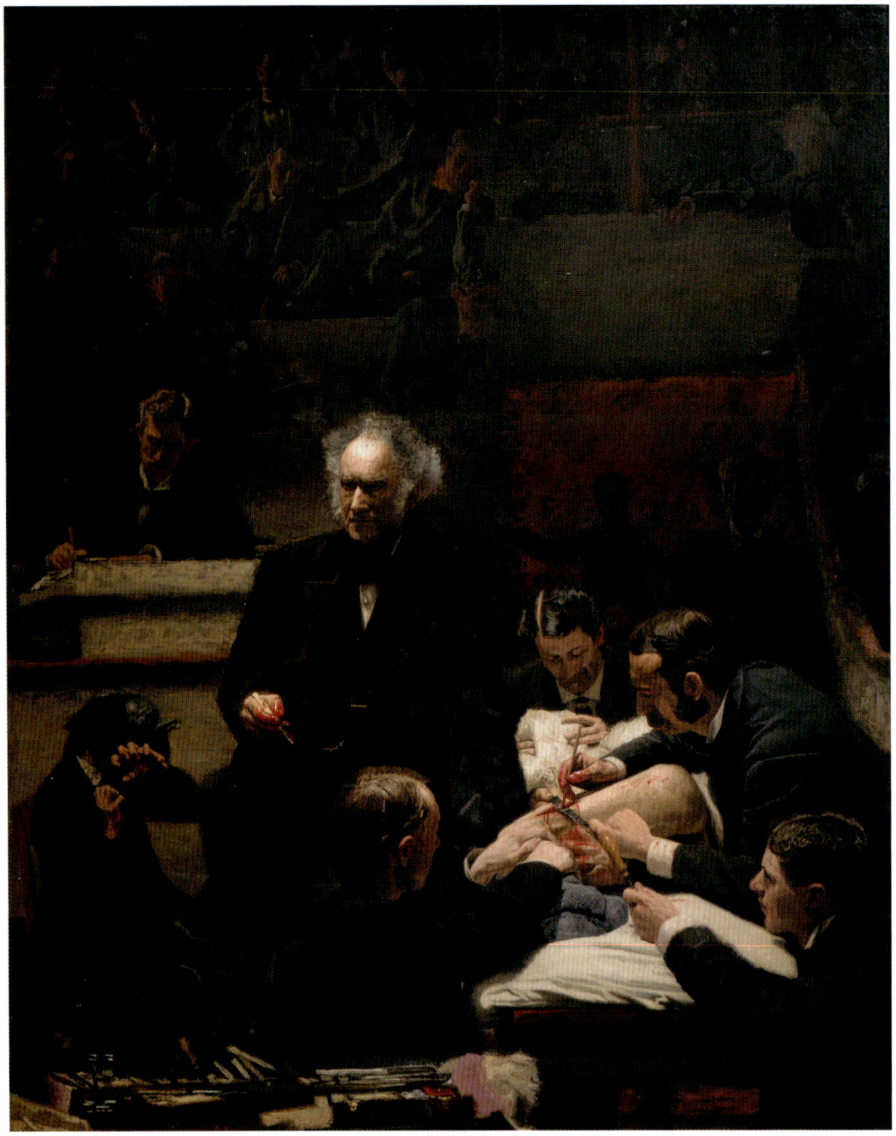

305 Thomas Eakins, *The Gross Clinic*, 1875, Philadelphia Museum of Art, Philadelphia

Eakins. He was determined to define the full, hair's-breadth exactitude of an operation for which Gross had become celebrated. The surgeon's assistants crowd round the exposed flesh, staring with the utmost concentration as they wield the instruments of their profession (see pl. 295). The precision so evident in their poses, as they hold their breath for fear of making a fateful slip, chimes with the orderliness of the appliances laid out so neatly in the fore-ground.

Gross himself stands apart from their zealous labours. Although the fresh blood on his hands proclaims his central involvement in the proceedings, he appears to pause for a moment and reflect on the activity which has been absorbing so much of his energy. He might be about to address his pupils, for Gross is carrying out his task in full view of a well-attended class. Eakins, however, relegates the students to a deeply shadowed region behind the surgeon, where their ascending ranks of wooden seats are scarcely visible in the pervasive gloom. The artist has included himself here on the far right, clasping a pen or pencil with eager fascination.[23] His implement's link with the scalpel wielded by the physician is surely intentional, for Eakins was fascinated by the connections between art and surgery.[24]

Even so, he ensures that his own dimly lit self-portrait does nothing to distract our attention from the all-important operation. Apart from the man in the doorway, who recalls the courtier in the penumbral recesses of Velázquez's *Las Meninas*, the most prominent member of the audience is the figure seated at a high desk, but he seems absorbed in writing rather than scrutinising the incision. Gross likewise appears preoccupied with his own thoughts (see pl. 305). As if painfully aware of the veiled woman with a wedding ring, who shields her eyes from the operation and claws the air with bony fingers,[25] the surgeon frowns. Perhaps he is pondering the terrible mystery of his command over the forces of life and death. Both Gross and, by extension, Eakins are conscious of the surgeon's god-like role. The blood smearing his index finger, thumb and scalpel could hardly be more down-to-earth in its glistening actuality. Yet the operating theatre's skylight illuminates his grey-white hair and whiskers with a spiritual radiance. A powerful undertow of religious feeling runs through this canvas, and the tenebrous atmosphere in the clinic is heavy with the burdensome responsibilities that Gross's expertise obliges him to shoulder.

Although Eakins believed that the *Gross Clinic* 'is very far better than anything I have ever done',[26] its pioneering realism worked against him. After submission to the selection committee of the Philadelphia Centennial Exhibition in 1876, his picture was rejected and placed instead in a medical exhibition staged by the United States Army Post Hospital.[27] His other five submitted works were hung in the main art exhibition, but the *Gross Clinic* was displayed in a ward encumbered with hospital bedding and furniture. It amounted to a humiliating snub. The painting had been deemed offensively frank, and the critic William Clark was incensed by the decision to exclude it. 'There is nothing so fine in the American section of the Art Department of the Exhibition', he complained,

> and it is a great pity that the squeamishness of the Selection Committee compelled the artist to find a place for it in the United States Hospital building. It is rumored that the blood on Dr. Gross's fingers made some of the members of the committee sick, but, judging from the quality of the works exhibited by them we fear that it was not the blood alone that made them sick. Artists have before now been known to sicken at the sight of pictures by younger men which they in their souls were compelled to acknowledge were beyond their emulation.[28]

Two years later, Eakins was enormously heartened by the decision of Jefferson Medical College to purchase the painting for a modest two hundred dollars. He had probably hoped from the outset that it would be acquired by Gross's own institution. In 1871 the alumni of the College had, after all, responded to the surgeon's suggestion that they should 'adorn the halls'[29] with portraits of its eminent teachers. The staff and students there did not react with squeamishness to the uncompromising veracity of an artist who, in his youth, had attended anatomy classes at a medical college as well as drawing at the Philadelphia Academy. Yet opposition to the *Gross Clinic* was far from over.

The full extent of Eakins's daring becomes clear when his canvas is compared with another large nineteenth-century painting of surgeons at work, Henri Gervex's *Before the Operation* (pl. 306). Proudly identifying himself with 'the painters who developed a love of reality',[30] Gervex counted Manet among his friends and won the admiration of Zola. But when he portrayed the great Parisian surgeon Jules-Emile Péan in his operating room at the Saint-Louis Hospital, the outcome entirely lacked Eakins's toughness and depth. Forceps in hand, Péan holds forth in lofty, well-lit surroundings. The appliances on the nearby table are defined with appropriate precision but everything appears sanitised to a fault. As for the young woman laid out on the sheet, her flowing tresses and exposed breasts serve only to titillate the viewer. For all its apparent realism, *Before the Operation* is a superficial exercise intended to gloss over the unsettling questions that Eakins insisted on raising in his picture.

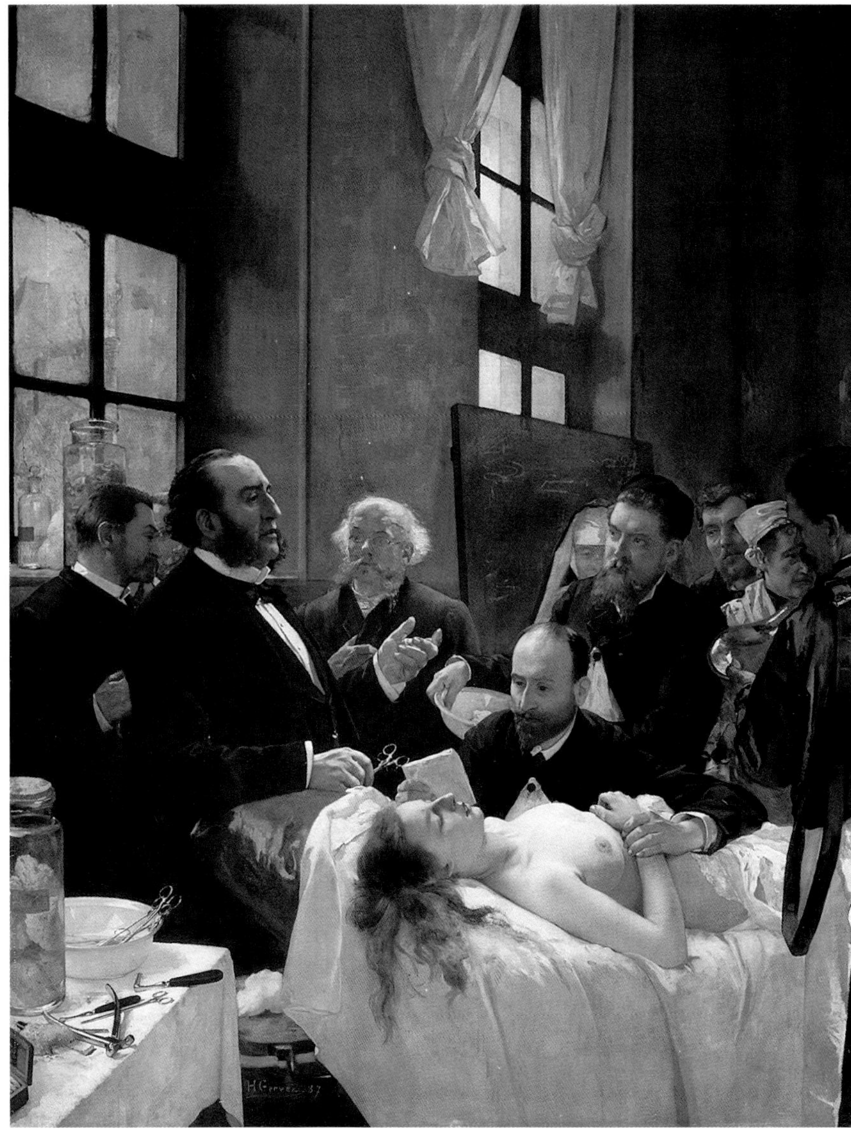

306 Henri Gervex, *Before the Operation*, 1887, Musée d'Orsay, Paris

He continued to pay a punitive price for his audacity. When the *Gross Clinic* was exhibited at New York's Society of American Artists in 1879, the critic of the *New York Daily Tribune* waxed apoplectic. After studying the picture, he wondered

> that it was ever painted, in the first place, and that it was ever exhibited, in the second . . . It is a picture that even strong men find it difficult to look at long, if they can look at it at all, and as for people with nerves and stomachs, the scene is so real that they might as well go to a dissecting-room and have done with it . . . No purpose is gained by this morbid exhibition, no lesson taught – the painter shows his skill and the spectator's gorge rises at it – that is all.[31]

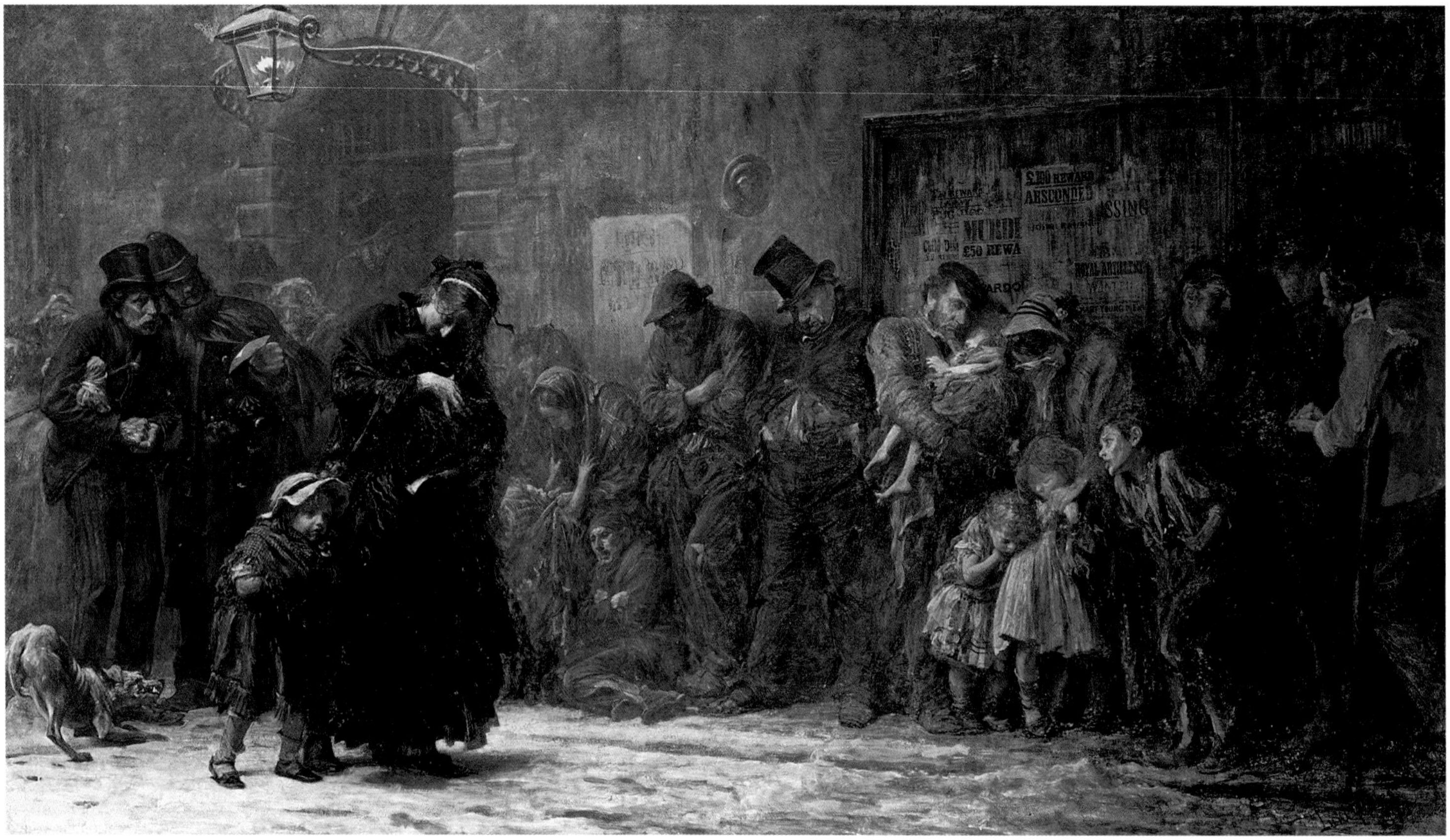

307 Luke Fildes, *Applicants for Admission to a Casual Ward*, 1874, Royal Holloway, University of London

Only the Medical College could fully appreciate Eakins's determination to identify with Gross's 'assertion of accomplishment and integrity',[32] as John Wilmerding described the intention behind this strange, troubled picture, caught so hauntingly between the urge to provide an objective account of the scene and an equally strong desire to explore its most disquieting spiritual implications.

Eakins never identified the patient in the *Gross Clinic*. But since most public operations were reserved for the working poor, the body laid out on the operating table probably belonged to one of Philadelphia's most impoverished citizens. Back in Victorian London, a young English artist likewise had the courage to scrutinise the plight of people unable to purchase proper medical care. Wandering at night around the poorest quarters of the city early in the 1870s, Luke Fildes was perturbed by the suffering he encountered. It led him to paint in 1874 a *tour de force* of nineteenth-century social realism, *Applicants for Admission to a Casual Ward* (pl. 307). A woman clutching her baby and accompanied by another child darkly dominates the foreground, staggering through the smog and filth of a metropolitan slum street. Soon she will be reduced to the wretched dependence of the figures lined up against the facade of the casual ward, hugging themselves for warmth and striving to protect their children against the bitter night air. All founded on direct observation by Fildes, these images of ragged victims amount to a bleak and crusading indictment of a society not yet ready to provide its working class with adequate welfare. In order to ram home his polemical intentions, Fildes exhibited the painting at the Royal Academy in 1874 with a quotation from a letter by Dickens, deploring the 'dumb, wet, silent horrors! Sphinxes set up against that dead wall, and none likely to be at the pains of solving them until the *general overthrow*.'[33] Confronted by such a scene, *The Times* upbraided Fildes for his 'unpleasant' pictures and lamented that 'painters do not more bear in mind the fact that their pictures are meant to adorn English living rooms'.[34]

That is why the most successful Victorian painting of a doctor showed a scene far removed from

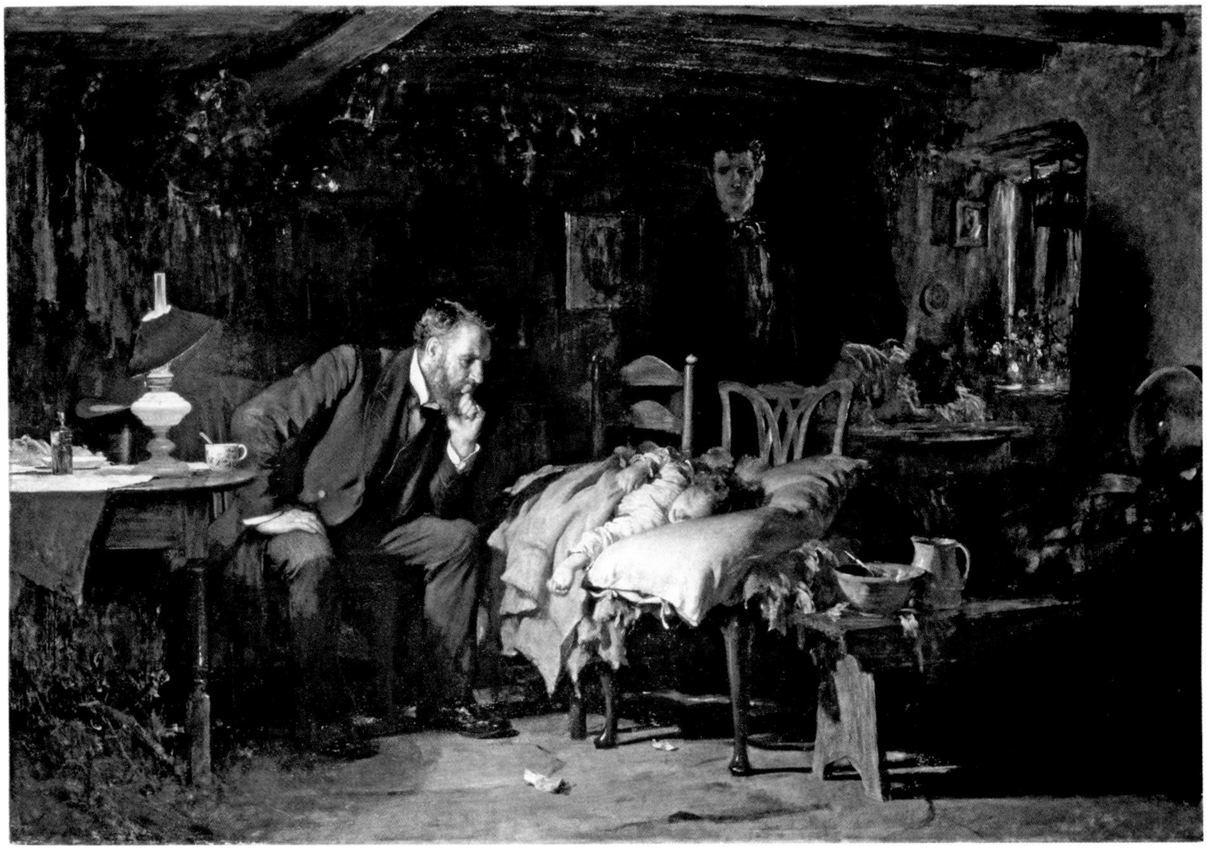

308 Luke Fildes, *The Doctor*, 1891, Tate, London

the gruelling urban impersonality of *Applicants*. Luke Fildes, by the 1890s an accomplished and sought-after Academy favourite equally adept at portraying society ladies and Venetian girls, was commissioned by Henry Tate to paint an English subject for a munificent fee of £3000. He left Fildes to select the subject, and the artist found himself remembering the death of his eldest son Paul on Christmas morning 1877. The family doctor's devotion to the boy had impressed Fildes immensely, helping him to cope with this traumatic tragedy. So he took Tate's invitation as the springboard for a large painting of a doctor attending a sick child in what *The Times* described as 'an English workman's home' (pl. 308).[35] After sketching cottages throughout England and Scotland, Fildes built in his London studio a full-size mock-up based on Devonshire fishermen's cottages at Hope Cove. Fildes himself dressed as a doctor and posed for photographs to help him decide on the seated, ruminative stance adopted by the professional model he eventually hired. According to the artist's son, his medical friends also visited the studio 'in relays', asking to sit for the figure, 'so that they could afterwards claim involvement with the noble picture'.[36]

When *The Doctor* was finally exhibited at the Royal Academy in 1891, it attracted crowds who hailed the canvas as the 'picture of the year'.[37] They warmed to the dramatic chiaroscuro of a nocturnal scene lit principally by a solitary lamp placed next to a medicine bottle and a cup. The child, supported by pillows on a couple of chairs, lies with arm outflung to signify suffering. But the bearded doctor reacts calmly and steadfastly, gazing at his patient and waiting for any signs of recovery. Judging by the stunned father, and the distraught attitude of the mother with her head buried in anguish on a table beyond, the outcome seems likely to be as distressing as the loss experienced by the Fildes family fourteen years before. However, Fildes had no intention of subjecting his audience to such pessimistic thoughts. Careful to include a secondary source of light beside the mother, he described how

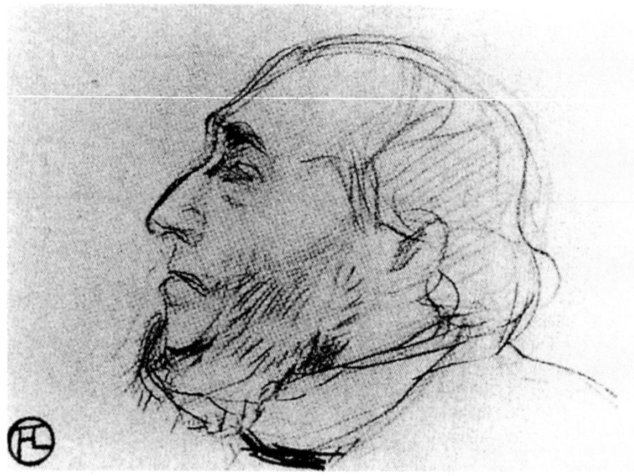

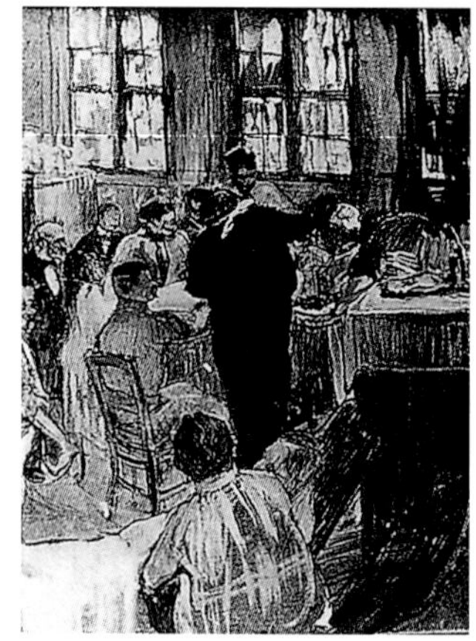

309 (*right*) Henri de Toulouse-Lautrec, Study of Jules-Emile Péan, *c.*1891, Private Collection

310 (*far right*) Henri de Toulouse-Lautrec, *Dr Péan Operating at the Hôpital International*, 1891, Private Collection

at the cottage window the dawn begins to steal in – the dawn that is the critical time of all deadly illnesses – and with it the parents again take hope into their hearts, the mother hiding her face to escape giving vent to her emotion, the father laying his hand on the shoulder of his wife in encouragement of the first glimmerings of the joy which is to follow.[38]

Such a reassuring explanation helped to ensure the prodigious success of *The Doctor*. When Agnew's issued a photogravure version of the picture in 1892, it sold more than a million copies and became the most popular print ever published by the firm. Pirated in the United States, it was widely sought there by people eager to possess an image of medical care more consoling than Eakins's heretical *Gross Clinic*. It appeared on postage stamps and, after Henry Tate gave it to the British nation along with the rest of his collection in 1894, swiftly became one of the most beloved paintings in the new Tate Gallery. Today, however, the *Doctor* seems sentimental compared with Eakins's unnerving canvas, now rightly regarded as a masterpiece of nineteenth-century American art.

Fildes's canvas also suffers in comparison with another portrayal of a physician produced during the same decade. It is the work of Henri de Toulouse-Lautrec, who in 1891 took a Paris flat in the rue Fontaine with his doctor friend Henri Bourges. Later the same year Lautrec's younger cousin Gabriel Tapié de Céleyran arrived in Paris as a medical student eager to complete his studies with the eminent surgeon Jules-Emile Péan. The prowess of this celebrated doctor had already been depicted in Henri Gervex's elaborate painting of 1887 and Lautrec quickly seized the opportunity to study Péan's work at first hand. Tapié de Céleyran later recalled that Lautrec, fascinated by 'all that squirms . . . lost little time in following me to the Hôpital Saint-Louis, where he was soon captivated by Péan's virtuosity. He went there every Saturday morning and filled up albums with notes and sketches.'[39] Lautrec drew swift, incisive studies of Péan's face, legs and feet (pl. 309). The surgeon, far from finding such attention a source of irritation, relished the artist's presence and welcomed observers so much that, as Julia Frey has pointed out, 'watching Péan operate was as much a ritual spectacle as going to the Comédie Française'.[40] Bluff, theatrical and totally assured, Péan was proud of his skill with the scalpel. He is now best remembered as the inventor of the forceps, but his stern insistence on high standards of hygiene also made a pioneering contribution to surgical excellence.

Lautrec was enthralled by the procedures he studied with such crisp avidity at the Saint-Louis Hospital. He would often declare that 'if I were not a painter, I would like to be a doctor'.[41] And Péan returned the compliment by harbouring dreams of becoming a painter. Lautrec mocked his elegantly attired cousin for wanting to 'adorn himself in the plumes of Péan',[42] whose addiction to immaculate dress suits and false shirt-fronts became legendary in the operating theatre. But before long, Lautrec's involvement with Péan led him to plan a full-scale painting of the eminent doctor in action (pl. 310). Many preliminary studies survive for this tall, vigorously executed image. The setting is the Hôpital

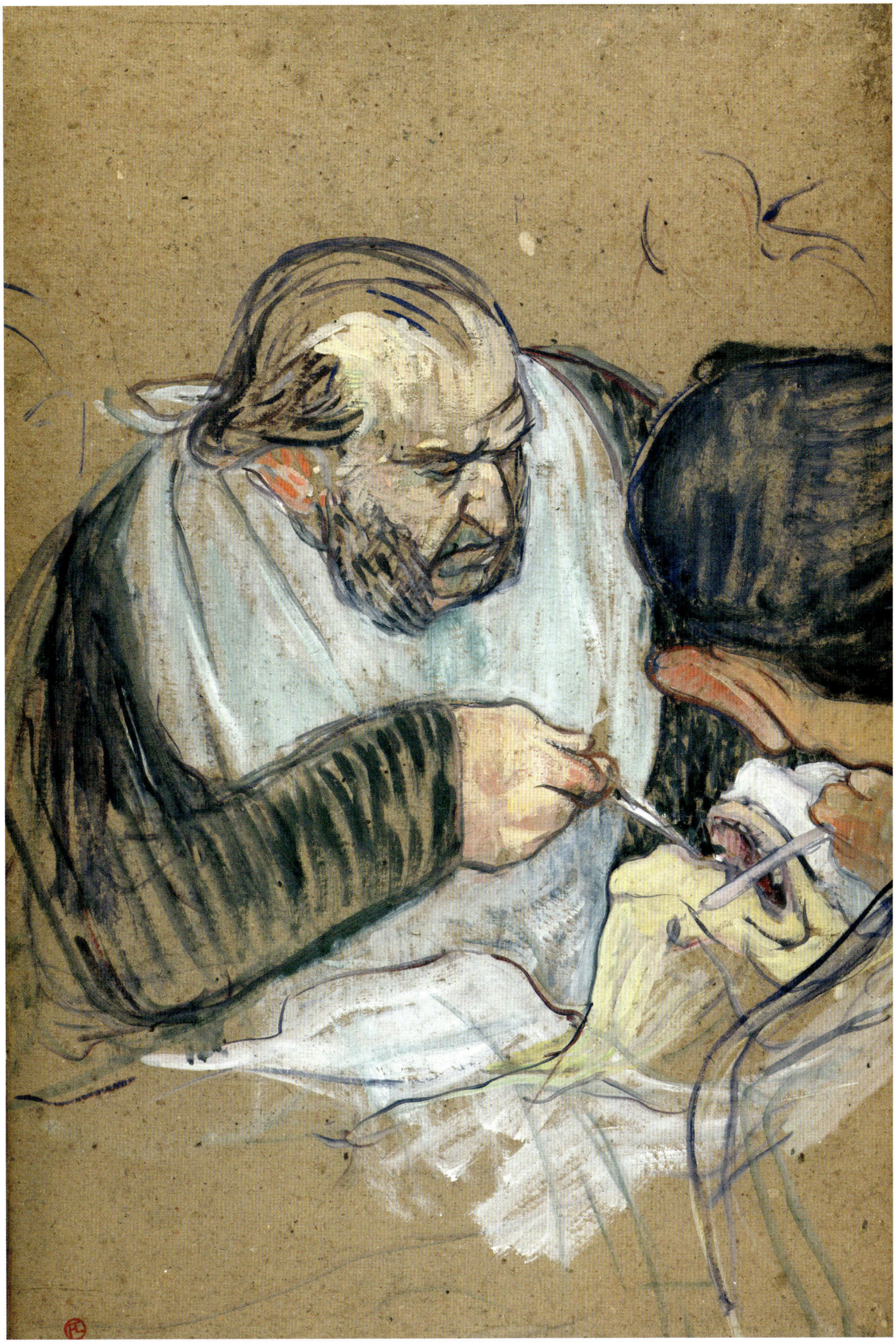

311 Henri de Toulouse-Lautrec, *Dr Péan Operating (A Tracheotomy Operation)*, 1891, Sterling & Francine Clark Art Institute, Williamstown

International, which the tireless Péan founded in 1892 after being obliged to retire from the municipal hospital at the age of sixty-two. Yet the high, luminous windows in this painting are reminiscent of the location painted by Gervex at the Hôpital Saint-Louis (see pl. 306). Lautrec also followed this precedent by showing Péan surrounded by observers gazing in awed concentration at the surgeon's performance. Unlike Gervex, though, Lautrec views Péan from behind. Typically unconventional, this decision might have ended up detracting from the doctor's formidable presence. His essential energy is nevertheless conveyed with vivid conviction in Lautrec's expressive silhouette, which summarises Péan's seasoned mastery. This was a surgeon who, according to Jules Renard, 'can rummage through an abdomen with the air of a man feeling in his pocket for small change'.[43] Yet there seemed nothing repellent about Péan's showmanship. 'It was amazing rather than horrific', recalled Maurice de Fleury, who described him as 'magnificent, imposing, Olympian . . . He did not much care whether anyone listened or not: what he wanted was to be seen at work: "Stand aside, gentlemen, let everyone see."'[44]

Even more revealing is Lautrec's smaller, close-up painting of *Dr Péan Operating* (pl. 311). It is an astonishingly stark and forceful image. All the impressive hospital surroundings have been jettisoned now, along with most of the observers. Only one assistant is retained, jutting in from the right edge with a curving ear that echoes the shape of the patient's parted mouth. The painting subsequently became known as *A Tracheotomy Operation* but Lautrec does not make clear whether the throat or the jaw is the focus of Péan's attention. The dynamism of the surgeon himself dominates the picture, as he prods his instrument deep inside the orifice gaping below. Péan's burliness is caught as he bends forward, his hefty shoulders swathed by an ample napkin. The whiteness of its fabric testifies to his pioneering emphasis on hygiene, as well as serving to isolate the doctor's face with dramatic intensity.

Lautrec stresses the bushy side whiskers, brusquely swept-back hair and frowning eyebrows. Péan appears as a tough veteran with a grimly downturned mouth, a man of peasant origins who thrives on the often exhausting demands of his profession. He addresses himself to the open mouth with gusto. Yet alongside his undoubted panache, Lautrec captures an authentic sense of concern. This surgeon is no brute, and cannot be accused of causing his patient unnecessary pain. Julia Frey suggests that Lautrec's 'operating-room works were representative of his fascination with all that was forbidden, hidden, organic, possibly disgusting – illness, vice, death'.[45] Yet this remarkable painting captures Péan's practised sensitivity and precision as well as his earthy ebullience. The surgeon appears determined to locate the precise point of pain, deal with it and thereby alleviate the suffering of the vulnerable patient laid out so trustingly beside him.

Back in *fin-de-siècle* London, a less visceral portrait of a surgeon was produced by Alfred Gilbert, who had become notorious with his Shaftesbury Memorial in Piccadilly Circus known as *Eros*. When the statue was unveiled in the summer of 1893, it provoked a national furore. Gilbert never fully recovered from the vituperation, and his enduring bitterness even led him to demand that the statue be melted down in order to finance the building of shelters for the homeless.[46] However, this searing experience did not prevent him from accepting, in the same year as the unveiling of *Eros*, another commission for a prominent London location. It came from the Board of Saint George's Hospital in Knightsbridge, who wanted to celebrate the centenary of John Hunter's death with a new bust (pl. 312) of the eminent eighteenth-century surgeon.

With typical procrastination, Gilbert did not finally deliver the completed bronze until 1899. But it is a spirited and sympathetic work, hailed by his biographer Richard Dorment as Gilbert's 'masterpiece in the half-length format'.[47] Liberated from the constraints of working from a sitter and striving for a likeness, Gilbert did not make the mistake of producing a remote and dutiful portrait of a man he never knew. On the contrary: *John Hunter* is instinct with wisdom, humour and intelligence. Hunter is giving a lecture, clutching an anatomical figure in one hand while pointing at it with the other. The contrast between the bald, sinewy nude and the surgeon himself could hardly be more extreme. Hunter rejoices in an ample mane of hair, and a soft hat is swept across his head with more than a hint of romantic dishevelment. Attired in neckcloth, suit and surgeon's gown, he is the epitome of stylishness. Although his furrowed face testifies to a life of hard study and application, Hunter's mouth widens in a smile. He is at the apex of his profession and a formidable sense of energy seems to run through the loose, animated folds of his gown. Its ample sleeves hang down freely from his wrists, as if intoxicated by the eloquence of this outstanding physician as he imparts knowledge to the would-be surgeons of the future. No wonder the Hospital eventually decided, after installing Gilbert's bronze in the board-room, that it should be given a more public location. When a new gate was erected in 1924 next to the main building, as an entrance to the Medical School, *John Hunter* was positioned above the portal as a flamboyant inspiration to staff and students passing underneath.[48]

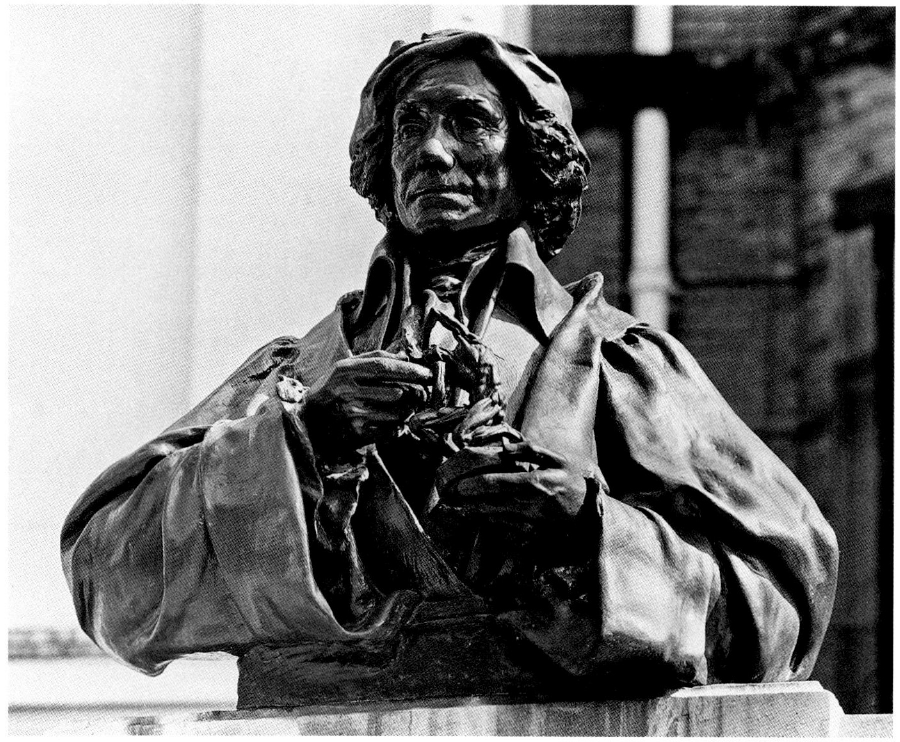

312 Alfred Gilbert, *John Hunter*, 1899, Saint George's Hospital Medical School, London

In the closing decades of the nineteenth century, ambitious attempts were made by a few other British hospitals to create chapels with richly wrought interiors. Nowhere more fervently than in Edinburgh, where the young, inexperienced yet ambitious artist Phoebe Anna Traquair gained a commission from a newly formed group of artists, clerics, academics and philanthropists. Determined to enhance the blighted surroundings of working-class people throughout the city, they founded the Edinburgh Social Union in 1885. They focused on the Old Town still urgently in need of rescue from impoverished squalor. As well as organising craft classes, where the local population could learn how to transform their own houses, the Social Union sought out professional painters capable of executing mural decorations in public buildings. Several images, long since destroyed, were executed for the wards of the Royal Infirmary. Traquair turned out to be the ideal choice for decorating a mortuary at the Royal Hospital for Sick Children in Lauriston Lane.

But she had no experience of working on an architectural scale. On the contrary: the Dublin-born artist specialised in illuminating manuscripts, variously inspired by the *Book of Kells*, the Psalms of David and William Blake's *Songs of Innocence and Experience*. Married to the Keeper of Natural History at the Edinburgh Museum of Science and Art, and the mother of three young children, she lacked professional status. Traquair received no fee for her work in the chapel. Only the money spent on materials was repaid to her, and it is a wonder that she managed to carry out such a major task when domestic duties claimed so much of her attention. W.B. Yeats claimed that she was 'forbidden to paint' by her husband and only produced the mural 'in stolen hours'.[49] She took two years to complete the decoration, struggling to overcome the limitations involved in converting a small, disused hospital coal-house. This top-lit interior would have posed a formidable challenge to even the most seasoned artist, but she had the backing of John Ritchie Findlay, the proprietor of *The Scotsman* newspaper, who was a member of the Social Union and a director of the hospital.[50] Moreover, the diminutive, impulsive and red-haired Traquair, who had received a proper art training at the Royal Dublin Society in the late 1860s, was determined to succeed.

She would have been aware of the need to think very carefully about the mortuary's *raison d'être*. The hospital ladies' committee declared that the transformation of its interior should be nothing 'extravagant or highly decorated but a suitable place where the bodies can be left reverently and lovingly for the parents before the burials'.[51] The presence of dead children meant that the mortuary was a supremely sensitive location, and Traquair took as her springboard a New Testament

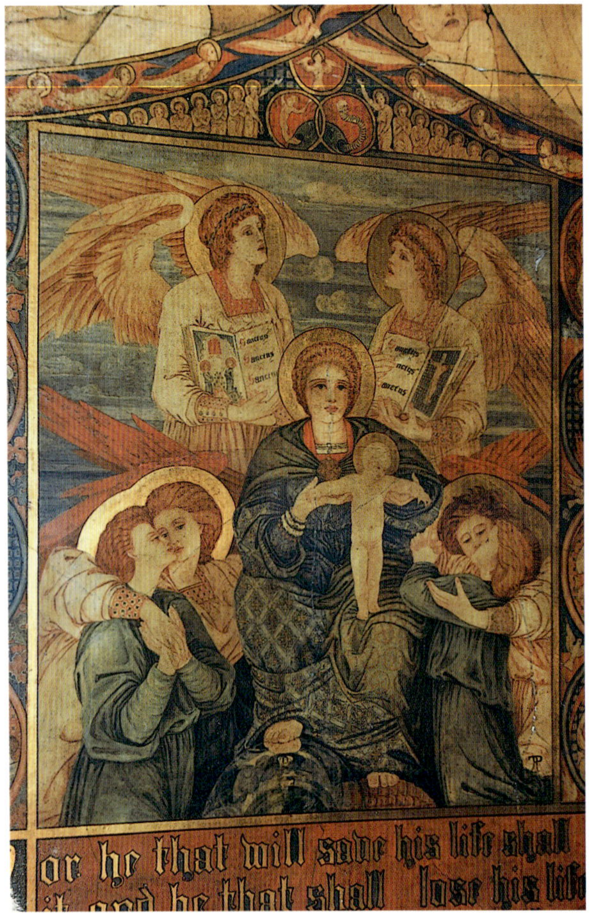

313 (*right*) Phoebe Anna Traquair, *Motherhood*, 1885–6, Royal Hospital for Sick Children, Mortuary Building, Edinburgh

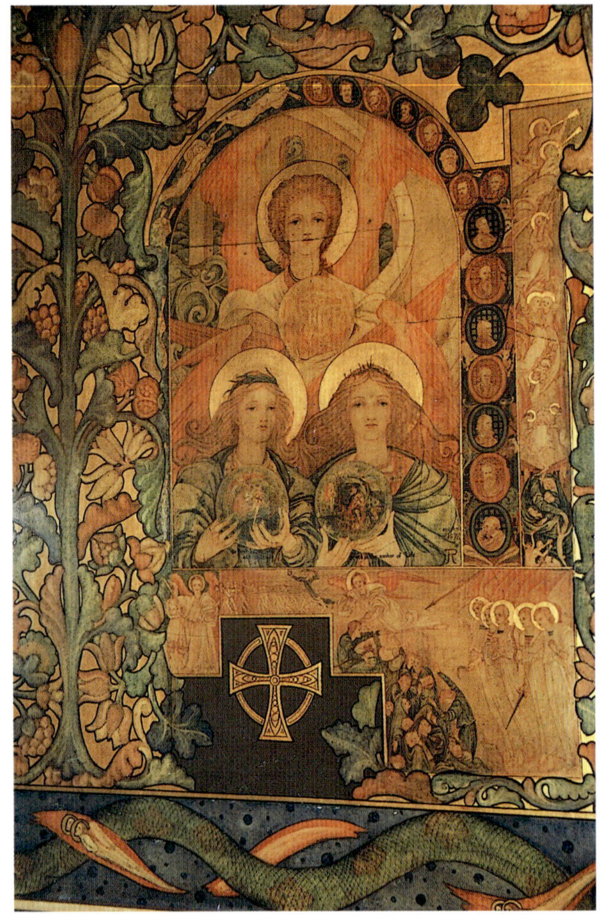

314 (*far right*) Phoebe Anna Traquair, *Three Angels*, 1885–6, Royal Hospital for Sick Children, Mortuary Building, Edinburgh

315 (*facing page*) Phoebe Anna Traquair, *The Days of Creation*, 1896–8, Royal Hospital for Sick Children, Mortuary Building, Edinburgh

response to bereavement. Her key quotation was from Matthew: 'For he that will save his life shall lose it and he shall lose his life for My sake, the same shall save it'.[52] This impassioned text was inscribed in grand Gothic script on a brilliant red backdrop, and further consolation for grieving parents was provided by the image above the inscription. Aptly entitled *Motherhood*, it depicted the Virgin with her infant and attendant angels holding illuminated books where the word 'Sanctus' is repeated like a blessing (pl. 313). Even so, Traquair was determined to ensure that the reality of suffering should not be shirked. The child standing on his mother's lap stretches out both his small, vulnerable arms. Although the Virgin supports them with her own hands, his attitude is inescapably prophetic of the martyrdom to come. Paintings of Christ on the cross are visible in the angels' books above, and elsewhere in the chapel the Crucifixion is presented as the gateway to eternal life.

Opposite *Motherhood*, a panel of three angels provided further cause for comfort (pl. 314). Gazing directly at the viewer, these divine figures clasp transparent globes containing small, exquisitely rendered scenes celebrating the journey of the spirit. In one, a holy knight takes on the Saint George-like role of defeating a dragon. Another globe shows a cross accompanied by a mass of spirits shouting for joy, and beneath the two lowest angels Traquair has inscribed two more consolatory quotations: 'Death is the author of life' and 'go forth be fruitful and multiply'. Executed in primary colours and gold reminiscent of her work with illuminated manuscripts, the chapel decorations also proclaim the influence of Eastern Orthodox paintings, Italian *quattrocento* artists and the work of Dante Gabriel Rossetti. Traquair was a frankly eclectic artist, and her interest in early feminism is reflected in her claim that the *Motherhood* panel was supposed to show 'Eve redeemed through Christ, or Nature redeemed through the incarnation of the Divine Spirit'.[53]

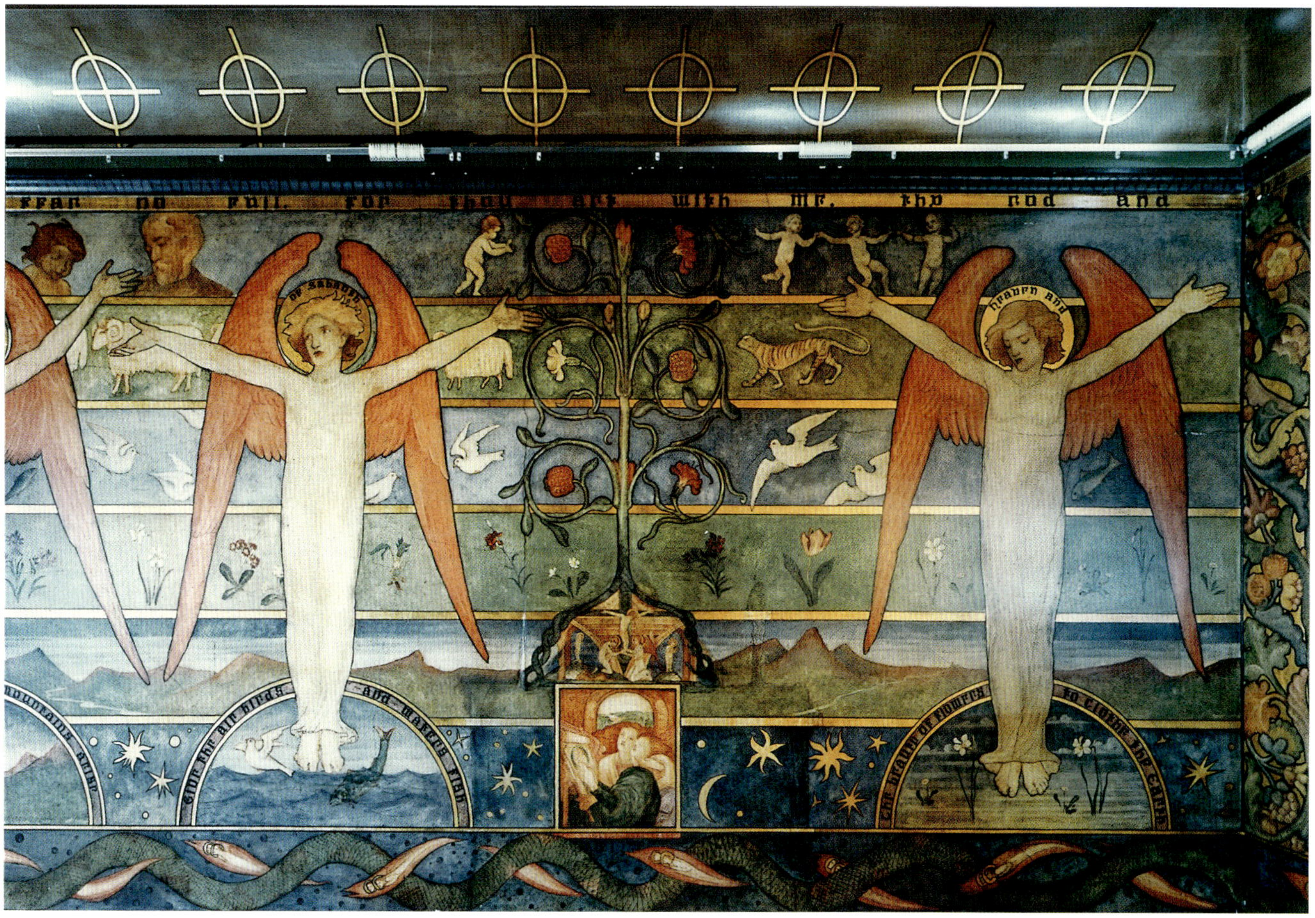

Soon after the murals were open to public view, they were hailed by the press as 'the most important and memorable portion of the art of the Social Union'.[54] Two years later, in 1889, Gerard Baldwin Brown in *The Scottish Art Review* declared that the chapel's interior was 'a piece of illumination enlarged' with the same 'curious elaboration of symbolic detail, the same fresh and cheerful appearance, the same refinement in drawing and execution'. Even Traquair, who was modest and retiring enough to claim that the prospect of a press article on her work was 'a more terrible thing than decorating a cathedral', must have been gratified by such a positive response. Baldwin Brown reported that 'the spirit of the work is evidently recognised by the mourners, often of the humblest class, who come here on occasions when the mortuary is in use'. He went on to comment that Traquair's decoration 'fails in architectural planning-out, though the work is on so small a scale that this is not a serious drawback'. Yet he had nothing but praise for Traquair's ability to emulate the vitality of medieval manuscripts. According to his indispensable account, 'the walls of this chapel, which measures twelve feet by eight, are covered with designs embodying allegories of human life, with especial reference to the growth of the human soul from infancy through mortal life and death to spiritual resurrection'. Then, with understandable fascination, Baldwin Brown focused on an astonishing aspect of these allegories:

> Round the walls of the chapel, above the dado, is painted in endless convolutions the serpent of eternity. In and out through the folds are seen passing the souls of men, which are given forth from the hands of the Creator on one side of the central picture at the altar end, and are finally received back as perfected by the same hands upon the other. We note that the souls, as they issue forth, seem as if asleep, and are enclosed in flames which appear to sweep them onward; but

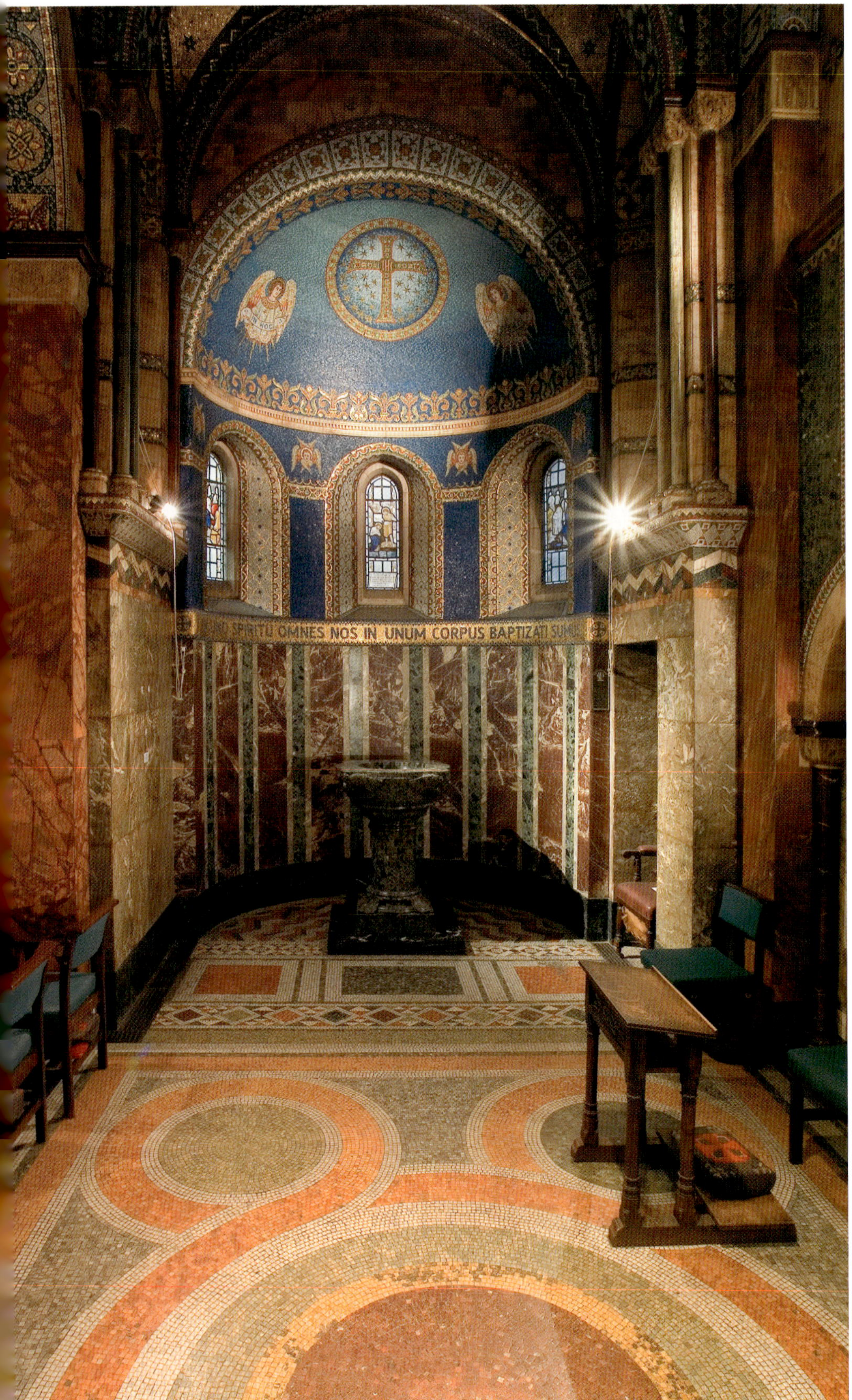

> on the return side these flames gradually develop into angel forms, embracing and bearing forward the now awakened souls, which here assume the features of some dear to the artist, or to the world, who had lately passed away.[55]

Parents and relatives visiting this intense, visionary mortuary at Lauriston Lane did not have long to appreciate Traquair's intricate, deeply considered and exquisitely executed decorations. Within five years of their completion, a disastrous outbreak of typhoid led to the hospital's demolition. The little mortuary remained for the time being, yet disrepair meant that the paintings were in danger of destruction from exposure to the weather.[56] Traquair was appalled. In 1891 she complained bitterly to her nephew about the plans to destroy her entire mural. 'They, the horrible Edinburgh little handful of bigots who form the directors of the hospital . . . want to pull it down', she wrote. 'I feel as if my pet child was to be murdered'.[57]

Happily, enough influential people agreed with her to mount a campaign to save the decorations. Some of the plaster murals were painstakingly transported by horse and cart to the new hospital mortuary at Rillbank, south of the Meadows. The four largest panels were sacrificed, because they could not be embedded in the walls, but Traquair painted revised alternatives in their place and was even able, during 1897–8, to paint large new sections for the interior (pl. 315). Dominated by six full-length angels with scarlet wings, painted on six horizontal bands representing the days of Creation, the east wall was intended above all as a celebration of childhood. Above the Seraphim with their outstretched arms, she included portraits of her husband Ramsay and daughter Hilda among the 'young men and maidens, old men and children' who all represented 'mankind'.[58] In the horizontal border below, where everyone could clearly see them, she painted a hallucinatory image of the undulating serpent of eternity, accompanied by souls 'mounting up to God . . . like thin flames'.[59] On the left of this visionary wall, a section of her mural was removed in the 1970s to make way for a grotesquely intrusive new door, but the rest of the Mortuary of the Royal Hospital for Sick Children still survives, testifying to the flair, resolve and redemptive faith of a woman who wanted to paint the 'departure and arrival of the spirit, the transfer from this life to the next'.[60]

316 John Loughborough Pearson, The new chapel at Middlesex Hospital, 1890

Edinburgh was not alone in wanting to combat the bare corridors and cheerless rooms at so many medical institutions. In Glasgow, the idealistic Kyrle Society was founded in 1883 'to bring the influences of natural and artistic beauty home to the people'.[61] Professor Thomas Martin Lindsay proudly announced that the Kyrle 'aims at giving infirmaries, poor-houses, sick children's hospitals, convalescent homes, such decorations as will rest the wearied eyes looking at the pure outlines and softly bright colours'.[62] In this respect, the Glasgow venture followed the initiative pursued by the first Kyrle Society, established in London six years before. Nothing now survives of the 'decorations for the typhoid fever wards of the London Fever Hospital', which consisted of 'twelve flower panels; and a screen, which forms the division between the two compartments of each ward, has been decorated with some tiles, the gift of a member of the society'.[63] Yet this wholly voluntary work was probably modest in terms of aesthetic achievement, especially when compared with the new chapel added to the Middlesex Hospital in London.

This lavish house of prayer was embellished with the most resplendent late Victorian ornamentation (pl. 316). John Loughborough Pearson, the notable architect whose most substantial work was Truro Cathedral, designed this small yet glowing space as a memorial to Major Alexander Ross MP, the former chairman of the board of governors. Within the Gothic chamber, seventeen different marbles were used to enhance an interior that Pearson insisted on supervising with exacting attention to minutiae. As well as designing the red-brick structure, he was responsible for the alabaster lectern, furnishings, pews and initial stained-glass windows. When the chapel was opened for use in 1891, staff and patients both found themselves worshipping in surroundings far more exalted than anything they had experienced at the Middlesex before.

Religious services were previously held either in the Board Room or the wards, and yet they now took place in a building where mosaic was lavishly deployed alongside the plethora of marble. In the baptistery, angels floated on a blue Italian-crafted mosaic inspired by Saint Mark's in Venice, and over the next couple of decades the chancel mosaics were supplemented by similar decorations on the upper reaches of the walls. The green marble font,

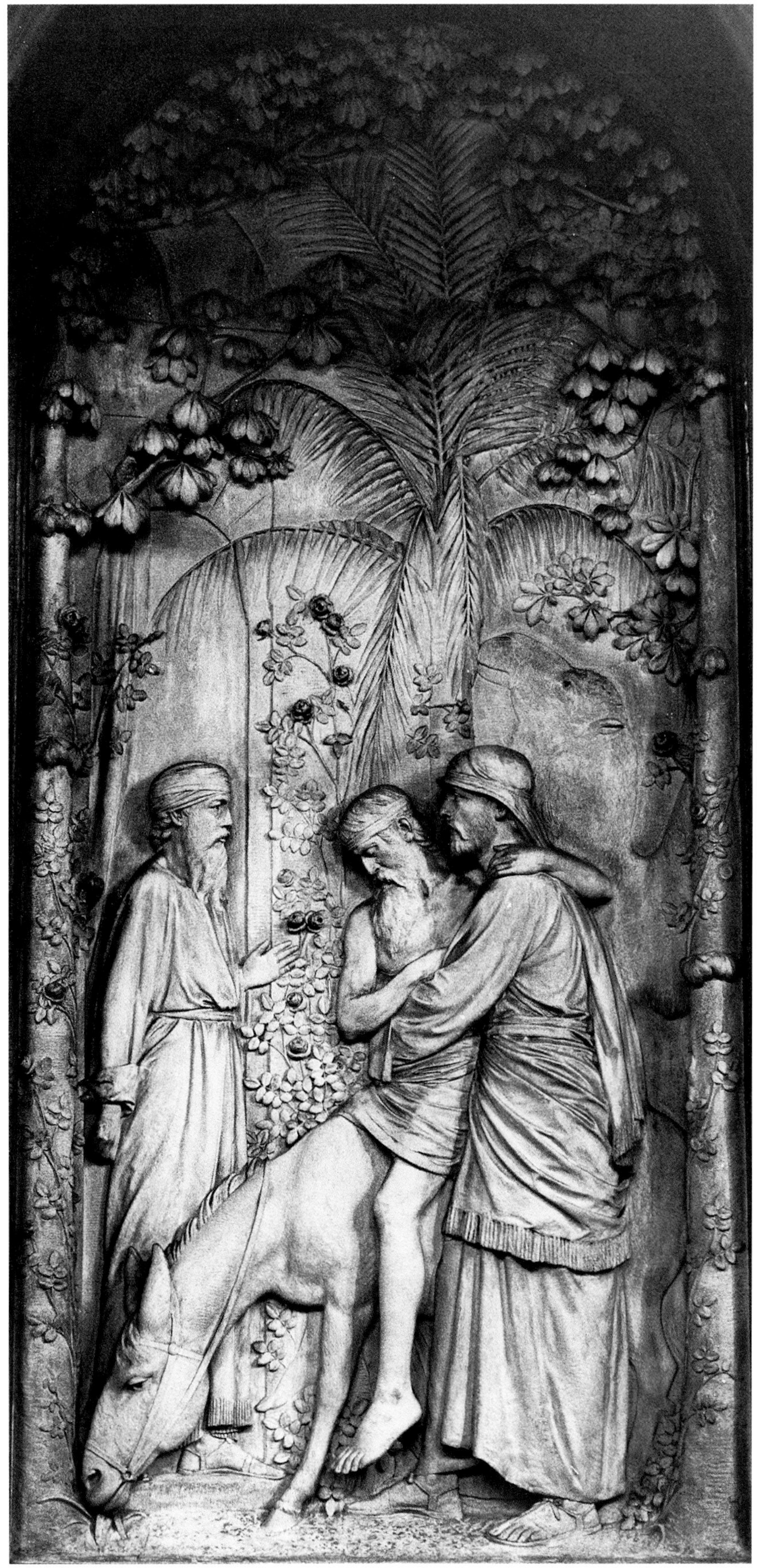

317 George Tinworth, *The Good Samaritan*, 1894, St Thomas's Hospital Chapel, London

adorned at its corners with symbols of the four Evangelists, was based on a prototype in Hagia Sophia in Istanbul. Like the rest of the fittings, it could be admired in the most favourable viewing conditions that an architect was then able to devise. For while much of the hospital still relied on gas appliances for illumination, Pearson ensured that his chapel glistened with jewel-like intensity by installing electric light throughout the interior.

Not to be outdone, the chapel at Saint Thomas's was soon provided with extensive sculptural additions. In 1894 the Archbishop of Canterbury unveiled a white terracotta bas-relief there as a memorial to Sarah Wardroper, the hospital's revered Matron for thirty-three years (pl. 317). George Tinworth designed this large Doulton panel, taking as his subject the *Good Samaritan* like Hogarth and Dadd before him (see pls 187 and 269). It was considered the most appropriate theme for a remarkable woman, selected by Florence Nightingale herself as the first Superintendent of the School of Nurses which she established at Saint Thomas's. Nightingale had chosen the hospital as the base for her Training School after a nationwide fund of £50,000 had been collected in tribute to her pioneering achievements. The inscription on the bas-relief records that Wardroper was 'the working leader in a great reform, quietly and peacably pursued, by which the care of the sick took its right place as a high and holy calling that enlists the noblest qualities of heart and mind, and turns to efficient use the intelligence, refinement, and devotion of good women'.

318 George Tinworth, *Ascension* reredos, 1899, St Thomas's Hospital chapel, London

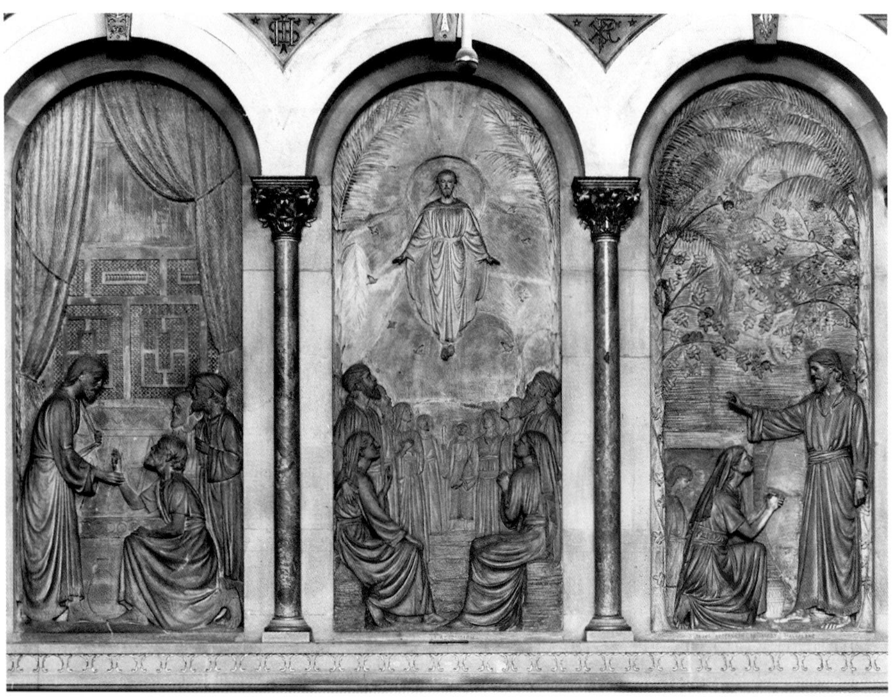

This elevation of the nursing profession was reinforced with the installation of a relief, on the same wall, depicting Nightingale holding a cup to the lips of a wounded soldier at the Crimea hospital. Then, in 1899, the sculpture of the chapel was crowned by the unveiling of a grand terracotta reredos, once again executed by Tinworth (pl. 318). Donated as a memorial by the family of Sir Henry Doulton, a long-standing governor and almoner of the hospital, its three panels contain at the centre an image of the Ascension intended to sustain generations of worshippers with its promise of miraculous regeneration after death.[64]

For all those British hospitals unable to rely on the generous endowments enjoyed by Middlesex and Saint Thomas's, the closing decade of the nineteenth century brought a remarkable surge in the production of an attractive, affordable new form of decoration. John Greene, who wrote a carefully researched study of the phenomenon, pointed out that 'the easily cleaned surfaces of glazed tiles were much in demand during the great public health drive to reduce infection in hospitals and public buildings'.[65] The popularity of tiles in the late Victorian period was directly inspired by Florence Nightingale, who had realised at Scutari that the quality of a hospital's environment was inextricably bound up with her patients' chances of recovery.

'Hospitals are a curse to civilisation', she had declared in her widely influential *Notes on Hospitals* of 1889, and she always emphasised the importance of the highest standards in hygiene. 'For all eating, drinking and washing vessels, and for other utensils', she insisted, 'the use of glass or earthenware is superior to that of tin or any other metal, on account of its greater cleanliness.'[66] Yet this gospel does not in itself account for the sudden proliferation of decorative tilework in hospitals during the final years of Victoria's reign. Although Nightingale was herself convinced that patients' minds as well as their bodies should be cared for in hospitals, where interior colours and exterior views of sky or garden were 'intimately connected with the reparative process', her disciples sometimes adopted a puritanical approach. The unblemished

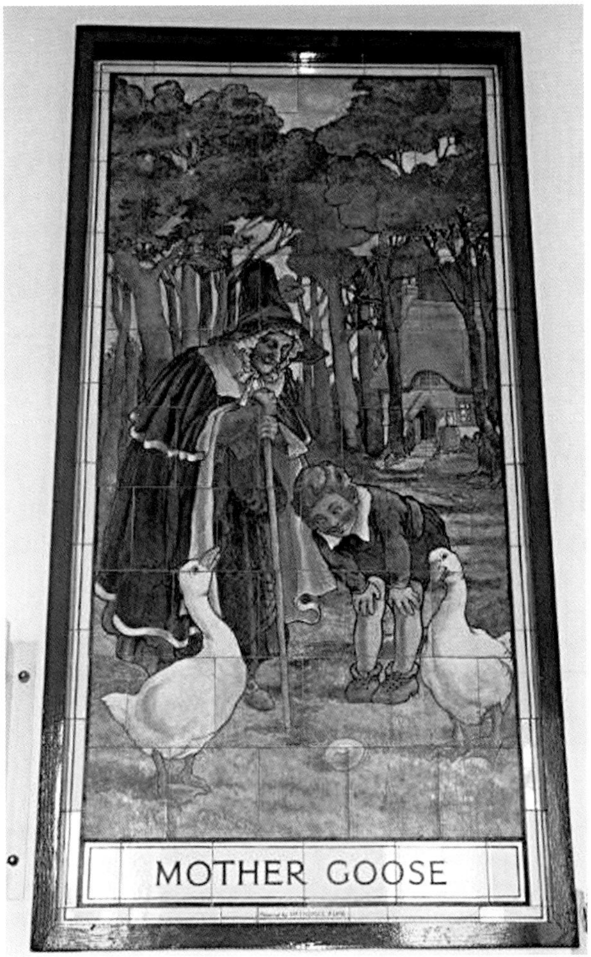

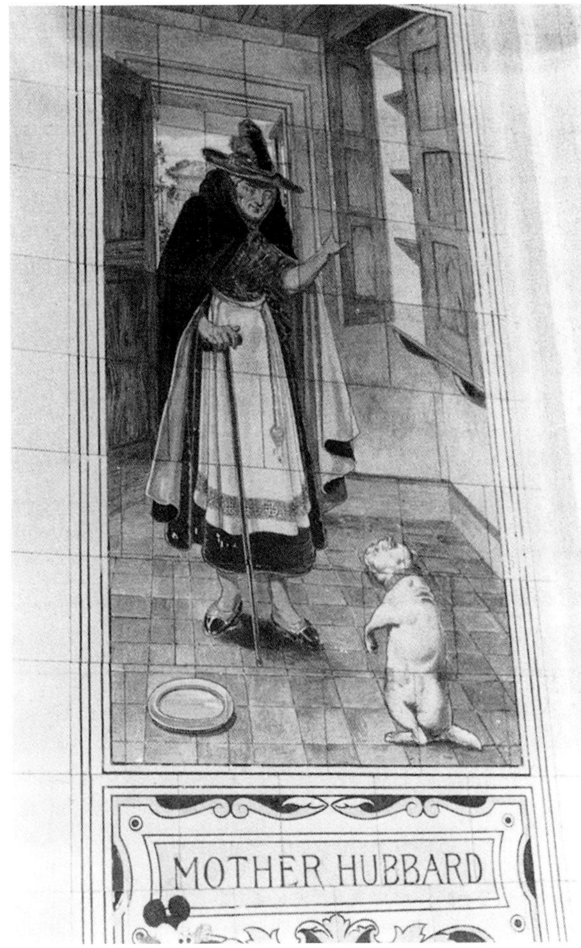

319 (*far left*) Percy Adams, Tile panels in Louisa Cary Children's Ward, Torbay Hospital, Torquay

320 (*left*) Philip Newman, Tile panels in Victoria Ward, Bedford General Hospital, 1898

probity of whiteness was often regarded as the ultimate aspiration, and in 1893 the hospital authority H. C. Burdett pronounced of water closets that 'the whole should be white, and no ornament of any kind should be permitted'.[67]

By that time, however, children's wards throughout the country were being animated by ceramic tile pictures of considerable merit. Half a century before, Samuel Wright and Herbert Minton had rediscovered the art of making encaustic tiles, and the subsequent enthusiasm for decorative tiling of all kinds eventually spread to children's hospitals not only in Britain, but also in India, New Zealand and other parts of the Empire.[68] They concentrate, sensibly enough, on nursery rhymes or fairy tales calculated to make the greatest appeal to their viewers. Now that many tile schemes have been moved from their original sites, to make way for demolition or remodelling of the interiors they first inhabited, it is easy to forget how intimately they were once related to the children's surroundings. At Torbay Hospital in Torquay, the Louisa Cary Children's Ward still possesses the twenty-one tile panels installed over the beds (pl. 319). Large enough to be relished from a considerable distance and set in a uniform green-and-white surround, they were designed by the architect Percy Adams whose firm, Adams, Holden and Pearson, donated four of the panels.[69] Their lively nursery-rhyme designs make an invaluable contribution to the ambience of the ward, for children are often the patients most in need of reassurance when confined to hospital.

Adams, in fact, was following his own precedent in earlier hospital tile schemes. He designed the Bedford General Hospital in 1898, when 'sixteen ladies' subscribed for a series of decorations on the walls of the Victoria Ward to celebrate the Queen's Jubilee (pl. 320). Philip Newman was responsible for designing what a commemorative booklet described as 'artistically painted panels illustrating

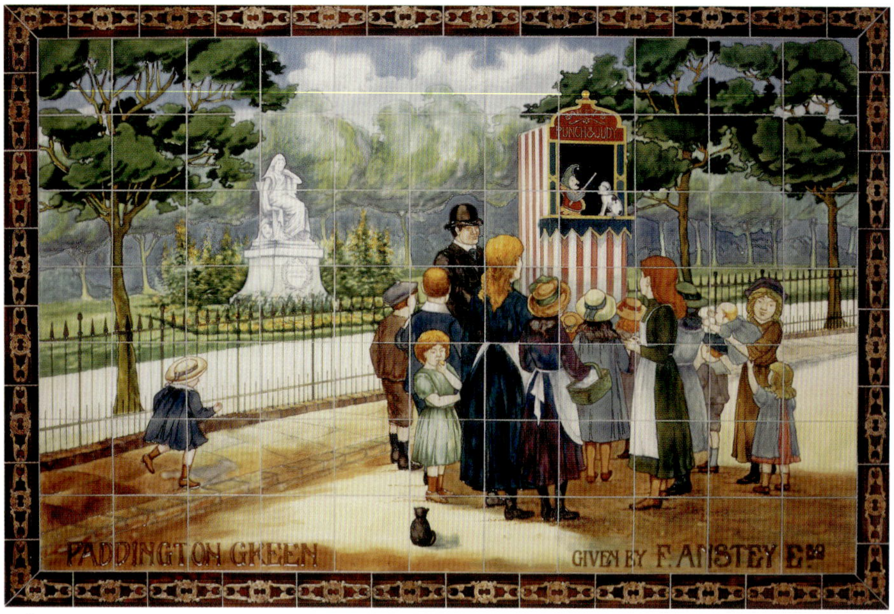

Old Nursery Rhymes and Tales'.[70] Installed above the 'sixteen cots' in the ward, they make up a highly impressive early example of tiling in a hospital. Like most other successful tile decorations of the period, they are carried out in a simplified, clear and bracing style, more indebted to contemporary poster design than to illustrated children's literature.

As Victorian hospitals underwent alterations and extensions, their tile schemes sometimes multiplied. One of the most spectacular and delightful examples of this burgeoning development was produced for Paddington Green Children's Hospital in London, where in 1895 a rebuilding programme prompted the installation of glazed nursery-rhyme tiles in the large Top Ward. Funded by a legacy 'left for the purpose by Miss Charlotte Jones, a valued servant for more than forty years',[71] it probably contained twenty pictures before a recent office

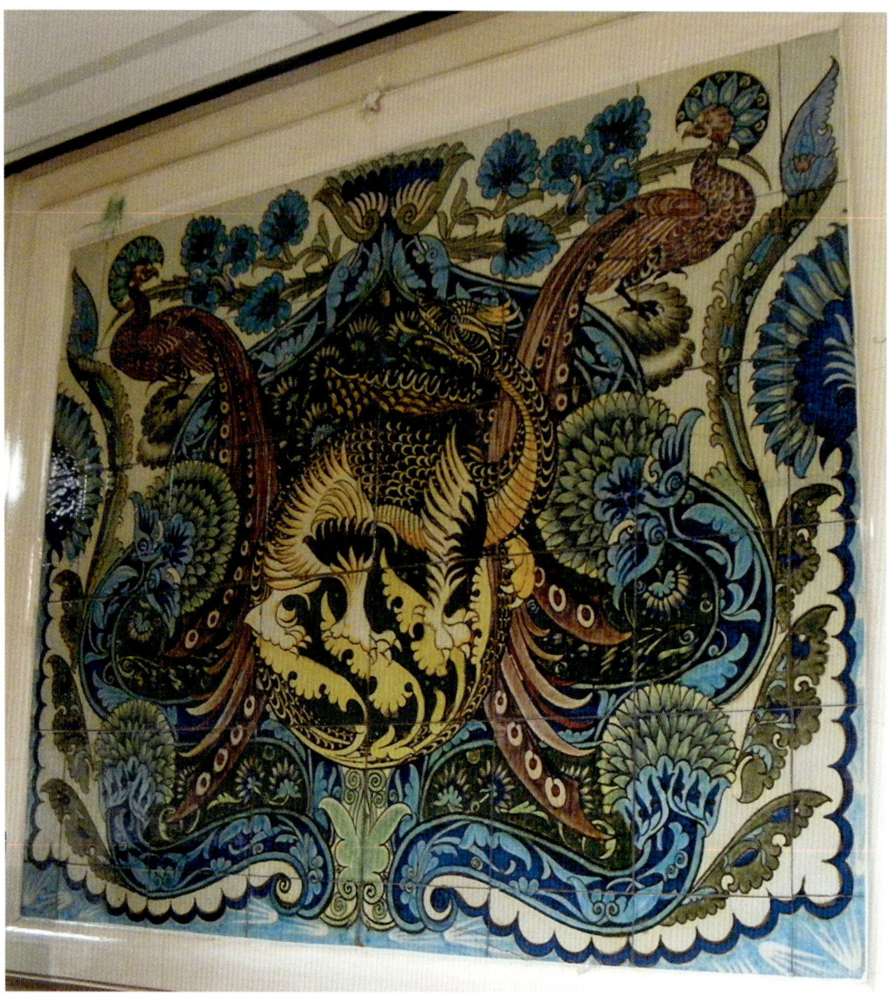

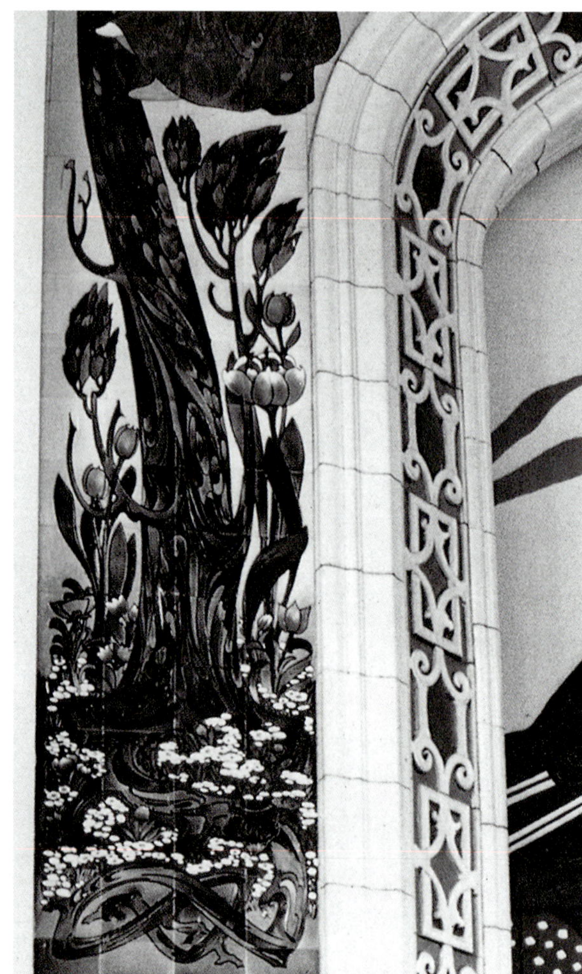

conversion hid all but two of them from view.[72] The original project proved so successful that a similar scheme was then begun in the Lower Ward, 'with subjects selected from the scriptures',[73] and more panels were installed whenever a new donor came forward with the appropriate funding. In 1895 each subscriber was expected to pay £20 for a panel, but the following year the entire decoration of the Small Ward with tile designs based on Aesop's Fables was financed by a generous donation of £500 from S. G. Holland, who gave the money in memory of his daughter.

Finally, and most remarkably of all, the Outpatients' Department at Paddington Green was embellished with fifteen panels when the architect Allen Munby designed its enlargement (pl. 321). A rare and intriguing rationale for the scheme can be found in the 1912 Hospital Committee Report, which claimed that the pictures representing 'children's games, nursery stories, country scenes etc . . . will serve three useful purposes, viz; to brighten and decorate the walls of the waiting room, to interest and distract the children from their sufferings: and also (the panels being washable) to reduce the cost of the annual cleaning'.[74] The outcome of this three-tiered enterprise, intended to provide aesthetic delight even as it hoped to alleviate children's fears and save money on the maintenance bill, was the finest sequence of decorations in the hospital. They have been admired so much since then by staff and patients alike that, when the building ceased to be a medical centre, the Outpatients' panels were transferred to the new District Hospital.

By no means all the tiling schemes installed during this productive period were meant for children. Perhaps the most exquisite surviving work, a tiled fireplace and overmantel by William de Morgan, was produced for the entrance hall of the King Edward VII building in Bristol Royal Infirmary (pl. 322). His sinuous, intertwining designs, derived from an ecstatic response to the flowers and leaves he interprets with such zest, gives the visitors a sense of irrepressible vitality from the moment they enter.

A similar source of inspiration galvanises the Art Nouveau decorations at Saint Nicholas Hospital in Gosforth, where the proscenium arch of the Recreation Hall Stage is surrounded by a swirling design in brilliantly coloured Doulton tiling (pl. 323). A pair of Pre-Raphaelite women attends the profusion of trees, flowers and birds inhabiting a paradisal region. W. J. Neatby, the architect who designed this unique and inventive scheme,[75] usually devoted his energies to decorative projects as prominent as Harrods Food Hall in London and the interior of Blackpool Tower. Working as an artist for Doulton's, he animated some of Britain's most celebrated public spaces with his headlong polychromatic fantasies. At Saint Nicholas in Gosforth, by contrast, Neatby's audience was restricted to the staff and patients of a mental hospital, but his design shows no sign of diminution compared with his work elsewhere. When the Recreation Hall was opened in May 1900, it became gratifyingly apparent that unstinting efforts had been made to provide its inhabitants with a decorative scheme capable of transporting them from their everyday surroundings into an alternative world, where the hospital's mundanity drops away and a seductive Eden becomes manifest for as long as they cared to look.

321 (*facing page, top*) Allen Munby, Tile panel in Outpatients' Department, Paddington Green Children's Hospital, London

322 (*facing page, bottom left*) William de Morgan, Tiled fireplace and overmantel, entrance hall, King Edward VII building, Bristol Royal Infirmary

323 (*facing page, bottom right*) W. J. Neatby, Doulton tiling, 1900, Recreation Hall Stage, St Nicholas Hospital, Gosforth

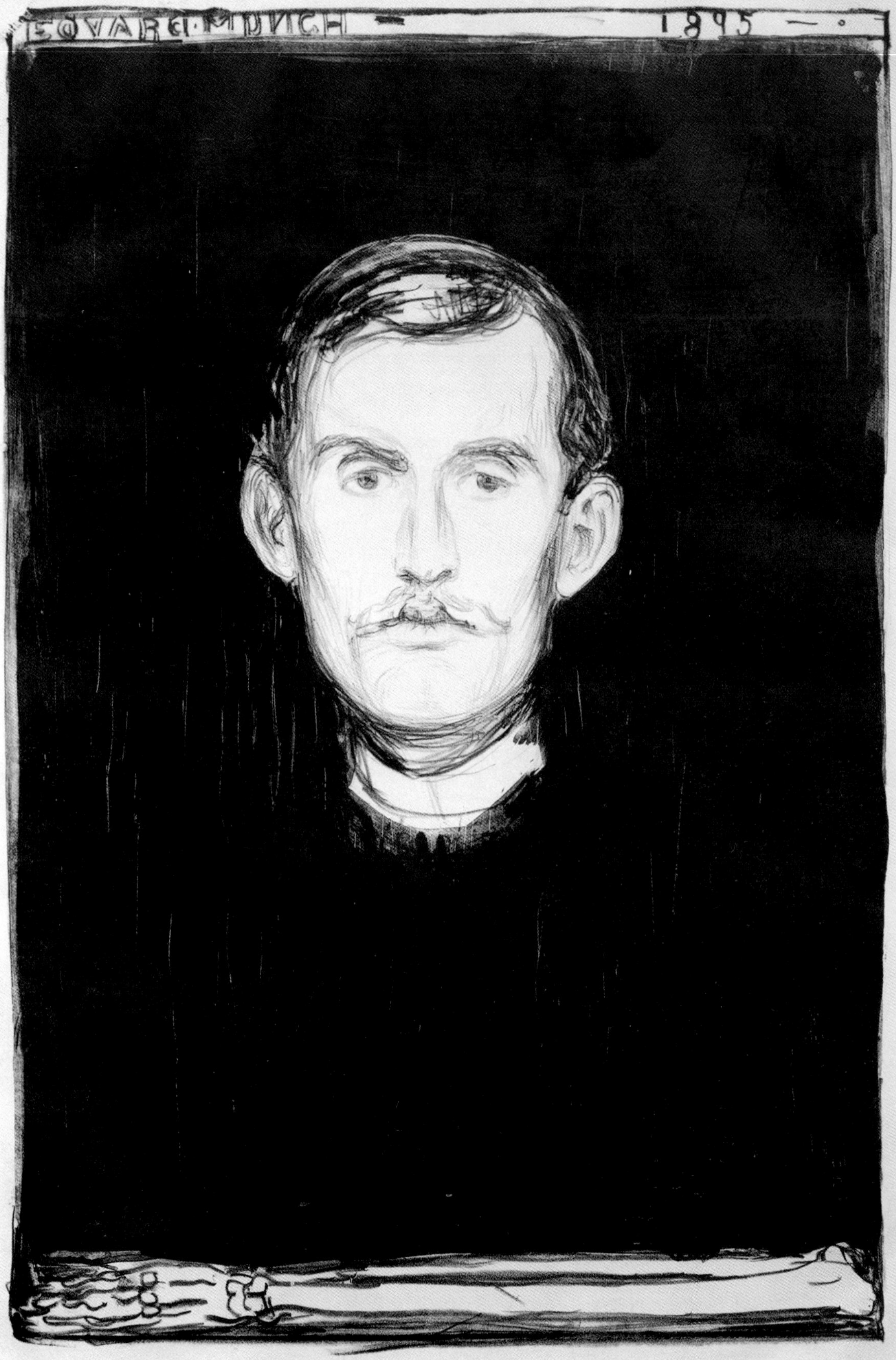
EDVARD MUNCH
1895

TWENTY-ONE
'I WANTED TO SCREAM'

Ever since his childhood, Edvard Munch had been confronted by the traumatic reality of fatal illness. His mother died of tuberculosis when Munch was only five, and nine years later his teenage sister Sophie succumbed to the same disease. The double loss left him exposed to the oppressive influence of his father, a neurotic military surgeon obsessed by discipline, religion and the need to destroy his son's unholy paintings of nude figures.[1] Death haunted Munch's vulnerable mind and sickly body thereafter, even though he lived to the age of eighty. Always psychologically intense, his work became preoccupied with bones beneath flesh, fatal stabbings and severed heads. In 1895 he produced a macabre *Self-portrait with Skeleton Arm* (pl. 324), and around the same time Munch drew himself as a sacrificial victim embraced by a long-haired Salome. All these alcohol-fuelled fantasies exhausted him and exacerbated his lung weakness so much that he spent several months in the Kornhaug sanatorium at Lillehammer at the turn of the century. A photograph survives of Munch standing there in the snow, buttoned up against the cold and his own agoraphobia (pl. 325). Although he adopts a resolute stance, the truth is that his fears were accelerating. And then, quite suddenly, they were transformed into brutal reality.

His affair with the heiress Tulla Larsen, who supported him financially while their relationship continued, had deteriorated when she announced their engagement without consulting him. Munch, who never married and had a horror of monogamy, broke up with Larsen. But she stalked him, accusing him of exploiting her in the most callous manner. 'She has spread horrible rumours about me', he complained. 'That I have lived on her; used her money then abandoned her like a heel. I heard that she had written letters to my family and told them that I had behaved like a scoundrel.'[2] Larsen went further, taking morphine and threatening to kill herself if Munch did not return. Finally, a female friend of Larsen's wrote him an urgent message in 1902, saying that she had just saved the distraught Larsen from a lethal overdose and claiming: 'she wants to die. She is in despair over you. Only you can save her. It's half past four now. If you want to speak to her, you must get the boat. Beside her bed I saw *two* empty vials of morphine.'[3]

What happened next is not clear. As Munch's latest biographer Sue Prideaux cautiously emphasised, only his diaries and letters survive to reconstruct the order of events: 'Tulla left no writings to put the case from the other side.'[4] Yet he certainly left his cottage in Aasgardstrand, made the boat-trip to her house and found Larsen laid out on her bed like a corpse. Candles were placed round her head, illuminating the red-gold tresses Munch had

324 (*facing page*) Edvard Munch, *Self-portrait with Skeleton Arm*, 1895, Kunsthalle, Hamburg

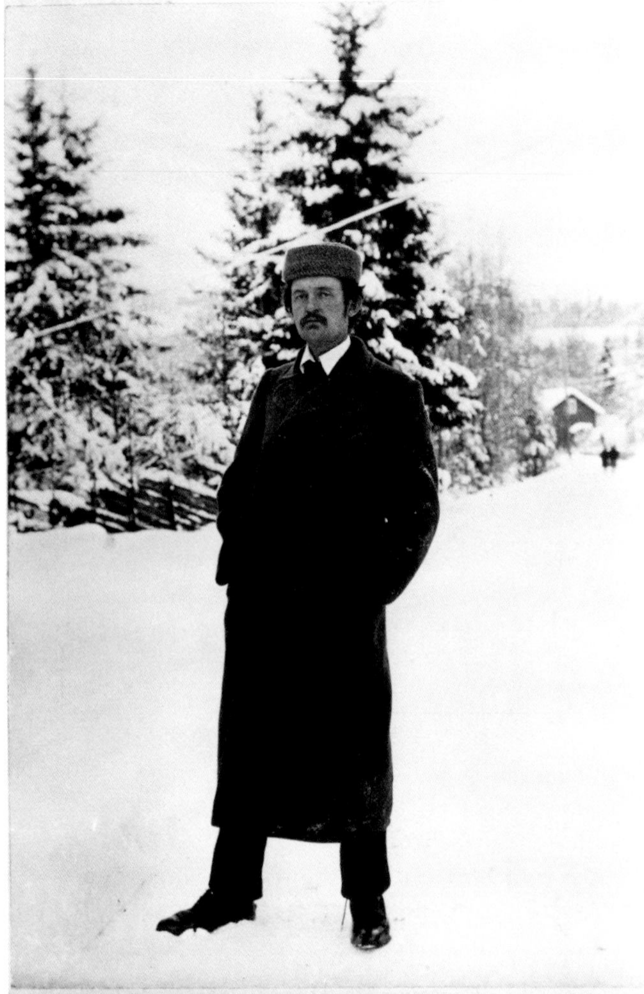

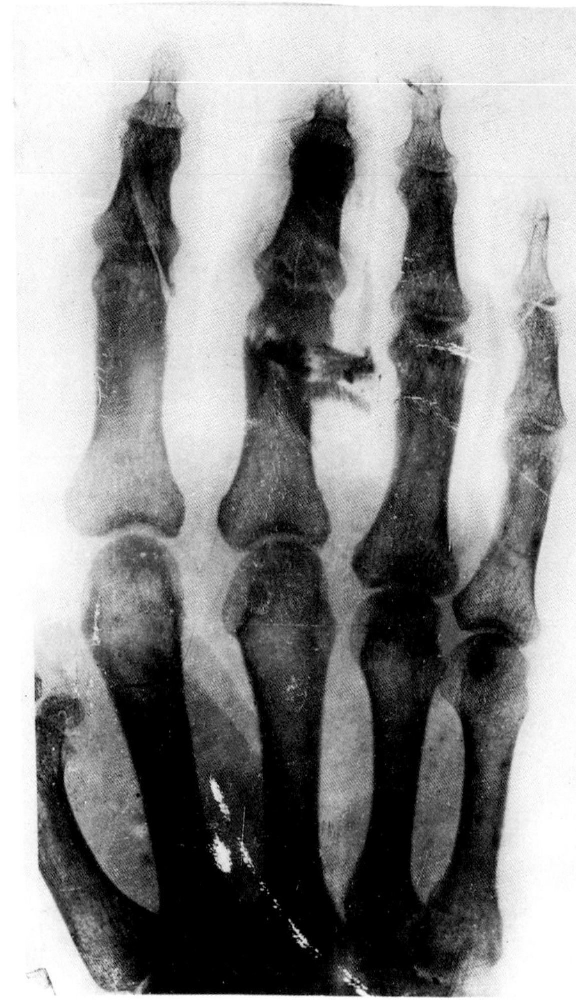

325 (*above left*) Photograph of Munch at Kornhaug sanatorium, Lillehammer, 1900

326 (*above right*) X-ray of Munch's injured hand, 1902

painted in some of his impassioned canvases, notably *The Dance of Life*. Larsen seems to have arranged a full-blown theatrical event for her ex-lover, and showed no difficulty in responding when he began explaining that 'the ill health that had stolen my youth made me afraid of starting a family'. According to Munch, she accused him of being 'easily manipulated' and her scornful laughter meant that 'my entire well-prepared speech vanished into thin air. The only thing I could think of was to say that we would speak no more of it – at which point she took to that dreadful sobbing again. My nerves were in shreds and the blood hammered at my temples in anger and despair – and compassion.'[5]

It is not known who had the gun, nor indeed who fired it, but a bullet certainly smashed into Munch's left hand, injuring it and shattering the middle finger. Munch claimed that, while he bled, she simply walked up and down the room before mopping the floor with a cloth. A doctor was eventually summoned and he despatched the wounded artist to hospital.

There Munch lay in the large open ward, as he had no money to pay for better care. Even so, he preferred having the company of others. 'The patients lay in two long rows . . . bed after bed. Iron beds with yellow blankets.' Munch noticed that he was flanked by 'a man with a broken leg, and on the other side a patient with infected sores. On the opposite side was a farmer who had been operated many times for cancer. His face was waxy yellow behind his black beard.' It could have been a desolate scene, yet Munch noticed with surprise that 'they talked to one another across the ward. There was a kind of gaiety amongst them, even those who were very sick.' He was even more intrigued when, in the evening, patients from other wards came visiting. A boy entered, showing off 'his newly-acquired wooden leg. He limped in on crutches. He and an elderly man from our ward practised walking. They laughed when things went wrong, and were very pleased with themselves when their efforts were successful. They looked so pathetic with their shoulders hunched up on their crutches.'[6]

Munch drew comfort from the realisation that his wound was 'nothing compared to the suffering of those lying here'.[7] He must also have been fascinated by X-rays taken of his injured hand on 12 September 1902, revealing skeletal images eerily reminiscent of his own work (pl. 326). Rediscovered only recently, they show the bullet lodged in his shattered finger. Munch's friend August Strindberg was so fascinated by these 'mystical rays' that he claimed to have invented them himself.[8] But Munch realised that the images fulfilled the uncanny prophecy he had made in *Self-Portrait with Skeleton Arm* seven years before (see pl. 324).

As for the operation itself, Munch subsequently painted a vivid and uninhibited image of himself laid out naked on a white sheet smeared with an alarming amount of blood (pl. 327). A nurse stands nearby holding a bowl while three surgical figures lurk ominously at a distance, as if reluctant to move forward and examine their patient. The red-faced man in the centre contrasts with the other two, who look strangely spectral. One of the figures, staring towards Munch, has a skull for a face. The uneasy, doom-laden mood is reinforced by rows of spectators gazing in through a large aperture. They help to give *On the Operating Table* its sense of tension. Munch was keenly aware of their grim, voyeur-like presence throughout the proceedings. He wrote a visceral account of the event 'in the brightly lit room', where 'the galleries on either side were filled with observers, just like theatre'. He even claimed to have 'recognised faces from the streets among

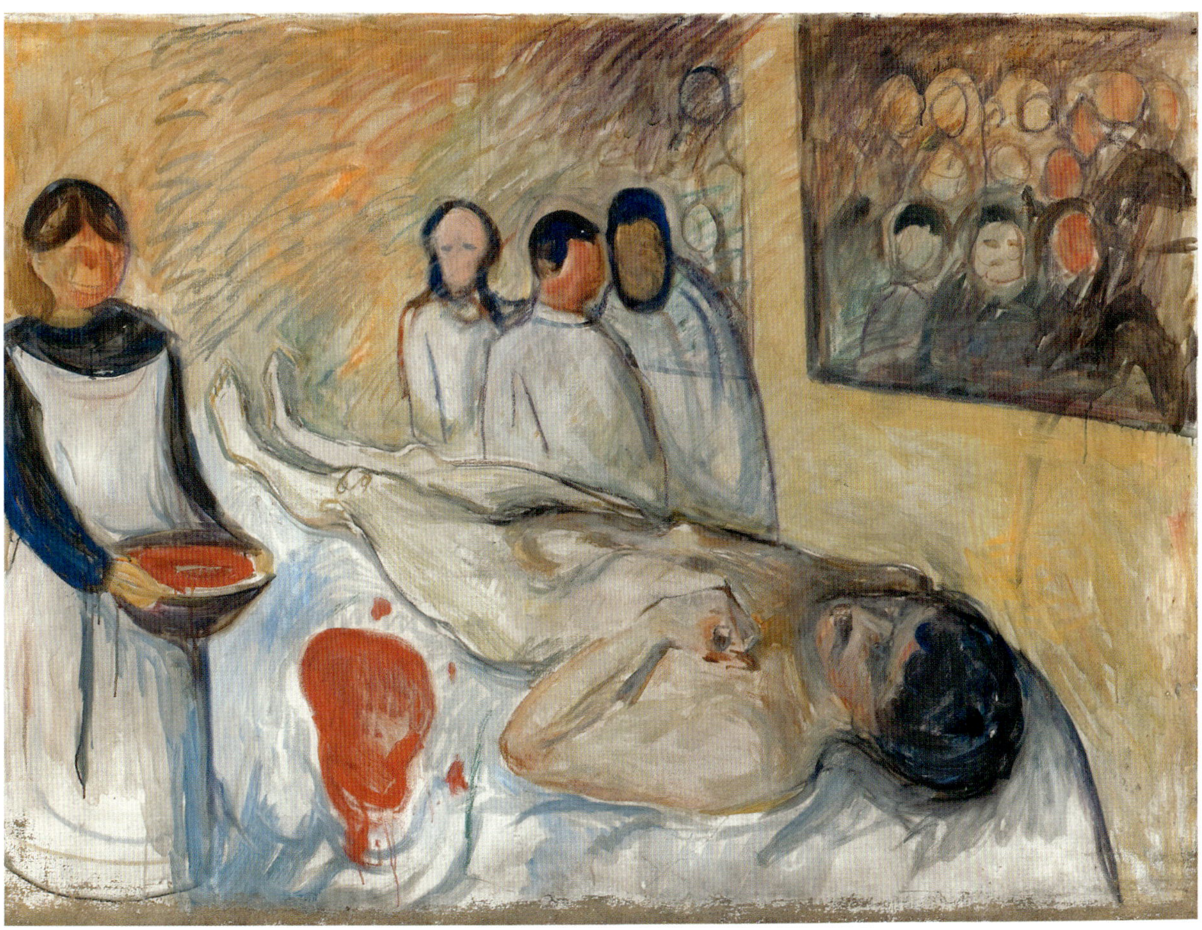

327 Edvard Munch, *On the Operating Table*, 1902–3, Munch Museum, Oslo

the female and male students',[9] and remained painfully conscious while the surgeon carried out his task. Having been asked by the anaesthetist if he would like chloroform, Munch said no: 'my heart condition will not permit it.' But the truth must be that he was determined to witness the scene, and commit it to memory:

> I watched as all the preparations were made, the knives that were brought out and the professor's every move. I felt the knife cut its way through the flesh, it scraped against the bones and blood gushed forth. The bullet had exploded, leaving the bones in splintered pieces which needed to be trimmed. Pieces of bone and lead were embedded in the flesh, and had to be removed. The operation lasted a long time. I saw my fingers and hand bloody and swollen like a glove. The pain caused sweat to form on my brow, I wanted to scream but the many eyes upon me forced me to clench my jaws together instead.[10]

Part of Munch's imagination must have been fascinated by the suffering he underwent on the operating table: as an artist he was, after all, involved with a lifelong struggle to come to terms with trauma. Even so, the physical and mental agony induced by surgery in 1902 should not be underestimated. Munch felt defiled by the procedures he witnessed. 'The flesh was cut, trimmed, pierced, sewn and the hand resembled a piece of chopped meat', he wrote. 'After an hour and a half the doctor announced, "Well, I hope that will do. The hand will not stand any more." ' Munch was wheeled back to the ward. 'My working hand would heal, I hoped. The days passed. I had a fever. The pain in the mangled hand was unbearable. When the doctor made his rounds I asked, "Will my hand heal? Will I be able to use it again?" "Yes, we hope so", replied the doctor.'[11] That optimism proved unfounded when Munch finally saw his mutilated flesh again. Writing in the third person, probably in an attempt to distance the anguish, he recalled the moment when

> his bandages were removed. He shuddered. A monstrosity – his once perfectly formed hand in perfect working order, was now dreadfully deformed. Deformed, disgusting and useless. He knocked it all the time, against furniture, on the tram. His once willing worker was no longer able to help him. He drank huge quantities of wine in order to deaden the pain. But at night he awoke and felt his hand. He lit the candle and stared at his poor deformed limb.[12]

As a result, Munch felt deeply alienated: 'He avoided people. Refused to eat together with anyone. Everybody stared at him, at his deformed hand.' Isolation turned to anger when he discovered that Tulla Larsen was, in reality, involved in a very close relationship with another painter, Arne Kavli. Apoplectic with rage, Munch found that 'his thoughts stormed in his head from morning till night. He whispered her name in hate; he clenched his fist at her, the alcohol made him sick. One evening in a restaurant, sitting drunkenly filled with rage, he noticed people looking at him and realised that he had been shaking his hand in the air.'[13]

Over the next few years, Munch was unable to put the disastrous affair with Larsen behind him. If anything, the bitter sense of resentment grew as he embarked on a series of paintings where a naked man is stretched out on a sheet next to an implacable, vengeful woman (pl. 328). He called these chilling and strident images *The Death of Marat*, pretending that the female executioner was Charlotte Corday. In reality, they are Munch's attempts to relive the shooting incident that left him permanently damaged. The brushstrokes take on a violence of their own as the mortified artist defines the contrast between his prone, horizontal corpse and Larsen's erect rigidity. Blood smears the sheet even more liberally than it did in his earlier canvas *On the Operating Table*. For the man is bleeding, now, from the heart as well as the hand.

He had good reason to feel gratified when the wealthy oculist Dr Max Linde, one of his early and more generous patrons, published a book with the visionary title *Munch and the Art of the Future* in 1903. The momentous words reflected the growing enthusiasm for Munch's work among the most avant-garde artists of the new generation. He claimed that the *Death of Marat*, 'the child conceived by me and my beloved', was not 'a masterpiece – it is more of an experiment'.[14] But young artists as audacious as the emergent German Expressionists admired Munch for a willingness to push his work far beyond accepted limits. In 1906 Emil Nolde declared that Munch's art 'acted upon

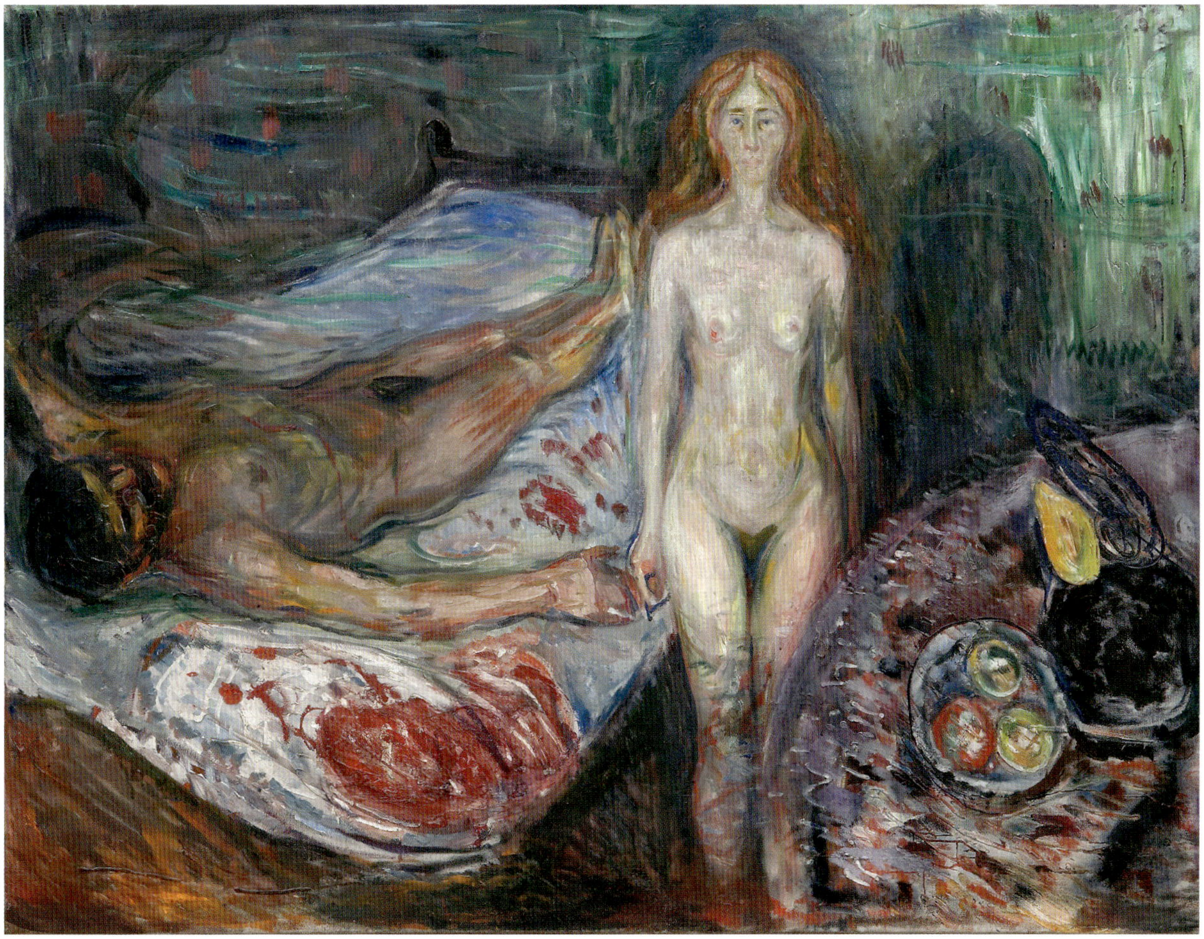

328 Edvard Munch, *The Death of Marat I*, 1907, Munch Museum, Oslo

us like an explosion . . . A hand slashing paint on the canvas as he does could sooner be imagined as wielding a knife or throwing a bomb.'[15]

Hailed by the young as a pioneering insurgent, Munch was invited to join the rebellious Die Brücke in Dresden as the group's revered mentor. He nevertheless found that his mental condition was deteriorating. Drunken brawls in restaurants became more common and he even threatened a fellow-guest at a spa hotel in Kosen with a pistol. Munch wrote to his aunt complaining that 'it was a long history in Berlin hospitals this winter with influenza – imagine if I'd had money troubles too!' He also reported that 'my finger is healing but it hurts all the time. It is not a pretty sight and it's not much use either but it does what it can – it's short and stiff.'[16] Despite his insistence on hiding the painful finger in a black leather sheath, he constantly found himself staring at this ugly reminder of the Larsen débâcle.

In 1908, alarmed by increasing attacks of numbness and paralysis, Munch travelled to Copenhagen in search of 'a nerve sanatorium'.[17] He became paranoid during the train-trip, and his delusions were undoubtedly envenomed by the memory of a doctor warning him that 'in the end it will go to your head. You will have a stroke.' Falling victim to panic, Munch recoiled from the 'tearing pains under my heart, terror in the morning, giddy when I stood up'.[18] Convinced that a gang of fiends was hunting him down, he visited a renowned Copenhagen clinic run by the psychotherapist Einar Brünning. After the interview, Brünning imagined that his fearful visitor would decide to stay for a course of treatment. But Munch fled, declaring that the eminent psychotherapist 'looked too serious'. Attempting to forget his troubles, he went on a drunken spree with a couple of friends. Terrifying voices assailed him at night, and they were so haunting that he longed for a revolver to shoot them. Then, quite suddenly, his attitude changed: 'I couldn't bear it any longer. "Take me to the clinic", I said.'[19]

Rather than returning to the institution run by Brünning, Munch went to a highly successful clinic at 21 Kochsveien, in the quiet, reassuring and well-foliated suburbs of Copenhagen. He may well have heard that Dr Daniel Jacobsen, its handsome and charismatic proprietor, was admired for his sympathetic treatment of artists. Jacobsen, who had previously worked in the city hospital before attending Charcot's celebrated lectures at La Salpêtrière in Paris, certainly achieved spectacular results with the best-selling yet suicidal Danish author Amelie Skram. Women patients always found him attractive, referring to him affectionately as 'Kissing Jacobsen'. But what would the proud and turbulent Munch make of such a man, when he harboured such a fear of insanity and its punitive treatment?

As it turned out, Jacobsen's charm lay at the centre of his appeal to Munch. Unlike the austere Brünning, he was able to empathise with his patients and deal with them in a consoling manner. Too lazy to concern himself much with radical theories, he concentrated instead on old-fashioned comfort and care. Intuitive rather than cerebral, Jacobsen was adept at distinguishing between hopelessly incurable cases and individuals capable of responding to his essentially benign regime at the clinic. He was correct in deciding that Munch, far from suffering an irredeemable malady, might well be helped towards recovery. Jacobsen was also right to diagnose the illness as *dementia paralytica* caused by the poisonous effects of acute alcoholism. Fortuitously, he had written a thesis in 1891 on *dementia paretica* in women, and the knowledge gained during his research played a decisive role in helping him to arrive at an accurate diagnosis of Munch. A decade later, Jacobsen classified his patient as a melancholic genius who, like Michelangelo, Goethe and Kirkegaard, suffered not from insanity but a 'manic-depressive psychosis'.[20] Munch was lucky: if a poorly informed doctor had examined him he might, as Sue Prideaux pointed out, have been 'treated for syphilis or for madness, in which case he might indeed have found himself locked up for life.'[21]

Avoiding the fate endured for so many years by Richard Dadd (see pl. 265), Munch slowly began savouring the attractions of an institution where the nurses, to his intense relief, were attractive and had smiles like 'a lily-of-the-valley'. He started eating in a far more healthy and regular way than hitherto. The food, he wrote, succeeded in 'putting flesh on the ends of my nerves'.[22] Heart massages proved equally effective, lulling him into a state where he no longer needed the cocktail of drugs prescribed by doctors in the past. At bedtime, the nurses only administered chloral. Nothing else was needed to give Munch the sleep that had often eluded him. At the beginning of his treatment he slept for eight days, and awoke to the reassuring sight of a nurse who slept on the sofa in his locked bedroom. At that stage, he still felt gloomy enough to ask himself 'were there voices in the street? My paralysis was better. Lying listening. What were they saying outside the door?' Munch thought he heard a man insisting 'he must be moved south'. Yet most of his feverish attention was focused on 'the window. Was it locked? I might have to escape through it. Down on the street – death. There were bars on the window – my last refuge was closed to me – death.'[23]

After a while, though, his delusions faded as the treatment took effect. Baths were crucial, for Jacobsen had written in his *Dementia* thesis that

> a most important ingredient in the cure is the bath in carbonic acid, but the following ingredients may also be added: iron, salt, soda, potash, sulphur, fir needles, certain flowers, the bark of the oak tree, malt and bran. If hallucinations are involved, a milk bath or a bath of bouillon may be used, or sometimes the unappetising bath in the blood of freshly slaughtered animals.[24]

Mercifully, Munch was confined to pine-needle and sun baths. Jacobsen must have guessed that his patient would respond hysterically to the sight of a bloodbath. The clinic's staff proved equally sensible when they applied electrical current to his brain. The voltage was weak and far less invasive than electro-convulsive therapy. So Munch submitted to it without complaint and even found that he savoured the experience. In a letter to his devoted aunt, he was prepared to admit that 'I have been rather short of electricity', and informed her that he had undergone 'Faradisation, Franklinisation and Galvanisation'.[25] He approved of them all and drew a lively ink caricature of Jacobsen with an elegant young nurse administering treatment

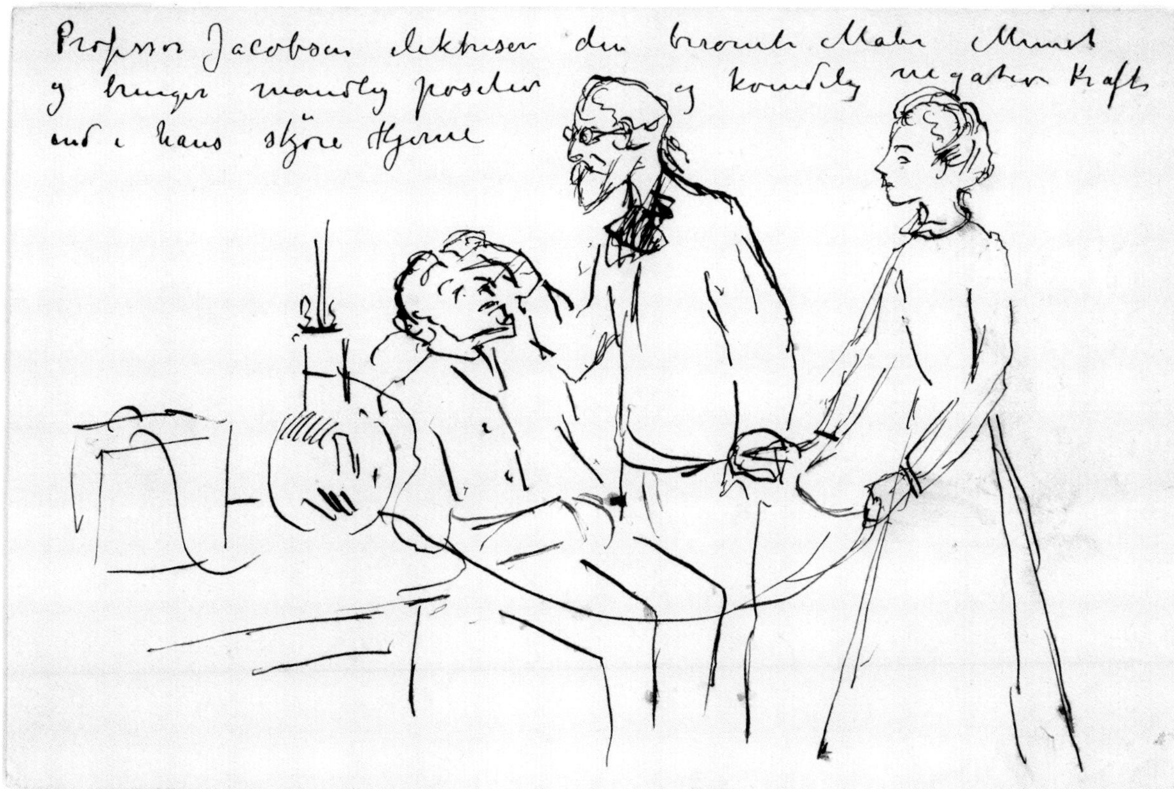

329 Edvard Munch, *Dr Daniel Jacobsen and Nurse Administering Treatment*, 1908, Munch Museum, Oslo

(pl. 329). While the nurse manipulates a wire attached to an appliance on the table, Munch leans back gratefully in his chair and allows the doctor to mop his sweaty brow. At the top of the drawing, an inscription proves that he still retained a self-mocking sense of satire: 'Professor Jacobsen passing electricity through the famous painter Edvard Munch, changing his crazy brain with the positive power of masculinity and the negative power of femininity.'

This little cartoon was probably one of the first images he made of life at the clinic. But Munch soon decided that he felt resilient enough to defy his nervous breakdown and embark on a programme of painting and writing as well. While realising that a return to art might reawaken some of his old neuroses, Munch understood that he should never aim at banishing them altogether. 'I don't want to get rid of illness, however unsympathetically I may depict it in my art', he wrote in a passage remarkable for its self-knowledge. Perhaps his conversations with Jacobsen had helped him to decide that 'my fear of life is necessary to me, as is my illness. Without anxiety and illness, I am a ship without a rudder. My art is grounded in reflections over being different to others. My sufferings are part of my self and my art. They are indistinguishable from me, and their destruction would destroy my art.'[26]

Perhaps, too, he took inspiration from the seminal example of van Gogh, whose work he greatly admired. Just as Vincent had insisted on continuing to produce art both at the Arles hospital and during his subsequent period of treatment at Saint-Rémy (see pls 279 and 291), so Munch steeled himself to perform a similar feat. 'During his short life, Van Gogh did not allow his flame to go out', Munch wrote later. 'Fire and embers were his brushes during the few years of his life, whilst he burned out for his art. I have thought, and wished, that in the long term, with more money at my disposal than he had – to follow in his footsteps. Not to let my flame die out, and with burning brush, to paint to the very end.'[27]

His most ambitious painting in the clinic was a grand, full-length portrait of Jacobsen himself. It may have been the doctor's idea, for the artist recalled that Jacobsen asked him during their initial consultation: 'What are you doing here?' Munch had replied tersely: 'Painting.' So the physician said:

330 (*right*) Photograph of Munch and Dr Jacobsen, 1909

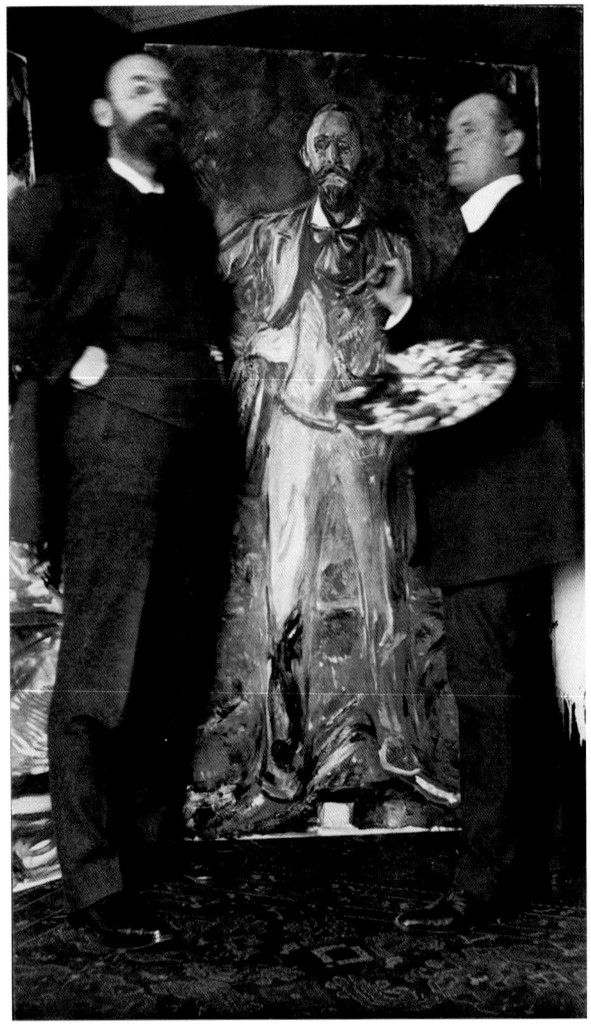

331 (*facing page*) Edvard Munch, *Dr Daniel Jacobsen*, 1909, Munch Museum, Oslo

'Well, paint me then.'[28] First of all, a black and white lithograph of his head was executed in preparation for the large oil. Sporting a white collar and full-blown cravat, the hirsute Jacobsen looks relatively genial in this swift, decisive print. It is a portrait of the doctor as charmer, but Munch had no intention of producing such a straightforward image when he set to work on the canvas. A fascinating photograph has survived of the two men standing next to the work in progress (pl. 330). Munch, dressed as formally as his sitter, gives no sign of being a dejected patient. He stands erect and sober, clean-shaven and clad in a crisp suit. The pigments splashed across the palette resting on his left arm could easily have besmirched the immaculate garment with unwanted colour. But Munch, who was capable of acting like an untamed bohemian, is determined in this context to present a respectable facade. He may even want to compete with Jacobsen, who adopts a more assertive pose and seems bent on appearing taller than his painter. The doctor was, at forty-six, two years older than Munch, and exudes a confident sense of medical authority.

Hence, no doubt, Munch's decision to give his sitter such an expansive stance in the finished painting (pl. 331). With arms akimbo, Jacobsen sweeps back his jacket and places his legs apart, with both feet projecting fiercely outwards. He looks ready for anything, and his facial expression is notably more severe than in the earlier lithograph. His gold watch-chain gleams as it describes an assured arc on his waistcoat, while Munch heightens the aura of virile vigour by making dramatic play with contrasts of light and dark. The doctor's jutting left arm is reduced to a triangle full of black paint, whereas his aggressively bunched right fist blazes with almost phosphorescent luminosity. Munch creates a substantial presence on the canvas without resorting to excessive detail. His brushwork summarises form, determined to retain the freshness and vitality of the artist's own touch. He slashes fiery colour at Jacobsen's face and body alike. The same streaked strokes are also allowed to pierce the shadows gathering so ominously behind the physician. While the upper half of the painting glows with flame-like scarlet and orange, the lower area threatens to engulf him in a sinister, strangely nocturnal region. Yet the entire picture is united by Munch's determination to retain an aura of heat throughout the canvas. For all the professional swagger exuded by Jacobsen, he is in danger of being consumed by the vehement colours seething all around him.

Munch drew immense, combative satisfaction from the ability to counter his sitter's dominant pose with a sense of menace. 'When I painted him I was the king', he explained, 'I controlled him who wanted to control me. During the process it came to me that there was no weakness in my art, it was stronger than him. It had not been destroyed. I told this to Professor Jacobsen when I painted his portrait.'[29] The doctor's response is not recorded, but he probably concluded that Munch's mental health was benefiting from the belief that the patient, not the physician, had become the victor in this dramatic battle of wills. Munch exulted as he made the extravagant claim that 'I have put him in the flames of hell. He stands looking down as a pope upon his white-clad nurses and us, the pale, sick ones.' So the psychiatric pontiff was being consigned to Hades, by an artist who even convinced himself that 'when I was painting him, Jacobsen begged for mercy and became gentle as a dove.'[30] Munch was patently indulging in wish-fulfilment, and there is no evidence that his physician felt at all threatened or subjugated by the experience of posing for such an openly competitive artist.

All the same, the result stands today as one of Munch's most powerful portraits. Its audacity baffled Jacobsen rather than unnerving him. He asked the opinion of another artist, Ludvig Karsten, and tried to pre-empt his verdict by gesturing at the canvas and saying 'frankly, I think he's pretty far gone, don't you?' Karsten, however, was a close friend of Munch's. Kneeling in front of the portrait, he closed his hands in an attitude of prayer and declared that 'it's pure genius'.[31] Jacobsen may have begun to think again after witnessing such an idolatrous response. His attitude undoubtedly altered when he heard the astonishing news that Norway had decided to honour Munch by awarding him the much coveted Order of Saint Olav (First Class). Established in 1847 by the King of Norway and Sweden in order to hail 'outstanding service to humanity', the Order was so prestigious that it transformed Munch from an outsider to a venerated cultural hero. His faithful patron Dr Linde wrote to congratulate him in frank disbelief: 'If anyone had said five or six years ago that this would happen, they would have been locked up in an asylum.'[32] Jacobsen, however, was profoundly impressed by the award and Munch reported with satisfaction that the nurses 'all admired my lovely brooch'. While viewing the receipt of royal honours with the scepticism of a passionate republican, he admitted that 'in this case I feel that it is as if a hand is reaching out from my home land'.[33]

Although the presentation of this high honour may have helped to speed Munch's recovery, he was not yet ready to consider leaving the clinic. Determined to resist any slavish dependence on Jacobsen, he nevertheless realised that the doctor was playing a significant part in freeing him from physical paralysis and mental turmoil. Munch wanted this beneficent process to continue, so that he could work towards a future life of 'tobacco-free cigars alcohol-free drinks and poison-free women'. Yet for

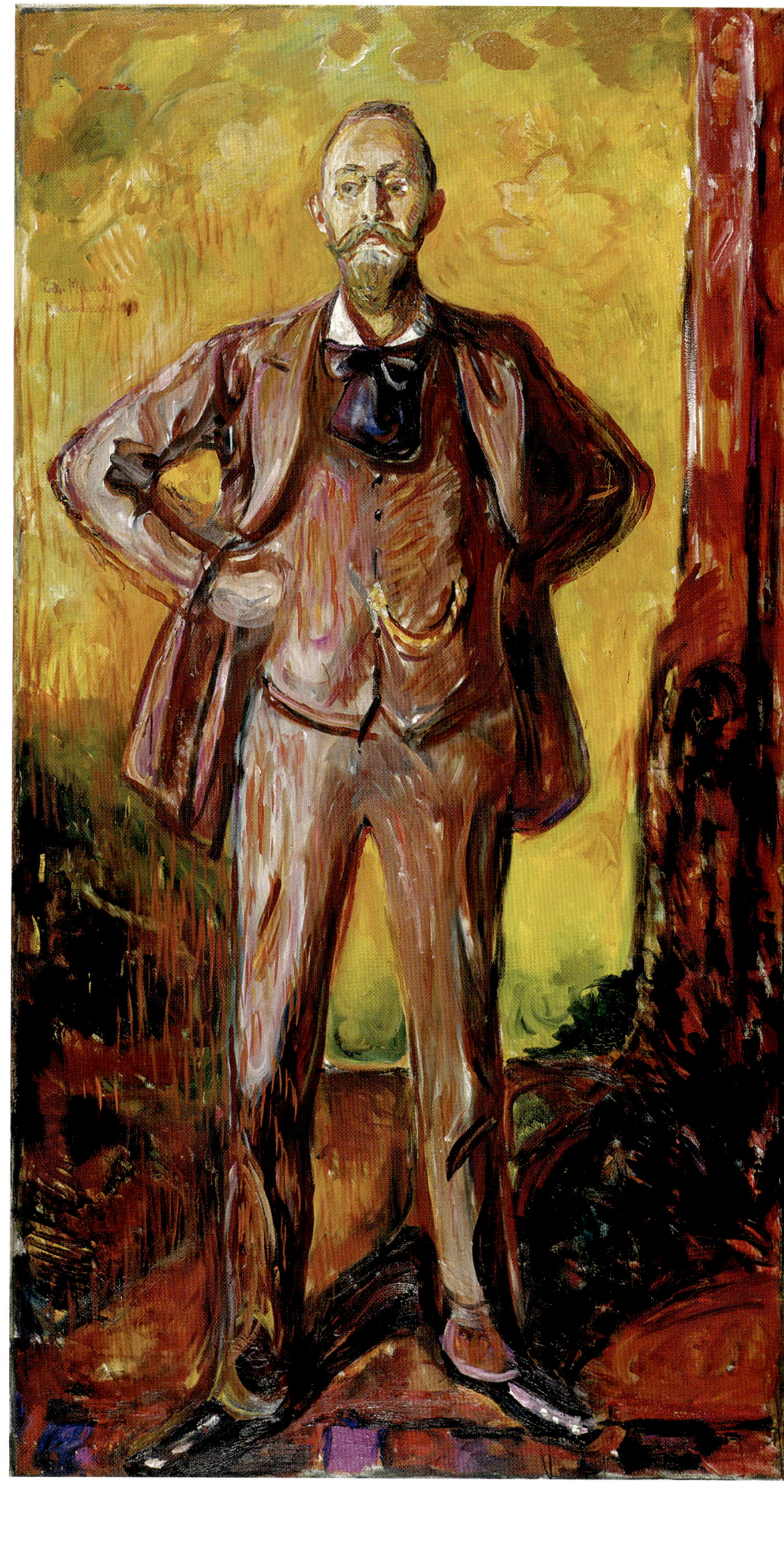

332 (*right*) Edvard Munch, *Alpha's Death*, 1908–9, Munch Museum, Oslo

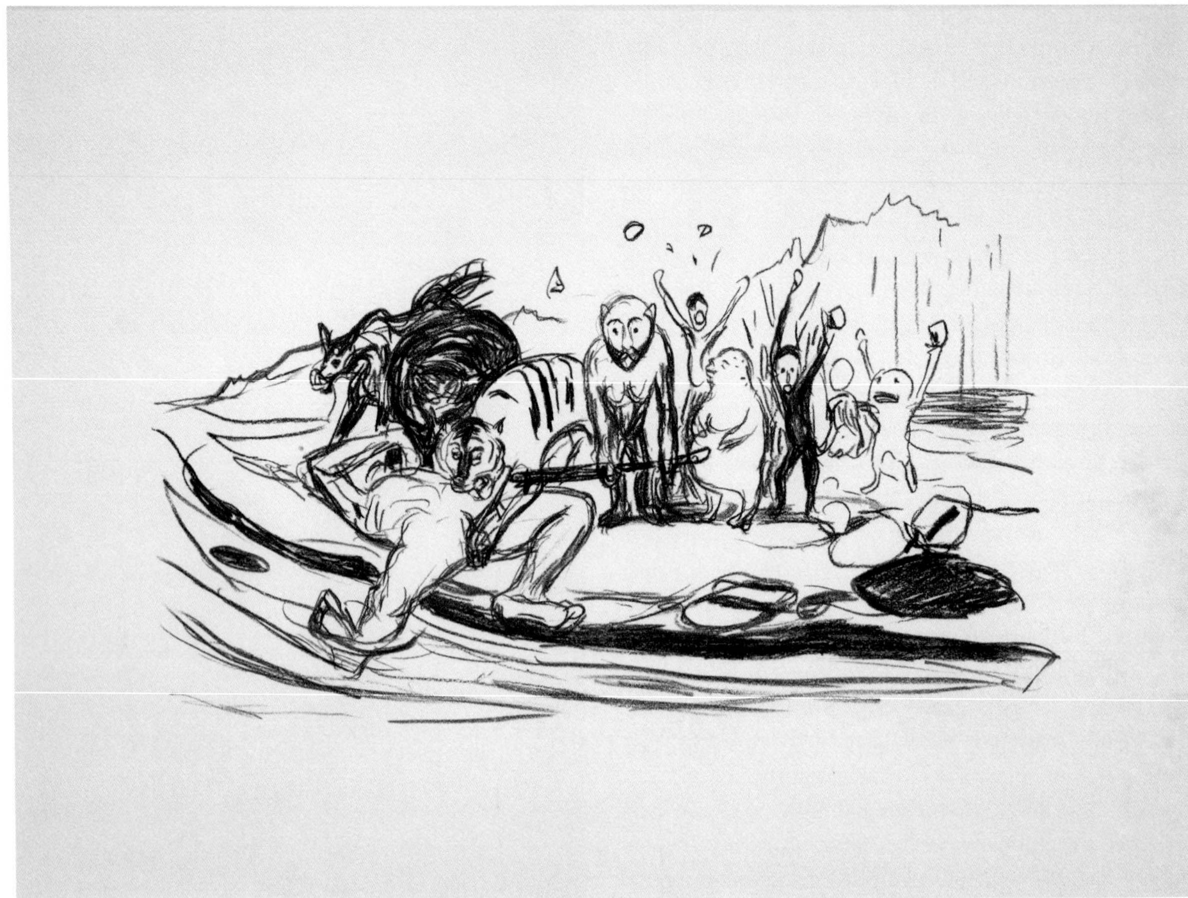

333 (*facing page*) Edvard Munch, *The Fatal Destiny* (photograph), 1907, Munch Museum, Oslo

the moment, he confessed in December 1908 to his friend the critic Jappe Nilssen that 'my mind is like a glass of cloudy water. I am now letting it stand to become clear again. I wonder what will happen when the dregs have settled on the bottom?'[34]

The problem of paying for a protracted stay in Jacobsen's expensive institution was solved when the newly appointed Director of Oslo's National Gallery purchased one of Munch's important early paintings for a substantial sum. Munch's relief from monetary worries must have strengthened his resolve and made him concentrate on pursuing the idea of recovery through creative work. As well as completing the ambitious Jacobsen portrait, he started writing a remarkably honest autobiographical text called *The Mad Poet's Diary*. Far more truthful than his previous memoirs, it was written in the third person. Munch intended the text as a corrective to his earlier writings, which he now considered 'rather naive and I notice a tendency to complain over my own cruel fate that seems to me rather unmanly. I probably wrote in that way to console myself.' Bent on distancing himself from self-pity, he even pretended that *The Mad Poet's Diary* consisted of 'records I have made, or notes I have received from a dear friend who slowly but surely became completely insane. I made his acquaintance at the Clinic in Copenhagen in 1908.'[35]

Both the text and the accompanying drawings were, even so, clearly centred on Munch's own life. He may have argued that 'I am making a study of the soul, as I can observe myself closely and use myself as an anatomical testing ground for this soul study . . . I have changed and exaggerated, and I have used others for these studies.'[36] But the incidents he wrote about are identifiably personal. He provides another account of the shooting with Tulla Larsen and for the first time takes responsibility for the incident: 'in a kind of unconscious otherworldly state he shoots himself in her presence. The shot wounds his arm and renders him a cripple.

The damage to his arm is a constant reminder and finally drives him to madness.' The references to a 'cripple' show that Munch has still failed to rid himself of his appetite for exaggeration. Yet he also admits with great honesty that 'he makes himself quite impossible in every way, acts brutally; gets drunk.'[37] This confessional drive must have helped him come to terms with his shortcomings in the privacy of the clinic.

The most impressive outcome of Munch's attempt to bring writing and drawing together was a creation myth entitled, initially, *The First Human Beings*. It was probably stimulated by a letter from Dr Linde, urging him to produce 'a series of drawings on the subject of your experiences in the unfamiliar realms of love. It will have a healing effect.'[38] The idea took wing in Munch's mind and he soon decided to rename it *Alpha and Omega* (pl. 332). His first draft was truly terrifying: humanity has been obliterated by an apocalypse, leaving behind only Alpha the first man and Omega the first woman. But the revised version is more biblical in tone. The couple live in harmony on an idyllic island until a serpent wriggles its way up Omega's body. Alpha slaughters the snake, yet he cannot prevent Omega falling in love with all the animals on the island, one after another. Then she escapes on the back of a fallow deer, leaving Alpha to act as a father figure for the 'small pigs, small serpents, small monkeys' and other animals who were all Omega's children. In a passage reminiscent of Munch's earlier painting *The Scream*, Alpha succumbs to madness: 'He ran along the seashore – sky and sea were the colour of blood. He heard footsteps in the air, and put his hands to his ears. Earth, sky and sea trembled, and he felt great fear.'

Terror turns to anger when, eventually, Alpha sees Omega returning. His reaction is ferocious: 'He struck Omega until she died. When he bent over her dead body and saw her face, he was terrified of her expression. It was the same expression she had worn in the forest when he had loved her most.'[39] Her children waste no time in taking revenge, attacking Alpha from behind and tearing him to pieces. So the legend proceeded, in the course of eighteen crayon drawings and the same number of written pages, from primordial bliss to sickening violence. Munch wanted the images to possess the simple, direct eloquence of paintings and carvings in prehistoric caves. Jacobsen was shocked by this murderous myth and ordered Munch to destroy *Alpha and Omega* in its entirety. But then the doctor relented, possibly because he realised how cathartic the work had been for his patient. So far as Munch was concerned, some malignant ghosts were ousted during this sustained bout of writing and drawing. He told Dr Linde that 'a strange feeling of peace came over me as I was working on that series – it was as though all the pain was leaving my body.'[40]

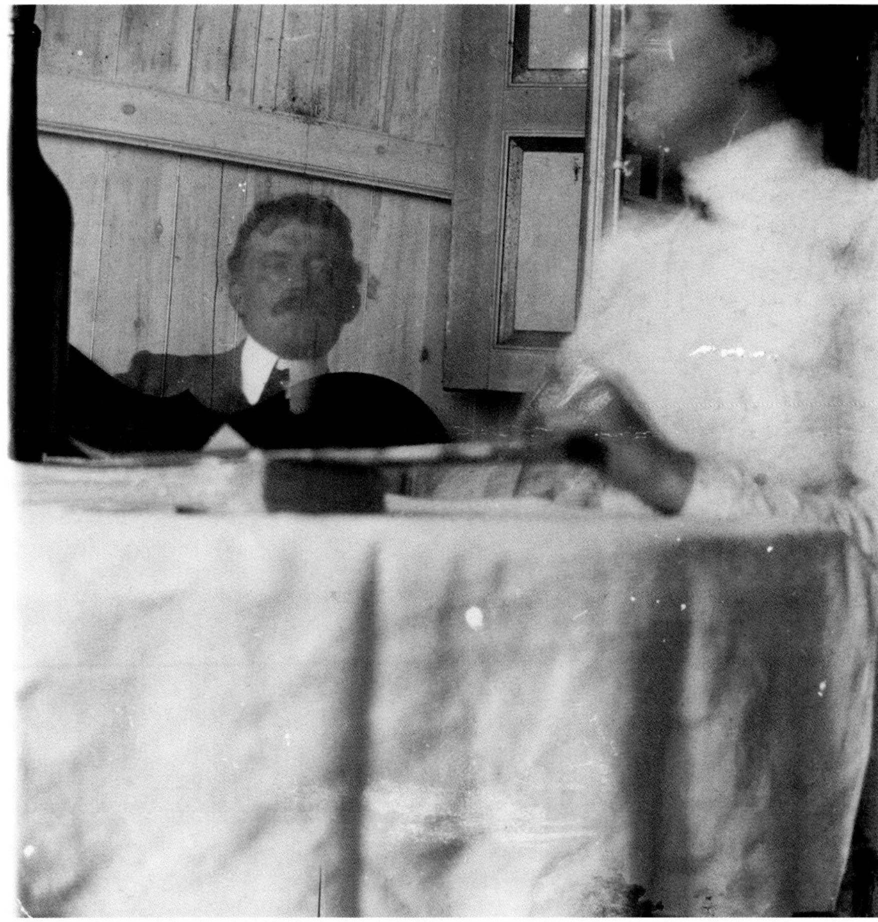

Not that Munch wanted to eradicate all the spirits who inhabited his speculative imagination. Another successful project undertaken in the clinic was a sequence of photographs taken with his Kodak camera. Earlier in his career, he had been keenly aware of photography's limitations compared with the innovative possibilities opened up by modern painters. 'The camera cannot compete with brush and canvas', he had declared, 'as long as it cannot be used in heaven and hell.'[41] Nevertheless, in 1902, just before his entanglement in the

334 (*right*) Edvard Munch, *The Sick Child* (photograph), *c.*1902, Munch Museum, Oslo

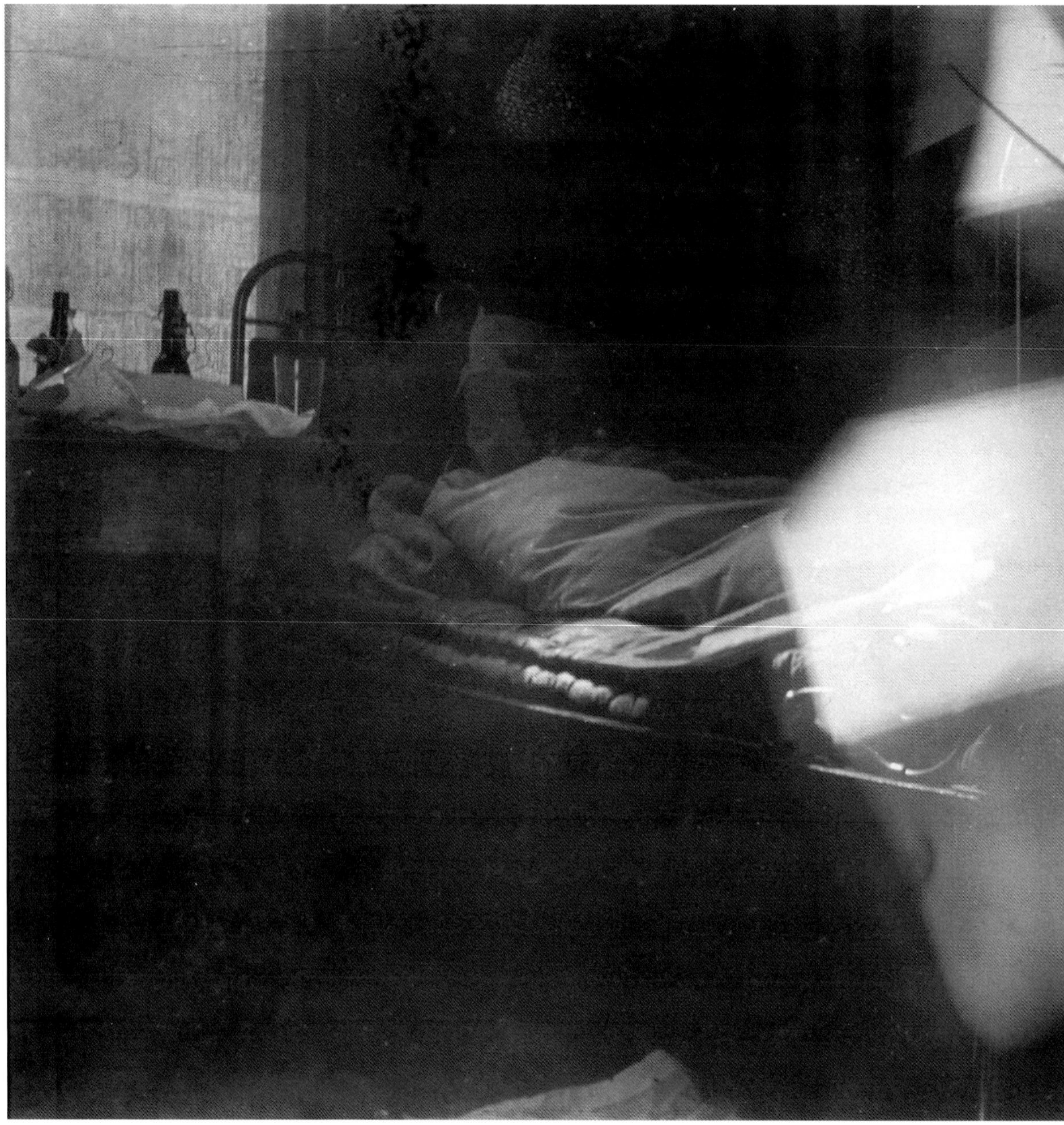

335 (*facing page*) Edvard Munch, *The Death of Marat* (photograph), 1908–9, Munch Museum, Oslo

shooting episode with Larsen, he had begun a series of photographs called *The Fatal Destiny*. They convinced him that his Kodak might be capable of conjuring a spirit world after all. In 1908 he resumed work on this highly experimental portfolio, aiming at images that hover between presence and absence. By moving the camera during its minute-long exposure, or moving his pose while the shot was being taken, he created a haunting series of self-portraits that seem to waver on the very edge of perception (pl. 333).

Such photographs convey the sense of fear and isolation that often assailed him in the clinic. They seem to arise from his conviction that corporeal solidity was about to fade, dissolving into the void. That is why he also tried to make photographic versions of paintings where illness and death had been his dominant themes. Munch recreated *The Sick Child*, playing the part of the ailing girl himself (pl. 334). He even wound a bed-sheet round his body in the clinic's bathroom, taking a photograph of himself laid out near a tub reminiscent of David's

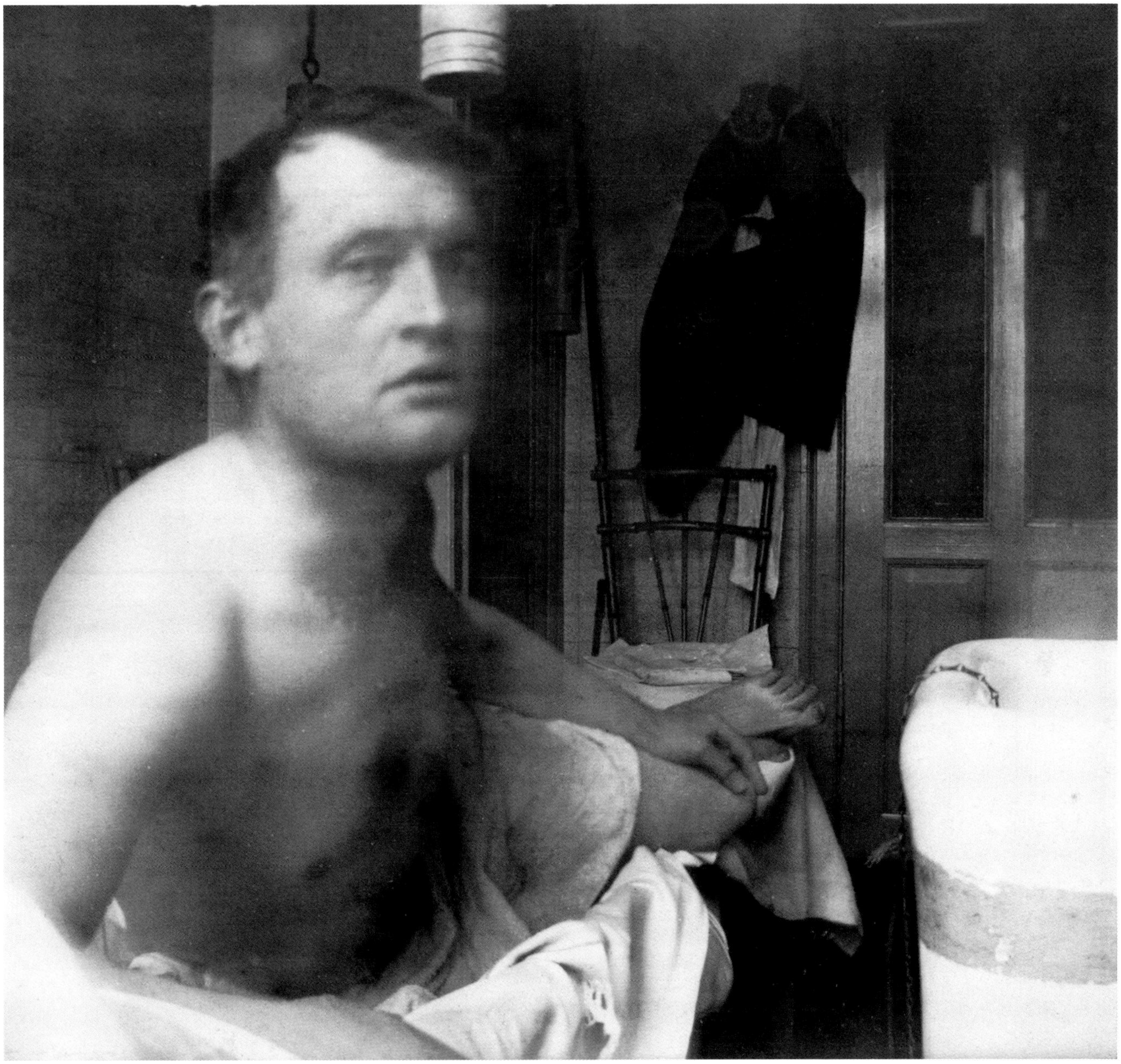

Death of Marat as well as Munch's own painted version of the murderous theme (pl. 335). However, the most eerie and unforced images show him walking past his paintings in a blurred form. It is as if he takes a journey through his life, from earlier canvases to more recent work (pl. 336). The artist's growth is charted, and in the most phantom-like photographs Munch's own body seems to melt into the pictures he had produced with brush and pigment. Is he suggesting that his work will outlive him and is therefore more substantial? Munch did not explain, but the idea of a fusion between the painter and his canvases is certainly explored in these grave, spiritual and very original photographs.

He even succeeded in persuading the clinic's nurses to participate. Whether or not they posed for his Kodak with Jacobsen's permission, the women appear willing to submit themselves to Munch's photographic experiments (pl. 337). Sometimes he was relatively restrained, arranging the nurses in variations on the theme of black and

336 (*right*) Edvard Munch, Munch walking past his paintings (photograph), Munch Museum, Oslo

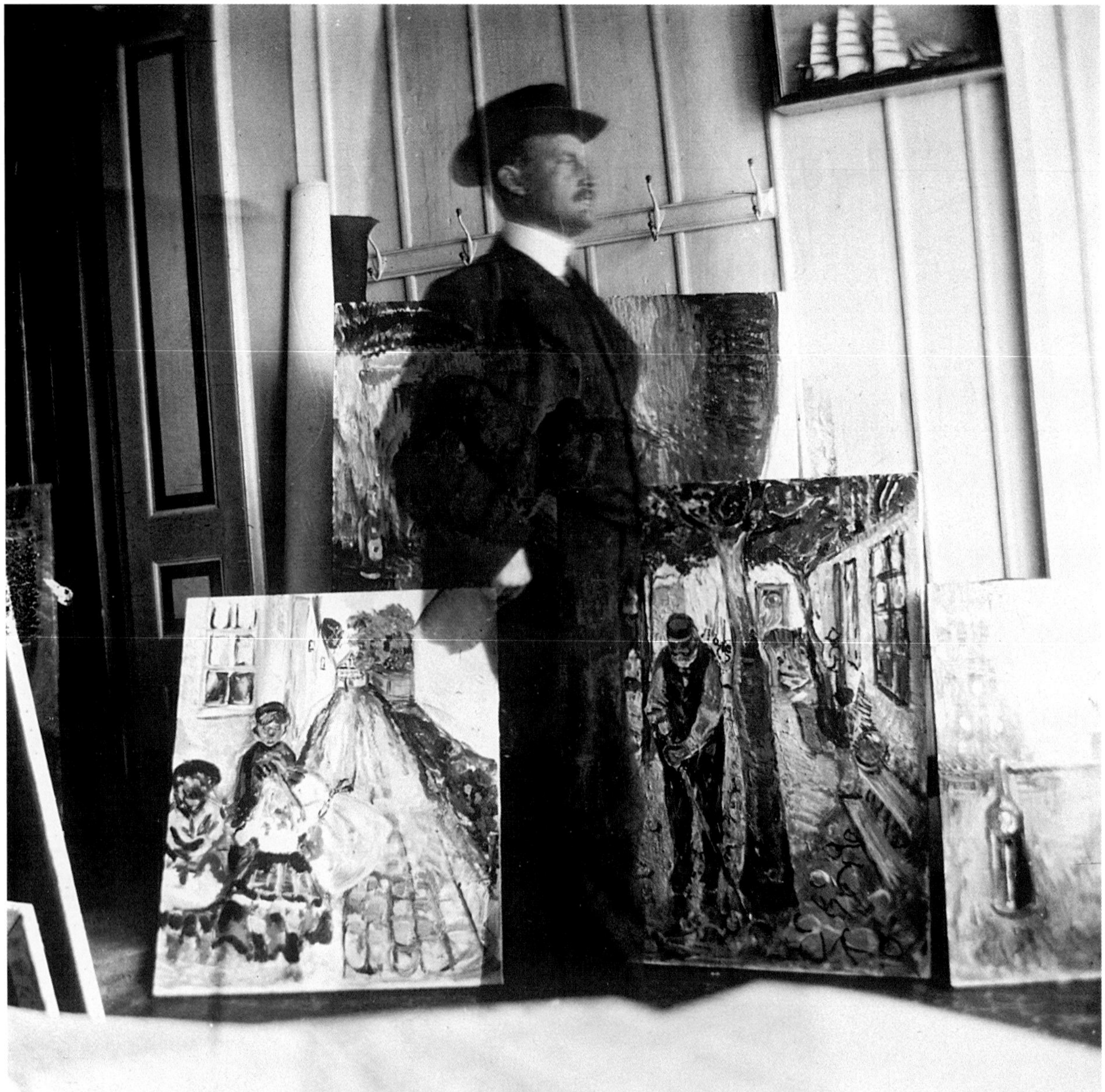

337 (*facing page, top*) Edvard Munch, Photograph of nurses, 1908–9, Munch Museum, Oslo

338 (*facing page, bottom*) Edvard Munch, Nurse posing as Sphinx, 1908–9, Munch Museum, Oslo

white uniforms. Just as he had explored extremes of light and dark in his painted portrait of Jacobsen (see pl. 331), so here a nurse dressed in black seems intended as a shadow cast by her white-uniformed companion. Munch was fascinated by these smudgy, phantom-like forms but he was still involved with the sexually desirable women who had appeared in his most seductive earlier paintings. Hence his decision to ask one nurse to copy the beguiling stance of the nude siren preening herself in an uninhibited canvas called *Sphinx (Woman in Three Stages)*. Perhaps to his surprise, the plump and homely figure agrees to his request with relish, smiling as she poses as a *femme fatale* for Munch's insatiable lens (pl. 338).

He must have realised that the nurse photographs ran the risk of incurring Jacobsen's displeasure. In his darkest moments, Munch wondered whether he would ever be allowed to escape from the institution: 'Don't you believe for a minute that it is easy to get out of such a clinic!' he wrote, complaining that 'when they ask you something, you don't answer the way you'd like to; instead you have to consider the question carefully and decide what they *want* you to say. If you don't come up with the exact answer you'll never get out.'[42] Nor was Munch convinced that he even wanted to leave the protection of Jacobsen's womb-like shelter. When he tried to go for a walk on his own outside the clinic, often to the neighbouring zoo where animals could be drawn, the old feelings of unbearable fear often assailed him once more.

For the moment, at least, he preferred to stay put in his bedroom-cum-studio. It was there that Munch painted a large, meditative and painfully revealing *Self-Portrait in Copenhagen*, where the middle-aged patient assesses his own condition with as much honesty as possible (pl. 339). Also known as *Self-Portrait in the Clinic*, it shows him seated in the room where he spent so much time working, sleeping and worrying. Unlike his most celebrated earlier painting of himself, the nocturnal and mysterious 1895 *Self-Portrait with Cigarette*, this new image specifies a considerable amount of information about his surroundings. The now unbarred window behind him looks ample and Munch includes a glimpse of the view beyond. Yet it does not promote a feeling of liberation. On the contrary: by summarising the facade of the building on the opposite side of the street, he creates a sense of claustrophobic enclosure. Perhaps he hoped to counter this entrapment by showing the window opening into his room. Sunlight appears to invade the wall behind him, and the horizontal streaks of orange blaze on an otherwise unpainted expanse of white canvas. Even so, those same streaks convey tension as well. They gather round his head with a disconcerting ferocity and the often straggling brushstrokes seem to echo the uncertainty inside his mind.

One side of his chair is set on fire by the same high-keyed colour. It contrasts with the dark sobriety of Munch's clothes, painted forcefully enough to establish him as a far more palpable presence than the ghostly figure in many of his contemporaneous photographs. This painting has also been called *Self-Portrait in a Blue Suit* and the garment certainly plays a potent role. In telling contrast to Munch's portrait of Jacobsen (see pl. 331), who opens up his jacket with an expansive gesture, the blue suit here is tightly buttoned up. Unlike the doctor, whose arms jut out at powerful diagonals, Munch allows his left arm to hang down. His right arm rests on the chair, suggesting that he needs its support. And his expression is sombre as he peers out at a future filled with uncertainty.

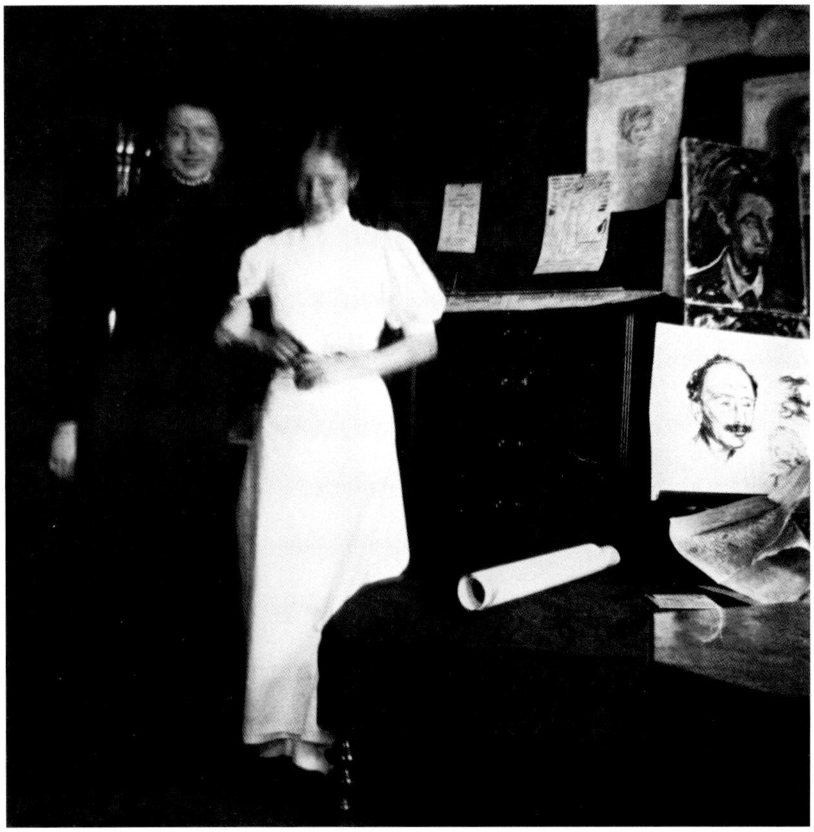

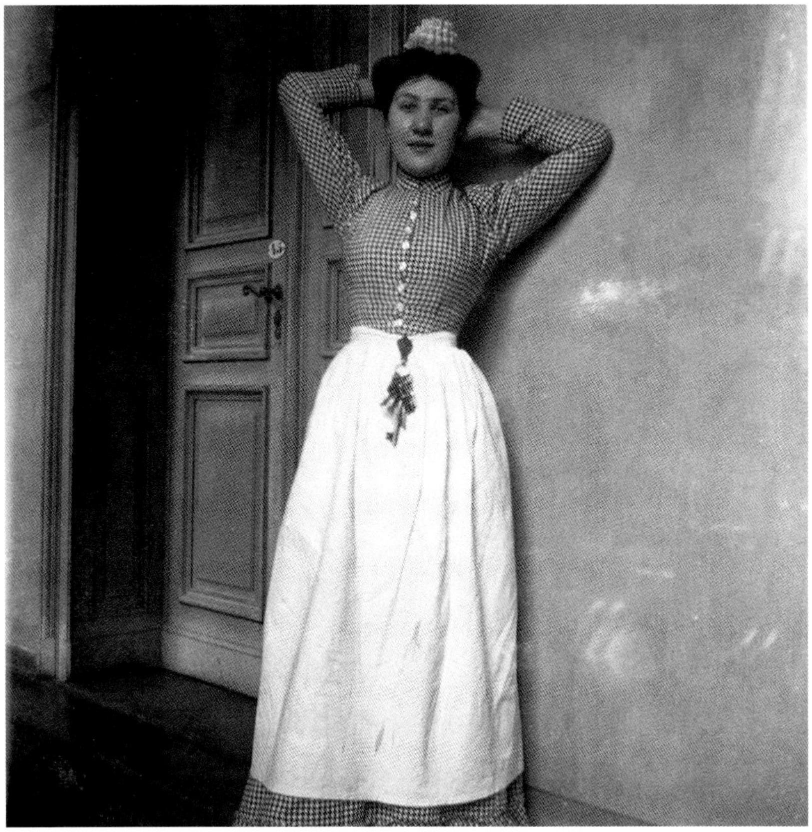

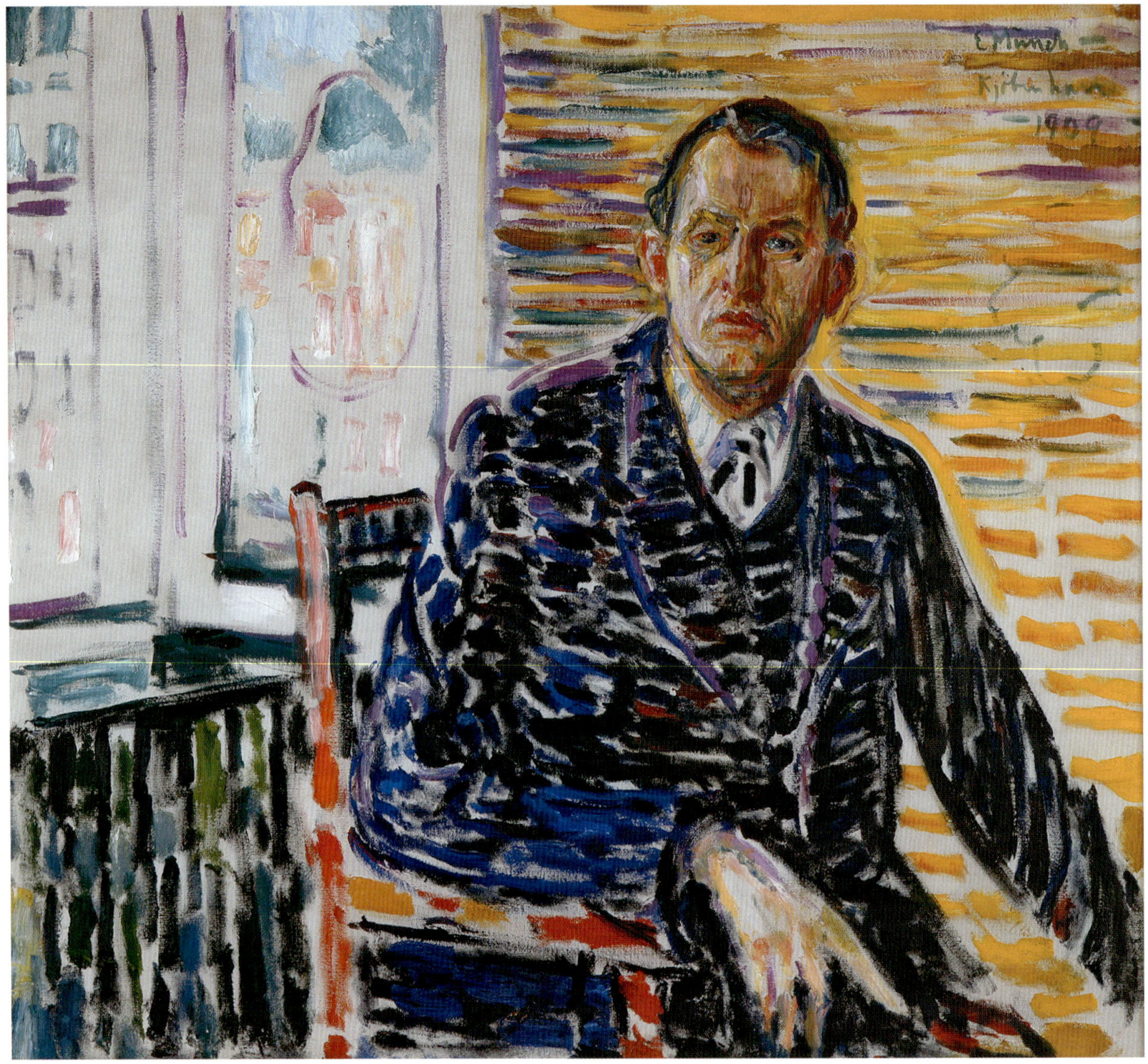

339 Edvard Munch, *Self-Portrait in Copenhagen*, 1909, Kunstmuseum, Bergen

He does, however, let the index finger of his right hand adopt a pointing pose. Its alertness is surely significant, standing out against the darkness behind and suggesting a determination to be positive. Munch may be buttoned up but there is something contained and decisive about his entire body now. He seems bent on sobering up, gaining control over his life and, above all, embarking on a sustained body of new work. The face still looks weary and he is clearly struggling to emerge from his ordeal. But resolve can be detected in his eyes and stubborn, downturned mouth. He appears to be preparing for action, and in a lithographic self-portrait made at the clinic Munch celebrates his decision to give up smoking. Clutching his final cigar before it is stubbed out for good, he stares defiantly through the smoke like a man on the edge of regaining some of his lost poise and charisma.

Eventually, in May 1909, he felt capable of returning home. His fear of leaving had receded and he asked his cousin Ludvig Ravensberg to assist him with preparations for the journey. As if to prove that his mischievous sense of humour had returned, Munch arrayed himself in a white tie and pinned on the St Olav's Cross before saying goodbye to the clinic's other patients. 'Peer Gynt', he announced with flamboyant irony, 'bids farewell to his fellow lunatics.'[43] He must have been surprised when Jacobsen enquired whether he could accompany the award-winning artist on his

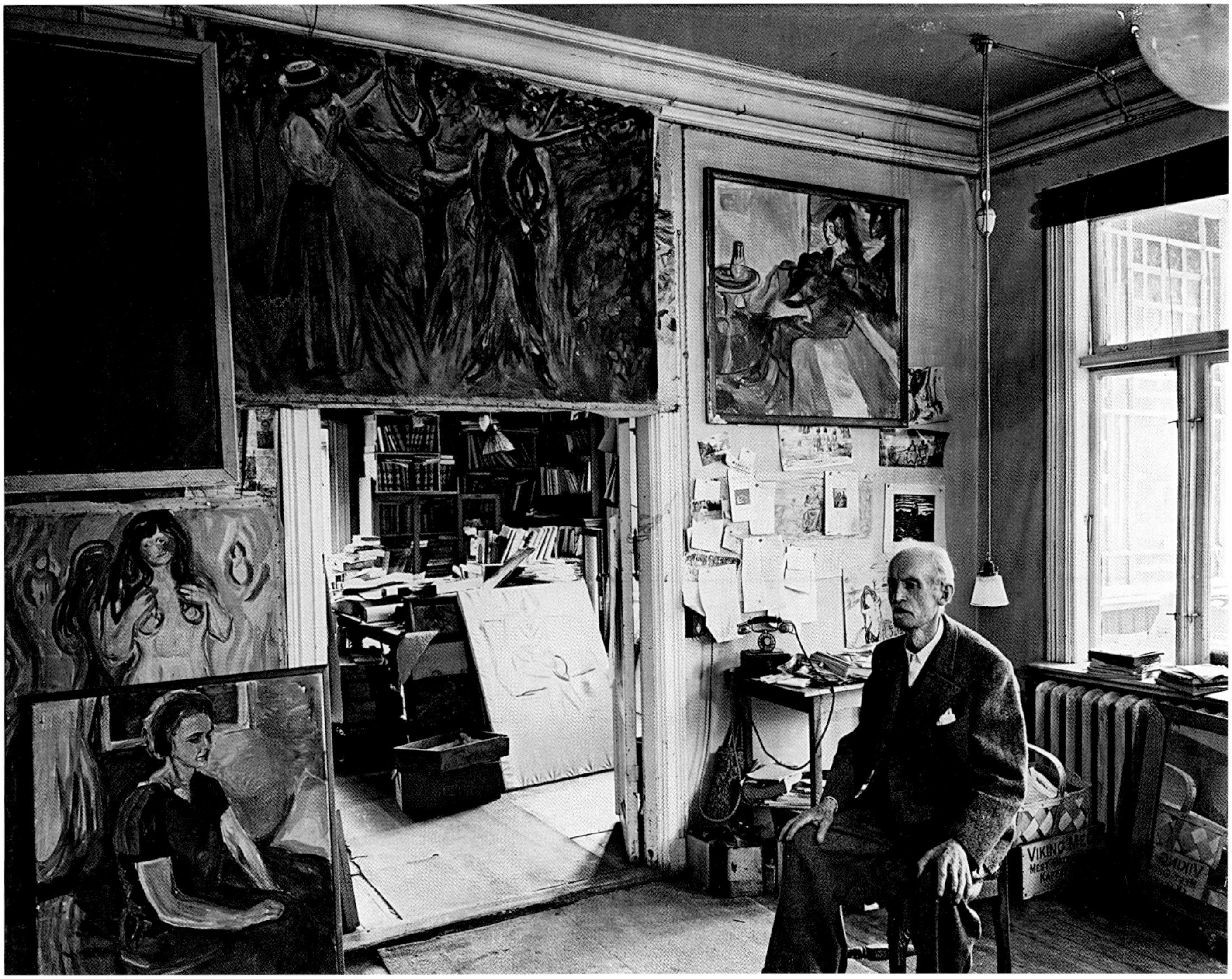

340 Edvard Munch, Photograph of Munch exposing his damaged finger, 1943

boat-trip back to Norway. The doctor may have entertained fantasies about benefiting from his proximity to such a renowned patient. Munch, however, failed to respond to Jacobsen's request

Nor did he show any desire to keep in contact with the doctor after his departure. When Jacobsen posted Munch several drawings mysteriously left behind in the clinic, he asked if they could be signed and returned to Copenhagen. Munch, however, simply kept the sketches, and did not recognise the doctor on the only occasion when they met in later years. Astonished and doubtless offended, Jacobsen identified himself. Munch stared at him, waving a hand across the physician's face before declaring: 'But you're a completely different colour this time.'[44]

The truth is that Jacobsen, for all his faults, deserves credit for helping Munch regain some degree of mental composure. Regaining his energy, he led a prolific life for more than three further decades after leaving the clinic. Yet he continued to insist on concealing the most disturbing sign of the violent incident that had done so much to unhinge his mind. After his death, more than forty gloves were discovered among his possessions. They had been used to sheathe his bullet-shattered finger, and only once could Munch bring himself to bring it out of hiding (pl. 340). Just before he died, the Kodak was used to take a single, elegiac photograph of the old man willing, at last, to expose his wound.

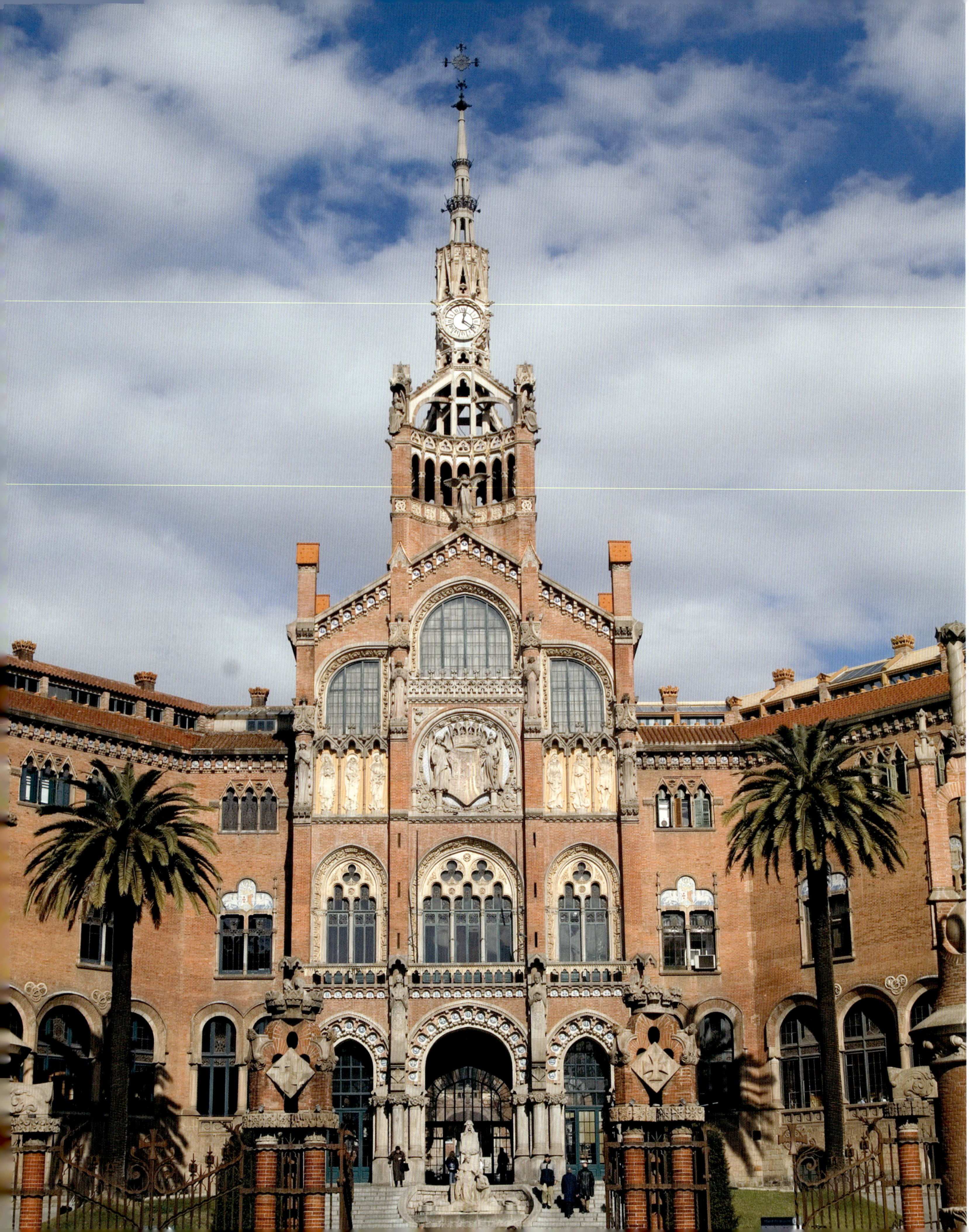

TWENTY-TWO
FROM EXUBERANT OPTIMISM TO THE TRAUMA OF WAR

The twentieth century's advance was marked, in burgeoning Barcelona, by a hospital embellished with ornament to a flamboyant degree. In 1902 work began on the Hospital de La Santa Creu i Sant Pau, an ebullient demonstration of Catalan culture's belief in the civic progress which economic expansion could bring about (pl. 341). Lluís Domènech i Montaner, the man responsible for this prodigious edifice, was the most outstanding member of a school of architects who flourished in Barcelona during the early years of the century. 'They became involved in the growth of political Catalanism and contributed to the ever more rapid construction and enlargement of the city', wrote Ignasi de Solà-Morales, 'and they developed a universal view of architecture: technically experimental; optimistic in its forms of decoration; expressing a positive conception of the totality of the work of art; and constructed specifically for the new institutions of society and for the new ruling classes.'[1]

These proponents of *modernista* architecture were frowned on by Gaudí and his followers, who rejected modern urban life in favour of a theological and unashamedly visionary alternative. The architect should, they believed, provide a militant antidote to the growing materialism of Western society, and Gaudí supported the Catholic Church's denunciation of the *modernista* heresy. Despite these divergent views, architects like Domènech were undoubtedly stimulated by the presence of Gaudí's genius. The turn of the century was a period of extraordinary richness in Barcelona's architectural development and the spirit of innovative vitality affected the Hospital de Sant Pau. It is not, in the final analysis, as spectacular in its adornment as Domènech's subsequent masterpiece the Palau de la Música, where the headlong facade is emblazoned with mosaics by Lluís Bru while the uninhibited auditorium appears to be supported by Pau Gargallo's winged horses as they soar across the elaborately carved ceiling. Yet the Hospital de Sant Pau is still a *tour de force* of impassioned *modernista* exuberance.

Intended to replace the old and insanitary Hospital of the Holy Cross, severely affected by a disastrous fire in 1887, Domènech's building was funded by a munificent bequest to the city by Catalan banker Pau Gil i Serra. Laid out in accordance with a plan 'that looks more like a city centre than a hospital', as Tim Benton observed,[2] the building grows from its central reception area into a range of forty-eight self-contained pavilions. They stress the paramount importance of isolating each ward as completely as possible from infection. Robert Hughes described how 'Domènech set out to make the enormous site – 360 acres, nine full

341 (*facing page*) Lluís Domènech i Montaner, Hospital de La Santa Creu i Sant Pau, Barcelona, built from 1902

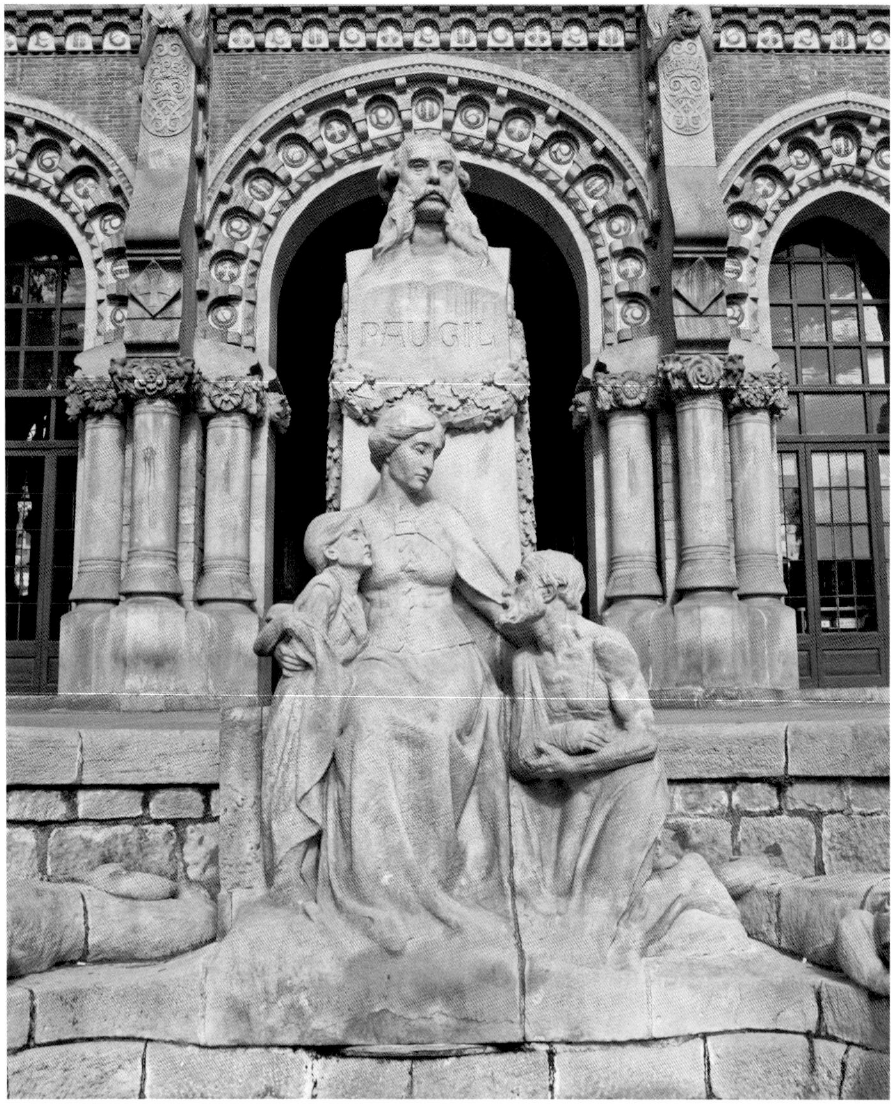

342 Eusebi Arnau and Pau Gargallo, Bust of Pau Gil, Hospital benefactor, Hospital de La Santa Creu i Sant Pau, Barcelona, built from 1902

blocks of the Eixample – a garden city within the grid city. He wanted, above all, to overcome the depressing, labyrinthine character that big general hospitals share with prisons. If the patients were to recover, they needed colour, an agreeable environment, fresh air, trees, a sense of ground underfoot.'[3]

A belief in the value of technology and experimentation is fused, here, with a more traditional respect for indigenous style. The new Hospital's facade, with its profusion of statuary both heraldic and ecclesiastical, exemplifies Domènech's irrepressible love of the decorative arts. Mosaic images enliven the frontage of the reception block with the history of the old Hospital, from the fifteenth century to the time of the calamitous fire. His willingness to produce an unfettered spectacle prevents the building from appearing academic in its attitude to the language of the past. Although Domènech was immensely learned and emphasised the need for historical study in his capacity as a Professor at the School of Architecture, he never deteriorated into sterile pedantry. His imagination was spirited enough to avoid revivalism for its own sake, and throughout the Hospital de Sant Pau the decorative elements are deployed with an impressive blend of delicacy and verve. If the carvings inside are *modernista* in spirit, Domènech eludes any attempt to classify his style. Praying stone figures rise between the interior archways, continuing the emphasis on carved symbolic statuary initiated outside, and the enhancement of spaces within the main building is executed in an infectiously animated manner. Domènech's sprightly building is charged, both within and without, by an implicit belief in the ability of modern medicine to aid and even transform the patients who benefited from its advances.

The heady sense of vivacity reached its playful climax in the sculpture, unleashing Domènech's uninhibited belief in the curative potential of art and architecture alike. His son, who completed the Hospital after Domènech's death, recalled how profoundly his father believed that if the most ordinary material 'was joined to the use of some rich material, even in small amounts, the thing acquired a character of richness, surprisingly so in view of its real price. So it was with the Hospital of Sant Pau, in which he thought that everything that could give a feeling of well-being to the sick was also a form of therapy.'[4] Hence his readiness to encourage a spirit of outright festivity in the building's embellishment.

Wisely, Domènech asked two like-minded artists to head the team responsible for sculpture: Eusebi Arnau and Pau Gargallo. Both they and a legion of assistants set to work with zeal. Wherever one walks in the Hospital de Sant Pau, images in stone and ceramics intoxicate the eye. On ground level, even the solemn carved bust of the benefactor Pau Gil is enlivened not only by his magnificently flowing side whiskers but also by two toads opening their mouths to gush water into the pool below (pl. 342). Further up the buildings, capitals surmounting columns sprout a profusion of flowers, insects and pullulating plant-life, while on the skyline, angels flaunt their curving wings as if

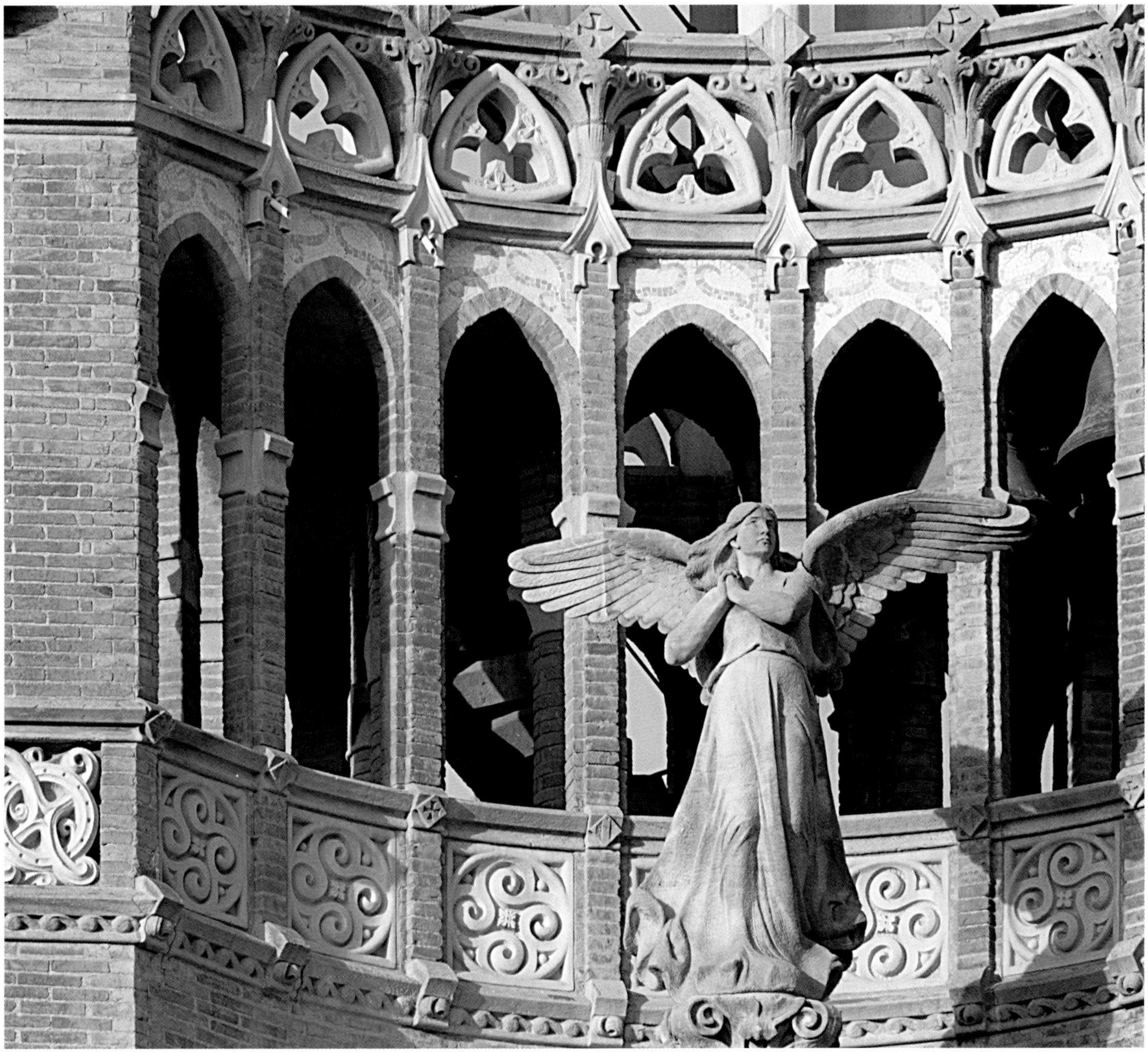

343 Eusebi Arnau and Pau Gargallo, Angel on the Hospital roof, Hospital de La Santa Creu i Sant Pau, Barcelona, built from 1902

poised to take flight (pl. 343). It all adds up to an overwhelmingly sensuous experience, celebrating a defiant spirit of fecundity and resilience in the face of even the most atrocious suffering.

This optimism was by no means universally shared. While the Hospital de Sant Pau was being constructed, Gustav Klimt found himself obliged to defend his immense painting of *Medicine* against critical vilification. Commissioned for the ceiling of the Festival Hall in the University of Vienna, the picture had already reached the stage of a composition study during the terminal years of the old century. Its powerful aura of *fin-de-siècle* melancholy was carried over intact to the final painting, which turned out to be dominated, paradoxically, by a mood of helplessness in the face of disease (pl. 344). Hygieia, the goddess of health, stands calm and erect in the foreground with the air of a priestess, holding her symbolic serpent and cup. Yet this gilded deity looks oddly detached from the people she is supposed to be helping. Indeed, she seems incapable of dealing effectively with the suffering swarms of humanity piled high above her. Although one naked woman stands apart from this agonised group, as if wishing to escape, her exhausted appearance suggests that nobody is able to escape the skeleton of Death lodged within the main huddle of figures.

The whole image expresses a profound feeling of despair in the face of affliction and mortality itself. Most of the University professors were offended by the fatalistic temper of Klimt's decorations, which

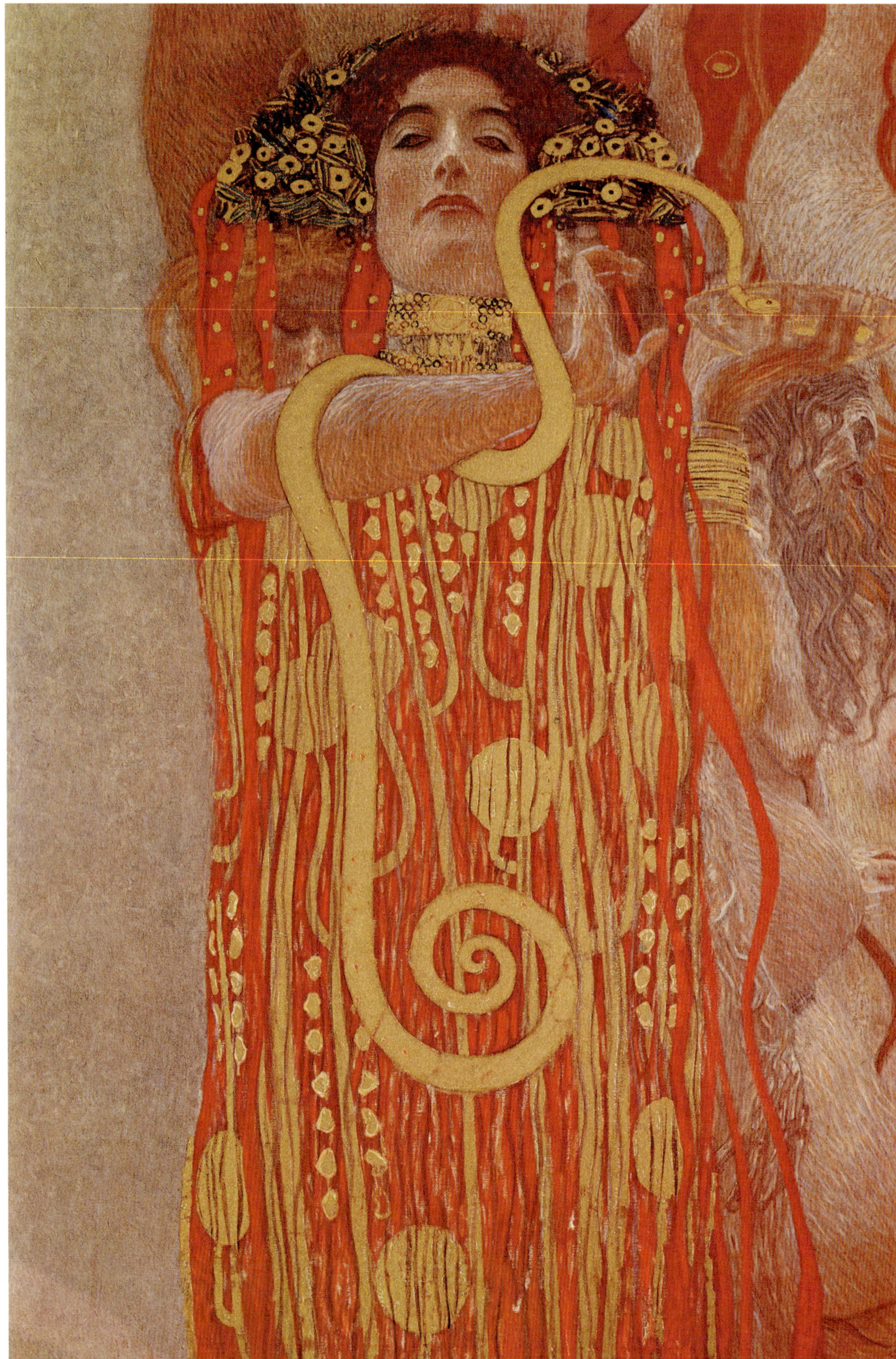

344 Gustav Klimt, *Medicine*, detail of Hygieia, 1900–07, University of Vienna, Destroyed in a fire at Castle Immendorf in 1945

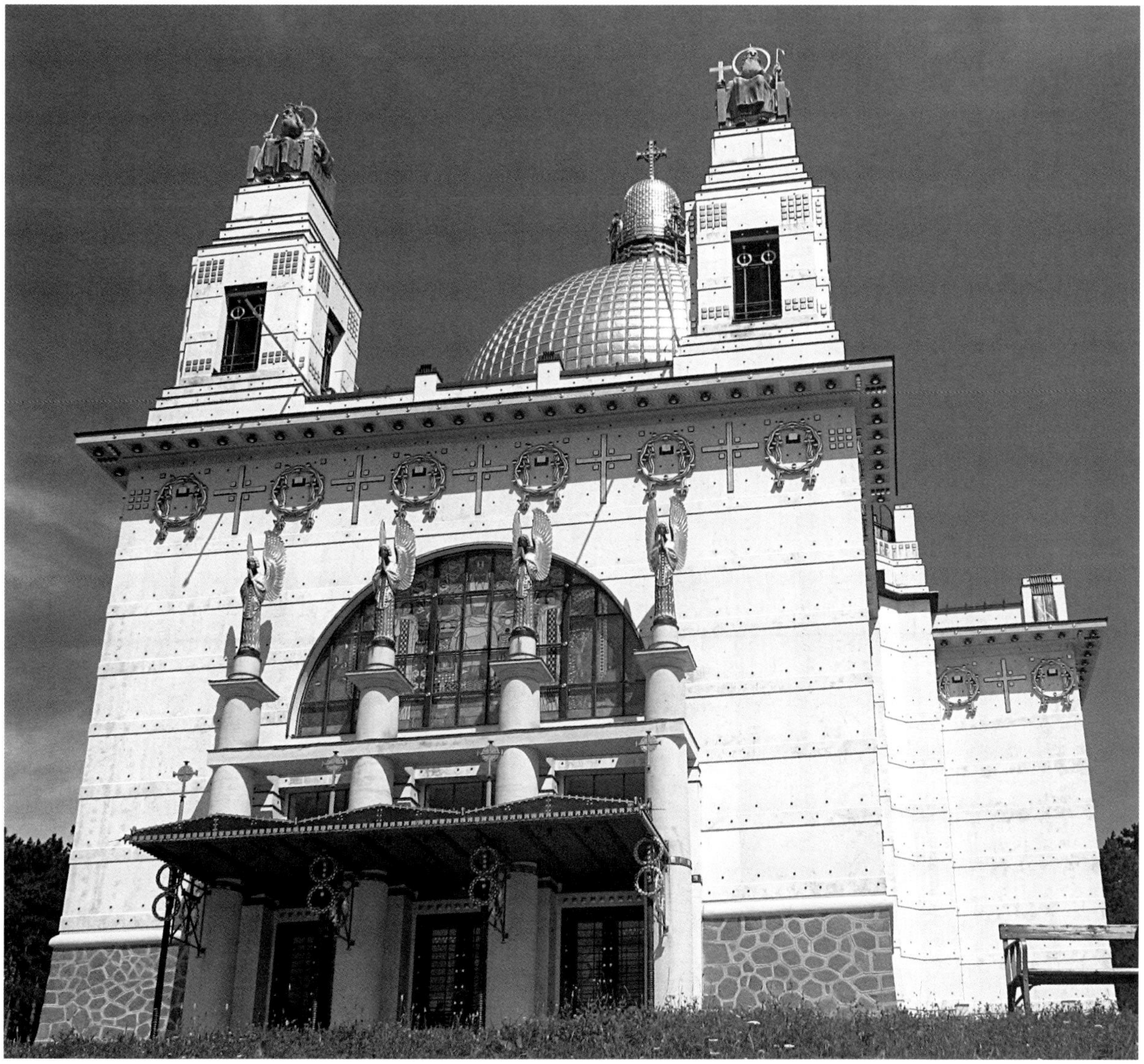

345 Richard Luksch, Saints Leopold and Severinus on towers and four angels above entrance, Church of St Leopold 'am Steinhof', Vienna, built 1904–7

included equally pessimistic interpretations of *Philosophy* and *Jurisprudence*.[5] They protested against the inference in *Medicine* that 'it is not medical progress that relieves human agony'[6] in a world overshadowed by the Nietzschian dynamic of eternal recurrence. Moreover, Karl Kraus claimed that he detected another layer of subversive meaning in the painting, acidly remarking that Klimt had produced an image 'in which the chaotic muddle of decrepit bodies symbolizes conditions at the General Hospital'.[7]

In September 1904, however, the foundation stone was laid for a Viennese building that proposed a vision of medical care more optimistic by far than Klimt's doomed allegory. His compatriot, Otto Wagner, had designed the immense and exalted church of St Leopold 'am Steinhof' for the patients of the Lower Austrian Institution and Sanatorium (pl. 345). Practical priorities were addressed with great seriousness and enlightened care throughout the church, so that its congregation benefited from excellent acoustics, ventilation, clear views of the altar and a sacristy for use as a treatment room should an emergency arise. Wagner's concern for the patients also led him to make the vestry available as a confessional for people with weak hearing, and he designed unusually short benches with room for a maximum of five, so that anyone afflicted by a sudden fit could be reached with ease, speed and quiet tact. Such considerations earned him formidable antagonism among Catholics, who condemned the church for its unduly secular atmosphere. Peter Vergo described how 'only the intervention of various highly placed personages, among them Dr Friedrich Piffl, Archbishop of Vienna, and Prince Liechtenstein, succeeded in quelling the architect's enemies'.[8]

The defence campaign was strengthened enormously when Wagner commissioned a complex and resplendent array of decorations by leading Secessionist artists. The exterior of the building, its white marble purity complemented by the gleam of a gilded dome acting as a burnished landmark for miles around, was further embellished by two prominent sculptors. Seated magisterially on each of the flanking towers are the patron saints of Lower Austria, Leopold and Severinus, who preside over their surroundings with massive certitude. The authority invested in them by their maker, Richard Luksch, contrasts felicitously with the altogether more ethereal character of the four elongated angels positioned above the principal entrance. Carried out in gilded copper, they clasp their hands in prayer while majestic wings curve up behind them in readiness for flight. Othmar Schimkowitz ensured that none of these graceful, attenuated figures disturbs the prevailing vertical thrust of the columns on which they rest. The angels appear to offer their blessings to anyone entering below, and inside the church all the decorative elements were used with similar devotional intent.

Determined to avoid using either canvas or what he acidly dismissed as 'the unreliable fresco technique which created so many difficulties',[9] Wagner insisted that the windows designed by Kolo Moser for the vault-crossing, organ-loft and side altars were carried out in a new mosaic technique. Composed of marble, glass, pottery and vitrified enamel, they enhanced both the splendour and the religious intensity of an airy interior where Wagner installed a vaulted ornamental ceiling within the dome. He had originally invited Moser to design the most important wall-mosaics in the church as well, extending above the high and side altars. Moser's study for the guardian angel over one of the side altars, fusing spiritual ardency with flamboyant patterning, suggests that the outcome would have been memorable (pl. 346). But his conversion to Protestantism led to a deterioration in relations with Wagner and the commission was never executed. Instead, the glass wall-mosaics above the side altars were designed by Rudolf Jettmar, while the most important decoration of all for the high altar, was given to Remigius Geyling (pl. 347). Its straightforward, even simple-minded organisation compares unfavourably with Moser's more sophisticated and intense imagination.

All the same, Geyling's towering image of a beneficent Christ, surrounded by his adoring followers, looks wholly at home in the interior it was

346 Kolo Moser, Study for guardian angel over side altar, 1904–5, Albertina, Vienna

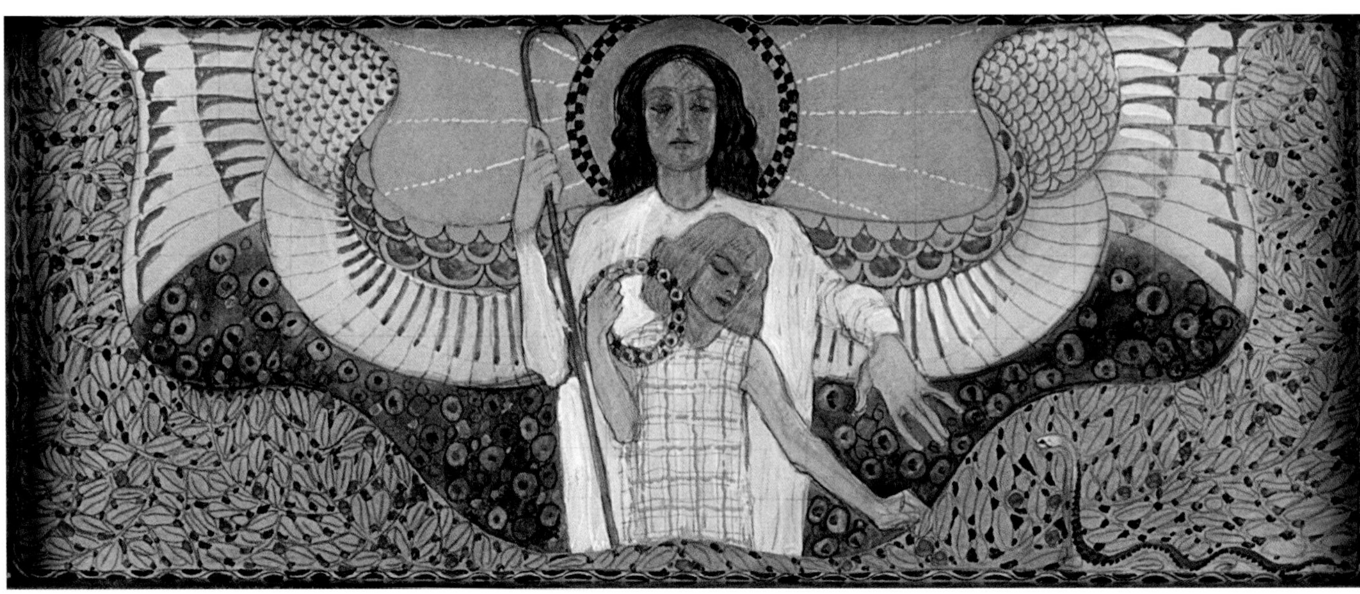

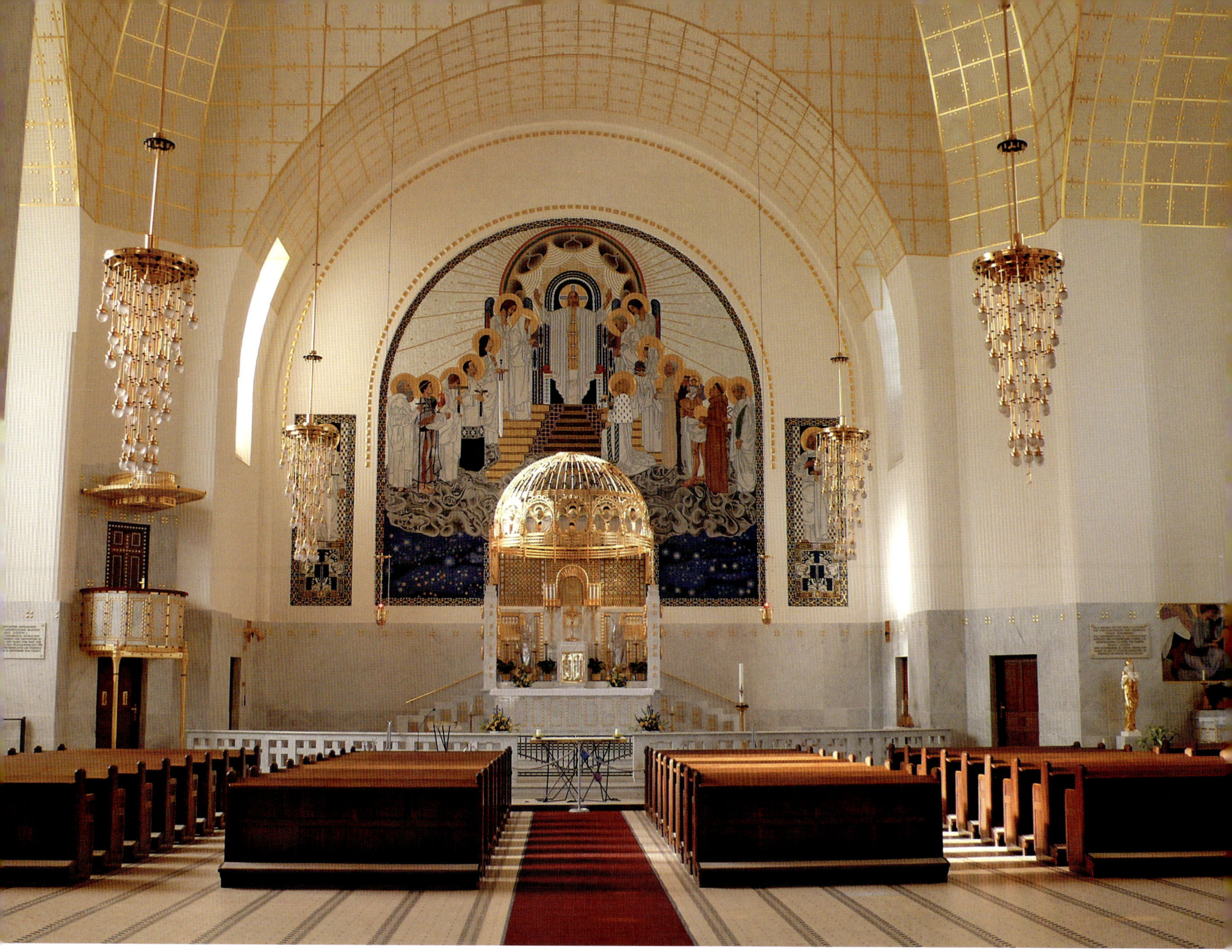

347 Remigius Geyling, Mosaic of Christ for high altar, Church of St Leopold 'am Steinhof', Vienna, built 1904–7

intended to enhance. Its predominantly pale colours accord well with the restraint Wagner exercised on the other walls, while the emphasis on flat pattern-making promotes a hieratic stillness thoroughly attuned to the rigorous delicacy of the architectural ornamentation elsewhere in the building. No wonder Archbishop Piffl declared, when he dedicated the altar mosaic, that 'I myself, when I entered the church, was literally seized by the monumental character of the building. I was overcome by the feeling: This is truly that holy place, of which it is written, Take off your shoes, leave all worldly thoughts behind you and turn to Him for whom this house of God was created!'[10] Many of the patients confronted by Wagner's beatific interior, with its air of reassuring protection culminating in Christ's outstretched and welcoming arms at the apex of Geyling's altar image, must surely have shared these sentiments and felt comforted.

Around the same time, Constantin Brancusi also suffered the mutilation of a work he had undertaken as a medical commission. In 1903, as a graduate of the Bucharest Academy of Fine Arts, he produced a plaster relief portrait of Dr Carol Davila, a distinguished army general and scientist who had founded the Military School of Medicine

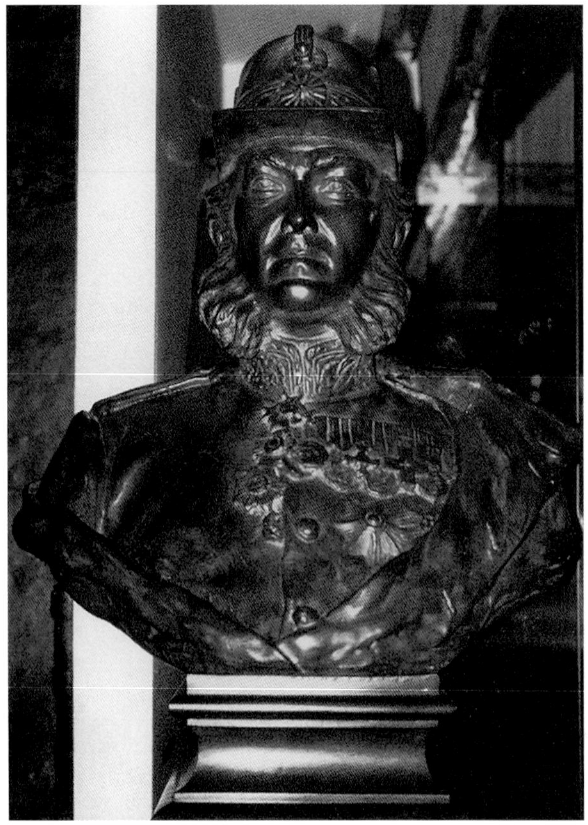

348 Constantin Brancusi, Bronze bust of Dr Carol Davila, 1912, Queen Elizabeth Military Hospital, Bucharest

in Bucharest. This preliminary image seems to have gratified his patrons at the Queen Elizabeth Military Hospital. Acting on a recommendation from another doctor, they commissioned Brancusi to make a plaster bust of the same sitter. Yet the bronze version was not installed in the hospital courtyard until 1912, for extensive alterations were inflicted on the plaster image after Brancusi had completed it and left Romania to settle in Paris (pl. 348). The military cap, which gave the plaster much of its vitality, was removed along with Dr Davila's arms. This truncated version of Brancusi's original portrait mortified the sculptor when he saw it on a visit to Bucharest in 1938. Quite understandably, he threatened legal action against the perpetrators of this unwarranted dismemberment, but by that time it was too late to register a protest: the plaster bust had vanished and only a photograph now testifies to Brancusi's original conception of the ill-fated Queen Elizabeth commission.[11]

Edouard Vuillard's major painting *The Surgeons*, commenced in 1912, has survived. At its centre is Dr Antonin Gosset, the eminent surgeon and urologist, engaged in an operation at his Parisian clinic on rue Antoine-Chantin. Vuillard, doubtless aware of Toulouse-Lautrec's earlier painting of Dr Péan (see pl. 311), produced with distemper and pastel a blanched, intense image where everyone – from the seated anaesthetist to the nurse with upraised arms – concentrates on the act of healing. A large basin in the foreground resembles a floodlight, and Vuillard did his utmost to illuminate the curative significance of a scene which impressed him profoundly when he witnessed it in May 1912. Unlike Munch's *On the Operating Table* (see pl. 327), Vuillard's painting opts for cool objectivity. The critic Claude Roger-Marx was right to emphasise how *The Surgeons* centres on

> the precious relations between so many shades of white: head-dresses, blouses, cloths, walls varnished with Ripolin, nickeled instruments; the lightness of the shadows, the character of hands and faces saturated with an aseptic atmosphere. Nurses, operator, and assistants are so many draped statues. A great white silence prevails, shot through with a sense of tragedy; but death and blood do not come into the picture, as they do in Rembrandt's.[12]

British hospitals of the period were occasionally prepared to furnish their exteriors with statuary. When a vast new Infirmary was erected in Glasgow between 1905 and 1915, the main entrance found itself crowned by a somnolent effigy of Queen Victoria, commemorating her reign in the most stolid and imperial manner. Most interiors were granted no imagery to offset their sparseness, however. Views of hospital rooms at this time are rare, but a photograph has survived of the Outpatients Waiting Hall at the Great Northern Central Hospital in 1912. Founded in 1856 to give medical care to the sick poor of north London, the building was relentlessly austere. No pictures were hung on the wall to alleviate the grimness of the Outpatients area, and just before the First World War broke out Wyndham Lewis lamented the fact that few opportunities presented themselves to artists eager to move outside the limits of the gallery. 'Formerly there were chapels, monasteries, and temples ready for the artist whose soul was too religious for his work to be mere entertainments and drawing-room pictures', he told a reporter in an angry interview headlined 'Rebel Art in Modern Life'. 'Today there is practically nothing. G. F. Watts offered to decorate Euston Station, and was refused. If I offered to decorate a working men's college or hospital I should meet with similar difficulties, no doubt.'[13]

By that time, though, a concerted attempt had been made to organise a pressure group capable of creating an awareness of the need for architectural decoration. In November 1911 Roger Fry, who had recently completed with several other young painters an ambitious post-impressionist mural scheme at a London school, met Charles Aitken, the Director of the National Gallery of British Art (later the Tate Gallery). A few days afterwards a committee was established, under the chairmanship of D. S. MacColl, 'to promote the practice of mural painting in schools, churches, hospitals, and other public institutions, more especially by young artists and students, a scheme long ago propounded by Mr Watts'. These courageous words appeared in an announcement in *The Times* the following February, when the committee launched an appeal for funds to subsidise painters interested in mural schemes.[14]

Their designs were supposed to be chosen from a special mural painting exhibition held at Crosby Hall, Chelsea, in June, when one reviewer declared that 'if it were common practice for public bodies and private persons, having a wall space to be decorated, to call in a painter to decorate it, painters would have both a business and a definite problem.'[15] Although the exhibition does not appear to have inspired the commissions it hoped for, Fry was set on tackling several projects with artists who shared his post-impressionist persuasion. Writing to Vanessa Bell in October 1911, he had already asked her: 'You will come and do my wall won't you . . . And the London Hospital and all the other jobs.'[16] By the following spring, when Fry and his painter-friends had formed themselves into the Mill Street Club, they decided 'to compete as a group' for a mural scheme at the Middlesex Hospital in central London, 'and to submit a communal decorative plan which included panels by each of the members'.[17]

The project came to nothing as a practical venture, and was soon superseded by Fry's formation of the Omega Workshops. All the same, the choice of the Middlesex Hospital proved prophetic. In 1915 the South African banker and collector Edmund Davis (later knighted), who had settled in London at the beginning of the century, offered to finance improvements to the Entrance Hall of the old hospital building. As well as forming a major collection of contemporary art which is now in Cape Town, Davis sat on the Board of the Middlesex for many years. He wanted to create a memorable decorative scheme at the hospital, and commissioned Frederick Cayley Robinson to paint four large pictures entitled 'Acts of Mercy' for the Entrance Hall. Perhaps Davis was aware of Cayley Robinson's activities as Artistic Adviser to the Haymarket Theatre in London, where he decorated the Upper Circle Bar with compositions owing a great deal to the French Symbolist tradition. Despite his retiring and dream-like demeanour, he had achieved considerable worldly success in 1911 with costume and set designs for Maurice Maeterlinck's admired play *The Blue Bird*. Only a year before completing the first of the Middlesex Hospital pictures, Cayley Robinson won a competition for a mural decoration in Dublin Art Gallery, so he was well prepared for Davis's commission.

His attenuated and hushed vision, which owes something to first-hand knowledge of Pierre Puvis de Chavannes and the Nabis acquired during his student days in Paris, was ideally suited to the earliest two Entrance Hall paintings. Indeed, he may have been able to dictate their theme, for his previous work reveals a distinct propensity to select subjects such as *The Foundling* and *The Little Child Found*.[18] The first two Middlesex canvases, quietly interlinked, are called *Orphans* (pls 349 and 350). They contain serene friezes of girls who file down a narrow staircase or sit at a low refectory table for their simple, orderly meal. The prevailing mood is tender yet melancholy. Some of the orphans gaze out towards the viewer, as if appealing for sympathy.

Each of the paintings is delicately organised, and the windows set high in the compositions intensify a persuasive feeling of monastic enclosure. These spotless and compliant figures, whose starched uniforms are redolent of a religious order, seem to be hidden safely below ground level – far away from the terrifying world of conflict referred to, however indirectly, in the other Entrance Hall paintings. Withdrawn and inviolate, the orphans occupy their sanctum with a humility bordering on placid resignation. Cayley Robinson's harmonious sensibility is at its most refined in the painting where a lamp glows softly on the table, irradiating nearby faces

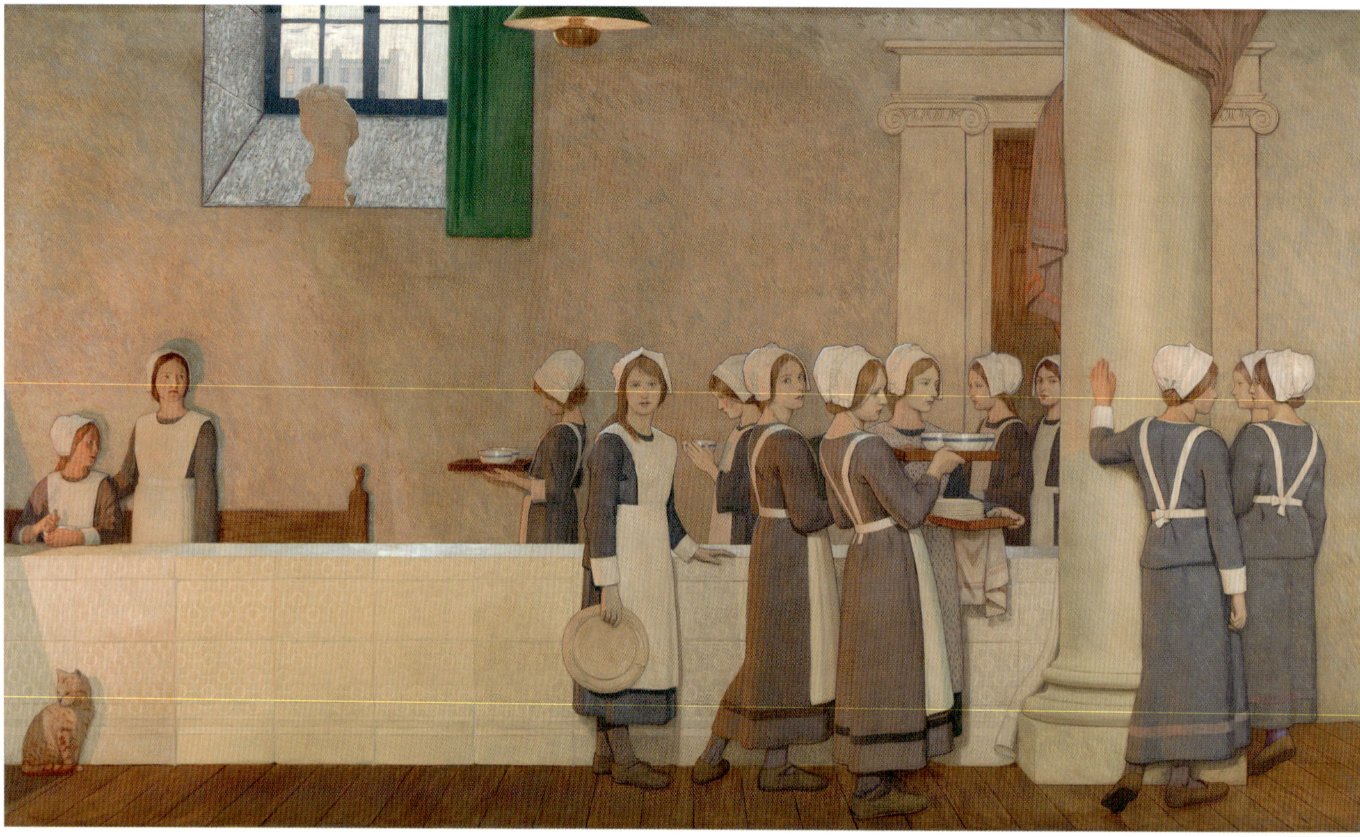

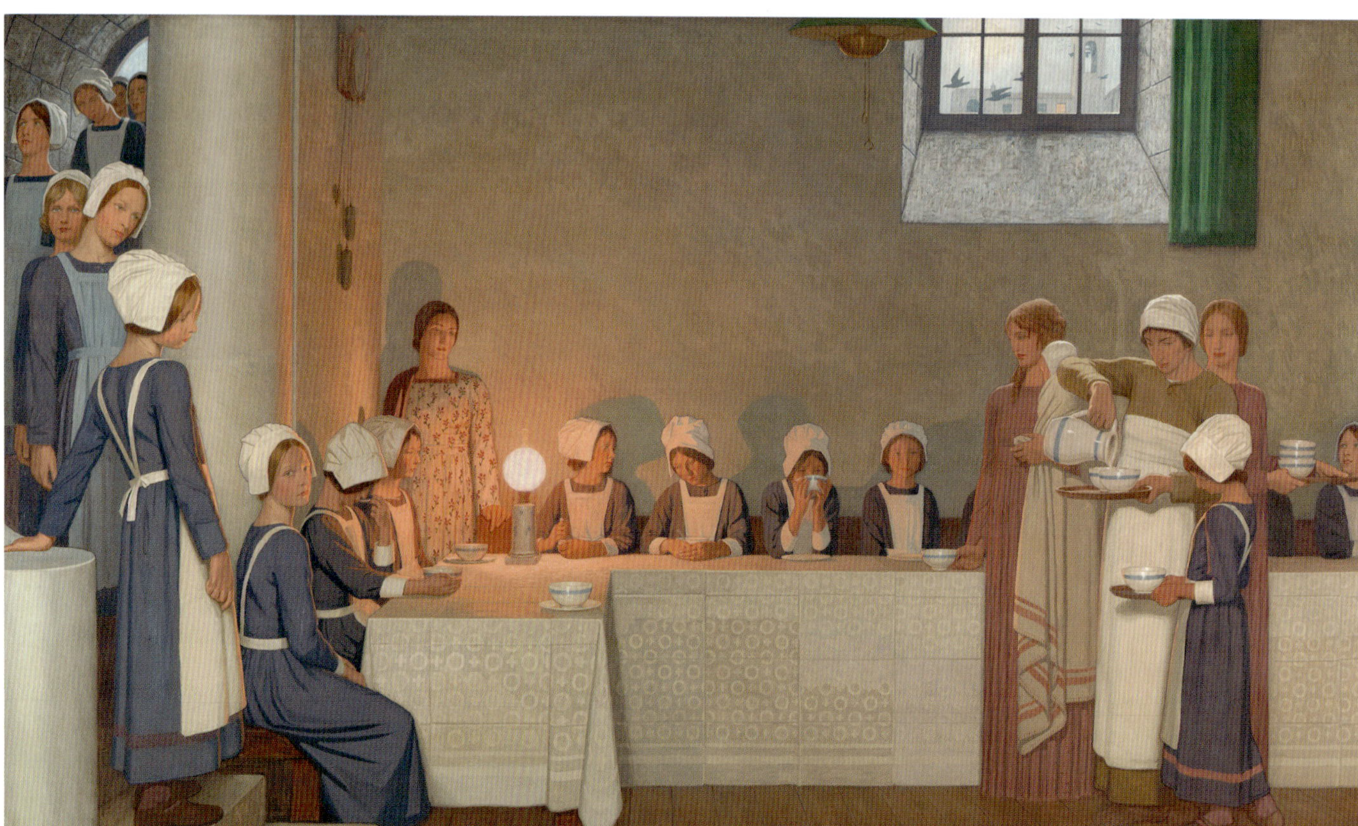

349 (*top*) and 350 (*bottom*) Frederick Cayley Robinson, *Orphans*, 1915, Wellcome Library, London

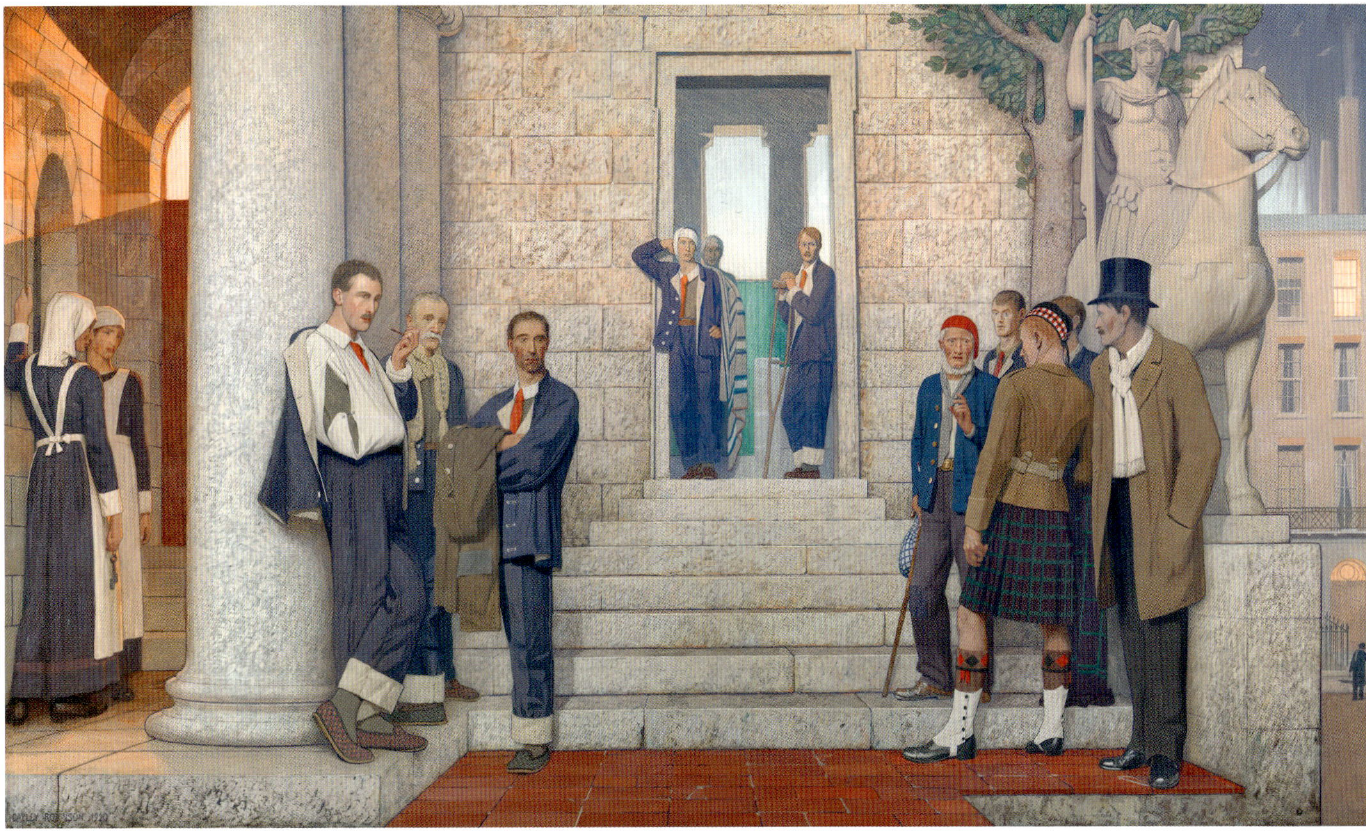

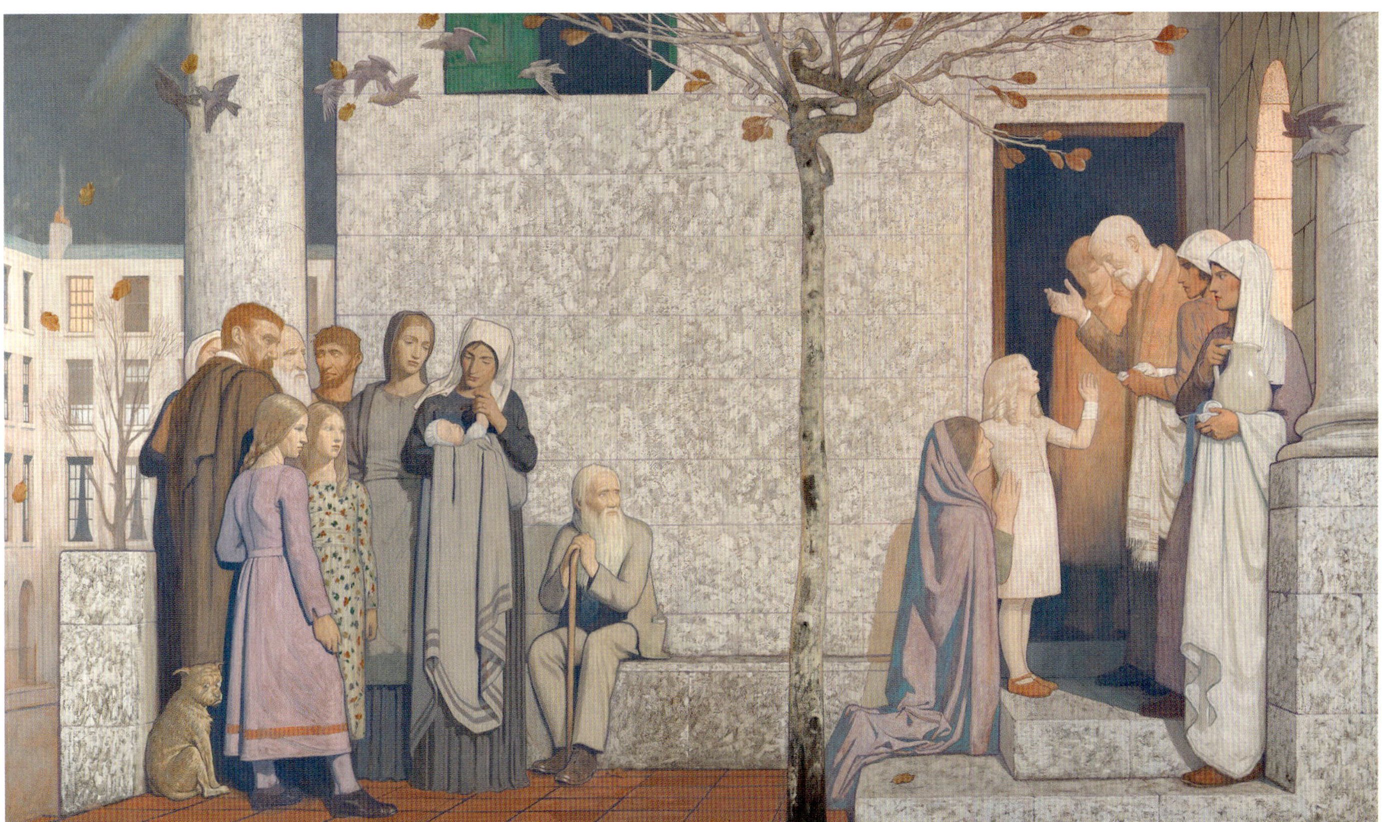

351 (*top*) and 352 (*bottom*) Frederick Cayley Robinson, *The Doctor*, left panel, top, 1920 and right panel, bottom 1916, Wellcome Library, London

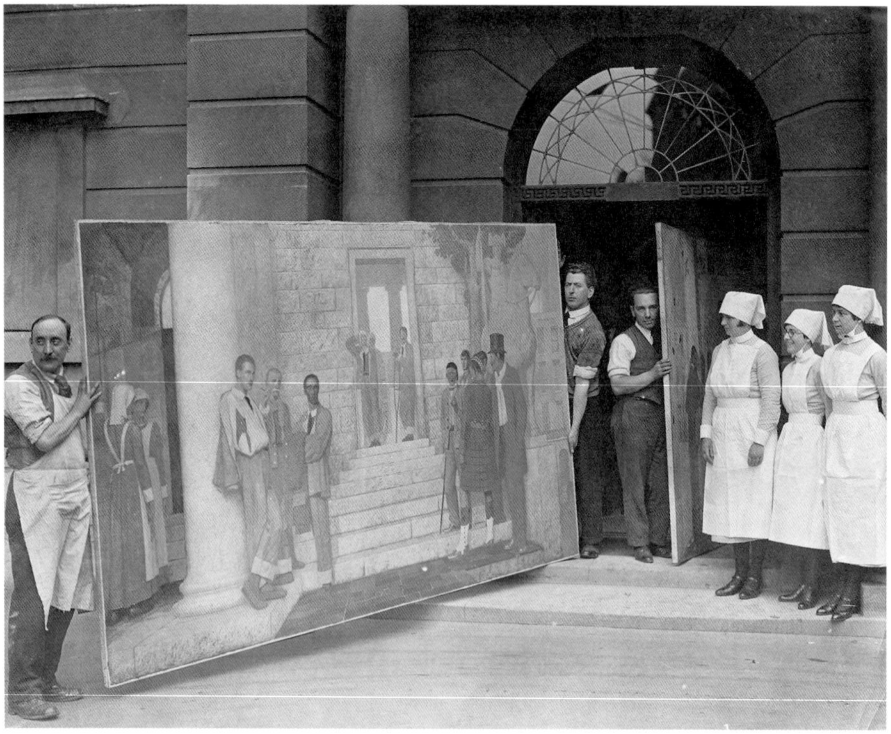

353 Photograph of Middlesex Hospital nurses watching the removal of Cayley Robinson's *The Doctor*, *c*.1930

with an almost visionary sense of beatitude. A maid pours milk into bowls with limpid blue-and-white stripes, and as the girls wait for their simple sustenance the scene takes on the heightened significance of an epiphany.

A similarly intense mood prevails in the other two Middlesex paintings, both called *The Doctor*. In the left-hand canvas, soldiers wounded or traumatised by war stand in front of the hospital looking stunned and haggard (pl. 351). Their slings and crutches show how well they are being treated, but their air of bewilderment is painfully clear. In the other painting (pl. 352), a bearded soldier resembling the artist himself stands among a group of equally still figures, who include an elderly man and a mother nursing her baby. Perhaps Cayley Robinson wanted to show how closely he identified with their suffering. Nearby, an isolated silver birch shedding its final leaves announces the imminent onset of winter. But beyond the tree a woman kneels to thank the doctor for helping her young, fair-haired daughter, who holds up her bandaged hand in a gesture of gratitude. Although the doctor himself looks old and exhausted by the long years of war, he responds to the girl with an almost religious devotion. It is a redemptive moment. As if to celebrate the girl's recovery, doves fly towards the nocturnal sky quickened by a spirit of soaring vitality.

Completed in 1920, the *Acts of Mercy* were widely admired by patients and staff, who ensured that the paintings were well cared-for when the old Middlesex building was demolished a decade later. A photograph survives of a *Doctor* canvas moving from the Entrance Hall while a row of attendant nurses stare at their departing picture with pride and regret (pl. 353). By this time, Cayley Robinson had died, but Davis, who eventually became Vice-President of the Hospital, ensured that the paintings were reinstated in similar, specially designed positions on the walls of the new Entrance Hall five years later. They remained there until 2007, constituting the most elaborate and quietly sustained painted decorations to be found in any early twentieth-century British hospital. Their uncertain future was secured when the Wellcome Trust acquired all four paintings for its Library in 2009.

A far less fortunate fate was inflicted on the defiantly profane decorations that Ernst Ludwig Kirchner carried out, during the Great War, in a remote location. Suffering from severe mental and physical exhaustion after active service, he found himself staying at the Kohnstamm sanatorium in Königstein, a small town sequestered in the Taunus Mountains north of Frankfurt. Here, probably during his initial stay in the spring of 1916, Kirchner responded positively to a suggestion by Dr Kohnstamm that he should paint a sequence of frescoes on the dining-hall ceiling. It was an ample arena, and the doctor thought that his debilitated patient might find therapeutic release in such a challenge.

The ceiling, where heavy beams divided the space into several grand areas for painting, appealed to the artist so powerfully that he 'wanted to divide up these fields into further smaller compositional groups, as in the Sistine Chapel'.[19] He had harboured leanings towards interior decorative schemes for many years and even in his weakened state Kirchner was prepared to take on this most prominent of sites in the sanatorium. Yet the proposal encountered formidable resistance from the other patients, anxious no doubt that such a vehement Expressionist rebel might produce a work unnerving enough to disturb their meal-times.

During the summer of 1916, when Kirchner returned to the sanatorium for a couple of months,

Dr Kohnstamm was nevertheless able to secure permission for an extensive project on the walls of the fountain-tower stairwell instead. In this more confined setting, where patients would not feel obliged to linger unless the paintings appealed to them, Kirchner executed five substantial panels in fresco *al secco*.[20] The misgivings harboured by the sanatorium's other inhabitants must have eased when they heard that he was intending to produce scenes inspired by bathing off idyllic Fehmarn. Kirchner could not, however, recapture the blitheness that had once prompted him to make paintings as celebratory as his 1912 *Striding into the Sea*. The intervention of a gruelling and traumatic war had affected him profoundly.[21] Whether or not he realised the extent of the decisive change in his imagination, the Königstein wall-paintings present a very different mood.

Sailing-boats and birds should have helped to ensure that cheerfulness prevails, and at first sight the naked figures seem to be savouring their island freedom. Yet signs of strain appear in the very first panel, where a diver's body is contorted with stiff-jointed harshness as he prepares to plunge into the sea. Next to him a man thrusts up an arm in either greeting or beseeching, an ambiguity that extends to the second panel. The woman who has wandered furthest into the sea raises both her arms, as if to wave at the diminutive figure in a distant boat. She might, alternatively, be gesturing more urgently, and Kirchner's terse, almost brutal handling of her body does nothing to allay the suspicion that she is about to give vent to alarm.

Since the frescoes were intended by Dr Kohnstamm to help his patient escape from the legacy of war trauma, Kirchner may have tried hard to concentrate on the most joyful and liberating aspects of his theme. Even so, the imaginative resources he brought to the task did not allow him to present an unqualified Fehmarn paradise. In the third panel, which shares with its counterparts a flat horizon for the sake of decorative unity, an enormous wave threatens to engulf the pair of female bathers (pl. 354). It should mark a moment of high excitement, and the small figure on the shore gesticulates with wonder at the spectacle, but Kirchner distorts his back so radically that he appears almost deformed. As for the women's faces, they register no obvious signs of pleasure while the wave gathers itself to overwhelm them with what Donald E. Gordon aptly described as its 'claw-like force'.[22]

The female bathers in the fourth, smaller panel seem unaffected by the waves as they gaze out of the picture, distracted perhaps by the drama in the previous scene (pl. 355). Even so, a seagull nearly brushes their heads with serrated wings as it flies low over them, and in the final panel this incipient violence becomes more overt. While two bathers splash their female companion who recoils, a trio

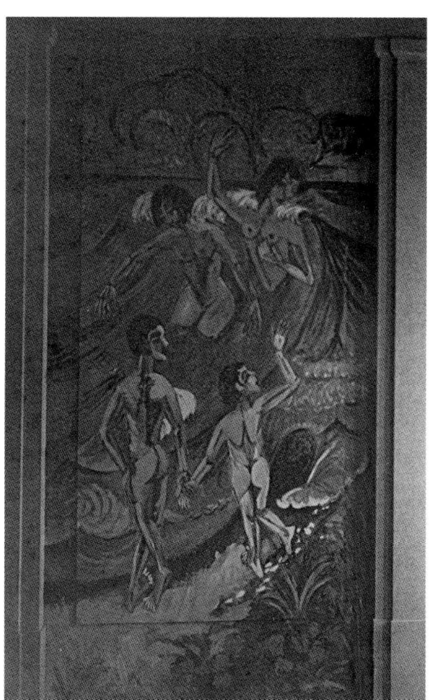

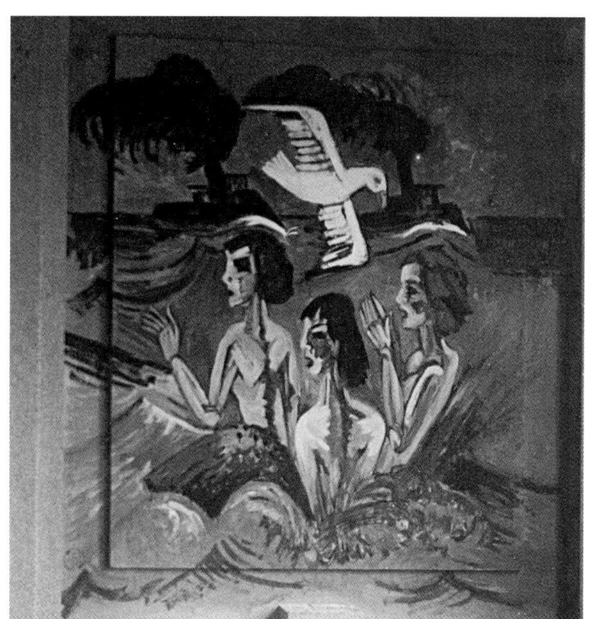

354 (*far left*) Ernst Ludwig Kirchner, Third stairwell panel at Kohnstamm sanatorium, *c.*1916, destroyed

355 (*left*) Ernst Ludwig Kirchner, Fourth stairwell panel at Kohnstamm sanatorium, *c.*1916, destroyed

356 Egon Schiele, *Gustav Klimt Dead*, 1918, Leopold Museum, Vienna

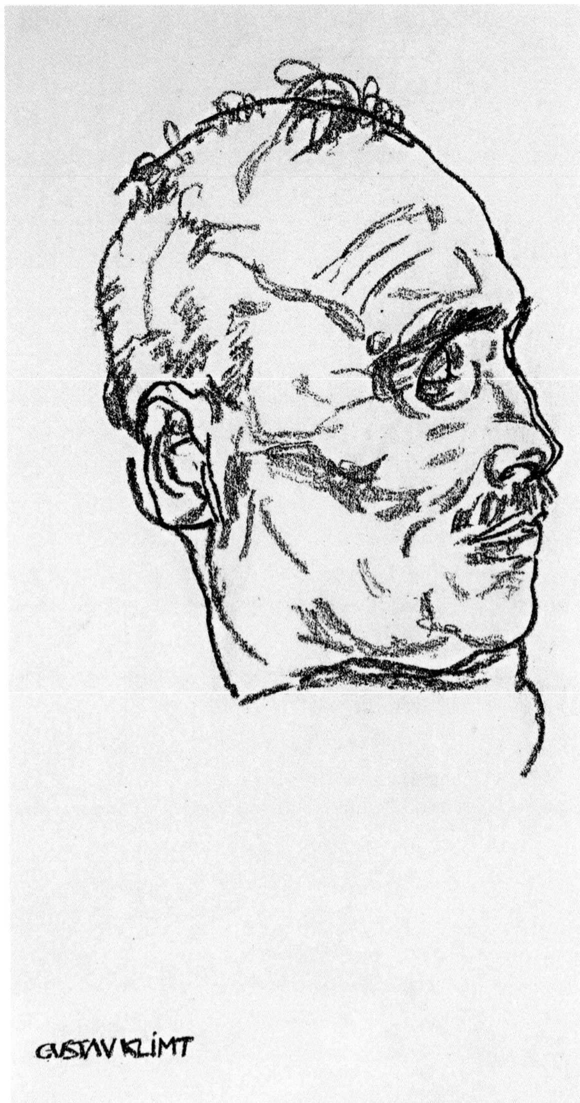

of seagulls join in the attack from the air. This time they look predatory, and the downcast expression on the woman's gaunt face indicates that something more than a lighthearted game is in progress. Even as he produced his most sustained achievement of 1916 on the stairwell walls, Kirchner could not rid himself of the haunted intimations of stress and aggression that beleaguered him during this intensely difficult period. Tragically, the entire fresco scheme was destroyed in 1938, the same year that deepening depression led the artist to commit suicide.[23]

For the most part, Egon Schiele had greater luck during the First World War. His precocious career continued to flourish and he was able to produce a surprising number of powerful paintings and drawings throughout the conflict. In 1918, however, Schiele's good fortune began to run out. Early in the year, Gustav Klimt, the senior Austrian artist whom he venerated above anyone else, succumbed to the epidemic of influenza sweeping the world. Klimt died on 6 February, and the very next day Schiele visited the corpse laid out in the hospital morgue of the Allgemeines Krankenhaus. He must have been shocked by the sight of the haggard Klimt wasted by disease. The shaving of the dead man's familiar beard made his face almost unrecognisable, but Schiele rallied sufficiently to make three incisive drawings in black chalk (pl. 356). Klimt's head seems to hover in a void, for Schiele did not bother to fill his paper with the drapes covering the body. Although he must have drawn all three images in a horizontal format, Schiele also insisted on inscribing and signing them as if they were to be viewed vertically. Perhaps he wanted to imply that Klimt's spirit, at least, would triumph over death and live on through his art. Nevertheless eight months later Schiele's defiant optimism swiftly evaporated. On 27 October, the distraught artist drew his own wife Edith as she lay dying of the same disease that had killed Klimt. Four days afterwards, Schiele himself succumbed to influenza at the age of only twenty-eight.

In Britain, the elaborate war artists scheme sponsored by the government decided that a small group of painters and draughtsmen should tackle medical themes. Most of the images they produced were based on photographs or models posed in the studio. That is one reason why Austin Osman Spare's large pastel of an *Operating Theatre, Endell Street, London* stands out: he visited the building itself, while the operation was in progress (pl. 357). The location makes this commission even more unusual, for Spare was sent to the only official military hospital run by British women during the Great War. Back in 1915, two former suffragettes, Dr Flora Murray and Dr Louisa Garrett Anderson (whose daughter Elizabeth became an outstanding doctor in her own right), were invited by the War Office to take control of a large military hospital in the capital. Male doctors of the Royal Army Medical Corps (RAMC) scorned the idea, and claimed that the women would never be able to cope with these unprecedented responsibilities. Yet Murray and Garrett Anderson gathered together a

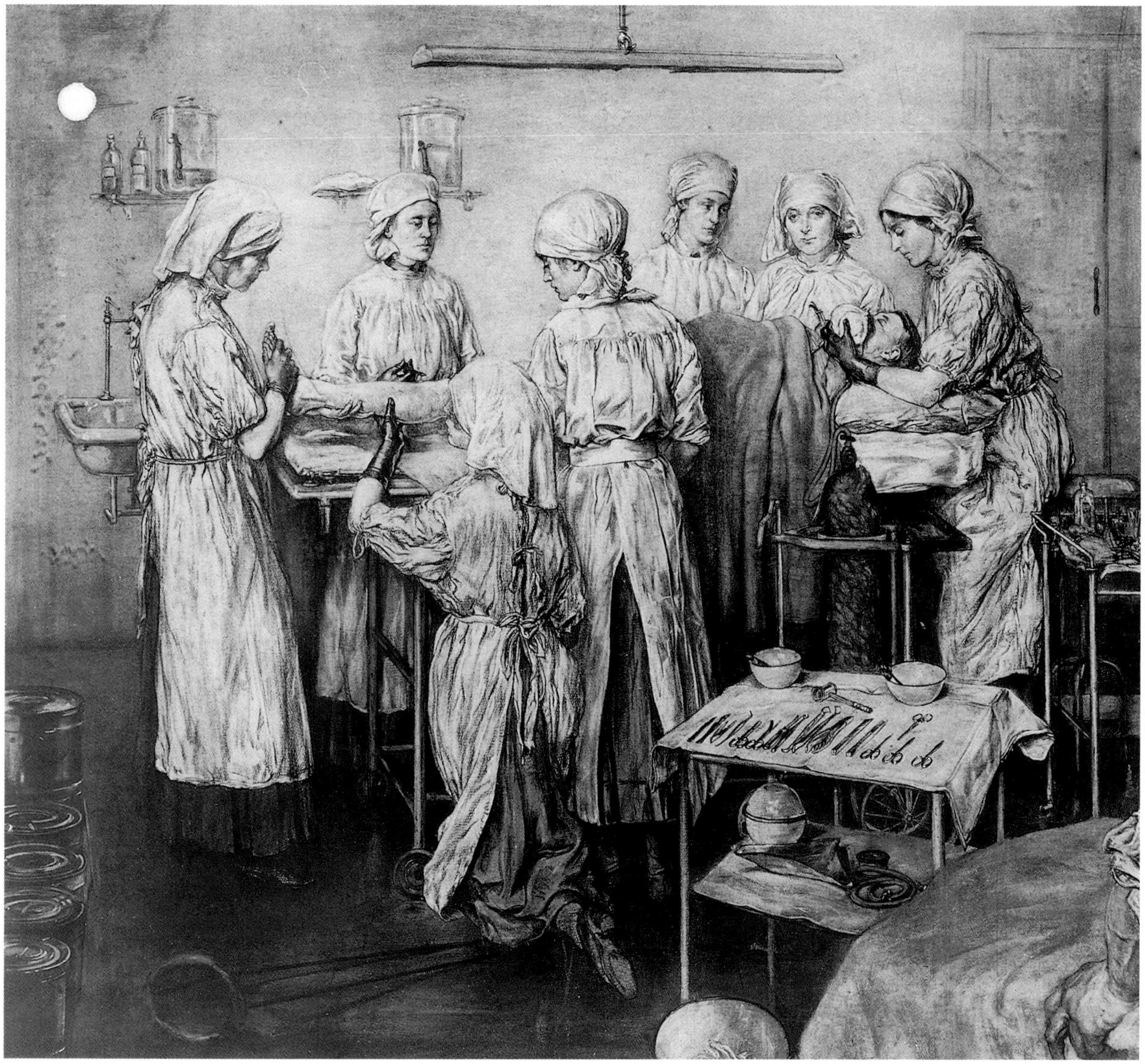

357 Austin Osman Spare, *Operating Theatre, Endell Street, London*, 1919, location unknown

group of like-minded feminists and ran the Endell Street Military Hospital with conspicuous success. Although none of them had previously been allowed to control such an institution, they dealt admirably with daunting quantities of severely injured men. By the time Armistice was declared, the sceptical male members of the RAMC acknowledged these pioneering women as professional equals. Spare was duly commissioned to celebrate their achievement by making his *Operating Theatre* pastel.

When the work was displayed at the Royal Academy in a 1919 exhibition of 'The Nation's War Paintings and other Records', one visitor admired it so much that a photograph was requested and duly taken. This is now the only surviving record of a pastel that became bitterly controversial, and soon vanished without trace. Aggressive discontent flared just after the exhibition closed in February 1920. Flora Murray sent an aggrieved letter to Colonel Brereton, who was in charge of the medical section at London's Imperial War Museum. After he failed to respond satisfactorily, she wrote again to Lady Norman, the chair of the women's section at the Museum. 'The picture does not pretend to have any artistic merit', stormed Dr Murray, incensed that its 'gross errors' had not been corrected. 'As it stands, the picture is a misrepresentation of the work of professional women', she went on, claiming that it was 'an object of ridicule'.

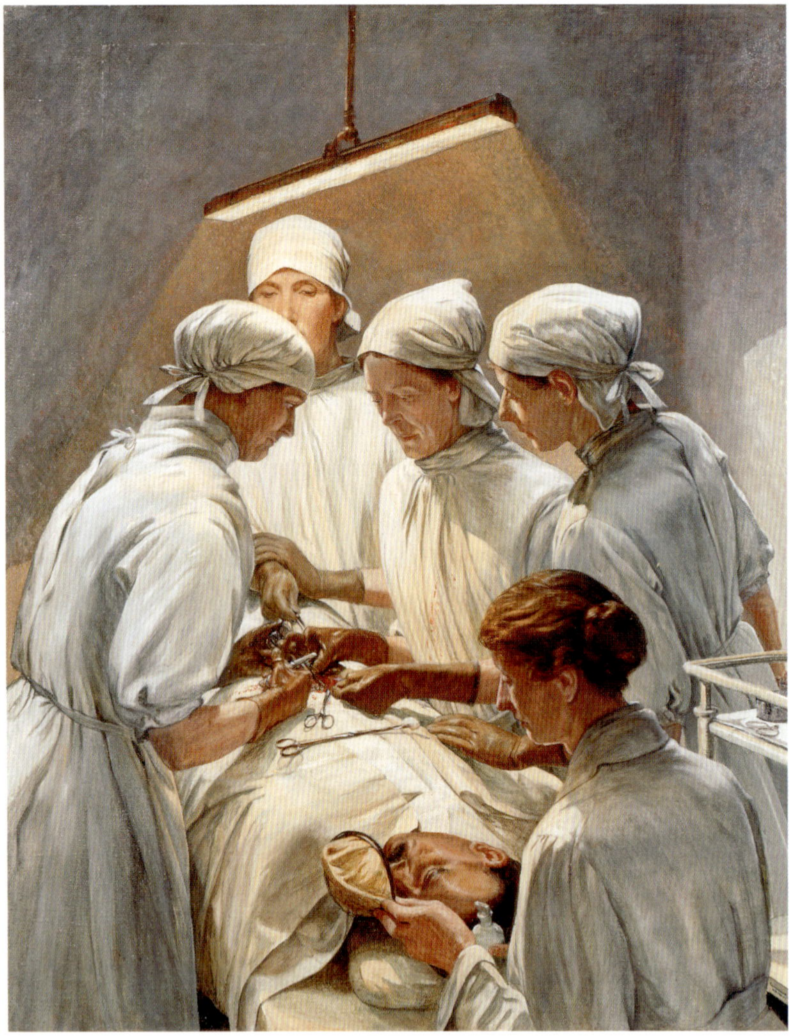

358 Francis Dodd, *An Operation at the Military Hospital, Endell Street* (Dr Louisa Garrett Anderson, Dr Flora Murray and Dr Winifred Buckley), 1921, Wellcome Library, London

According to Murray, 'it is very painful to all those of us who worked at Endell Street to see such a picture hung. We would rather have no record of our work than a false record; and Dr Garrett Anderson and I must earnestly ask you to do all you can to have this picture destroyed.'[24]

Lady Norman and her sub-committee reacted far more sympathetically than Colonel Brereton. She informed Spare that his pastel could not be exhibited again unless alterations were carried out, getting rid of 'inaccuracies' that made the picture 'look ludicrous to the technical mind'. The astounded artist was asked to 'cut the floor off the picture so as to remove the various things so out of place in an operating room, such as the couch, Thomas's splint, the sterilising drums and the kneeling figure of the nurse, all of which, Dr Garrett Anderson points out, would not be seen in an operating room, and would indicate a serious professional breach of the most ordinary surgical practice.'[25] When he received the letter, Spare responded with unconcealed anger. 'I *cannot* consent to the suggested mutilation of my picture', he declared, before insisting that while the pastel was in progress the women doctors had 'ample opportunity' to 'offer suggestions or criticisms, which I should have been only too glad to receive, providing always, that my conception as an artist was not infringed thereby: – but I wish to say very clearly that I actually saw at Endell Street *everything* I have put into my picture.'[26]

Spare need not have bothered to protest. Lady Norman had predicted his response and asked Henry Tonks, the Slade School Professor, to recommend another artist. That is why Francis Dodd was invited to produce an alternative image of the Endell Street women at work. He eventually consented, visiting the Hospital to study the closed-down operating theatre, as well as making portraits of the surgeons and anaesthetist. The eventual painting, completed in 1921, concentrates on five figures alone (pl. 358). Lit dramatically from above, it jettisons all the surroundings that had excited such furious condemnation in the earlier pastel. However, Jennian F. Geddes, who has researched this controversy in detail and studied contemporary photographs of the Hospital, now argues that Spare's picture 'faithfully represents' the operating theatre. Since he probably depicted a leg operation, 'a nurse might well have been kneeling in order to momentarily support the leg, the couch presumably was the one on which the patient came to theatre, and it is unlikely that Spare would have invented the presence of sterilising drums.'[27]

Why, therefore, were the Endell Street doctors so aggrieved, to the extent that Spare's offending pastel found itself discarded by the Imperial War Museum and banished to the Royal Herbert Hospital in Woolwich, where it disappeared altogether? Geddes can only conclude that the women's violent reaction reveals insecurity: 'despite the remarkable success of their hospital and their acknowledged contribution to the war effort, they knew that there was still some way to go before they would be accepted by the medical profession at large, particularly in the field of surgery. They obviously felt they could not risk their work being seen as having anything less than the highest possible standards.'[28]

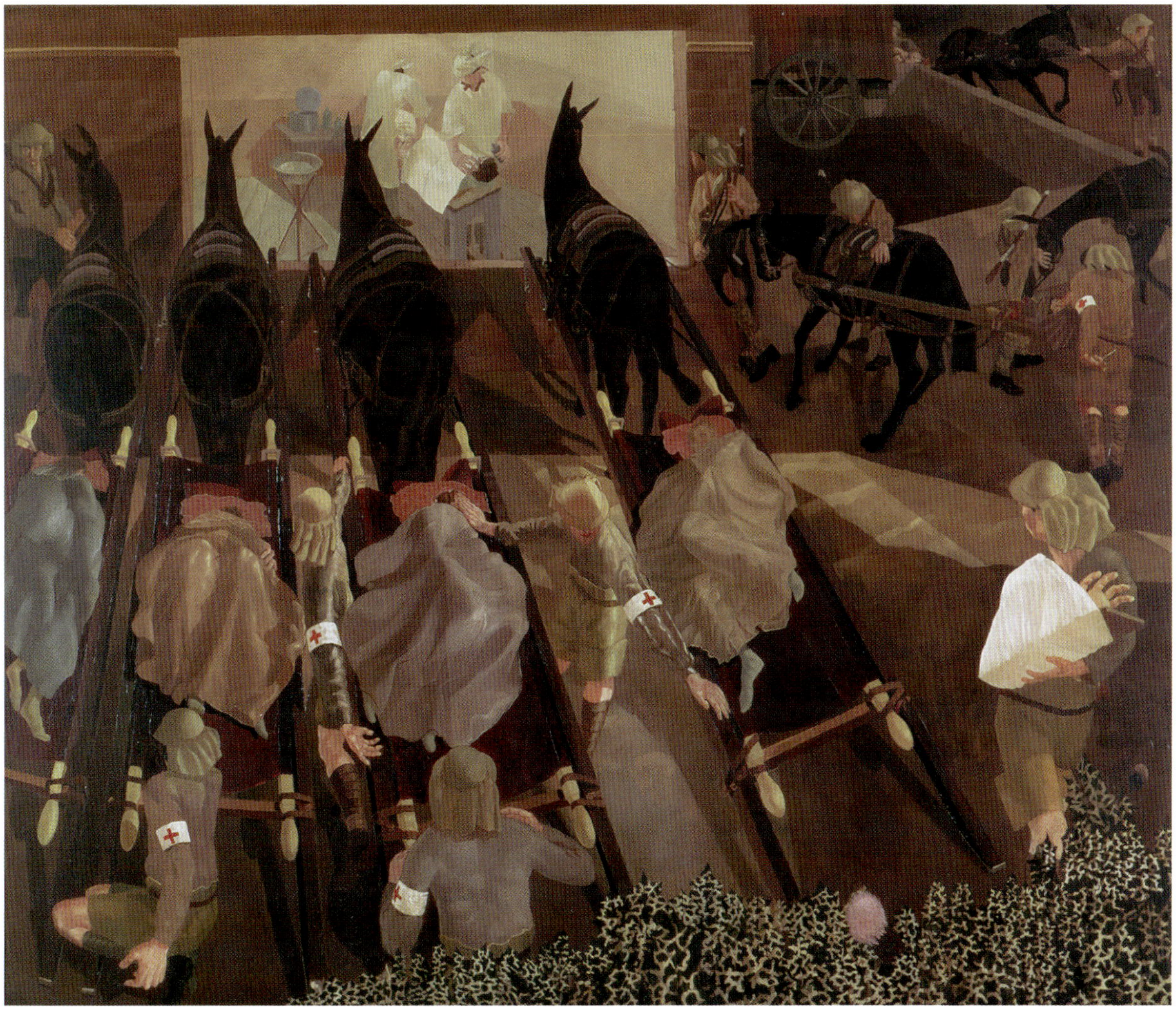

359 Stanley Spencer, *Travoys arriving with Wounded at a Dressing Station at Smol, Macedonia*, 1919, Imperial War Museum, London

Long before this furore erupted, Stanley Spencer began to hatch a more elaborate plan at a hospital in Bristol. Enlisted in the RAMC and stationed at Beaufort War Hospital, a former lunatic asylum taken over by the army for war casualties, he began almost at once to conceive a monumental cycle of paintings based on his momentous experiences there. 'I am still thinking about the hospital, which the more I think about, the more it inspires me', he wrote to a friend in July 1916.

> I am determined that when I get a chance, I am going to do some wonderful things – a whole lot of big frescoes. Of the square pictures, there will be the 'Convoy' – (I have that alright). The operation (and that). Then the narrow panels – a nurse (Oh such a beauty for that), an orderly (very good). . . . Think of the different things there are in a hospital, a storesman, an engineer, a carpenter, a surgeon – (I have that and it exasperates me not to be able to do it) . . . What will be wonderful . . . [are] the places where things [were] going on, and all is still and quiet and then, outside, all tumult and hurry.[29]

Spencer's immediate urgency abated once he realised how difficult it would be to secure a building for such an epic task, but the ambition revived in 1921 when he was given a commission to paint a mural in Steep village hall. Although the project came to nothing, his lively drawing for the scheme of floor-scrubbing and washing soldiers played an important part in his memorial chapel decorations at Burghclere several years later. A small pencil and wash sketch, for one of the panels on the chapel walls, offers a tantalising hint of the way he might have painted a large-scale

360 Stanley Spencer, *Convoy of Wounded Soldiers arriving at Beaufort Hospital Gates*, 1927, Sandham Memorial Chapel, Burghclere, Hampshire

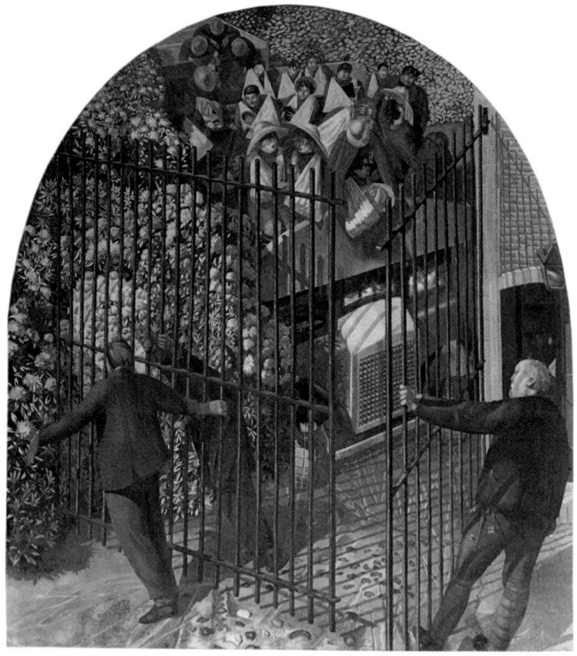

image of a hospital operation. The idea had been growing in his mind since 1916 when, after witnessing just such a scene at Bristol, he admitted that

> I should love to do a fresco of an operation . . . and have the incision in the belly in the middle of the picture, and all the forceps radiating from it like this [small sketch] . . . How mysterious the hands look – wonderfully intense. There was something very classical about the whole operation . . . What is so wonderful, also, is the stillness in the theatre, and outside the swift, silent steps of those 'fetching and carrying'. I would like to do a figure on either side of the operation, of a nurse and a man with a frock bringing sterilisers. This does not sound much but leave it to me.[30]

In the event, the only painting of an operation that Spencer managed to carry out was a small yet potent passage in his great First World War canvas, an official government commission called *Travoys arriving with Wounded at a Dressing Station at Smol, Macedonia* (pl. 359).[31] Everything in this elegiac composition leads up, through the bodies of injured or dying soldiers huddled on their stretchers in billowing blankets, to the warmly lit room beyond. Here a surgeon attempts to bring comfort and relief, his hands echoing the reassuring gestures of the Red Cross orderlies who gently press their palms and fingers down on the suffering figures waiting to be examined. The operating theatre, a small Greek church converted for the purpose, is given a sacred significance. Always ready to dis-

361 Stanley Spencer, *Scrubbing Floors*, 1927, Sandham Memorial Chapel, Burghclere, Hampshire

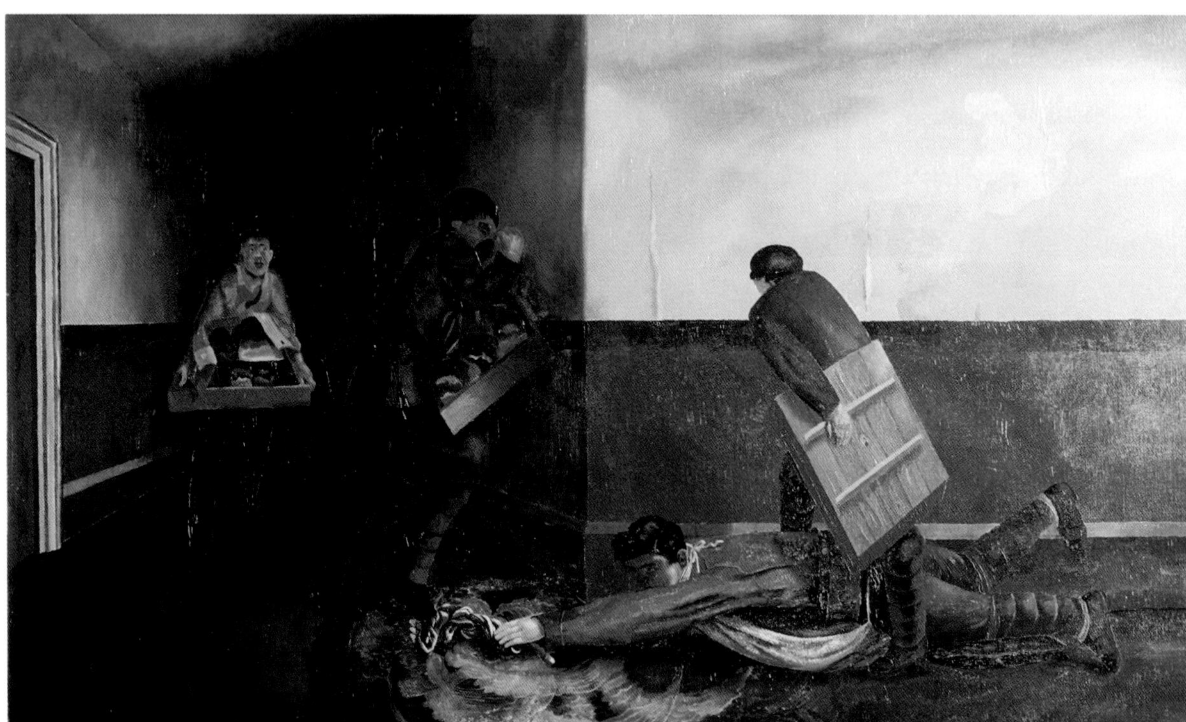

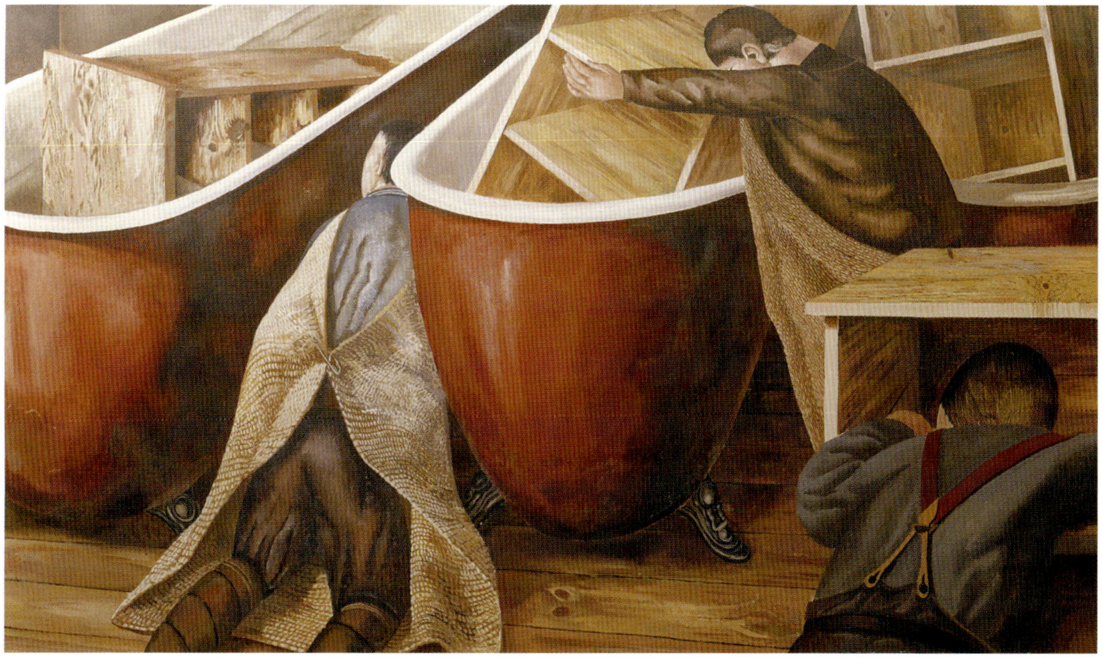

362 Stanley Spencer, *Washing Lockers*, 1920, Sandham Memorial Chapel, Burghclere, Hampshire

cover the religious in the everyday, Spencer shows a characteristic desire to counter the suffering of war through his sturdily compassionate art.

The same aim prevails, with still more moving effect, in the Burghclere cycle. The first picture to be painted in this small, deliberately Giottesque chapel after it was built in 1927 was the large *Convoy of Wounded Soldiers arriving at Beaufort Hospital Gates* (pl. 360). Here the opening of the gates, which Spencer remembered were 'as massive and as high as the gates of hell',[32] acts as an implicit pictorial invitation to explore the chapel itself. A potentially grim scene is transformed into a beneficent alternative by the introduction of burgeoning rhododendrons crowding in on the soldiers with their overwhelming richness of blossom. A similar sense of salvation runs through all the other hospital scenes in the chapel, discovering an exalted meaning within the most quotidian images of medical life. Whether scrubbing the floor, carrying out ablutions, sorting kitbags and laundry, filling tea urns or eating bread-and-butter sandwiches at teatime in a ward, memories of his time at the Beaufort War Hospital fill many of these paintings with celebrations of communal activity (pl. 361).

Yet perhaps the most revealing of these tributes to the War Hospital can be found in a 'predella' picture called *Washing Lockers*, where Spencer depicted his younger self kneeling between the immense shiny baths (pl. 362). Isolated and protected from the frenetic activity around him, he was able there to work undisturbed. Spencer revealed the full significance of this quirky shelter when he wrote on a preliminary drawing that it showed 'me scrubbing: I say "me", because I have only to mentally place myself between the baths to feel at once inspired.'[33] If Spencer had ever received a commission to decorate a hospital, he would undoubtedly have carried it out with an unusual amount of fervent, redemptive conviction.

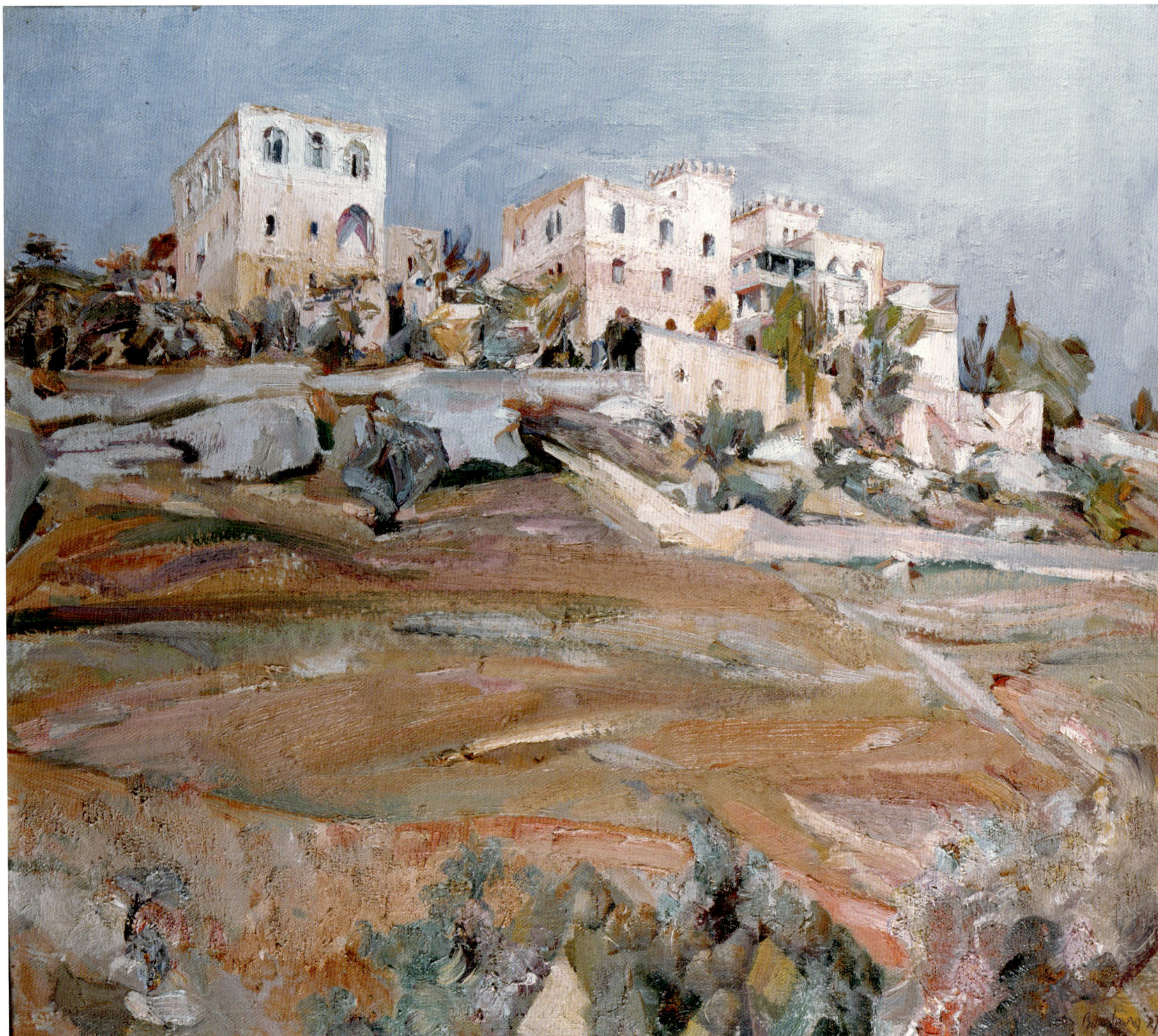

TWENTY-THREE
'A MEGAPHONE FOR HEALTH'

In Palestine, where he had settled for a few years to escape the crushing indifference of the British art establishment, David Bomberg was heartened by a hospital commission. Dr Strathearn, the Warden of the Ophthalmic Hospital of the Order of St John, asked him in 1927 to paint the building for £100 (pl. 363). It was, in his view, an immensely sympathetic subject. Bomberg had been fascinated by the challenge of studying the relationship between architecture and landscape ever since he first made the long journey from London to Jerusalem four years earlier. The fact that it was a hospital dedicated to the treatment of eyesight may also have meant much to an artist who, in his Palestine work, relied on a keen and exacting scrutiny of the scenes he observed with such zeal.[1]

All the same, the commission did not prove easy to carry out. For Bomberg was determined to set the Order of St John's building in the context of the countryside it inhabited. 'First of all', recalled his wife Alice, 'I must meet the Turkish notable who owned the land near where the Eye Hospital was built and get his consent to us fixing the tent in his field.' Then, having opted for settling in 'an empty house near the field', work began outdoors in arduous, high-summer temperatures. 'We were tormented with flies', Alice remembered, 'and I had to stand by David while he unscrewed the top of the particular colour he was using at the moment and quickly screwed the cap on again while chasing the flies away.'[2]

However taxing the conditions, they also encouraged Bomberg to achieve a greater breadth and freedom of handling than he had deployed in his previous Palestine work. After painting the hospital on the hill in a relatively naturalistic manner, he experienced great difficulty in depicting the group of olive trees in the foreground. 'Still we stood in the sunshine with flies buzzing around us until the day David got exasperated', wrote Alice, describing how he 'took his brush and casually rubbed out the paint he had been putting on so meticulously.'[3] The act of obliteration proved momentous. It had a liberating effect, prompting Bomberg to deal with the whole area in a vigorously manipulated impasto that anticipates the free, impassioned handling he would develop in his subsequent career. Here it dramatises the contrast between nature and architecture, stressing the tension between the ordered, rational structure of the hospital building and the parched wildness of the surrounding terrain.

By a felicitous coincidence, another important British artist was given a Palestine-linked commission by an ophthalmic institution only a few years later. In 1934 Eric Gill received an invitation to

363 (*facing page*) David Bomberg, *The Ophthalmic Hospital of the Order of St John*, 1927, Museum of the Order of Saint John, London

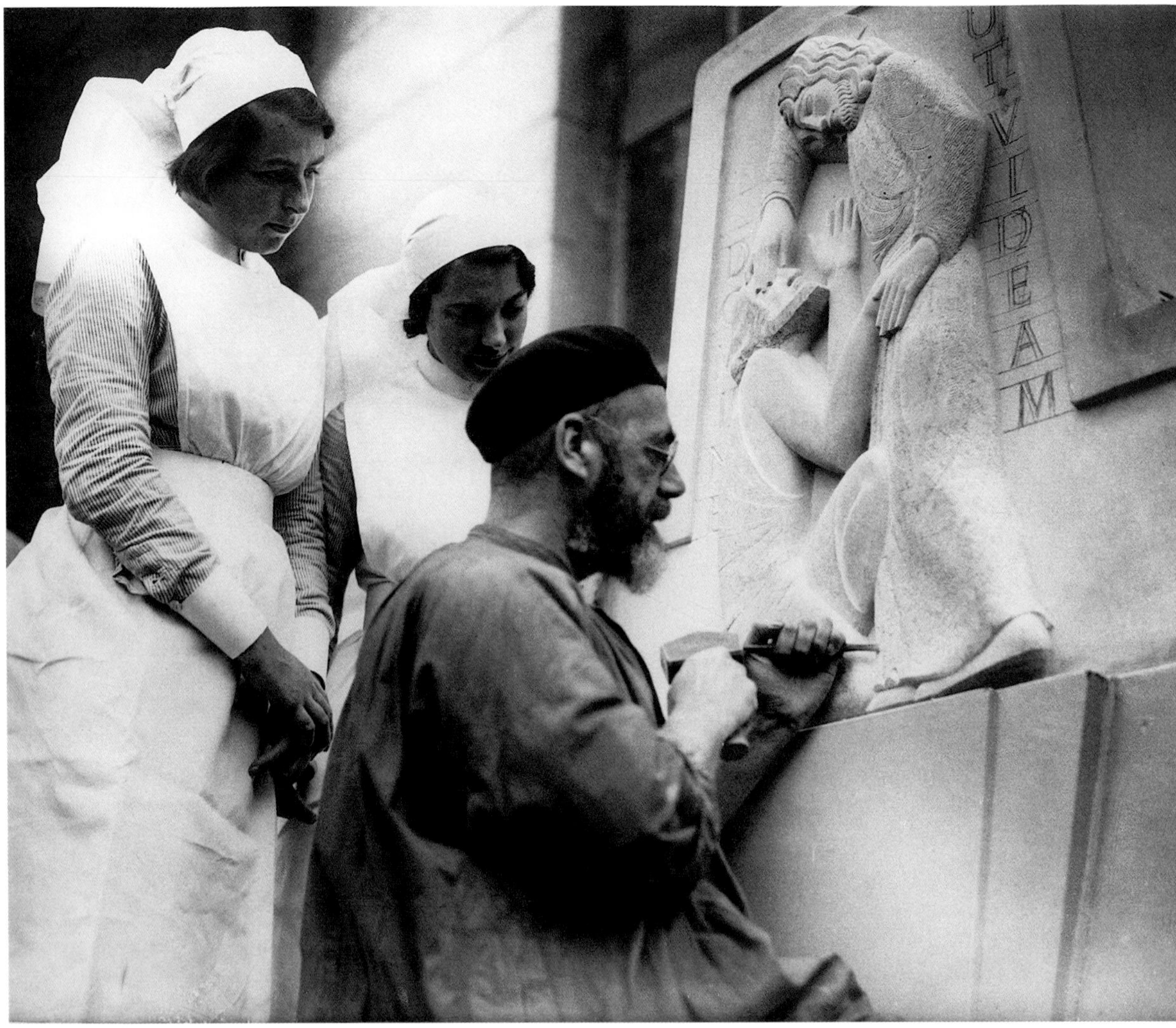

364 Photograph of Nurses at Moorfields Eye Hospital watching Eric Gill carving *Christ Giving Sight to Bartimaeus*, 1934

carve a half-relief image over the entrance to Moorfields Eye Hospital's extension in east London. Working on site between August and September, he recorded that the sculpture was intended 'as a gift to the Hospital!'[4] His strong religious convictions probably influenced the decision to depict *Christ Giving Sight to Bartimaeus*, and a contemporary photograph shows the sculptor chiselling beside an audience of appreciative nurses (pl. 364). He doubtless told them that Bartimaeus was among the blind beggars of Jericho whom Christ healed on his final journey to Jerusalem. Gill would also have explained the significance of the Latin inscription incised on either side of the figures: 'Lord, that I might see', a heartfelt quotation from the New Testament.[5]

Although the finished work is small enough to be dwarfed by the building around it, Gill turns the cramped dimensions of the Portland stone to expressive account (pl. 365): for the two figures are bound together by their unusually intense involvement in the miracle. Rather than standing at a dignified distance from Bartimaeus, Christ shows no hesitation in closing in on the blind man with a complete lack of inhibition. Their legs touch as he concentrates on the task, and the yearning Bartimaeus is allowed to grasp his saviour's waist in a surprisingly intimate manner. His other hand thrusts upwards, fingers splayed in exclamation at the unexpectedness of the event. Christ, by contrast, plunges his fingers purposefully down, pressing them onto the eyes of a man who appears astonished by such direct, firmly administered physical contact from a spiritual leader.

A few years later, Gill was able to pursue this intimacy of feeling on a more prominent hospital site.

In November 1937 he executed a careful preparatory drawing of the *Good Samaritan* for a carving commissioned by A.H. Gardner, the architect of Coventry and Warwickshire Hospital's new ward and administration block. Destined for a space above the building's main entrance, where Gill executed it *in situ* the following year,[6] the stone relief required simple forms that could be seen and understood from a considerable distance. So Gill focused on the two principal figures, isolated in profile on a bare plinth where no room is left for attendant animals or landscape (pl. 366). Just as at Moorfields, the humane, redemptive contact between protector and victim is the only theme explored here.

Unlike the interpretations of the same subject painted by Hogarth and Dadd for other hospitals (see pls 187 and 269), Gill's image brings the two men into the closest possible proximity. The Samaritan kneels in order to let the inert figure rest against his body. He cradles the wounded man like a child, clasping his thigh with one hand while the other props up his back. At the same time, the Samaritan leans his head towards the victim, so that their two faces – one bearded and elderly, the other young and clean-shaven – draw very near to each other. The resemblance to a *Pietà* group is surely deliberate, for Gill seems eager to stress the parental, loving role assumed by the Samaritan. Moreover, the victim's limp and attenuated body, much more helpless than the well-built men painted by Hogarth and Dadd, emphasises the magnitude of the task confronting his comforter.

Only three years after its completion, the vulnerability of Gill's naked figure was accentuated by damage inflicted on the lower part of his right leg by a Nazi bombing raid. It was the most devastating of the attacks on Coventry, carried out at night despite a large red cross of lights displayed on the hospital roof. Half the in-patient accommodation was destroyed in this brutal raid, along with several wards. The hospital, starved of water, sewerage, electricity and windows, nevertheless received at least three hundred casualties during the night. And surgeons insisted on continuing their operations without electricity or even a roof to protect them. The same blitz attack completely destroyed another relief, either of the *Good Shepherd* or *St Martin and the Beggar*, carved by Gill for the rear of the Hospital.[7] Severely cracked and in parts fragmented, the *Good Samaritan* was moved to a new position on the exterior of the physiotherapy block, built in 1957. Here, in its battered state, the sculpture was soon regarded as 'the hospital's war memorial'[8] but its fragile condition does not impair the work's fundamental meaning. For Gill surely wanted to imply, through the exceptional tenderness of this carving, that the staff of Coventry Hospital would do well to emulate the compassionate devotion extended by the Samaritan to the forlorn and broken figure lying in his arms.

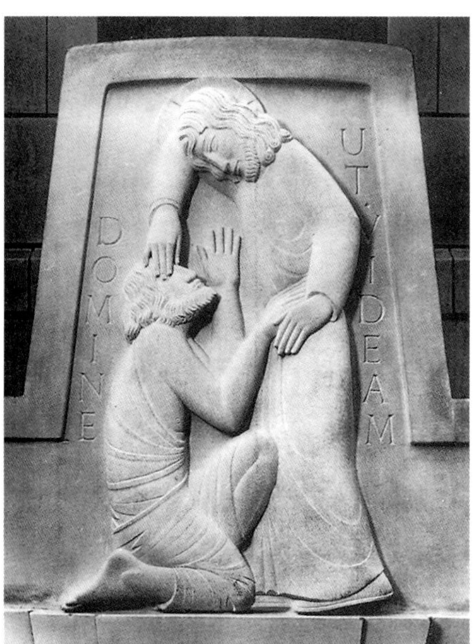

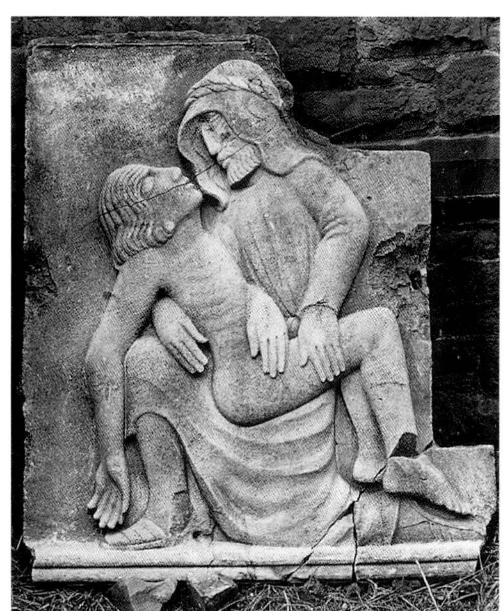

365 (*far left*) Eric Gill, *Christ Giving Sight to Bartimaeus*, 1934, Moorfields Eye Hospital, London

366 (*left*) Eric Gill, *The Good Samaritan*, 1938, sold by Sotheby's July 2007, originally carved for main entrance of Coventry Hospital

367 (*right*) Eric Gill, *Madonna and Child*, 1939, Leahurst Hostel, Braintree

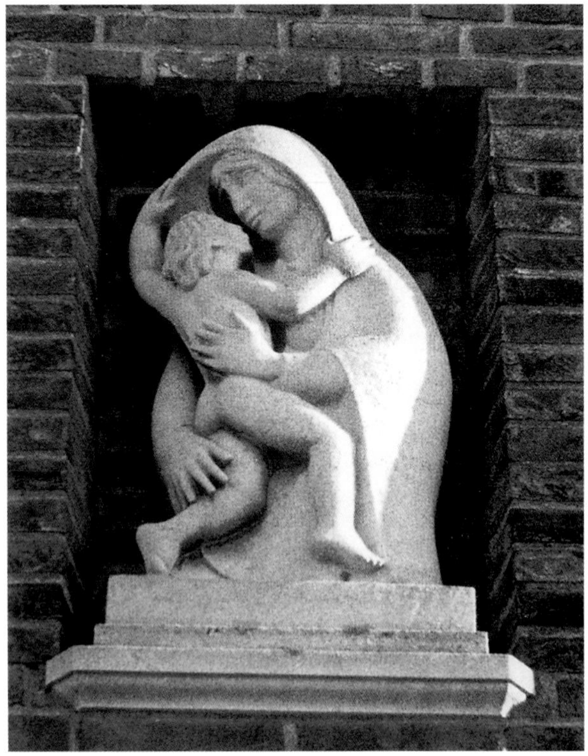

368 (*below*) Julien Dillen, *Monument to Georges Brugmann*, 1923, Brugmann University Hospital, Brussels

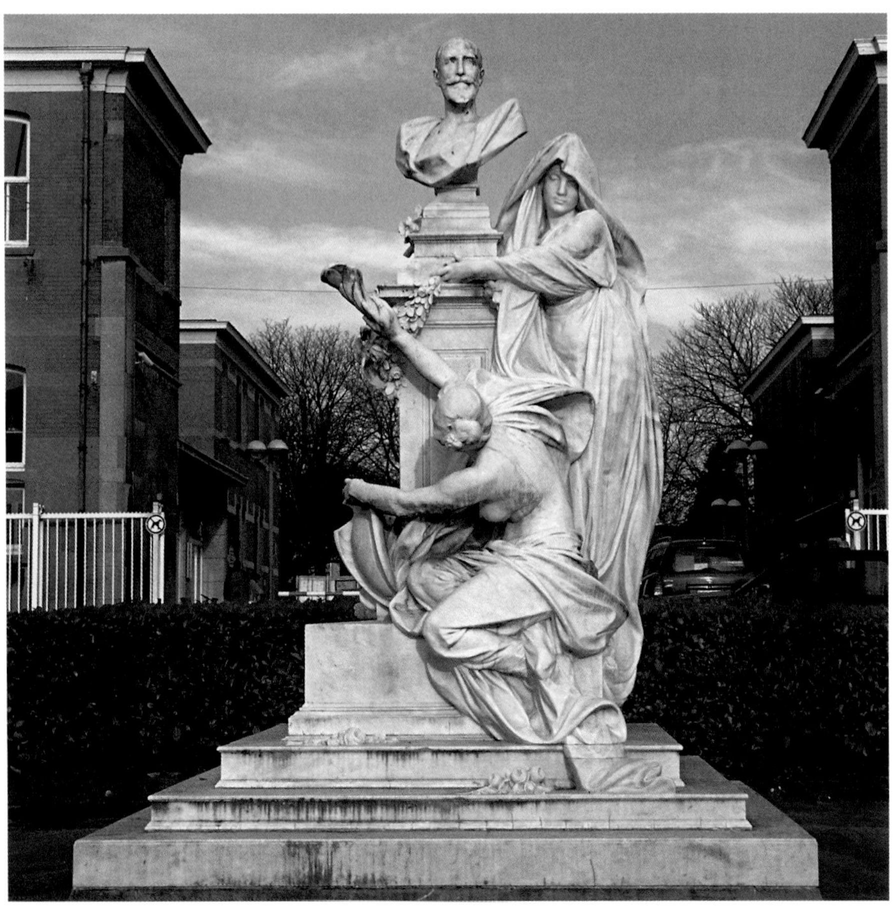

Hence, perhaps, his willingness to execute one further hospital-related work, a *Madonna and Child* completed only a year before his untimely death in 1940 (pl. 367). The commission came from the architect E. Vincent Harris, who was designing a new hostel for nurses at Braintree in Essex. Like the previous hospital carvings for London and Coventry, Gill's new sculpture was intended to be placed above an exterior door. Unlike its predecessors, this Portland stone group was largely carved in his studio and now occupies a niche in a brick facade. Only in the final stages did Gill journey to Braintree and cut the inscription, crest and monogram on site. Two months before, on New Year's Day 1939, he had told a friend that 'at present I'm struggling to finish a Madonna & Child',[9] but no sign of strain can be detected in the completed carving.

On the contrary: this modest work is one of the most assured of his final pieces and takes the theme of physical intimacy to a still greater extreme. Far from sitting with complacent formality on his mother's lap, the Christ Child surges towards her and, with an ardent gesture, lifts the Virgin's hood. He seems determined, above all, to kiss her lips. After a while, though, the very impulsiveness of his movement suggests that he may be seeking shelter as well. He presses his body so urgently against her that a hint of desperation can be felt, and the Madonna responds by enfolding him with protective, loving hands.

On the whole, however, hospital commissions during the inter-war period lacked this sense of strong, personal engagement. All too often, the role of art was restricted to grandiloquent monuments outside the building, lauding the generosity of its wealthy benefactor. When the great Art Nouveau pioneer Victor Horta designed the Brugmann University Hospital near Brussels, he created a pavilion-based structure in an extensive campus setting. Although it provoked initial controversy at the royal opening in 1923, the building came to be widely admired throughout Europe. Yet the only notable art-work was Julien Dillens's monument to Georges Brugmann (pl. 368), who had bequeathed ten million francs to the Brussels Conseil Général des Hospices more than three decades before. Occupying a prominent open-air site in front of the main entrance, this supremely pompous sculpture glorifies one man's beneficence rather than acknowledging the wider needs of the staff and patients inside the building.

Artists in England continued to be fascinated by hospital themes. The nineteen-year-old Lucian Freud found himself, after developing tonsilitis, in the Emergency Medical Services Hospital at Ashridge. Once his tonsils had been removed, he went home and painted a small canvas of an adolescent recovering in a *Hospital Ward* (pl. 369). While a nurse patrols beyond, the patient gazes out at us with sedative-heavy eyes. Yet he manages to smile woozily, and the water plant on his blanket counteracts the institutional gloom.

So did one of London's most radical and audacious hospital buildings. Berthold Lubetkin and Tecton were asked to design a Health Centre for Finsbury (pl. 370). The structure, ranked among Lubetkin's great achievements by the time it was completed in 1938, served one of the city's highly deprived areas. All the Borough's dispersed health facilities, ranging from a dental clinic and a solarium to a disinfection station and a foot clinic, were moved out of their old, substandard premises and placed in this central location. Lubetkin responded to the Borough's forward-looking desire for a far-ranging improvement in health care by producing what he saw as a 'megaphone for health'.[10] With its two wings thrusting out from a central axis, the streamlined new building seemed to be broadcasting the merits of its services with all the vigour of a loudhailer. The clarity and boldness announced in the exterior was carried into the Reception Hall, too. Its light and spacious identity, more reminiscent of a 1930s seaside pavilion than a claustrophobic hospital, promoted a much needed sense of well-being. The different clinics housed in the Health Centre were organised with similar lucidity and, as Nicholas Bullock pointed out, 'the relationship of structure to the arrangement of spaces ensures a valuable flexibility in planning'.[11]

The vast mural designed by Gordon Cullen for the Reception Hall emphasised, with outspoken and optimistic brio, the various forms of assistance on offer in the building. Cullen also took on a cru-

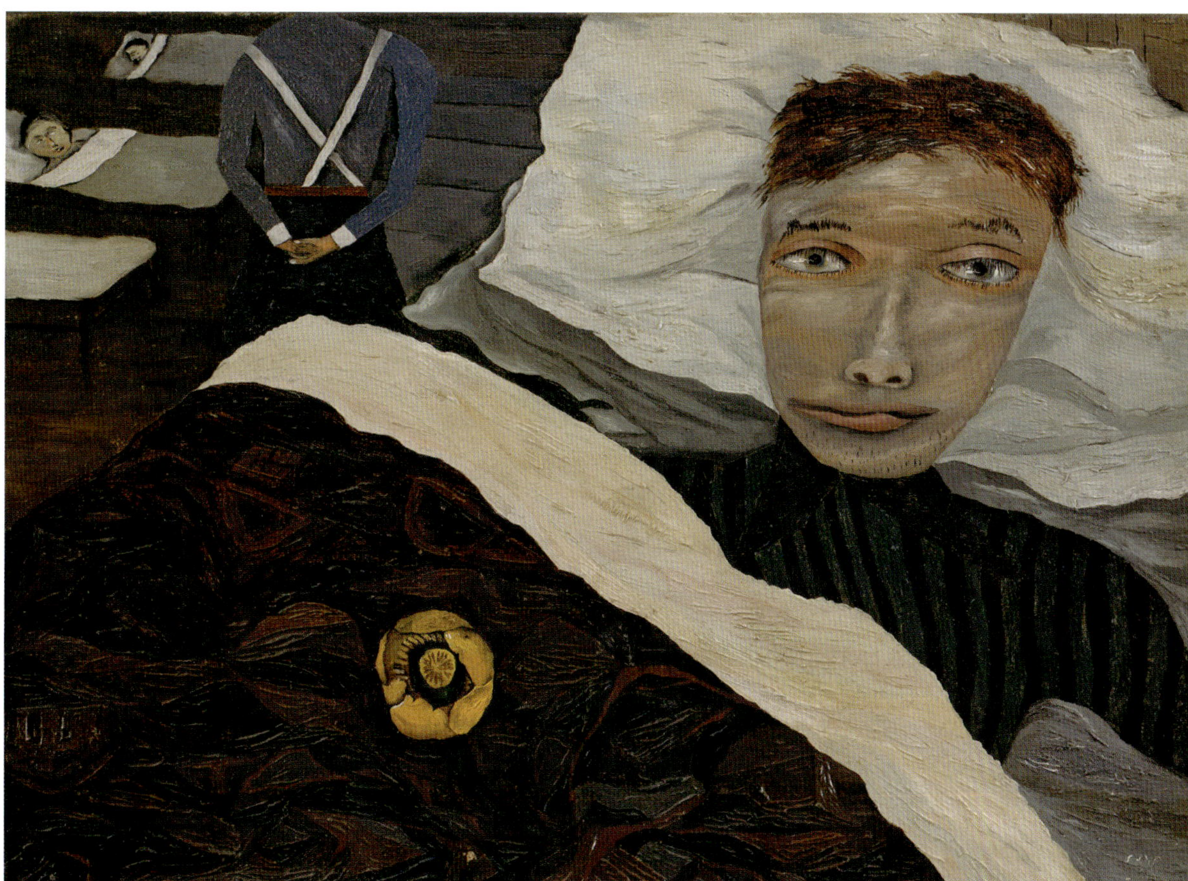

369 Lucian Freud, *Hospital Ward*, 1941, Chatsworth House, Derbyshire

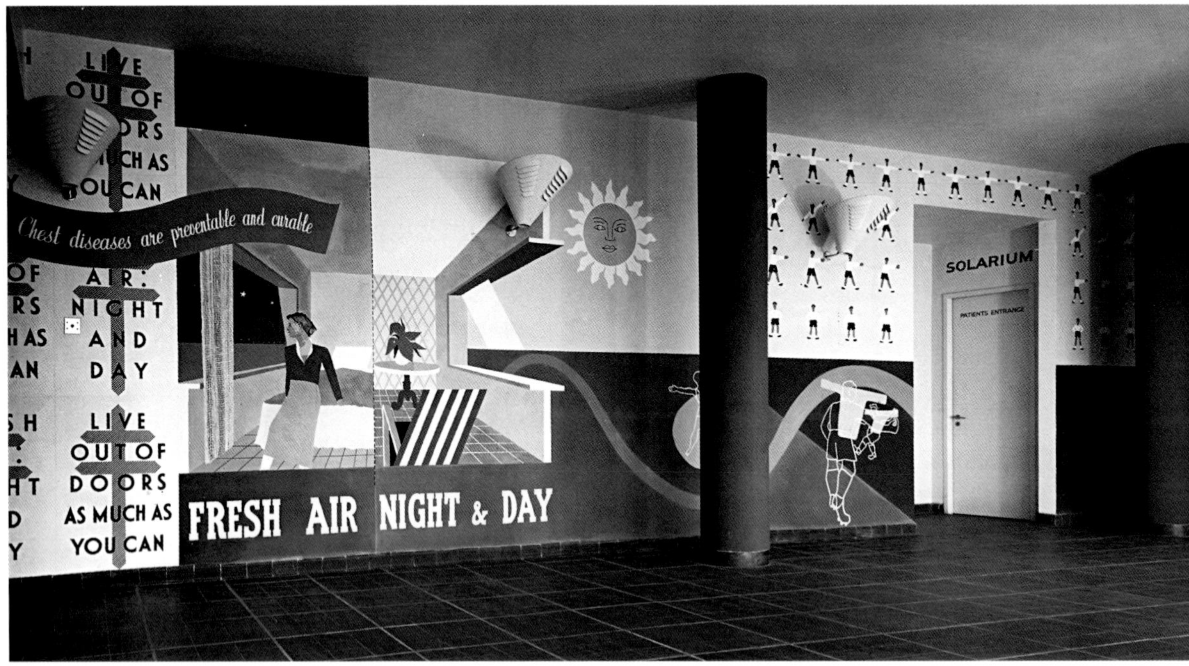

370 Gordon Cullen, Mural for Reception Hall in Finsbury Health Centre, London, 1938

sading and prescriptive role. He made the mural announce, in capital letters worthy of the brashest newspaper headline, the importance of 'FRESH AIR NIGHT & DAY'. Above this slogan, redolent of forward thinking between the wars, a healthy young woman stares out of her modernist bedroom at an unpolluted nocturnal sky. She is juxtaposed with the pleasures of a Corbusian terrace lit by a cheerful sun. 'Chest diseases are preventable and curable' proclaims a festive banner undulating through the mural, while another inscription descends in a vertical progression as it exhorts patients to 'LIVE OUT OF DOORS AS MUCH AS YOU CAN'.

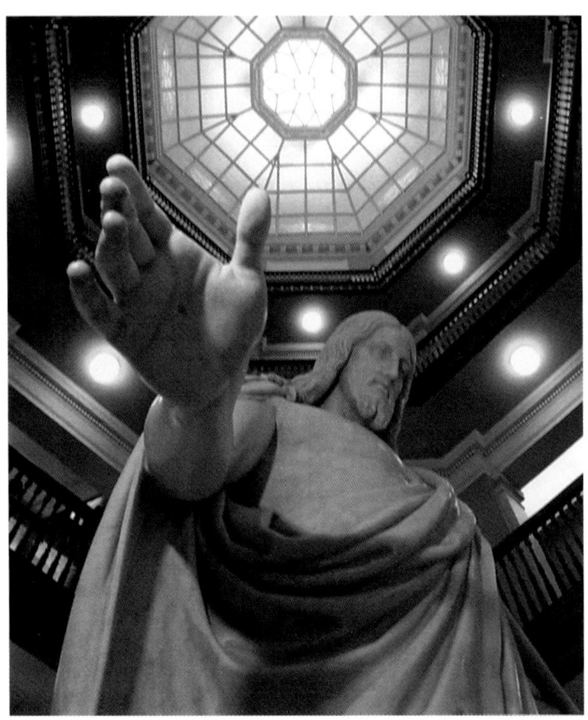

371 Bertel Thorvaldsen, *Christus Consolator*, replica, 1890, Johns Hopkins Hospital, Baltimore

The whole wall looks more like a billboard or a medical announcement than a work of art, and it is tempting to lament that Lubetkin did not commission a more substantial, lasting image for his building. Around the same time he did, after all, invite Henry Moore to make an alcove carving for his outstanding block of flats at High Point in north London. The outcome, although never installed in its intended space, was a masterly elmwood *Reclining Figure* which can be included with confidence among Moore's formidable achievements.[12] The stylish zest of the Health Centre did, nevertheless, complement the vivacity of the design that Lubetkin bestowed with such enthusiasm on his Finsbury building. It quickly came to be regarded as a landmark in modern medical architecture.

While Gordon Cullen was prepared to employ the technique and rhetoric of advertising, in order to promote the message supported by the Health Centre, a clear commitment to the role of painting and sculpture in public spaces was reasserted across the Atlantic. For the administrators of the WPA Federal Art Project gave employment to artists throughout the United States, and a number of them devoted their energies to projects in hospitals. The range of styles and subjects nurtured by the Project was wide, but the finest of them had no intention of returning to the pious conservatism of the nineteenth century. Back then, art in American hospitals was usually expected to carry a powerful religious charge. When the Baltimore businessman Johns Hopkins donated several million dollars for a splendid new hospital in the city, spiritual priorities were at the forefront of his concerns. Even though he insisted on the high calibre of the surgeons and physicians who would staff his exemplary building, the donor was also at pains to recommend the beneficial 'influences of religion . . . upon the whole management of the Hospital'.[13] In order to honour this special request, a speaker at the dedicatory opening of the building in 1889 voiced the hope that a benefactor would present a copy of Bertel Thorvaldsen's carving *Christus Consolator* as a reminder to staff, students and patients alike 'that over this institution rests the perpetual benediction of Christian charity, the constant spirit of "good will to man" '.[14]

This wish was granted two years later, when a majestic full-size replica of Thorvaldsen's statue in the Frue Kirk, Copenhagen, was installed in the central reception hall of the neo-Gothic administration building (pl. 371). Originally lit from the lantern of the dome high above it, the towering robed figure has remained in position with his arm extended in blessing ever since. Cleaning women have been photographed kneeling in prayer in front of it before starting their work for the day, and its immense calm still exerts a reassuring influence on the patients: 'When I was first brought to this hospital as a very little girl', remembered one Baltimore resident, 'I was scared of the doctors, of what they would do to me. But then I thought, "*He's* on *my* side, and he's bigger'n *they* are!" '[15]

Such pious and tradition-laden priorities were far removed from the hopes motivating Walter Quirt, who was described as a 'social surrealist' when he worked for the WPA scheme between 1935 and 1943. At Bellevue Hospital, New York, he painted two elaborate mural panels in tempera for the psychiatry lecture room in 1937 (pl. 372). They

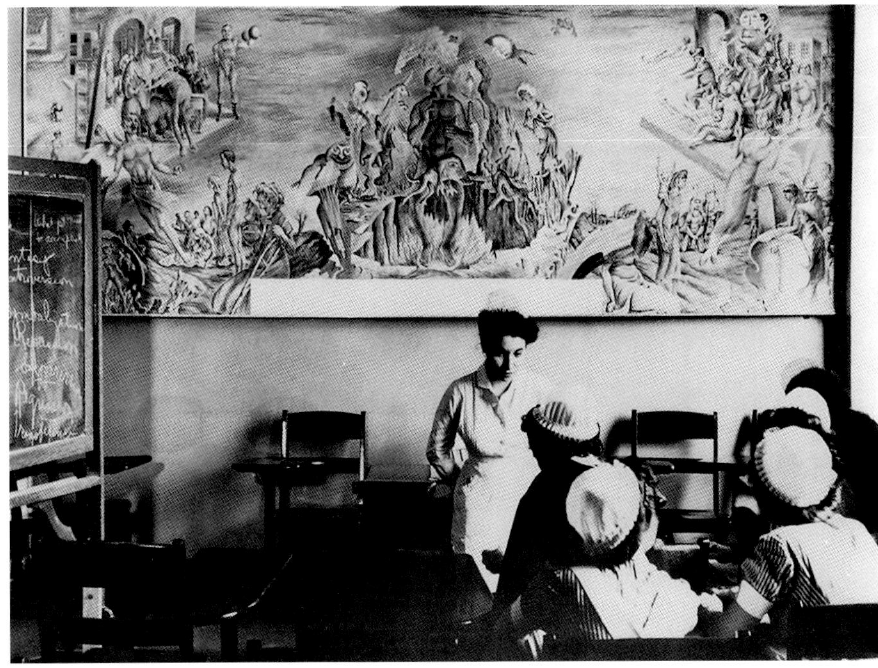

372 Walter Quirt, *The Growth of Medicine from Primitive Times* at Bellevue Hospital, New York, 1937, destroyed

interpreted the unwieldy theme of the *Growth of Medicine from Primitive Times* and could easily have degenerated into a laboured, pedantic depiction of historical events, but Quirt believed defiantly that the modern painter needed to escape from a literal representation of the allotted theme. 'The artist who deals in social content would be correct in assuming that what he does interests the spectator', Quirt wrote in an essay, *On Mural Painting*,

> if he could and would put into his mural all his doubts and conflicts, his philosophy and fantasy, all the release that the subject originally gave him. But between the original feeling stimulated by the subject and its final execution there is a tremendous gap, and it is this gap that really contains the vital content. The artist usually consciously censors his work and carefully gives a cut and dried version of a given theme . . . What he fails to put in are all his feelings and doubts. Thus the finished work has clearly written across it the dictum, 'Accept me and my sociological views completely, or not at all.' This can result in only one thing, blocking the audience from participating in the mural.[16]

As his Bellevue panels demonstrate, Quirt arrived at a more subconscious level of awareness. Although they appear to have been destroyed later, like many of the WPA images, photographs of the

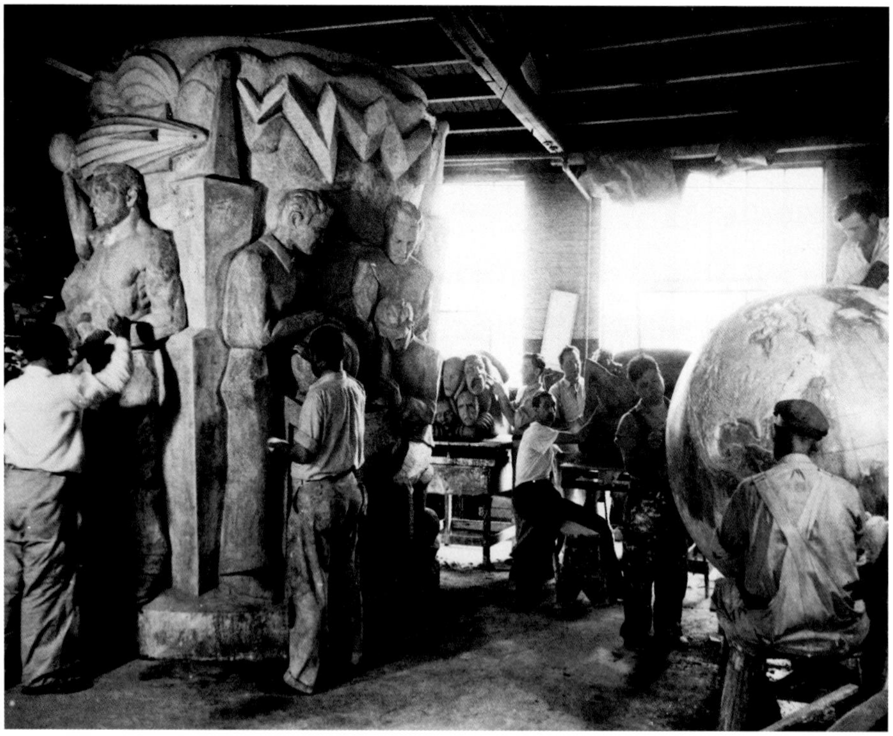

373 Waylande Gregory at work on *Light Dispelling Darkness*, 2 June 1937

paintings reveal that he developed a language aimed at a synthesis of Surrealism and a more indigenous American tradition. The powerful influences of Salvador Dalí, Max Ernst and Yves Tanguy are crossed with Thomas Hart Benton, and Quirt set both panels in a landscape of the mind almost as fanciful, in its way, as the dream-haunted territory defined by Hieronymus Bosch (see pl. 119). Areas of extreme perspectival recession, where ruined architecture evokes de Chirico-like presentiments of melancholy and decay, alternate with passages of complex foreground incident where the epic scope of Quirt's brief threatens to choke the compositions with a surfeit of detail. They are eclectic paintings, yet the precision of their execution is matched by the evident sincerity of his attempt to provide the Bellevue's psychiatry lecture room with images centrally related to the professional work carried out there.

He certainly hoped that the murals would be instrumental in eliciting a sense of therapeutic liberation. 'The fact that people generally do have a fantasy life, that this fantasy life constantly demands release, and that our fantasy worlds are all pretty similar', he wrote, 'offers us the key with which to unlock the emotional responses of people.' Yet it could only be attained if the muralist was prepared to participate in the process. 'What the artist must learn to do to evoke this response is to learn to release his own fantasies, release them completely and uninhibitedly, free from self-censorship and intellectualization whether they revolve around a factual problem or an imaginary one, for . . . art is a language of the emotions.'[17] Quirt seems to have met with the approval of the staff who worked in the psychiatry lecture room. According to the muralist Lou Block, who contrasted the paintings with the purely decorative murals 'in the lobby of the building [where] the embellishments are an adjunct to the architecture', Quirt's images served 'a directly functional' purpose. Here, in a space 'where lectures on psychiatry and the kindred subjects which have to do with the treatment of mentally disturbed individuals are given', his tempera panels were aimed at 'an audience whose interests are of a scientific order and his theme is entirely bound in with the functions of the room. The officials of the hospital find the subject matter of the mural accurately documented with a definite educational value and an aid to the work which is carried on in this room.'[18]

Other mural schemes for medical institutions demonstrate that 'social surrealism' was not the only stylistic option open to the WPA painter. If Quirt's visionary language was deemed suitable for a psychiatric unit, Darrel Austin employed a more heroic form of figuration in the four panels he produced for the Medical School of the University of Oregon in Portland. One of these lost images, symbolising the *Evolution of Education*, concentrated on the straightforward rhetoric of aspiration. The uplifted arms, straining towards a beneficent godlike figure personifying a teacher of omniscient authority, owe much to the Mexican muralists who exerted such a mesmeric influence on North American painting at that time.

A related form of heroism characterises the colossal ceramic fountain designed by Waylande Gregory for the grounds of the Roosevelt Hospital in New Brunswick (pl. 373). Prompted by his realisation that the site bordered the place where Edison had invented the incandescent lamp, Gregory chose as his subject *Light Dispelling Darkness*. 'I wanted to interpret this theme, not only in its scientific meaning', he explained, 'but in the broader sense of "Enlightenment Destroying Ignorance".'[19] Gregory, who in his student days had made monumental decorations for several buildings in Kansas City, was also conscious of the severe unemployment afflicting the area. It had formerly been at the centre of the thriving ceramic district of New Jersey. Encouraged by the WPA, who wanted to find work for the redundant artisans, he made every effort to use 'the materials and facilities of the local ceramic industry' in his fountain scheme. 'I found that the nucleus of men on the sculpture project in New Jersey consisted of ornamental modelers and plaster molders all formerly employed by the terra-cotta industry', Gregory wrote. 'I therefore decided to use terracotta and molded concrete aggregate in this fountain. Although these men had no experience executing sculptures directly in terra-cotta clay, they were quick to learn the important lesson of adhering to true sculptural forms as related to the purpose of the work and the nature and function of the material.' The fountain has since been moved,[20] but a photograph taken in the New York Federal Arts Project's sculpture studio shows work in progress on the over-life-size figures who served an almost caryatid-like function at the base of the sculpture. Zigzag lines expressive of electric energy crackle above their heads with Art Deco vivacity, while a vast global form on the right of the photograph indicates that Gregory saw the triumph of light over darkness as a force capable of transforming the world.

Gregory went on to create the enormous *Fountain of the Atom* for the entrance of the New York World's Fair in 1939, around the time when Albert Sumter Kelley was completing his WPA mural cycle for the children's ward of Lincoln Hospital in New York (pls 374–5). These sprightly canvases were clearly intended to delight the young patients, and they could well have succeeded in their aim. Working in an idiom that combined meticulous naturalism with passages of surprising fluency, Kelley celebrated the earthbound antics of the elephants as jauntily as the airborne performers swinging from their trapezes across the circus top. Playful and innocent, the murals belong to a strain in WPA painting that reflected what Francis V. O'Connor called 'a longing for a bucolic, or just a plain, peaceful, uncluttered past that is now lost'.[21] Although no hint can be detected in Kelley's work of the seedy side of circus life in the 1930s, his determination to concentrate on acrobatic *élan* constituted a well-judged response to the needs of the children in the Lincoln Hospital's ward.

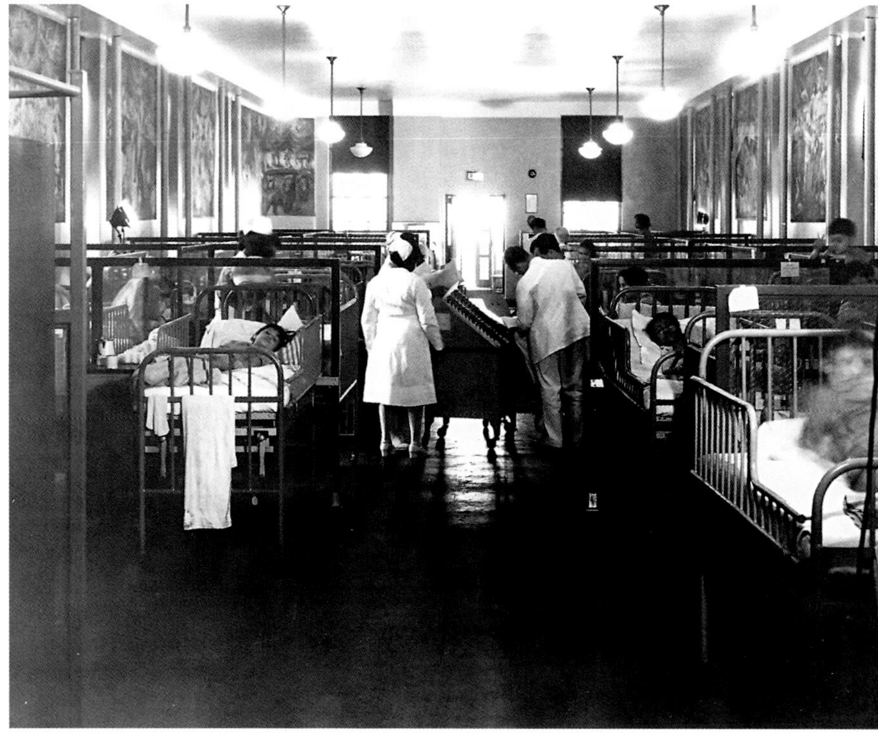

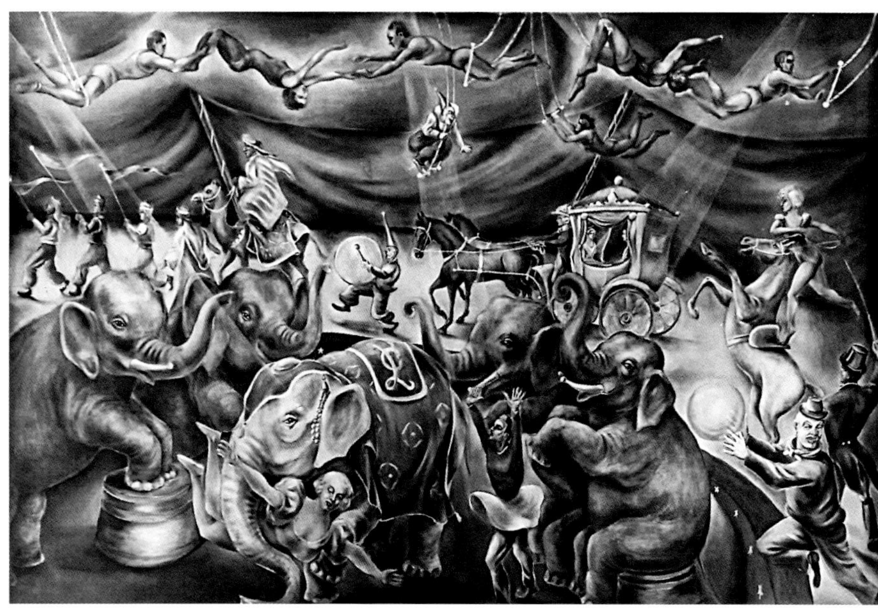

374 *(top)* Albert Sumter Kelley, Mural Cycle for Children's ward, Lincoln Hospital, New York, *c.*1939, destroyed

375 *(bottom)* Albert Sumter Kelley, *Circus Parade*, part of Mural Cycle for Children's ward, Lincoln Hospital, New York, *c.*1939, destroyed

The accessible figurative style employed by Kelley did not always ensure popularity for hospital decorations. A more abstract approach could also win favour, as Ilya Bolotowsky discovered while he was employed by the mural division of the Federal Arts Project. In 1940, he received a com-

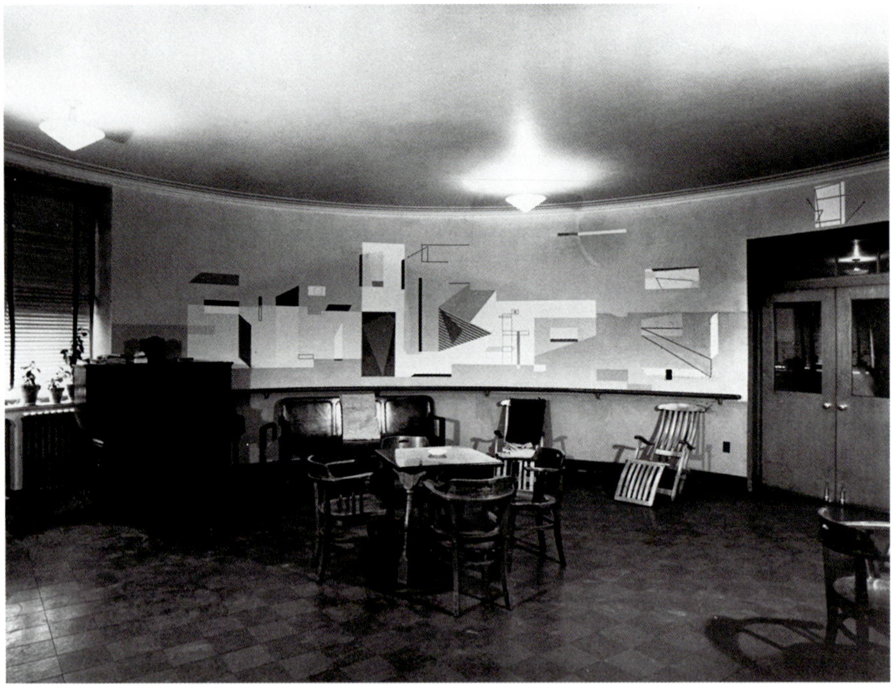

mission to execute a wall-painting for the Men's Day Room of the Chronic Diseases Hospital on Welfare Island, New York. It had previously been decorated with 'a photomural of girls in bathing suits. The confined men, aroused by the sight of the scantily clad females, had defaced the photomural with pornographic graffiti.'[22] Understandably, Bolotowsky found the Day Room 'rather depressing' when he visited it.[23] So he contemplated how to provide its occupants with an image they would respect rather than vandalise.

The opportunity provided here was daunting in scale: the oil painting, executed on canvas and then attached to a curving wall, extended fifteen metres along the Day Room. Bolotowsky, however, had already gained considerable experience of large-scale decorations in his two previous murals for the Federal Art Project, working under the supervision of his fellow-abstractionist Burgoyne Diller.[24] So the hospital commission was carried out with com-

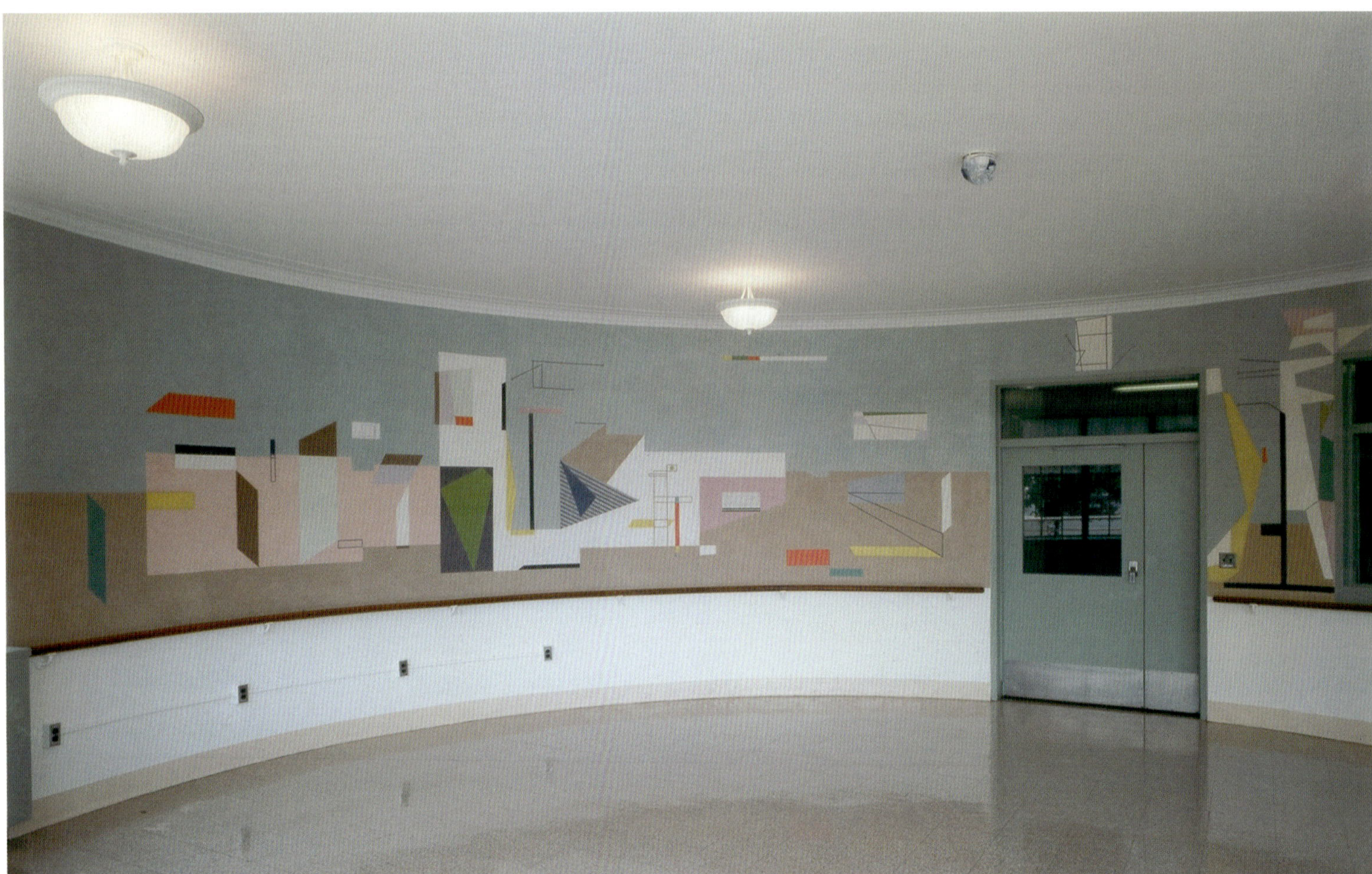

mendable assurance. Since the wall was divided horizontally by a handrail, beneath which chairs were likely to be placed, he restricted the lower section of the mural to a plain expanse of grey-brown. Although it might have become dull in the hands of another painter, photographs of the original mural disclose that he treated this band of uninterrupted colour as an expanse of water (pl. 376).

Bolotowsky's solution was ingenious, leaving him free to produce images above the handrail evocative of sailing. He called the mural *Abstraction* and its schematic organisation certainly accords well with the style of an artist who in 1936 had become a co-founder of the American Abstract Artists Association. Yet his mature neo-plastic manner, much indebted to the example of Mondrian, only emerged after the Second World War. In 1940 he was still prepared to allow blue-and-green references to sail reflections, keels and rudder forms into the otherwise austere structure of his mural. Even if these boat shapes might not have been readily recognisable to the men in the Day Room, they seem to have approved of Bolotowsky's painting and refrained from vandalising it.

The artist himself felt very enthusiastic about the Day Room venture. He saw it as an opportunity to liberate 'a very unusually beautiful' interior space. Bolotowsky argued, in a thoughtful statement submitted to the New York City WPA/FAP Mural Division, that the room's 'roundness might give some patients a feeling of being walled-in and fenced off from the rest of the world. Therefore, in the mural I have sought to create a feeling of a free, open space. . . The shapes of the doors and windows all around the day room have been woven into the design. . . Since straight lines are the most restful things to contemplate, this mural is of straight lines and geometric shapes. The day room, its architecture, and its mural form one plastic unit.'

Sadly, the mural suffered from neglect after the war and it was painted over. Although Bolotowsky started recreating it in 1981, he died the same year before completing his task. But subsequently, when the hospital was renamed the Coler-Goldwater Specialty Hospital and Nursing Facility, on what is now Roosevelt Island, the mural was indeed restored with invaluable help from the artist's son Andrew Bolotowsky. Seven coats of over-painting were removed with the aid of chisels and solvent paste, before areas missing from the original mural were carefully painted-in. The result, completed in 2001 (pl. 377), discloses just how well Bolotowsky had used his Suprematist-influenced abstraction to give the Day Room its distilled serenity and poise.

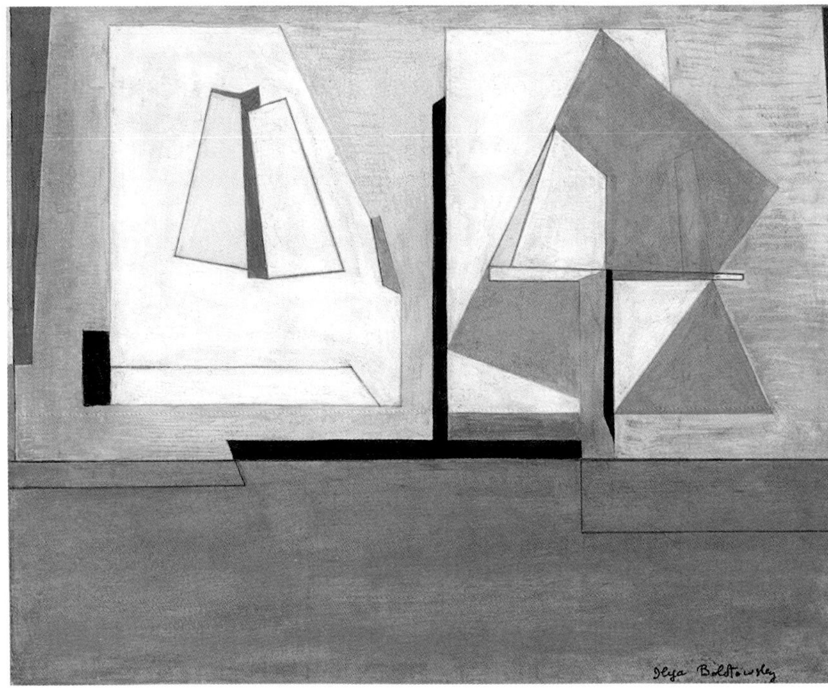

378 (*above*) Ilya Bolotowsky, *Sailing*, Study for second Men's Day Room mural, Chronic Diseases Hospital, Welfare Island, New York, 1940, Yale University Art Gallery, New Haven

Back in the 1940s, realising that the mural 'kept the patients quiet',[25] the Doctors' Committee members were sufficiently gratified to commission another decoration from the artist. Although it was never carried out, sketches approved by the doctors propose an image close in feeling to its predecessor. A nautical scene can once more be discerned in the taut, angular disposition of a tempera design for the mural's left section,[26] and at its centre is a mast-like form clearly reliant on the language of De Stijl painting (pl. 378). Evoking once again the bulk of distant ships, the mural would have taken its viewers away from their institutional confines and presented them with an open-air alternative, serene in its emphasis on maritime activity in surroundings unruffled by disturbance of any kind. However, Bolotowsky's inability to execute this second Day Room mural underlines the limited opportunities then available to artists in the US. Their frustrations become all the more palpable when set against the contemporaneous flowering of public commissions in Mexico, where hospitals across the nation became transformed by painters of exceptional ambition, dynamism and tenacity.

376 (*facing page, top*) Ilya Bolotowsky, *Abstraction*, wall painting for Men's Day Room (B11), Hospital for Chronic Diseases, Welfare Island, New York, 1940–41, in original situ

377 (*facing page, bottom*) Ilya Bolotowsky, *Abstraction*, 1940–41, restored 2001, Coler-Goldwater Memorial Hospital, New York

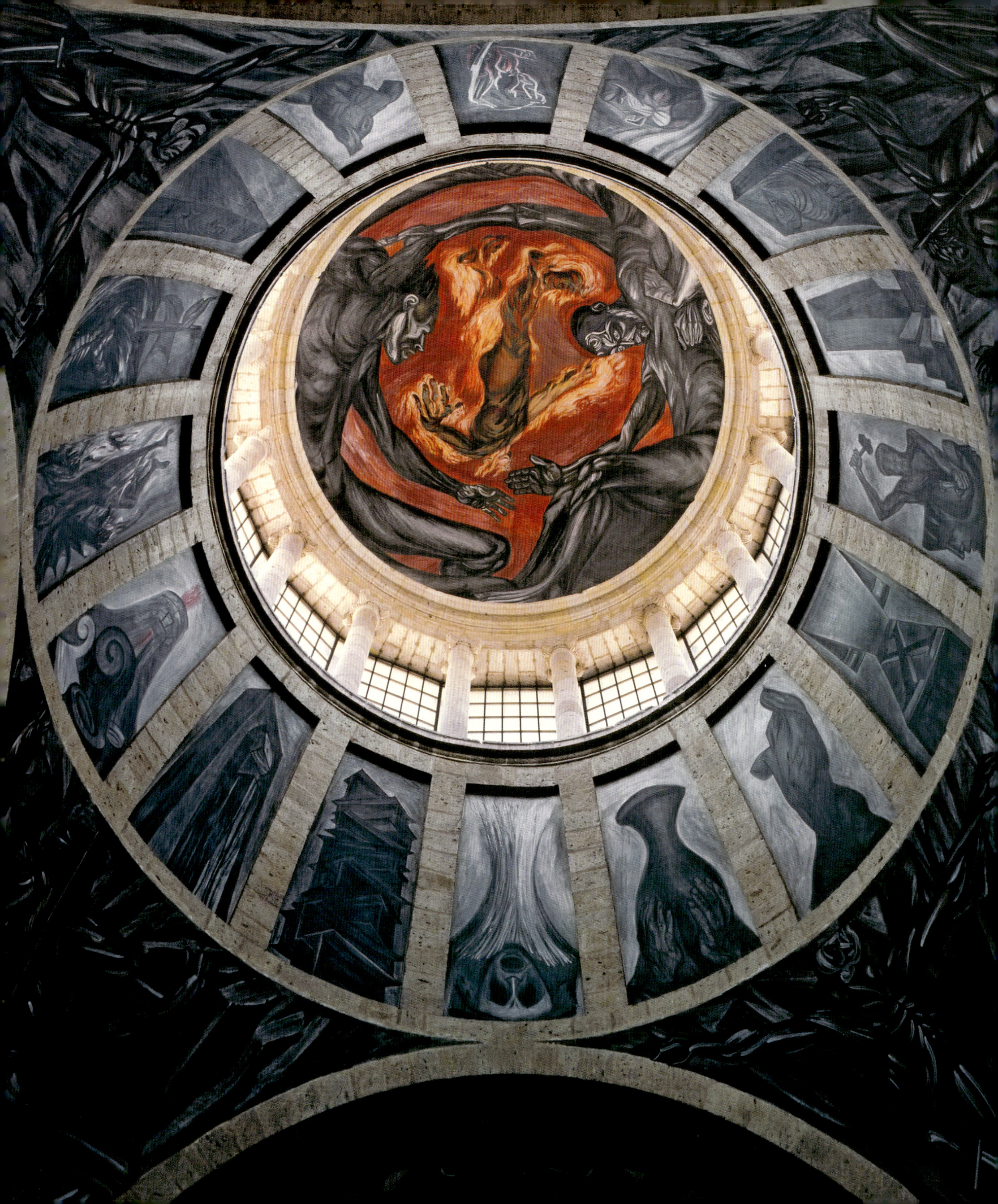

TWENTY-FOUR
THE MEXICAN REVOLUTION

Stimulated beyond measure by patrons willing to let muralists flourish on the grandest scale imaginable, artists in twentieth-century Mexico brought about an efflorescence of public decorations. Of the three most prominent painters active during the great age of mural painting, José Clemente Orozco was an unpredictable choice to carry out a major hospital commission (pl. 379). His work, after all, is characterised by a refusal to avoid the harrowing aspects of life. He did not soften his attitude after accepting, in the late 1930s, an invitation from Don Everado Topete to produce an extensive mural scheme for the Hospicio Cabañas in Guadalajara, the capital city of the state where he was born.

Diego Rivera, the irrepressible optimist, would have been the most congenial artist for such a task, and many years later he executed a typically benevolent painting for the Hospital de la Raza in Mexico City (see pl. 397). Yet Orozco, who took on the Hospicio Cabañas commission with wholehearted conviction and turned it into the most impressive of all his mural projects, was incapable of making images that soothe the eye. Contrasting him with his contemporary, Antonio Rodríguez argued that 'Rivera raises idols, Orozco destroys them. Rivera's *leitmotiv* is construction, Orozco's is fire, destruction and chaos. To the former everything live is important – a flower, a woman's breasts or a landscape – whereas the latter seems able to respond only to drama, tragedy or mourning.'[1]

Nor was this dark vision merely a temperamental indulgence on Orozco's part. He believed that the best way to counter the negative side of existence was to confront it in the most direct manner. Turning away from destructive themes would have been tantamount, for him, to accepting their existence. Orozco was obsessed by the need to forge an art that honestly and powerfully reflected the contradictions, complexities and disillusionments riddling contemporary Mexican society. Having assisted the armed revolution with his caricatures, he then found outspoken fault with those responsible for implementing the revolutionary victory. Orozco never aligned himself with the Mexican Communist party, as did Rivera and David Alfaro Siqueiros. His view of Mexico's working people veered from warm understanding to outright despair, and the volatility of his vision is the hallmark of a man whose extreme sensitivity found itself battered by the exhilarating yet traumatic character of Mexican life during that turbulent period.[2]

At the cruciform church of the Hospicio Cabañas, formerly the city's orphanage, Orozco displayed his stringent and deeply troubled imagination in all its uncomfortable rawness. Having spent the previous two years working on mural

379 (*facing page*) José Clemente Orozco, Cupola of Hospicio Cabañas, Guadalajara, 1936–9

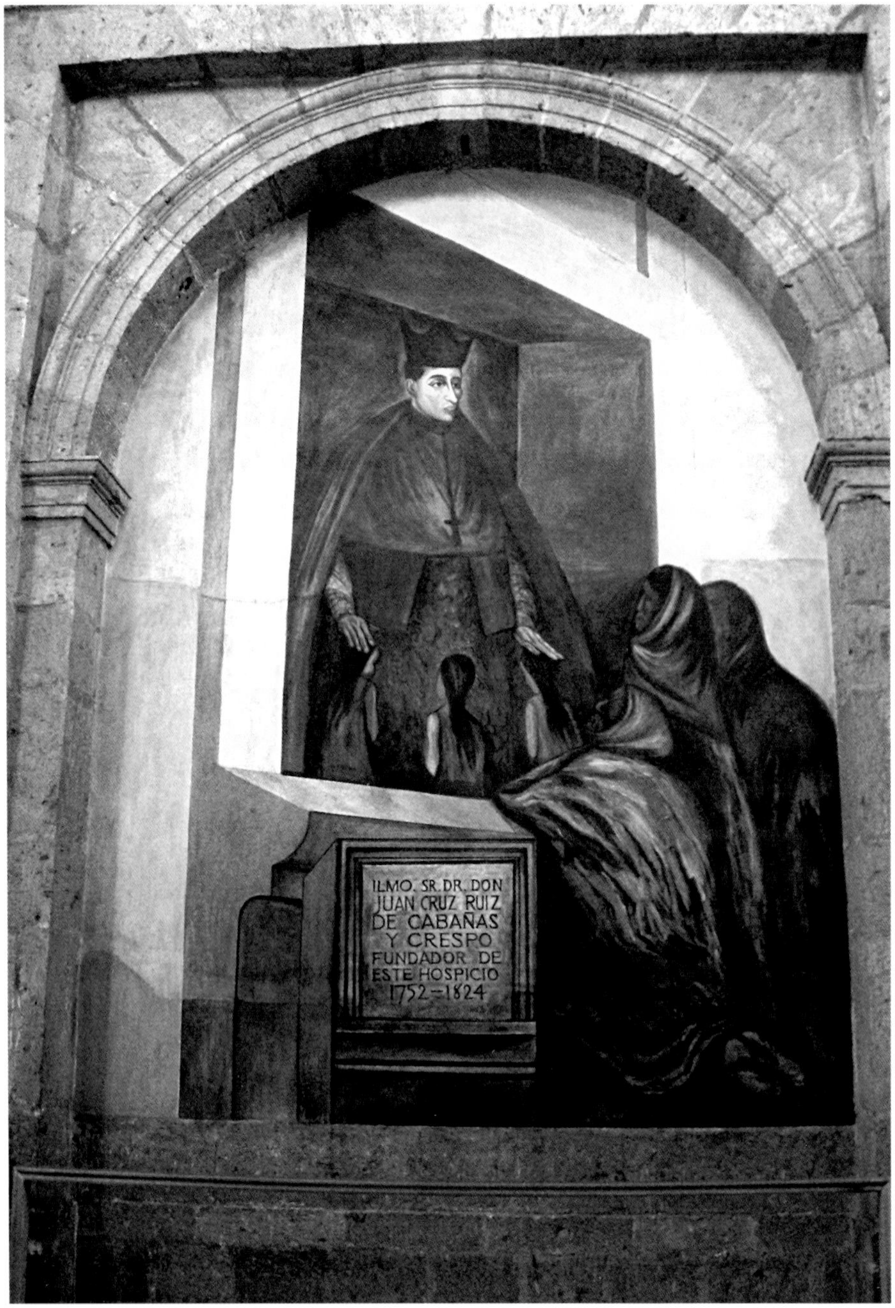
ILMO. SR. DR. DON
JUAN CRUZ RUIZ
DE CABAÑAS
Y CRESPO
FUNDADOR DE
ESTE HOSPICIO
1752–1824

380 José Clemente Orozco, *Bishop Juan Cruz Ruiz de Cabanas Welcoming Women at Hospicio Cabañas*, 1936–9, Hospicio Cabañas, Guadalajara

schemes in other prominent Guadalajara locations, the University and the Palacio de Gobierno, he arrived at the Hospicio as an artist who had already given vent to rasping images of history as a Joycean nightmare. Like Stephen Daedalus, the agonised masses who seethe, implore and suffer on the walls of these earlier cycles are struggling to awake from a protracted torment. Orozco was determined to stress how difficult such a phoenix-like resurgence would be, and many of the images he produced there have a virulence that assails the spectator in a manner calculated to overwhelm or even terrify. Only in the uppermost sections of the murals does he offer any hint of hope, and even here the meaning is ambivalent. At the Palacio de Gobierno, Hidalgo towers above the pullulating hordes like a harbinger of Mexico's future striving for independence. Yet Orozco presents the white-haired colossus as fierce and vengeful, his right fist thrusting out of the picture space in an aggressive form that dramatises the violence involved in overthrowing tyrannical oppression.

Far from deciding that he had exorcised this tragic interpretation of history, and using the Hospicio commission to elaborate an alternative, Orozco deepened and intensified the same tumultuous vision on 1200 square metres of walls, vaults and cupola. The deconsecrated Hospicio church presented him with epic opportunities to develop these themes on the grandest scale, and he met the challenge with a furious, uncompromising energy. Only in one of the murals does serenity prevail. The founder of the orphanage, Bishop Juan Cruz Ruiz de Cabañas, is shown at the Hospicio's entrance to welcome the huddle of ragged, exhausted women who hope for his assistance (pl. 380). They are generalised enough in their massive cloaks to symbolise the whole of humanity in travail, desperate for the solace and protection that the Hospicio can provide. One old woman leans an elbow thankfully on the ledge surmounting a plinth with a formal inscription about the bishop. It makes clear that the institution has been offering care for more than a century, and the long-term priorities of the Hospicio are underlined by Orozco's decision to include three orphan girls who press forward to receive the prelate's benediction. They kneel close enough to be partially enfolded in robes almost as capacious and reassuring as the cloak worn by El Greco's *Madonna of Charity* at the Illescas Hospital (see pl. 103). Bishop Cabañas responds to the urgency implicit in these waif-like figures by pressing his hands very firmly on their bowed heads. The particularity of the consoling gesture made by his attenuated fingers is, at the same time, allied with an awareness of his responsibilities in their largest sense. His gaze is deliberately directed away from the children and the women behind them towards a more distant perspective, thereby signifying that he took into account the needs of the entire popu-

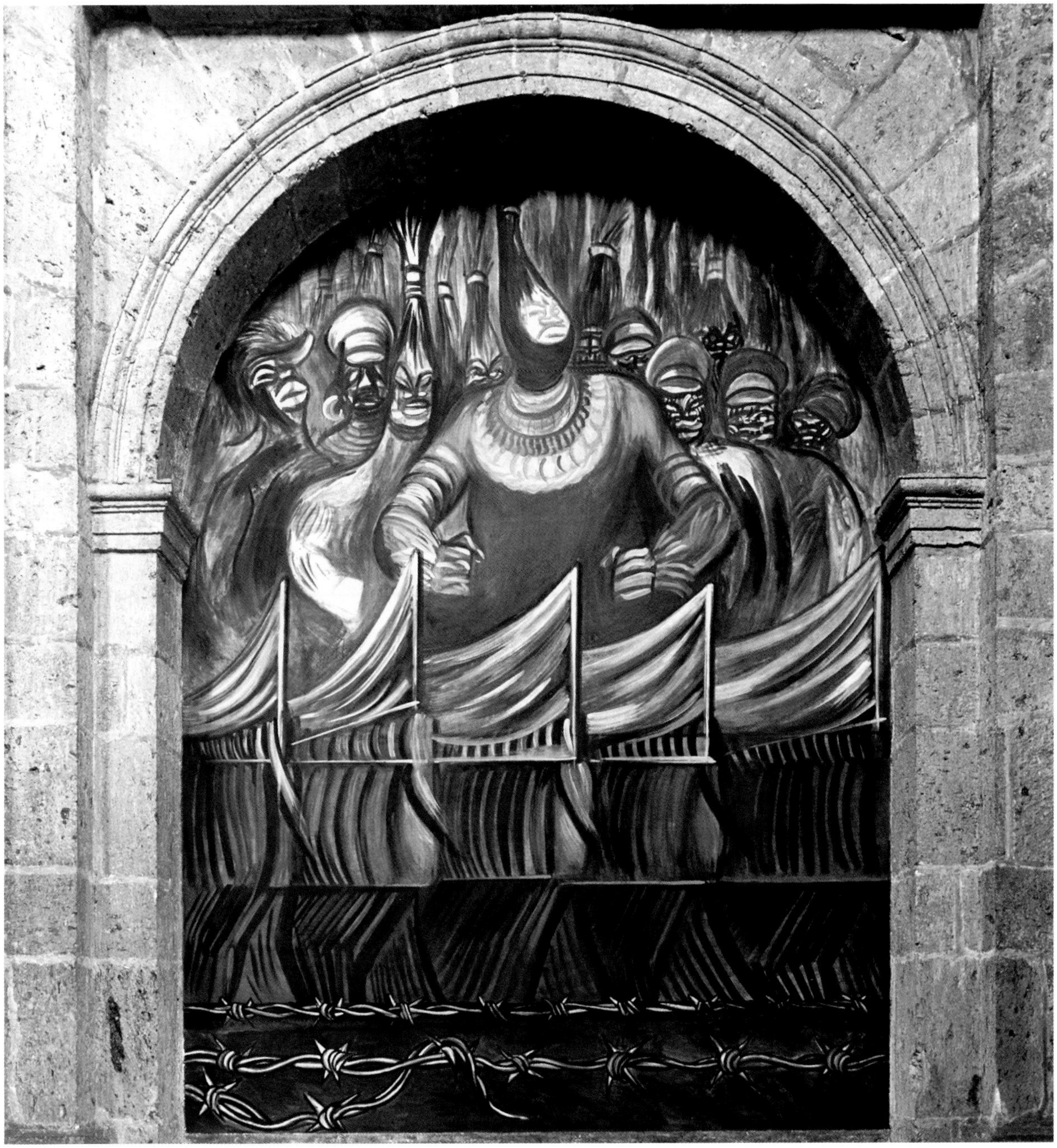

381 José Clemente Orozco, *The Dictators*, 1936–9, Hospicio Cabañas, Guadalajara

lace even as his hands bless two of the Hospicio's inhabitants.

This painting provides a rare moment of calm in a scheme otherwise preoccupied with images of apocalyptic upheaval. Opposite the picture with the bishop, Orozco executed an unyielding mural of the *Dictators* where a cluster of grotesque thugs preside over a march-past by ranks of identical, anonymous supporters, bearing flags yet bereft of individual thought (pl. 381). Most of Orozco's decorations in the church leap out from their surfaces like phantasms personifying the dangers that assail people hoping for the bishop's protection. Unlike his previous Guadalajara mural projects, which concentrated on contemporary subjects, he deals here with the polarities of idealism and disillusion in the context of Mexico's troubled history.

Vehement, looming and invariably macabre, the agents of conquest promise in one sense to liberate the nation from barbarity; but the triumphant

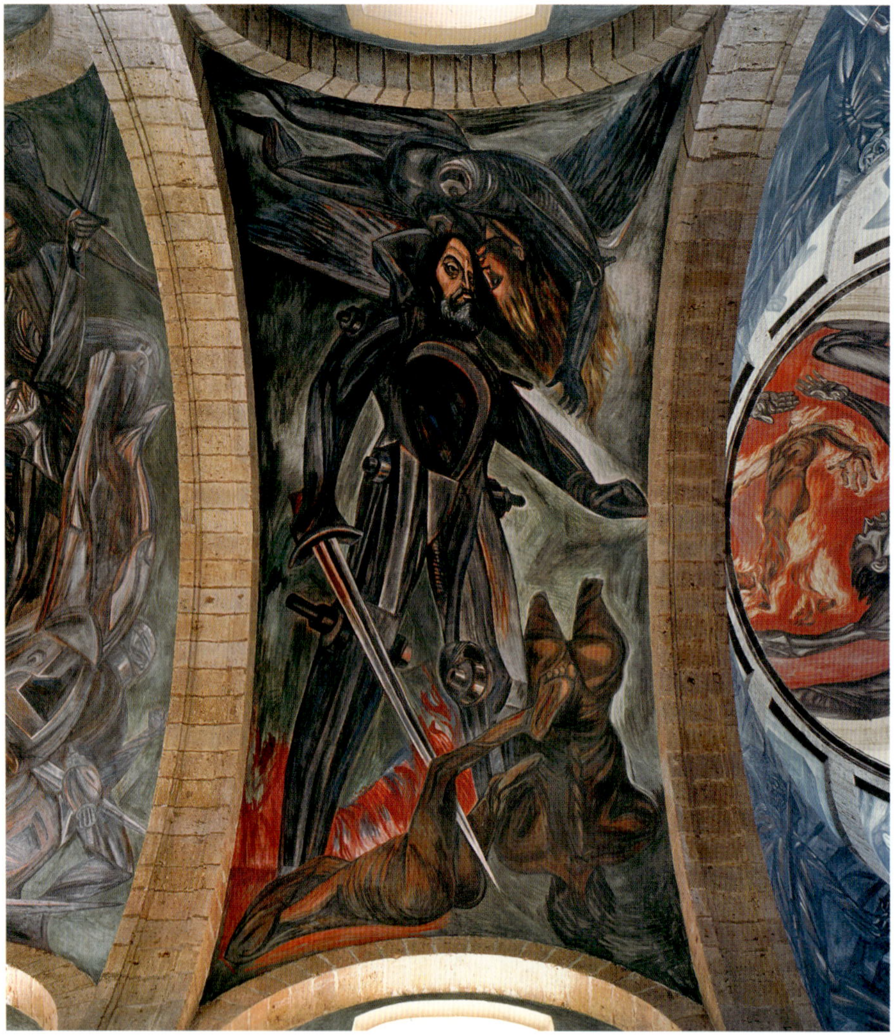

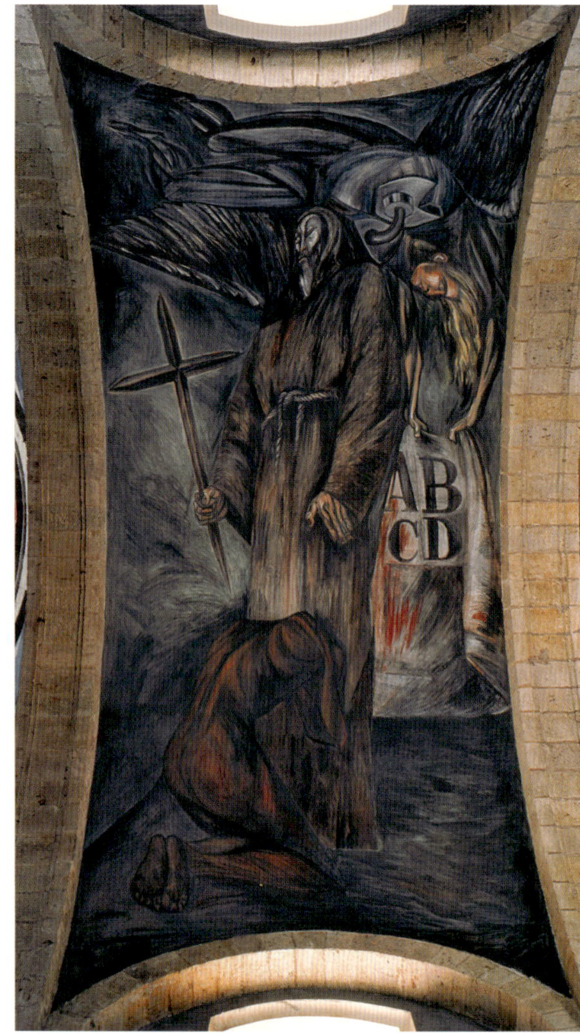

382 (*above left*) José Clemente Orozco, *Cortés the Executioner*, 1936–9, Hospicio Cabañas, Guadalajara

383 (*above right*) José Clemente Orozco, *Franciscan Monk with Crucifix*, 1936–9, Hospicio Cabañas, Guadalajara

conquistador Cortés is shown in one especially ominous painting as a grim-faced executioner brandishing a fearful sword (pl. 382). Shining horribly in the light, it threatens to slice through the naked body sprawled ignominiously on the blood-drenched earth. Cortés is guided by God, who communicates through the agency of the angel twisting dynamically through the sky to whisper in Cortés's ear. The angel's inverted position suggests, however, that the messenger may in some sense distort the divine communication, and the limbs of this winged courier are hinged with bolts redolent of a robot. They resemble the conquistador's armoured legs bestriding the land subjugated by his overweening army.

Here lies the paradox at the centre of the Hospicio decorations. Although Orozco pays tribute in the murals over the nave doors to the civilising influence of Cervantes and El Greco, a painter whose work surely played a substantial role in helping to develop Orozco's own impassioned style, the conquest itself is presented as a disturbing and dehumanised event. The Spanish King Philip II is seen as a pugnacious initiator of the conflict, grimly grasping a cross hefty enough to be used as a weapon. Moreover, in the enormous mural depicting the struggle at its height, one invader's horse sprouts a pair of heads while the steeds around him are metamorphosing into mechanisms devoid of any urges other than the brutalised desire to exterminate. Painted at a time when the world was about to be embroiled in a war more destructive and far-reaching than the campaigns conducted by Cortés, Orozco's images appear to contain references to modern conflict. They are fused with the historical conquest in order to express the artist's

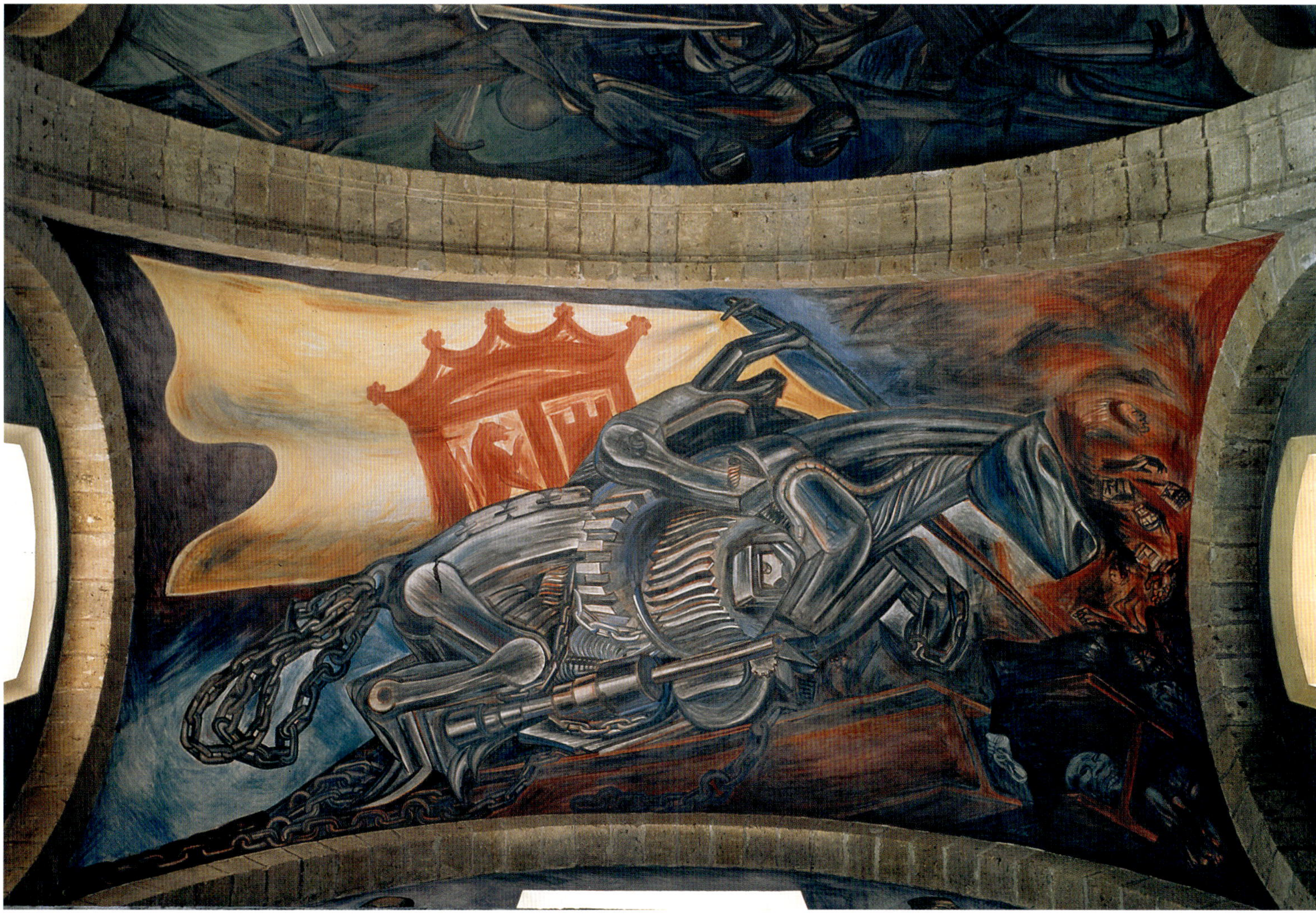

384 José Clemente Orozco, *Mechanical Horse*, 1936–9, Hospicio Cabañas, Guadalajara

belief that violent struggle is, in essence, unchanging. He abominated war so much that the murals convey an unmistakeable horror even as they confirm the conquistador's prowess.

The Hospicio scheme presents the colonising Franciscan monks in a generally favourable light, emphasising the protective role they played among the Mexican natives. It stresses as well the cultural benefits that the conquest brought to a country previously bedevilled by cruel, often bestial rituals. But Orozco was obsessed by duality and his depiction of Cortés's triumphant progress through the ravaged land is riddled with misgivings. One powerful image, which echoes the Cortés mural by showing a Franciscan priest backed by a mechanistic angel of God (pl. 383), dramatises the imposition of Christian religion on the Indians. Pale, haughty and omnipotent, the monk looms over the subjugated native with a crucifix that bears a disconcerting resemblance to Cortés's sword. 'As a painter', Orozco once explained, 'I take and accept the good and bad in man, I take it as being part of one unit. I believe that in everything, in men and in things, there are good and bad sides. This is the way the artist must confront problems, which he uses as raw materials for his creations.'[3]

Hence the alarming menace that runs through his interpretation of the conquest, prophesying the machine-like devastation of global conflict in the modern period. This link between historical and contemporary war reaches its apogee in the mural called *Mechanical Horse* (pl. 384). The conquistadorial mount has undergone a disturbing transformation, changing from an animal into a tank-like structure powered by an engine replete with cogs, pistons and shafts, and brandishing a 'tail' made of

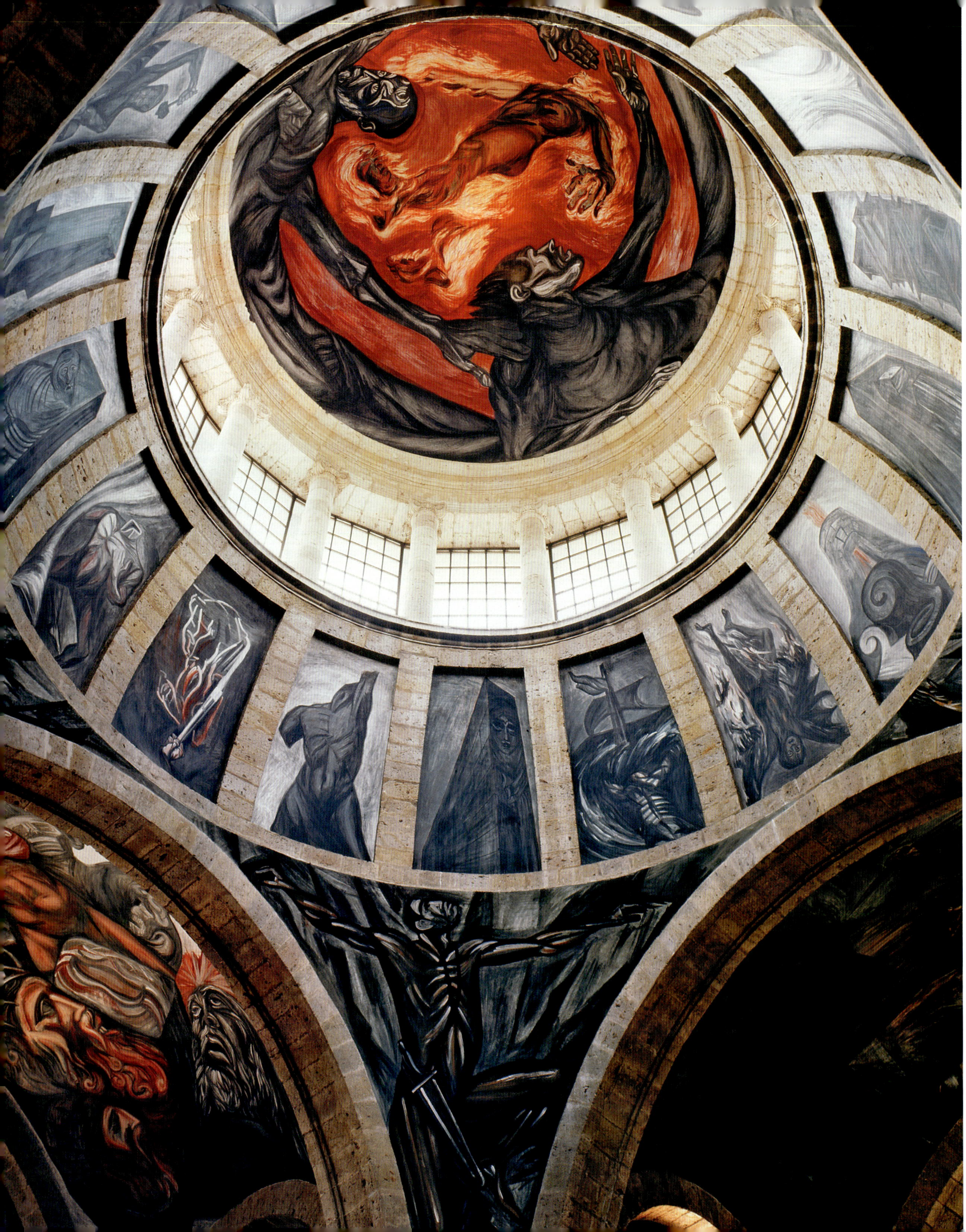

heavy chains. On its back, the heraldic banner bearing the lion and tower of Castile looks frankly anachronistic on this mechanical version of Yeats's 'rough beast',[4] slouching over a landscape that Orozco equated with the increasingly strife-ridden Europe of 1939.

Just as Orozco had reserved the most positive elements for the highest reaches of his previous Guadalajara schemes, so he allowed himself to become rather more optimistic when tackling the climax of the Hospicio murals: a cupola some fourteen metres in diameter. In the rest of the church he had, on the whole, restricted his palette to a sombre range. When Guillermo Lemus later restored the murals, he came across a test-run by the artist employing ten distinct shades of black, while the lighter colours that Orozco did admit to the lower reaches of the decoration still signified the tarnished, bloody stains of battle rather than anything more exuberant. In the top of the cupola, however, he suddenly gave rein to more inflammatory hues, gaining in forcefulness by contrasting so completely with the subdued colours below. Orozco leads the viewer towards these orgiastic heights by degrees, commencing with armed men climbing up the spandrels towards the light-filled bowl beyond (pl. 385). The rifles and other weapons weigh their bodies down, making the ascent even more arduous than it would otherwise have been. But these figures are sufficiently sinewy and aspirant to arrive at the summit, even if their path is formidably steep and they throw back their heads in awed acknowledgement of the ordeal confronting them.

The images immediately above are not calculated to instil confidence (pl. 385). A circle of recessed paintings awaits them, bearing forms as harshly defined as the baleful patriarch swinging his hammer in preparation for a blow on his chisel. Some of the murals in this forbidding circle are confined to inanimate objects, like the stack of industrial units stretching their oppressive angularity into a sky almost obliterated by their bulk. Their machine-age starkness is palpable, yet their impassivity stops short of the horror and distress conveyed in the paintings where figures dominate the compositions. One of them reveals himself, with a peremptory sweep of the curtain, as a headless apparition, ready to participate in some grotesque ceremony. Nearby another decapitated body, this time more akin to a statue, lifts the trunks of amputated arms in the air, while a further painting is filled with the blazing form of a winged figure plummeting headlong through the air. Despite the references to painting, sculpture and construction incorporated in this circle, Orozco's temperamental scepticism gives the entire sequence an embattled character.

It is a relief to discover that these sombre murals are succeeded, higher up, by an array of windows irradiating the bowl of the cupola with light (pl. 385). The affirmative nature of this incendiary scene can be gauged by comparing it with Orozco's earlier interpretation of the Prometheus myth. There, at Pomona College in California, he showed the gigantic protagonist stealing the sacred fire from the gods. But instead of enlightening the crowds gathered beneath him, Prometheus struggles mournfully to retain his prize while the people beseech him to emancipate them without discernible faith that their cries will be answered. A similar sense of strain is detectable round the lower edges of the Hospicio cupola, where outsize figures in vivid electric blue strive to arise from their recumbent position. They reach across to grasp one another's hands without success, and Orozco invests one bearded figure with a frowning intensity reminiscent of a saint in a forbidding medieval icon. The power of this hieratic head is reinforced by the spontaneously applied brushstrokes that give his features much of their mesmeric vigour. Orozco was capable of great improvisatory boldness when he worked, and Antonio Rodríguez once marvelled at the demonic panache of his mark-making. Watching the muralist busily painting the ceiling of the Iglesia de Jesús in Mexico City, Rodríguez described how,

> with a brush which he had attached to a stick in order to enlarge the swing of his strokes, Orozco worked like one possessed. He did not paint like Diego Rivera, as if he were fondling the wall with his brush, he painted with energetic swings of his only arm, as if the brush were a weapon. When I saw Orozco painting I always felt as if I were witnessing a fight. And his fight was really a struggle against the limitations of art, against himself, against society which, for all his denials, he was for ever castigating.[5]

Nowhere in Orozco's work is this audacious handling of paint more compelling than in the Hospi-

385 *(facing page)* José Clemente Orozco, Armed men climbing towards the recessed paintings in the cupola, 1936–9, Hospicio Cabañas, Guadalajara

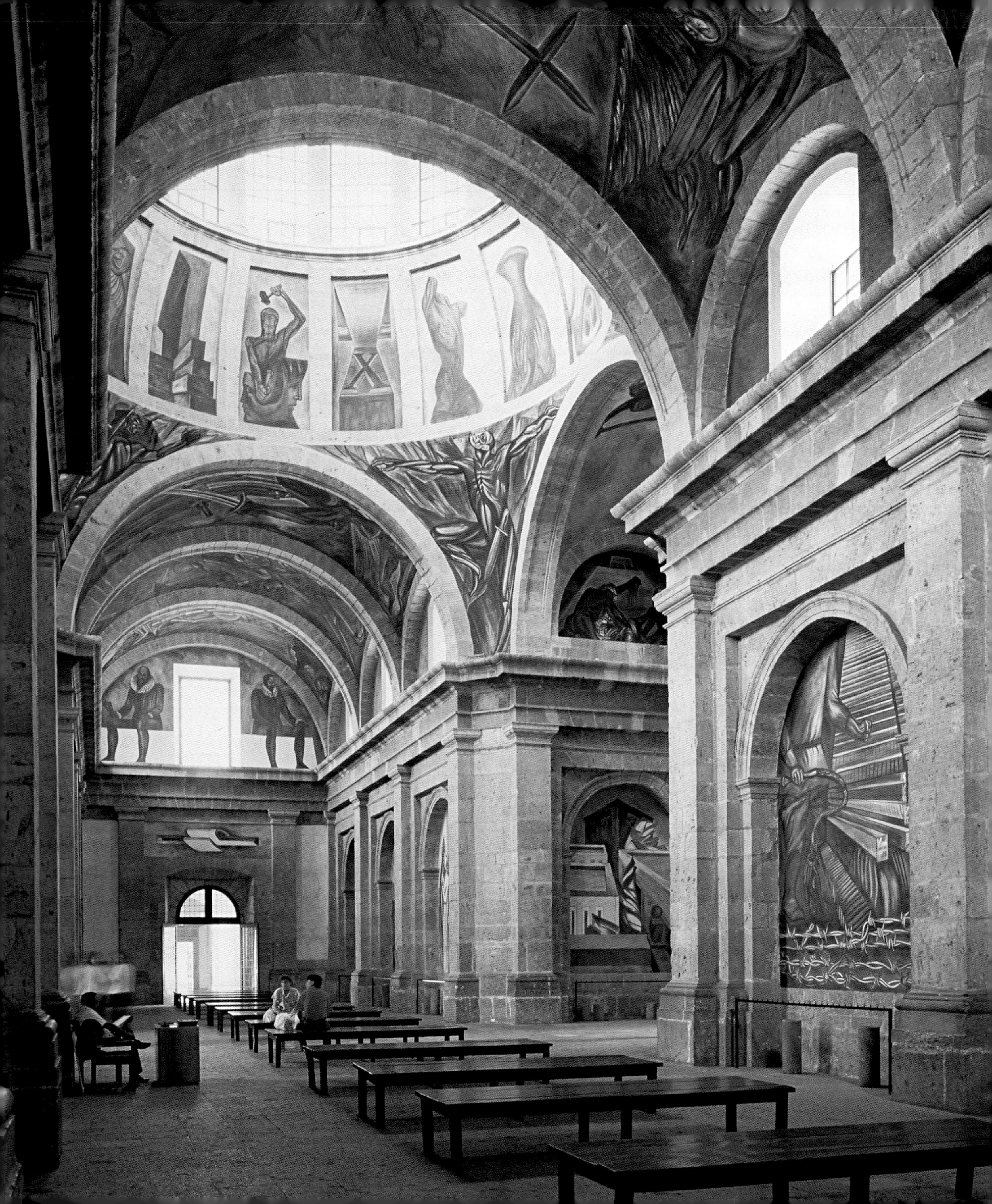

cio's cupola. For the Promethean figure at the centre of the composition has become *The Man of Fire*, consumed by tongues of orange flames that will soon reduce his body to ashes (pls 379 and 387). As in much of Orozco's work, the meaning of this torch-like apotheosis is ambiguous to the point of enigma. The artist never explained what he intended, and in one sense it must be seen as an image of imminent disintegration. But he chose to depict the moment before immolation, when the burning hero still achieves a spectacular grandeur. The flames raging round feet, arms and head have not yet destroyed the rest of his flesh, and so his muscular presence still asserts itself in the scorching red air. The flames lend him a savage magnificence as he leaves earthly constraints behind. Painted with a vivacity matching the dynamism that Prometheus relied on to steal the fire from Olympus, he ascends into space like a man released at last from all burdens.

After the melancholy commotion, futility and devastation so evident in the lower murals at the Hospicio, the verve of this blazing airborne demigod is cathartic indeed. Having acquainted humanity with fire and the arts, and then become engulfed in a conflagration intended by Orozco as a warning against the perils of self-destruction, the Promethean figure propels himself towards heaven with an authority that gives the entire Hospicio sequence a final glimpse of freedom, renewal and hope. Achieved despite everything that the evil forces of negation were allowed to perpetrate below, his purified release seems all the more impressive because it is so hard-won.

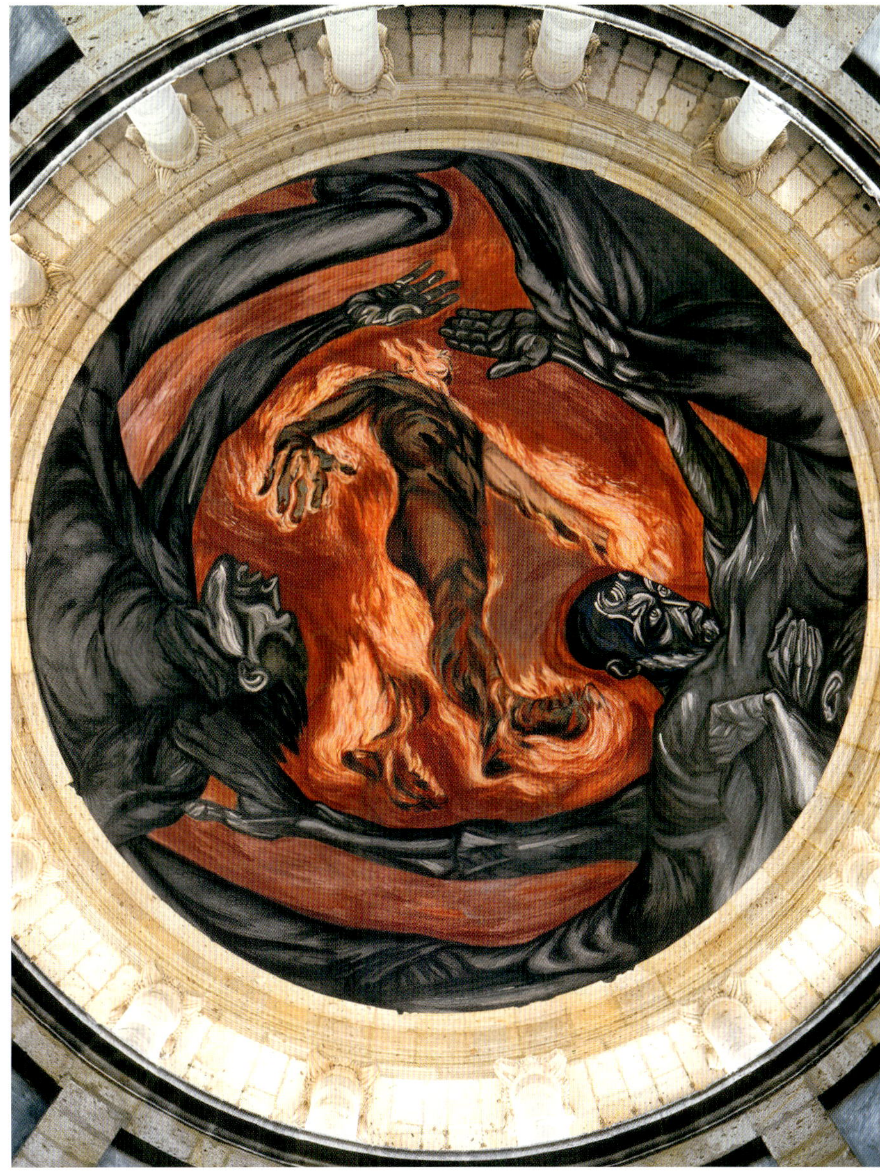

387 *(above)* José Clemente Orozco, *The Man of Fire*, 1936–9, Hospicio Cabañas, Guadalajara

No direct relationship can be discerned between the Hospicio's former function and most of the murals here (pl. 386). Although Orozco went out of his way to paint the institution's founding bishop (see pl. 380), as well as a dedicatory wall panel showing the Hospicio Cabañas itself, the rest of his sequence refers to the 'health of the nation' only in the widest sense. Diego Rivera, by contrast, was willing to place medical themes at the heart of his frescoes, notably in the imposing image he created for the Hospital de la Raza towards the end of his prolific career (see pl. 397). Before then, he had dealt with curative concerns on a couple of occasions. At the Secretariat of Health and Public Assistance, an idiosyncratic building designed in early Mexican Art Deco style by Carlos Obregón Santacelia, he was invited in 1929 to decorate the main ceiling and wall areas of the conference room.

Santacelia, a confirmed devotee of Rivera's work and the man who later invited him to paint an outstanding mural in the Hotel del Prado,[6] was responsible for the Secretariat commission. Having spent much of the decade labouring on the immense task of decorating the Ministry of Education, where he and his assistants completed an astounding total of 235 separate fresco sections, Rivera must have regarded the Secretariat project as a relatively simple affair. Although he designed four stained-glass windows elsewhere in the building and painted two frieze-like frescoes called

386 *(facing page)* Windows irradiating cupola with light, Hospicio Cabañas, Guadalajara

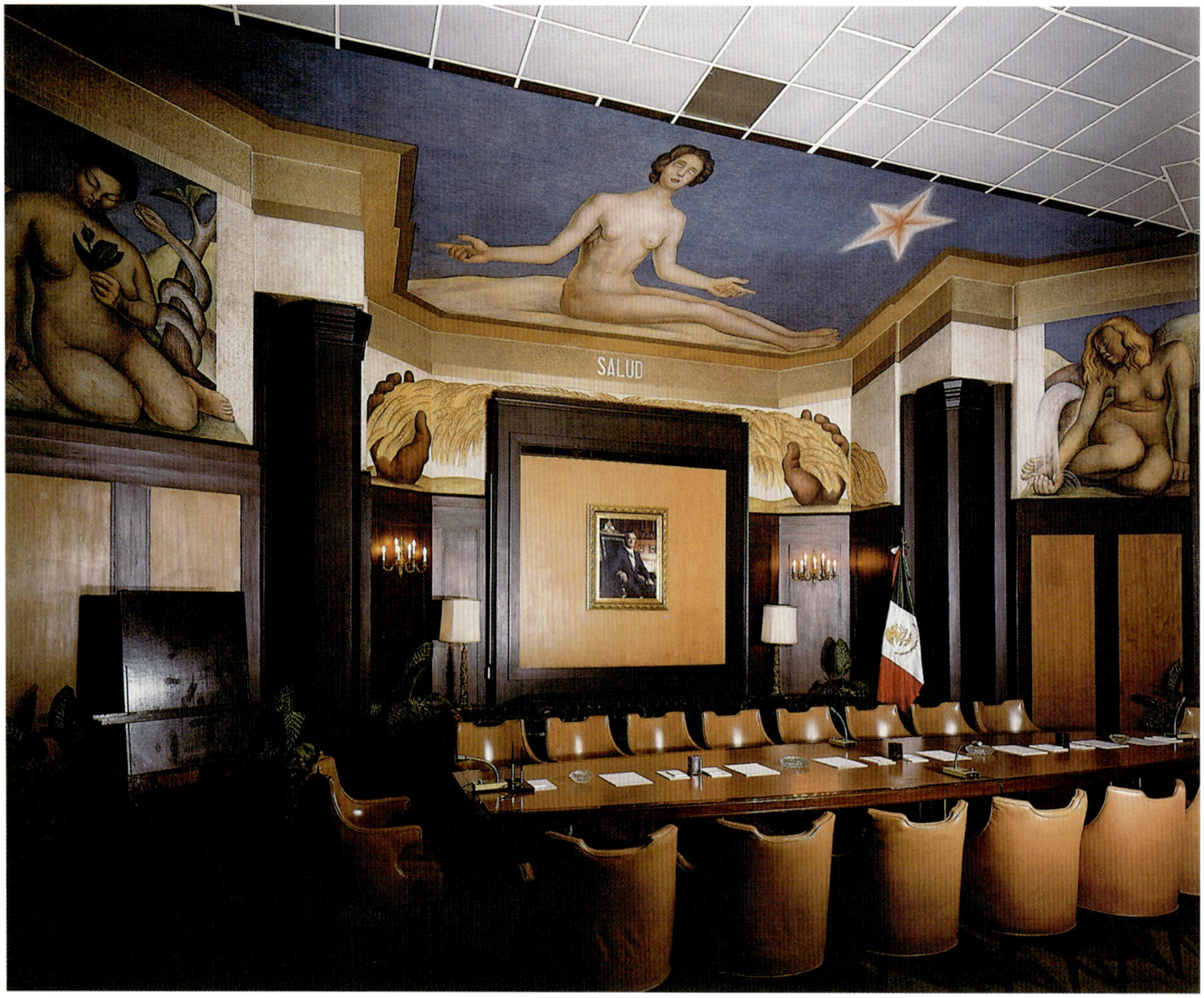

388 Diego Rivera, *Knowledge*, *Purity*, *Health*, 1929, Secretariat of Health and Public Assistance, Mexico

Microbiology and *Education and Prophylaxis* for the Pavilion of Laboratories on the far side of the central court,[7] the conference room was the most important interior scheme he carried out here. Continuing to employ the monumental classicising language he had earlier developed for the chapel of the National Autonomous University of Chapingo, Rivera concentrated principally on six female nudes personifying 'Purity, Continence, Health, Life, Strength and Knowledge'.

They gave him the chance to indulge his love of painting voluptuous women, and the sensuality of these bodies is their most outstanding characteristic. However, Rivera has taken them out of the traditional boudoir setting, where many nineteenth-century male artists preferred to locate their models, and placed them in the Mexican landscape at its most primordial. *Knowledge*, who sits among bare hills while the symbolic serpent whispers in her ear, embodies instinctive rather than cerebral wisdom (pl. 388). The rounded contours of her ample form are redolent, in themselves, of a natural equilibrium at one with the equally swollen terrain behind her. *Purity*, on the other side of the eccentrically shaped wall, is just as content, holding out her hand to catch the almost crystalline water pouring from a nearby rock. Her body is like a landscape, ranging from the soft hummocks of her breasts to the curving plain of her belly and then burgeoning into thighs as generously proportioned as mountains. These sculptural nudes, which show Rivera's awareness of the even more massive neo-classical women painted earlier in the decade by Picasso, exude the sense of physical well-being that the Secretariat aimed to promote among the Mexican people.

In the smaller frescoes running round the room, the link between humanity and the germinating natural order is reinforced. Budding flowers rise from the earth with a freshness and innocence that seem to announce a new beginning for the world. Alongside, humanity's need to nurture organic growth is represented by a sequence of hands. They extend from the land like plants, and grasp in their powerful fingers glowing ears of corn and sunflower blossoms.

On the polygonal ceiling *Health* presides over these images of fruition like a wholesome deity (pl. 388). Extending her left leg in a curve that precisely echoes the lie of the horizon beyond, she points to the flanking images of *Knowledge* and *Purity* with unaffected gestures. The terrain has by this time assumed less significance, reduced to a thin stretch of ground at the lower edge of the panel. An undefiled azure sky takes up most of the space behind her, as befits a ceiling decoration. And in the largest of the frescoes, the conference room is completely opened out to the air where a figure representing *Life* floats free of the earth altogether (pl. 389).

Liberated by her own glowing health, she hovers in the blue like a swimmer savouring the liberty her limbs have been granted. One historian speculated that, 'as a literary precedent for this transformation, one could think that Homer's story of the Sirens, those omniscient half-birds, half-women, who were turned into exemplars of female beauty by Hellenistic artists, was not beyond the reach of Rivera's roving imagination.'[8] Homer may well have helped to form the image of *Life*, but her body has no need of assistance from the birds in order to maintain its accord with an elemental region where the sun and moon are her only companions.

Rivera's appreciation of medical care's importance would have been profoundly affected by his relationship with Frida Kahlo, whom he married while working on the Secretariat scheme. For her achievement as an artist grows even more astonishing when we realise how hard she had to battle against the fragility of her own broken body. Her childhood was blighted by the onset of polio, permanently afflicting her right leg. But a greater ordeal began when, at the age of eighteen, she became the victim of a traffic accident. The year was 1925, and Kahlo sustained serious injuries when a street car collided with her school bus. A metal handrail was thrust into her stomach, 'the way a

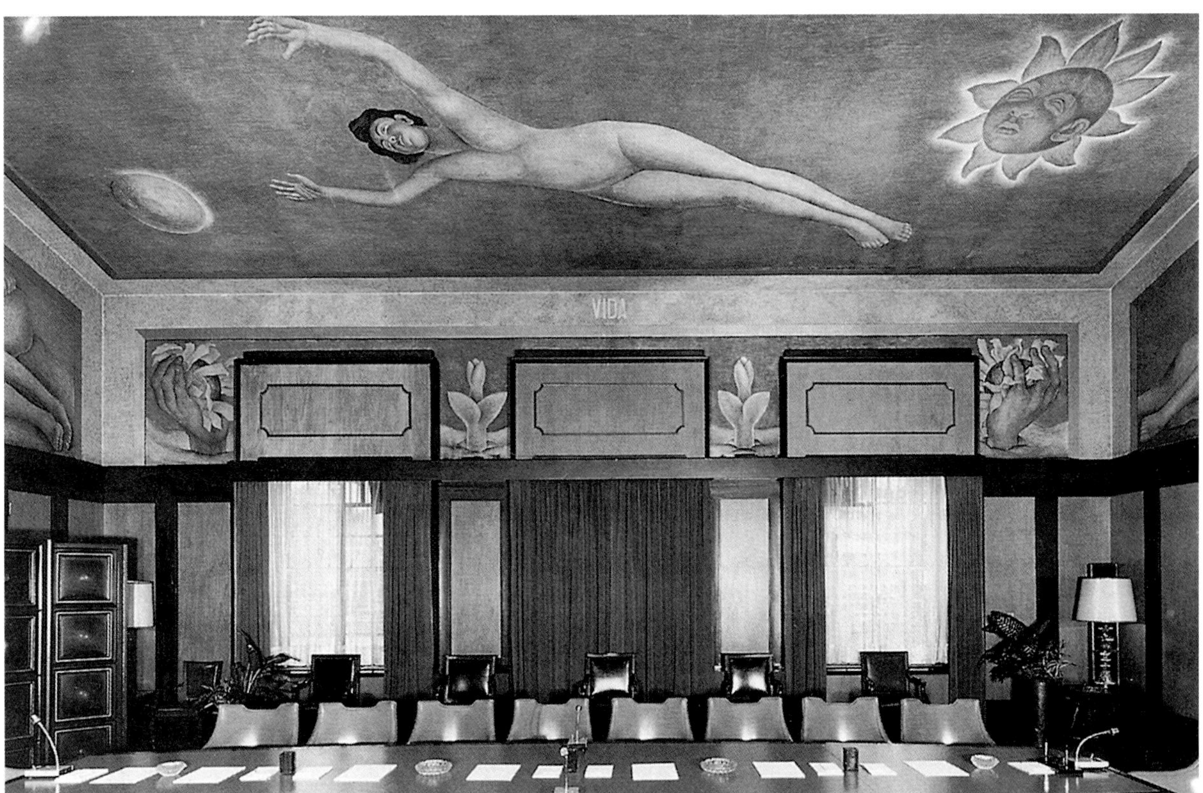

389 Diego Rivera, *Life*, 1929, Secretariat of Health and Public Assistance, Mexico

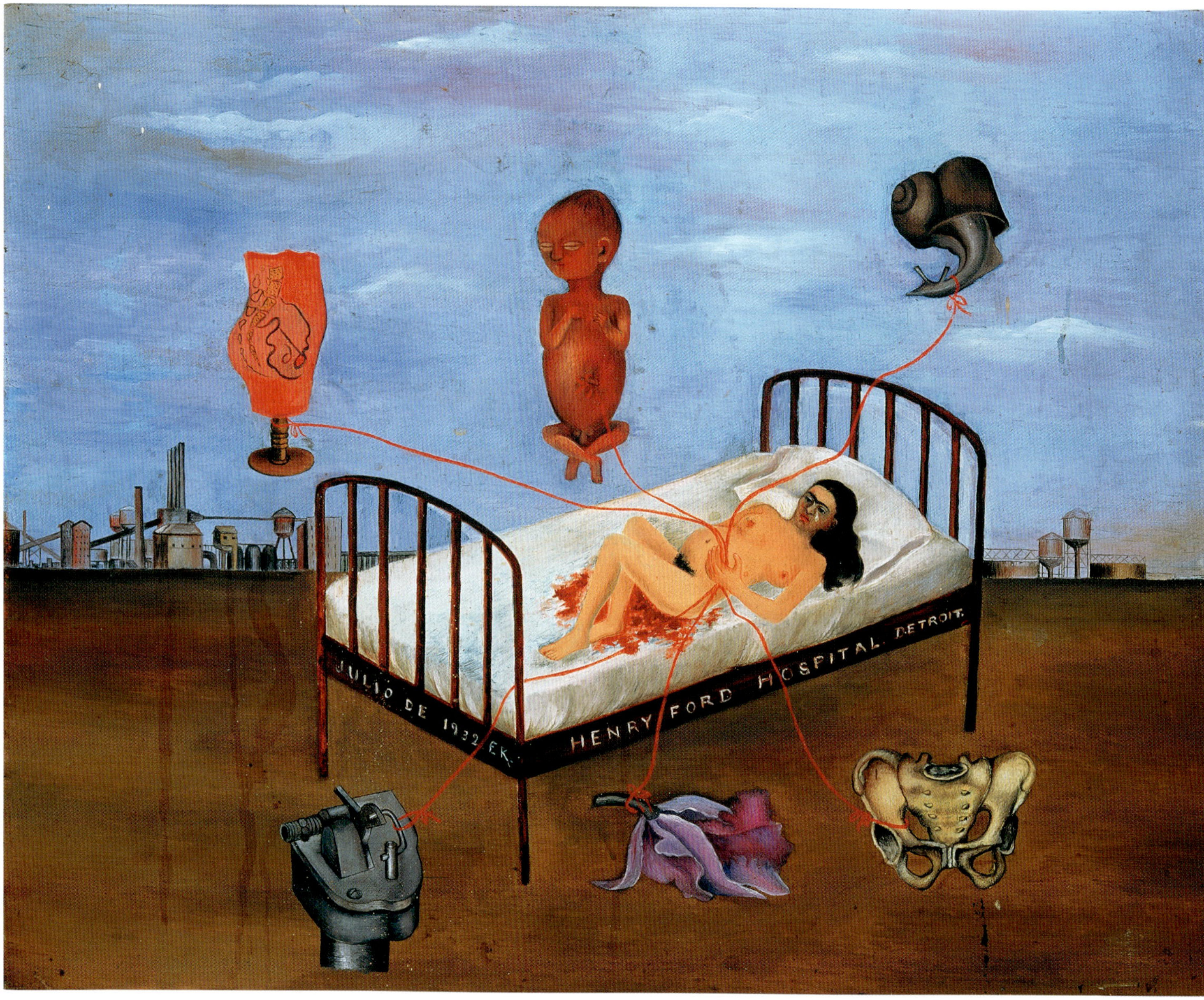

390 Frida Kahlo, *Henry Ford Hospital*, 1932, Fundacion Dolores Olmedo, Mexico City

sword pierces a bull'. For the rest of her life she struggled to sustain a body made desperately frail by extensive fractures in her spine, a shattered pelvis, collarbone, ribs and a broken foot that was eventually amputated.

Her parlous state of health could hardly have been further removed from the robust wholeness of the nudes painted by Rivera in the conference room. Such a tragedy might well have overwhelmed a less strong-willed adolescent, but Kahlo was determined to survive. Intelligent and resourceful, she abandoned her ambition to study medicine and instead began to paint. In this respect, the accident and prolonged convalescence proved the making of her. Deciding that she was 'bored as hell in bed', she taught herself to use brushes and employed a special easel that enabled her to paint lying down.

Her health, however, remained frail. Kahlo once wrily commented that 'I hold the record for operations.'[9] In 1930 she was forced to have an abortion and two years later suffered a dangerous miscarriage in Detroit. At the time, her husband was engaged on an elaborate mural scheme for the city's Institute of Arts, filling the walls of the garden court with images of energetic activity in factories

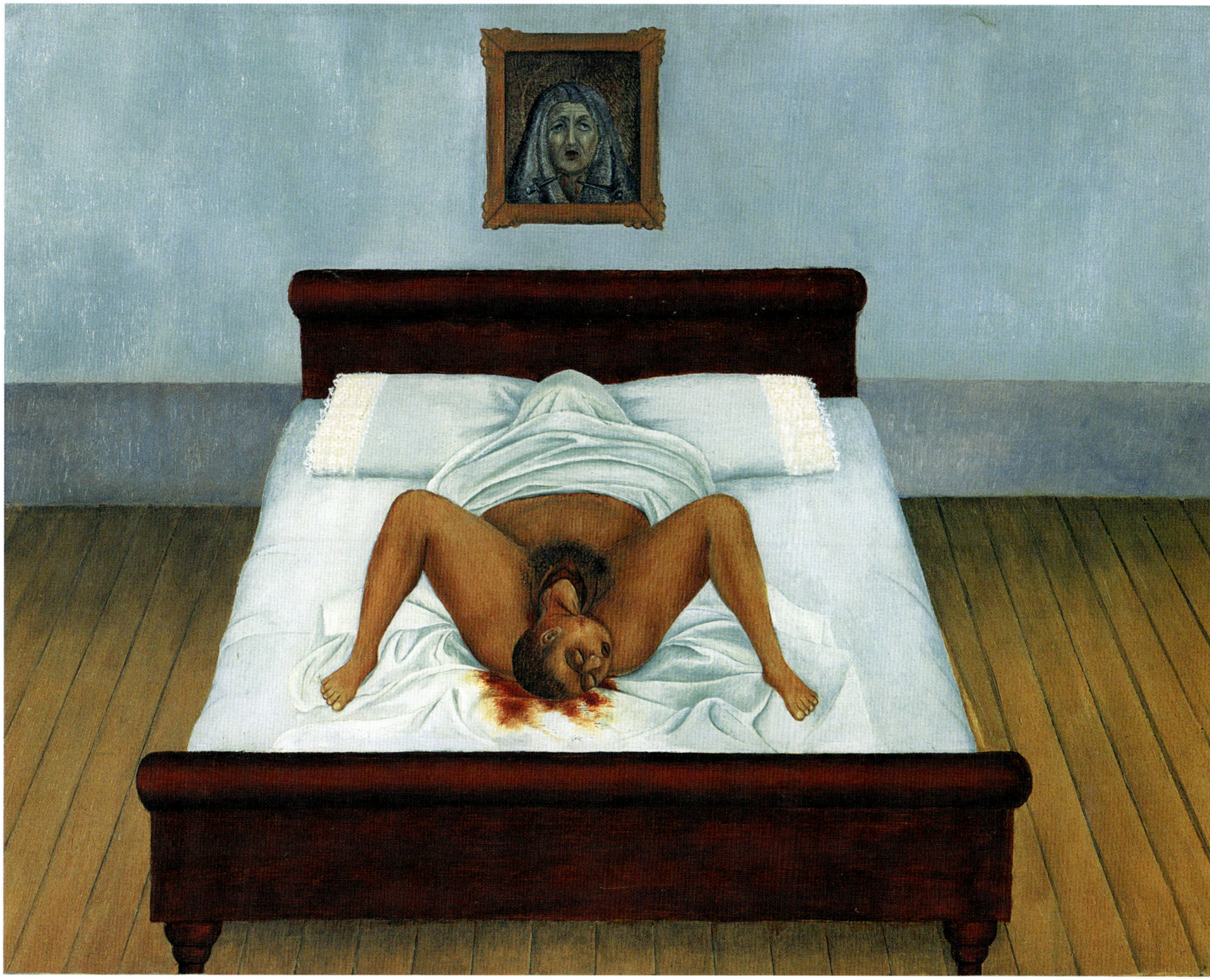

391 Frida Kahlo, *My Birth*, 1932, Private Collection

and Ford automobile assembly plants. Yet Kahlo was confined to a bed at Henry Ford Hospital, and soon gave its name to a poignant little painting of her travail (pl. 390). Executed in a blend of Surrealism and Mexican folk art that she made her own, the panel shows the weeping Kahlo stranded on a blood-spattered bed and holding her still-swollen stomach. The industrialised world of Detroit is relegated to an insignificant skyline, but its uninhabited sterility contributes to the mournful mood of a picture filled with references to loneliness and loss. Kahlo confronts her predicament in solitude, while the ghost of the foetus hangs in space, cross-legged and helpless, above a forbidding hospital bed. So do a diverse assortment of other forms, including a pelvic bone, a female abdomen and an orchid resembling a uterus. Over the bedhead, Kahlo even paints a snail to symbolise the excruciating slowness of the miscarriage she had endured. On the barren ground beneath sits the metallic, glinting instrument used at Henry Ford Hospital to sterilise utensils.

The loss of her second baby may have made Kahlo lament her infertility, but it liberated her as a painter. And 1932 turned out to be her *annus mirabilis*. For she also produced an equally intense

392 (*facing page*) Frida Kahlo, *The Broken Column*, 1944, Fundacion Dolores Olmedo, Mexico City

and traumatic picture called *My Birth*, the product not only of her miscarriage but her mother's death a few months later (pl. 391). This time, the only image above the bed is a *mater dolorosa*, and she cannot save the woman whose identity is hidden by a sheet covering her face and torso. She could be Kahlo's mother or the artist herself, yet there is no mistaking the dead child whose head and neck jut out of the woman's exposed vagina. It is Kahlo, lying on a blood-smeared sheet. The bareness of the floorboards surging up at either side of the bed contribute to the desolate mood. So does the scroll, unfurled at the base of the painting yet devoid of any consoling inscription. God seems absent in this bleak room, where death prevails and all hope of new life is brutally extinguished.

Between 1925 and her death almost three decades later, Kahlo was obliged to endure about thirty operations. No wonder that a friend once commented that 'she lived dying'. Many of her paintings were executed in hospital, focusing on images of her agony, dreams and fantasies about miraculous recovery. 'In some respects her painting was a form of therapy', wrote Laura Mulvey and Peter Wollen, 'a way of coping with pain, warding off despair and regaining control over the image of her crushed and broken body. Painting brought pleasure, hope and power over herself. It made possible both a triumphant reassertion of narcissism and a symbolization of her pain and suffering.'[10]

Until André Breton encouraged Kahlo to exhibit these deeply cathartic images, she worked essentially for herself. She was fortified not only by the satisfaction they gave her, but also by her love of the popular ex-voto paintings that Mexicans hung in church as a thank-offering for surviving mishap or serious illness. Kahlo collected these images, executed on tin in great quantities during the nineteenth century especially, and displayed them in her native home, the distinctive 'Blue House'. They offered her consolation, and a painting of her own called *Marxism Can Cure the Sick* consciously adopted the ex-voto format. In place of the saint, god or Virgin to be found at the top of the traditional prototype, Kahlo placed the bearded face of Marx. Below, the centre of the picture is dominated by the artist casting her crutches aside. Although her chest is still strapped in by a formidable surgical corset, she adopts here a more optimistic stance than the gory figures who reveal their afflictions on ex-voto paintings.

Such hopeful images are rare in Kahlo's confessional, fear-haunted art. In an unusually grand, imposing canvas called *The Two Fridas*, painted in 1939 when she and Rivera were divorced, the seated Kahlo on the left is shown with her heart ripped apart. An artery drips blood onto her lap, defiling the whiteness of her dress. Yet her face remains proud, resolute and defiant, like the Frida in *Tree of Hope, Keep Firm* who wears a red Tehuana costume and remains defiant beside another Kahlo lying on the hospital trolley, her back slashed by the surgeon's knife. As for the woman resembling Kahlo who sleeps in a picture called *The Dream*, she is obsessed by the skeletal apparition reclining on top of her bed, festooned with explosives that might at any instant blow both himself and the artist into oblivion.

Understandably, Kahlo was preoccupied with the feeling that her entire existence might be threatened by imminent collapse. She conveyed this presentiment with the greatest intensity in a harrowing image called *The Broken Column* (pl. 392). Here the bands encircling the artist's torso have not prevented a wide fissure from splitting her body from neck to navel. The darkness within contains a solitary classical column, sustaining her posture and propping up her proud head with an Ionic order just beneath her chin. The column is severely cracked in several places, however, just as the arid landscape beyond is gouged with rifts. Kahlo's feeling that the fundamental structure of her being was fatally undermined is here given unforgettable, gruelling expression. Tears spatter her cheeks as she struggles to withstand the agony inflicted both by the shattered spinal column and by the harsh nails, piercing her flesh like reminders of Christ's mortification on the cross.

Kahlo's dependence on her doctor's advice, and on any medical advances that might have helped to alleviate the continual battle against pain, was a central reality in her life. By 1950 her health had declined so severely that she was obliged, after discovering that four toes on her right foot were black on the ends, to spend a whole year at the English Hospital in Mexico City, undergoing a traumatic sequence of no less than seven separate operations on her spine. The anguish she endured, especially when advised to submit to amputation, was har-

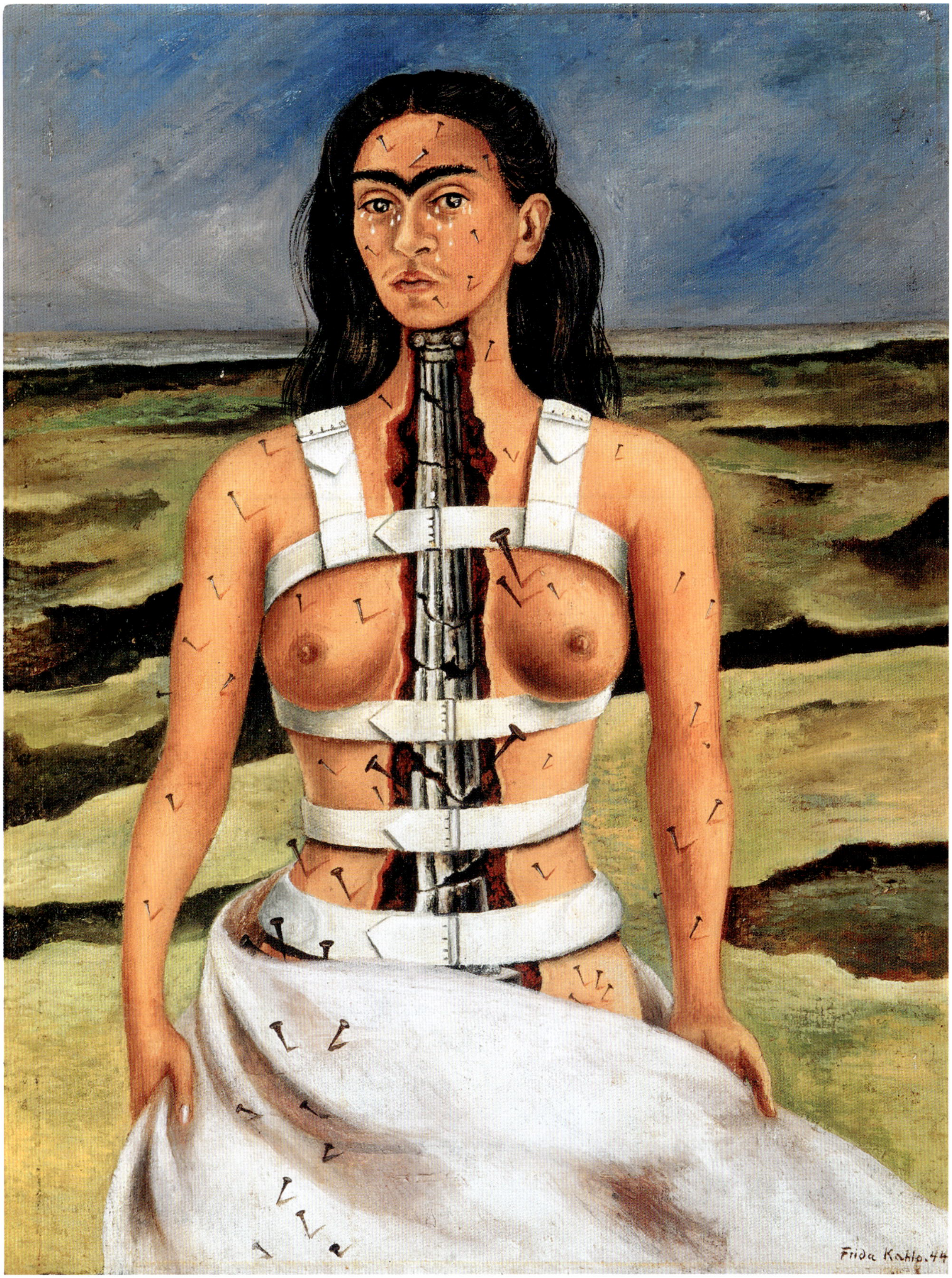
Frida Kahlo.44

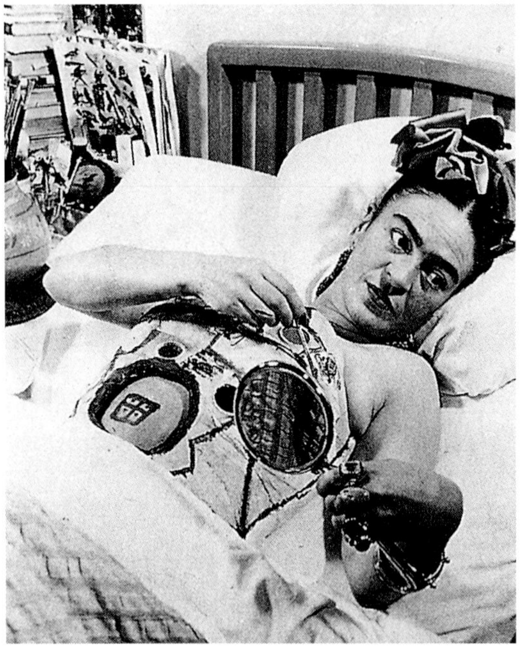

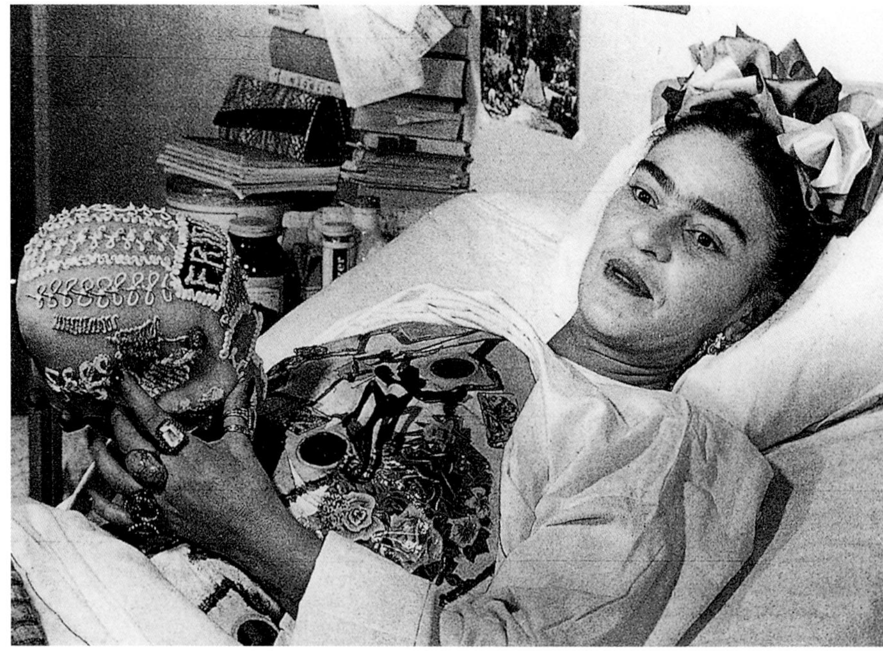

393 (*above left*) Photograph of Frida Kahlo in hospital painting decorated plaster corset, 1950–51

394 (*above right*) Photograph of Frida Kahlo in hospital, clutching a sugar skull with her name on it, 1950–51

rowing. 'They are driving me crazy and making me desperate', she wrote to Dr Leo Eloesser, the Chief of Service at San Francisco Hospital and a thoracic surgeon whom Kahlo had first consulted in 1930. 'What should I do? It is as if I am being turned into an idiot and I am very tired of this fucking foot and I would like to be painting and not worrying about so many problems. But, it can't be helped, I have to be miserable until the situation is resolved.'[11] Dr Eloesser was her most trusted doctor and lifelong friend. In 1931 she had affectionately painted his portrait and nine years later Kahlo dedicated a disturbing self-portrait to him, where she bleeds from wounds pierced in her skin by a necklace of thorns reminiscent of Christ's Passion. The inscription testifies that 'I painted my portrait in the year 1940 for Dr Eloesser, my doctor and my best friend. With all love, Frida Kahlo'. She must have later wished that he was with her in Mexico City, helping her to survive the gruelling operations at the English Hospital.

On the whole, Kahlo kept the misery to herself. Matilde, her sister, described how 'she has been through a real Calvary', especially when her spine developed an abscess after an operation. Kahlo became known in hospital for her stoicism. Matilde reported that, after 'they operated for a second time', her corset became 'as dirty as a pigsty since she is secreting through her back, it smells like a dead dog and these "senores" say that the wound is not closing'.[12] Kahlo, however, was admired by the nurses for her extraordinary gaiety. 'She never complained', wrote Dr Velasco y Polo. 'She never said this is badly done. She stood it all a little bit *a la Mexicana*, suffering, but without protesting.'[13] Whenever Kahlo felt well enough, she staged exuberant puppet shows with her feet. Visiting relatives and friends would be invited to peer through a hole in her plaster cast at the festering wound. She once showed her defiance by announcing, after the arrival of a bone taken from a corpse, that 'I feel like shooting my way out of this hospital and starting my own revolution'.[14]

Above all, though, Kahlo retained her sanity by transforming her hospital room into an artist's haven. Festooned with brilliantly coloured candelabra symbolising the tree of life, and wax doves painted white with paper wings heralding the advent of peace, her surroundings were instrumental in helping to raise her spirits. She laughed at death by decorating the room with skulls made of candy, and a photograph shows her clutching a sugar skull with her name inscribed on it (pl. 394). She ensured that pots of paint and brushes clustered in a jar sat on her bedside table. Whenever doctors insisted that her paints were taken away, Kahlo resorted to decorating her plaster corset with lipstick and iodine (pl. 393). She encouraged visitors to participate in the transformation of other corsets as well, letting them sign their names and cover the grim plaster surfaces with life-affirming photographs, feathers, pebbles and mirrors.

Kahlo was indomitable. Even after enduring six operations she felt energetic enough to ask the doctors' permission for a special easel to be fixed to her hospital bed. With its help, she discovered how to paint in a remarkably sustained manner for several hours a day. Juan Gunzmán took a moving photograph of her at work on an ambitious, highly formal painting called *The Kahlo Family Portrait*. Commenced several years before and left incomplete, it assembles the artist's relatives in a region divided between earth and sky. Portraying these solemn ranks of siblings, parents and remote forebears must have given her immense consolation at a time when she knew that her own health was disintegrating irrevocably. The ability to work sustained her, and she succeeded in adding her sisters, niece and nephew to the pictorial ensemble. 'When I leave the hospital two months from now', Kahlo declared, 'there are three things I want to do: paint, paint, paint.'[15]

Before going home, however, she insisted on dispensing hilarity and irreverence to everyone who came across her. Noticing one day that Dr Velasco y Polo was accompanied by an attractive young woman, Kahlo exclaimed: 'Lend her to me! I'll smoke that one myself!' Recalling with affection the artist's prodigious vivacity, he described how Kahlo 'liked to talk about medicine, politics, her father, Diego, sex, free love, the evils of Catholicism'.[16] Above all, visitors cherished her willingness to empathise with them. Even when emerging from anaesthesia after an operation, she delighted in the company of friends and asked them about their own afflictions. Sometimes Kahlo would cry when people told her of their problems. She often voiced concern about her fellow patients, as if they were more gravely stricken than she believed herself to be. 'She did not concentrate on herself', remembered Fanny Rabel. 'One did not feel her miseries and conflicts when one was with her. She was full of interest in others and in the outside world. She would say, "Tell me things. Tell me about your childhood."'[17] Young visitors fascinated her more than anyone. She allowed an Indian boy called Vidal Nicolas to stand by the bed and watch her paint. Although he was only nine, Kahlo became convinced that the boy would himself become an outstanding artist. 'He has great talent', she announced, 'and I am going to pay for all his education and send him to the San Carlos Academy.'[18]

She did not live long enough to discover if her prediction was correct. But in 1951, three years before her death at the age of forty-seven, Kahlo managed to paint a poignant tribute to the man who had carried out these perilous operations. Dr Juan Farill (pl. 395), who suffered from leg and foot ailments that forced him for a long time to rely on crutches, was among the most outstanding Mexican surgeons in this period. He combined orthopaedic expertise with a genuine, far-reaching concern for impoverished children. If their parents could not afford to pay for treatment at the special hospital he had founded, Dr Farill would waive their fees. Kahlo trusted him completely, nicknaming him *chulito* (cutie) and always obeying his instructions.

395 Photograph of Frida Kahlo and Dr Farill with Kahlo's *Self-Portrait with the Portrait of Dr Farill*, 1951

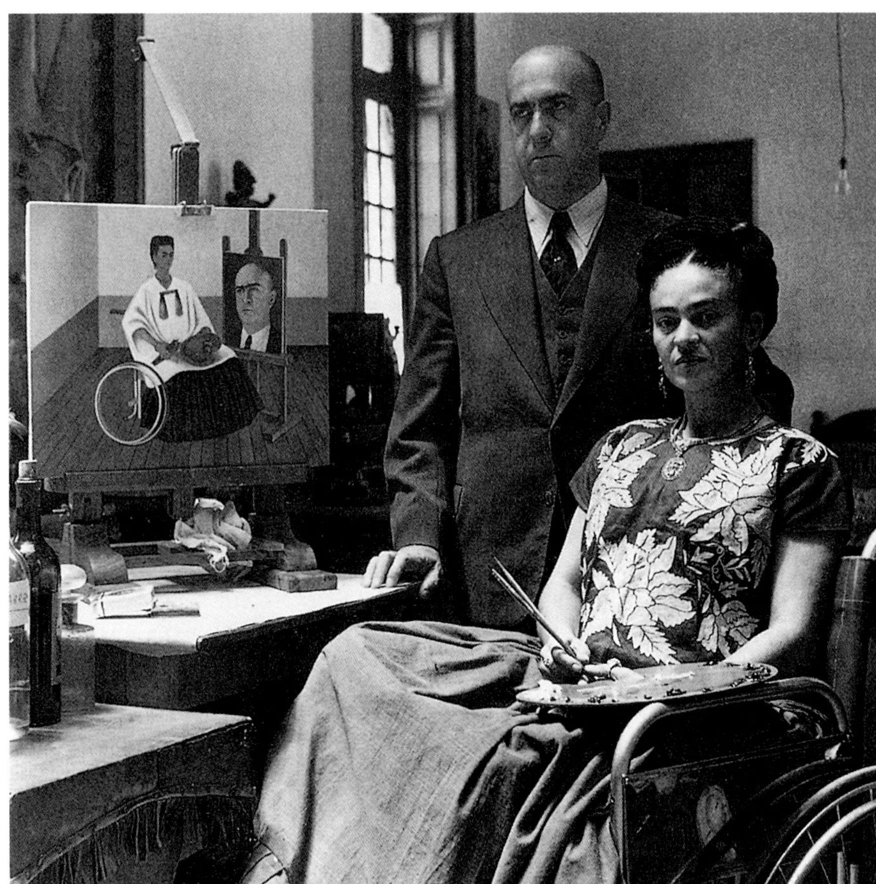

She conveyed the full extent of her regard for his care in *Self-Portrait with the Portrait of Dr Farill* (see pl. 395). Convalescing at home after a sequence of bone grafts on her spinal column, the fragile artist is now confined to a wheelchair and clutches a bundle of brushes dripping blood onto her otherwise immaculate white smock. Dr Farill is not personally present in the bare room, with its clinical walls and exposed floorboards, so the painting lacks the extraordinary physical intimacy defined by Goya in his comparable *Self-Portrait with Doctor Arrieta* (see pl. 256). Kahlo appears much more reserved than the openly troubled Goya, probably because she had long ago learned to cope with her ailments by cultivating stoical resilience. Yet her dependence on Dr Farill is still apparent, largely through the strange disparity in scale between her tiny head and his far larger features in the painted portrait on the easel.

Filling this canvas with the grandeur of a political leader's face displayed on a public building, he exudes a calm authority and patience that Kahlo, presumably, found reassuring. Hayden Herrera rightly pointed out that this small panel is 'a secular *retablo*, with Frida the saved victim of a narrowly escaped danger and Dr. Farill taking the place of the holy image'.[19] Although her manner may seem distant, an underlying affection for the doctor is signified by the heart-shaped palette held in her diminutive fingers. To stress the cardiac analogy, the form of a real heart is painted on the palette's surface in all its anatomical detail. As well as suggesting that Kahlo paints 'from the heart', this disquieting image seems to be reminding Dr Farill that her survival depends heavily on his care, expertise and good judgement.

'Dr. Farill saved me', Kahlo wrote in her diary after she had been

> sick for a year. He gave me back the joy of life. I am still in a wheelchair and I do not know if soon I will be able to walk again. I have a plaster cast, which, in spite of being a frightful bore, helps my spine feel better. I do not have pains. Only a weariness . . . and as is natural, often desperation. A desperation that no words can describe. Nevertheless, I want to live. I already have begun to paint the little painting that I am going to give Dr Farill and that I am doing with all my affection for him.[20]

In the end, not even the wise and devoted Farill could enable his determined patient to reach her half-century. Yet Kahlo's paintings have survived, testifying at every step to the courage, resolve and defiant originality of a woman whose work was for long overshadowed by the provocative, heroic, fiercely left-wing and controversial art produced by her husband. Kahlo's small-scale, highly autobiographical images could hardly be further removed from the epic and mythical sweep of Rivera's monumental offerings. But her stubborn and insistent vision is increasingly admired, and the extent of Kahlo's hospital ordeals makes her determination to keep on working still more admirable.

No wonder Rivera did his utmost to honour the advance of medical knowledge in the work he produced. During the 1940s he addressed himself, with an extraordinary amount of meticulous dedication, to the task of painting two large images for the Instituto Nacional de Cardiologia in Mexico City (pl. 396). Now installed in the Centro Medico Nacional, where they embellish the foyer of the auditorium in a multi-building complex embracing a hospital and training centre for advanced treatment of heart disease, they were originally executed for an institute more concerned with research into cardiac matters. Hence the overriding emphasis in the *History of Cardiology*, which led Rivera to fill both panels with an abundance of references to great pioneers in the field. His alarmed awareness of Kahlo's vulnerable health may help to account for the exceptional zeal he displayed when researching the subject. Dr Ignacio Chávez provided him with historical details about research into the heart and circulation of the blood, and proposed suitable candidates for portraits of the most prominent specialists. Yet Rivera wanted to find out more, undertaking so exhaustive a study of cardiology's development over the centuries that he furnished himself with a formidable knowledge of the subject. Antonio Rodríguez recalled that 'I happened to hear [Rivera] discuss the subject with an eminent cardiologist, who was astonished to hear him talk as if he too were a specialist.'[21]

The cornucopia of information absorbed by Rivera did, unfortunately, lead him to crowd both panels with an intolerable excess of figures. While his earlier frescoes in the Secretariat of Health and Public Assistance were characterised by simplicity, unadorned emphasis on form and refusal to clutter the composition with superfluous details (see pls 388–9), the *History of Cardiology* reveals the other, more garrulous side of Rivera's imagination. The only passage in the main sections of the paintings to avoid this persistent *horror vacui* is the burning of Michel Servet, the Spanish anatomist and theologian who was martyred in 1533 for advancing heretical theories about blood circulation. Rivera's anger was aroused by such senseless brutality. He made room for a generous representation of the flames devouring Servet's scorched body and the volumes of his writings piled beneath. Perhaps Rivera's interest in the pictorial drama of this episode was quickened by memories of Orozco's *Man of Fire* (see pl. 387), at the top of the cupola at the Hospicio Cabañas. If he had invested the rest of his panels with a similar excitement, they would have been far more compelling works of art. But a spirit of worthy diligence overtook him and the writhing fire gave way to a conscientious yet dull assembly of pioneers like Harvey and Laennec.

Since a hundred specialists and patients had to be crammed into the panels, Rivera tried to articulate their proliferating forms with an elaborate curving structure reminiscent of the lecture theatres where many of them might have taught. The ramps, steps and walls ought to flow through the designs with the ease of blood passing through the channels of the heart itself. Instead of clarifying matters, however, this stage scenery only adds to the sense of confusion. The plethora of names and dates inscribed on every available surface further reinforces the feeling of pedantic overkill. Rivera appears bent on supplying the Instituto with a wearyingly comprehensive encyclopaedia rather than a concise imaginative vision. As the parade of life-size figures approaches the twentieth century at the top of the second panel, it grows progressively more tedious and respectable.

He should have taken his cue from the four grisailles beneath the panels, where the cardiology practised in China, Greece, Africa and Anahuac is defined with cool, limpid simplicity . They evince a readiness to leave generous areas of the composition uninhabited, thereby enabling the figures to establish themselves with an identity unhampered by tiresome incidentals. Maybe the very intensity of Rivera's engagement with the history of his allotted theme blinded him to the dangers of over-elaboration. Neither of the main panels can be counted among his successful works, although the seriousness with which he approached the commission did earn him the unqualified praise of the Instituto's founder. He declared that

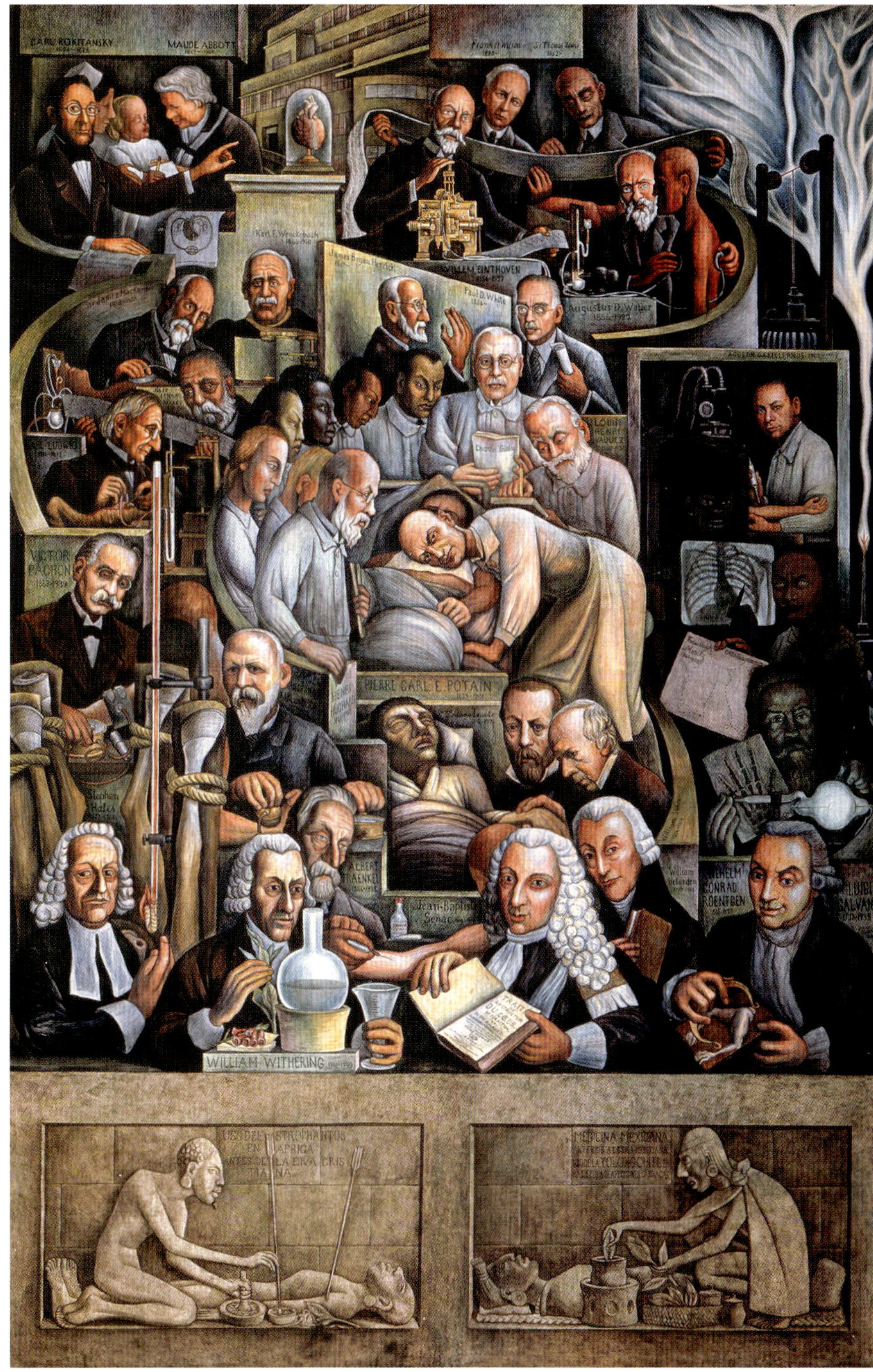

396 Diego Rivera, *The History of Cardiology* (one of two panels), 1943–4, Instituto Nacional de Cardiologia, Mexico City

> Rivera's work has great historical value because he groups, harmonizes and fuses into a single impulse the various schools in the history of

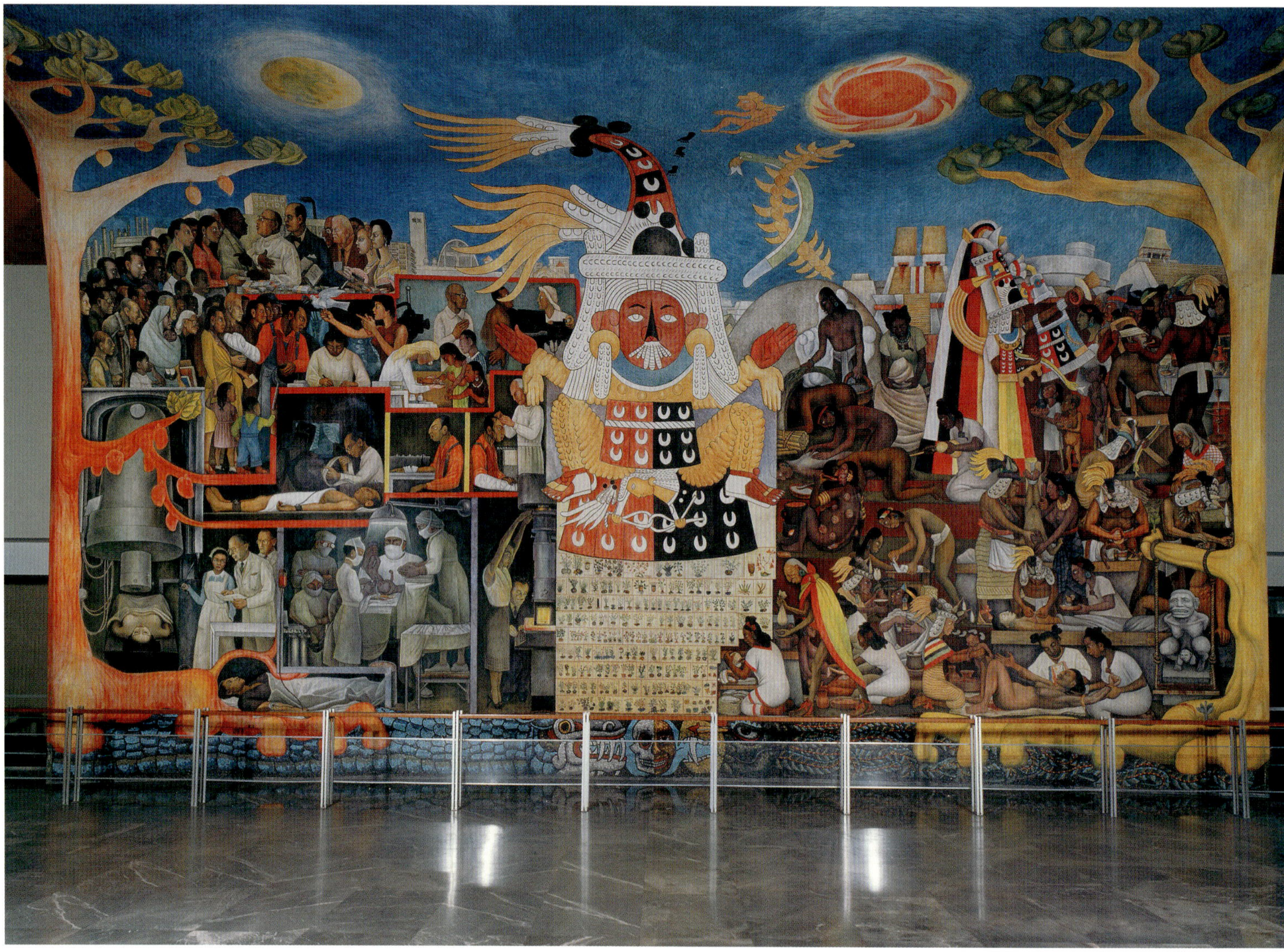

397 Diego Rivera, *The History of Medicine in Mexico: The People's Demand for Better Health*, 1953, Hospital de la Raza, Mexico City

cardiology. But it also has a higher and more imponderable quality: its educational value for future generations. It teaches a lesson in humility by evoking the heroic past. The voice of the masters of yesterday retains its stimulating power; the call of tradition formed through the centuries urges us to go on. The young, passing these murals on their way to the theatres, will become familiar with the great thinkers and, knowing them, will look on them with reverence and try to carry on with their good work.[22]

The 'educational value' referred to in this encomium suggests one reason why Rivera's cardiology murals are burdened by the 'reverence' they seek so earnestly to induce: he may have been urged by his patrons to clutter his work with an excess of historical references. However, a subsequent hospital commission made spectacular amends for the shortcomings of his work in the Instituto. Invited by the Hospital de la Raza to produce a vast fresco for the foyer above the main entrance stairway, he did not allow the complexity of the theme to cramp his innate exuberance (pl. 397). The subject, the *History of Medicine in Mexico: The People's Demand for Better Health*, invited him once again to delve into the minutiae of the past. Yet the country's pre-Columbian history had provided Rivera with rich inspiration before, and the indigenous tradition of his own nation stimulated him more rewardingly than the international survey of cardiologists. Fortified by material so close to his heart, he resisted any urge that he or his patrons may have possessed to produce a dutiful illustration of medical heroes.

The enticing surface at his disposal, a projecting concave wall which bends up and out in a parabolic curve over the floor of the foyer, doubtless spurred him to place an enormous Aztec deity at the mural's centre. Tlazoltéotl is based on a facsimile of an early sixteenth-century illustrated manuscript, the Codex Borbonicus,[23] and Rivera remained faithful to the original appearance of the goddess. Fantastically attired in an elaborate cotton head-dress and a garment of flayed human skin, she wears outsize ear pendants and displays a blackened nose with utter impassivity. At the top of her head-dress sprout exotic tendrils that undulate in the sky, as if waving to the sun and moon hanging there with vaguely human features.

Their joint cosmic presence recalls the mural of *Life* painted by Rivera a quarter of a century earlier for the Secretariat of Public Health (see pl. 389), where a naked woman flung her arms joyfully across the heavens with sun and moon in equal attendance. The link between the two frescoes may have been intentional, for Tlazoltéotl was the goddess of life. She aroused great hostility and revulsion among Spanish settlers in the sixteenth century, who were disturbed by her reputation as the 'goddess of repulsive things', the 'mistress of lust' and the 'absorber of filth'. Yet all these names reflected her healthy ability to accept and forgive even the most obscene sins when people came to her with their confessions. The sinner was purged by contact with this infinitely sympathetic deity, exclaiming: 'In your presence I bare myself and cast away all my shameful deeds, however many I may have committed.' Relieved of guilt and shame, the sinner was then free to relish the pleasures of life, assisted again by the goddess, who encouraged sexual union and even condoned orgiastic excess.

Tlazoltéotl was on the side of love and health, so it is easy to understand why Rivera should have considered her an ideal focus for his hospital mural. She was able to cure the sick, and place under her divine protection the healers who looked after the natives of Mexico in pre-Conquest times. Beneath her body, no less than eighty-four species of medicinal plant are arrayed on a painted tablet. Proclaiming the efficacy of herbal treatment with encyclopaedic pride, it is placed symbolically above a mask divided between life and death. For Rivera's mural is on the side of recovery, and the mosaic serpents flanking the mask flow back into the two tree-like forms framing the fresco's main wall with their affirmations of growth.

One yellow and the other predominantly blood-red, these immense forms are reminiscent of enormous arteries. Drawing strength from their proximity to the sun and moon respectively, they extend their sustaining presence into the composition. The yellow tree on the right side of the mural thrusts out a phallic branch, terminating in a budding plant similar to the shoots that Rivera painted for the Secretariat conference room (see pl. 388). This time, however, the plant is subservient to the penile form, which uses its proud stiffness to act as a support for the ropes of a swing. Within the ropes, a figure of Tlazoltéotl crouches in the act of childbirth (pl. 398). Similar to the carving that inspired Kahlo to paint her *Childbirth* twenty-one years before (see pl. 391), the goddess here survives to produce a healthy baby. At the same time, she presides over the moment of birth experienced with such joy by a native woman lying on the ground nearby. In pointed contrast to the goddess's solitude and straining posture, the mother relaxes in the care of two white-clothed helpers who smile and

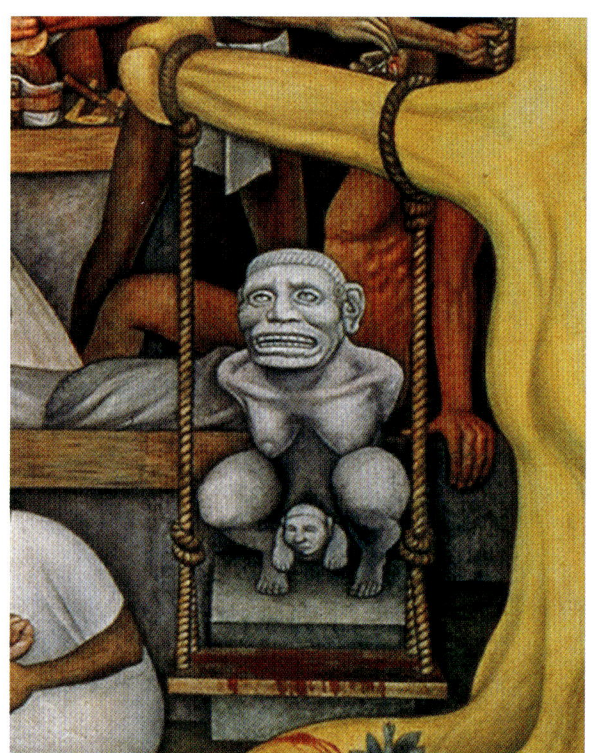

398 Detail of pl. 397, Aztec figure of Tlazoltéotl in childbirth

support the back of her head. She holds out an ecstatic arm towards the newborn boy. Rivera has depicted him with tender accuracy as a helpless little figure, head lolling on shoulder while an Aztec woman holds him up for delighted inspection.

The entire scene exudes gentle fulfilment, and the same compassionate spirit flows through this entire section of the fresco. For the pre-Columbian treatment of illness is depicted here, by an artist who clearly viewed it as a golden age of communal support and solicitude. By no means all the incidents it contains are as happy as the childbirth scene. The figure immediately above the fulfilled mother lies in a blanched and enfeebled trance, while a healer carries out intricate sewing on an incision he has made. Further up, a howling boy hangs inverted from bound feet as a woman examines his teeth, and behind them a muscular surgeon is conducting a major operation on a patient's skull. On the left of the section, a woman with a distended stomach sips a potion presumably intended to cure her of the boils erupting all over her back, as extensive as the putrefied swellings on the afflicted man's body in Grünewald's *Temptation of Saint Anthony* (see pl. 73). Nearby another woman kneels on the step to be purged by an enema, while a patient above is swathed in a white shroud signifying death.

399 Detail of pl. 397, The goddess Izcuitl

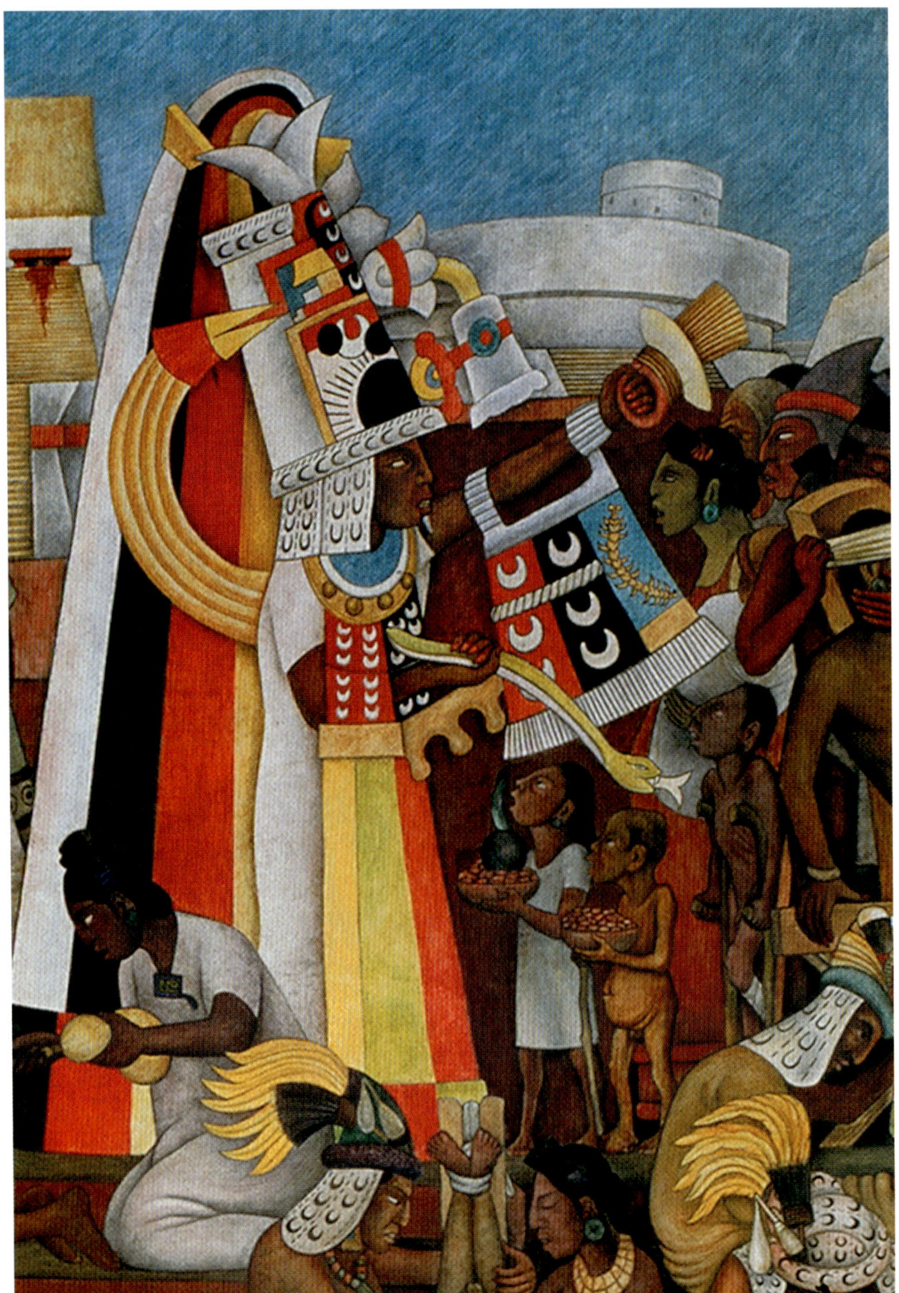

Rivera does not pretend that pain has been ousted from the scene, or that medical success is guaranteed in all cases. But he does imply, through flowing rhythms no less than a persistent emphasis on figures bending over their patients with graceful concentration, that healing in pre-Columbian times was achieved with the utmost concern. Moreover, the incessant bandaging, extracting, massaging and bathing seen all over this section is undertaken with the blessing of the deity standing near the top of the steps (pl. 399). Here the goddess Izcuitl, barely distinguishable from the symbolic fire spirals, intertwined serpents and cosmic nebulae adorning her hieratic form, offers spiritual potency. Her force is honoured by the disabled children who bring offerings of food, staring up with an awe that acknowledges just how much their civilisation depends on the deities' benevolence.

To move on from this highly idealised image of historic Mexico to the other side of the mural, where modern medical science is depicted (pl. 400), is to exchange direct physical contact for an altogether cooler and more impersonal alternative. No gods can be discerned here, and the fluent curvilinear organisation of the right section gives way to a more angular structure. Here different operations are separated from each other in cell-like rooms. Yet the uppermost area of this clinical world represents, in principle at least, a development Rivera ought to have approved. Instead of a god, the white-coated figure of a bespectacled physician

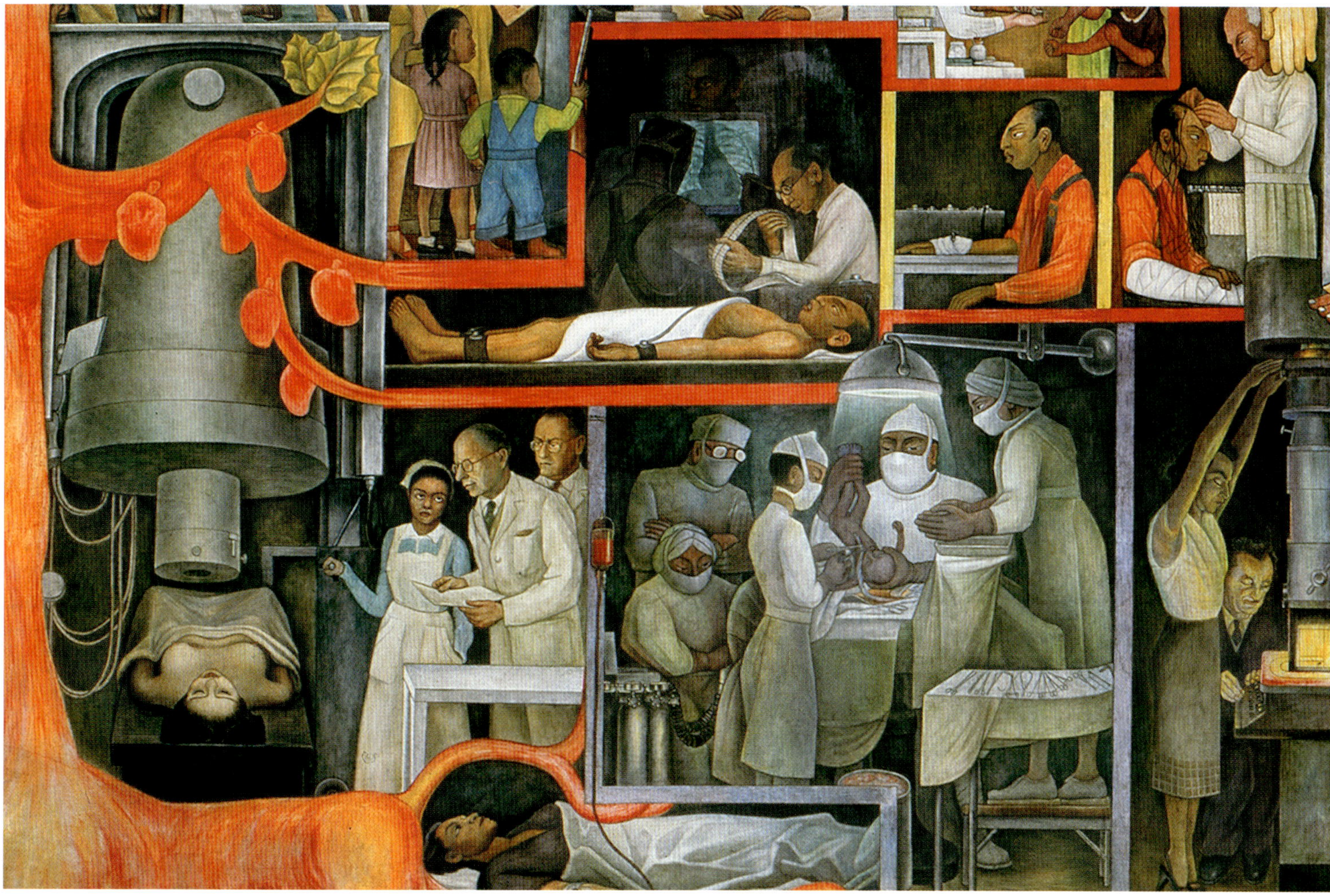

400 Detail of pl. 397

receives the poor people. He is able to inform them that they no longer have to pay for medical care. Behind him stand the practitioners of private medicine, fanning their money as they stare with indignant, thwarted greed at the state's intervention.

The scene below them is, nevertheless, far from idyllic. However much Rivera supported the introduction of Mexico's national health system, he could not prevent himself from viewing its implementation with misgivings. The immense machine bearing down on the recumbent woman is both aggressive and sinister, threatening to crush her with its weight in a space where she is divorced from the nurse and specialists in attendance. Childbirth is taking place next door, but it could hardly be more removed from the relaxation of its pre-Columbian counterpart on the other side of the fresco. Now the mother is nowhere to be seen and masked attendants, lit by the glare of an electric lamp, display no emotion while cutting the baby's cord with utter efficiency.

As he painted the other scenes in this unsettling cross section of a modern hospital, Rivera appears to have been asking himself and his audience, 'what have we lost by allowing the technology of medicine to dominate healing so completely?' When working on the mural he began to receive treatment for the cancer that eventually caused his own death, and personal experience of up-to-date examination and treatment techniques might well inform the unease in his vision of modern medical prowess. In the darkened room where a man lies awaiting the results of his tests, he seems marooned in clinical isolation. The doctors attending him are far too absorbed in a scrutiny of his X-ray and heart recordings to pay him the attention enjoyed by the pre-Columbian patient. No wonder the man whose head is festooned with

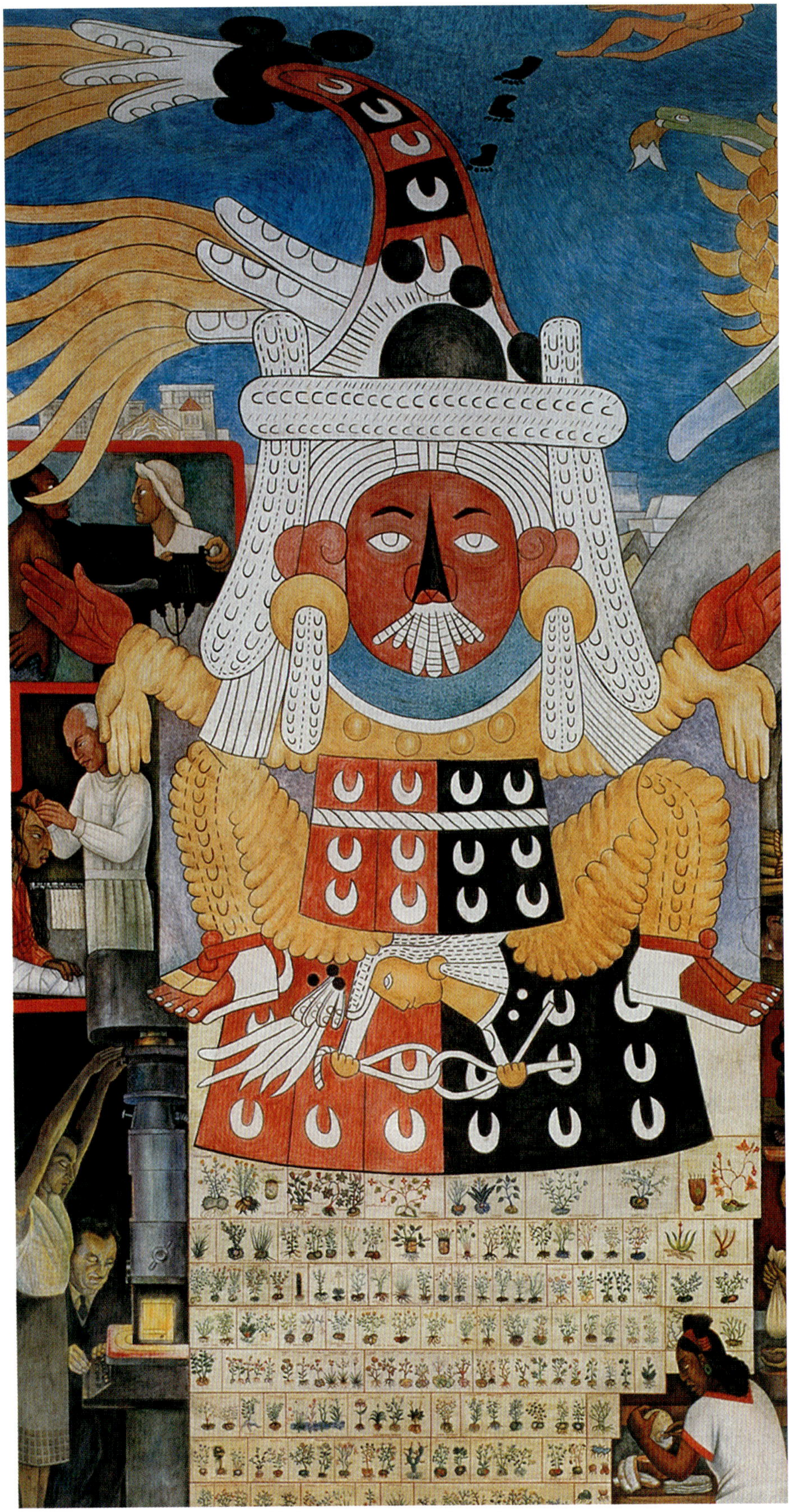

electrodes looks apprehensive. Caught up in a world where machines are relied on for every diagnosis, and where the doctor has become little more than a silent engineer monitoring the results of scientific tests, the patient's sense of alienation is profound. Rivera sums up the malaise in the reclining form of a young woman at the base of the design. Her arm is attached to a life-giving transfusion of blood suspended from a wall, but she is denied access to the reassuring presence of other human beings. They are too busy administering their gleaming instruments and, because this patient has no need of technology, she finds herself abandoned in a claustrophobic cell eerily akin to a tomb.

Rivera's infatuation with Mexico's past, a love he shared with Kahlo, led him to present a naively romanticised view of traditional healing in the Hospital de la Raza mural. His celebration of pre-Columbian life was of a piece with his insistence on employing the encaustic method with so much enthusiasm that the innovatory David Alfaro Siqueiros mocked him for producing 'Egyptian frescoes'.[24] Rivera did not mind this satire. For him, the ideals of the Mexican Revolution were inextricably bound up with defining a national culture, which entailed a rediscovery and revaluation of the country's indigenous heritage. However much Rivera may have recognised the rational value of a national health service equipped with streamlined machines, the sixty-seven-year-old equated such inventions with a new political climate which aroused his scepticism. Post-war Mexico was busily engaged in transforming its economy along Western capitalist lines, modernising the country and welcoming a new, semi-abstract style of mural painting practised by Rufino Tamayo. While stressing that 'Rivera took no public stand against these developments', Stanton Catlin explained that the grand old man of revolutionary art 'could not have been sympathetic, ideologically or artistically, to this turn of affairs. As the international modernizing trend developed, it seems altogether probable that he dug in his heels and insistently continued to uphold his traditional indigenist, popular, and anti-capitalist social-revolutionary point of view.'[25]

Seen from the perspective of today, Rivera's mural appears prescient in its stubborn desire to question what might have been sacrificed with the wholesale acceptance of medical technology. For all his late affiliation with Soviet Communism, he remained a humanist, always on the side of the individual's need for the sustenance that direct contact between people can alone provide. The festive presence of Tlazoltéotl in his mural is not just an archaeological caprice (pl. 401): Rivera placed it at the heart of his painting as an embodiment of life-affirming values, enlivening the interior of the capital city's most modern hospital with an exuberance that draws on the oldest sources of healing power in Mexican society. Blazing with unbridled colour and an unshakeable faith in time-honoured curative principles, the goddess raises her hands to bless everyone who approaches this invigorating fresco in search of sustenance.

401 (*facing page*) Detail of pl. 397

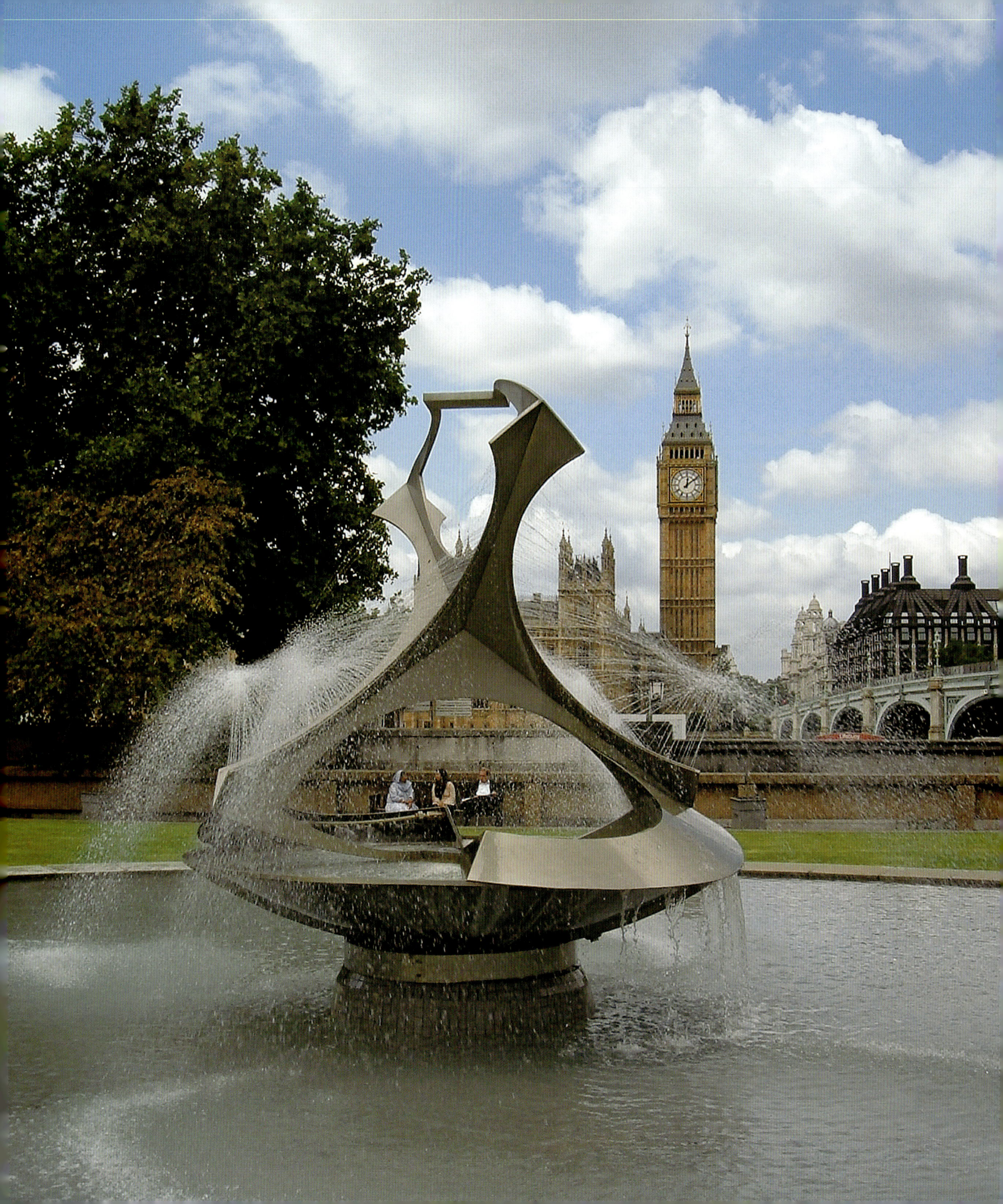

TWENTY-FIVE
'FOR THE NEEDS OF THEIR OWN SPIRIT'

Throughout the long years of the Second World War, Antonin Artaud was confined to French hospitals, struggling with mental instability and obsessive patterns of behaviour. Before the Nazi offensive commenced, he had been returned in a straitjacket to Le Havre by Irish authorities disturbed by his irrational state of mind. Artaud was gripped by an apparently unshakeable belief that the world would soon come to an end. His family in France were disturbed and terrified by the enraged letters he had sent them during his trip to Ireland. Many of the messages were besmirched by cigarette burns and cosmic symbols. With hindsight, however, these unnerving documents can be seen as proof of his new-found involvement with visual expression.

Artaud's psychological illness was so acute that, after internment at Le Havre, he was sent to a hospital at Ville-Evrard for four years. It was an appalling institution, blighted by wartime neglect. His desperate pleas to escape were finally answered when, in 1943, the poet Robert Desnos managed to organise his transfer to a far more congenial hospital at Rodez. Here, Artaud came under the care of the enlightened Dr Gaston Ferdière, a psychiatrist whose fascination with Surrealism, poetry and collecting the art of mentally ill patients ensured that Artaud's art soon began to flourish. Like Dadd, van Gogh, Munch, Kirchner and Kahlo before him, he was encouraged to find ways of giving even his most anguished sense of alienation a cathartic visual form.

Artaud had spent most of his eruptive career exploring the possibilities for revolt in writing, acting and drama. Yet everything he tried to do was haunted by the fear of insanity. Preoccupied above all with the threat of an inner void, he attempted in the early 1920s to write poetry and regarded the outcome as 'the shreds that I have managed to snatch from complete nothingness'.[1] He became involved with the Surrealists, trained as an actor and began writing reviews of art exhibitions, advocating ideas that heralded his subsequent championship of expressive intensity. His most influential period began in 1926, when he joined forces with the playwright Roger Vitrac and the essayist Robert Aron in founding the Alfred Jarry Theatre. Inspired by the violence and erotic obsessions he had discovered in Balthus's paintings, Artaud concentrated on a form of drama directly assaulting the audience's nerves and senses. In subsequent years it led to his invention of a Theatre of Cruelty, a hugely influential development where everything – bodily gesture, stage sets, language and sound – centred on shocking viewers into a new, therapeutic awareness of their repressed selves. Artaud's own

402 (facing page) Naum Gabo, *Revolving Torsion, Fountain*, 1972–3, St Thomas's Hospital, London

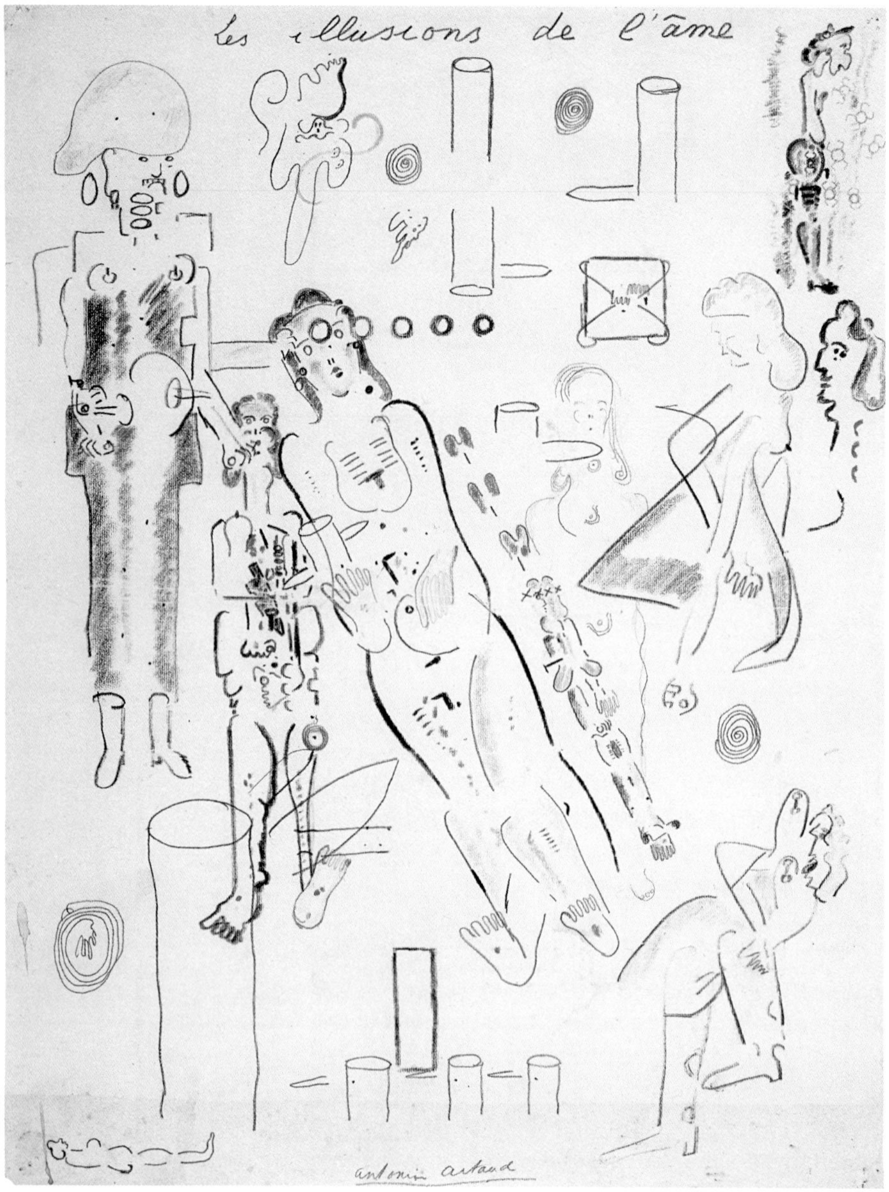

403 Antonin Artaud, *Les Illusions de l'âme*, 1946, Musée Nationale d'Art moderne, Centre Georges Pompidou, Paris

1935 production of his play *The Cenci*, armed with a provocative set designed by Balthus, failed to attract audiences in Paris after vilification by theatre critics. Mortified by its failure, Artaud escaped to Mexico and struggled unsuccessfully to overcome a debilitating heroin addiction. Nothing could prevent his breakdown during the doomed trip to Ireland in 1937.

Even when he was moved to the hospital at Rodez six years later, Dr Ferdière subjected him to a gruelling sequence of electro-convulsive treatments. They succeeded only in heightening Artaud's fundamental fear of the abyss and caused him to break a vertebra in a shock-induced fall. So he wrote a pleading letter to the psychiatrist Jacques Latrémolière who had administered this brutal treatment at Rodez. Claiming that electric shock 'reduces me to despair', Artaud described how

> it takes away my memory, it dulls my mind and my heart, it turns me into someone who is absent and who knows he is absent and sees himself for weeks in pursuit of his being, like a dead man alongside a living man who is no longer himself, but who insists on the dead man being present even though he can no longer enter into him.

He stressed that, after the last series of electro-convulsive treatments, 'I remained throughout the months of August and September absolutely incapable of working, thinking, and *feeling that I was alive*. Each time it brings on those horrible splinterings of the personality.'[2]

Despite this 'living agony',[3] Artaud was fortified by his experiments with drawing. He had first experimented with pencil, charcoal and chalk back in 1915, when his short-lived period of military service led to excruciating headaches, extreme mood-swings and debilitating depression. Placed for two years under the care of Dr Dardel at Neufchatel in Switzerland, he responded eagerly to the suggestion that drawing might aid his recovery. He produced, among other things, his first surviving self-portrait. After moving to Paris in 1920, though, Artaud put drawing aside and only resumed when Frédéric Delanglade, a Surrealist artist hiding from the Nazis under Dr Ferdière's protection at Rodez hospital , encouraged him. The initial drawings were made in 1944 and the following February Artaud started using school exercise books to produce a complex, free-ranging work now known under the collective title 'Cahiers de Rodez'.

Interspersed with lists, and verbal explanations which Dr Ferdière asked him to write, these extraordinary works were described by Artaud himself as *dessin-écrits*. Memories of his Mexican trip, when he had studied in particular the ritual ceremonies of the Tarahumaras tribe, surfaced in images and phrases scattered across the paper's surface (pl. 403). Human body-parts are accompanied by skulls, coffins, guns and other reminders of death's inescapability. Although sexual organs are often specified, eroticism is always countered by the threat of dismemberment and obliteration. Artaud's sense of humour lends the work a paradoxical vitality. He even called one page of drawings, signs and words *The Machine of Being or Drawing to be Looked at Cockeyed* (pl. 404). However, plenty of evidence in this image suggests that he was still struggling to recover from the gruesome aftermath of his electric shock trauma. Many of the figures seem reminiscent of actors embroiled in some bizarre performance, and visitors to Rodez were astonished when Artaud suddenly indulged in bouts of 'speaking with tongues' accompanied by macabre dances and singing.

The therapeutic effect of producing the 'Cahiers de Rodez' cannot be doubted. Ferdière and his colleagues at the hospital were gratified by their patient's progress throughout 1945. He became more stable, and increasingly voiced an urgent desire to be released from the institution. Many artists, including Giacometti and Picasso, contributed works of art to raise funds to give Artaud financial security. So a home was found for him, run by Dr Delmas, at Ivry in the Parisian suburbs. He moved there in 1946 and while using it as a base Artaud soon reverted to his old bohemian existence in the café society of Saint-Germain. Abandoning the 'Cahier de Rodez', he began producing intense portraits of his friends. On one level, these pencil and red chalk studies were more conventional in their rapt observation than his previous *dessins-écrits*. But on another level their violence soon became overt, as Artaud subjected the faces of Mania Oïfer, Minouche Pastier and Henri Pichette to eruptive distortions. In some, notably a 1947 portrait of Arthur Adamov, he allowed scrawled words to resume their old expressive force within the overall image. When Artaud set about drawing some haggard self-portraits, he unleashed a destructive power that disturbed friends who watched him feverishly at work (pl. 405).

Not long before Artaud's death from an anal tumour in March 1948, Jean Dequeker had the unnerving experience of witnessing his ferocious attack on a large sheet of white paper. Here, Artaud had already

> drawn the abstract outlines of a face, and in these barely sketched traits, where he had placed black blotches, apparitions of the future, with no mirror for reflection, I saw him create his double, as though in a crucible at the price of nameless torture and cruelty. He worked with rage, broke crayon after crayon, enduring the throes of his own exorcism. Amid cries and the most feverish poems which ever emanated from the spleen of a tortured being, he cursed and cast spells on a nation of obstinate worms; when, suddenly taking on reality, his face appeared.

Dequeker never forgot the haunted image that emerged there:

> It was the ghastly lucidity of Artaud's creation of himself, the horrible mask of all enslaved hori-

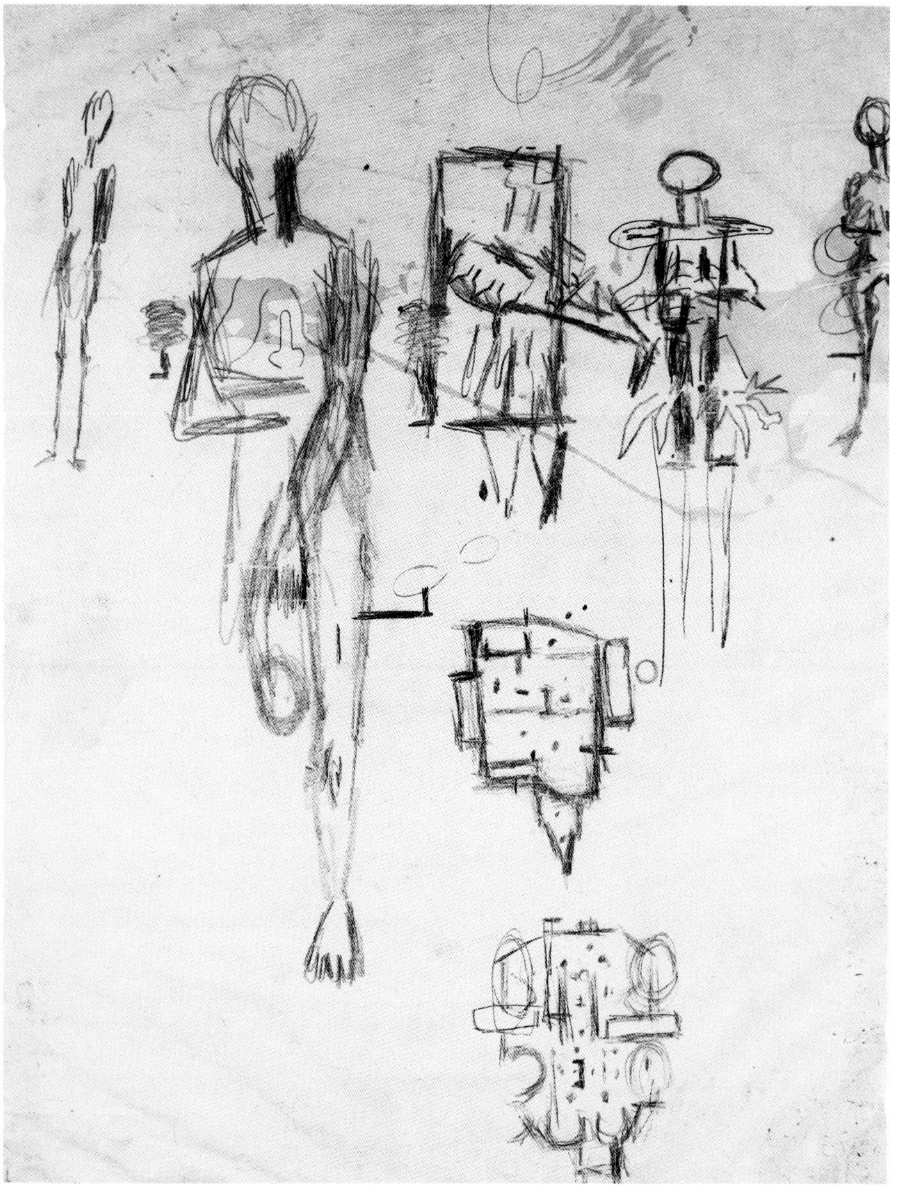

404 Antonin Artaud, *The Machine of Being or Drawing to be Looked at Cockeyed*, 1946, Musée Nationale d'Art moderne, Centre Georges Pompidou, Paris

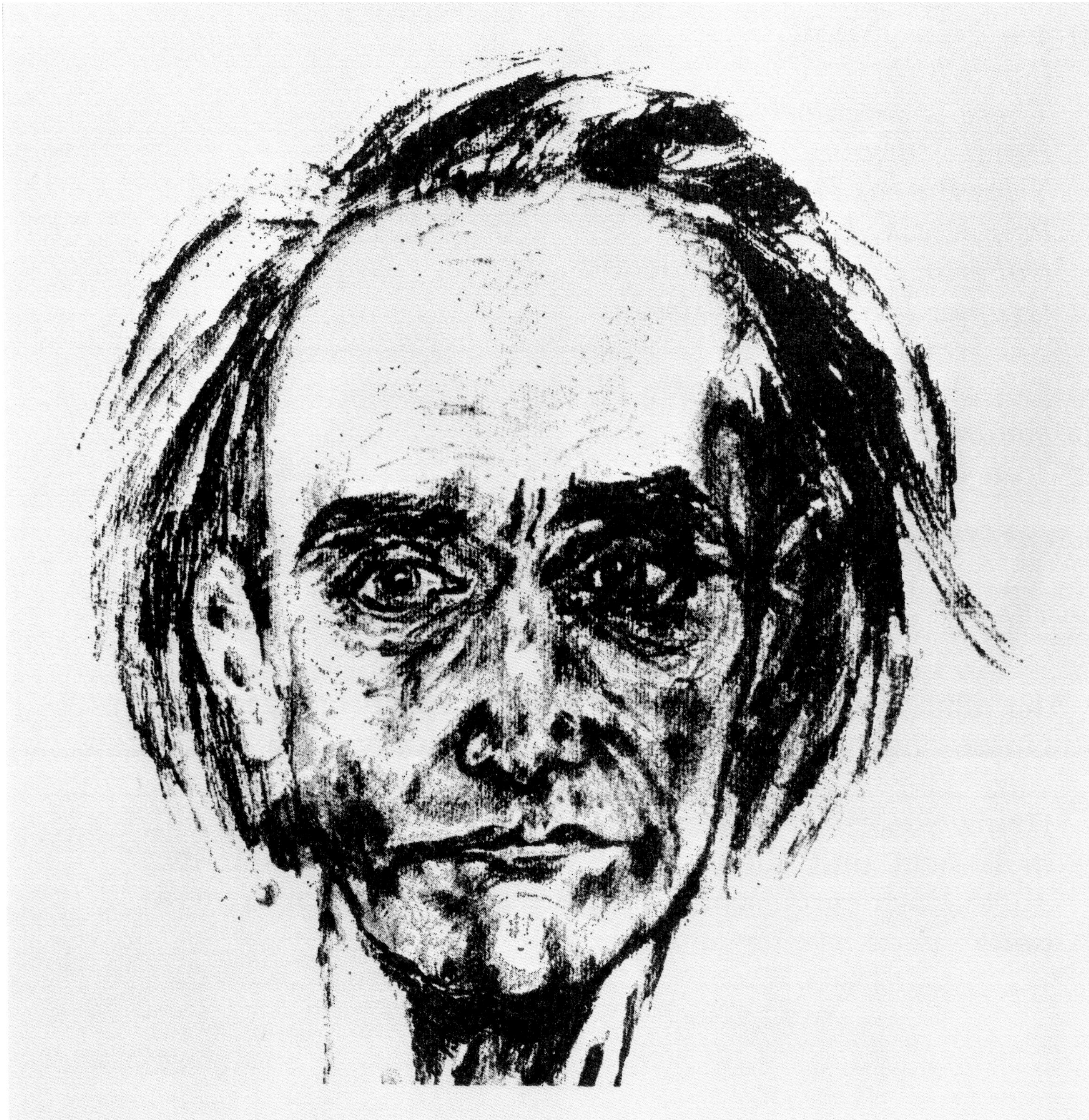

zons, thrown out to challenge the feeble means and mediocre technique of the painters of reality (those who look at themselves in mirrors). And when the face had become a symbolic identity with his own face, when its dark image was displayed before him, the tragic destiny of the actor was fulfilled . . . With the creative rage which made him burst the bolts of reality and all the locks of the surreal, I have seen him blindly put out the eyes of his own image. For that was what being a visionary was to him: to look with the pupils' blackness at the reality of the other side of things.[4]

This deeply visceral involvement with the physical act of drawing connects Artaud's work as an artist with his earlier experiments as a playwright, theatre director and performer. In the catalogue accompanying his 1947 solo exhibition at the Galerie Pierre in Paris, *Portraits et Dessins*, he stressed the need for 'barbarity and disorder' and the creative use of accident. Nevertheless he viewed this drastic fusion of art and assault in a positive, even beneficent light: 'the human face bears in effect a kind of perpetual death on its countenance. It is precisely up to the painter to save this face by restoring its personal features.'[5] Artaud saw himself as an artist who had refused to be silenced by psychiatric treatment in hospitals. Far from feeling grateful to the doctors who had helped him, he attacked them for trying to impose their own medical norm on the artist's 'superior lucidity'.[6] In this respect, his anger was roused above all by the reaction to a van Gogh exhibition at the Orangerie. Infuriated with a psychiatrist who described Vincent as 'a degenerate',[7] Artaud asked:

> And what is an authentic madman? A man who has preferred to go mad in the sense that society understands it, rather than forfeit a certain superior idea of human honour. This is how society has had strangled in her asylums all those she has wanted to get rid of or protect herself against those who have refused to become her accomplices to certain lofty obscenities. For a madman is also a man society does not want to hear, whom it wants to prevent from uttering unbearable truths.[8]

Soon after publishing this polemic, in a 1947 text called 'Van Gogh, the Man Suicided by Society', Artaud found his condemnation borne out by the response to an impassioned voice and sound performance he recorded for radio. This profoundly disruptive work, filled with screams, unaccountable silences and multiple voices speaking in bizarre accents, was banned by the radio company just before its transmission. Recoiling from Artaud's uninhibited obsession with sexuality, death and the void, the executives took fright and decided that they could not broadcast an outburst summed up by the defiantly pagan aggression of its title: 'To Have Done With the Judgement of God.'[9] Yet Artaud was unrepentant. Right up to his premature death he continued to believe that 'no one has ever written, painted, sculpted, modelled, built, or invented except literally to get out of hell'.[10]

Given a longer life, Artaud would surely have deplored the medical establishment's failure to engage with the vitality of innovative art in the post-war world. Extensive reconstruction of hospitals across Europe should have given painters and sculptors a wealth of opportunities to work in the new buildings. Yet hardly anyone was prepared to commission on the Mexican scale. The priorities of clinical functionalism left little room for debate about the putative role of painting and sculpture. In Britain, the first sign of a renewed relationship between art and medical institutions came from Barbara Hepworth's chance contact with a surgeon. After her daughter Sarah suffered a prolonged and serious illness,[11] a friendship developed between the sculptor and Norman Capener, the specialist who had operated on the girl. In the summer of 1947, realising that Hepworth's fascination with the structure of the human body might predispose her to find stimulus in observing an operation, he proposed that she attend one at the Princess Elizabeth Orthopaedic Hospital in Exeter. She responded to the surgeon's felicitous suggestion with alacrity, and the experience proved so compelling that Hepworth observed further operations at the National Orthopaedic Hospital and the London Clinic.

In aesthetic terms, the outcome was far removed from her previous involvement with art in a medical context. More than twenty years earlier, when still a student, Hepworth had made a proposal for a 'panel sculpture' over the main entrance of a hospital.[12] Produced while she was at the Royal College of Art and submitted as an entry for the Rome scholarship in 1924, this academic exercise

405 (*facing page*) Antonin Artaud, *Self-Portrait*, 1948, Private Collection

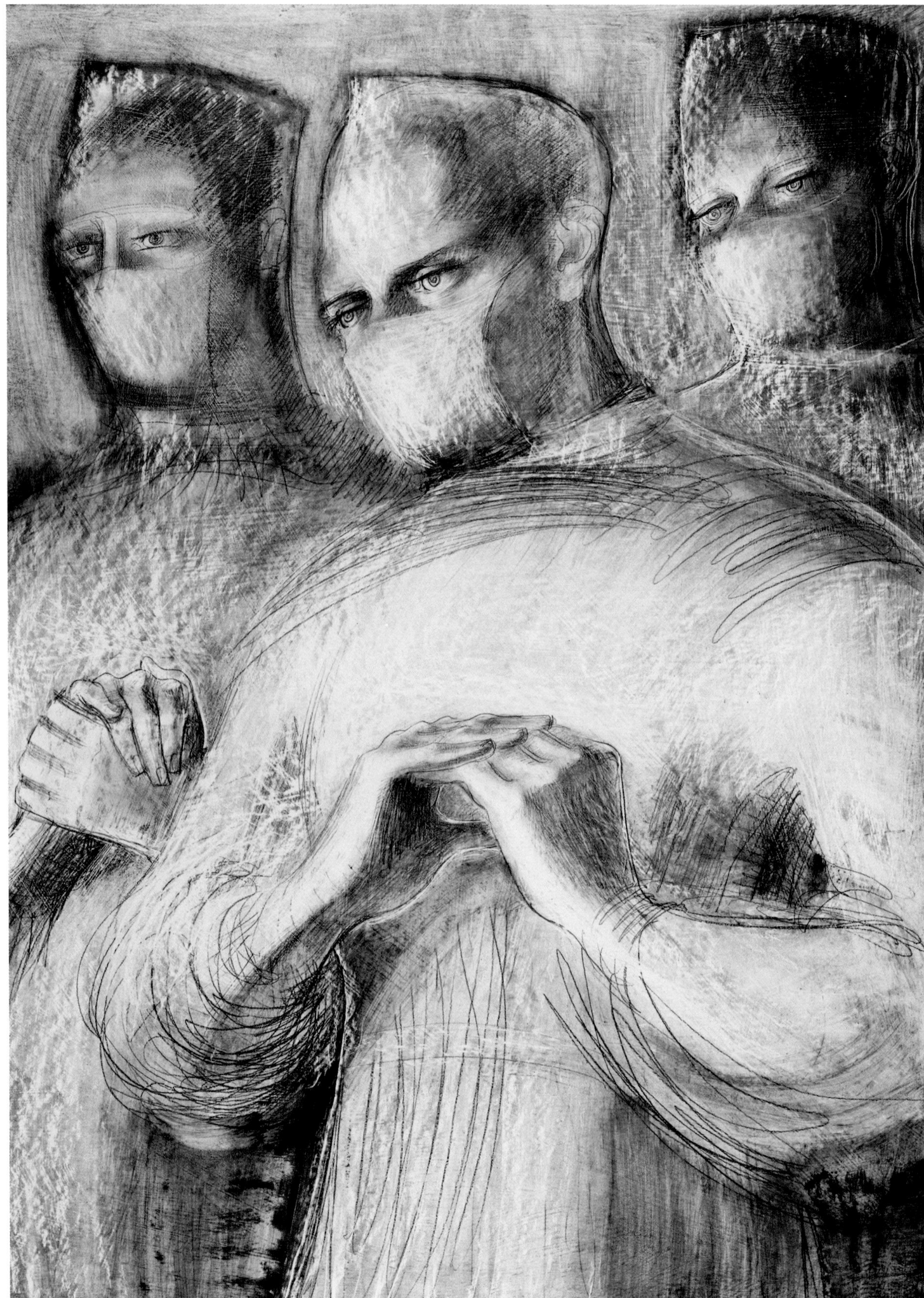

gives no hint of the woman who would soon play such a major part in revitalising contemporary British sculpture. Nor did she take the project further, realising no doubt that its tame allegiance to precedent would lead nowhere. Yet Hepworth's youthful reliance on a very unadventurous interpretation of a religious theme, where the central figure of Christ is dutifully surrounded by adult and child applicants, was replaced by her far more impressive response to the hospital theme in the late 1940s.

Armed with a pen and a sterilised pad, she made notes while a number of leading surgeons carried out intricate bone operations. Having expected to dislike the spectacle, she found it captivating. 'From the moment when I entered the operating theatre I became completely absorbed by two things', she recalled;

> first, the extraordinary beauty of purpose and co-ordination between human beings all dedicated to the saving of life, and the way that unity of idea and purpose dictated a perfection of concentration, movement, and gesture; and secondly by the way this special grace (grace of mind and body) induced a spontaneous space composition, an articulated and animated kind of abstract sculpture very close to what I had been seeking in my own work.[13]

Extending over two years, the experience that Hepworth gained in operating theatres generated a body of work among the finest and most moving of all her drawings. Curiously, they could be said to fulfil the ambition outlined three decades earlier by Stanley Spencer, who had disclosed in 1916 his desire to 'do a fresco of an operation' catching the 'classical' quality of the scene, the 'wonderfully intense' hands and the 'stillness in the theatre'.[14] Hepworth's drawings could also be seen as celebrations of the National Health Service, inaugurated in July 1948 after several years of planning by Britain's radical Labour government.[15] Yet her interpretations are still highly personal in feeling. Several, made from memory in oil and pencil immediately after scrutinising the operation, do not show surgeons in action. One particularly commanding study, *Skiagram*, focuses on the moment of preparation, when a triumvirate of masked figures flex their fingers in readiness for the testing activity ahead of them (pl. 406). Their eyes are defined with special precision, by the point of a pencil almost as sharp as a scalpel itself, while the pupils concentrate on the problem in hand with laser-like probity. Another drawing, executed with a delicacy worthy of a *quattrocento* Florentine draughtsman, defines the gentle flow of a theatre sister's drapery as it creases in response to the belt tied round her waist.

Most of these studies, however, share Toulouse-Lautrec's desire to reveal the surgeon in action –

406 (*facing page*) Barbara Hepworth, *Skiagram*, 1949, Private Collection

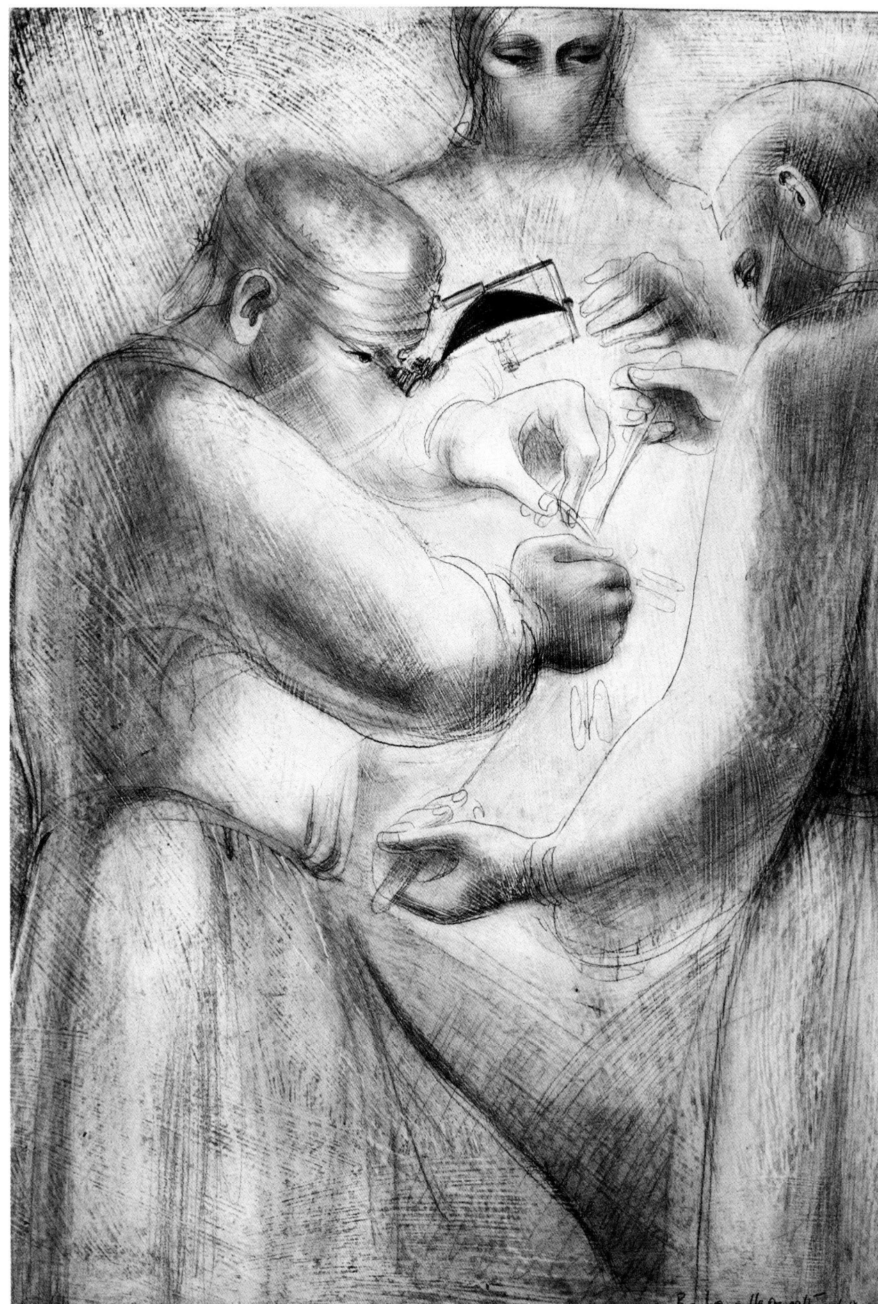

407 (*below*) Barbara Hepworth, *Fenestration of the Ear, The Magnifying Glass Stage 2*, 1948, Bolton Museum and Art Gallery, Lancashire

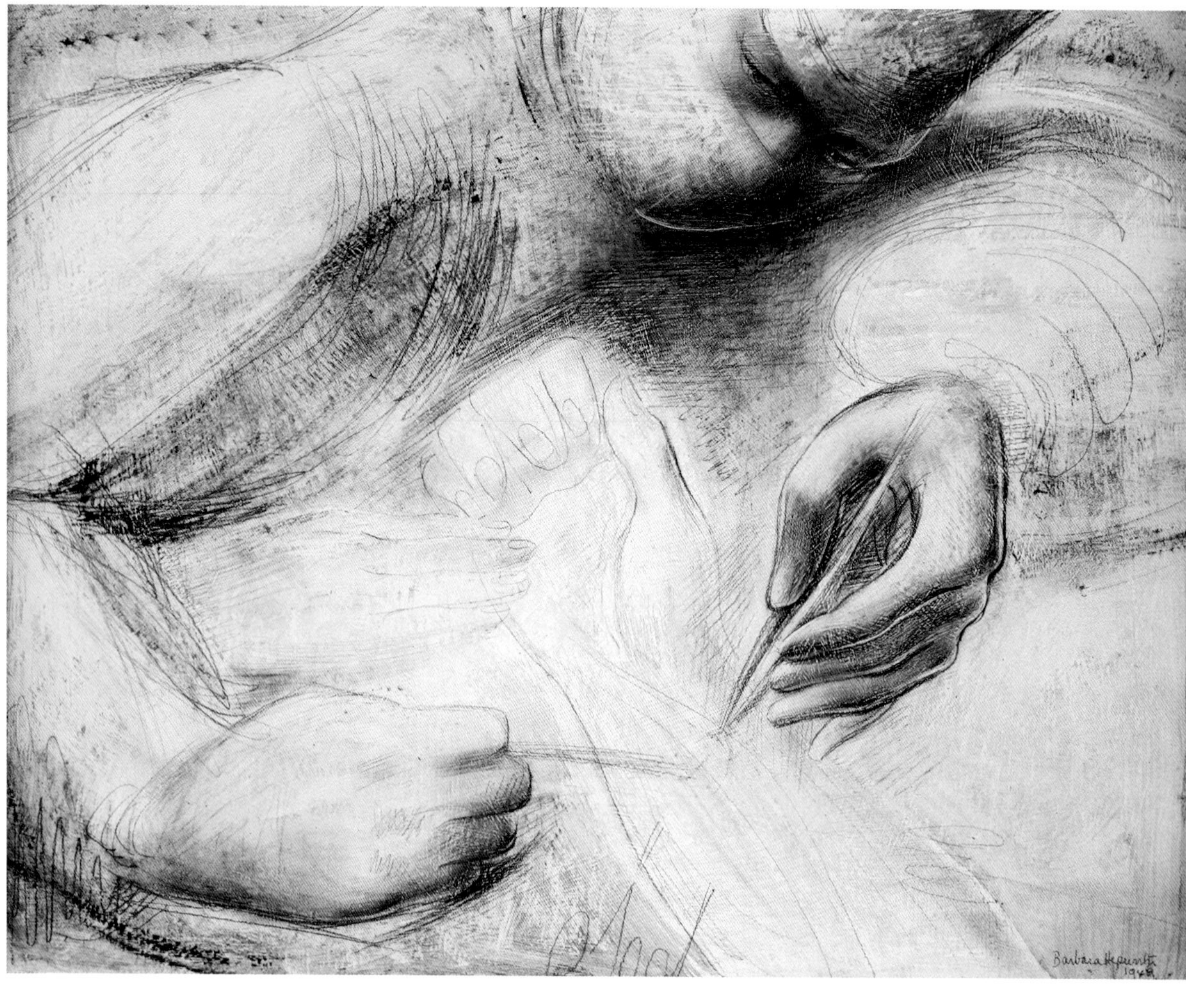

408 Barbara Hepworth, *The Hands and the Arm*, 1948, Private Collection

first of all bending over the patient with a scalpel held expertly between thumb and index finger, and then preparing to make the initial incision in a body.

Several of the drawings stress the communal aspect of an operation: the interdependence between one set of hands and another as they work together, in a state of utter concentration and poise. Especially dramatic are the *Fenestration of the Ear* images, where the leading London Clinic surgeon E. R. Garnett Passe, accompanied by his assistant Dr John Seymour and the theatre sister Margaret Moir,[16] perform a mastoidectomy and gain access to the inner ear with the aid of a hammer and other instruments (pl. 407). But perhaps the most arresting are studies like *The Hands and the Arm* (pl. 408), where the surgeon leans at a commanding angle over the patient's outflung wrist and cuts into the inert flesh with absolute, needle-fine exactitude. These paradoxically reassuring images are a long way from the callous butchery satirised in eighteenth-century drawings of operations (see pls 210 and 211). Hepworth, who brought a carver's knowledge and apprehension to the task of interpreting surgical finesse, was in awe of the activities she witnessed. 'A particularly beautiful example of the difference between physical and spiritual animation can be observed in a delicate operation on the human hand by a great surgeon', she declared.

> The anatomy of the unconscious hand exposed and manipulated by the conscious hand with the scalpel, expresses vividly the creative inspiration of superb co-ordination in contrast to the unconscious mechanism. The basic tenderness of the large and small form, or mother and child, proclaims a rhythm of composition which is in contrast to the slapping and pushing of tired mother

and frustrated child through faults in our way of living and unresolved social conditions.[17]

Soon after Hepworth's sacramental operating theatre drawings came to an end in 1949, a long-established London hospital decided to acquire a major painting for its chapel. However, the choice fell on the art of the past rather than the present. In 1950 the Special Trustees of Westminster Hospital purchased, through the active interest of Canon Christopher Hildyard, a large Veronese altarpiece, *The Resurrection* (pl. 409). It was placed in the chapel 'as a source of comfort and inspiration',[18] thereby returning the picture to the religious context it had originally inhabited in Venice. For Veronese's canvas formed part of a series of altarpieces and organ shutters painted around 1578 for the Church of San Jacopo di Murano. The ensemble was dispersed in the second half of the eighteenth century and the *Resurrection* then became part of the Lonsdale collection at Lowther Castle until its acquisition by Colnaghi's of London in 1947. Although the extent of studio participation in the painting has been debated by scholars, Terisio Pignatti is now firmly convinced of its autograph status.[19] Understanding of Veronese's late style has increased significantly in recent years, and the *Resurrection* can today be seen as a dramatic example of the poetic freedom with which the ageing master deployed loose brushwork and a light that breaks up his colour in order to generate a wild, brooding emotion. While the soldiers are restricted to a penumbral region, mystical brightness is allowed to irradiate the white cloth draped over the coffin. Christ has discarded it as he rises to the sky, but there is none of the overwhelming triumph that enlivens Ricci's interpretation of the theme in Chelsea Royal Hospital (see pl. 165). The ascending figure still conveys the sadness of suffering in his haggard face, even as he clasps a victorious banner with one hand and raises the other in the direction of his Father in heaven. His return from death is hard-won, here, and Veronese makes no attempt to minimise the travail that Christ has undergone.

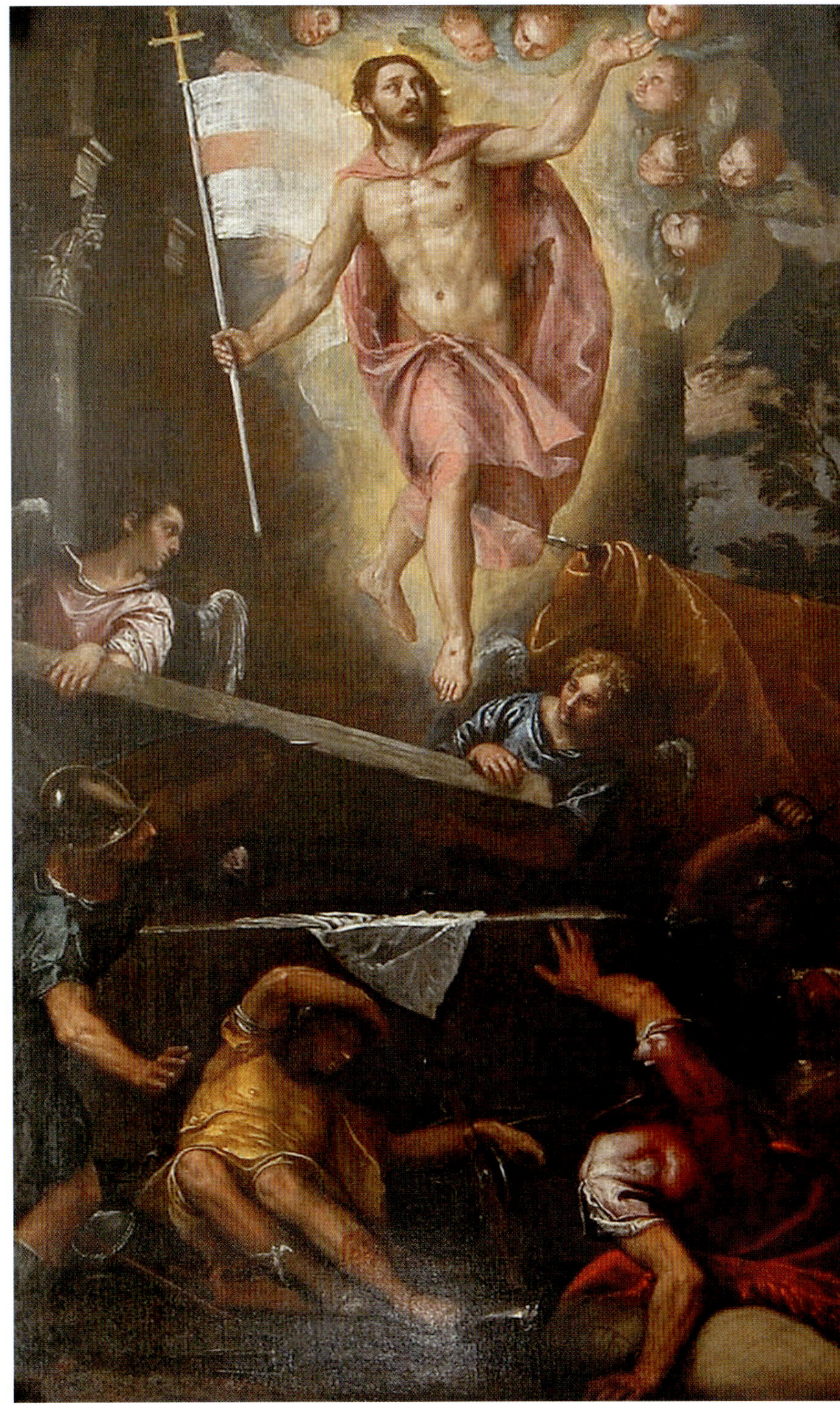

409 Paolo Veronese, *The Resurrection*, c.1580, Chelsea and Westminster Hospital, London

Remarkable though this acquisition was by the Westminster Trustees, it did not lead to a matching demonstration of support for contemporary art in British hospitals. Most of their interiors remained uncompromisingly grim, and in 1952 L. S. Lowry produced an image of desolation bordering on outright despair (pl. 410). Commissioned by Ancoats Hospital Medical Committee to paint a picture of the building's Outpatients Hall in Manchester, he did not hesitate to reveal the disconsolate ugliness of a place that intensified the anxieties

410 (*right*) L.S.Lowry, *Outpatients Hall, Ancoats Hospital*, 1952, The Manchester Museum, University of Manchester

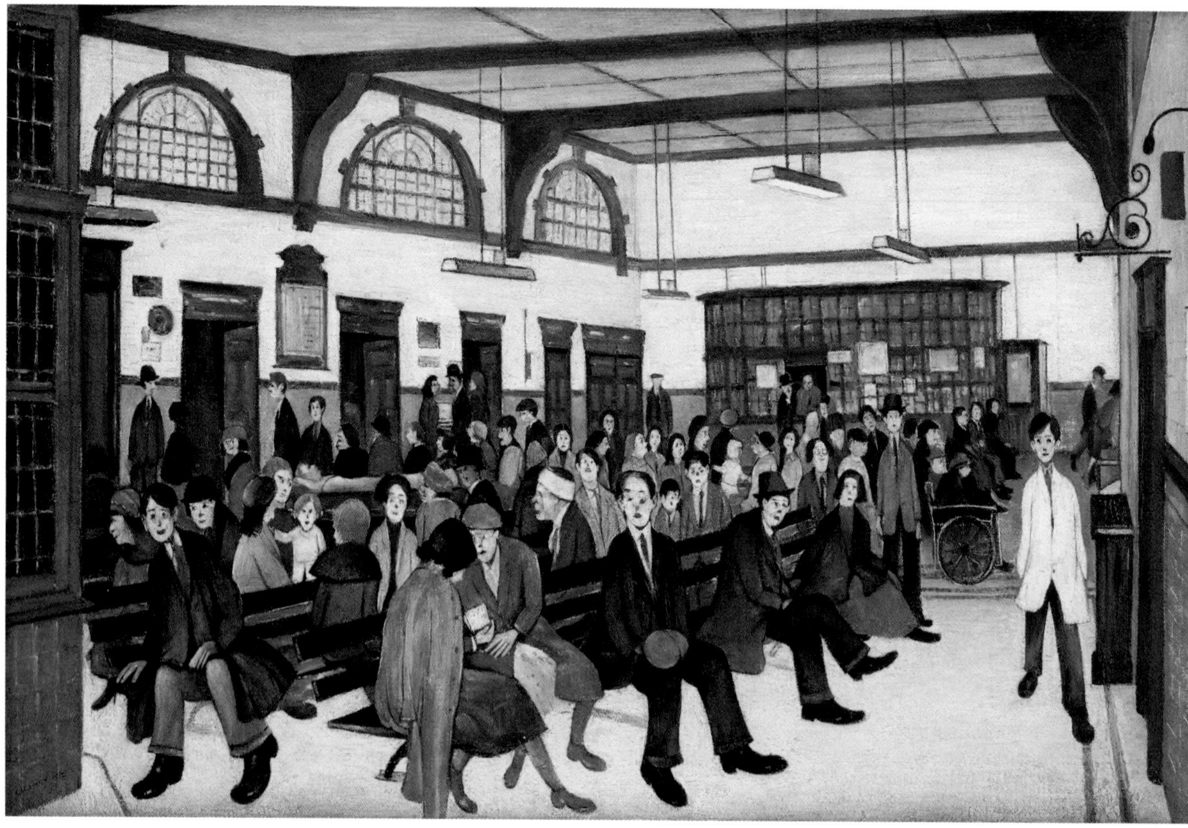

411 (*facing page*) Fernand Léger, *La Fleur Qui Marche*, 1952, Albright Knox Gallery, Buffalo, NY

of Mancunians obliged to endure its drab depression. Lowry, who knew how to disclose the loneliness of the individual even when he depicted the urban crowd at its most proliferating, defines the acute sense of isolation assailing each of the patients assembled in this gloomy interior. The interminable waiting experienced by its inhabitants is made still more irksome by the surroundings they are forced to contemplate. Only the white-coated doctor retains a semblance of cheerfulness in this dispiriting locale, and he is set apart from the cluster of dazed, forlorn figures condemned to sit on the hard wooden benches. Some stare at the patient passing on a trolley, while most make no attempt to alleviate their alienation by conversing with neighbours. No wonder the Ancoats committee eventually presented Lowry's painting to the local art gallery: the image he had produced was probably too disturbing to be hung in the hospital for long.

During the austere decade after the Second World War ended, even the most reverential works were capable of incurring official disapproval and condemned as a waste of public money. But nothing could prevent the irrepressible Fernand Léger from adopting a boldly simplified blitheness in his immense exterior decoration for the Memorial Hospital at Saint-Lô in Normandy. Built as a tribute to the American role in the liberation of France after D-Day, the Hospital was one of the final projects undertaken by Léger before his death. He began preparing colour studies for the Saint-Lô venture in 1954 and managed to complete an exuberant maquette for a ceramic sculpture as well (pl. 411). Called *La Fleur Qui Marche*, it advances with infectious vitality towards the onlooker. Leaves and petals explode from the central heart in an outburst of *joie de vivre* and, without straining the transition from flower to human, Léger makes the forms undergo a convincing metamorphosis. This 'Flower' really does resemble a child walking impetuously forward, legs bending and arms flung out in a gesture of unqualified welcome. At the same time the sculpture's floral character is retained, so that an expansive feeling of organic growth fills the ceramic with animation.

Léger's innate faith in the future was ideally suited to a hospital commission and he never allowed his optimism to be thwarted by the anxieties of the post-war world. His passionate belief in the importance of working for public locations intensified as he grew older, making him embrace a variety of major commissions during the last years of his life. They were all charged with his desire to move away, finally, from the angular, machine-like severity of his earlier art, and the Saint-Lô sculpture was no exception. Indeed, it embodied Léger's yearning for a restorative union between humanity and nature more explicitly, perhaps, than anything else he produced. 'The earth is round, so why try to play it square?' he asked in his text for *The Circus*. 'Beneath the sun and beneath the moon, in the clouds that sail gently by, everything is going round. Children dance in a ring . . . Roundness is free; it has no beginning and no end.'[20]

The sense of playfulness is infectious in *La Fleur*, anticipating the even more outspoken exhilaration of his large ceramic sculpture posthumously installed in the grounds of the Léger Museum at Biot.[21] He was determined, at Saint-Lô, that the tragedy of war should be superseded by an undaunted faith in the future. Although he had fought in the First World War and suffered from the disastrous impact of its successor, his condemnation of the waste of human life at the Vienna Peace Congress in 1952 did not affect the serenity of his war memorial work. A few years before the Saint-Lô project, Léger decorated a memorial crypt at Bastogne in Belgium with designs that remain, as Sarah Wilson pointed out, 'conspicuously non-sectarian'.[22] When the building was completed in the autumn of 1950, an American flag was flying in front of the facade.[23]

A similar motif emblazons Léger's mural for Saint-Lô, where the Stars and Stripes unfurl between dates marking the onset and close of the Second World War (pl. 412). His willingness to celebrate the US in this unequivocal way may have been heightened by the fact that he found refuge there during the war years. The flag motif at Saint-Lô was in this respect a personal offering of thanks, and it allowed him to indulge his love of heraldic boldness in pattern-making. It also excluded any disturbing references to catastrophic loss of life in the recent conflict, in a decoration conspicuous for its desire to offer redemptive images of alliance and peace – most notably in the monumental hand

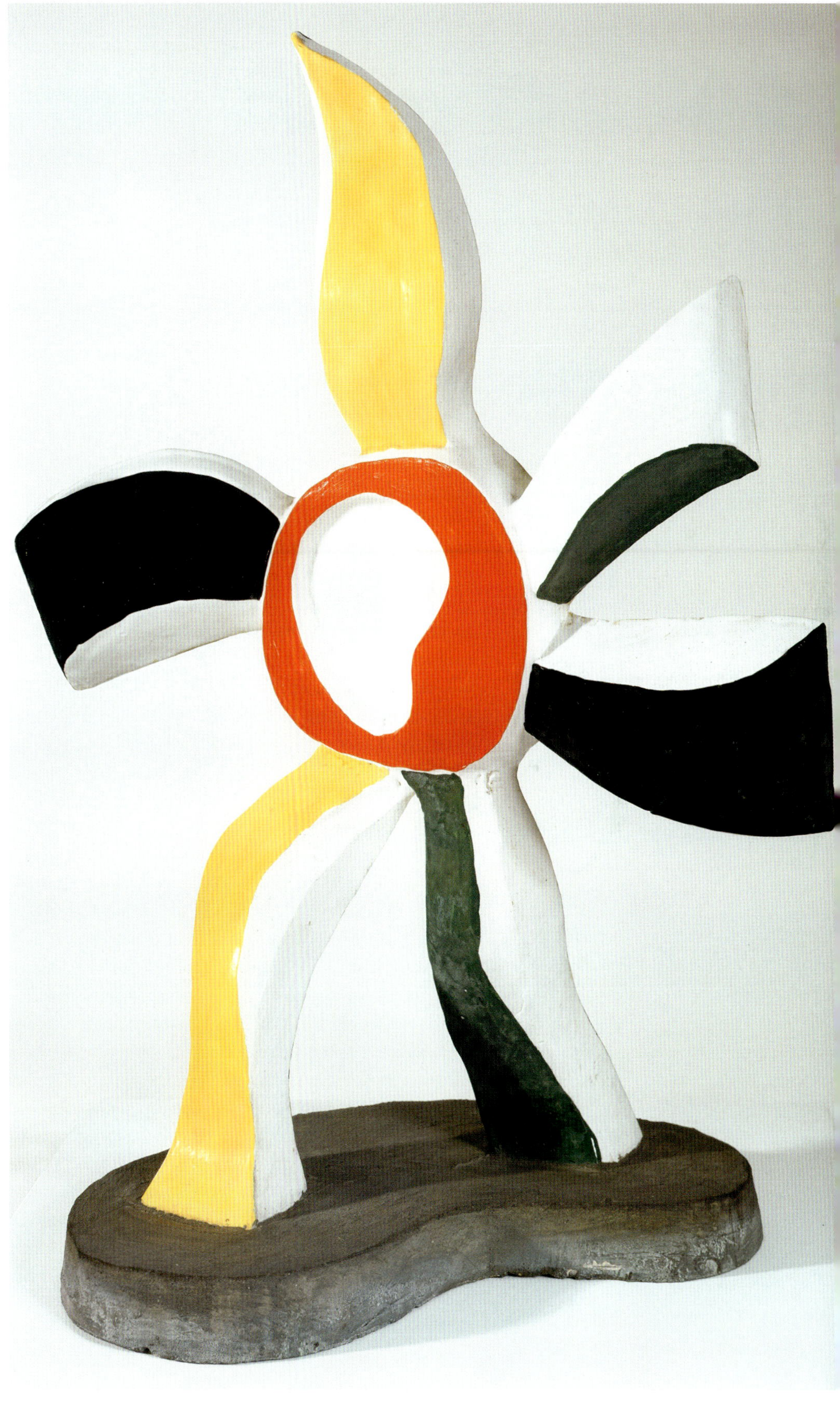

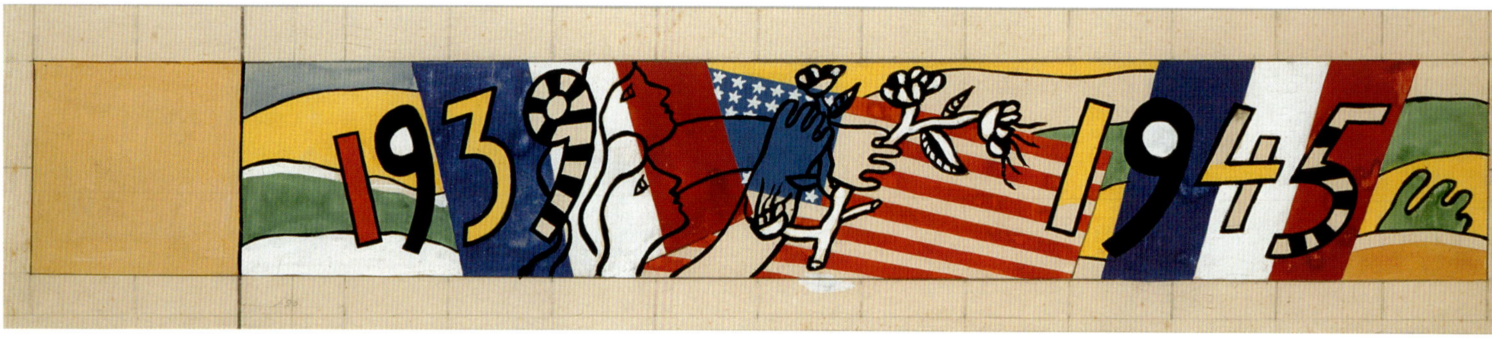

412 Fernand Léger, maquette for Mural for Memorial Hospital, Saint-Lô, *c.*1955, Musée National Fernand Léger, Biot

stretching across the wall while clutching a plant symbolic of fresh growth.

Léger's untimely death in August 1955 robbed him of the opportunity to bring his work for the Hospital to completion. But it was still carried out, in accordance with his preliminary studies, soon afterwards. It thereby became a memorial to the artist as well as the soldiers who had died in France during the battle for liberation. While it cannot be ranked among the most inventive of Léger's late architectural projects, its uninhibited modernity created a stimulating precedent for post-war artists who shared his commitment to working in public spaces beyond the gallery. Moreover, the Hospital building would itself prove even more influential in architectural circles. John Weeks, a prominent designer of hospitals in Britain, remembered that 'in 1948 only one hospital, at St-Lô in northern France, seemed to have any message for the designers of post-war hospitals in Europe'.[24] Its architect, Paul Nelson, divided hospital accommodation for the first time into major zones: the repetitive and non-repetitive. The former, confined to the wards, was placed in the tower, while the latter's departments were placed in a single-storey structure on ground level and interspersed with courtyards. This simple yet flexible model was persuasive enough to be emulated throughout the world.

John Weeks was himself at the forefront of an important initiative in post-war Britain to encourage collaboration between artists and architects of similar persuasion. In 1956 Mary Martin joined forces with Weeks and Kenneth Martin to produce one of the pavilions in the historic exhibition 'This Is Tomorrow'. Held at the Whitechapel Art Gallery in London, it displayed the contributions of twelve groups of artists and architects, some of whom (notably Richard Hamilton) anticipated the emergence of Pop Art. But Mary Martin aspired to a more purified and abstract ideal, producing 'a series of "minimal" reliefs integral to the architecture'[25] of her pavilion. In a review of the exhibition, *The Times*'s critic declared that 'any tendency towards a synthesis based on collaboration of this kind between the more vigorous and imaginative of our artists is, of course, of immediate importance to the general public; however highbrow it looks at the moment it is bound sooner or later to reflect upon the world of houses, cars, and clothes, the world outside art.'[26]

This prophecy was accurate, for Mary Martin's collaboration in 'This Is Tomorrow' led a year later to an architectural commission from the firm of Llewelyn Davies Weeks. She was invited to make a wall-screen for Musgrave Park Hospital, Belfast, and set about her task with a typical blend of thoughtfulness and enthusiasm. Weeks ensured that her steel and plaster relief was installed in a specially built, freestanding brick wall placed just inside the main entrance. The maquette Martin produced for the screen demonstrates that the wall, constructed as she put it 'brick on brick without artificial support other than occasional horizontal wire mesh', was an integral part of the work from the outset. Although the final double-sided work looks predominantly rectilinear in structure, she was inspired by the idea of a waterfall (pl. 413). 'Both architects and I felt that the wall must have a hole or holes in it to allow space to flow freely through it', she wrote, adding that 'it is also free standing for the same reason.' Much of the work's tension derives from the contrast between the plaster areas, painted with white emulsion, and their stainless steel neighbours. According to Martin, the steel was 'polished with a satin finish so that it would not give a mirror reflection but would give the feel of water gliding over a surface, or, in the case of the strong verticals, suspended in a jet. The grain of the polish is vertical throughout but it gives off horizontal lights in the same way as water pouring down a vertical surface.'[27] Martin arrived at the waterfall after searching for a symbol that would convey her awareness of

> the architecture, my own work, the function of the building and the fact that all who worked in it or were patients in it would be concerned with building living organisms . . . A consistent squiggle representing the wall appeared in all the drawings I made on the spot beforehand. It corresponded with the Chinese symbol of life. 'Life' in the Encyclopaedia Britannica is compared to 'a river which flows upwards'. Remembering Gaudí who built many models of cathedrals upside down I jumped to the idea of a waterfall. Very apt to Belfast, which is full of waterfalls. When I later found that in Central America an altar of human sacrifice was discovered carved with the same symbol it seemed to me to be even more appropriate to a surgical unit.[28]

In the end, though, her clean-cut, resolutely abstract *Wall Screen* has little in common with either Gaudí or the imagery that Diego Rivera derived from similar sources of South American inspiration (see pl. 397). With its D-shaped apertures breaking the emphasis on rectangular order, this lucid relief presents a variety of aspects to viewers passing by on the entrance side or scrutinising it from the staircase leading to the first floor. The fact that it is also visible from the full length of the wards on either side testifies to the important role played by the screen in the life of the hospital. It exemplifies, too, Martin's belief that 'the artist should . . . have an understanding of, and a capacity to enter into, architecture, without

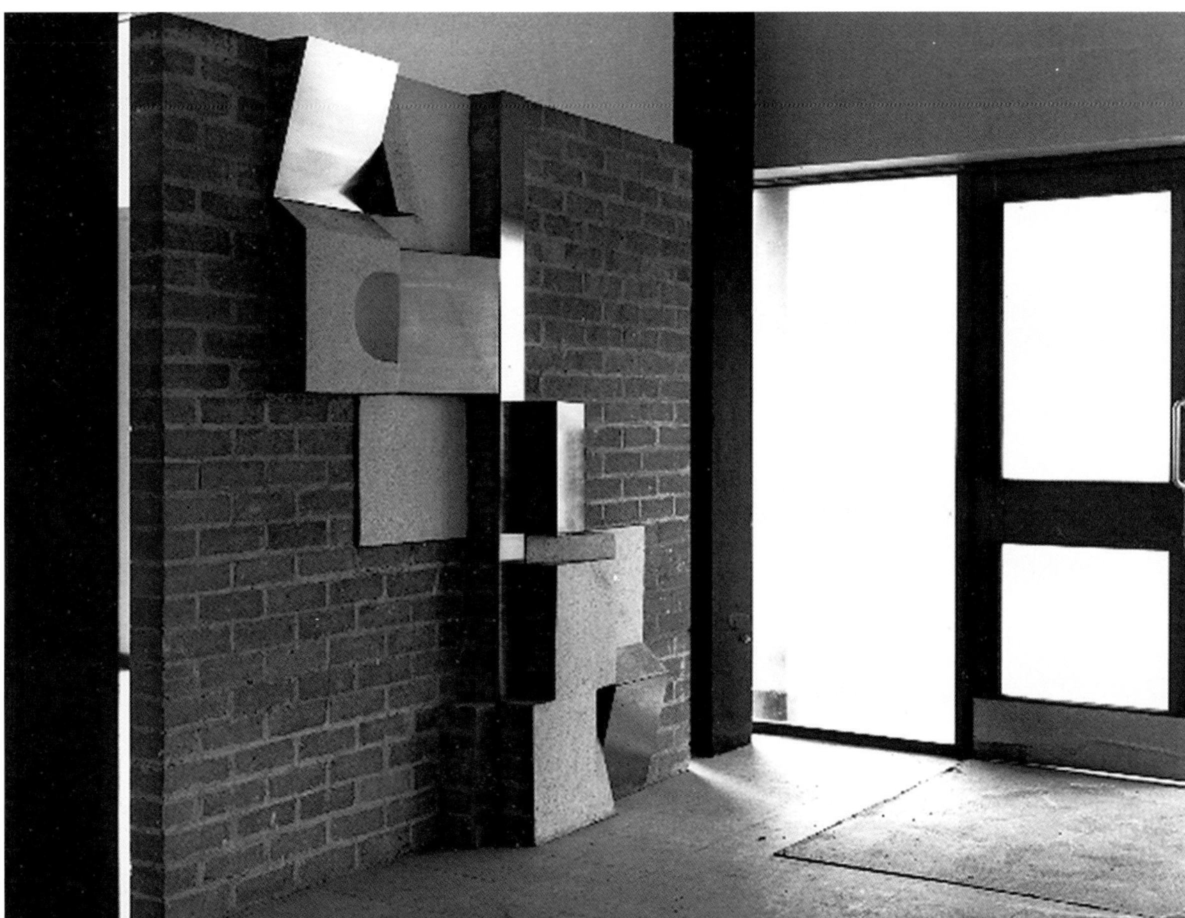

413 Mary Martin, *Wall Screen* at Musgrave Park Hospital, Belfast, 1957

destroying it, or dominating it, or distracting from it; an ability to crystallize it in an art which is a simple statement on the personal scale so that the work becomes a comprehensible symbol of the building itself, a part of the architecture but not architecture.'[29]

The precedent established by Martin and Weeks may have helped to provide Northern Ireland with another memorable hospital decoration a few years later. The architectural firm of Yorke, Rosenberg and Mardall was engaged on the Altnagelvin Hospital in Londonderry, and Eugene Rosenberg approached two artists with strong roots in the region to make ambitious works for the institution that opened its doors in 1962 as Britain's first newly built National Health Hospital. F. E. McWilliam, who had been born in County Down, was delighted to receive a commission to make a large, elongated bronze figure for the entrance (pl. 414). The Northern Ireland Hospital Authority wanted it to represent Macha, the mythical Celtic princess who is supposed to have founded the first Irish hospital back in 300 BC. As a young sculptor before the Second World War, McWilliam had been a carver of wildly distorted images. But by this time he was working in a more figurative idiom, and his *Princess Macha* exudes a spirit of attenuated beneficence as she extends her arms in a gesture poised half way between welcoming and blessing.

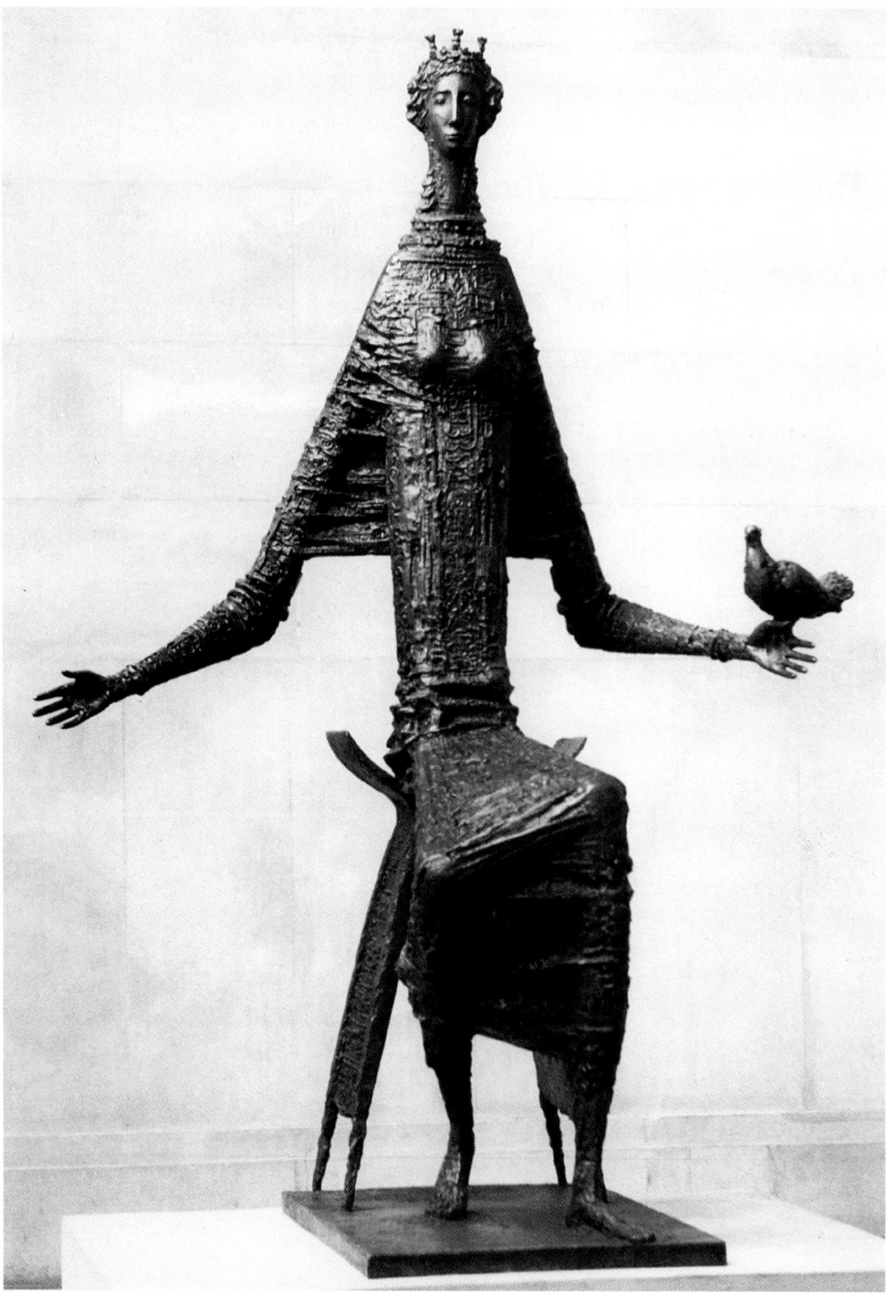

414 F. E. McWilliam, *Princess Macha*, 1957, Altnagelvin Hospital, Londonderry

William Scott, the other artist chosen by Rosenberg for Altnagelvin, adopted a far more abstract approach. He was offered an expanse of straight wall in the Hospital's entrance hall. Although lacking previous experience in public work on the grand scale, Scott warmed to the proposal. He was an appropriate choice in terms of his origins: born in Scotland, he had returned with his family at the age of eleven to his father's home town of Enniskillen and later studied at Belfast College of Art. Moreover, Scott felt ready for such a monumental task. He had just entered a second phase of abstract painting, which prompted him to evolve a style well suited to immense dimensions. *Morning in Mykonos*, executed just before the Altnagelvin mural, employs great blocks of colour and elementally drawn forms in a painting reliant on Scott's response to the light and architecture of Greece.

Scott would, however, have been incapable of producing a work that fulfilled the bizarre expectations defined by the local Hospitals Authority. Its secretary insisted that the mural should contain specific references to Londonderry, 'including the traditional shirt factories, naval associations, the apprentice boys of course and . . . recent organisations including cadets, boy scouts, girl guides and others'.[30] Scott's unwillingness to produce such a painting would have been backed by Rosenberg, an enlightened supporter of adventurous new art.[31] Mercifully, since the mural was a gift to Altnagelvin

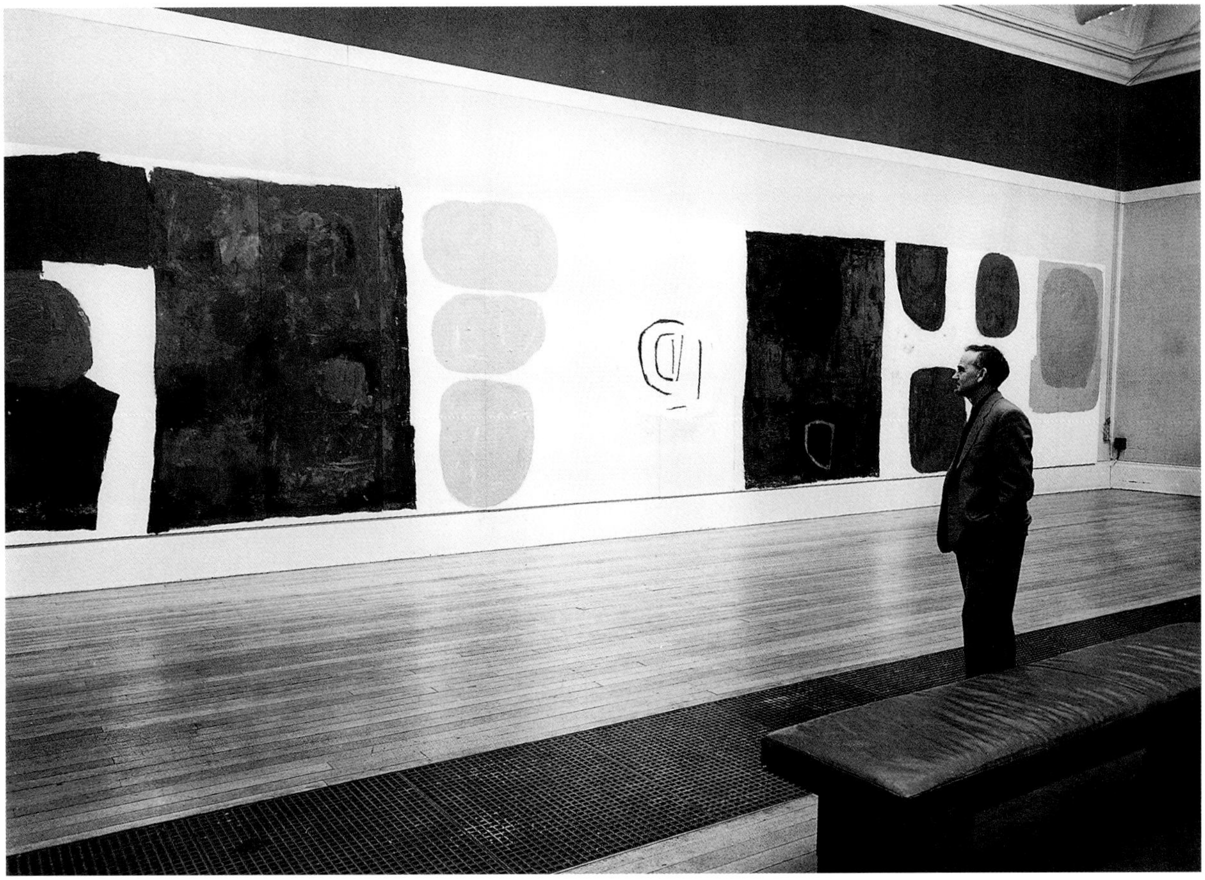

415 Photo of William Scott in front of *Altnagelvin Mural*, 1959–61, at the Tate Gallery, London, where it was shown before being installed at the Altnagelvin Hospital, Londonderry

from the Hospital's architects and engineers, they were able to disregard the secretary's requirements. Rosenberg recalled how Scott was 'given carte blanche after we had discussed the problem with him to ensure the right scale was kept' (pl. 415).[32]

Rosenberg might have suggested *The Four Seasons* as the mural's title, and Norbert Lynton wondered if it was 'in any way a response to the news'[33] that Mark Rothko had recently accepted an invitation to paint some ambitious, mural-like canvases for The Four Seasons restaurant in the Seagram Building, New York. Intriguingly, Rothko visited Scott's Somerset studio while the latter was painting his Altnagelvin panels in 1959. The two men, who had similar hopes for the viability of abstract language in contemporary painting, would have found much to discuss. Scott also took Rothko and his wife on a visit to Bath, where they explored the city's architecture. After his return to Manhattan, Rothko wrote to Scott thanking him 'for your warm friendship, our talks, and the day at Somerset which is memorable to me'. After making clear how much he admired Scott's 'beautiful murals in the shed', Rothko expressed the 'hope that there is gratification for you in the way they are being used'. But he also revealed that

> I looked again at my paintings and then visited the place for which they were destined. It seemed clear to me at once that the two are not for each other . . . The decision was easy and inevitable. What is depressing is the thought that there is really no place for them. Where in this world are the edifices which share the motives from which our pictures are painted?[34]

Ultimately, Rothko decided that the answer to his despairing question lay in a public museum, and donated his nine magisterial paintings to the Tate Gallery.[35] Scott, by contrast, was content to imagine his painting installed in a building dedicated to caring for the people of Londonderry. The boldness of his preliminary studies for the panels, executed in gouache on card around 1960 (pl. 416), show how reliant he had become on a few simpli-

416 William Scott, Gouache study for *Altnagelvin Mural*, 1960, Private Collection, UK

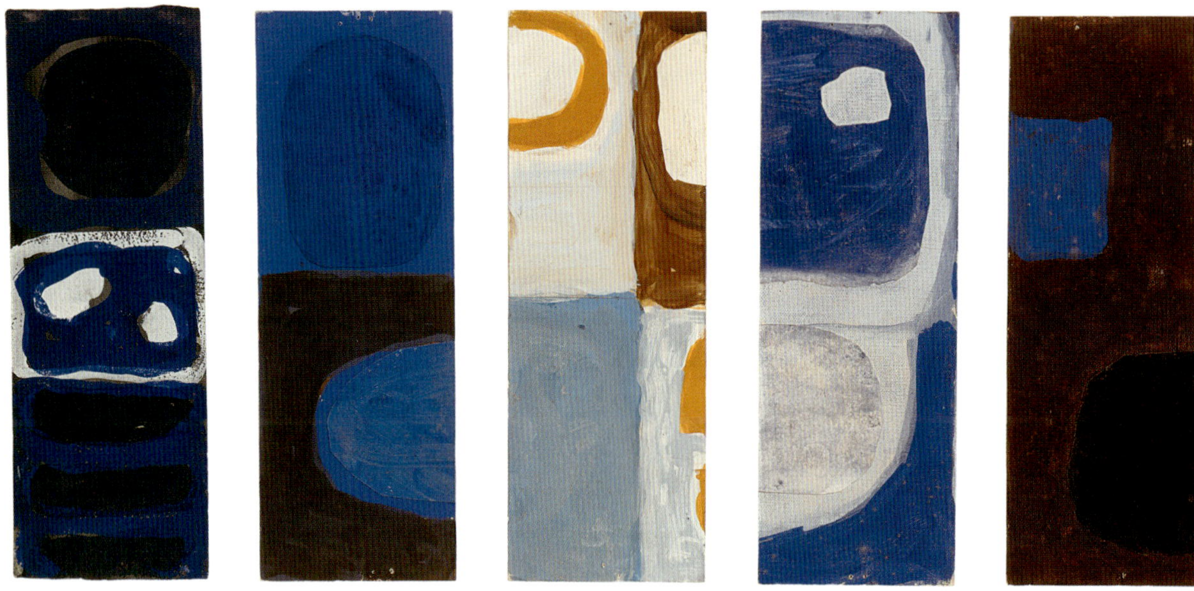

fied forms. As an artist particularly alive to the texture of stone walls, and windows that dissolve the barrier between outside and inside, he felt at home in the space provided by the Hospital. Looking back on his work of this period, Scott described how 'the pictures were now larger and a process of elimination again took place – hardly with my awareness. I had returned to a new phase of abstraction with the difference that I was now prepared to leave larger areas of undisturbed colour.'[36]

Altnagelvin must have hastened this development, convincing Scott that the 'larger areas' could be permitted to inhabit the mural without undue distraction (pl. 417). They certainly dominate the vast dimensions of the wall, even if the forms vary considerably as our eyes traverse the full width of the panels. Linear elements are flanked by immense fields of colour, ranging from dark verticals redolent of primordial boulders to rounded, warmer expanses possessing a strong, luminous power. Scott indulged in a range of mark-making from scoring and scribbling to a pronounced emphasis on impasto. He was content to let the episodic structure of the mural generate its own meanings, unaided by any representational clues. 'I no longer worry about whether a painting is about something or not', he wrote later; 'I am only concerned with the expectation from a flat surface of an illusion.'[37]

Such a belief, and its uncompromising implementation in the Altnagelvin panels themselves, guaranteed a largely hostile reception when they were unveiled in February 1962. According to a report in the *Belfast Telegraph*, 'Scott's work was immediately condemned as "awful" and "ridiculous"'.[38] One doctor was so incensed that he wanted the patients' comforts fund to supply the money for a screen to be installed in front of the paintings. The fact that Scott, like McWilliam, came from a Protestant family only intensified the vituperation in Londonderry, a largely Catholic city. Among the Hospital staff the sense of dismay was palpable: few of them 'really understood'[39] the offending work. By 1967 Sir John Heygate, who admired Scott's art, protested to the Altnagelvin authorities about the public notices attached to the mural. It was still resented by certain members of the Hospital team, who refused to let the Scott's work establish an unforced relationship with the building's other occupants. In this respect, it is a pity that the Altnagelvin executives did not share Rothko's faith in the ability of adventurous modern painting, over time, to sustain and enrich the viewer's innermost being. 'If I must place my trust somewhere', Rothko once wrote, 'I would invest it in the psyche of sensitive observers who are free of the conventions of understanding. I would have no apprehensions about the use they would make of the pictures for the needs of their own spirit. For if

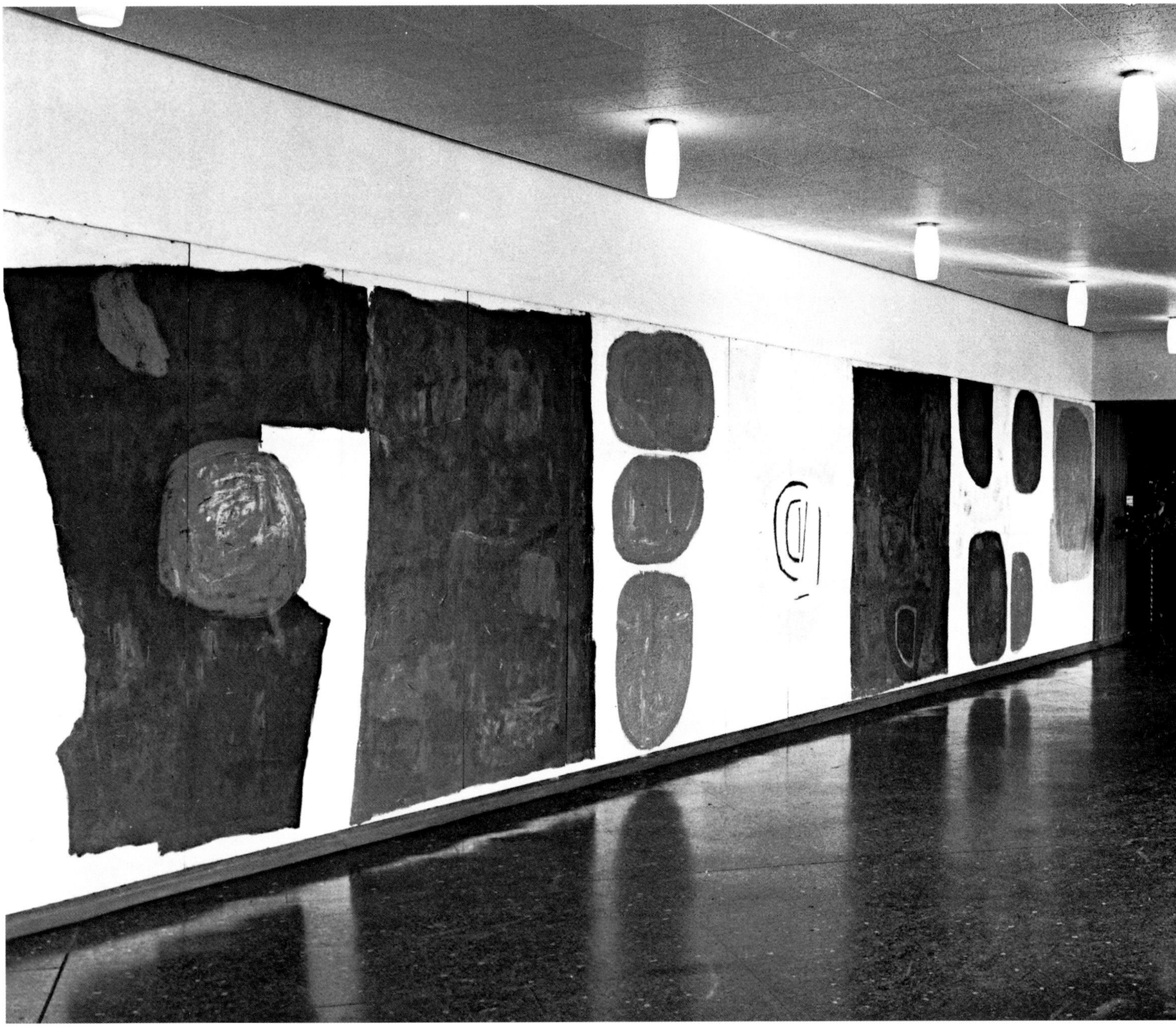

there is both need and spirit, there is bound to be a real transaction.'[40]

The challenge originally provided by the great expanse of wall at Altnagelvin's entrance hall stimulated Scott to produce a work without precedent in his oeuvre. But even that epic painting is dwarfed by the scale of the Chagall stained-glass windows installed in the synagogue of the Hadassah-Hebrew University Medical Centre in Israel in February 1962 (pl. 418). Built on a plateau in the Judaean Hills overlooking the ancient monastery of Ein Kerem, where Saint John the Baptist is believed to have been born, this streamlined concrete structure contains a hospital, a medical school and a nursing school. Joseph Neufeld's spectacular design replaced the old Jerusalem Hospital on Mount Scopus, and the six-hundred-bed building for patients benefits from the presence of an internationally respected medical faculty. Its emphasis on planned efficiency and academic prowess was

417 William Scott, *Altnagelvin Mural*, 1959–61, Altnagelvin Hospital, Londonderry

418 Marc Chagall, Stained-glass windows in the synagogue of the Hadassah University Medical Centre, Jerusalem, dedicated in 1962

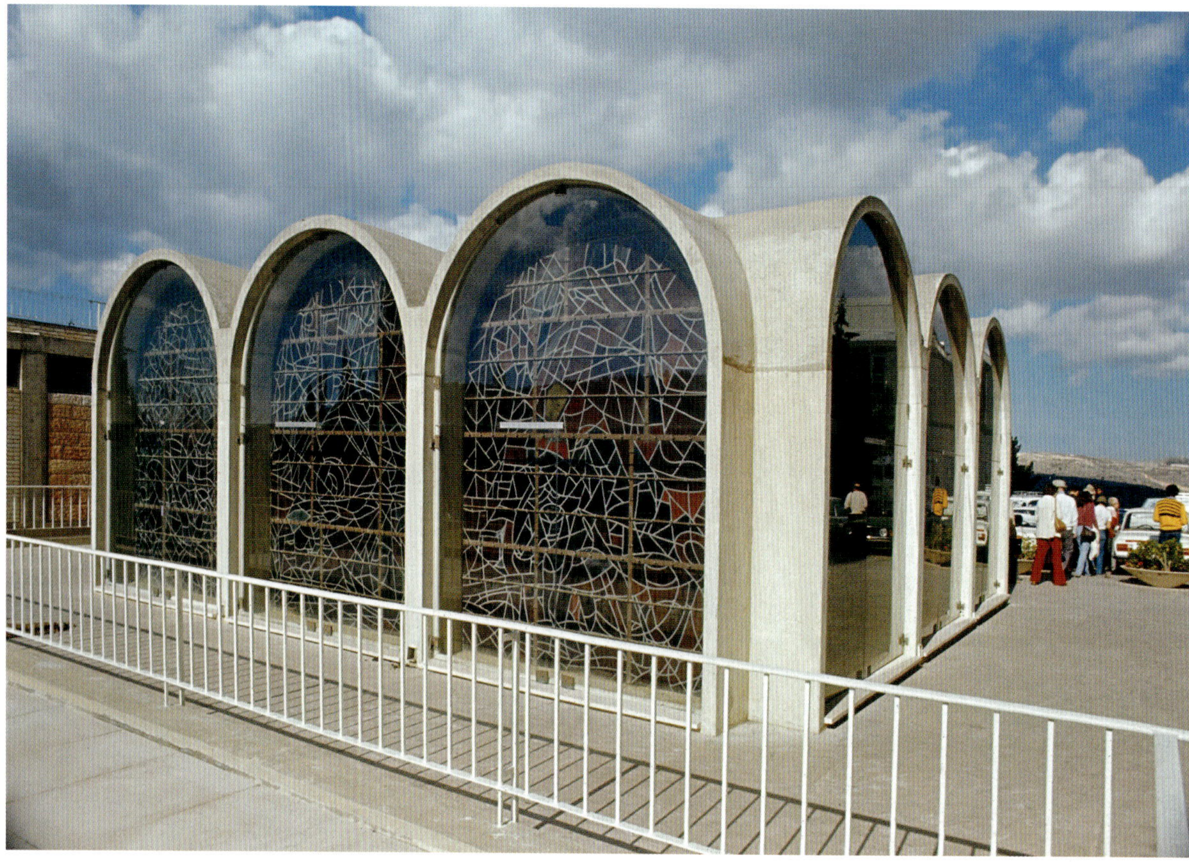

accompanied, from the outset, by a desire to give art an arresting role at the very heart of the institution's synagogue. Accordingly, in the summer of 1959, Neufeld and Dr Miriam Freund, the National President of Hadassah, visited Chagall in Paris. They invited him to design twelve stained-glass panels, each over three metres high, for the round-arched windows of the synagogue's lantern-turret. Rearing above the roof of the Hospital, the windows were intended to act as a beacon in the surrounding countryside.

Chagall, excited by the potential of such a venture, imagined the stained-glass panels as a sequence of fiery, translucent jewels set in 'a crown offered to the Jewish Queen'.[41] He had been involved with the medium ever since a visit to Chartres in the summer of 1952, when a thorough exploration of the medieval windows from outside as well as within helped to convince him that stained glass lent itself to his particular vision. He was also aware, no doubt, that both Léger and Matisse had recently executed memorable stained-glass schemes for religious settings at Audincourt and Vence respectively, thereby proving that adventurous painters could find liberating possibilities for colour in this most traditional of media. After carrying out a commission to decorate the baptistery at Assy, where he installed among other works a pair of light *grisaille* angels, Chagall ventured further at the Cathedral of Saint Etienne, Metz. It occupied him for a number of years, but he was obliged at Metz to work with Roger Bissière and Jacques Villon rather than producing a scheme entirely on his own. He felt that his experiments there were 'still only an embryo, but now I am beginning to sense all the possibilities'.[42]

So the Jerusalem commission arrived at a propitious moment, enabling him to develop his involvement with stained glass on a larger and more unified architectural scale than before. Working on the ambulatory windows at Metz had affected his approach to painting on canvas, prompting him to strive for an ever more luminous palette. But the Jerusalem venture led him to find, in stained glass, a medium that yielded finer results than many of his contemporaneous paintings. The softness and sentimentality always threatening to impair Chagall's later pictures becomes far less cloying in his window designs. Translated into glass, his deployment of colour grows more brilliant and pure, aided by the techniques he evolved through his collaboration with the Rheims-based stained-glass specialist Charles Marq. Determined to realise Chagall's vision of how the ensemble should appear in the synagogue, Marq discovered a method of making pure white lend particular vibrancy to the colours. Since it no longer became necessary to employ lead as a dividing agent between each colour, Chagall was able to escape from the confining effect it can exert on the forms in a window. Instead of imprisoning, Chagall found that he could arrange the lead separations in broader, more dynamic curves that often end up spanning an entire design. Chagall's insistence on personally brushing *grisaille* figures and shadows onto the glass before the firing also added to the windows' vitality.

A further stimulus was provided by the biblical starting point on which the iconography of the Jerusalem cycle is based. Chagall felt exhilarated by the whole notion of exploring the subject proposed by Neufeld and Freund: the twelve tribes of Israel, ranged in trios on each side of the lantern-turret. His recent paintings had been dealing with thematic cycles in immense sequences inspired by biblical sources, and the verses concluding both Genesis and Deutoronomy, where the twelve tribes of Israel are blessed by Jacob and Moses respectively, possess a lyrical intensity. Jacob's benedictions became especially momentous when reiterated by the dying Moses, who blessed the tribes as they were preparing to enter the land of Canaan. The disposition of the windows in the lantern-turret, with three panels on each of the four walls round the tabernacle, echoes the placing of the tribes themselves, who camped in trios to guard the Ark at its four principal points.

Another artist might have felt hampered by the obligation to adhere to the Mosaic injunction banning the depiction of the human figure. Chagall, however, rose blithely above this stricture. Just as he had always felt free to defy earthbound limits in his work, where people often float far beyond normal gravitational constraints, so he believed that animals, fish and the elements deserved to occupy a special place in his pictorial hierarchy. He understood why Paul Claudel, in a 1937 essay on the importance of revitalising the stained-glass tradition in twentieth-century art, had issued this challenge: 'Why not make use of all the ideas with which nature provides us – trees, foliage, the sea, all kinds of animals . . . All of them have a spiritual significance.'[43] Chagall had long been accustomed to investing animals with human

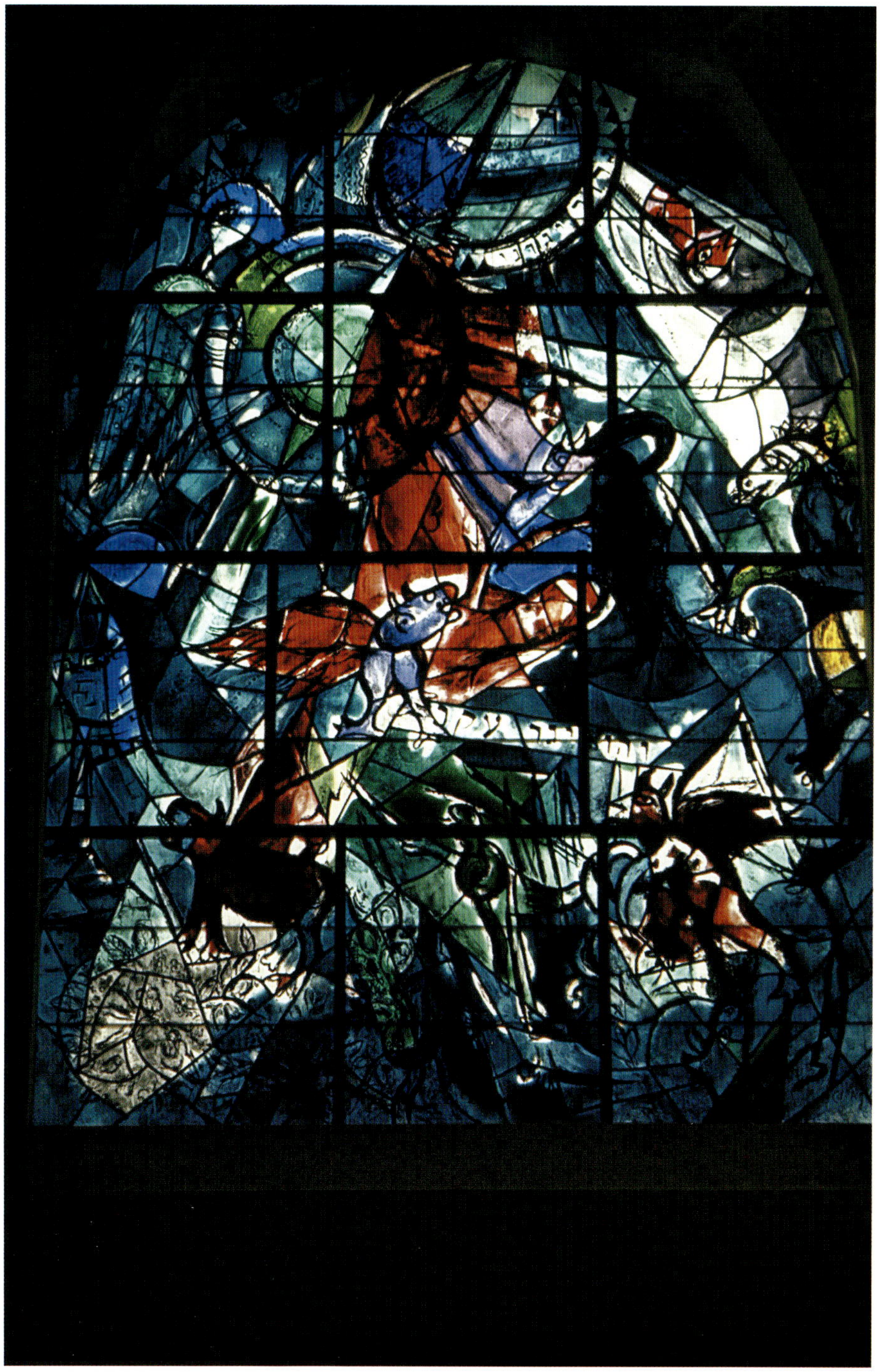

419 Marc Chagall, *The Tribe of Gad*, 1962, synagogue of the Hadassah University Medical Centre, Jerusalem

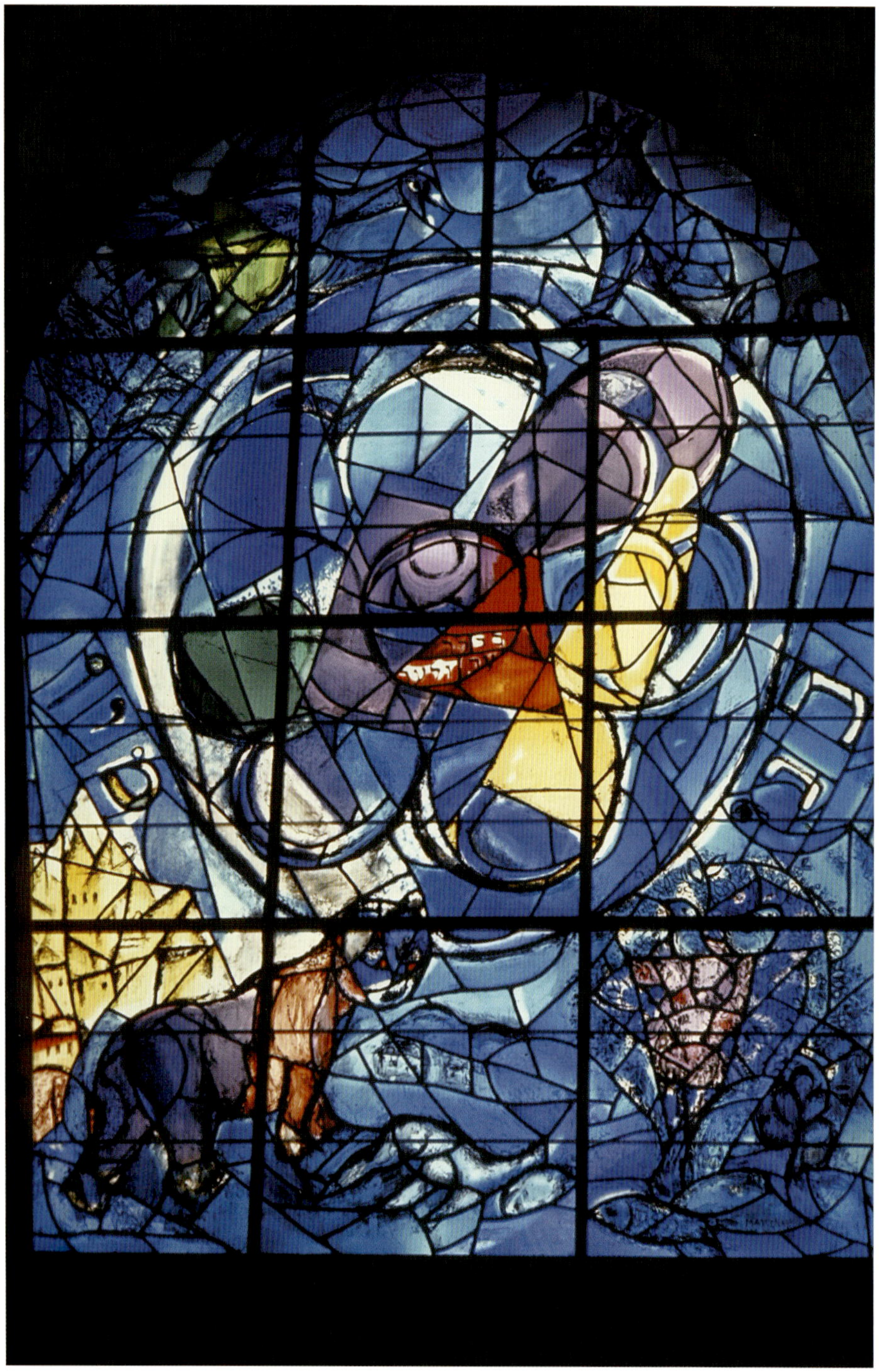

420 Marc Chagall, *The Tribe of Benjamin*, 1962, synagogue of the Hadassah University Medical Centre, Jerusalem

characteristics, and he deployed this instinctive anthropomorphism without any strain throughout the Jerusalem scheme.

Such a strategy seems particularly apposite in this context, for Chagall's iconography honours the ancient connection between the tribes of Israel and the twelve signs of the Zodiac. Avoiding the human presence became a source of inspiration rather than a hindrance here, encouraging him to aim at a freewheeling cosmic dimension where elemental rhythms course across all the windows he created. The power of light is, nevertheless, predominant. Its incandescence becomes ecstatic enough to carry a redemptive charge, confirming the significance of the Israeli tribes' arrival in the Promised Land. The pertinence of such a theme for patients in a Jerusalem hospital need hardly be laboured, and Chagall ensured that the windows of their synagogue are ablaze with the most affirmative vision he could provide.

The first window of the cycle, representing Reuben in cerulean blue, sets about this unifying aim with conspicuous zest. Although Jacob considered Reuben to be 'unstable as water',[44] the ascending birds and joyful fish both seem to exult in the advent of a potent sun. However, the next window on the east wall, dedicated to the cruel Simeon, unleashes a more penumbral and melancholy blue as injured doves escape from a world of destruction. Chagall was not afraid to depict violent, even apocalyptic forces in his scheme, which acknowledges the ever-present threat of global devastation even as it seeks the fundamental source of hope. Levi, in contrast, restores us in the third east-wall window to a universe animated by a clear yellow light, where animals and birds alike leap and soar delightedly above the Torah amid its protective circle of candles.

A great burst of crimson ushers in the south wall, heralding Judah the 'lion's whelp'[45] on a window dominated by outsize hands clasping the royal crown. Chagall incorporated his signature in Hebrew characters here, doubtless to emphasise that the crown image was centrally important in his conception of the sequence. The moods prevailing in these windows are, however, as volatile as the images emblazoning the previous wall. Zebulun, 'at the haven of the sea',[46] introduces a turbulent vermilion that threatens the ship, and only modulates it with the violet streaks cast on the water by a setting sun. In the final south-wall design this menacing mood gives way to a salutary and refreshing alternative – the soft green of spring, allowing Issachar the 'strong ass'[47] to loll lazily in flower-strewn fields.

Only for a moment does Chagall permit the scheme to bask in this mellow paradise. On the west wall his windows surge into invigorating motion once again, with the brilliant red lion-cub Dan leaping on an ultramarine ground. Nor does the neighbouring panel offer relief after this aggressive burst of energy. On the contrary: Gad is the most openly explosive of all the windows (pl. 419), erupting with images of conflict between beasts who snarl and lunge in a deep green region envenomed by an almost bloody red. Everything in this cacophonous design appears to be at war, exemplifying Chagall's readiness to admit the existence of the most evil impulses in the world he has imagined here. By doing so, he remains faithful to the spirit of his source, for the Hebrew Bible is itself never loath to explore humanity's destructive impulses. Yet he also delights in celebrating life, and the rainbow magnificence of Asher brings the west wall to a gleaming conclusion on its sensuous emerald ground.

If Asher is alive with the ascending motion of birds above a blazing seven-branched candelabrum, the first window on the north wall returns our gaze to earth. Naphtali directs the viewer, through the agency of another bird descending over a wind-tossed tree, to a sleepy hind stretched out on the ground below. The lemon colour predominating in this panel accentuates the mood of sated indolence, and nothing else on this final wall destroys the sense of well-being. Lemon turns to gold in the window dedicated to Joseph 'the fruitful bough',[48] who is shown on the point of aiming his arrow. The gesture might seem belligerent in a different context, but here takes on a beneficent role among the burgeoning fruit and blossoms of a land given over to nature's abundance. Animals graze without fear of assault, and in the ultimate window called Benjamin all God's creatures are brought together on a triumphant, pellucid blue ground (pl. 420). The revolving form in the centre of the Benjamin design evokes the grandeur of a rose window from the Gothic cathedrals that Chagall greatly admired. It brings together all twelve of Jacob's sons, the tribes of Israel, in a satisfying resolution of the emotions explored by the rest of this ambitious cycle. The threat of universal catastrophe gives way, in the end, to the promise of redemption in a temple of light fit for the building it irradiates with flamboyant conviction.

Nothing, finally, could be more felicitous than the setting enjoyed by Naum Gabo's *Revolving Torsion, Fountain*, which inhabits a spacious riverside location outside St Thomas's Hospital in London (see pl. 402). Looking at the sculpture today, with the Houses of Parliament forming a resplendent backdrop across the Thames, it is hard to believe that Gabo had no specific setting in mind when he started work on the piece. But he built the first model in the early 1960s without any such idea (pl. 421). Nor did he know who would be prepared to finance its realisation on the grand scale. For a while, the bronze *Torsion (Project for a Fountain)* looked as if it might never attain the fulfilment Gabo desired, remaining instead a symbol of the immense difficulties he often encountered in his efforts 'to dedicate myself to the task of making constructivism into a public art'.[49] The *Torsion* form had, after all, originated many years before, and stayed alive in his imagination as an idea pregnant with possibilities. In 1976 he told his friend Lewis Mumford that the fountain scheme was 'a dream which I have been carrying with me ever since 1929 and before',[50] and the plastic model he made at that time remained carefully preserved.

Gabo executed this model at the end of a heroic decade, which he had ushered in with the *Realistic Manifesto*'s announcement that 'art should attend us everywhere that life flows and acts . . . at the bench, at the table, at work, at rest, at play; on working days and holidays . . . at home and on the road . . . in order that the flame to live should not extinguish in mankind'.[51] He published those optimistic words with his brother Antoine Pevsner in Moscow, at a momentous stage in Russian history when Gabo imagined that sculpture might play a central part in a new society. Subsequent developments in his native country, culminating in the Stalinist determination to crush all hope of nurturing adventurous art, frustrated these grand schemes irretrievably. The emigrant Gabo, moving from Berlin and Paris to London and finally the US, enjoyed only limited success in his attempts to achieve the ambitious public aims defined in the *Realistic Manifesto*.

He must, therefore, have been elated in 1968 when Norman Reid, then the Director of the Tate Gallery, returned from a visit to Gabo in America fired with the idea of building the large version of *Revolving Torsion, Fountain*.[52] 'I put the idea to Eugene Rosenberg', remembered Reid, 'knowing his dedication to the siting of works of art in public places and that he had in his own collection a sculpture by Gabo which he had bought many years before.'[53] It was an inspired suggestion. Reid had the pleasure of experiencing 'at first hand the benign explosiveness of Eugene Rosenberg's enthusiasm in fulfilment of an idea'. Then immersed in the rebuilding of bomb-damaged St Thomas's Hospital, Rosenberg persuaded the collector Alistair McAlpine to pay for the making of the fountain. 'With two such volatile characters as Gabo and Rosenberg I anticipated a bumpy ride', admitted Reid, 'but in fact all went remarkably smoothly.'[54]

Gabo lost little time in collaborating with two construction and metalworking companies on the stainless steel structure. He followed the form of his 1929 plastic model with great fidelity, realising no doubt that the small sculpture he had initiated so long ago would form an excellent basis for the monumental statement he wanted to produce. As Steven Nash explained, 'the fact that Gabo could freely return to earlier ideas for certain of [his] sculptures, or repeat compositions in later, multiple originals, indicates that he did not think of his work in terms of art-historical phases. Rather, it was all part of an on-going process in which worthy ideas never lost their relevance.'[55] However, the contribution made by water changed the character of the work. Not only did it set the upper section into revolving motion, thereby implementing the kinetic energy latent in the spiralling form of the initial model. It also introduced, through the carefully orchestrated jets of water, an irrepressible linear dimension that parallelled the incorporation of lines in his string sculpture.

421 Photograph of Naum Gabo with *Torsion (Project for a Fountain)*, 1965, now owned by Tate, London

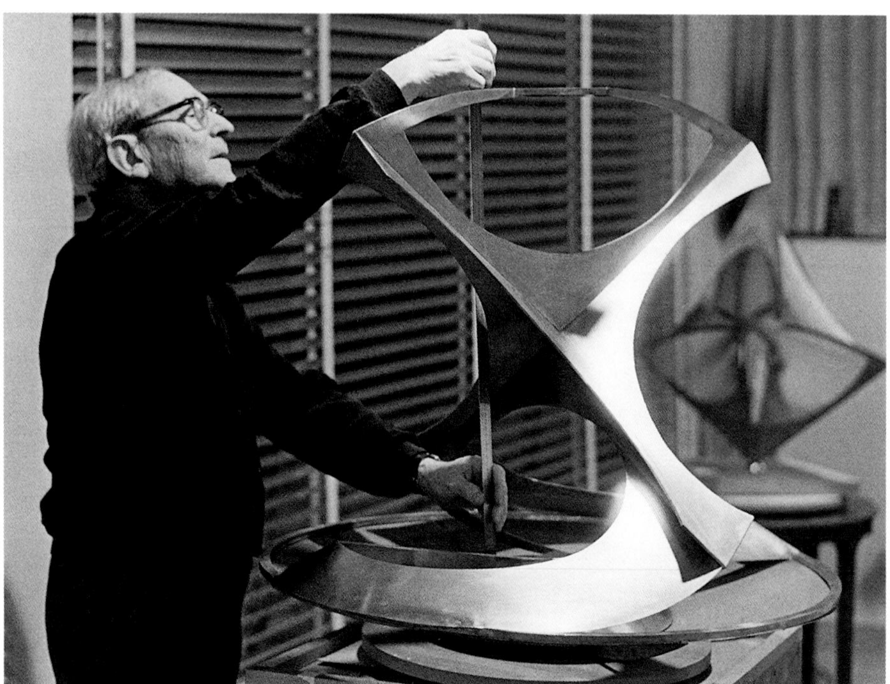

Nevertheless, the project could only be brought to successful fruition with a site large enough to contain an ample stretch of water. So Rosenberg persuaded the Special Trustees at St Thomas's to provide a generous stretch of hospital garden on the south bank of the Thames, between the building's main entrance and Westminster Bridge. Apart from the excellence of the location, St Thomas's boasted a tradition of distinguished art-works extending back to the time when Thomas Cartwright carved his remarkable figures for the old Hospital late in the seventeenth century (see pls 148–51). Rosenberg had likewise ensured that pictures embellished the interior of the new hospital at every turn. Norman Reid was impressed by the way they 'have become completely integrated into the life of the hospital – an art gallery which is open to the public twenty-four hours every day'.[56] The fortuitous advent of Gabo's sculpture therefore represented the culmination of Rosenberg's enthusiasm for art in hospitals, and the Tate Gallery was more than happy to place *Revolving Torsion, Fountain* on permanent loan to St Thomas's (pl. 422).

Late in 1975, two years before his death at the age of eighty-seven, the infirm Gabo travelled from the United States to London for the installing of what would prove to be his final public sculpture. He was able to see the gleaming structure set into spectacular yet delicate motion and spurt thin jets of water from the outer edges of its ribs, shooting a fine tracery of lines in a timed pattern that harmonises with the motion of the sculpture's upper half (see pl. 402). The sharp-edged angularity of its steel components is held in elegant tautness, contrasting with the softer and more rounded playfulness of the water. The jets erupt with festive abandon around the stern, tensely balanced core of the sculpture, countering its sinuous solidity with the evanescence of spray caught by the prevailing Thames-side winds. Patients and staff fortunate enough to look down on this graceful fountain from the Hospital's windows surely never tire of its intricate permutations, while the modernity of Gabo's materials and form-language

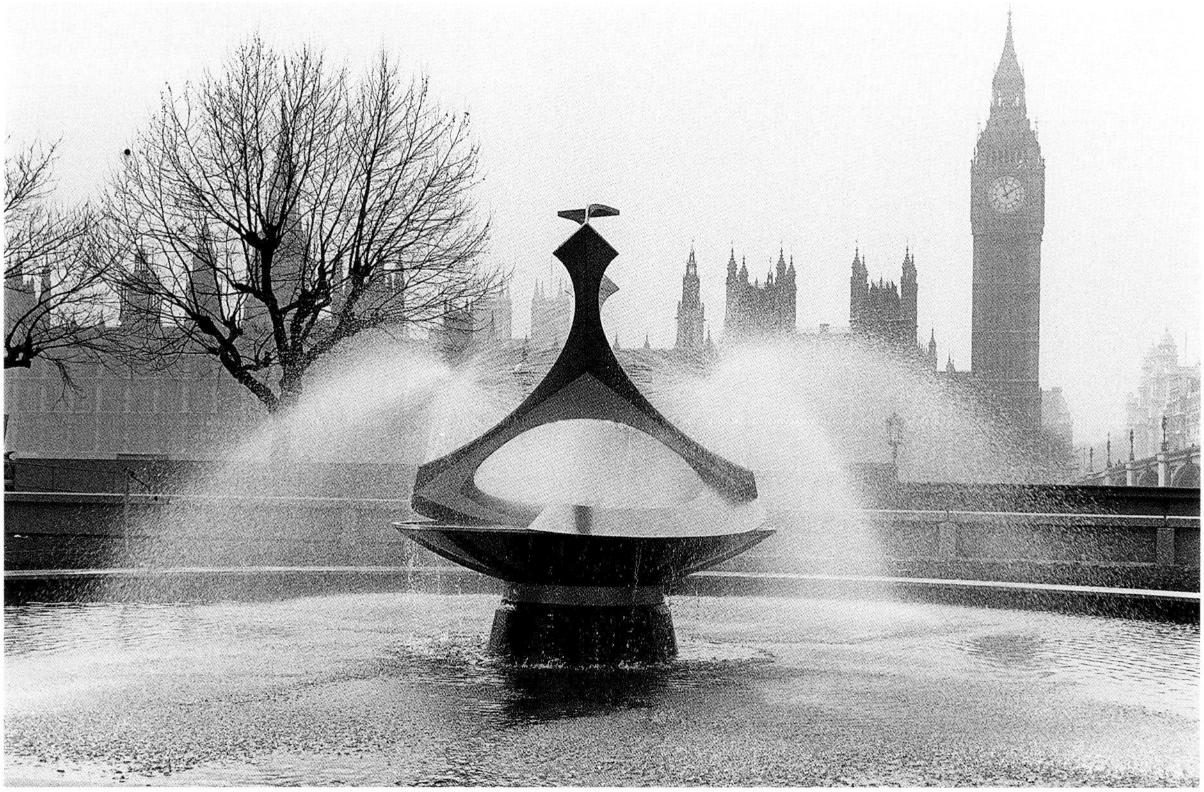

422 Naum Gabo, *Revolving Torsion, Fountain* 1972–3, outside St Thomas's Hospital, London

offers an implicit, courteous challenge to the Victorian authority of Big Ben across the river.

The setting could hardly be more felicitous, enhancing a joyful work that celebrates Gabo's lifelong commitment to the belief that sculpture can fulfil a role far beyond the boundaries of the museum. Installed almost five hundred years after the della Robbia medallions were placed on the facade of Brunelleschi's Innocenti building in Florence, Gabo's fountain demonstrates the modern artist's continuing ability to provide hospital inhabitants with inexhaustible nourishment for what Mark Rothko called, in a resonant phrase, 'the needs of their own spirit'.[57]

NOTES

INTRODUCTION

1 See Richard Cork, 'Pictures of Health: Six Leading Artists have donated Prints', *Telegraph Weekend Magazine* (21 October 1989).
2 Florence Nightingale, *Notes on Hospitals* (London 1859) p. 16.
3 Henri de Toulouse-Lautrec in Numa Baragnon, 'Toulouse-Lautrec chez Péan', *Chronique médicale* (15 February 1902) p. 98.
4 Toulouse-Lautrec quoted by Jules Renard, diary entry, 26 November 1894, in Julia Frey, *Toulouse-Lautrec: A Life* (London 1994) p. 399.
5 Vincent van Gogh quoted by Ronald Pickvance, *Van Gogh in Saint-Rémy and Auvers* (New York 1986) p. 89.

ONE SALVATION IN SIENA

1 See George Rosen, *Madness in Society* (New York 1968) pp. 116–17.
2 Ivan Illich, *Limits to Medicine. Medical Nemesis: The Expropriation of Health* (London 1976; 1984 ed.) p. 162.
3 John Summerson, *The Architecture of the Eighteenth Century* (London 1986) p. 127.
4 Lorenzo Ghiberti, quoted by Andrew Martindale, *Simone Martini: Complete Edition* (Oxford 1988) p. 43.
5 In the 1448 contract for Sano di Pietro's additions to the altar in the Capella de' Nove, in *ibid.*, p. 203.
6 According to the 1448 contract, in *ibid.*
7 See M. Eisenberg, *Burlington Magazine* CXXIII (1981) for a complete account of this commission.
8 Diana Norman, *Siena and the Virgin: Art and Politics in a Late Medieval City State* (New Haven and London 1999) p. 101.
9 L. Banchi (ed.) *Statuti senesi scritti in volgare ne' secoli XIII e XIV. Vol. 3: Statuto delle Spedale di Siena* (Bologna 1877) p. 233.
10 Saint Bernardino, *Le prediche volgari dette nella piazza del Campo l'anno MCCCCXXVII* 3 vols (Siena 1880–88) vol. III p. 323.
11 See Carl Brandon Strehlke, 'Art and Culture in Renaissance Siena', in Keith Christiansen, Laurence B. Kanter and Carl Brandon Strehlke (eds), *Painting in Renaissance Siena 1420–1500* (New York 1988), where he points out (p. 47) that the ordinance of 1433 made clear that the charitable activities of the hospital 'were now being regulated by the commune itself'.
12 John Pope-Hennessy, *Sienese Quattrocento Painting* (Oxford and London 1947) p. 15.
13 See e.g. Domenico's *Madonna and Child before a Hedge of Roses*, now in the John G. Johnson Art Collection, Philadelphia.
14 See Carl Brandon Strehlke, 'Madonna of Mercy', in Christiansen *et al.*, *Painting in Renaissance Siena*, pp. 254–7.
15 *Ibid.*, p. 254.
16 Henk W. van Os, *Vecchietta and the Sacristy of the Siena Hospital Church: A Study of Renaissance Religious Symbolism*, trans. Eva Biesta (Maarssen 1974) pp. 1–15.
17 *Ibid.*
18 John Pope-Hennessy argued that *The Risen Christ* also shows an awareness of Donatello's bronze *David* and his figures of Daniel and Giustina in Padua; *Italian Renaissance Sculpture* (London 2000 ed.) vol. II p. 218.

TWO MADONNA OF MERCY

1 See James R. Banker, 'The Altarpiece of the Confraternity of Santa Maria della Misericordia in Borgo Sansepolcro', *Piero della Francesca and His Legacy*, ed. Marilyn Aronberg Lavin (Hanover, N.H., 1995) pp. 21, 24.
2 See James R. Banker, 'Piero della Francesca, il fratello Don Francesco di Benedetto e Francesco dal Borgo', *Prospettiva* 68 (1992) pp. 54–6.
3 Ivano Ricci, *La fraternità di S. Bartolomeo* (Sansepolcro 1936) pp. 19–20.
4 See Amintore Fanfani, 'La beneficenza in un commune toscana dal XIII al XV secolo', in Fanfani, *Saggi di storia economica italiana* (Milan 1936) pp. 37–82.
5 Matthew 25: 34–7.
6 Diane Cole Ahl, 'The Misericordia Polyptych', in *The Cambridge Companion to Piero della Francesca*, ed. Jeryldene M. Wood (Cambridge 2002) p. 19.
7 See esp. John Henderson, 'The Flagellant Movement and Flagellant Confraternities in Central Italy, 1260–1400', *Studies in Church History* 15 (1978) pp. 147–61.
8 See Ronald Lightbown, *Piero della Francesca* (New York 1992) p. 285.
9 Giuliana Maggini and Luigi Andreini (eds), *Laudario della Compagnia di S. Maria della Notte* (Sansepolcro 1979) pp. 180–81. The song, preserved in a book owned by Sansepolcro's Museo Civico, is dated 1449.
10 The contract is translated in D.S. Chambers, *Patrons and Artists in the Italian Renaissance* (Columbia 1971) pp. 52–3.
11 See Eugenio Battisti, *Piero della Francesca* 2

vols (Milan 1971) vol. II p. 427.
12 *Ibid.*, pp. 427–9.
13 Masaccio's Pisa Altarpiece was painted in 1426 for the family burial chapel of Giuliano di Colino degli Scarsi. It was dismembered around 1590 and the surviving panels are now in different museums.
14 See esp. Fra Angelico's *Cortona Triptych*, painted during the late 1430s for the church of San Domenico. Since Cortona is relatively near Sansepolcro, Piero would surely have seen the painting *in situ*.
15 Maggini and Andreini, *Laudario* p. 130.
16 I Corinthians 12: 14–26.

THREE THE HARROWING OF HELL

1 Nicholas Rolin, document dated 4 August 1443, trans. in Dirk De Vos, *Rogier van der Weyden: The Complete Works* (New York 1999) pp. 133–4.
2 *Ibid.*
3 *Ibid.*
4 *Ibid.*, p. 262.
5 'I suspect that the considerable workshop input in the painting was the result of time pressures, too many commissions or possibly even the temporary absence of the master (the trip to Italy in 1450?)', *ibid.*, p. 252.
6 Dedication quoted in Nicole Veronee-Verhaegen, *L'Hôtel-Dieu de Beaune*, intro. Pierre Quarré (Brussels 1973) p. xi.
7 Bryan Little, *The Life and Work of James Gibbs 1682–1754* (London 1955) p. 82.
8 Rolin in Vos, *Rogier van der Weyden*, pp. 133–4.
9 Lorne Campbell, *Van der Weyden* (London 1979), p. 81, points out that, 'though the scales were originally drawn with the figure representing sins ascending', it may have finally 'been considered more appropriate that the figure representing sins should descend towards hell'.
10 John D. Thompson and Grace Goldin, *The Hospital: A Social and Architectural History* (New Haven and London 1975) p. 24.
11 Martin Davies, *Rogier van der Weyden* (Oxford 1972) p. 19.
12 Margaret Whinney, *Rogier van der Weyden* (London 1966) p. 5.
13 Matthew 25: 31–46.

FOUR RESCUING THE ORPHANS

1 For a detailed account of the Innocenti's genesis, see Howard Saalman, *Filippo Brunelleschi: The Buildings* (London 1993) pp. 36–9.
2 Quoted by Eugenio Battisti, *Brunelleschi: The Complete Work* (London 1981) p. 47.
3 Frederick Hartt, *History of Italian Renaissance Art* (London 1970; new rev. ed. 1987) p. 146.
4 According to John Pope-Hennessy, *The Study and Criticism of Italian Sculpture* (New York 1980) p. 177.
5 Ten of the medallions are by Andrea della Robbia but the other four (two at each end) are imitations.
6 Battisti, *Brunelleschi* p. 46.
7 E.M. Forster, *A Room with a View* (London 1908; pb ed. 1958) p. 23.
8 Nikolaus Pevsner, *An Outline of European Architecture* (Harmondsworth 1943; 5th ed. 1958) p. 130.
9 A similar interpretation is offered in Janice Elliott's novel *The Italian Lesson* (London 1985; pb 1987) pp. 117–18.
10 Chellini quoted by Horst W. Janson, 'Giovanni Chellini's *Libro* and Donatello', *Studien zur Toskanischen Kunst: Festschrift L.H. Heydenreich* (Munich 1964) p. 131.
11 Fra Bernardo di Francesco, 1488 contract, quoted by Michael Baxandall, *Painting and Experience in Fifteenth Century Italy* (Oxford 1978) p. 6.
12 B. Hatfield Strens, 'L'Arrivo del trittico Portinari a Firenze', *Commentari* 19 (1968) pp. 315–19.
13 See Raymond de Roover, *The Rise and Decline of the Medici Bank, 1397–1494* (Cambridge 1963) p. 357.
14 Margaret L. Koster, 'New Documentation for the Portinari Altar-piece', *Burlington Magazine* (March 2003) pp. 164–79.
15 Max J. Friedländer, *Early Netherlandish Painting from Van Eyck to Bruegel* (London 1956) p. 40.
16 Vincent van Gogh to Theo van Gogh, 25 July 1888, quoted by Douglas W. Druick and Peter Kort Zegers, *Van Gogh and Gauguin: The Studio of the South* (London 2001) p. 121.
17 Koster, 'New Documentation', p. 171.
18 Erwin Panofsky, *Early Netherlandish Painting* (Princeton 1953) p. 333.
19 See Andrée Hayum, *The Isenheim Altarpiece: God's Medicine and the Painter's Vision* (Princeton 1989).
20 Robert Walker, 'The Demon of the Portinari Altarpiece', *Art Bulletin* 42 (1960) pp. 218–19.
21 See Jacobus de Voragine, *The Golden Legend*, trans. W. Granger Ryan (Princeton 1993) pp. 37–43. See also Ruth Mellinkoff, *The Devil at Isenheim: Reflections of Popular Belief in Grünewald's Altarpiece* (Berkeley, Cal., 1988).
22 Saint Augustine quoted in Voragine and Granger Ryan, *op. cit.*
23 Koster, 'New Documentation', pp. 177–8, argued that the exterior wings were designed by van der Goes but painted by his workshop.

FIVE THE BLOOD OF THE MARTYRS

1 The restoration of St John's was carried out in 1911–13, when the tympanum was completed by the sculptor Remi Rooms.
2 Only in the late 1970s did all the hospital services leave the old site.
3 There are now plans to re-instal the Memling paintings in the hospital church.
4 Hilde Lobelle-Caluwe, the author of *Memlingmuseum Bruges* (Brussels 1987) and the Director of O.C.M.W. Musen-Bruges, wrote to the author (15 July 1987): 'this is a complete mystery for us, no mentions in the records, no contract, no payments, for the four paintings made for St. John's'.
5 The story was largely discredited by W.H.J. Weale's pioneering researches in the hospital archives.
6 The other two works by Memling in the hospital are *Portrait of a Woman or the Sibylla Sambetha* and *Diptych with the Virgin and Martin van Nieuwenhove*. They both came in 1815 from Saint Julian's Hospice in Bruges.
7 Saint Wilgeforte wanted to remain a virgin and deterred her suitor by growing a beard. She was crucified by her enraged father.
8 Lobelle-Caluwe, *Memlingmuseum* p. 61.
9 The hospital's original patron saint was Saint John the Evangelist but he was later joined in special esteem by Saint John the Baptist.
10 Lobelle-Caluwe, *Memlingmuseum* p. 51.
11 Weale, *Hans Memlinc* [*sic*] p. 37.
12 See M. Guillaume-Linephty, *La Chasse de Sainte Ursule* (Paris 1958) p. 11.
13 Pieter Pourbus quoted by K.B. McFarlane, *Hans Memling* (Oxford 1971) p. 34 n. 26.
14 Friedländer, *Early Netherlandish Painting* p. 46.

SIX THE BURNING SICKNESS

1 Horst Ziermann, *Matthias Grünewald* (Munich, London and New York 2001) p. 78.
2 For a pioneering account of the curative ambitions behind the altarpiece, see E. Ruhmer, *Grünewald: The Paintings* (London 1958) pp. 118–20.
3 J.K. Huysmans, *Trois primitifs* trans. Robert Baldick, in Ruhmer, *Grünewald* p. 19.
4 *Ibid.*, p. 20.
5 Dom Félibien quoted by Huysmans, *ibid.*, p. 21.
6 Ziermann, *Grünewald* p. 149.
7 For a detailed analysis of the three different 'views' offered by the polyptych as it opened out, see *ibid.*, pp. 82–152.
8 Dr Richet quoted by Huysmans, *Trois primitifs* p. 20.
9 *Ibid.*
10 For Andrée Hayum's book see ch. 4 n. 19. She had previously published an important essay, 'The Meaning and Function of the Isenheim Altarpiece: The Hospital Context Revisited', *Art Bulletin* (1977) pp. 501–17.
11 Albert Chatelet argued his case at the 'Table Ronde' on Grünewald in 1974 and Christian Heck's analysis of the ground-plans appeared in 'Les bâtiments de l'ancienne préceptorie des Antonins d'Issenheim', *Le Retable d'Issenheim et la sculpture au nord des Alpes à la fin du moyen age: Actes du colloque de Colmar 2–3 novembre 1987, réunis et présentés par Christian Heck*

(Colmar 1989) pp. 128–39.
12 Ziermann, *Grünewald* pp. 104–5.
13 Jean Gebser, *Ursprung und Gegenwart* (Stuttgart 1949) p. 235.
14 Huysmans, *Trois primitifs* pp. 24–5.
15 Georg Sheja, *The Isenheim Altarpiece* (New York 1969) p. 66.
16 Wilhelm Waetzoldt, *Dürer and his Times* (London 1955) pp. 24, 25.
17 Dürer quoted by Alistair Smith, *Albrecht Altdorfer: Christ taking Leave of his Mother* (London 1983) p. 12.
18 Barnett Newman, unedited transcript of a taped interview with Alan Solomon and Lane Slate, 20 May 1966, p. 7, quoted by Mark Godfrey, 'Barnett Newman's "Stations of the Cross" and the Memory of the Holocaust', in *Reconsidering Barnett Newman*, ed. Melissa Ho (New Haven and London 2005) p. 52.

SEVEN PORTRAYING THE PATIENTS

1 See A. Ferrajoli, 'Un testamento dello scultore Pietro Torrigiani e ricerche sopra alcune sue opere', *Bollettino d'arte* IX (1915) pp. 181–92. See also M. Cammerer (ed.), 'New Documents for Pietro Torrigiano and Other Early Cinquecento Florentine Sculptors Active in Italy and England', *Kunst des Cinquecento in der Toskana* (Munich 1992) pp. 108–38.
2 George Orwell, 'How the Poor Die', *Collected Essays* (London 1961) pp. 349–50.
3 Leonardo da Vinci quoted by Martin Kemp, *Leonardo da Vinci: The Marvellous Works of Nature and Man* (London, pb 1989) p. 257.
4 Leonardo quoted by Charles Nicholl, *Leonardo da Vinci: The Flights of the Mind* (London 2004) p. 241.
5 *Ibid.*, p. 419.
6 *Ibid.*
7 Kemp, *Leonardo: Marvellous Works* pp. 257–8.
8 Nicholl, *Leonardo* p. 422.
9 *Ibid.*
10 Kenneth Clark, *Leonardo da Vinci* (Harmondsworth, rev. ed. 1958) p. 121.
11 Leonardo quoted in *ibid.*
12 Nicholl, *Leonardo* p. 444.
13 Paolo Giovio quoted in *ibid.*, pp. 443–4.
14 Vasari quoted in *ibid.*, p. 443.
15 Leonardo quoted in *ibid.*, p. 445.
16 *Ibid.*, p. 443.
17 *Ibid.*, p. 479.
18 *Ibid.*, p. 241.
19 *Ibid.*, p. 481.
20 *Ibid.*, p. 483.
21 Vasari quoted in *ibid.*
22 Antonio de Beatis quoted in *ibid.*, pp. 490–91.
23 Pontormo's age, according to Luciano Berti, entry on *Hospital Scene*, *Frescoes from Florence*, exh. cat. Hayward Gallery (London 1969) p. 198.
24 S.J. Freedberg quoted in *ibid.*
25 G. Gaeta Bertela, *Luca, Andrea, Giovanni Della Robbia* (London n.d.) p. 22.
26 After leaving Frankfurt, Elsheimer stayed in Venice from 1598 to 1600, when he moved to Rome.
27 See Ken Arnold, Lindsay Granshaw and Denna Jones, *Saving Bodies Saving Souls: Hospitals in History*, exh. cat., Wellcome Trust History of Medicine Gallery (London 1997) p. 23.
28 Elizabeth of Hungary quoted by Anne L. Austin, *History of Nursing Source Book* (New York 1957) p. 90.
29 Keith Andrews, 'Once More Elsheimer', *Burlington Magazine* (March 1979) p. 172.
30 Voragine, *Golden Legend* p. 681.
31 For a detailed account of the Crociferi Hospital's history, see Silvia Lunardon, *Hospitale S. Mariae Cruciferorum* (Venice 1984).
32 The Pieter de Coster painting shows *Venice comforted by Faith at the Virgin's Feet*.
33 Lunardon, *Hospitale S. Mariae* p. 185.
34 S.J. Freedberg, *Painting in Italy 1500 to 1600* (Harmondsworth 1971; new ed. 1983) p. 561.

EIGHT VISIONS OF REDEMPTION

1 See William B. Jordan, catalogue entry 43 in *El Greco of Toledo* (Boston 1982) p. 249.
2 Illescas administrators quoted by Alfonso E. Pérez Sánchez, 'On the Reconstruction of El Greco's Dispersed Altarpieces', *ibid.*, p. 168.
3 *Ibid.*
4 Enriqueta Harris, 'A Decorative Scheme by El Greco', *Burlington Magazine* LXXII (1938) pp. 154–64.
5 Ellis Waterhouse, *El Greco* (London 1965) p. 5.
6 El Greco quoted by Jonathan Brown, 'El Greco and Toledo', *El Greco of Toledo* p. 127.
7 *Ibid.*, p. 107.
8 For a detailed account of the Illescas scheme, see Susan G. Barnes, 'El Greco and the Decoration of the Church of Charity, Illescas', in Jonathan Brown (ed.), *Figures of Thought: El Greco as Interpreter of History, Tradition, and Ideas* (Washington, D.C., 1982).
9 Pedro Salazar de Mendoza quoted by Richard L. Kagan, 'The Toledo of El Greco', *El Greco of Toledo*, p. 65.
10 El Greco quoted by Jordan, catalogue entry 55, *ibid.*, p. 256.
11 See Richard G. Mann, *El Greco and his Patrons: Three Major Projects* (Cambridge 1986).
12 Hospital inventory quoted by Pérez Sánchez, 'On the Reconstruction' p. 174.
13 *Ibid.*
14 See Keith Christiansen, catalogue entry 60 in David Davies (ed.), *El Greco* (London 2003) p. 210.
15 The young Picasso encountered *The Opening of the Fifth Seal* when it was owned by the Paris-based Spanish painter Ignacio Zuloaga. It is widely believed to have influenced *Les Demoiselles d'Avignon* (1907). Jackson Pollock sketched *The Opening of the Fifth Seal*: see Katharine Baetjer, Lisa Mintz Messinger and Nan Rosenthal, *The Jackson Pollock Sketchbooks in The Metropolitan Museum of Art* (New York 1997).
16 Revelation 6, 9–11.
17 See Mann, *El Greco* pp. 112, 136.

NINE THE ANATOMIST'S KNIFE AND REGENTS' CHARITY

1 Simon Schama, *The Embarrassment of Riches: An Interpretation of Dutch Culture in the Golden Age* (London 1987) p. 576.
2 Jakob Rosenberg, *Rembrandt: Life and Work* (Harvard 1948; London 1968) p. 132.
3 See John Rowlands, *Holbein: The Paintings of Hans Holbein The Younger. Complete Edition* (Oxford 1985) p. 148.
4 Dr Tulp quoted by Gary Schwartz, *Rembrandt: His Life, his Paintings* (Harmondsworth 1985) p. 143.
5 Joost van den Vondel, 'On the dissection of the human body', translated into Dutch by V.F. Plemp, quoted by Schwartz, *Rembrandt* p. 144.
6 In *The National Gallery. January 1969–December 1970* (London 1971) p. 34, the Nonnius portrait is presumed to have been painted either 'in the second half of the 1620s . . . or soon after his [Rubens's] return to Antwerp in 1630'.
7 According to the records of the Anatomy Theatre in Amsterdam, 'on January 28th 1656, there was punished with the rope Joris Fonteijn of Diest, who by the worshipful lords of the law court was granted to us as an anatomical specimen. On the 29th Dr. Joan Deyman made his first demonstration on him in the Anatomy Theatre, three lessons altogether.' Complete entry quoted by Christopher Brown, *Rembrandt: The Master and his Workshop* (London 1991) p. 264.
8 For other precedents, see *ibid.*, pp. 265–6.
9 According to Dr William Schupbach of the Wellcome Institute for the History of Medicine, London, Deyman's gesture with the scalpel is 'a punning reference to the scythe as a *vanitas*-motif'; quoted in *ibid.*, p. 266.
10 See William S. Heckscher, *Rembrandt's Anatomy Lesson of Dr. Nicolaas Tulp* (New York 1958).
11 According to Zacarias Conrad von Uffenbach, *Merkwürdige Reisen durch Niedersachsen: Holland und Engelland*, 1753.
12 See *Masters of Seventeenth-Century Dutch Genre Painting* exh. cat. (Philadelphia, Berlin and London 1984) p. 313.
13 Jean Leymarie, *Dutch Painting*, trans. Stuart Gilbert (London 1977) p. 98.
14 As Seymour Slive points out in *Frans Hals* (London 1989) p. 284, this map 'is the only one known in his oeuvre'.
15 Document quoted by N.S. Trivas, *The Paintings of Frans Hals* (London 1941) p. 9.
16 R.H. Wilenski, *Dutch Painting* (London 1928; rev. ed. 1945) p. 77.

17 See H. P. Baard, *Frans Halsmuseum: Municipal Art Gallery at Haarlem* (Haarlem 1960) p. 3.
18 Schama, *Embarrassment* pp. 576–7.
19 John Berger, *About Looking* (London 1980) pp. 169–70.

TEN FIGHTING THE PLAGUE

1 See Jesús Maria Granero, SJ, *D. Miguel de Mañara: un caballero sevillano del siglo XVII* (Seville 1963).
2 Antonio Dominguez Ortiz, 'Murillo's Seville', in Jane Martineau (ed.), *Bartolomé Esteban Murillo* (London 1982) pp. 30–31.
3 F. Morales Padrón, *Memorias de Seville (noticias sobre el siglo XVII)* (Cordoba 1981) p. 142.
4 See Nicholas Turner and Carol Plazzotta, *Drawings by Guercino from British Collections* (London 1991) pp. 146–51.
5 Numbers 20: 3, 6–8, 11.
6 See George Parsons Lathrop's shocked reaction in his *Spanish Vistas* (1883), quoted by Suzanne L. Stratton-Pruitt, 'Murillo in America', *Bartolomé Esteban Murillo (1617–1682): Paintings from American Collections* (New York 2002) p. 102.
7 The remaining pair of paintings in Murillo's cycle are *Abraham visited by the Three Angels* and the *Liberation of Saint Peter*.
8 John 5: 2–8.
9 *Ibid.*
10 *Ibid.*
11 *Ibid.*
12 Some historians argue that the other *Prodigal Son* images were executed well before the Caridad painting. Others believe that they were produced as late as 1670.
13 For Murillo's extensive use of children in his work, see Xanthe Brooke and Peter Cherry, *Murillo: Scenes of Childhood* (London 2001).
14 Luke 15: 22.
15 Quoted by Diego Angulo Iñiguez, 'Murillo: His Life and Work', in Martineau, *Murillo* p. 24.
16 *Ibid.*
17 F. A. Wright, (ed.), *Select Letters of St. Jerome* (London 1933) p. 323.
18 See Iñiguez, 'Murillo', in Martineau, *Murillo* p. 24.
19 See Stratton-Pruitt, 'Murillo in America', pp. 100–01.
20 For full context, see Sybille Ebert-Schifferer, *Still Life: A History* (New York 1999).
21 Georges Bataille, *Story of the Eye*, trans. Joachim Neugroschal (1928; Harmondsworth 1987) p. 57.

ELEVEN FRENZY, BEDLAM AND 'THE CRIPPLES'

1 Thompson and Goldin, *Hospital* p. 79.
2 M. Groseley quoted by Patricia Allderidge, *Cibber's Figures from the Gates of Bedlam* (London 1977) n.p.
3 Christopher Smart quoted in *ibid.*
4 From the inscription on the engraving of the new Hospital by Robert White, 1676–7.
5 Thompson and Goldin, *Hospital* p. 69.
6 Quoted by Edward G. O'Donaghue, *The Story of Bethlehem Hospital* (London 1914) p. 238.
7 Quoted in *ibid.*, pp. 282–3.
8 William Wordsworth, *The Prelude* Book VII, 127–33.
9 Sydney Smirke quoted by Allderidge, *Cibber's Figures* n.p.
10 Bethlem museum's archivist quoted in *ibid.*
11 Crispin Fisher, 'St Thomas Perambulations Part I', *St Thomas's Hospital Gazette* (Winter 1985) p. 102.
12 Ward notice quoted by Benjamin Golding, *An Historical Account of St Thomas's Hospital, Southwark* (London 1819) p. 138.
13 Hospitals' joint order of 1569 quoted by Thomas Rogers Forbes, *Chronicle from Aldgate: Life and Death in Shakespeare's London* (New Haven 1971) p. 177.
14 Fisher, 'St Thomas Perambulations', p. 103.
15 F. G. Parsons, 'The Statues in St Thomas's Hospital and their Associations', *St Thomas's Hospital Gazette* XXXIV (1933) p. 317.

TWELVE SHELTER FOR SOLDIERS

1 Anthony Blunt, *Art and Architecture in France 1500–1700* 5th ed, rev. Richard Beresford (New Haven and London 1999) p. 231.
2 Quoted by Jean-Marcel Humbert and Lionel Dumarche, *The Tomb of Napoleon and The Hôtel des Invalides* (Paris 1988) p. 26.
3 *Ibid.*, p. 28.
4 Pilon's original organ-case was severely damaged by an explosion at the end of the eighteenth century and later restored.
5 A glass panel now effectively seals off the two churches from each other.
6 See Antoine Schnapper, *Jean Jouvenet 1644–1717 et la peinture d'histoire à Paris* (Paris 1974).
7 Quoted by Louis Hautecoeur, 'Avant-propos', in *Les Invalides: trois siècles d'histoire* ed. René Baillargeat (Paris 1974) p. 21.
8 Quoted by Edward McParland, 'Royal Hospital, Kilmainham, Co. Dublin – I', *Country Life*, 9 May 1985.
9 James Malton, *A picturesque & descriptive view of the city of Dublin* (London 1799) quoted in *ibid.*
10 Thomas Wilson, *An account of the foundation of the Royal Hospital of King Charles the Second* (Dublin 1713).
11 From a reference in the minute books of the governors of the Royal Hospital, 11 December 1699, National Archive, Dublin.
12 McParland, 'Royal Hospital'.
13 For Tabary's identity, see Edward McParland, *Public Architecture in Ireland 1680–1760* (New Haven and London 2001) p. 68.
14 Quoted by Edward McParland, 'Royal Hospital, Kilmainham, Co. Dublin – II', *Country Life*, 16 May 1985.
15 See Christine Stevenson, *Medicine and Magnificence: British Hospital and Asylum Architecture 1660–1815* (New Haven and London 2000) p. 32.
16 Jeffrey Daniels, *Burlington Magazine* (July 1974) pp. 421–2.
17 Ellis Waterhouse, *Painting in Britain 1530 to 1790* (Harmondsworth 1953) p. 92.
18 See Edward Croft-Murray, *Decorative Painting in England 1537–1837. Vol. 2: The 18th and Early 19th Centuries* (London 1970) p. 16.
19 Jeffrey Daniels, *Sebastiano Ricci* (Hove 1976) p. 55.
20 Matthew 28: 2–4.
21 See C. G. T. Dean, *The Royal Hospital Chelsea* (London 1950) pp. 138, 222.
22 John Evelyn underlined the religous emphasis of the Hospital when he wrote that the men at Chelsea were subject to 'Laws & Orders . . . in every respect as strickt as in any religious Convent'; 27 January 1682 *Diary*, ed. E. S. de Beer (Oxford 1955) IV pp. 269–70.

THIRTEEN SAVING THE SEAMEN

1 Summerson, *Architecture of the Eighteenth Century* p. 127.
2 Marcus Faulkner, *An Historical and Descriptive Account of the Royal Hospital . . . at Chelsea* (London 1805) p. 46.
3 P. Newell, *Greenwich Hospital: A Royal Foundation 1692–1983* (Greenwich 1984) p. 8.
4 In *Hawksmoor* (London 1977) p. 24, Kerry Downes observed of Hawksmoor's Greenwich designs: 'In particular there is a sheet of careful studies (plan, elevation and section) for the east end of the Hall, datable 1697; the vocabulary of detail is Wren's, and in a drawing of this kind Hawksmoor must have been working very closely with Wren.'
5 Nicholas Hawksmoor quoted by Westby Percival-Prescott, 'Thornhill at Greenwich', *Ingrid and Other Studies* (London 1978) p. 47.
6 Greenwich Hospital governors quoted by Lindsay Stainton and Christopher White, *Drawing in England from Hilliard to Hogarth* (London 1987) p. 233.
7 Greenwich Hospital governors quoted by Jacob Simon, *English Baroque Sketches* exh. cat. (Twickenham, Surrey, 1974) n.p. (under 'Thornhill').
8 Paul Nash, *Outline: An Autobiography and Other Writings* (London 1949) p. 42.
9 Greenwich Hospital Council quoted by Percival-Prescott, 'Thornhill', p. 56.
10 Kenneth Clark, *Civilisation: A Personal View* (London 1969) p. 215.
11 Thornhill quoted by Stainton and White, *Drawing in England* p. 41.
12 Charles Mitchell, 'Benjamin West's "Death of Wolfe" and the Popular History Piece', *Journal*

of the Warburg Institute VII (1944) pp. 25–6.

13 Thornhill quoted by Stainton and White, *Drawing in England* p. 234.

14 Hogarth's opinion was supported by the writer of an admiring French guide sold at the Hospital: *Description de l'Hôpital Royal pour les marins, Greenwich* (London 1851).

15 See John Bold, *Greenwich: An Architectural History of the Royal Hospital for Seamen and the Queen's House* (New Haven and London 2000) p. 119.

16 *Meekness* and *Hope* flank the entrance to the chapel, while *Charity* and *Faith* flank the large outside door. *Meekness* is dated 1790.

17 The Acts of the Apostles 28: 2.

18 *Ibid.*, 3–4.

19 Death at sea was the subject of West's grand Nelson pediment at Greenwich, 1812.

FOURTEEN THE GOOD SAMARITAN AND CORAM'S FOUNDLINGS

1 Jenny Uglow, *Hogarth: A Life and a World* (London 1997) p. 4.

2 Ronald Paulson, *The Art of Hogarth* (London 1975) p. 13.

3 Little, *Life and Work of Gibbs* p. 114.

4 Lynda Moss, 'Paintings, Patients and Propaganda', *Art and Artists* (April 1986) p. 16.

5 Bart's General Plan, reproduced as fig. 153 in Thompson and Goldin, *Hospital* p. 148.

6 St Bartholomew's Hospital Archives, Ha 1 /11, p. 129.

7 A suggestion made by Michael Snodin, *Rococo: Art and Design in Hogarth's England* (London 1984) p. 69.

8 See Lawrence Gowing, *Hogarth* (London 1971) p. 40.

9 See Ronald Paulson, *Hogarth: His Life. Art, and Times* (New Haven and London 1971) pp. 378–86.

10 Illich, *Limits to Medicine* p. 163.

11 Peter Quennell, *Hogarth's Progress* (London 1955) p. 143.

12 The Raphael prototype is the crippled figure in the *Healing of the Lame Man*.

13 Hogarth quoted by Quennell, p. 143.

14 St Bartholomew's Hospital Archives, Ha 1/11, p. 173.

15 Horace Walpole quoted in *The Story of the Thomas Coram Foundation for Children* (London n.d.) p. 5.

16 Thomas Coram quoted in Quennell, *Hogarth's Progress* p. 164.

17 Lampoon quoted in H.F.B. Compston, *Thomas Coram* (London 1918).

18 Dr Brocklesby quoted in *Story of the Coram Foundation* p. 6.

19 *Ibid.*, p. 7.

20 Hogarth quoted by Gowing, *Hogarth* p. 55.

21 See John Brownlow, *The History and Design of the Foundling Hospital* (London 1858).

22 Ellis Waterhouse quoted by Elizabeth Einberg, *Manners and Morals: Hogarth and British Painting 1700–1760* (London 1987) p. 175.

23 Marc-Antoine Laugier, *Essai sur l'architecture* (Paris 1755) pp. 169–70.

24 See D. Gibbs, *Emblems, Tokens and Tickets of the London Hospital and The London Hospital Medical College* (London 1985).

25 Matthew 25: 4.

26 André Rouquet, *The Present State of the Arts in England* (London 1755) p. 24.

27 John Brownlow, *Memoranda: or. Chronicles of the Foundling Hospital . . . &tc* (London 1847) p. 15.

28 See George Vertue, 'Vertue Note Books III', *Walpole Society* XXII (1933–4) p. 134.

29 Coram quoted in Brownlow, *History and Design* pp. 20–21.

30 Exodus 2: 6, 7.

31 Brian Allen, *Francis Hayman* (New Haven and London 1987) p. 120.

32 Vertue, 'Vertue Note Books III', p. 135.

33 *Ibid.*

34 John Hayes, *Thomas Gainsborough* (London 1980) p. 19.

35 Gainsborough is supposed, according to Vertue in 1751, to have painted two more roundels for the Court Room but neither of them has been found.

36 Rysbrack's election took place in March 1745.

37 Vertue quoted by M.I. Webb, *Michael Rysbrack Sculptor* (London 1954) p. 135.

38 Michael Rysbrack, 7 April 1761, quoted *ibid.*, p. 205.

39 Vertue quoted *ibid.*, p. 132.

40 'Vertue Note Books III', p. 135.

41 See Terry Friedman, *James Gibbs* (New Haven and London 1984) p. 210.

42 See Alastair Smart, *Allan Ramsay 1713–1784* (Edinburgh 1992) p. 4.

43 John Pringle, *Observations on the Nature and Cure of Hospital and Jayl-Fevers* (London 1750) p. 8.

44 Richard Mead, *A Discourse on the Plague* (London 1721) pp. 186–7.

45 Jonathan Richardson quoted by Smart, *Allan Ramsay* p. 4.

46 George II quoted in *Story of the Coram Foundation*, p. 10.

FIFTEEN BENEFACTORS, DOCTORS AND QUACKS

1 F.G. Parsons, 'The Statues in St Thomas's Hospital and their Associations', *St Thomas's Hospital Gazette* XXXIV (1933) p. 325.

2 Minute dated 20 June 1701, quoted by Crispin Fisher, 'St Thomas Perambulations Part I', *St Thomas's Hospital Gazette* (Winter 1985) pp. 102–3.

3 The statue, presented to Charles II by his retainer Tobias Rustat, was bronzed in 1787.

4 The portrait of Edward VI, originally full-length, is now three-quarter-length and no longer attributed to Holbein. It is preserved in the Royal Collection.

5 George Vertue, *Notebooks 1713–46* (London 1934) XXII p. 94. Scheemakers's statue is stone, coloured in imitation of bronze.

6 Margaret Whinney, *Sculpture in Britain 1530–1830* (London 1988 ed.) p. 465, describes *Sickness* as a 'study' for the Guy monument but *Sickness* is called a 'copy' in Helen Valentine, *From Reynolds to Lawrence: The First Sixty Years of the Royal Academy of Arts and its Collections* (London 1991) p. 22.

7 Celina Fox, *Londoners* (London 1987) p. 237.

8 *Ibid.*, p. 239.

9 Gowing, *Hogarth* p. 67.

10 Hogarth quoted *ibid.*, p. 69.

11 See M. Dorothy George, *Hogarth to Cruickshank: Social Change in Graphic Satire* (London 1967) p. 36.

12 Sir John Hawkins, *Life of Johnson* (London 1787) p. 238n.

13 See Susan Jenkins, *Compton Verney Handbook* (Compton Verney House Trust 2004) p. 140.

14 John Collier, *Human Passions Delineated* (London 1773).

15 See John Hayes, *Rowlandson Watercolours and Drawings* (London 1972) pp. 28–9.

16 Whinney, *Sculpture in Britain* p. 105.

17 Philippa Bishop, Susan Sloman and Amina Wright, *Pickpocketing the Rich: Portrait Painting in Bath 1720–1800* (Bath 2002) p. 39.

18 Hospital governors quoted in Mary Holbrook, 'Painters in Bath in the Eighteenth Century', *Apollo* (November 1973) p. 50.

19 *Sporting Magazine* (July 1808).

20 John Burton, *Essay towards a Complete New System of Midwifery*, etchings by George Stubbs (London 1751) preface.

21 Nicholas Penny (ed.) *Reynolds* (London 1986) p. 316.

22 *Ibid.*, p. 317.

23 See Christopher Green (ed.) *Art Made Modern: Roger Fry's Vision of Art* (London 1999) p. 202.

24 Roger Fry, 'The Old Masters at Burlington House', *Athenaeum* (20 January 1906).

25 Joseph Moser, 'Vestiges, Collected and Recollected, by Joseph Moser, Esq', *European Magazine* XIII (July–December 1803).

26 Reynolds's portrait is based largely on a picture by Mason Chamberlin.

27 The suggestion about Ramsay and Chardin is made by Smart, *Allan Ramsay 1713–1784* (Edinburgh 1992) p. 139.

28 Most recently by Wendy Moore in the title of her biography *The Knife Man: The Extraordinary Life and Times of John Hunter, Father of Modern Surgery* (London 2005).

29 After extensive redesign, London's Hunterian Museum reopened in February 2005.

30 Royal Academy announcement quoted by Ian McIntyre, *Joshua Reynolds: The Life and Times of the First President of the Royal Academy* (London, pb 2004) p. 472.

31 Thomas Gainsborough to an unknown recipient, c. April 1788, in John Hayes (ed.) *The Letters of Thomas Gainsborough* (New Haven and London 2001) p. 170.
32 Gainsborough to Robert Bowyer, 1 May 1788, *ibid.*, p. 172.
33 See David Mannings, *Sir Joshua Reynolds: A Complete Catalogue of his Paintings: Text* (New Haven and London 2000) p. 272.
34 Orwell, 'How The Poor Die', p. 350.
35 George, *Hogarth to Cruikshank* p. 95, records that 'out of a number of vaccination prints between 1801 and 1812 only one is Jennerian'.
36 See Draper Hill, *Fashionable Contrasts: Caricatures by James Gillray* (London 1966) p. 174.
37 Dr Adams, *Morbid Poisons* (London 1795) p. 134.

SIXTEEN ENFANTS-TROUVÉS, LYING-IN AND MUSIC-MAKING

1 See Homan Potterton, *Venetian Seventeenth Century Painting* (London 1979) p. 103.
2 These canvases depict Apostles and Fathers of the Church, which may explain why Gregorio Lazzarini's biographer Vincenzo da Canal in 1732 praised the 'Apostles' which Tiepolo had, he maintained, painted for the Ospedaletto. Scholars have recently proposed that Tiepolo himself may have been responsible for at least one of them.
3 Vincenzo da Canal quoted by Antonio Morassi, *G. B. Tiepolo: His Life and Work* (London 1955) p. 8.
4 Michael Levey, *Giambattista Tiepolo: His Life and Art* (New Haven and London 1986) p. 11.
5 Now in the Musée des Beaux-Arts, Tours.
6 *Letters from Georgian Ireland: The Correspondence of Mary Delany, 1731–68* ed. Angélique Day (Belfast 1991) p. 264.
7 Noreen Casey, 'Architecture and Decoration' in I. C. Ross (ed.) *Public Virtue, Public Love: The Early Years of the Dublin Lying-in Hospital* (Dublin 1986) p. 68.
8 McParland, *Public Architecture in Ireland* p. 83.
9 National Archive Dublin, Rotunda Hospital Dublin papers, DUB.22.
10 *A sermon intended to have been preached at the publick opening of the Chappel of the lying-in hospital . . . Dublin* (Dublin 1759) p. 21.
11 Bartholomew Mosse quoted by McParland, *Public Architecture* p. 87.
12 National Archive Dublin, Rotunda Hospital papers, DUB.22.
13 Hugh Honour, *The Companion Guide to Venice* (London 1965; 1977 ed.) p. 79.
14 Morassi, *Tiepolo* p. 30.
15 Pietro Gradenigo quoted in *ibid.*
16 The facade of the Pietà church was only finished in 1906, not entirely in accordance with Massari's plans.
17 Rousseau quoted by Milton Grundy, *Venice: An Anthology Guide*, preface John Julius Norwich (London 1971; 1985 ed.) p. 119.
18 For a detailed account of the Ospedaletto's musical activities, see Virginio Fagotto (ed.) *Arte e Musica all'Ospedaletto* (Venice 1978), esp. his essay, pp. 17–22.

SEVENTEEN PESTILENCE AND PHYSIOGNOMY OF MADNESS

1 Antoine Schnapper, *David* (New York 1982) p. 50.
2 Philip Conisbee, *Painting in Eighteenth-Century France* (Oxford 1981) p. 72.
3 See M. Pötzl-Malikova, *Franz Xaver Messerschmidt* (Vienna and Munich 1982) for a catalogue raisonné of the sculptor's work.
4 Friedrich Nicolai, 'Recollection of a Meeting with Messerschmidt in Pressburg in 1781', *Franz Xaver Messerschmidt: Character-Heads 1770–1783* (London n.d.) pp. 14–16.
5 *Ibid.*, p. 16.
6 Ernst Kris, 'Die Charakter-Köpfe des F.X. Messerschmidt' (1932), Eng. trans. in *Psychoanalytic Explorations in Art* (New York 1952).
7 Margaret and Rudolf Wittkower, *Born Under Saturn* (London 1963).
8 See Jill Lloyd's illuminating essay, 'Character-heads', in *Messerschmidt: Character-Heads* pp. 4–13.
9 The 3-vol. English version of Lavater's *Physiognomy* was published between 1789 and 1798.
10 Juliet Wilson-Bareau, *Goya: Truth and Fantasy. The Small Paintings* (New Haven and London 1994) p. 200.
11 Goya to Iriarte, 7 January 1794, British Library, London.
12 Sarah Symmons, *Goya* (London 1977) p. 71.
13 Anita Brookner, *Look At Me* (London 1983) p. 9.
14 See Xavier de Salas, *Goya* (London 1979) p. 156.
15 Trans. in Symmons, *Goya* p. 89.
16 Lorenz Eitner, *Géricault: His Life and Work* (London 1982) p. 245.
17 See Patrick Noon, *Constable to Delacroix: British Art and the French Romantics* (London 2003) p. 162.
18 Etienne-Jean Georget, *De la physiologie du système nerveux* (Paris 1821) vol. I, p. 345.
19 See Denise Aimé-Azam, *Mazeppa: Géricault et son temps* (Paris 1956) p. 226.
20 Jean-Etienne-Dominique Esquirol, *Des maladies mentales considérées sous les rapports médicals, hygièniques et médico-legaux* (Paris 1838) vol. II p. 167.
21 Alexander Morison cited in R. Hunter and I. Macalpine, *Three Hundred Years of Psychiatry* (London 1963) p. 737.
22 Charles Clément, *Géricault: étude biographique et critique* (Paris 1879 3rd ed.) p. 130.
23 In *Géricault* (Bristol 1966) p. 8, Francis Haskell referred to Géricault's 'cool sympathy'.
24 Charles Cockerell quoted by Germain Bazin, *Théodore Géricault: étude critique et catalogue raisonné* 7 vols (Paris 1987–94) vol. I p. 65.
25 See Duncan Macmillan, 'Géricault et Charles Bell', *Géricault* (Paris 1996) pp. 449–66.

EIGHTEEN 'CLASSED AMONG THE DEAD'

1 *Quarterly Review*, CI (1857) pp. 361–2.
2 *Art Union* (October 1843) p. 267.
3 Sir Alexander Morison quoted in a National Galleries of Scotland bulletin (1980, no. 6) marking the rediscovery of Dadd's portrait of Morison at the Royal College of Physicians of Edinburgh.
4 Gow's encounter with Dadd reported in *Art Union* (May 1845) p. 137.
5 Patricia Allderidge, *The Late Richard Dadd 1817–1886* (London 1974) pp. 28–9.
6 J. E. Johnson to Sir Alexander Morison, 5 May 1856, archives of Bridewell Royal Hospital, quoted *ibid.*, p. 35.
7 William Charles Hood case-books, archives of Bethlem Royal Hospital, quoted *ibid.*, p. 30.
8 Hood's Dadd works are listed in Christie's sale catalogue, 28 March 1870.
9 The painting is now in the Andrew Lloyd Webber collection.
10 'Her Majesty's Pleasure, The Parricide's Story', *The World* (26 December 1877) p. 13.
11 G.A. Sala, 'A Visit to the Royal Hospital of Bethlehem', *Illustrated London News* (24 March 1860) p. 291.
12 William Michael Rossetti, *Some Reminiscences of William Michael Rossetti* (London 1906) I, pp. 269–70.
13 According to Allderidge, *Late Richard Dadd* p. 125, 'it is possible that the date . . . should really be 1857 or 1858–64'. The picture is inscribed on its verso: 'The Fairy Feller's Master-Stroke – Painted for G.H. Haydon. Esqre by Rd. Dadd quasi – 1855–64.' The word 'quasi' may indicate that Dadd could not remember when he began work on the painting.
14 All quotations from the poem, written in 1865 and entitled 'Elimination of a Picture & Its Subject – Called the Feller's Master Stroke', are taken from *ibid.*, pp. 127–9.
15 Richard Dadd quoted by Simon Wilson, *Tate Gallery: An Illustrated Companion* (London 1989) p. 77.
16 *The World* (26 December 1877).
17 *Ibid.*
18 Sir Hugh Orange to Ian Phillips, 12 February 1946, quoted by Allderidge, *Late Richard Dadd* p. 137.
19 The portrait is signed, inscribed and dated (indistinctly) 1874.
20 *The World* (26 December 1877).
21 Mary Ann Dadd to Catherine (Carter) Dadd, 31 January 1886, quoted by Allderidge, *Late Richard Dadd* p. 33.
22 *The World* (26 December 1877).

NINETEEN 'ACUTE MENTAL DERANGEMENT'

1 Dr Théophile Peyron quoted by Susan Alyson Stein (ed.) *Van Gogh: A Retrospective* (New York 1986) pp. 151–2.
2 For a detailed account of the two painters' relationship, see Druick and Zegers, *Van Gogh and Gauguin.*
3 Vincent to Wil [helmina, his sister], June–July 1888, quoted by Lawrence and Elisabeth Hanson, *Portrait of Vincent: A Van Gogh Biography* (London 1955) p. 248.
4 Dr Frédéric Salles quoted *ibid.*, p. 251.
5 *Ibid.*
6 Signac to Theo, March 1889, *ibid.*, p. 253.
7 According to the catalogue *French Paintings from the USSR: Watteau to Matisse* (London 1988) p. 82, the Rey portrait was painted in January 1889 and at once presented, 'as a souvenir', to the sitter.
8 Dr Félix Rey, interview with Max Braumann, *Kunst und Kunstler* 1928.
9 Vincent to Signac, March 1889, quoted by Hanson, *Portrait of Vincent* p. 256.
10 Vincent to Theo, quoted *ibid.*
11 Brochure for the asylum *Maison de Santé de Saint-Rémy-de-Provence* c. 1865, republished in Stein, *Van Gogh* pp. 147–50.
12 Peyron to Theo, 26 May 1889, *ibid.*, p. 152.
13 *Ibid.*
14 Vincent to Theo, n.d., beginning of April 1889, in Mark Roskill (ed.), *The Letters of Vincent Van Gogh* (London 1963) pp. 315–16.
15 The other painting is *Lilacs*, now in the Hermitage Museum, St Petersburg.
16 Vincent to Theo, quoted by Ronald Pickvance, *Van Gogh in Saint-Rémy and Auvers* (New York 1986) p. 81.
17 Félix Fénéon quoted *ibid.*
18 The lost painting, *A Corner of the Asylum Garden*, is reproduced *ibid.*, p. 82.
19 Vincent quoted *ibid.*, p. 85.
20 Pickvance, *ibid.*, p. 93, relates the idea to van Gogh's earlier plan for a triptych of Arles orchards.
21 Vincent to Theo, 22 May 1889, in Stein, *Van Gogh* p. 155.
22 Vincent quoted by Pickvance, *Van Gogh in Saint-Rémy* p. 89.
23 Vincent to Theo, 22 May 1889, in Stein, *Van Gogh* pp. 153–4.
24 Quoted by Pickvance, *Van Gogh in Saint-Rémy* p. 94.
25 *Ibid.*, p. 134.
26 *Ibid.*, p. 135.
27 *Ibid.*, p. 141.
28 *Ibid.*
29 *Ibid.*, c. 3 September 1889, p. 127.
30 Vincent to Theo, early September 1889, in Roskill, *Letters* p. 323.
31 Mme Trabuc's portrait was supposed lost for many years and as late as 1986 Pickvance, *Van Gogh in Saint-Rémy* p. 127, declared that its location remained unknown. However, Judy Sund, 'Famine to Feast: Portrait Making at St.-Rémy and Auvers', in *Van Gogh Face To Face: The Portraits* (Detroit 2000), pp. 192–4, reproduces it in colour, discusses it in detail and clears up the mystery by noting that it belongs to the State Hermitage Museum, St Petersburg.
32 Vincent to Theo, early September 1889, in Roskill, *Letters* p. 323.
33 Vincent to Theo, 12 October 1889, in Pickvance, *Van Gogh in Saint-Rémy* p. 143.
34 Vincent to Bernard, 22 November 1889, in *ibid.*, pp. 146–7.
35 Vincent to Wil, 9 May 1889, in Hanson, *Portrait of Vincent* pp. 259–60.
36 *Ibid.*, p. 267.
37 Vincent to the Ginouxes, January 1890, in *ibid.*, p. 272.
38 Vincent to Theo, April 1890, in *ibid.*, p. 274.
39 *Ibid.*, pp. 274–5.
40 Vincent to his mother and Wil, April 1890, in *ibid.*, p. 274.
41 Vincent to Wil, June 1890, in *ibid.*
42 *Ibid.*, p. 289.

TWENTY VICTORIAN VALUES

1 Florence Nightingale posed for Barrett while he was working on *The Mission of Mercy.*
2 Christopher Wood pointed out, in *Victorian Panorama: Paintings of Victorian Life* (London 1976) p. 230, that there are, perhaps surprisingly, few pictures of Florence Nightingale to be found anywhere.
3 For a full account of Seacole in the Crimea, see Jane Robinson, *Mary Seacole: The Charismatic Black Nurse who became a Heroine of the Crimea* (London 2005).
4 Florence Nightingale quoted by Helen Rappaport, 'The Invitation that never came: Mary Seacole after the Crimea', *History Today* (February 2005) p. 12.
5 Helen Rappaport quoted by Charlotte Higgins, 'Historic Portrait of Crimean War Nurse Unveiled', *Guardian* (11 January 2005).
6 The portrait went on view for the first time in public at the National Portrait Gallery, London, in January 2005.
7 *London Review* (1 September 1860).
8 One of the benefactors, Lt Col. Hyde, also commissioned his portrait from Emma Brownlow; see Benedict Nicolson, *The Treasures of the Foundling Hospital* (Oxford 1972).
9 These pictures were first exhibited in 1852 and 1853 respectively.
10 Pamela Gerrish Nunn, *Victorian Women Artists* (London 1987) p. 161.
11 In *Dickens: A Life* (Oxford 1979) p. 278, Norman and Jeanne MacKenzie point out that *Little Dorrit* exemplified his growing belief that 'childhood is the only phase of life on which the shades of the prison house have not closed'.
12 George Augustus Sala published nine essays on Hogarth in *The Cornhill Magazine* during the course of 1860. See Rosemary Treble's detailed entry on Ward's painting in *Great Victorian Pictures: Their Paths to Fame* exh. cat. (London 1978) pp. 84–5.
13 *Art Journal* (May 1863) p. 97.
14 Roubiliac's original bust is owned by the Royal College of Physicians.
15 Parsons, 'Statues in St Thomas's Hospital', p. 318.
16 *Ibid.*, p. 320.
17 F.T. Palgrave, *Essays on Art* (London and Cambridge 1866) pp. 119, 91.
18 See Mary S. Watts, *George Frederick Watts: The Annals of an Artist's Life* (London 1912) vol. 1 p. 217.
19 Barbara Bryant, *G. F. Watts Portraits: Fame and Beauty in Victorian Society* (London 2004) p. 144.
20 Tom Taylor in *The Times* (6 June 1865).
21 Marc Simpson, 'The 1870s', in *Thomas Eakins*, organised by Darrel Sewell (Philadelphia 2001) p. 32.
22 See Julie S. Berkowitz, *'Adorn the Halls': The History of the Art Collection at Thomas Jefferson University* (Philadelphia 1999) p. 175.
23 Kathleen A. Foster, *Thomas Eakins Rediscovered: Charles Bregler's Thomas Eakins Collection at the Pennsylvania Academy of the Fine Arts* (New Haven 1997) pp. 108–9, identifies a photograph as a probable source for this self-portrait.
24 See Michael Fried, *Realism, Writing, Disfiguration: On Thomas Eakins and Stephen Crane* (Chicago and London 1987).
25 The woman is unknown but some contemporary critics identified her as Eakins's mother.
26 Thomas Eakins to Earl Shinn, 13 April 1875, Richard T. Cadbury Papers, Friends Historical Library, Swarthmore College, Pa.
27 See Gordon Hendricks, 'Thomas Eakins's Gross Clinic', *Art Bulletin* LI (March 1969) pp. 57–64.
28 William Clark, *Evening Telegraph*, (16 June 1876).
29 See Berkowitz, 'Adorn the Halls' pp. 24–6.
30 Quoted by Stéphane Guégan in Serge Lemoine (ed.) *Paintings in the Musée d'Orsay* (London, new ed. 2004) p. 494.
31 *New York Daily Tribune* (22 March 1879).
32 John Wilmerding, *American Art* (Harmondsworth 1976) p. 139.
33 Charles Dickens quoted in *Royal Academy* 1874, p. 22.
34 *The Times* quoted by Wood, *Victorian Panorama* p. 53. *The Times* was commenting on Fildes's equally harrowing *The Widower*, exhibited at the Royal Academy in 1876.
35 *The Times* (2 May 1891).
36 Fildes's son quoted by Treble, *Great Victorian Pictures* p. 36.
37 *The Times*, (2 May 1891).
38 Luke Fildes quoted by Wilson, *Tate Gallery* p. 90.

39 Gabriel Tapié de Céleyran, 'Toulouse-Lautrec et ses rélations médicales', *La Chronique médicale* (1 December 1922) p. 355.
40 Julia Frey, *Toulouse-Lautrec: A Life* (London 1994) p. 290.
41 Henri de Toulouse-Lautrec quoted by Numa Baragnon, 'Toulouse-Lautrec chez Péan', *Chronique médicale* (15 February 1902) p. 98.
42 Lautrec quoted by Henri Perruchot, *Toulouse-Lautrec* (London 1960) p. 214.
43 Jules Renard, *Journal, 1887–1910* ed. L. Guichard and G. Sigaux (Paris, new ed. 1984) pp. 239–40.
44 Horace Brianchon (pseudonym of Dr Maurice de Fleury) *Nos Grands Médécins d'aujourd'hui* (Paris 1891) p. 316.
45 Frey, *Toulouse-Lautrec* p. 291.
46 See Richard Dorment, *Alfred Gilbert: Sculptor and Goldsmith* (London 1986) p. 138.
47 *Ibid.*, p. 171.
48 In 1980 St George's Hospital, together with Gilbert's *John Hunter*, moved to Tooting in south London.
49 Yeats made this assertion in 1906; see Elizabeth Cumming, *Phoebe Anna Traquair 1852–1936* (Edinburgh 2005) p. 22.
50 Findlay was also the benefactor of the Scottish National Portrait Gallery, whose first curator, John Miller Gray, was an enthusiastic patron of Traquair's illuminated work.
51 See Cumming, *Traquair* p. 20.
52 Matthew 16: 25.
53 Phoebe Traquair quoted in Cumming, *Traquair* p. 22.
54 Quoted *ibid.*, p. 20.
55 Gerard Baldwin Brown, 'Some Recent Efforts in Mural Decoration', *Scottish Art Review* (January 1889).
56 See Cumming, *Traquair* p. 59.
57 Phoebe Anna Traquair, letter to her nephew Willie, 1891, Scottish National Library, Edinburgh.
58 See Cumming, *Traquair* p. 59.
59 Dante Gabriel Rossetti, *The Blessed Damozel* illuminated by Traquair in 1897–8.
60 Cumming, *Traquair* p. 22.
61 Glasgow Kyrle Society report, 1883–4, Mitchell Library, Glasgow.
62 Thomas Martin Lindsay, *Kyrle Societies and their Work* (Glasgow 1883) p. 15.
63 *Ibid.*, p. 7.
64 The other two panels in Tinworth's reredos at Saint Thomas's depict *The Conversion of Saint Thomas the Apostle* and *Christ and Saint Mary Magdalene*.
65 John Greene, 'Introduction' to *Brightening the Long Days: Hospital Tile Pictures* (Gloucester 1987) p. xiii.
66 Nightingale, *Notes on Hospitals* p. 16.
67 H.C. Burdett, *Hospitals and Asylums of the World* (London 1893) vol. IV p. 26.
68 Greene, 'Introduction', pp. 76–8, provides details of tiling schemes in the Sassoon Hospital, Poona, India; the Southland Hospital, Kew, Invercargill, New Zealand; and the Wellington Hospital, Newtown, Wellington, New Zealand.
69 See *ibid.*, pp. 58–9.
70 *Bedford County Hospital: A Commemorative Booklet*, c. 1898.
71 Paddington Green Children's Hospital, *Annual Report* for 1895.
72 See Greene, 'Introduction', p. 33.
73 Paddington Green *Annual Report*, 1895.
74 *Paddington Green Children's Hospital Committee Report*, 1912.
75 Greene, 'Introduction', p. 50, pointed out that 'the choice of a Doulton tiling scheme [at St Nicholas] may have been connected with a Doulton tiling plan for Newcastle Royal Infirmary around the same time. The leading personalities of St. Nicholas Hospital were also prominent in the Royal Infirmary fund raising.'

TWENTY-ONE 'I WANTED TO SCREAM'

1 See Ludwig Ravensberg, 'Ludwig Ravensbergs Dagbok', 7 October 1909, Munch Museum, Oslo.
2 Edvard Munch quoted by Sue Prideaux, *Edvard Munch: Behind the Scream* (New Haven and London 2005) p. 221.
3 Cecilie Dahl to Edvard Munch, 23 August 1902, Munch Museum.
4 Sue Prideaux, 'Beneath the Skin', *RA Magazine* (Autumn 2005) p. 47.
5 Munch quoted by Prideaux, *Munch*, p. 222.
6 Munch quoted by Poul Erik Tøjner, *Munch in his own Words* (Munich 2001) p. 190.
7 *Ibid.*, p. 191.
8 Frederick Delius, 'Recollections of Strindberg', *The Sackbut* 1 8 (1920) pp. 353–4.
9 Tøjner, *Munch in his own Words*, p. 191.
10 See Prideaux, *Munch*, p. 223.
11 *Ibid.*
12 See Tøjner, *Munch*, p. 192.
13 See Prideaux, *Munch*, p. 224.
14 Munch to Christian Gierloff, 19 March 1908, Munch Museum.
15 Emil Nolde quoted in Ragna Stang, *Munch/Nolde: The Relationship of their Art* (London 1969) p. 6.
16 Edvard Munch, *Edvard Munchs Brev. Familien* (Oslo 1949) p. 174.
17 Munch to Ludwig Ravensberg, Munch Museum.
18 See Prideaux, *Munch*, p. 246.
19 *Ibid.*
20 Daniel Jacobsen, *Sindsyg – ikke Syndsyg?* (Copenhagen 1918).
21 Prideaux, *Munch*, p. 249.
22 *Ibid.*, p. 250.
23 *Ibid.*, pp. 249–50.
24 Daniel Jacobsen, '*Dementia paretica* in women', thesis (Copenhagen 1891).
25 Prideaux, *Munch*, p. 250.
26 *Ibid.*, p. 251.
27 Munch, 23 October 1933, quoted by Tøjner, *Munch*, p. 149.
28 Prideaux, *Munch*, p. 250.
29 Edvard Munch, 'Looking Back', note, n.d., Munch Museum.
30 Prideaux, *Munch*, p. 251.
31 *Ibid.*
32 *Ibid.*, pp. 259–60.
33 Munch to Jappe Nilssen, 27 October 1908, Munch Museum.
34 Munch to Nilssen, 27 December 1908, Munch Museum.
35 Munch, note in Munch Museum.
36 *Ibid.*
37 Edvard Munch, *The Mad Poet's Diary*, after 1908.
38 Prideaux, *Munch*, p. 258.
39 See Gerd Woll *et al.*, *Alpha and Omega* (Oslo 1981).
40 Edvard Munch, 'Tilbakeblikk', p. 3, Munch Museum.
41 Munch quoted by Lisa Appignanesi, 'Up Close and Personal', *RA Magazine* (Autumn 2005) p. 40.
42 Munch quoted in Rolf E. Stenerson, *Close-Up of a Genius* (Oslo 1946) p. 34.
43 Munch liked in particular his fellow-patient Anders Wilhelm Holm, the Danish writer.
44 Eigil H. Brünniche, 'Edvard Munch og to Danske Leger', *Statens Museum for Kunst Arbok* (Oslo 1992).

TWENTY-TWO FROM EXUBERANT OPTIMISM TO THE TRAUMA OF WAR

1 Ignasi de Solà-Morales, 'Modernista Architecture', *Homage to Barcelona: The City and its Art 1888–1936* exh. cat. (London 1985) p. 115.
2 Tim Benton, 'Spain: Modernismo in Catalonia', *Art Nouveau Architecture*, ed. Frank Russell (London 1979; new ed. 1983) p. 58.
3 Robert Hughes, *Barcelona* (London 1992) pp. 401–2.
4 Lluís Domènech's son quoted *ibid.*, p. 403.
5 The decorations were all destroyed at Schloss Immendorf in 1945.
6 Werner Hofmann, *Gustav Klimt* (London 1972) p. 23.
7 Karl Kraus quoted by Christian Nebehay, *Gustav Klimt* (Vienna 1969) p. 254.
8 Peter Vergo, *Art in Vienna 1898–1918* (Oxford 1975; 2nd ed. 1981) p. 109.
9 Otto Wagner quoted by Vergo, *op. cit.* p. 108.
10 Archbishop Piffl quoted by J.A. Lux, *Otto Wagner* (Munich 1914) p. 78.
11 By 1909 Brancusi had decided that he could no longer 'make anybody's portrait because I cannot lend it that special thing that would make it resemble the model: life'; quoted by Anna C. Chave, *Constantin Brancusi: Shifting the Bases of Art* (New Haven and London 1993) pp. 23–5.

12 Claude Roger-Marx, *Vuillard: His Life and Work* (New York 1946) pp. 79–80.
13 Wyndham Lewis, interview with 'M.M.B.', *Daily News and Leader* (7 April 1914).
14 *The Times* (5 February 1912).
15 *Ibid.* (4 June 1912).
16 Roger Fry to Vanessa Bell, 12 October 1911, in Denys Sutton (ed.) *Letters of Roger Fry* (London 1972) vol. 1 p. 352.
17 Judith Collins, *The Omega Workshops* (London 1983) p. 21.
18 See David Brown, 'Introduction', in *Frederick Cayley Robinson ARA* exh. cat. (London 1977).
19 Kirchner quoted by Donald E. Gordon, *Ernst Ludwig Kirchner* (Cambridge, Mass., 1968) p. 106.
20 The stairwell scheme was first mentioned by Kirchner when he wrote to Dr Carl Hagemann on 27 June 1916.
21 Roland Scotti, 'War, Art and Crisis: Ernst Ludwig Kirchner 1914–1918', in *Ernst Ludwig Kirchner: The Dresden and Berlin Years*, ed. Jill Lloyd and Magdalena M. Moeller (London 2003), p. 27, maintains that Kirchner 'induced a physical and mental condition in himself (through alcohol and drug abuse, as we now know, doubtless with an additional component of malingering, and very much in his own interests) that would necessarily lead to an early discharge from military service'.
22 Gordon, *Kirchner* p. 106.
23 The Nazi 'Degenerate Art' campaign was a key factor in driving Kirchner to take his own life.
24 Flora Murray to Lady Norman, 3 March 1920, London, Imperial War Museum, Central Archive, Papers of the Women's Work Subcommittee: Correspondence.
25 Lady Norman to Austin Spare, 22 May 1920, London, Imperial War Museum, Department of Art, Correspondence with First World War Artists.
26 Austin Spare to Lady Norman, 29 May 1920, *ibid.*
27 Jennian F. Geddes, 'Artistic Integrity and Feminist Spin: A Spat at the Endell Street Military Hospital', *Burlington Magazine* (September 2005) p. 618.
28 *Ibid.*
29 Stanley Spencer to James Wood, 27 July 1916; quoted by Richard Carline, *Stanley Spencer at War* (London 1978) p. 59.
30 Spencer to Desmond Chute, May 1916, Stanley Spencer Gallery Collection, Cookham.
31 For a full account of this painting, and Spencer's subsequent chapel at Burghclere, see Richard Cork, *A Bitter Truth: Avant-Garde Art and the Great War* (New Haven and London 1994) pp. 227–8 and 296–300.
32 Stanley Spencer, memoir written in 1918, Tate Archive, London.
33 Spencer quoted by Carline, *Spencer at War* p. 182.

TWENTY-THREE 'A MEGAPHONE FOR HEALTH'

1 For a full account of Bomberg's sojourn in Palestine, see Richard Cork, *David Bomberg* (New Haven and London 1987) ch. 6.
2 Alice Mayes, 'The Young Bomberg 1914–1925', memoir, November 1972, p. 59, Tate Archive, London.
3 *Ibid.*
4 Eric Gill's ledgers, quoted by Judith Collins, *Eric Gill: The Sculpture. A Catalogue Raisonné* (London 1998) p. 190.
5 Luke 18: 41.
6 Although the drawing is dated 1937, Gill had still not finished the sculpture when he wrote to Graham Carey on 15 September 1938: 'I have some carving to do on a Hospital at Coventry'; Walter Shewring (ed.) *Letters of Eric Gill* (London 1947) p. 408. He travelled to Coventry the following month.
7 According to the Herbert Art Gallery's 'Survey of Public Art in Coventry' (1980) p. 35, Gill 'had been commissioned to carve two panels, one for the front of the building and one for the rear. The second panel, of the Good Shepherd, or possibly of St Martin and the Beggar, was destroyed as a result of the air-raid on the hospital in 1941.'
8 *Ibid.*
9 Eric Gill to Graham Carey, 1 January 1939, in Shewring, *Letters* p. 413.
10 Berthold Lubetkin quoted by Peter Coe and Malcolm Reading, *Lubetkin and Tecton: Architecture and Social Commitment* (London and Bristol 1981) p. 143.
11 Nicholas Bullock, *Circle: Constructive Art in Britain 1934–40* ed. Jeremy Lewison, exh. cat. (Cambridge 1982) p. 85.
12 See Richard Cork, 'An Art of the Open Air: Moore's Major Public Sculpture', in Susan Compton, Richard Cork and Peter Fuller, *Henry Moore* exh. cat. (London 1988) p. 17.
13 Johns Hopkins quoted in *Hospital Plans: Five Essays* (New York 1875) p. xvii.
14 *Address at the Opening of the Hospital, May 7, 1889* (Baltimore, Md., 1889) p. 67.
15 Quoted by Thompson and Goldin, *Hospital* p. 187.
16 Walter Quirt, 'On Mural Painting', in *Art for the Millions: Essays from the 1930s by Artists and Administrators of the WPA Federal Art Project* ed. Francis V. O'Connor (Boston 1975 ed.) p. 78.
17 *Ibid.*, p. 81.
18 Lou Block, 'Murals for Use', in *ibid.*, p. 81.
19 Waylande Gregory, 'Planning a Public Fountain', in *ibid.*, p. 94.
20 *Ibid.*, pp. 94–5.
21 Francis V. O'Connor, 'Introduction', *ibid.*, p. 22.
22 Rosalind Bengelsdorf Browne, 'The American Abstract Artists and the WPA Federal Art Project', *The New Deal Art Projects: An Anthology of Memoirs*, ed. Francis V. O'Connor (Washington, D.C., 1972) p. 234.
23 Ilya Bolotowsky, 'On Neoplasticism and my own Work: A Memoir', *Leonardo* II 3 (1969) p. 225.
24 Bolotowsky's mural for the Williamsburg Housing Project, begun in 1936 and since destroyed, was one of the first abstract murals produced in the US.
25 Browne, 'American Abstract Artists', p. 234.
26 Although Bolotowsky's tempera design is simply called *Untitled*, it has been identified as a study for the unexecuted hospital mural; see R.L. Herbert, S.L. Apter and E.K. Kenney (eds), *The Société Anonyme and the Dreier Bequest at Yale University: A Catalogue Raisonné* (New Haven 1984) p. 78.

TWENTY-FOUR THE MEXICAN REVOLUTION

1 Antonio Rodríguez, *A History of Mexican Mural Painting* (London 1969) p. 311.
2 Some critics have accused Orozco of blatant inconsistency and even outright muddle, but Desmond Rochfort argued that 'the contradictions within Orozco's work are dialectical and calculated. They are not confused, and are neither dogmatic nor monolithic'; 'A Terrible Beauty: Orozco's Murals in Guadalajara 1936–1939', *¡Orozco! 1883–1949* (Oxford 1980) p. 74.
3 José Clemente Orozco, interview with Antonio Rodríguez, 1946, quoted by Rodríguez, *History of Mexican Mural Painting* p. 357.
4 In his poem 'The Second Coming', W.B. Yeats asked: 'And what rough beast, its hour come round at last, / Slouches towards Bethlehem to be born?'
5 See Rodríguez, *History of Mexican Mural Painting* p. 353.
6 The Hotel del Prado, at one stage severely damaged in a Mexico City earthquake, was designed by Santacelia.
7 The Pavilion of Laboratories frescoes are dedicated 'To the memory of Dr Francis Javier de Balmes and the Mexican children who, with smallpox vaccine in their arms, sailed from Acapulco for the Philippines on February 5, 1805, to provide material necessary to prevent the disease.'
8 Stanton L. Catlin, 'Mural Census', in *Diego Rivera: A Retrospective* (New York and London 1987) p. 275.
9 Frida Kahlo quoted by Laura Mulvey and Peter Wollen, *Frida Kahlo and Tina Modotti* exh. cat. (London 1982) p. 6.
10 *Ibid.*, p. 25.
11 Frida Kahlo to Dr Leo Eloesser, 11 February 1950, quoted by Hayden Herrera, *Frida: A Biography of Frida Kahlo* (London 1998 ed.) p. 385.
12 Matilde Kahlo to Eloesser, mid-April 1950, in *ibid.*, p. 386.

13 Dr Velasco y Polo, private interview, in *ibid.*, p. 388.
14 *Ibid.*
15 Kahlo quoted by Lozano, dispatch to *Time* (9 November 1950).
16 Dr Velasco y Polo, private interview, in Herrera, *Frida* pp. 389–90.
17 Fanny Rabel, private interview, in *ibid.*, p. 390.
18 Kahlo quoted by Lozano, *Time* (9 November 1950).
19 Herrera, *Frida* p. 391.
20 Frida Kahlo, 1951 diary, in *ibid.*, p. 392.
21 Rodríguez, *History of Mexican Mural Painting* pp. 272–305.
22 Instituto's founder quoted in *ibid.*, p. 305.
23 The Codex Borbonicus is now in the Bibliothèque de l'Assemblée Nationale, Paris.
24 David Alfaro Siqueiros quoted by Rodríguez, *op. cit.* p. 309.
25 Catlin, 'Mural Census', pp. 322–3.

TWENTY-FIVE 'FOR THE NEEDS OF THEIR OWN SPIRIT'

1 Antonin Artaud in Jack Hirshman (ed.), *Artaud Anthology* (San Francisco 1965) p. 8.
2 Artaud in Susan Sontag (ed.), *Antonin Artaud: Selected Writings* (New York 1976) p. 438.
3 *Ibid.*
4 Jean Dequeker, 'Birth of the Image' from 'Antonin Artaud ou la Santé des poètes', *La Tour de Feu* LXIII–IV (1959), trans. Sarah Wilson in *Aftermath* exh. cat. (London 1982) p. 122.
5 Antonin Artaud, 'Le Visage humain', *Portraits et dessins par Antonin Artaud* exh. cat. (Paris 1947).
6 Antonin Artaud, 'Van Gogh, the Man Suicided by Society' (Paris 1947), in Sontag, *Artaud* pp. 483–514.
7 Dr Joachim Beer, see John MacGregor, *The Discovery of the Art of the Insane* (Princeton 1989) p. 284.
8 Artaud, 'Van Gogh'.
9 See Stephen Barber, 'A Foundry of the Figure: Antonin Artaud', *Artforum* (September 1987) pp. 88–95.
10 Artaud, 'Van Gogh'.
11 Sarah suffered from osteomyelitis; see Matthew Gale and Chris Stephens, *Barbara Hepworth: Works in the Tate Gallery Collection and the Barbara Hepworth Museum St Ives* (London 1999) p. 110.
12 The 'panel sculpture' was reproduced in the *Daily Chronicle* (7 March 1925).
13 Barbara Hepworth, quoted by Alan Bowness, 'Introduction', *Barbara Hepworth Drawings from a Sculptor's Landscape* (London 1966) p. 22.
14 Stanley Spencer to Desmond Chute, May 1916, Stanley Spencer Gallery Collection, Cookham.
15 See Chris Stephens, 'From Constructivism to Reconstruction: Hepworth in the 1940s', in David Thistlewood (ed.), *Barbara Hepworth Reconsidered* (Liverpool 1996) pp. 140–42.
16 Margaret Moir later became Hepworth's secretary and recalled how Hepworth 'came to the London Clinic on several occasions in the space of two or three weeks, each time a Fenestration Operation was being performed . . . She did brief sketches during these visits, at all stages of the operation'; letter to the Tate Gallery, 13 June 1978.
17 *Barbara Hepworth Drawings*, p. 22.
18 Terisio Pignatti, entry on Veronese's *Resurrection* in *Art Commerce Scholarship* exh. cat. (London 1984) p. 97.
19 Pignatti claims, *ibid.*, that studio collaboration in *The Resurrection* is 'limited to areas of minor importance such as the cherubs and foliage in the upper right'.
20 Fernand Léger, 'Comment Je Conçois La Figure', *Fonctions de la peinture* (Paris 1965) p. 153.
21 The full-scale version of *La Fleur Qui Marche*, measuring 165 × 132 × 147 cm, is in the Musée National d'Art Moderne, Paris.
22 Sarah Wilson, 'Fernand Léger: Art and Politics 1935–1955', in *Fernand Léger: The Later Years* exh. cat. (London 1987) p. 72.
23 The photograph appeared in *Art d'Aujourd'hui* (October 1950).
24 John Weeks, 'Forty Years of Hospital Buildings', *HD* (February 1988) p. 23.
25 Michael Compton, 'Introduction', in *Mary Martin*, exh. cat. (London 1984) p. 18.
26 *The Times* (9 August 1956).
27 Mary Martin, 'The Waterfall', 1957, in *Mary Martin*, p. 27.
28 Mary Martin, 'Artist and Architect', 1957, *ibid.*, p. 26.
29 *Ibid.*
30 Hospitals Authority quoted by Norbert Lynton, *William Scott* (London 2004) p. 227.
31 For a full account of Rosenberg's enthusiasm for art, see Eugene Rosenberg, *Architect's Choice: Art in Architecture in Great Britain since 1945* text by Richard Cork (London 1992).
32 See Rósín Kennedy, 'Art for the Public: William Scott and F. E. McWilliam at Altnagelvin', *Irish Arts Review Yearbook* XVIII (2002) pp. 55–61.
33 Lynton, *Scott* p. 263. The William Scott Foundation now prefers to call it *Altnagelvin Mural* because *The Four Seasons* may not have been 'a title of which Scott approved'. Letter to Yale University Press, 4 July 2011.
34 Mark Rothko to William Scott, 14 December 1959, William Scott Archives, in *ibid.*
35 The nine paintings were presented by Rothko to the Tate in 1968 and 1969.
36 Scott quoted in Alan Bowness, *William Scott: Paintings, Drawings and Gouaches 1938–71* exh. cat. (London 1972) p. 77.
37 *Ibid.*
38 *Belfast Telegraph* (28 February 1962).
39 *Ibid.*
40 Mark Rothko to Katherine Kuh, quoted by Michael Compton, 'Mark Rothko, the Subjects of the Artist', in *Mark Rothko* exh. cat. (London 1987) p. 58.
41 Jean Leymarie, *Marc Chagall: The Jerusalem Windows* (London 1968) p. vii.
42 *Ibid.*, p. xi.
43 Paul Claudel quoted in *ibid.*, p. xiii.
44 *Ibid.*, p. 1.
45 *Ibid.*, p. 31.
46 *Ibid.*, p. 41.
47 *Ibid.*, p. 51.
48 *Ibid.*, p. 101.
49 Naum Gabo to Herbert Read, 4 January 1952, Gabo Papers, Beinecke Library.
50 Gabo to Lewis Mumford, 29 October 1976, *ibid.*
51 The *Realistic Manifesto* was first published in Moscow in August 1920. An English translation of the complete text is in *Naum Gabo: The Constructive Idea* exh. cat. (London 1988) pp. 52–4.
52 For a detailed account of the project's progress, see 'Naum Gabo talks to David Thompson', *Art Monthly* (February 1977) pp. 10–13.
53 Norman Reid, 'Foreword', in Rosenberg, *Architect's Choice*, p. 7.
54 *Ibid.*
55 Steven A. Nash, 'Naum Gabo: Sculptures of Purity and Possibility', in Steven A. Nash and Jorn Merkert (eds) *Naum Gabo: Sixty Years of Constructivism* (Munich 1985) p. 43.
56 Reid, 'Foreword', p. 7.
57 Rothko quoted by Compton, 'Mark Rothko', p. 58.

SELECT BIBLIOGRAPHY

Adams, Dr. *Morbid Poisons* (London 1795).
Adamson, Edward. *Art as Healing* (London 1984).
Address at the Opening of the Hospital, May 7, 1889 (Baltimore, Md., 1889).
Ahl, Diane Cohl. 'The Misericordia Polyptych', in *The Cambridge Companion to Piero della Francesca*, ed. Jeryldene M. Wood (Cambridge 2002).
Aimé-Azam, Denise. *Mazeppa: Géricault et son temps* (Paris 1956).
Ajmar-Wollheim, Marta, and Flora Dennis. *At Home in Renaissance Italy* (London 2006).
Alcantara, Isabel, and Sandra Egnolff. *Frida Kahlo and Diego Rivera* (Munich, London and New York 1999).
Allderidge, Patricia. *The Late Richard Dadd 1817–1886* (London 1974).
—. *Cibber's Figures from the Gates of Bedlam* (London 1977).
Allen, Brian. *Francis Hayman* (New Haven and London 1987).
Andersson, Christiane. 'The Isenheim Altarpiece: God's Medicine and the Painter's Vision', *Burlington Magazine* (September 1991).
Andrews, Keith. 'Once More Elsheimer', *Burlington Magazine* (March 1979).
Arnold, Catharine. *Bedlam: London and its Mad* (London 2008).
Arnold, Ken. *Cabinets for the Curious: Looking back at Early English Museums* (Aldershot 2006).
— and Olsen D. (eds). *Medicine Man: The Forgotten History of Henry Wellcome* (London 2003).
—, Lindsay Granshaw and Denna Jones. *Saving Bodies Saving Souls: Hospitals in History* exh. cat. (London 1997).
Art in Hospitals (London, King Edward's Hospital Fund, n.d.).
Artaud, Antonin. *The Theatre and its Double*. 1938, trans. Mary C. Richards (New York 1958).
—. 'Le Visage humain', *Portraits et dessins par Antonin Artaud* (Paris 1947).
—. 'Van Gogh, the Man Suicided by Society' (1947), trans. in Susan Sontag (ed.). *Antonin Artaud: Selected Writings* (New York 1976).
Attenborough, Richard. 'Foreword', in *Arts for Health: A Vision of Caring Environments* (Manchester 1989).
Aubry, Françoise, and Jos Vandenbreeden (eds). *Horta: Art Nouveau to Modernism* (Ghent 1996).
Austin, Anne L. *History of Nursing Source Book* (New York 1957).
Baard, H.P. *Frans Halsmuseum: Municipal Art Gallery at Haarlem* (Haarlem 1960).
Banchi, L. (ed.). *Statuti senesi scritti in volgare ne'secoli XIII e XIV*. Vol. III: *Statuto dello Spedale di Siena* (Bologna 1877).
Banker, James R. 'Piero della Francesca, il fratello Don Francesco di Benedetto e Francesco dal Borgo', *Prospettiva* LXVIII (1992).
—. 'The Altarpiece of the Confraternity of Santa Maria della Misericordia in Borgo Sansepolcro', *Piero della Francesca and His Legacy*, ed. Marilyn Aronberg Lavin (Hanover, N.H., 1995).
Baragnon, Numa. 'Toulouse-Lautrec chez Péan', *Chronique médicale* (15 February 1902).
Barber, Stephen. 'A Foundry of the Figure: Antonin Artaud', *Artforum* (September 1987) pp. 88–95.
—. *Antonin Artaud: Blows and Bombs* (New York 1993).
Barnes, Susan G. 'El Greco and the Decoration of the Church of Charity, Illescas', in Jonathan Brown (ed.). *Figures of Thought: El Greco as Interpreter of History, Tradition, and Ideas* (Washington, D.C., 1982).
Baron, J.H. 'How to beautify your old hospital', *British Medical Journal* (29 September 1984).
—. 'Art in Hospitals and for the Disadvantaged in New York and London', *The Lancet* (20/27 December 1986).
—. 'Hogarth and Hospitals', *The Lancet* (26 December 1987).
—. 'Frederick Cayley Robinson's "Acts of Mercy" Murals at the Middlesex Hospital, London', *British Medical Journal* (Clinical Research ed. 1994).
—. 'Art in Hospitals: The Fitzpatrick Lecture 1994', *Journal of the Royal College of Physicians of London* (March/April 1995).
— and Lesley Greene. 'Art in Hospitals: Funding Works of Art in New Hospitals', *British Medical Journal* (22–29 December 1984).
—, Megan Hadden and Midge Palley. *St Charles Hospital Works of Art* (London 1984).
Bataille, Georges. *Story of the Eye* trans. Joachim Neugroschal (1928; Harmondsworth 1987).
Battisti, Eugenio. *Piero della Francesca* 2 vols (Milan 1971).
—. *Brunelleschi: The Complete Work* (London 1981).
Baxandall, Michael. *Painting and Experience in Fifteenth Century Italy* (Oxford 1978).
Bazin, Germain. *Théodore Géricault: étude critique et catalogue raisonné* 7 vols (Paris 1987–1994).
Bedford County Hospital: A Commemorative Booklet (1898).
Bellucci, Gualtiero, and Piero Torriti. *Santa Maria della Scala in Siena: l'ospedale dai mille anni* (Genoa 1991).
Bennet, Glin. *The Wound and the Doctor: Healing, Technology and Power in Modern Medicine* (London 1987).
Bennett, Bonnie A., and David G. Wilkins. *Donatello* (Oxford 1984).
Benton, Tim. 'Spain: Modernismo in Catalonia', in *Art Nouveau Architecture*, ed. Frank Russell (London 1979; new ed. 1983).
Berger, John. *About Looking* (London 1980).
Berkowitz, Julie S. *'Adorn the Halls': The History of the Art Collection at Thomas Jefferson University* (Philadelphia 1999).
Berman, Greta, Leslie King-Hammond, Gerald Monroe and Francis V. O'Connor. *A New Deal for Public Art: Murals from Federal Work Programs* exh. cat. (New York 1993).
Bernardino, Saint. *Le prediche volgari dette nella piazza del Campo l'anno MCCCCXXVII* 3 vols (Siena 1880–888).
Bertela, G. Gaeta. *Luca, Andrea, Giovanni Della Robbia* (London, n.d.).
Bertelli, Carlo. *Piero della Francesca* (New Haven and London 1992).

Berthoud, Roger. *The Life of Henry Moore* (London 1987).
Berti, Luciano. *Frescoes from Florence* (London 1969).
Biesboer, Pieter, Friso Lammertse and Fred G. Meijer. *Painting Family: The De Brays, Master Painters of 17th Century Holland* (London 2008).
Bilbey, Diane, with Marjorie Trusted. *British Sculpture 1470 to 2000* (London 2002).
Bishop, Philippa, Susan Sloman and Amina Wright. *Pickpocketing the Rich: Portrait Painting in Bath 1720–1800* (Bath 2002).
Black, Peter (ed.). *Art, Medicine and the Enlightenment: The Art Collections of William Hunter in the Hunterian Museum and Art Gallery* (London 2007).
Blackshaw, Gemma, and Leslie Topp (eds). *Madness and Modernity: Mental Illness and the Visual Arts in Vienna 1900* (London 2009).
Blunt, Anthony. *Art and Architecture in France 1500–1700* 5th ed., rev. by Richard Beresford (New Haven and London 1999).
Bold, John. *Greenwich: An Architectural History of the Royal Hospital for Seamen and the Queen's House* (New Haven and London 2000).
Bolotowsky, Ilya. 'On Neoplasticism and my own Work: A Memoir', *Leonardo 2* 3 (1969).
Borchert, Till-Holger. *Memling and the Art of Portraiture* (London 2005).
Bostridge, Mark. *Florence Nightingale: The Woman and her Legend* (London 2008).
Boswell, John. *The Kindness of Strangers: The Abandonment of Children in Western Europe from Late Antiquity to the Renaissance* (London 1988).
Bourke, Joanna. *Fear: A Cultural History* (London 2005).
Bovey, Alixe. *Tacuinum Sanitatis: An Early Renaissance Guide to Health* (London 2005).
Bowe, Nicola Gordon, and Elizabeth Cumming. *The Arts and Crafts Movements in Dublin and Edinburgh 1885–1925* (Dublin 1998).
Bowness, Alan. 'Introduction', in *Barbara Hepworth: Drawings from a Sculptor's Landscape* (London 1966).
—. *William Scott: Paintings, Drawings and Gouaches 1938–1971* (London 1972).
Bowness, Sophie, and James Holland-Hibbert. *Barbara Hepworth: Drawings from the 1940s* (London 2005).
Brianchon, Horace [Dr Maurice de Fleury]. *Nos Grands Medecins d'aujourd'hui* (Paris 1891).
Brooke, Xanthe, and David Crombie. *Henry VIII Revealed: Holbein's Portrait and its Legacy* (London 2003).
— and Peter Cherry. *Murillo: Scenes of Childhood* (London 2001).
Brookner, Anita. *Jacques-Louis David* (London 1980).
Brown, Christopher. *Rembrandt: The Master and his Workshop* (London 1991).
Brown, David. 'Introduction', in *Frederick Cayley Robinson* exh. cat. (London 1977).
Brown, Gerard Baldwin. 'Some Recent Efforts in Mural Decoration', *Scottish Art Review* (January 1889).
Brown, Jonathan. 'El Greco and Toledo', *El Greco of Toledo* (Boston 1982).
— (ed.). *Figures of Thought: El Greco as Interpreter of History, Tradition and Ideas* (Washington, D.C., 1982).
Browne, Rosalind Bengelsdorf. 'The American Abstract Artists and the WPA Federal Art Project', *The New Deal Art Projects: An Anthology of Memoirs*, ed. Francis V. O'Connor (Washington, D.C., 1972).
Brownlow, John. *Memoranda: or, Chronicles of the Foundling Hospital . . . &tc* (London 1847).
—. *The History and Design of the Foundling Hospital* (London 1858).
Bruillot, Dominique, and Alain Roels. *Beaune et ses hospices* (Parcours 1996).
Brünniche, Eigil H. 'Edvard Munch og to Danske Leger', *Statens Museum for Kunst Arbok* (Oslo 1992).
Bryant, Barbara. *G.F. Watts Portraits: Fame and Beauty in Victorian Society* (London 2004).
Buckling, Maraike (ed.). *The Fantastic Heads of Franz Xaver Messerschmidt* (Munich 2006).
Bullock, Nicholas. *Circle: Constructive Art in Britain 1934–40* ed. Jeremy Lewison, exh. cat. (Cambridge 1982).
Burdett, H.C. *Hospitals and Asylums of the World* (London 1893).
Burton, John. *Essay towards a Complete New System of Midwifery* etchings by George Stubbs (London 1751).
Bynum, W.F., and Roy Porter. *Medical Fringe and Medical Orthodoxy 1750–1850* (London 1987).
Calderhead, James. *Hospitals for People: A Look at Some New Buildings in England* (London 1975).
Callen, Anthea. *Angel in the Studio: Women in the Arts and Crafts Movement 1870–1914* (London 1979).
Calne, Roy. 'The Art and Science of Surgery: Hunterian Oration 1989' (London, Royal College of Surgeons, 1989).
Cameron, H.C. *Mr Guy's Hospital 1726–1948* (London 1954).
Cammerer, M. (ed.). *Kunst des Cinquecento in der Toskana* (Munich 1992).
Campbell, Lorne. *Van der Weyden* (London 1979).
Cardini, Franco. *Europe 1492: Portrait of a Continent Five Hundred Years Ago* (New York and Oxford 1989).
Carli, Enzo. *Sienese Painting* (London 1983).
Carline, Richard. *Stanley Spencer at War* (London 1978).
Casey, Noreen. 'Architecture and Decoration', in *Public Virtue, Public Love: The Early Years of the Dublin Lying-in Hospital*, ed. I.C. Ross (Dublin 1986).
Catlin, Stanton L. 'Mural Census', *Diego Rivera: A Retrospective* (New York and London 1987).
Céleyran, Gabriel Tapié de. 'Toulouse-Lautrec et ses relations médicales', *La Chronique médicale* (1 December 1922).
Chambers, D.S. *Patrons and Artists in the Italian Renaissance* (Columbia, N.Y., 1971).
Chave, Anna C. *Constantin Brancusi: Shifting the Bases of Art* (New Haven and London 1993).
Christian, John (ed.). *The Last Romantics: The Romantic Tradition in British Art* (London 1989).
Christiansen, Keith, Laurence B. Kanter and Carl Brandon Strehlke (eds). *Painting in Renaissance Siena 1420–1500* (New York 1988).
— (ed.). *Giambattista Tiepolo* (London 1996).
Clair, Jean. *Vienne 1880–1938: L'apocalypse joyeuse* (Paris 1986).
—. *L'âme au corps: arts et sciences 1793–1993* (Paris 1994).
—. *Mélancolie: génie et folie en occident* (Paris 2005).
Clark, Kenneth. *Civilisation: A Personal View* (London 1969).
Clark Kennedy, A.E. *The London* Vol. 1: *1740–1840* (London 1962).
Clarke, Michael (ed.). *Velázquez in Seville* exh. cat. (Edinburgh 1996).
Clegg, Elizabeth. *Art, Design and Architecture in Central Europe 1890–1920* (New Haven and London 2006).
Clément, Charles. *Géricault: étude biographique et critique* (Paris 1879 3rd ed.).
Cocke, Richard. *Veronese* (London 1980).
Coe, Peter, and Malcolm Reading. *Lubetkin and Tecton: Architecture and Social Commitment* (London and Bristol 1981).
Cogeval, Guy, with Kimberley Jones, Laurence des Cars and MaryAnne Stevens. *Edouard Vuillard* (London 2004).
Cole, Bruce. *Sienese Painting from its Origins to the Fifteenth Century* (New York 1980).
Coles, Peter. *Manchester Hospitals' Arts Project* (London 1981).
—. *Art in the National Health Service: A Report by the DHSS* (London 1983).
—. *The Arts in a Health District* (London, DHSS, n.d.).
Collier, John. *Human Passions Delineated* (London 1773).
Collins, Judith. *The Omega Workshops* (London 1983).
—. *Eric Gill: The Sculpture. A Catalogue Raisonné* (London 1998).
Compston, H.F.B. *Thomas Coram* (London 1918).
Compton, Michael. 'Introduction', in *Mary Martin* (London 1984).
—. 'Mark Rothko, the Subjects of the Artist', in *Mark Rothko* exh. cat. (London 1987).
Compton, Susan, Richard Cork and Peter Fuller. *Henry Moore* exh. cat. (London 1988).
Conisbee, Philip. *Painting in Eighteenth-Century France* (Oxford 1981).
The Story of the Thomas Coram Foundation for Children (London n.d.).
Cork, Richard. *Art Beyond the Gallery in Early 20th Century England* (New Haven and London 1985).
—. *David Bomberg* (New Haven and London 1987).
—. 'For the Needs of their own Spirit: Art in Hospitals', in *Art for Public Places: Critical Essays* (Winchester 1989).
—. 'Towards a New Alliance', in Eugene Rosenberg, *Architect's Choice: Art in Architecture in Great Britain since 1945* (London 1992).
—. *A Bitter Truth: Avant-Garde Art and the Great War* (New Haven and London 1994).
—. 'Pictures of Health: Six Leading Artists have donated Prints', *Telegraph Weekend Magazine* (21 October 1989).
—. 'Hannah Collins at Colindale', *New Spirit, New Sculpture, New Money: Art in the 1980s* (New Haven and London 2003).
—. *Wild Thing: Epstein, Gaudier-Brzeska, Gill* (London 2009).
—. 'Calligraphy of Light', in *Rebecca Salter: Into the Light of Things*, ed. Gillian Forrester (London and New Haven 2011).
Croft-Murray, Edward. *Decorative Painting in England 1537–1837* Vol. 2: *The 18th and Early 19th Centuries* (London 1970).
Cruickshank, Dan. *The Secret History of Georgian London* (London 2009).
Cumming, Elizabeth. *The Arts and Crafts Movement in Edinburgh 1880–1930* (Edinburgh 1985).
—. *Phoebe Anna Traquair 1852–1936* exh. cat. (Edinburgh 1993).
—. 'Patterns of Life: The Art and Design of Phoebe Anna Traquair and Mary Seton Watts', in *Women Artists and the Decorative Arts 1880–1935: The Gender of Ornament* ed. Bridget Elliott and Janice Helland (London 2002).
—. *Phoebe Anna Traquair 1852–1936* (Edinburgh 2005).
Dabrowski, Magdalena, and Rudolf Leopold. *Egon Schiele* (New York 1997).
Daniels, Jeffery. *Sebastiano Ricci* (Hove 1976).
Davies, David (ed.). *El Greco* (London 2003).
Davies, Martin. *Rogier van der Weyden* (Oxford 1972).
Dean, C.G.T. *The Royal Hospital Chelsea* (London 1950).

Dejardin, Ian A. C., Desmond Shawe-Taylor and Giles Waterfield. *Rembrandt to Gainsborough: Masterpieces from Dulwich Picture Gallery* (London 1999).
Delaney, Mary. See *Letters from Georgian Ireland*.
Dequeker, Jean. 'Birth of the Image', from 'Antonin Artaud ou la santé des poètes', *La Tour de feu* LXIII–IV (1959).
Description de l'Hôpital royal pour les marins, Greenwich (London 1851).
Dexter, Emma, and Tanya Barson (eds). *Frida Kahlo* (London 2005).
Dormandy, Thomas. *The Worst of Evils: The Fight against Pain* (New Haven and London 2006).
Dorment, Richard. *Alfred Gilbert: Sculptor and Goldsmith* (London 1986).
Douglas, R. Langton. *Piero di Cosimo* (Chicago 1946).
Downes, Kerry. *Hawksmoor* (London 1977).
Downs, Linda Bank. *Diego Rivera: The Detroit Industry Murals* (New York and London 1999).
Druick, Douglas W., and Peter Kort Zegers. *Van Gogh and Gauguin: The Studio of the South* (London 2001).
Ebert-Schifferer, Sybille. *Still Life: A History* (New York 1999).
Egerton, Judy. *George Stubbs: Anatomist and Animal Painter* (London 1976).
Einberg, Elizabeth. *Manners and Morals: Hogarth and British Painting 1700–1760* (London 1987).
Eitner, Lorenz. *Géricault: His Life and Work* (London 1982).
Ekkart, Rudi, and Quentin Buvelot. *Dutch Portraits: The Age of Rembrandt and Frans Hals* (London 2007).
Emery, Alan E. H., and Marcia L. H. Emery. *Medicine and Art* (London 2003).
Erffa, Helmut von, and Allen Staley. *The Paintings of Benjamin West* (New Haven and London 1986).
Esquirol, Jean-Etienne-Dominique. *Des maladies mentales considérées sous les rapports médicals, hygiéniques et médico-legaux, II* (Paris 1838).
Esterly, David. *Grinling Gibbons and the Art of Carving* (London 1998).
Evelyn, John. *Diary*, ed. E. S. de Beer (Oxford 1955) vol. 4.
Fagotto, Virginio (ed.). *Arte e musica all'Ospedaletto* (Venice 1978).
Fanfani, Amintore. 'La beneficenza in un commune toscana dal XIII al XV secolo', *Saggi di storia economica italiana* (Milan 1936).
Faulkner, Marcus. *An Historical and Descriptive Account of the Royal Hospital . . . at Chelsea* (London 1805).
Feghelm, Dagmar. *I, Goya* (Munich, London and New York 2001).
Fenton, James. *School of Genius: A History of the Royal Academy of Arts* (London 2006).
Ferrajoli, A. 'Un testamento dello scultore Pietro Torrigiani e ricerche sopra alcune sue opere' *Bolletino d'arte* IX (1915) pp. 181–92.
Fisher, Crispin. 'St Thomas Perambulations Part I', *St Thomas's Hospital Gazette* (Winter 1985).
Forbes, Thomas Rogers. *Chronicles from Aldgate: Life and Death in Shakespeare's London* (New Haven 1971).
Forster, E. M. *A Room with a View* (London 1908).
Foster, Kathleen A. *Thomas Eakins Rediscovered: Charles Bregler's Thomas Eakins Collection at the Pennsylvania Academy of the Fine Arts* (New Haven 1997).
Foucault, Michel. *The Birth of the Clinic* trans. A. M. Sheridan (London 2003 ed.).
—. *History of Madness* (London 2006).
Fox, Celina. *Londoners* (London 1987).
Freedberg, S.J. *Painting in Italy 1500 to 1600* (Harmondsworth 1971; new ed. 1983).
Frey, Julia. *Toulouse-Lautrec: A Life* (London 1994).
Fried, Michael. *Realism, Writing, Disfiguration: On Thomas Eakins and Stephen Crane* (Chicago and London 1987).
Friedländer, Max J. *Early Netherlandish Painting from Van Eyck to Breughel* (London 1956).
Friedman, Terry. *James Gibbs* (New Haven and London 1984).
Fry, Roger. 'The Old Masters at Burlington House', *Athenaeum* (20 January 1906).
'Naum Gabo talks to David Thompson', *Art Monthly* (February 1977) pp. 10–13.
Naum Gabo: The Constructive Idea exh. cat. (London 1988).
Gale, Matthew, and Chris Stephens. *Barbara Hepworth: Works in the Tate Gallery Collection and the Barbara Hepworth Museum St Ives* (London 1999).
Gayford, Martin. *The Yellow House: Van Gogh, Gauguin and Nine Turbulent Weeks in Arles* (London 2006).
Gebser, Jean. *Ursprung und Gegenwart* (Stuttgart 1949).
Geddes, Jennian F. 'Artistic Integrity and Feminist Spin: A Spat at the Endell Street Military Hospital', *Burlington Magazine* (September 2005).
George, M. Dorothy. *Hogarth to Cruickshank: Social Change in Graphic Satire* (London 1967).
Georget, Etienne-Jean. *De la physiologie du système nerveux* (Paris 1821).
Gibbs, D. *Emblems, Tokens and Tickets of the London Hospital and the London Hospital Medical College* (London 1985).
Girouard, Mark. *The English Town* (New Haven and London 1990).
Godfrey, Mark. 'Barnett Newman's "Stations of the Cross" and the Memory of the Holocaust', *Reconsidering Barnett Newman*, ed. Melissa Ho (New Haven and London 2005).
Golding, Benjamin. *An Historical Account of St Thomas's Hospital, Southwark* (London 1819).
Gordon, Donald E. *Ernst Ludwig Kirchner* (Cambridge, Mass., 1968).
Gowing, Lawrence. *Hogarth* (London 1971).
Granero, Jesús Maria, SJ. *D. Miguel de Mañara: un caballero sevillano del siglio XVII* (Seville 1963).
Granshaw, Lindsay, and Roy Porter (eds). *The Hospital in History* (London 1989).
Green, Christopher (ed.). *Art Made Modern: Roger Fry's Vision of Art* (London 1999).
Greene, John. *Brightening the Long Days: Hospital Tile Pictures* (Gloucester 1987).
Greene, Lesley. *Art in Hospitals: A Guide* (London 1989).
Greenlaw, Lavinia. *Signs and Humours: The Poetry of Medicine* (London 2007).
Grimberg, Salomon. *I Will Never Forget You . . . Frida Kahlo to Nickolas Muray* (London 2005).
Gronberg, Tag. *Vienna: City of Modernity 1890–1914* (Bern 2007).
Grouvel, F. *Memling* (Paris 1968).
Gruffyd, Bodfan. *Landscape Architecture for New Hospitals* (London 1967).
Grundy, Milton. *Venice: An Anthology Guide* preface John Julius Norwich (London 1971; 1985 ed.).
Guégan, Stéphane. *Paintings in the Musée d'Orsay* (London 2004).
Guillaume-Linephty, M. *La Chasse de Sainte Ursule* (Paris 1958).
Haldane, Duncan, and Susan Loppert (eds). *The Arts in Health Care: Learning from Experience* (London 1999).
Hamilton, Richard. Statement in *Four Rooms* exh. cat. (London 1984).
Hanson, Lawrence, and Elisabeth. *Portrait of Vincent: A Van Gogh Biography* (London 1955).
Harris, Enriqueta. 'A Decorative Scheme by El Greco', *Burlington Magazine* LXXII (1938) pp. 154–64.
Hartt, Frederick. *History of Italian Renaissance Art* (London 1970; new rev. ed. 1987).
Haskell, Francis. *Géricault* (Bristol 1966).
Hautecoeur, Louis. 'Avant-propos', in *Les Invalides: trois siècles d'histoire*, ed. René Baillargeat (Paris 1974).
Hawkins, Sir John. *Life of Johnson* (London 1787).
Hayes, John. *Rowlandson Watercolours and Drawings* (London 1972).
—. *Thomas Gainsborough* (London 1980).
— (ed.). *The Letters of Thomas Gainsborough* (New Haven and London 2001).
Hayum, Andrée. 'The Meaning and Function of the Isenheim Altarpiece: The Hospital Context Revisited', *Art Bulletin* (1977) pp. 501–17.
—. *The Isenheim Altarpiece: God's Medicine and the Painter's Vision* (Princeton 1989).
The Healing Touch: 500 Years of Scots in Sickness and Health (Edinburgh 2005).
Heck, Christian. 'Les bâtiments de l'ancienne préceptorie des Antonins d'Issenheim', *Le Retable d'Issenheim et la sculpture au nord des Alpes à la fin du moyen age: Actes du colloque de Colmar 2–3 novembre 1987, réunis et présentés par Christian Heck* (Colmar 1989) pp. 128–39.
Heckscher, William S. *Rembrandt's Anatomy of Dr. Nicolaas Tulp* (New York 1958).
Henderson, John. 'The Flagellant Movement and Flagellant Confraternities in Central Italy, 1260–1400', *Studies in Church History* 15 (1978) pp. 147–61.
—. *The Renaissance Hospital: Healing the Body and Healing the Soul* (New Haven and London 2006).
Hendricks, Gordon. 'Thomas Eakins's Gross Clinic', *Art Bulletin* LI (March 1969) pp. 57–64.
Herbert R. L., Apter S. L., and Kenney E. K. (eds). *The Société Anonyme and the Dreier Bequest at Yale University: A Catalogue Raisonné* (New Haven 1984).
Herrera, Hayden. *Frida: A Biography of Frida Kahlo* (London 1989).
Heugten, Sjraar van. *Van Gogh Draughtsman: The Masterpieces* (Amsterdam 2005).
Higgie, Jennifer. *Bedlam* (New York and Berlin 2006).
Hill, Draper. *Fashionable Contrasts: Caricatures by James Gillray* (London 1966).
Hirshman, Jack (ed.). *Artaud Anthology* (San Francisco 1965).
Hofmann, Werner. *Gustav Klimt* (London 1972).
Holbrook, Mary. 'Painters in Bath in the Eighteenth Century', *Apollo* (November 1973).
Honour, Hugh. *The Companion Guide to Venice* (London 1965; 1977 ed.).
Hook, Judith. *Siena: A City and its History* (London 1979).
Hooreweder, Carlos van. *Hans Memling* (Bruges 1984).
—. *Hans Memling in the Hospital of St John, Bruges* (Bruges 1993).
Horton, Richard. *Second Opinion: Doctors, Disease and Decisions in Modern Medicine* (London 2003).
Hosking, Sarah, and Liz Haggard. *Healing the Hospital Environment: Design, Management and Maintenance of Healthcare Premises* (London 1999).
Hospital Audiences, Inc. *The Healing Role of the Arts: Working Papers* (New York 1978).

The Hospital of St Cross and St Cross Church (Andover 1993).
Hospital Plans: Five Essays (New York 1875).
Howard, Deborah. *The Architectural History of Venice* (New Haven and London, rev. and enlarged ed. 2002).
Hughes, Robert. *Barcelona* (London 1992).
—. *Goya* (London 2004).
Humbert, Jean-Marcel, and Lionel Dumarche. *The Tomb of Napoleon and the Hôtel des Invalides* (Paris 1988).
Hunter, R., and I. Macalpine. *Three Hundred Years of Psychiatry* (London 1963).
Husslein-Arco, Agnes. *Tony Cragg. Franz Xaver Messerschmidt* (Vienna 2008).
Huysmans, J.-K. *Trois primitifs* trans. Robert Baldick, in E. Ruhmer, *Grünewald: The Paintings* (London 1958).
Hyslop, Roy. *Art in Hospitals: Conference Report* DHSS (London 1983).
Illich, Ivan. *Limits to Medicine, Medical Nemesis: The Expropriation of Health* (London 1976; 1984 ed.).
Iñiguez, Diego Angulo. 'Murillo: His Life and Work', *Bartolomé Esteban Murillo* (London 1982).
Ives, Colta, Susan Alyson Stein, Sjraar van Heugten and Marije Vellekoop. *Vincent Van Gogh: The Drawings* (New Haven and London 2005).
Jansen, Leo, Hans Luijten and Nienke Bakker (eds) Vincent van Gogh - The Letters: The Complete Illustrated and Annotated Edition (Amsterdam and London 2009) 6 vols.
Jason, Horst W. 'Giovanni Chellini's *Libro* and Donatello', *Studien zur Toskanischen Kunst: Festschrift L. H. Heydenreich* (Munich 1964).
Jencks, Charles, and Edwin Heathcote. *The Architecture of Hope: Maggie's Cancer Caring Centres* (London 2010).
Jenkins, Susan. *Compton Verney Handbook* (Compton Verney House Trust 2004).
Jordan, William B. Catalogue entries in *El Greco of Toledo* (Boston 1982).
Junquera, Juan Jose. *The Black Paintings of Goya* (London 2003).
Kagan, Richard L. 'The Toledo of El Greco', *El Greco of Toledo* (Boston 1982).
Kemp, Martin. *Cima da Conegliano* (Bristol 1967).
—. *Leonardo da Vinci: The Marvellous Works of Nature and Man* (London, pb 1989).
—. *Leonardo da Vinci: Experience, Experiment and Design* (London 2006).
— and Marina Wallace. *Spectacular Bodies: The Art and Science of the Human Body from Leonardo to Now* exh. cat. (London 2000).
Kennedy, Rósín. 'Art for the Public: William Scott and F. E. McWilliam at Altnagelvin', *Irish Arts Review Yearbook* XVIII (2002) pp. 55–61.
Kiers, Judijke, and Fieke Tissink. *The Golden Age of Dutch Art* (London 2000).
Kiple, Kenneth F. *Plague, Pox and Pestilence: Disease in History* (London 1997).
Klessmann, Rüdiger. *Adam Elsheimer 1578–1610* with contributions from Emilie E. S. Gordenker and Christian Tico Seifert (Edinburgh and London 2006).
Koster, Margaret L. 'New Documentation for the Portinari Altar-piece', *Burlington Magazine* (March 2003) pp. 164–79.
Kris, Ernst. *Psychoanalytic Explorations in Art* (New York 1952).
Kuhl, Isabel. *I, van Gogh* (Munich, London and New York 2005).
Larner, Melissa, James Peto and Nadine Monem (eds). *War and Medicine* (London 2008).
Laugier, Marc-Antoine. *Essai sur l'architecture* (Paris 1755).
Lauts, Jan. *Domenico Ghirlandaio* (Vienna 1943).
Léger, Fernand. 'Comment je conçois la figure', *Fonctions de la peinture* (Paris 1965).
Lemoine, Serge (ed.). *Paintings in the Musée d'Orsay* (London, new ed. 2004).
Letters from Georgian Ireland: The Correspondence of Mary Delany, 1731–68 ed. Angelique Day (Belfast 1991).
Levey, Michael. *Painting in XVIII Century Venice* (London 1959).
—. *Giambattista Tiepolo. His Life and Art* (New Haven and London 1986).
Lewis, Wyndham. Interview with 'M.M.B.', *Daily News and Leader* (7 April 1914).
Leymarie, Jean. *Marc Chagall: The Jerusalem Windows* (London 1968).
—. *Dutch Painting* trans. Stuart Gilbert (London 1977).
Lightbown, Ronald. *Piero della Francesca* (New York 1992).
Little, Bryan. *The Life and Work of James Gibbs 1682–1754* (London 1955).
Livingstone, Karen, and Linda Parry (eds). *International Arts and Crafts* (London 2005).
Llewellyn, Nigel. *The Art of Death: Visual Culture in the English Death Ritual, c. 1500–c. 1800* (London 1991).
Llosa, Mario Vargas. *The Perpetual Orgy* (London 1987).
Lloyd, Jill, *et al. Franz Xaver Messerschmidt: Character-Heads 1770–1783* (London n.d.).
— and Magdalena M. Moeller (eds). *Ernst Ludwig Kirchner: The Dresden and Berlin Years* (London 2003).
Lobelle-Caluwe, Hilde. *Memlingmuseum Bruges* (Brussels 1987).
Loppert, Susan, and Tamsin Dillon. *Don't Worry: An Exhibition of Specially Commissioned Works at Chelsea & Westminster Hospital* (London 2000).
Lunardon, Silvia. *Hospitale S. Mariae Cruciferorum* (Venice 1984).
Lux, J. A. *Otto Wagner* (Munich 1914).
Lynton, Norbert. *Willliam Scott* (London 2004).
MacCarthy, Fiona. *Eric Gill* (London 1989).
McClure, Ruth K. *Coram's Children: The London Foundling Hospital in the Eighteenth Century* (New Haven and London 1981).
MacDonald, Helen. *Human Remains: Dissection and its Histories* (New Haven and London 2006).
McFarlane, K. B. *Hans Memling* (Oxford 1971).
MacGregor, John. *The Discovery of the Art of the Insane* (Princeton 1989).
McIntyre, Ian. *Joshua Reynolds: The Life and Times of the First President of the Royal Academy* (London, pb ed. 2004).
MacKenzie, Norman and Jeanne. *Dickens: A Life* (Oxford 1979).
Macmillan, Duncan. *Scottish Art 1460–1990* (Edinburgh 1990).
—. 'Géricault et Charles Bell', *Géricault* (Paris 1996) pp. 449–66.
McParland, Edward. 'Royal Hospital, Kilmainham, Co. Dublin – I', *Country Life* (9 May 1985).
—. 'Royal Hospital, Kilmainham, Co. Dublin – II', *Country Life* (16 May 1985).
—. *Public Architecture in Ireland 1680–1760* (New Haven and London 2001).
Maggini, Giuliana, and Luigi Andreini (eds). *Laudario della Compagnia di S. Maria della Notte* (Sansepolcro 1979).
Malton, James. *A picturesque & descriptive view of the city of Dublin* (London 1799).
Mann, Richard G. *El Greco and his Patrons: Three Major Projects* (Cambridge 1986).
Mannings, David. *Sir Joshua Reynolds: A Complete Catalogue of his Paintings: Text* (New Haven and London 2000).
Marteau, R., and C. Marq. *Les Vitraux de Chagall, 1957–1970* (Paris 1972).
Martin, Mary. 'The Waterfall', 1957, in *Mary Martin* exh. cat. (London 1984).
—. 'Artist and Architect', 1957 in *Mary Martin* exh. cat. (London 1984).
Martindale, Andrew. *Simone Martini: Complete Edition* (Oxford 1988).
Mayhew, Edgar de N. *Sketches by Thornhill in the V&A* (London 1967).
Mead, Richard. *A Discourse on the Plague* (London 1721).
Medvei, N. C., and J. C. Thornton (eds). *The Royal Hospital, Saint Bartholomew 1123–1973* (London 1974).
Mellinkoff, Ruth. *The Devil at Isenheim: Reflections of Popular Belief in Grünewald's Altarpiece* (Berkeley, Cal., 1988).
Mellor, David Alan. *The Art of Robyn Denny* (London 2002).
Merot, Alain. *French Painting in the Seventeenth Century* (New Haven and London 1995).
Millard, Graham. *Commissioning Hospital Buildings* (London 1975).
Mitchell, Charles. 'Benjamin West's "Death of Wolfe" and the Popular History Piece', *Journal of the Warburg Institute* VII (1944).
Moore, Wendy. *The Knife Man: The Extraordinary Life and Times of John Hunter, Father of Modern Surgery* (London 2005).
Morassi, Antonio. *G. B. Tiepolo: His Life and Work* (London 1955).
Morris, Frances. *Paris Post-War: Art and Existentialism 1945–55* (London 1993).
Moscoso, Javier. *Pain: Passion, Compassion, Sensibility* (London 2004).
Moser, Joseph. 'Vestiges, Collected and Recollected, by Joseph Moser, Esq', *European Magazine* XIII (July–December 1803).
Moss, Lynda. 'Paintings, Patients and Propaganda', *Art and Artists* (April 1986).
—. 'The Arts as Healing Agents in Recovery from Operation: A Critical Review', *Theoretical Surgery* I (1986).
Mulvey, Laura, and Peter Wollen. *Frida Kahlo and Tina Modotti* exh. cat. (London 1982).
Munch, Edvard. *Edvard Munchs Brev. Familien* (Oslo 1949).
Muray, Nickolas. *I Will Never Forget You . . .* (London 2005).
Murray, Flora. *Women as Army Surgeons, Being the History of the Women's Hospital Corps in Paris, Wimereux and Endell Street, September 1914–October 1919* (London 1920).
Nash, Paul. *Outline: An Autobiography and Other Writings* (London 1949).
Nash, Steven A., and Jorn Merkert (eds). *Naum Gabo: Sixty Years of Constructivism* (Munich 1985).
Natter, Tobias, and Christoph Grunenberg (eds). *Gustav Klimt: Painting, Design and Modern Life* (London 2008).
Nebehay, Christian. *Gustav Klimt* (Vienna 1969).
Newman, G. F. *The Nation's Health* (Granada 1983).
Nicholl, Charles. *Leonardo da Vinci: The Flights of the Mind* (London 2004).
Nicolai, Friedrich. 'Recollection of a Meeting with Messerschmidt in Pressburg in 1781', *Franz Xaver Messerschmidt: Character-Heads 1770–1783* (London n.d.).

Nicolson, Benedict. *The Treasures of the Foundling Hospital* (Oxford 1972).
Nightingale, Florence. *Notes on Hospitals* (London 1859).
Noon, Patrick. *Constable to Delacroix: British Art and the French Romantics* (London 2003).
Norman, Diana. *Siena and the Virgin: Art and Politics in a Late Medieval City State* (New Haven and London 1999).
North, John. *The Ambassadors' Secret: Holbein and the World of the Renaissance* (London and New York 2002).
Nunn, Pamela Gerrish. *Victorian Women Artists* (London 1987).
O'Connor, Francis V. (ed.). *Art for the Millions: Essays from the 1930s by Artists and Administrators of the WPA Federal Art Project* (Boston 1975 ed.).
O'Donaghue, Edward G. *The Story of Bethlehem Hospital* (London 1914).
Olding, Simon. *Medical and Scientific Collections in London* (London 1987).
Ortiz, Antonio Dominguez. 'Murillo's Seville', *Bartolomé Esteban Murillo* (London 1982).
Orwell, George. 'How the Poor Die', *Collected Essays* (London 1961).
Os, Henk W. van. *Vecchietta and the Sacristy of the Siena Hospital Church: A Study of Renaissance Religious Symbolism* trans. Eva Biesta (Maarssen 1974).
Oursel, Raymond. *L'Hôtel-Dieu de Beaune* (Lyon 1968).
Paddington Green Children's Hospital: Annual Report for 1895.
— *Committee Report, 1912*.
Padrón, F. Morales. *Memorias de Seville (noticias sobre el siglo XVII)* (Cordoba 1981).
Palgrave, F.T. *Essays on Art* (London and Cambridge 1866).
Panofsky, Erwin. *Early Netherlandish Painting* (Princeton 1953).
Parsons, F.G. 'The Statues in St Thomas's Hospital and their Associations', *St Thomas's Hospital Gazette* XXXIV (1933).
Parsons, Gerald. *Siena, Civil Religion and the Sienese* (London 2005).
Paulson, Ronald. *Hogarth: His Life, Art, and Times* (New Haven and London 1971).
—. *The Art of Hogarth* (London 1975).
Penny, Nicholas (ed.). *Reynolds* (London 1986).
—. 'Journey to Arezzo', *London Review of Books* (17 April 2003).
Percival-Prescott, Westby. 'Thornhill at Greenwich', *Ingrid and Other Studies* (London 1978).
Perruchot, Henri. *Toulouse-Lautrec* (London 1960).
Petherbridge, Deanna. *Art for Architecture: A Handbook on Commissioning* (London 1987).
Pevsner, Nikolaus. *An Outline of European Architecture* (Harmondsworth 1943; 5th ed. 1958).
Phillips, Elaine. *A Short History of the Great Hospital Norwich* (Norwich, 1999).
Pickvance, Ronald. *Van Gogh in Saint-Rémy and Auvers* (New York 1986).
Pignatti, Terisio. Catalogue entry on Veronese's *Resurrection*, in *Art Commerce Scholarship* exh. cat. (London 1984).
Pinault, C. 'Les activités de Santa Maria della Scala à travers le statut de 1318 et des fresques', *Medicina nei secoli* (2002).
Pope-Hennessy, John. *Giovanni di Paolo 1403–1483* (London 1937).
—. *Sienese Quattrocento Painting* (Oxford and London 1947).
—. *Italian Renaissance Sculpture* (Oxford and London 1958) vol. 2 (London 2000 ed.).
—. *The Study and Criticism of Italian Sculpture* (New York 1980).
—. *Luca della Robbia* (Oxford 1980).
Porter, Roy. *The Greatest Benefit to Mankind: A Medical History of Humanity from Antiquity to the Present* (London 1997).
—. *Flesh in the Age of Reason* (London 2003).
—. *Madmen: A Social History of Mad-Houses, Mad-Doctors and Lunatics* (London 2005).
— and Andrew Wear. *Problems and Methods in the History of Medicine* (London 1987).
Postle, Martin (ed.). *Joshua Reynolds: The Creation of Celebrity* (London 2005).
Potterton, Homan. *Venetian Seventeenth Century Painting* (London 1979).
Pötzl-Malikova, M. *Franz Xaver Messerschmidt* (Vienna and Munich 1982).
Poulden, S. *The Arts in Hospitals* conference report (Manchester 1981).
Powers, Alan. 'Wards and Walls', *Country Life* (17 March 1988).
Poynter, F.N.L. (ed.). *The Evolution of Hospitals in Britain* (London 1964).
Prideaux, Sue. *Edvard Munch: Behind the Scream* (New Haven and London 2005).
Pringle, John. *Observations on the Nature and Cure of Hospital and Jayl-Fevers* (London 1750).
Quennell, Peter. *Hogarth's Progress* (London 1955).
Quiney, Anthony. *Town Houses of Medieval Britain* (New Haven and London 2003).
Rappaport, Helen. 'The Invitation that never came: Mary Seacole after the Crimea', *History Today* (February 2005).
Rawcliffe, C. *Medicine and Society in Later Medieval England* (Stroud 1995).
—. *Medicine for the Soul: The Life, Death and Resurrection of an English Medieval Hospital: St Giles's, Norwich, c. 1249–1550* (Stroud 1999).
Renard, Jules. *Journal, 1887–1910* ed. L. Guichard and G. Sigaux (Paris, new ed. 1984).
Ricci, Ivano. *La fraternità di S. Bartolomeo* (Sansepolcro 1936).
Rifkin, Benjamin A., Michael J. Ackerman and Judith Folkenberg. *Human Anatomy: Depicting the Body from the Renaissance to Today* (London 2006).
Riley-Smith, Jonathan. *Hospitallers: The History of the Order of St John* (London 1999).
Robinson, Jane. *Mary Seacole: The Charismatic Black Nurse who became a Heroine of the Crimea* (London 2005).
Rochfort, Desmond. 'A Terrible Beauty: Orozco's Murals in Guadalajara 1936–1939', *¡Orozco! 1883–1949* (Oxford, 1980).
—. *The Murals of Diego Rivera* (London 1987).
Rodríguez, Antonio. *A History of Mexican Mural Painting* (London 1969).
Roger-Marx, Claude. *Vuillard: His Life and Work* (New York 1946).
Roover, Raymond de. *The Rise and Decline of the Medici Bank, 1397–1494* (Cambridge 1963).
Rosen, George. *Madness in Society* (New York 1968).
Rosenberg, Jakob. *Rembrandt: Life and Work* (Harvard 1948; London 1968).
Rosenthal, Michael. *The Art of Thomas Gainsborough: A Little Business of the Eye* (New Haven and London 1999).
—. *William Hogarth* (London 2005).
Roskill, Mark (ed.). *The Letters of Vincent Van Gogh* (London 1963).
Rossetti, William Michael. *Some Reminiscences of William Michael Rossetti* (London 1906).
Rouquet, André. *The Present State of the Arts in England* (London 1755).
Rowlands, John. *Holbein: The Paintings of Hans Holbein The Younger. Complete Edition* (Oxford 1985).
The Royal Hospital Chelsea (London 1985).
Ruhmer, E. *Grünewald: The Paintings* (London 1958).
Russell, David. *Scenes from Bedlam: A History of Caring for the Mentally Ill at Bethlem Royal Hospital and the Maudsley* (London 1997).
Russell, Frank (ed.), *Art Nouveau Architecture* (London 1979).
Saalman, Howard. *Filippo Brunelleschi: The Buildings* (London 1993).
Sala, G.A. 'A Visit to the Royal Hospital of Bethlehem', *Illustrated London News* (24 March 1860) p. 291.
Salas, Xavier de. *Goya* (London 1979).
Sales, J.E.L. 'William Hogarth's View of Medical Practice', *St Bartholomew's Hospital Journal* (1972).
Salomon, Antoine, and Guy Cogeval (eds). *Edouard Vuillard: Critical Catalogue of Paintings and Pastels* (Milan and London 2005).
Sánchez, Alfonso E. Pérez. 'On the Reconstruction of El Greco's Dispersed Altarpieces', in *El Greco of Toledo* (Boston 1982).
Sandblom, Philip. *Creativity and Disease: How Illness affects Literature, Art and Music* (New York and London, rev. 8th ed. 1995).
Sanders, R. 'William Hogarth (1697–1764)', *St Bartholomew's Hospital Journal* (1964).
Sass, Louis A. *Madness and Modernism: Insanity in the Light of Modern Art, Literature and Thought* (London 1992).
Schama, Simon. *The Embarrassment of Riches: An Interpretation of Dutch Culture in the Golden Age* (London 1987).
Scheja, Georg. *The Isenheim Altarpiece* (New York 1969).
Scherf, Guilhem (ed.). *Franz Xaver Messerschmidt: From NeoClassicism to Expressionism, 1736–1783* (New York and Paris 2010).
Schnapper, Antoine. *Jean Jouvenet 1644–1717 et la peinture d'histoire à Paris* (Paris 1974).
—. *David* (New York 1982).
Schupbach, William. 'Un Ex-voto di R. Pistoni del 1872', *KOS* I 6 (1984).
—. *Acts of Mercy: The Middlesex Hospital Paintings by Frederick Cayley Robinson (1862–1927)* (London 2009).
Schwartz, Gary. *Rembrandt: His Life, his Paintings* (Harmondsworth 1985).
Scull, Andrew. *The Most Solitary of Afflictions: Madness and Society in Britain, 1700–1900* (London 1993).
—. *Social Order/Mental Disorder: Anglo-American Psychiatry in Historical Perspective* (London 1989).
—. *Madhouse: A Tragic Tale of Megalomania and Modern Medicine* (New Haven and London 2005).
Senior, Peter, and Jonathan Croall. *Helping to Heal: The Arts in Health Care* (London 1993).
A sermon intended to have been preached at the publick opening of the Chappel of the lying-in hospital . . . Dublin (Dublin 1759).
Shaw, C.D., and W.R.Winterton. *The Middlesex Hospital* (London n.d.).
Shewring, Walter (ed.). *Letters of Eric Gill* (London 1947).
Simon, Jacob. *English Baroque Sketches* exh. cat. (Twickenham, Surrey, 1974).
Simpson, Marc. 'The 1870s' in *Thomas Eakins* (Philadelphia 2001).
Slive, Seymour (ed.). *Frans Hals* (London 1989).
Smart, Alastair. *Allan Ramsay 1713–1784* (Edinburgh 1992).
Smets, Irene. *St John's Hospital Bruges* (Ghent-Amsterdam 2001).
Smith, Alistair. *Albrecht Altdorfer: Christ taking Leave of his Mother* (London 1983).

Snodin, Michael. *Rococo: Art and Design in Hogarth's England* (London 1984).
— and Nigel Llewellyn. *Baroque: Style in the Age of Magnificence* (London 2009).
Solà-Morales, Ignasi. 'Modernista Architecture', *Homage to Barcelona: The City and its Art 1888–1936* exh. cat. (London 1985).
Somers-Cocks, Anna. 'Reprieve for Acts of Mercy', *Art Newspaper* (January 2008).
Sontag, Susan (ed.). *Antonin Artaud: Selected Writings* (New York 1976).
Spivey, Nigel. *Enduring Creation: Art, Pain and Fortitude* (London 2001).
Stainton, Lindsay, and Christopher White. *Drawing in England from Hilliard to Hogarth* (London 1987).
Stang, Ragna. *Munch/Nolde: The Relationship of their Art* (London 1969).
Stein, Susan Alyson (ed.). *Van Gogh: A Retrospective* (New York 1986).
Stenerson, Rolf E. *Close-up of a Genius* (Oslo 1946).
Stevens, MaryAnne. 'Frederick Cayley Robinson', *The Connoisseur* (September 1977).
Stevenson, Christine. *Medicine and Magnificence: British Hospital and Asylum Architecture 1660–1815* (New Haven and London 2000).
Stewart, Michael. 'Introduction', in *Forty Years of British Art from the Collection of Paintings in Hospitals* exh. cat. (London 1987).
The Story of the Thomas Coram Foundation for Children (London n.d.).
Stratton-Pruitt, Suzanne. 'Murillo in America', *Bartolomé Esteban Murillo (1617–1682): Paintings from American Collections* (New York 2002).
Strens, B. Hatfield. 'L'Arrivo del trittico Portinari a Firenze', *Commentari* XIX (1968).
Summerson, John. *The Architecture of the Eighteenth Century* (London 1968).
Sund, Judy. 'Famine to Feast: Portrait Making at St.-Rémy and Auvers', in *Van Gogh Face To Face: The Portraits* (Detroit 2000).
Sutton, Denys (ed.). *Letters of Roger Fry* (London 1972) vol. I.
Sutton, Peter C. *Masters of Seventeenth-Century Dutch Genre Painting* (London 1984).
Symmons, Sarah. *Goya* (London 1977).
Syson, Luke. *Renaissance Siena: Art for a City* (London 2007).
Szczeklik, Andrzej. *Catharsis: On the Art of Medicine* (Chicago 2007).
Tait, J. 'William Hogarth and the Pictures he painted in St Bartholomew's Hospital', *St Bartholomew's Hospital Journal* (1954).
Tempesti, Anna Forlani. *Pontormo* (Milan 1965).
Thevenin, Paule. *Antonin Artaud: Portraits et dessins* (Paris 1968).
Thistlewood, David (ed.). *Barbara Hepworth Reconsidered* (Liverpool 1996).
Thompson, John D., and Grace Goldin. *The Hospital: A Social and Architectural History* (New Haven and London 1975).
Tøjner, Poul Erik. *Munch in his own Words* (Munich 2001).
Tooby, Michael, and Simon Morley. *William Scott Paintings and Drawings* (London and Dublin 1998).
Topp, Leslie. *Architecture and Truth in Fin-de-Siècle Vienna* (Cambridge 2004).
—. James Moran and Jonathan Andrews (eds). *Madness, Architecture and the Built Environment: Psychiatric Spaces in Historical Context* (New York and London 2007).
Tovell, Ruth Massey. *Roger van der Weyden and the Flémalle Enigma* (Toronto 1955).
Townsend, Eleanor. *Death and Art: Europe 1200–1530* (London 2009).
Townsend, Peter (ed.). *Art within Reach* (London 1984).
Treble, Rosemary. *Great Victorian Pictures: Their Paths to Fame* exh. cat. (London 1978).
Trevor-Roper, Hugh. *Europe's Physician: The Various Life of Sir Theodore de Mayerne* (New Haven and London 2006).
Trivas, N. S. *The Paintings of Frans Hals* (London 1941).
Tromans, Nicholas (ed.). *The Lure of the East: British Orientalist Painting* (London 2008).
—. *Richard Dadd: The Artist and the Asylum* (London 2011).
Turner, Nicholas, and Carol Plazzotta. *Drawings by Guercino from British Collections* (London 1991).
Uglow, Jenny. *Hogarth: A Life and a World* (London 1997).
Valdivieso, Enrique. *Juan de Valdés Leal* (Seville 1988).
Valentine, Helen. *From Reynolds to Lawrence: The First Sixty Years of the Royal Academy of Arts and its Collections* (London 1991).
Venturi, Adolfo. *Paolo Veronese* (Milan 1928).
Vergo, Peter. *Art in Vienna 1898–1918* (Oxford 1975; 2nd ed. 1981).
Veronee-Verhaegen, Nicole. *L'Hôtel-Dieu de Beaune* (Brussels 1973).
Vertue, George. 'Vertue Note Books III', *Walpole Society* XXII (1933–4).
—. *Notebooks 1713–46* (London 1934) vol. XXII.
Viatte, Germain, and Sarah Wilson. *Aftermath: France 1945–54. New Images of Man* (London 1982).
Virdis, Caterina Limentani, and Mari Pietrogiovanna. *Gothic and Renaissance Altarpieces* (London 2002).
A Vision of History: The Wellcome Institute for the History of Medicine (London 1987).
Voragine, Jacobus de. *The Golden Legend* trans. W. Granger Ryan (Princeton 1993).
Vos, Dirk de. *Rogier van der Weyden: The Complete Works* (New York 1999).
Waddingham, Malcolm R. *Adam Elsheimer* (Bristol 1966).
Waetzoldt, Wilhelm. *Dürer and his Times* (London 1955).
Wagner, Anne Middleton. *Mother Stone: The Vitality of Modern British Sculpture* (New Haven and London 2005).
Wagner, Gillian. *Thomas Coram, Gent.* (Woodbridge 2004).
Walker, Robert. 'The Demon of the Portinari Altarpiece', *Art Bulletin* XLII (1960).
Warner, Malcolm, and Robin Blake. *Stubbs and the Horse* with an essay by Lance Mayer and Gay Myers (New Haven and London 2004).
Waterhouse, Ellis. *Painting in Britain 1530 to 1790* (Harmondsworth 1953).
—. *El Greco* (London 1965).
Watts, Mary S. *George Frederick Watts: The Annals of an Artist's Life* (London 1912).
Webb, M. I. *Michael Rysbrack Sculptor* (London 1954).
Webster, Mary. *Johan Zoffany 1733–1810* (London 1976).
Wedd, Kit. *The Foundling Museum* (London 2004).
Weeks, John. 'Forty Years of Hospital Building', *HD* (February 1988).
Wellcome Institute for the History of Medicine: A Brief Description (London 1985).
Whinney, Margaret. *Sculpture in Britain 1530 to 1830* (London 1988 ed.).
—. *Rogier van der Weyden* (London 1966).
Wilenski, R. H. *Dutch Painting* (London 1928; rev. ed. 1945).
Willsdon, C. A. P. *Mural Painting in Britain 1840–1940: Image and Meaning* (Oxford 2000).
Wilmerding, John. *American Art* (Harmondsworth 1976).
Wilson, Sarah. 'Fernand Léger: Art and Politics 1935–1955', in *Fernand Léger: The Later Years* exh. cat. (London 1987).
—. 'Introduction' and 'Saint-Germain-des-Prés: Antifascism, Occupation and Postwar Paris' in *Paris: Capital of the Arts 1900–1968* exh. cat. (London 2002).
Wilson, Simon. *Tate Gallery: An Illustrated Companion* (London 1989).
Wilson, Thomas. *An account of the foundation of the Royal Hospital of King Charles the Second* (Dublin 1713).
Wilson-Bareau, Juliet. *Goya: Truth and Fantasy. The Small Paintings* (New Haven and London 1994).
Wine, Humphrey, Jon and Linda Whiteley and Alain Gerard. *Tradition and Revolution in French Art 1700–1880. Paintings and Drawings from Lille* exh. cat. (London 1993).
Wittkower, Margaret and Rudolf. *Born Under Saturn* (London 1963).
Wohl, Hellmut. *The Paintings of Domenico Veneziano ca. 1410–1461* (Oxford 1980).
Woll, Gerd, *et al. Alpha and Omega* (Oslo 1981).
Wood, Christopher. *Victorian Panorama: Paintings of Victorian Life* (London 1976).
Wood, Jeryldene M. (ed.). *The Cambridge Guide to Piero della Francesca* (Cambridge 2002).
Woodham-Smith, Cecil. *Florence Nightingale 1820–1910* (London 1950).
Wright, F. A. (ed.). *Select Letters of St Jerome* (London 1933).
Wullschlager, Jackie. *Chagall: Love and Exile* (London 2008).
Yorke, Malcolm. *Eric Gill: Man of Flesh and Spirit* (London 1981).
Ziermann, Horst. *Matthias Grünewald* (Munich, London and New York 2001).

UNPUBLISHED MATERIAL

Baron, J. H. Ms and archive of research on Art in London Hospitals, now donated to Goldsmiths Library, London.
Naum Gabo Papers, Beinecke Rare Book and Manuscript Library, Yale University.
Heighton, Luke. 'Exhibiting Madness, Art and the Asylum: The Creation and Exhibition of Images by Psychiatric Hospital Patients in Vienna, 1890–1914' (doctoral thesis, University of London, Birkbeck College, 2008).
Imrie, Nicola J. 'The Architecture and Culture of Sanatoria for Nervous Ailments in the Austro-Hungarian Empire, 1890–1914' (doctoral thesis, University of London, Birkbeck College, 2008).
Imperial War Museum, London, Central Archive, Department of Art, Correspondence with First World War Artists
Mayes, Alice. 'The Young Bomberg 1914–1925', memoir, November 1972. Tate Archive, London.
'A Picture for Health', transcript of a BBC documentary on art in hospitals, written and presented by Richard Cork, produced by Judith Bumpus, broadcast on Radio 4, 11 November 1985. Now in British Library, London.
Wieber, Sabine. 'Nervous Bodies and Femmes Fragile: Sculpting the Sanatorium in Vienna 1900', forthcoming.

PHOTOGRAPH CREDITS

Every effort has been made by the publisher to trace copyright holders.

akg-images: 83, 110, 116, 123, 153, 248, 249, 250, 256, 261, 281, 284, 285, 286, 292, 293, 324, 405; akg-images/De Agostini Picture Library: 8, 239; akg-images/Maurice Babey: 121; akg-images/Bible Land Pictures: 418; akg-images/Bildarchiv Monheim: 163; akg-images/David Borland: 343; akg-images/Cameraphoto: 91, 92; Hervé Champollion/akg-images: 27, 29, 127, 229; akg-images/Electa: 228, 231; akg-images/André Held: 279, 280; akg-images/John Hios: 108; akg-images/Erich Lessing: 57c, 240, 266, 287, 291, 358; akg-images/Joseph Martin: 154; akg-images/James Morris: 181, 209; Album/Oronoz/akg-images: 126, 128, 131, 134, 135, 254; akg-images/Sambraus: 341, 342; akg-images/Jürgen Sorges: 161; Alinari Archives, Florence – Reproduced with the permission of The Ospedale of S. Maria della Scala. Photographer: Tatge, George for Alinari: 4, 9, 11; Collection Amsterdam Museum: 113, 117, 118; Archives de l'AP-HP: 232; Reinier van Arkel groep: 141; Ashmolean Museum, University of Oxford: 213, 230; Bergen Art Museum, Rasmus Meyers collection. Photo: Werner Zellien: 339; © Bethlem Art and History Collections Trust: 142, 144, 145, 264, 265, 268, 269, 272, 273, 274, 275, 276; bpk/Skulpturensammlung und Museum für Byzantinische Kunst, SMB/Jörg P. Anders: 143; © Birmingham Museums and Art Gallery: 223; Photography by Michael Bodycomb: 253; The Bridgeman Art Library: 2, 36, 37, 95, 105, 136, 189, 190, 191, 193, 194, 195, 196, 197, 198, 199, 202, 203, 227, 243, 283, 288, 290, 307, 311, 359, 407; Alinari/The Bridgeman Art Library: frontispiece, 6; John Bethell/The Bridgeman Art Library: 168, 169, 170; James Brittain/The Bridgeman Art Library: 174, 176, 179, 180, 182; Cameraphoto Arte Venezia/ The Bridgeman Art Library: 94; Jorge Contreras Chacel/The Bridgeman Art Library: 391; Reproduced by permission of Chatsworth Settlement Trustees/The Bridgeman Art Library: 369; © Chetham's Library, Manchester, UK/The Bridgeman Art Library: 215; © Coram in the care of the Foundling Museum, London/ The Bridgeman Art Library: 299, 300, 301, 302; Giraudon/The Bridgeman Art Library: 71, 107, 238, 257, 258; Gillian Jason Modern & Contemporary Art/The Bridgeman Art Library: 408; © Paul Maeyaert/The Bridgeman Art Library: 26, 28, 30, 31, 32a, 32b, 32c, 33, 34a, 34b, 35; © Philip Mould Ltd, London/The Bridgeman Art Library: 226; © Royal Hospital Chelsea, London, UK/ The Bridgeman Art Library: 296; By permission of the William Salt Library, Stafford/The Bridgeman Art Library: 205; Roger-Viollet, Paris/The Bridgeman Art Library: 155; Peter Willi/The Bridgeman Art Library: 124, 125; © Courtesy of the Worshipful Company of Barbers/The Bridgeman Art Library: 112; © Trustees of the British Museum: 171, 217, 252; Fondazione IRCCS Ca' Granda: 130; Chelsea and Westminster Health Charity: 409; © Country Life: 406; © The Courtauld Institute of Art, London: 183, 303, 312; Conway Library, The Courtauld Institute of Art, London: 317; Photographic Survey, The Courtauld Institute of Art, London. Private collection: 234; Photograph courtesy of the Witt Library, The Courtauld Institute of Art, London: 233, 318; By Permission of the Trustees of Dulwich Picture Gallery: 166; © Coram in the care of the Foundling Museum: 192, 201, 204; Frans Hals Museum, Haarlem: 122; © Fundació Institut Amatller d'Art Hispànic. Arxiu Mas: 137; David Rubinger/Getty Images: 419, 420; Old Royal Naval College. Photographer: Roger M Stevens ARPS: 172, 177, 178; © Guy's and St Thomas' Charity: 148, 149, 150, 151, 208; Heritage Tile Conservation Ltd: 321; © The Hunterian, University of Glasgow 2011: 225; Courtesy of the Huntington Art Collections, San Marino, California: 218; Photo © IWM (image 3095): 357; Indianapolis Museum of Art: 200; Irish Museum of Modern Art: 162; Photograph 24 x18 cm, Kirchner Museum Davos, www.kirchnermuseum.ch: 354, 355; © Leeds Museum and Galleries (City Art Gallery): 364; Leopold Museum, Vienna: 356; Musée Brugge © Lukas-Art in Flanders vxw: 55, 56; © Estate of F. E. McWilliam, 2011: 414; © Manchester City Galleries: 184; The Estate of Mary Martin: 413; © Munch Museum: 333, 334, 335, 336, 337, 338; Kristiania Røntgeninstitut, Kristiania (Oslo), copy in Munch Museum, Oslo: 326; © Munch Museum/Munch Ellingsen Group: 327, 328, 329, 332; Ragnvald Væring, copy in the Munch Museum, Oslo: 340; Unknown photographer, copy in Munch Museum, Oslo: 325, 330; Courtesy of The Municipal Art Society of New York: 376; Courtesy of The Municipal Art Society of New York and conservator Luca Bonetti: 377; © The National Gallery, London: 115; © National Maritime Museum, Greenwich, UK: 173; © National Portrait Gallery, London: 297, 298; © NTPL/Roy Fox: 360, 361, 362; Museum of Order St John, London: 363; The Pierpont Morgan Library, New York. III, 35; photography by Graham Haber, 2011: 210; Public Design Commission of the City of New York, New York, New York, USA: 374, 375; Dell & Wainwright/RIBA Library Photographs Collection: 370; © RMN/Gérard Biot: 412; © RMN/René-Gabriel Ojéda: 245; © Collection Centre Pompidou, Dist. RMN/Philippe Migeat: 403, 404; © Royal Academy of Arts, London; photographer: P. Highnam: 206; The Royal Collection © 2011 Her Majesty Queen Elizabeth II: 86, 185; © Royal College of Physicians: 219, 224; © The Royal College of

Surgeons of England: 222; Laura Curnock, RNHRD: 220; © St Bartholomew's Hospital Archives: 186, 187, 188; © 2010. Photo Scala, Florence: 3, 5, 7, 13, 14, 15, 16, 17, 18, 19, 20, 21, 24, 25, 38, 39, 40, 41, 42, 45, 46, 54, 57a, 57b, 58, 59a, 59b, 60, 61, 62, 63, 64, 65, 66, 67, 68, 70, 72, 73, 74, 75, 76, 77, 78, 79, 80, 81, 82, 84, 85, 89, 99, 100, 101, 102, 103, 104, 106, 106, 114, 119, 132, 138, 139, 241, 247, 255, 259, 262, 331; © 2011. Photo Scala, Florence: 23; © 2010. Photo Scala, Florence – courtesy of the Ministero Beni e Att. Culturali: 10, 12, 22, 47, 48, 49, 50, 51, 52, 53, 88; © 2010. De Agostini Picture Library/Scala, Florence: 97, 160; © 2010. Photo Albright Knox Art Gallery/Art Resource/Scala, Florence: 411; © 2010. Photo Art Resource/Bob Schalwijk/Scala, Florence: 379, 381, 382, 383, 384, 385, 386, 387, 390, 392, 397, 398, 399, 400, 401; © 2010. Photo Austrian Archives/Scala, Florence: 344; © 2010. Cameraphoto/Scala, Florence: 93; © 2010. Photo Scala, Florence/Heritage Images: 146, 211, 212, 278; © 2010. Photo Ann Ronan/Heritage Images/Scala, Florence: 87; © 2010. Image copyright The Metropolitan Museum of Art/Art Resource/Scala, Florence: 96, 109; © 2010. Copyright The National Gallery, London/Scala, Florence: 69, 133, 214; © 2010. Photo The Philadelphia Museum of Art/Art Resource/Scala, Florence: 120, 295, 305; © 2010. White Images/Scala, Florence: 156, 244, 246, 263, 306; © 2011. White Images/Scala, Florence: 242; © William Scott Foundation 2011: 416; © William Scott Foundation 2012, photographer: Browne: 417; © William Scott Foundation 2010; photographer Bill Warhust (The Times): 415; Federal Art Project, Photographic Division Collection, Archives of American Art, Smithsonian Institution: 373; © Tate, London 2009: 267, 270, 308; © Tate, London 2011: 1; UCLH NHS Foundation Trust Archives: 207, 316, 353; © Victoria and Albert Museum, London: 43, 44, 175, 251, 271; Wellcome Library, London: 90, 111, 147, 221, 349, 350, 351, 352; The Whitworth Art Gallery, The University of Manchester: 410; © Annual/Wikimedia Commons: 129; © Doris Antony/Wikimedia Commons: 345; © Alejandro Linares Garcia/Wikimedia Commons: 380; © Marie-Lan Nguyen/Wikimedia Commons: 145, 158, 159; © Welleschik/Wikimedia Commons: 347; Yale University, Harvey Cushing/John Hay Whitney Medical Library: 216.

COPYRIGHT CREDITS

© ADAGP, Paris and DACS, London 2011: 348, 403, 404, 405, 411, 412; © Estate of Ilya Bolotowsky/DACS, London/VAGA, NY 2011: 376, 377, 378; © The Estate of David Bomberg. All Rights Reserved, DACS 2011: 363; Chagall®/© ADAGP, Paris and DACS, London 2011: 419, 420; © DACS 2011: 379, 380, 381, 382, 383, 384, 385, 386, 387; © The Lucian Freud Archive: 369; Bowness, Hepworth Estate: 406, 407, 408; © The Estate of L.S. Lowry. All Rights Reserved, DACS 2011: 410; © Estate of F. E. McWilliam, 2011: 414; The Estate of Mary Martin: 413; © Munch Museum/Munch – Ellingsen Group, BONO, Oslo/DACS, London 2011: 324, 327, 328, 329, 331, 332, 339; © 2011 Banco de México Diego Rivera Frida Kahlo Museums Trust, Mexico, D.F./DACS: 388, 389, 390, 391, 392, 393, 394, 395, 396, 397, 398, 399, 400, 401; © The Estate of Stanley Spencer 2011. All rights reserved DACS: 360, 361, 362.

INDEX

NOTE: Page numbers in italics refer to an illustration. Names containing prepositions are indexed under the last element of the name, e.g. Gogh, Vincent van, except for Italian names containing 'della'; these are indexed under the prefix in the D sequence, e.g. della Robbia, Andrea.